Nuclear Medicine and Immunology

Sara Harsini · Abass Alavi
Nima Rezaei

Editors

Nuclear Medicine and Immunology

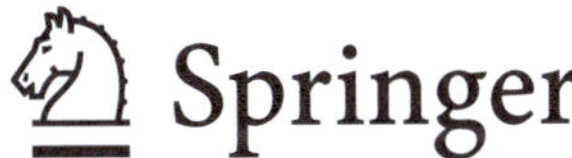 Springer

Editors
Sara Harsini
Department of Nuclear Medicine
Tehran University of Medical Sciences
Tehran
Iran

Abass Alavi
Department of Radiology
University of Pennsylvania
Philadelphia, PA
USA

Nima Rezaei
Research Center for Immunodeficiencies
Tehran University of Medical Sciences
Tehran
Iran

ISBN 978-3-030-81263-8   ISBN 978-3-030-81261-4   (eBook)
https://doi.org/10.1007/978-3-030-81261-4

This Springer imprint is published by the registered company Springer Nature Switzerland AG
The registered company address is: Gewerbestrasse 11, 6330 Cham, Switzerland

To Masoud and Zohreh
For their endless, unconditional love and support…

Sara

To my mother, Fatemeh
For sacrifices she has made to make my life most rewarding…

Abass

To my daughters, Ariana and Arnika
With wishes to have a better world for the new generation to live…

Nima

Preface

The fields of Nuclear Medicine and Immunology are tightly inter-related, and the close interaction between these disciplines has led to introducing many novel methodologies for detecting infection and inflammation, radioimmunoimaging, and radioimmunotherapy.

Molecular imaging with PET and SPECT is increasingly employed to detect, characterize, and monitor the course of the disease activity in the setting of inflammatory disorders of known and unknown etiologies. Moreover, the recent developments in hybrid multimodality imaging techniques make a combined assessment of molecular biology and the related structural alterations possible. Such synergic approach leads to better diagnostic accuracy in many settings. Various radiopharmaceuticals and radiolabeled preparations have been introduced to image inflammation. Among the imaging techniques currently used in practice, PET/CT imaging has been proven to be of great value for the detection of inflammation and has become the centerpiece of several research and clinical initiatives during the last several years. This very powerful technique will play an increasingly important role in the management of patients with inflammatory conditions in the future.

Molecular imaging techniques have gained great recognition for managing patients with a variety of infections, and this has also dramatically gained interest among researchers and clinicians in recent years. Applying these novel approaches has allowed a better understanding of the underlying pathophysiology of many infections. These molecular imaging-based techniques offer unique opportunities to better understand infection-related processes from those of sterile inflammatory conditions. These discoveries have been of great value in selecting the best anatomic site for biopsy and, most importantly, in monitoring response to treatment. These radiotracer-based imaging modalities have positioned themselves as important and key players for diagnosing and monitoring a variety of infectious and inflammatory disorders.

Similarly, the role of standard and modern radiotracer-based imaging techniques in the diagnosis and treatment of cancers has grown exponentially during the past two decades. These rapid changes have been fueled by advances that have been made in better understanding of tumor biology, on the one hand, and the synthesis of novel agents that target specific sites for both diagnostic and therapeutic purposes, on the other. The eradication of cancer remains a vexing problem despite recent advances in better understanding of the molecular basis of many malignancies. One major therapeutic approach involves selective targeting of radiolabeled preparations to the cancer-associated cell surface antigen sites by monoclonal antibodies. Although radioimmunotherapy (RIT) approaches have been investigated for several decades, the cumulative advances in cancer biology, antibody engineering, and radiochemistry in the past decade have markedly enhanced the ability of RIT to produce durable remissions of multiple cancer types. The rapid development of medical and bioengineering technology and introduction of novel theragnostic probes to recognize tumor microenvironment have allowed shifting from labeled antibodies to some small-molecule ligands for cancer applications in the future.

Advances that have been made in so many scientific domains have shown that collaborative efforts between immunology and molecular imaging experts are very timely and will substantially enhance the role of this very important discipline in medicine in the near future.

This multidisciplinary book reviews the state of the art with respect to applications of radiotracer-based procedures for the detection of infection and inflammation, radioimmunoimaging, radioimmunotherapy, interaction among these disciplines and the future prospects. After an overview of the interconnections between nuclear medicine and immunology in Chap. 1, the nuclear imaging of endogenous markers of lymphocyte response is explained in Chap. 2, followed by the radioimaging of activated T cells in Chap. 3. Imaging of infection and inflammation using gallium, indium-111-labeled leukocytes, technetium-99m-HMPAO-labeled leukocytes, and 2-[^{18}F]fluoro-2-deoxy-D-glucose are separately described in Chaps. 4–7, respectively. Next, the role of 2-[^{18}F]fluoro-2-deoxy-D-glucose PET in the fever of unknown origin is reviewed in Chap. 8. Tumor targeting agents are explained in Chap. 9, followed by a description of tumor architecture and targeted delivery provided in Chap. 10. Chapter 11 focuses on radionuclide therapy and immunomodulation. Translational development and testing of theranostics in combination with immunotherapies are explained in Chap. 12. Meanwhile, Chaps. 13 and 14 explain radioimmunotherapy and radiolabeled antibodies used for cancer radioimmunotherapy. Subsequently, Chap. 15 presents the dosimetric principles of targeted radiotherapy and radioimmunotherapy. Theranostics of hematologic disorders are explicated in Chap. 16. In addition, radioimmunotherapy for acute leukemia (Chap. 17), targeted radionuclide therapy and immunotherapy for prostate cancer (Chap. 18), and radioimmunotherapy and targeted radiotherapy for squamous cell carcinoma of the head and neck (Chap. 19) are individually described in the following chapters. Chapter 20 enlightens the use of PET in evaluating the efficacy of immunotherapy in oncology. Finally, by allocating the final chapter to the evolving opportunities for the development of new therapeutic agents, this book comes to its end.

This book is the result of the valuable contribution of more than 50 scientists from well-known universities/institutes worldwide. We would like to hereby acknowledge the expertise of all contributors and express our gratitude for their willingness to devote a considerable amount of time and effort in preparing the respective chapters. During the editorial process, the sad news reached us of the untimely death of one of our contributors, professor Sanjiv Sam Gambhir. Sam was an internationally recognized pioneer in advancing techniques for molecular imaging and early cancer detection. His innovations have, undoubtedly, founded modern medicine's approach to early disease diagnostics and will continue to guide the future of precision health. He will be greatly missed.

We hope that this book will be welcomed by researchers and clinicians who wish to have an updated reference source that is related to these interconnected disciplines.

Tehran, Iran   Sara Harsini
Philadelphia, PA   Abass Alavi
Tehran, Iran   Nima Rezaei

Acknowledgment

We would like to thank Sina Harsini for his technical contribution to the project, without which completion of this book would not have been possible.

Contents

Introduction on Nuclear Medicine and Immunology

Sara Harsini, Abass Alavi, and Nima Rezaei

Contents

S. Harsini (✉)
Department of Nuclear Medicine, Tehran University of Medical Sciences, Tehran, Iran

Association of Nuclear Medicine and Molecular Imaging (ANMMI), Universal Scientific Education and Research Network (USERN), Tehran, Iran
e-mail: sharsini@bccrc.ca

A. Alavi
Department of Radiology, Hospital of the University of Pennsylvania, Philadelphia, PA, USA

University of Pennsylvania, Philadelphia, PA, USA
e-mail: abass.alavi@uphs.upenn.edu

N. Rezaei
Research Center for Immunodeficiencies, Children's Medical Center, Tehran University of Medical Sciences, Tehran, Iran

Network of Immunity in Infection, Malignancy and Autoimmunity (NIIMA), Universal Scientific Education and Research Network (USERN), Tehran, Iran

Department of Immunology, School of Medicine, Tehran University of Medical Sciences, Tehran, Iran
e-mail: rezaei_nima@tums.ac.ir

© Springer Nature Switzerland AG 2022
S. Harsini et al. (eds.), *Nuclear Medicine and Immunology*,
https://doi.org/10.1007/978-3-030-81261-4_1

1.1 The Immune System: Building Blocks and Mechanisms

Considering the ultimate aim of the human body to survive, human immune response, whether preplanned, i.e., innate immunity, or partly planned, i.e., adaptive or acquired immune reactions, has evolved to counteract changes of uncertain nature. Immunity refers to the body's resistance to changes, mediated by the collection of molecules, cells, and tissues regarded as the immune system. The coordinated reaction of these molecules and cells to the unwelcome factor of change is termed as immune response. In this manner, important physiologic functions of the immune system are not only to prevent or eradicate infections caused by invading pathogens but also to provide protection against the growth of some tumors, participate in the clearance of dead cells, and initiate tissue repair. It is of note that this system can also recognize, respond to, and injure cells and induce pathologic inflammation. Human immunity follows main principles of action to detect the threatening factor early and activate response systems; set the stage for an effective, least interfering, response with normal body function; activate long-term survival and adaptation signals and natural repair systems; and finally to dismiss the response in a timely manner and learn from the experience if necessary.

Immune aspects of human physiology and pathology are now the prevailing notion in research, day-to-day practice, and therapeutic modalities used by clinicians. In an effort made by researchers in basic science and clinical medicine to untangle the complex trails by which human immune response is regulated by and controls many functions of a living creature, the immune system has been suggested as the executive actor in almost every defense mechanism of the human body to respond to threats. Since a 24-h alert system is required to exercise the proper scenario of action to counteract changes, the effector cells of the immune system are therefore distributed in a tightly regulated manner throughout the body and over time. The immune system has conventionally been defined by introducing these mediators, cells, and organs involved in immune responses and then by categorizing the responses into innate and adaptive responses.

The division of pluripotent hematopoietic stem cells resident in the bone marrow produces two types of progenitor cells, common lymphoid progenitor, which in turn gives rise to T cells and B cells and then would differentiate into activated T cells and effector plasma cells, respectively, and common myeloid progenitor, generating two progenitor cells at later stages, namely, granulocyte/macrophage progenitor and megakaryocyte/erythrocyte progenitor, the former of which gives rise to circulating granulocytes such as neutrophils; eosinophils; basophils; unknown precursors; monocytes that will differentiate into mast cells, macrophages, and immature dendritic cells (DCs) once migrating into tissues; and immature DCs that will mature in lymph nodes, while the latter turns into megakaryocyte and erythroblast lineages, resulting in the generation of platelets and erythrocytes, respectively [1].

While every cell and organ in the body is endowed with a nonspecific defense system, there are accumulations of lymphoid tissue shaping systematized organs with a lead role in human immunity, termed as central (or primary) and peripheral (or secondary) lymphoid organs, in charge of training lymphocytes, fostering immune interactions, and providing long-term reservoirs for memory cells residence. Lymphocyte proliferation, selection, clonal expansion, and maturation occur in central lymphoid organs, that is, bone marrow (B cells) and thymus (T cells) [1]. The differentiated lymphocytes enter into the bloodstream and then migrate to the peripheral lymphoid organs including the lymph nodes, spleen, and mucosa-associated lymphoid tissues, which harbor expansion of mature lymphocytes and facilitation of acquired immune response via exclusive structural delicacies. Lymph fluid-filled lymphatics facilitate the transportation of antigens to lymph nodes and recirculation of activated lymphocytes to the blood.

When pathogens invade the body, the ancient gatekeeper, innate immunity, provides immediate protection and elicits responses in a nonspecific manner, followed by slower but more specific responses against pathogens provided by the adaptive immunity. While the adaptive immunity, as a relatively modern immunity, is restricted to vertebrates, the observation of similar mechanisms underlying innate immune recognition in different species provides evidence that the innate immune mechanisms are highly conserved throughout evolution. An everlasting struggle with frequently changing and rapidly reproducing microbial pathogens is assumed to shape the evolution of the human immune system. Although not able to make specific responses against pathogens, the innate immune system can discriminate between self and non-self following the systematic interaction of germline-encoded pattern recognition receptors (PRRs) with pathogen-associated molecular patterns (PAMPs) [2]. Such pattern recognition is based on, but not confined to, identification of peptides, carbohydrates, as well as pathogen-associated nucleic acid segments [3]. Recognition of infectious non-self agents by PRRs results in the development of effector cells contributing to the initiation of the inflammatory response from polymorphonuclear leukocytes along with mast cells, macrophages, and natural killer (NK) cells [4].

It is on the adaptive immunity to continue efforts to distinguish self and non-self in case of the innate immunity failure to effectively resolve the infection. The innate immunity employs antigen-presenting cells (APCs), particularly costimulatory molecules cluster of differentiation (CD)80 and CD86 expressing DCs, to introduce the infectious agent to the adaptive immune system. The adaptive immune system, unlike the innate immunity using receptors fixed in the genome, is armed with a full repertoire of antigen receptors built up from random gene segment rearrangements [5], the distribution of which over the effector cells, i.e., activated T cells and antibody-producing cells, enables the adaptive immunity to specifically recognize pathogens and associated proteins, carbohydrates, lipids, and nucleic acids whereby the immunological memory is made [4]. The properties of adaptive immune responses, including specificity, diversity, memory, clonal expansion, specialization,

contraction and homeostasis, and nonreactivity to self, are pivotal for the effectiveness of responses in fighting against pathogens.

1.1.1 Inflammation

Inflammation is the transitory and ongoing nonspecific effort of injured cells, including, but not confined to, vascular response, i.e., vasodilation, increased permeability, and activation of endothelial cells, followed by a cellular response, with increased leukocyte chemotaxis, adhesion, and transmigration into extracellular tissue, in order to communicate the danger signal, on the spot, to the first-line innate mechanisms to diminish the invasion hazards. A full-armed stimulation of defense and repair mechanisms, as well as involvement of the pathogen-specific acquired immune responses, can ensue. Infection, tissue necrosis, foreign bodies, aseptic trauma with or without necrosis, and hypersensitivity to a sustained assault or autoantigens in the case of inflammatory disorders could all be the triggers for inflammation. An array of plasma proteins (complement system, vasoactive mediators, cytokines, antimicrobial peptides such as defensins and cathelicidins), circulating and infiltrating leukocytes (polymorphonuclear leukocytes, macrophages/monocytes, lymphocytes, etc.), and even the endothelial lining of the vessels and indolent cells of the parenchyma are highly active players of inflammation.

The first to encounter the products of tissue assault are resident phagocytes, epithelial cells, dendritic cells, and based on whether endothelial damage is present, platelets, which recognize the danger via the PAMP receptors, leading to the production of a multitude of danger signals such as proinflammatory cytokines. Their response to histamine, thrombin, interleukin (IL)-1, IL-6, and tumor necrosis factor (TNF)-α, via the production of chemotactic agents, further expedites leukocyte transmigration. The allocation of leukocytes to the damage site is further facilitated by the endothelial expression of adhesion and selectin molecules and their interaction with a wide array of surface integrin and cell adhesion molecules on leukocytes. Ingestion of microorganisms and dead cells and the subsequent secretion of reactive oxygen and nitrogen species, extracellular digestive enzymes, and products of lipoxygenase cascade such as leukotrienes and prostaglandins, by activated indigenous or infiltrated phagocytes, along with the complement system and antibody response, shape the main body of chemical mediators of inflammation.

After the stage has been set for the specific recognition of the antigens and their presentation to T cells by antigen-presenting cells, the face of inflammatory response changes in a way that antigen-specific T cells, macrophages, circulating plasma cells, and memory B cells act as leading characters in a durative inflammation. Although the principal goal of the inflammatory response is to recruit immune cells to the site of the invasion, failure to eliminate the pathogen from the site of entry, failure to dismiss the response, and excessive response to a benign pathogen result in the formation of different immune diseases.

1.1.2 Infection

Infectious agents were the initial factors historically drawing our attention to the immune system. The self/non-self paradigm that reigned the knowledge of immunology for years was a direct revelation from years of investigating host defense against microbes [6].

In response to an extracellular pathogen, for instance, infiltration of neutrophils, chemoattraction of distinct populations of leukocytes, and secretion of TNF-α, IL-1, IL-6, nitrous oxide, and proteases take place, followed by the presentation of parts of the degraded pathogen on the surface major histocompatibility complex (MHC) receptors of macrophages, dendritic cells, along with other tissue-specific and nonspecific APCs. In order for appropriate interaction of APCs and lymphocytes to occur, an intricate system of surface receptors and chemokines regulates lymphocyte circulation and makes sure that the painstakingly selected mature T and B lymphocytes travel in a nonstop trip, trafficking in and out of secondary lymphoid organs, and take proper homing signals to the sites where the interaction of immune cells mainly takes place. The primary signal for lymphocyte activation could be provided by the recognition of antigens via immunoglobulin (Ig) or T cell receptor (TCR). T cells binding with moderate to low avidity to MHC/antigen complex do not receive maturation signal, as a consequence of the negative selection of lymphocyte in bone marrow and thymus, unless elicited by costimulatory molecules, generally from activated APCs providing the secondary signal. The innate immune response stimulates APCs for more proficient phagocytosis and antigen presentation to T cells, expressing costimulatory molecules and IL-2 necessary for T cell proliferation and differentiation.

1.1.3 Immuno-Oncology

Footprints from the immune system could be unearthed in many aspects of cancer pathogenesis. The host immune system shows a complex interaction with tumor cells through the activation of innate and adaptive immune mechanisms. Cancer is not only characterized by the genetic mechanisms resulting in transformed cells with a senseless tendency to proliferate but also as an everyday challenge of the body with cells that undergo subtle yet malignant mutations and intracellular alterations. Unless transformed cells are thoroughly eradicated by a competent immune system, sporadic tumor cells manage to survive and may enter an equilibrium phase during which editing occurs. Immunologically sculpted tumors eventually begin to grow progressively, establish an immunosuppressive tumor microenvironment, and become clinically evident [7]. The identification of the tumor's ability to selectively and efficiently defeat components of the immune system in favor of its longevity and invasion puts a further spin on the fundamental role of immunity in cancer [8].

The immune system has three primary roles in preventing tumors, through the elimination or suppression of viral infections, thus protecting the host from virus-induced tumors; interference with the establishment of an inflammatory environment conducive to tumorigenesis by timely eliminating the pathogens and inflammation; and specific identification and elimination of tumor cells in the light of their expression of tumor-specific antigens or molecules induced by cellular stress, also referred to as tumor immune surveillance. It is now apprehended that once the tumor develops, the immune response against it is generally dominated by tolerance or regulation, not by effective immunity. Immune elimination of malignant cells releases tumor-specific antigens and danger signals and builds a tumor-edited immunity. The field of tumor immunology has focused on determining the types of tumor antigens (commonly classified into a couple of categories including products of diverse mutated genes, products of oncogenes or mutated tumor suppressor genes, aberrantly expressed proteins, and viral antigens), against which the immune system reacts, the nature of the immune responses, and introducing strategies for maximally enhancing antitumor immunity.

The advent of drugs targeting the cutting-edge knowledge of immune culprits of cancer and tumor-specific antigens has deeply changed the paradigms and needs of clinicians and brought hope for effective cancer immunotherapy for tumor suppression or even tumor ablation [9]. In recent years, several approaches using immune checkpoint inhibitors, therapeutic antibodies, therapeutic vaccines, and immune-modulating agents have been a trending topic in cancer research, some providing promising results. The efforts to unleash the immune system against tumors are paying off, and the numbers of available immunotherapeutic drugs are rapidly increasing; however, it is yet to be determined as to which patients do benefit from the expensive immunotherapy.

The development of immune checkpoint inhibitors (ICIs) is raising the highest interest as a revolutionary milestone in the field of immune-oncology due to the demonstration of their efficacy in the treatment of relapsed/refractory lymphomas and other tumors such as melanoma and lung cancer [10–12]. ICIs reinvigorate anti-tumor immune responses by interfering with co-inhibitory signaling pathways and promote immune-mediated destruction of tumor cells. The immune system is regulated by a complex system including multiple checkpoints controlling the homeostasis. T lymphocytes are the immune system agents in charge of identifying and eliminating tumor cells. Autoimmunity is prevented in normal conditions by the interaction of molecules called programmed cell death protein 1 (PD-1), expressed by T lymphocyte and programmed death ligand (PD-L1 and PD-L2) expressed by normal cells. One strategy of cancerous cells to escape detection is through camouflaging themselves with a shield of programmed death ligands, thus blocking immune response by T lymphocytes, making them capable of rapid proliferation [13]. Binding of lymphocytes' PD-1 receptors to the PD-L1 on the tumor cells abolishes their capacity to attack. The antibodies blocking PD-1 from the immune system cells or PD-L1 from the tumor cells constitute immuno-therapeutic drugs, such as nivolumab and pembrolizumab, culminating in the regain of lymphocytes' defense potential. The PD-1/PD-L1 checkpoint and the cytotoxic T-lymphocyte-associated protein 4 (CTLA-4) checkpoint are the most extensively studied targets for more efficacious cancer immunotherapy, particularly in non-small cell lung cancer (NSCLC) [14, 15]. The expression of PD-L1 by tumor microenvironment can stand as a biomarker to predict the response to immunotherapy keeping in mind that tumors with low levels of PD-L1 expression will not respond to these drugs.

The use of IL-2 and the adoptive transfer of antitumor T cells grown in IL-2 denoted the first effective immunotherapies for cancer in humans [16], extensively investigated in several tumors such as melanoma [17], renal cell carcinoma [18], and squamous cell carcinomas of the head and neck [19]. Other examples include recombinant interferon-2b in hairy cell leukemia, multiple myeloma, chronic myelogenous leukemia, follicular lymphoma, and as adjuvant therapy in malignant melanoma [20]; toll-like receptor agonist imiquimod administered to treat various skin cancers including squamous cell carcinoma, basal cell carcinoma, cutaneous T cell lymphoma, and lentigo maligna melanoma [21]; as well as Calmette-Guerin bacillus as the gold standard adjuvant treatment of high-risk non-muscle invasive bladder cancer [22].

1.2 Nuclear Medicine in Immune-Mediated Conditions

Nuclear medicine is a branch of medicine using radionuclides to noninvasively characterize diseases, allowing a precise and early diagnosis and treatment. Functional diagnostic applications rely on the ability of radiopharmaceuticals to concentrate in pathological tissues and to emit radiations subsequently exposed by external detectors and then recorded. The molecules and cells involved in the pathogenic process could be visualized by means of the molecular imaging techniques and then be used to guide clinicians to the best therapeutic approach and follow its efficacy for each patient, thereby improving therapy response and circumventing high costs of patient management. Therapeutic strategies use a selective concentration of radiopharmaceutical agents in pathological tissues and utilize the radiations to demolish them. Bearing in mind the fact that available radiopharmaceuticals identify specific target molecules, this specificity could be used for therapeutic outcomes by substituting diagnostic isotopes with therapeutic ones.

Nuclear medicine imaging techniques comprise two-dimensional scintigraphy, three-dimensional single-photon emission computed tomography (SPECT), and positron emission tomography (PET), and hybrid techniques combining computed tomography (CT) or magnetic resonance imaging (MRI) scans with SPECT or PET, which might allow us to determine the target molecules expressed at certain locations, to make an early diagnosis, and to decide the best therapy in a diversity of pathologies by targeting the complex and various pathways involved in the diseases. The implementation of the hybrid techniques, in particular, provides high sensitivity, which together with the increased development of new radiopharmaceutical agents have made feasible the targeting of specific molecules and cells expressed in the lesions that are of clinical significance for therapy decision-making and follow-up. Utilization of such new imaging techniques along with the advent of molecular genetics, molecular pathophysiology, and advances in bioinformatics and health data has opened eyes to more pieces of the puzzle of diseases of the human body and shed light over novel etiologic factors of disorders.

Several radiolabeled molecules, such as peptides, cytokines, monoclonal antibodies (mAbs) and their fragments, and radiolabeled immune cells have shown promising results to recognize pathological inflammatory sites. Considering the diverse biological characteristics and thus heterogeneous behaviors and responses to treatment of different lesions even in the same patient, it is not a daring notion that having several radiolabeled probes available to specifically target various molecular pathways involved in the inflammatory process and tumor biology might pave the path for the transition from personalized medicine to the concept of "lesion-specific" medicine.

1.2.1 Infectious Diseases

Radiolabeled white blood cell (WBC) scintigraphy, using both technetium-99m (^{99m}Tc) and indium-111 (^{111}In), is the nuclear medicine gold standard examination for imaging of infection/inflammation, covering several indications such as osteomyelitis, prosthetic joint infections, or implantable cardiac device infections. Although this procedure is limited by some disadvantages such as a cumbersome procedure of cellular labeling, high costs related to equipment and training, and the need to acquire images at different time points, making it inconvenient for the patient and logistically problematic for the nuclear medicine department, no radiopharmaceutical was able to compete with it, and thus the SPECT-based radiolabeled WBC is the most commonly used in clinical practice. However, the discovery of a radiopharmaceutical to be utilized as an alternative to radiolabeled WBCs would have a huge impact on the management of patients affected by infectious diseases. Monoclonal antibodies (mAbs) directed against specific antigens expressed on the surface of granulocytes, such as [^{99m}Tc]Tc-besilesomab (Scintimun®), have been propounded as an alternative to WBC [23–25]. The administration of mAbs, although seemed a valid alternative to be used in osteomyelitis, is further limited by the possibility to develop human anti-mouse antibodies (HAMAs), thus warranting the use of humanized versions with high costs of production. It should be also noted that the lack of anatomical landmarks on planar images stands as a limiting factor of both radiolabeled WBC and mAbs, usually necessitating SPECT/CT scans to evaluate the precise location of the uptake and to assess the extent of the infective process in many specific clinical indications.

Gallium-67 (^{67}Ga) citrate is a radiopharmaceutical able to bind to molecules chelating iron such as transferrin glycoproteins, lactoferrin, and bacterial siderophore that has been widely used to image inflammation, infection, and solid tumors [26]. This radiotracer, accumulating in inflammatory or fast proliferating sites, showed a very high sensitivity in imaging fever of unknown origin (FUO). Although [^{67}Ga]Ga-citrate might still find application in FUO, sarcoidosis, spinal discitis, or vertebral osteomyelitis, it is generally considered obsolete and has been replaced by 2-[^{18}F]fluoro-2-deoxy-D-glucose (2-[^{18}F]FDG) PET/CT in centers with access to a PET/CT scanner.

PET imaging of infection has gained prominence in infective and inflammatory diseases over the last decade and is likely to be validated in more clinical contexts in the future. 2-[^{18}F]FDG is the most prevailing PET tracer used in the evaluation of site-specific bacterial, fungal, parasitic, and viral infections such as spondylodiscitis, infection in certain groups of patients like those with diabetes, neutropenia, or prosthetic devices [27–30]. Although logistically easier and quicker to perform, 2-[^{18}F]FDG has gained a prominent role in some indications such as spon-

dylodiscitis, vasculitis, FUO, or bacteremia; this modality is not specific and therefore not able to discriminate infection from inflammation [31]. In an attempt to overcome this limitation, other PET tracers have been examined by taking advantage of differences in microorganisms and mammalian biochemical processes [32]. Gallium-68 (^{68}Ga) citrate is also a nonspecific tracer accumulating in non-infectious inflammation, tested in some infections. The use of the ^{68}Ga-based radioisotopes has been gaining a reputation in the last decade with some being used in infection imaging or have the potential to be used. In procedures where a longer half-life is desirable, other PET tracers such as copper-64 (^{64}Cu) and zirconium-89 (^{89}Zr) have been used in infection imaging. Other compounds have also been labeled using fluorine-18 (^{18}F) for infection imaging. The establishment of PET/MRI may open a new chapter in infection imaging, particularly making soft-tissue delineation easier. The utility of microorganism-specific tracers is also being explored. Many of these tracers are at the preclinical stage of development requiring extensive research for their clinical application. The search for an ideal PET tracer, easy to prepare, able to distinguish infection from inflammation, cheap, able to detect both resistant and susceptible species, and not requiring handling of blood products, is still ongoing.

Moreover, both the WBC scintigraphy and 2-[^{18}F]FDG PET/CT have offered a unique possibility to monitor the response to treatment of infection. Keeping in mind the higher spatial resolution and better ability to quantify tracer uptake of PET imaging, white blood cells have been labeled with PET radiotracers to take advantage of the properties of PET imaging; however, challenges in PET labeling of WBC as well as the brief half-life of fluorine-18, making it impossible to obtain images at a late time point often essential in diagnosing an infection, have not allowed WBC PET to supplant WBC SPECT in the clinical practice.

Nuclear medicine also offers a wide array of radiopharmaceuticals with different targets in order to define the etiology, once the infection is stated. For this purpose, certain antibiotics, antimicrobial peptides, and antiviral and antifungal medications have been tested in preclinical animal models, [^{99m}Tc]Tc-ciprofloxacin (Infecton®) binding to topoisomerase IV and DNA gyrase expressed by proliferating bacteria targeting Gram-positive, Gram-negative, and anaerobic bacteria [31, 33]; cephalosporins, fluoroquinolones, and other antimicrobial peptides, e.g., [^{99m}Tc]Tc-ubiquicidin (UBI); [^{99m}Tc] Tc-fluconazole binding to cytochrome 450 of the microorganism [34]; and [^{18}F]fluoro-5-ethyl-1beta-D-arabinofuranosyluracil ([^{18}F] FEAU) identifying an enzyme produced by herpes simplex virus [35], to name but a few. There are still many concerns about the use of these agents for imaging purposes. Furthermore, the lack of standardization among these studies makes drawing appropriate conclusions about the potential of these antibiotics and anti-microbial peptides very challenging.

1.2.2 Inflammatory Diseases

By targeting specific interleukins, chemokines, interferons, natural ligands, or antigens expressed by particular cells, nuclear imaging techniques offer the possibility to assess the presence of T or B lymphocytes. Some examples include IL-2, radiolabeled with both gamma emitters (technetium-99m, iodine-123) and positron emitters (fluorine-18), extensively evaluated for imaging activated T lymphocytes in a multitude of chronic inflammatory and autoimmune diseases such as type 1 diabetes, inflammatory bowel disease, thyroiditis, and Sjögren's syndrome [36–40]; mAbs and their fragments, including anti-TNF (Infliximab®) and anti-CD20 expressed by B-lymphocytes (Rituximab®), radiolabeled with technetium-99m, iodine-123 or indium-111 for SPECT imaging in both the diagnostic setting and for a prognostic evaluation of treatment response in patients with rheumatoid arthritis [41–44]; somatostatin (SST) analogues radiolabeled with technetium-99m or indium-111 for SPECT imaging frequently used for diagnosis and treatment monitoring by targeting somatostatin receptors (SSTRs) on the surface of activated lymphocytes and fibroblasts in patients affected by rheumatoid arthritis, Sjögren's syndrome, and other chronic inflammatory diseases [45]; as well as gallium-68 (^{68}Ga)-conjugated octreotide/octreotate peptides (-TOC, -NOC, -TATE), also targeting SSTRs as an alternative to gamma-camera studies, providing high-quality images with an improved resolution in comparison with SPECT [46].

1.2.3 Radioimmunoimaging

Radioimmunoimaging refers to the use of radio-labeled antibodies and/or fragments for the in vivo recognition of cancer and other diseases. The development of its key component, antibodies, dates back to the beginning of the twentieth century when Ehrlich brought up the "magic bullet" idea to seek out and eradicate the spirochete of syphilis without affecting normal tissues. Radionuclide-labeled antibodies for the purpose of detecting neoplasms were pioneered by Pressman and Keighley in 1948 [47], followed by several other attempts. However, the potential clinical success of these approaches has been limited by inadequate specificity of labeled antibodies, in part due to their polyclonal origin. The hybridoma technology, firstly introduced by Kohler and Milstein in 1975, made the production of a defined specificity of mAbs possible in unlimited quantities to practically bind to any antigen. However, several constraints, such as the appearance of HAMA due to the murine origin, laborious and time-consuming mAbs production technology, as well as the impracticality of the production of the high-affinity antibody to a particular antigen in small mammals like mice, limit their clinical applications.

Nowadays, the advent of recombinant DNA technology and antibody engineering has made possible the cloning and successful expression of the antibody genes as a fragment in bacteria and other types of cells, also enabling the retention of the intact antigen-binding site (paratope) while diminishing the size of the antibody molecule, expression of the functional antibody and their fusion in bacteria, production of sufficient homogenous protein for diagnostic and therapeutic aims, and the production of a huge variety of genetically engineered antibodies including antigen-binding (Fab) fragments, Fv (variable domain) fragments, or scFv (single-chain fragment variable) antibodies [48]. As times are evolving and new technologies are constantly emerging, the minimized antibody molecules, such as bivalent antibodies, multivalent antibodies, domain antibodies, affibodies, nanobodies, and anticalins, have been provided as building blocks for the construction of new recombinant proteins; nevertheless, these promising imaging agents still have a long way to translate to the clinic.

Since the first radioimmunoimaging study with a radiolabeled antibody targeting carcinoembryonic antigen (CEA) preclinically and in humans in 1974 and 1978, respectively, performed by Dr. Goldenberg [49, 50], unremitting preclinical and clinical studies at various stages have been carried out with the hope of detecting promising targets which are intended to be readily accessible, highly overexpressed only within the desired target tissue, with minimal shedding or secretion from the cell surface, circulation in the blood, and residence in the interstitial compartment. Well-studied molecular patterns against which radiolabeled mAbs have been developed include PD-1, PD-L1, prostate-specific membrane antigen (PSMA), CD20, folate receptor (FR), epidermal growth factor receptor 2 (HER2), and epidermal growth factor receptor (EGFR) (for reference, see [51]). This area of study is still regarded as one of the hot topics in nuclear medicine; however, there are many problems to be solved for clinical application as yet.

1.3 Radioimmunotherapy

Radioimmunotherapy (RIT) refers to a molecular targeted radionuclide therapy using appropriately radiolabeled antibodies to deliver low-dose irradiation from radionuclides to tumor cells by antibodies binding to tumor antigens, thus involving both immunological and radiobiological processes in the cytotoxic mechanisms. In recent years, an immense interest has been posed on RIT following the wide success of immunotherapy and targeted radionuclide therapy. The radionuclides' insensitivity to multidrug resistance, feasibility of simultaneous localization of the tumor via radioimmunoscintigraphy [52, 53], and sterilization of those cancer cells not expressing targeted antigens through "cross-fire" phenomenon (i.e., fatal effects on nearby normal cells not expressing tumor antigens, due to the ranges of ionizing radiations in the tissue being much larger than a typical cell size) [54] account for some of the added advantages of RIT over the mAbs labeled with toxins or drugs. However, a multitude of challenges such as the possible suboptimal pharmacokinetics and biodistribution of the mAb carriers, possible decay of radionuclide-conjugated mAbs prior to reaching the cancerous cells, and possible perturbation of mAb antigen-binding site by the conjugates have made the road to the success of RIT not easy to navigate [55].

Since the first clinical attempt by Beierwaltes in 1951 to assess the therapeutic potential of iodine-131-labeled rabbit antibodies in 14 patients with metastatic melanoma, which reported the complete remission in one patient [56], numerous studies have been carried out till the breakthrough for RIT in 2002, when ibritumomab tiuxetan (Zevalin, murine CD20 mAb conjugated to yttrium-90) had been approved by the US Food and Drug Administration (FDA) [57], followed by the approval of another radioimmunoconjugate, iodine-131-tositumomab (Bexxar), in 2003 [58]. Despite the extensive research efforts made in the recent past, most of the success achieved by radioimmunotherapy is still more notable in hematological malignancies compared to solid tumors. Selection of the ideal targeting antibody and cell surface antigen, preferably expressed at a high, uniform density on the surface of all malignant cells, but not on normal cells or in the bloodstream, is crucial to the success of RIT. Moreover, the success of this therapeutic program is highly dependent on the delivery of an adequate amount of radiolabeled monoclonal antibodies to the target lesions, e.g., by using a suitable radionuclide with satisfactory half-life and path length, using pretargeting, augmenting dosimetry, increasing the immunoreactivity of the antigen, selecting the route of administration, and using novel chelators.

To examine the possible clinical benefit of combinations of RIT with other modes of therapy, such as chemotherapy and/or immunotherapy, to maximize the cytotoxic effect of one's indigenous immune cells would be an interesting topic to be worked on in the future.

1.4 Evaluation of Tumor Response to Immunotherapy

Imaging specialists have to make huge efforts to develop strict criteria to evaluate response to immunotherapy and preferably as early as possible to provide important information for therapy decision-making and allow cessation of therapy in non-responders to avoid further side effects and to keep the economic burden at the lowest level possible. Atypical tumor response patterns that do not belong to four known patterns of response, namely, complete response, partial response, stable disease, or progression, can be observed with immunotherapeutic agents and make the therapeutic evaluation of these treatments challenging. Such atypical response patterns include pseudoprogression, characterized by an apparent increase in the size of lesions or the visualization of new lesions due to the initial T-cell tumor infiltration, disconnected to the tumor cell proliferation, and followed by a response [59–61], as well as dissociated responses, defined as shrinkage of some lesions with concomitant growth in some others. Due to these atypical responses, classical tools for response assessment, such as the Response Evaluation Criteria in Solid Tumors (RECIST) or the PET Response Criteria in Solid Tumors (PERCIST), which are mainly based on the fact that the appearance of new lesions and/or an increase in lesions' size following treatment reveals therapeutic failure and progression, can be limited in the assessment of therapeutic response to the immune checkpoint inhibitors [59, 62].

In order not to misinterpret the post-therapy images and misdiagnose between progressive disease and inflammation, a modification of the anatomical and morphological scales has been suggested, resulting in at least four modified criteria, including irRC (immune-related response criteria) [59], irRECIST (immune-related RECIST) [63], iRECIST (immune RECIST) [61], and imRECIST (immune-modified RECIST) [64].

The misleading impact of new lesions' formation and the increased lesions' size, known as pseudoprogression, on the therapeutic evaluation in radiological imaging is not the only caveat to confront while evaluating patients' response to immunotherapy; it is of note that the 2-[^{18}F]FDG PET metabolic evaluation can also be misleading since 2-[^{18}F]FDG might nonspecifically accumulate as a result of the inflammatory response displacing neutrophils, macrophages, and activated T cells to the tumor site [65]. In an effort to rectify this issue, a number of modified scales have been proposed in nuclear medicine for therapeutic evaluation by 2-[^{18}F]FDG PET of solid tumors treated by immune checkpoint inhibitors, comprising PECRIT (PET/CT Criteria for the early prediction of Response to Immune checkpoint inhibitor Therapy) [66], PERCIMT (PET Response Evaluation Criteria for Immunotherapy) [67], imPERCIST5 (immunotherapy-modified PERCIST up to five lesions) [68], and iPERCIST (immune PERCIST) [69], which are quite different and, thus, require standardization [70]. Considering different response patterns observed in hematological malignancies, scales different than solid tumors are required. The modified Lugano criteria have been recommended with the establishment of lymphoma response to immuno-modulatory therapy criteria (LYRIC) for lymphomas [71]. More details on the abovementioned criteria and their existing constraints are discussed in Chap. 20.

Bearing in mind the fact that not every patient receiving immuno-radiopharmaceuticals will respond to the treatment, nuclear medicine and molecular imaging can play a central role to identify proper biomarkers necessary to predict response to immunotherapy and improve patients' selection.

1.5 Concluding Remarks

In this chapter, we have summarized the immune system, its main building blocks, its innate and adaptive arms, and the role it plays in the development and/or elimination of inflammation, infection, and malignancy. Moreover, there are links between the fields of nuclear medicine and immunology projecting as the procedures for the detection of infection, inflammation and malignancy, radioimmunoimaging, and radioimmunotherapy. Several efforts made in the field of nuclear medicine in recent decades have made it possible to evaluate, in vitro or in vivo in some instances, many molecules playing a central role in the development of infectious, inflammatory, and oncological diseases. The application of molecular imaging techniques may set the stage to assess the expression of the specific molecular targets at the disease site and quantify their presence, resulting in a better understanding of the pathogenesis and cellular network of the infective/inflammatory or neoplastic diseases and thus providing an indispensable tool for an individualized therapy decision-making. In this manner, nuclear medicine imaging contributes in a decisive way to broaden the knowledge, particularly on cancer management and cancer response to treatment, providing several functional data, which also lead to cost-effectiveness. This would permit ideally to change in the near future the approach of treating immune-mediated conditions, cancer care in particular, by selecting the right personalized therapy for the right patient, unraveling the immunological basis of disease pathogenesis and reasons of resistance to treatments received, and laying the foundations to get around them.

References

1. Shlomchik MJ. Immunobiology: the immune system in health and disease. New York: Garland Science; 2005.
2. Akira S, Uematsu S, Takeuchi O. Pathogen recognition and innate immunity. Cell. 2006;124(4):783–801.
3. Rezaei N. Therapeutic targeting of pattern-recognition receptors. Int Immunopharmacol. 2006;6(6):863–9.
4. Janeway CA Jr, Medzhitov R. Innate immune recognition. Annu Rev Immunol. 2002;20(1):197–216.
5. Medzhitov R, Janeway CA. Innate immunity: the virtues of a nonclonal system of recognition. Cell. 1997;91(3):295–8.
6. Matzinger P. The danger model: a renewed sense of self. Science. 2002;296(5566):301–5.
7. Mittal D, Gubin MM, Schreiber RD, Smyth MJ. New insights into cancer immunoediting and its three component phases—elimination, equilibrium and escape. Curr Opin Immunol. 2014;27:16–25.
8. Grivennikov SI, Greten FR, Karin M. Immunity, inflammation, and cancer. Cell. 2010;140(6):883–99.
9. Kantoff PW, Higano CS, Shore ND, Berger ER, Small EJ, Penson DF, et al. Sipuleucel-T immunotherapy for castration-resistant prostate cancer. N Engl J Med. 2010;363(5):411–22.
10. Kirienko M, Sollini M, Chiti A. Hodgkin lymphoma and imaging in the era of anti-PD-1/PD-L1 therapy. Clin Transl Imaging. 2018;6(6):417–27.
11. Ciarmiello A, Fonti R, Giovacchini G, Del Vecchio S. Imaging of immunotherapy response in non-small cell lung cancer: challenges and perspectives. Clin Transl Imaging. 2018;6(6):483–5.
12. Vaz SC, Capacho AS, Oliveira FP, Gil N, Barros CT, Parreira A, et al. Radiopharmacology and molecular imaging of PD-L1 expression in cancer. Clin Transl Imaging. 2018;6(6):429–39.
13. Gordon SR, Maute RL, Dulken BW, Hutter G, George BM, McCracken MN, et al. PD-1 expression by tumour-associated macrophages inhibits phagocytosis and tumour immunity. Nature. 2017;545(7655):495–9.
14. Evangelista L, de Jong M, del Vecchio S, Cai W. The new era of cancer immunotherapy: what can molecular imaging do to help? New York: Springer; 2017.
15. Zappa C, Mousa SA. Non-small cell lung cancer: current treatment and future advances. Transl Lung Cancer Res. 2016;5(3):288.
16. Rosenberg SA. IL-2: the first effective immunotherapy for human cancer. J Immunol. 2014;192(12):5451–8.
17. Signore A, Annovazzi A, Barone R, Bonanno E, D'Alessandria C, Chianelli M, et al. 99mTc-interleukin-2 scintigraphy as a potential tool for evaluating tumor-infiltrating lymphocytes in melanoma lesions: a validation study. J Nucl Med. 2004;45(10):1647–52.
18. Renard V, Staelens L, Signore A, Van Belle S, Dierckx R, Van De Wiele C. Iodine-123-interleukin-2 scintigraphy in metastatic hypernephroma: a pilot study. Q J Nucl Med Mol Imaging. 2007;51(4):352.
19. Loose D, Signore A, Staelens L, Bulcke KV, Vermeersch H, Dierckx RA, et al. (123)I-Interleukin-2 uptake in squamous cell carcinoma of the head and neck carcinoma. Eur J Nucl Med Mol Imaging. 2008;35(2):281–6.
20. Borden EC. Interferons α and β in cancer: therapeutic opportunities from new insights. Nat Rev Drug Discov. 2019;18(3):219–34.
21. Huen AO, Rook AH. Toll receptor agonist therapy of skin cancer and cutaneous T-cell lymphoma. Curr Opin Oncol. 2014;26(2):237–44.

22. Herr HW, Morales A. History of bacillus Calmette-Guerin and bladder cancer: an immunotherapy success story. J Urol. 2008;179(1):53–6.

23. Ruf J, Oeser C, Amthauer H. Clinical role of anti-granulocyte MoAb versus radiolabeled white blood cells. Q J Nucl Med Mol Imaging. 2010;54(6):599.

24. Chianelli M, Boerman O, Malviya G, Galli F, Oyen W, Signore A. Receptor binding ligands to image infection. Curr Pharm Des. 2008;14(31):3316–25.

25. Malherbe C, Dupont A-C, Maia S, Venel Y, Erra B, Santiago-Ribeiro M-J, et al. Estimation of the added value of 99mTc-HMPAO labelled white blood cells scintigraphy for the diagnosis of infectious foci. Q J Nucl Med Mol Imaging. 2019;63(4):371–8.

26. Anghileri L, Heidbreder M. On the mechanism of accumulation of 67Ga by tumors. Oncology. 1977;34(2):74–7.

27. Ammann RW, Stumpe KD, Grimm F, Deplazes P, Huber S, Bertogg K, et al. Outcome after discontinuing long-term benzimidazole treatment in 11 patients with non-resectable alveolar echinococcosis with negative FDG-PET/CT and anti-EmII/3-10 serology. PLoS Negl Trop Dis. 2015;9(9):e0003964.

28. Ankrah AO, Sathekge MM, Dierckx RA, Glaudemans AW. Imaging fungal infections in children. Clin Transl Imaging. 2016;4(1):57–72.

29. Sathekge M, Maes A, Van de Wiele C, editors. FDG-PET imaging in HIV infection and tuberculosis, Seminars in nuclear medicine. Amsterdam: Elsevier; 2013.

30. Glaudemans AW, Signore A. FDG-PET/CT in infections: the imaging method of choice? Eur J Nucl Med Mol Imaging. 2010;37(10):1986–91.

31. Glaudemans AW, de Vries EF, Galli F, Dierckx RA, Slart RH, Signore A. The use of F-FDG-PET/CT for diagnosis and treatment monitoring of inflammatory and infectious diseases. Clin Dev Immunol. 2013;2013:623036.

32. Auletta S, Varani M, Horvat R, Galli F, Signore A, Hess S. PET radiopharmaceuticals for specific bacteria imaging: a systematic review. J Clin Med. 2019;8(2):197.

33. Auletta S, Galli F, Lauri C, Martinelli D, Santino I, Signore A. Imaging bacteria with radiolabelled quinolones, cephalosporins and siderophores for imaging infection: a systematic review. Clin Transl Imaging. 2016;4(4):229–52.

34. Agrawal SG, Mather SJ. Pathogen identification by nuclear imaging–almost there? Eur J Nucl Med Mol Imaging. 2012;39(7):1173–4.

35. Buursma AR, Rutgers V, Hospers GA, Mulder NH, Vaalburg W, de Vries EF. 18F-FEAU as a radiotracer for herpes simplex virus thymidine kinase gene expression: in-vitro comparison with other PET tracers. Nucl Med Commun. 2006;27(1):25–30.

36. Di Gialleonardo V, Signore A, Glaudemans AW, Dierckx RA, De Vries EF. N-(4-18F-fluorobenzoyl) interleukin-2 for PET of human-activated T lymphocytes. J Nucl Med. 2012;53(5):679–86.

37. D'Alessandria C, Di Gialleonardo V, Chianelli M, Mather SJ, de Vries EF, Scopinaro F, et al. Synthesis and optimization of the labeling procedure of 99m Tc-HYNIC-interleukin-2 for in vivo imaging of activated T lymphocytes. Mol Imaging Biol. 2010;12(5):539–46.

38. Signore A, Chianelli M, Ronga G, Pozzilli P, Beverley P. In vivo labelling of activated T lymphocytes by iv injection of 123I-IL2 for detection of insulitis in type 1 diabetes. Prog Clin Biol Res. 1990;355:229–38.

39. Annovazzi A, Biancone L, Caviglia R, Chianelli M, Capriotti G, Mather SJ, et al. 99m Tc-interleukin-2 and 99m Tc-HMPAO granulocyte scintigraphy in patients with inactive Crohn's disease. Eur J Nucl Med Mol Imaging. 2003;30(3):374–82.

40. Chianelli M, Parisella M, Visalli N, Mather S, D'Alessandria C, Pozzilli P, et al. Pancreatic scintigraphy with 99mTc-interleukin-2 at diagnosis of type 1 diabetes and after 1 year of nicotinamide therapy. Diabetes Metab Res Rev. 2008;24(2):115–22.

41. Horton SC, Emery P. Biological therapy for rheumatoid arthritis: where are we now? London: MA Healthcare; 2012.

42. Malviya G, Signore A, Lagana B, Dierckx R. Radiolabelled peptides and monoclonal antibodies for therapy decision making in inflammatory diseases. Curr Pharm Des. 2008;14(24):2401–14.

43. Iodice V, Laganà B, Lauri C, Capriotti G, Germano V, D'amelio R, et al. Imaging B lymphocytes in autoimmune inflammatory diseases. Q J Nucl Med Mol Imaging. 2014;58(3):258–68.

44. Conti F, Ceccarelli F, Priori R, Iagnocco A, Signore A, Valesini G. Intra-articular infliximab in patients with rheumatoid arthritis and psoriatic arthritis with monoarthritis resistant to local glucocorticoids. Clinical efficacy extended to patients on systemic anti-tumour necrosis factor α. Ann Rheum Dis. 2008;67(12):1787–90.

45. Vanhagen P, Markusse H, Lamberts S, Kwekkeboom DJ, Reubi J-C, Krenning E. Somatostatin receptor imaging. The presence of somatostatin receptors in rheumatoid arthritis. Arthritis Rheum. 1994;37(10):1521–7.

46. Signore A, Lauri C, Auletta S, Anzola K, Galli F, Casali M, et al. Immuno-imaging to predict treatment response in infection, inflammation and oncology. J Clin Med. 2019;8(5):681.

47. Pressman D, Keighley G. The zone of activity of antibodies as determined by the use of radioactive tracers; the zone of activity of nephritoxic antikidney serum. J Immunol. 1948;59(2):141–6.

48. Hust M, Jostock T, Menzel C, Voedisch B, Mohr A, Brenneis M, et al. Single chain Fab (scFab) fragment. BMC Biotechnol. 2007;7(1):1–15.

49. Goldenberg DM, Preston DF, Primus FJ, Hansen HJ. Photoscan localization of GW-39 tumors in hamsters using radiolabeled anticarcinoembryonic antigen immunoglobulin G. Cancer Res. 1974;34(1):1–9.

50. Goldenberg DM, DeLand F, Kim E, Bennett S, Primus FJ, van Nagell JR Jr, et al. Use of radio-labeled anti-

bodies to carcinoembryonic antigen for the detection and localization of diverse cancers by external photoscanning. N Engl J Med. 1978;298(25):1384–8.

51. Harsini S, Rezaei N. Cancer imaging with radiolabeled monoclonal antibodies. In: Cancer immunology. Cham: Springer; 2020. p. 739–60.

52. Baum R, Hoer G, Lorenz M, Senekowitsch R, Albrecht M. Clinical results of immunoscintigraphy and radioimmunotherapy. Nuklearmedizin. 1987;26(2):68–78.

53. Perkins A, Baum R. Immunoscintigraphy and immunotherapy 1988 Report of the 3rd IRIST Meeting, Frankfurt/Main, March 1988. Int J Biol Markers. 1988;3(4):265–72.

54. Dixon K. The radiation biology of radioimmunotherapy. Nucl Med Commun. 2003;24(9):951–7.

55. Wu AM, Senter PD. Arming antibodies: prospects and challenges for immunoconjugates. Nat Biotechnol. 2005;23(9):1137–46.

56. Beierwaltes W. Radioiodine-labelled compounds previously or currently used for tumour localization. Meeting on Tumour Localization with Radioactive Agents; 1976.

57. Borghaei H, Schilder RJ, editors. Safety and efficacy of radioimmunotherapy with yttrium 90 ibritumomab tiuxetan (Zevalin), Seminars in nuclear medicine. Amsterdam: Elsevier; 2004.

58. Friedberg JW, Fisher RI. Iodine-131 tositumomab (Bexxar®): radioimmunoconjugate therapy for indolent and transformed B-cell non-Hodgkin's lymphoma. Expert Rev Anticancer Ther. 2004;4(1):18–26.

59. Wolchok JD, Hoos A, O'Day S, Weber JS, Hamid O, Lebbé C, et al. Guidelines for the evaluation of immune therapy activity in solid tumors: immune-related response criteria. Clin Cancer Res. 2009;15(23):7412–20.

60. Borcoman E, Kanjanapan Y, Champiat S, Kato S, Servois V, Kurzrock R, et al. Novel patterns of response under immunotherapy. Ann Oncol. 2019;30(3):385–96.

61. Seymour L, Bogaerts J, Perrone A, Ford R, Schwartz LH, Mandrekar S, et al. iRECIST: guidelines for response criteria for use in trials testing immunotherapeutics. Lancet Oncol. 2017;18(3):e143–e52.

62. Humbert O, Cadour N, Paquet M, Schiappa R, Poudenx M, Chardin D, et al. 18 FDG PET/CT in the early assessment of non-small cell lung cancer response to immunotherapy: frequency and clinical significance of atypical evolutive patterns. Eur J Nucl Med Mol Imaging. 2020;47(5):1158–67.

63. Nishino M, Giobbie-Hurder A, Gargano M, Suda M, Ramaiya NH, Hodi FS. Developing a common language for tumor response to immunotherapy: immune-related response criteria using unidimensional measurements. Clin Cancer Res. 2013;19(14):3936–43.

64. Hodi FS, Ballinger M, Lyons B, Soria J-C, Nishino M, Tabernero J, et al. Immune-modified response evaluation criteria in solid tumors (imRECIST): refining guidelines to assess the clinical benefit of cancer immunotherapy. J Clin Oncol. 2018;36(9):850–8.

65. Rossi S, Castello A, Toschi L, Lopci E. Immunotherapy in non-small-cell lung cancer: potential predictors of response and new strategies to assess activity. Immunotherapy. 2018;10(9):797–805.

66. Cho SY, Lipson EJ, Im H-J, Rowe SP, Gonzalez EM, Blackford A, et al. Prediction of response to immune checkpoint inhibitor therapy using early-time-point 18F-FDG PET/CT imaging in patients with advanced melanoma. J Nucl Med. 2017;58(9):1421–8.

67. Anwar H, Sachpekidis C, Winkler J, Kopp-Schneider A, Haberkorn U, Hassel JC, et al. Absolute number of new lesions on 18 F-FDG PET/CT is more predictive of clinical response than SUV changes in metastatic melanoma patients receiving ipilimumab. Eur J Nucl Med Mol Imaging. 2018;45(3):376–83.

68. Ito K, Teng R, Schöder H, Humm JL, Ni A, Michaud L, et al. 18F-FDG PET/CT for monitoring of ipilimumab therapy in patients with metastatic melanoma. J Nucl Med. 2019;60(3):335–41.

69. Goldfarb L, Duchemann B, Chouahnia K, Zelek L, Soussan M. Monitoring anti-PD-1-based immunotherapy in non-small cell lung cancer with FDG PET: introduction of iPERCIST. EJNMMI Res. 2019;9(1):8.

70. Evangelista L, De Rimini ML, Bianchi A, Schillaci O. Immunotherapy and 18F-FDG PET/CT: standardised procedures are needed. New York: Springer; 2019.

71. Cheson BD, Ansell S, Schwartz L, Gordon LI, Advani R, Jacene HA, et al. Refinement of the Lugano Classification lymphoma response criteria in the era of immunomodulatory therapy. Blood. 2016;128(21):2489–96.

Nuclear Imaging of Endogenous Markers of Lymphocyte Response

2

Israt S. Alam, Travis M. Shaffer, and Sanjiv S. Gambhir

Contents

I. S. Alam · T. M. Shaffer
Department of Radiology, and Molecular
Imaging Program at Stanford (MIPS),
Stanford University School of Medicine,
Stanford, CA, USA
e-mail: israt@stanford.edu

S. S. Gambhir (✉)
Department of Radiology, and Molecular
Imaging Program at Stanford (MIPS),
Stanford University School of Medicine,
Stanford, CA, USA

Department of Bioengineering, Bio-X,
Stanford University, Stanford, CA, USA
e-mail: sgambhir@stanford.edu

© Springer Nature Switzerland AG 2022
S. Harsini et al. (eds.), *Nuclear Medicine and Immunology*,
https://doi.org/10.1007/978-3-030-81261-4_2

2.1   Introduction

The need to image immune cells and their functional states has largely been motivated by the wider application of immunotherapies and due to mounting experimental and clinical evidence for their role in the pathogenesis of certain diseases. Conventional immune monitoring methods such as profiling of peripheral blood using multiplexed tools like flow cytometry, mass cytometry, and cytokine analyses are minimally invasive and allow for serial sampling of immune related biomarkers but ultimately lack spatial information. On the other hand, biopsies that enable histological analyses of immune infiltrate within tissues are invasive and are unable to capture tissue heterogeneity or whole-body information. Conventional imaging protocols that provide anatomical information have limited utility in early and sensitive measurements of the immune response, thus mobilizing the imaging community to develop superior molecular imaging approaches.

The immune response involves the activation, coordination, and deployment of multiple immune cell subsets and their signaling molecules to protect us from pathogens and aberrant cells. Broadly divided into two arms, the innate and the adaptive system, these synergize and communicate extensively to ensure that an appropriate and complimentary response to a particular stressor is launched. The innate system represents the first line of defense comprising of physical, chemical, and biological barriers to infection. A hallmark of this system is that innate immune cells have the ability to respond to pathogens in a rapid, transient manner, through the recognition of conserved molecular patterns found in microorganisms [1]. In contrast, adaptive immunity is characterized by a delayed onset. A hallmark of this response is the specificity required for antigen recognition which occurs through specific cell surface receptors on adaptive immune cells. Rapid clonal expansion and the capacity

for immunological memory are further attributes of the adaptive system which enable the host to launch faster responses upon subsequent exposure to the antigen.

All immune cells are derived from hematopoietic stem cell precursors in the bone marrow. These pluripotent cells give rise to more specialized cells known as the common myeloid and the common lymphoid progenitors. The majority of innate immune cells such as neutrophils, dendritic cells (DCs), and macrophages derive from the myeloid progenitor. While neutrophils can kill pathogens directly, DCs engage and activate the adaptive immune system by acting as antigen-presenting cells (APCs) [2], and macrophages are able to fulfil both functions. The common lymphoid progenitor gives rise to lymphocytes, comprised of T lymphocytes (T cells), B lymphocytes (B cells), and natural killer (NK) cells. Cumulatively lymphocytes can represent 20–40% of total leukocytes and play critical roles in the immune response. T cells and B cells are morphologically similar and articulate the adaptive response, specifically cell-mediated and humoral adaptive responses, respectively. NK cells have the predominant morphology of large, granular lymphocytes and constitute an important part of innate immunity. Lymphocytes have high specificity and potency and thus are optimal targets for treating disease. This therapeutic focus catalyzes the need for quantitative, clinically applicable lymphocyte imaging tools.

The unprecedented success of cancer immunotherapies such as immune checkpoint blockade [3], cancer vaccines [4], and adoptive cell therapies [5] has served to highlight the critical role lymphocytes, particularly activated T cells, have in the killing of aberrant cells [6]. Conventional anatomical imaging using computed tomography (CT) and magnetic resonance imaging (MRI) along with response criteria originally established for chemotherapy and radiotherapy assessment, have struggled to predict anti-cancer immune responses. In particular, distinguishing disease progression from pseudoprogression, an initial increase in tumor size resulting from immune cell influx and usually a positive indicator of immunotherapy (IOT) outcome, using anatomical imaging or 2-[18F]fluoro-2-deoxy-d-glucose ([^{18}F]FDG)–PET, has been challenging [7, 8]. Current immune response evaluation criteria developed specifically for solid tumors undergoing IOT protocols require at least 9–12 weeks before follow-up and assessment of therapeutic efficacy is possible [9, 10]. Clinicians need superior methods to confirm true response *early* on in treatment. Despite impressive clinical responses in scenarios where all first-line treatments have failed, IOT response rates can vary drastically, with only a subset of patients responding favorably [11]. The specific readouts that immune cell imaging could provide for early assessment of IOT efficacy include global monitoring of immune cell homing, tumor infiltration, activation, proliferation, dysfunction, and immune-related adverse effects (irAEs) that have been extensively reviewed elsewhere [12–14]. With the increasing number of newly approved IOTs and many more in the drug development pipeline, there is a critical unmet need for superior tools that can accurately capture these behaviors in vivo to monitor therapeutic efficacy more effectively.

In parallel to the growth of cancer IOTs, the role of immune cells as principal drivers of inflammatory events in infection, allergy, and autoimmunity are better understood today. B and T cells are heavily implicated in autoimmune diseases, a diverse group of mostly chronic disorders that are characterized by a loss of self-tolerance. The resulting abnormal immune responses often culminate in the destruction of normal tissues as observed in type I diabetes [15], multiple sclerosis (MS) [16], inflammatory bowel diseases (IBD) [17], and systemic lupus crythematosus (SLE) [18]. Collectively, these pathologies are a significant cause of morbidity and mortality and globally are on the rise, highlighting the need for adequate tools to monitor underlying immune activity and disease progression. The field of transplantation also has the potential to benefit from longitudinal immune imaging protocols since allogenic immune responses represent the most frequent cause of transplant-related complications, observed in solid organ transplant rejection [19, 20] and in recipients of hematopoietic cell transplantation (HCT) whom frequently develop graft versus host disease (GvHD) [21]. Monitoring early activation, migration, and tissue-specific infiltration of immune cells through imaging has the potential to determine the prognostic significance of these events and facilitate early intervention.

Though planar bioluminescence and intravital microscopy have greatly informed our current knowledge of immune cell behaviors in the preclinical setting [22–24], nuclear imaging has emerged as an ideal, clinically relevant modality for noninvasive detection of immune responses. Lymphocytes are highly mobile, migrating between different compartments of differentiation, immunosurveillance, and activation, thus requiring whole-body imaging such as nuclear imaging to capture the vast immune geography. Within the nuclear imaging modalities, positron emission tomography (PET) has added potential over single photon emission computed tomography (SPECT) due to its superior sensitivity and quantitative capabilities. These criteria are ideal for immune imaging where relatively small numbers of immune cells may be distributed within a large volume [25]. By far the most common approach for PET imaging of immune cells has been through the direct targeting of endogenous immune biomarkers that are either present constitutively or upregulated during immune responses. These markers can be imaged by direct injection of a radiolabeled probe with specificity for the biomarker and bypass the need for isolation or ex vivo manipulation of immune cells.

In this chapter, we first broadly discuss the different types of endogenous biomarkers that can be targeted for immune imaging. Next we review endogenous biomarker-targeted nuclear imaging probes that have been developed specifically for visualization of each of the lymphocyte populations. Undoubtedly the mostly widely imaged immune population to date has been T cells, for which we provide a comprehensive overview of probes that have been developed to specifically image distinct T cell functional states. This is followed by a discussion of B cell imaging probes that have been developed targeting specific lineage receptors. Next we provide an overview of NK cell imaging strategies reported to date and the increasing demand for improved monitoring of these cells as they emerge as a highly promising candidate in cancer IOT. We evaluate these imaging probes for their ability to visualize each of the lymphocyte populations, their strengths and limitations. Finally, we discuss priority focus areas for the field of immune imaging and developments that are on the horizon for enhancing the capabilities of this rapidly evolving field.

2.2 Strategies for Imaging Endogenous Immune Biomarkers

The immunoimaging toolbox has grown exponentially in the last decade fueled in part by improvements in radiometal availability, radiochemistry, and probe development [26]. Broadly, ideal characteristics for general labeling of any immune cell includes facile radiolabeling, an imaging probe that is biologically inert, demonstrates high metabolic stability in vivo, possesses optimal pharmacokinetics, and is compatible and safe for human translation. Here we introduce endogenous biomarkers which may be present on the immune cell surface, reside intracellularly, or be secreted, that can be targeted to probe lymphocyte responses in vivo. We further discuss the merits and challenges of these strategies compared to direct and indirect labeling methods that require ex vivo manipulation of cells.

2.2.1 Cell Surface Immune Markers

Targeting endogenous cell surface markers has gained considerable traction in the immune-imaging field due to advances in immunobiology that have led to the characterization of multiple immune-specific, cell surface membrane proteins known as cluster of differentiation (CD) molecules. CD markers can be reflective of cell lineage, differentiation, and the activation status of cells and often fulfil important functions, acting as receptors or ligands capable of downstream signaling. While immunophenotyping of cells using multiplexed tools such as flow cytometry involves assaying several CD markers in parallel, nuclear imaging approaches to date have targeted a single CD marker at a time. Lymphocyte-associated cell surface CD markers that have been imaged to date are summarized in Table 2.1.

By far the most popular approach to image surface immune markers has depended on antibodies. ImmunoPET, the use of antibodies and smaller antibody fragments radiolabeled with PET isotopes, combines the ultra-high specificity and affinity antibodies have for antigen recognition, with the superior sensitivity of PET [27]. Originally used to target tumor-associated antigens, immunoPET is a swiftly expanding imaging approach that has been extended to other applications and has benefited from the growing repertoire of FDA-approved monoclonal antibody therapies. In addition, standard radiochemistries are now available, where intact antibodies and their fragments can be modified with bifunctional chelates and subsequently radiolabeled with relative ease [27].

Design considerations for immunoPET probes are highly dependent on the application and imaging requirements. The choice of vector (the biological targeting entity) significantly impacts the pharmacokinetics of the final probe and consequently the optimal imaging timepoint, choice of radiometal, and associated bifunctional chelate. Full-size monoclonal antibodies (mAbs) exhibit slower penetration into tissues and long blood residence times due to their large size (~150 kDa), often requiring the patient to return to the clinic for imaging for optimal target: background ratios (4–7 days post-tracer injection). Thus, full-size mAbs pair well with longer-lived isotopes such as zirconium-89 (^{89}Zr, $t_{1/2}$ = 3.3 days). Imaging with ^{89}Zr-labeled full-size mAbs is however associated with high radiation doses (a function of the long half-life, frequency of high-energy non-positron emissions and the slow clearance of the vector). To overcome these limitations, smaller engineered antibody fragments including minibodies (~75 kDa) and diabodies (~50 kDa) have been developed, which exhibit rapid uptake into target sites and clearance. The removal of constant domains of the immunoglobulin heavy chain that also constitutes the Fc region significantly reduces non-specific binding of the vector to Fc receptors on other immune cells [28, 29]. With the serum half-life reduced from weeks (for full antibodies) to hours, the rapid kinetics of smaller fragments like diabodies makes them amenable to labeling and same-day imaging with short-lived isotopes like fluorine-18 (^{18}F, $t_{1/2}$ = 110 min) and gallium-68 (^{68}Ga, $t_{1/2}$ = 68 min) [30, 31].

In parallel antibody and antibody fragments from other species like camelid and shark are also under active evaluation for immunoPET applications due to their small size [32, 33]. Single-domain antibodies (sdAbs) that are considered the smallest (~15 kDa), naturally derived antigen-binding fragment of an antibody have been developed to improve tissue penetration and clearance rates [34]. Specifically, those derived from heavy chain only IgG antibodies from camelid (also known as VHHs or nanobodies) have shown utility in immune imaging applications [32, 35–37]. VHH domains also exhibit low immunogenicity, likely due to the high sequence identity with human type 3 VH domains. It is worth noting that smaller fragments can exhibit reduced stability and low overall uptake into target sites, a function of their monovalent binding and rapid clearance [38, 39]. Finally, advances in de novo protein and chemical engineering platforms have further expanded the toolbox of potential immune imaging probes and facilitated the development of alternate protein scaffolds such as fibronec-

Table 2.1 Endogenous biomarkers for nuclear imaging of lymphocytes and their associated probes

Biomarker	Biomarker location and type	Biomarker imaging-development stage	Nuclear imaging probes	Species reactivity of probe	Comments
CD3	Cell surface lineage marker	Preclinical	[^{89}Zr]Zr-DFO-CD3-mAb [87, 279]	Murine	• CD3 may undergo down-regulation during T cell activation • Targeting CD3 can modulate T cell subsets in vivo (e.g, reduce CD4+ T cells and stimulate CD8+ T cells)
CD8	Cell surface lineage marker	Clinical	[^{89}Zr]Zr-malDFO-CD8-cDb [91, 102, 280]	Murine	• Multiple ongoing clinical imaging studies using the CD8-targeted minibody [^{89}Zr]Zr-DFO-IAB22M2C: NCT03107663 NCT03802123 NCT03610061
			[^{64}Cu]Cu-NOTA-CD8-Mb [90]	Murine	
			[^{89}Zr]Zr-DFO-CD8-VHH-XI8 [282]	Murine	
			[^{89}Zr]Zr-DFO-IAB22M2C [97, 283]	Human	
CD4	Cell surface lineage marker	Clinical	[^{99m}Tc]Tc-HYNIC-CD4-Fab [101]	Human	• CD4-targeted antibody fragments exhibit improved kinetics compared to full antibodies and warrant clinical evaluation with PET particularly for autoimmune disease diagnosis and therapy monitoring
			[^{64}Cu]Cu-NOTA-CD4-F(ab') 2 [103]	Murine	
			[^{89}Zr]Zr-malDFO-CD4-cDb [89]	Murine	
CD7	Cell surface lineage marker	Preclinical	[^{89}Zr]Zr-DFO-CD7-F(ab') 2 [284]	Human	• CD7 targeting with full IgG or F(ab')2 advantageously did not modulate T cell activity
CD25 (IL-2 receptor alphachain)	Cell surface activation marker	Clinical	[^{99m}Tc]Tc-HYNIC-IL-2 [106, 115]	Human	• CD25 is a broad immune activation marker • May also be upregulated on hematological tumor cells
			[^{18}F]FB-IL-2 [107]	Human	
CD69	Cell surface activation marker	Preclinical	[^{64}Cu]Cu-NOAGA-CD69-mAb [121]	Murine	• CD69 is an early activation marker and may have a narrow window of expression
OX40 (CD134)	Cell surface activation marker	Preclinical	[^{64}Cu]Cu-DOTA-OX40-mAb [104, 4]	Murine	• OX40 expression is skewed toward CD4+ T cells versus CD8+ T cells
ICOS (CD278)	Cell surface activation marker	Preclinical	[^{89}Zr]Zr-DFO-ICOS-mAb [128]	Murine	• ICOS is highly upregulated on both activated CD4+ and CD8+ T cells
HKs	Intracellular metabolic enzyme–glycolysis	Clinical	2-[^{18}F]FDG [143, 50]	Murine/human	• GLUT expression increases during immune activation and mediates 2-[^{18}F]FDG uptake into cells • 2-[^{18}F]FDG has low specificity for visualizing T cell specific responses

(continued)

Table 2.1 (continued)

Biomarker	Function	Stage	Probe	Species	Notes
TK1	Intracellular metabolic enzyme-DNA synthesis	Clinical	[^{18}F]FLT [152, 154]	Murine/human	• High levels of endogenous thymidine in rodents and humans leads to low levels of [^{18}F]FLT accumulation and limits the overall sensitivity
dCK	Intracellular metabolic enzyme-DNA synthesis	Clinical	[^{18}F]FAC [156, 158, 161], [^{18}F]CFA [159, 160]	Murine/human	• [^{18}F]FAC undergoes rapid catabolism in humans, [^{18}F]-CFA is more stable and suitable for human use
dGK	Intracellular metabolic enzyme-DNA synthesis	Clinical	[^{18}F]F-AraG [167-169]	Murine/human	• [^{18}F]F-AraG is predominantly metabolized by dGK but may also reflect dCK activity
Granzyme B	Secreted marker of CD8+ T cell cytotoxicity	Preclinical	[^{68}Ga]Ga-NOTA-GZP [55, 171]	Murine	• The peptide probe [^{68}Ga]Ga-NOTA-GZP binds to the secreted granzyme B compartment • Secreted molecules pose challenges for imaging due to target dilution • Biomarker is also present within intracellular granules (inaccessible to probe)
IFN γ	Secreted marker of CD8+ T cell cytotoxicity	Preclinical	[^{89}Zr]Zr-DFO-IFNγ-mAb [56]	Murine	• [^{89}Zr]Zr-DFO-IFNγ-mAb was shown to bind to surface of tumor cells via their IFNγ-receptor expression
PD-1 (CD279)	Cell surface marker for inhibition and control	Clinical	[^{64}Cu]Cu-NOTA-PD-1-mAb [285]	Murine	• [^{89}Zr]Zr-DFO-nivolumab is feasible and safe in humans. Uptake correlated with PD-1 expression on lymphocytic aggregates detected in tumor biopsies from non-small cell lung cancer patients
			[^{64}Cu]Cu-DOTA/[^{89}Zr]Zr-DFO-pembrolizumab [286, 185]	Human	
			[^{89}Zr]Zr-DFO-nivolumab [287, 191]	Human	
CTLA-4 (CD152)	Cell surface marker for inhibition and control	Clinical	[^{64}Cu]Cu-DOTA-CTLA-4-mAb [288]	Murine	A phase 2 trial with [^{89}Zr]Zr-ipilimumab in metastatic melanoma patients is currently underway: NCT03313323
			[^{64}Cu]Cu-DOTA-ipilimumab [187]	Human	
			[^{64}Cu]Cu-DOTA-CTLA-4-mAb and [^{64}Cu]Cu-DOTA-CTLA-4-F(ab')$_2$ [289]	Human	
CD19	Cell surface lineage marker	Preclinical	[^{64}Cu]Cu-DOTA-CD19-mAb [237]	Murine	CD19 targeted imaging has the potential to detect a broader range of B cell subsets than CD20
CD20	Cell surface lineage marker	Clinical	[^{89}Zr]Zr-Df-rituximab [290, 210-212, 291]	Human	• CD20 has been most commonly been imaged with rituximab, a chimeric mouse/human antibody mAb therapy approved for treatment of B cell malignancies and rheumatoid arthritis
			[^{64}Cu]Cu-DOTA-rituximab [78]	Human	
			[^{124}I]I-GA-cDb, [^{124}I]I-GA-cMb [^{89}Zr]Zr-GA-cDb, [^{89}Zr]Zr-GA-cMb [224]	Human	
			[^{64}Cu]Cu-DOTA-FN3(CD20) [40]	Human	
			[^{124}I]I-CD20-scFv-Fc, [^{124}I]I-CD20-Mb, [^{64}Cu]Cu-DOTA-CD20-Mb [292]	Human	
			[^{177}Lu]Lu-DTPA-sdAb 9079, [^{68}Ga]Ga-NOTA-sdAb 9079 [228]	Human	
CD56	Cell surface lineage marker	Preclinical	[^{99m}Tc]Tc-HYNIC-CD56-mAb [262]	Human	• While CD56 is a useful marker for peripheral human NK cells (defined as CD3-, CD56+), it is also expressed on other cell types and some cancers
NKp30	Cell surface activation marker	Preclinical	^{64}Cu-NKp30-mAb, ^{89}Zr-NKp30-mAb[264]	Human	• While NKp30 is a specific marker for human NK cells, the relatively low expression (2000-3000 receptors per cell) may preclude its use as a diagnostic target
NKp46	Cell surface activation marker	Preclinical	^{64}Cu-NKp46-mAb, ^{89}Zr-NKp46-mAb [265]	Human	• NKp46 is expressed on both human andmurine NK cells, allowing for the use ofimmunocompetent murine models for preclinical optimization

Endogenous markers associated with T lymphocytes (white cells), B lymphocytes (blue cells), and natural killer cells (purple cells) and their associated probes imaged to date. Common acronyms for biomarkers: *CD* cluster of differentiation marker, *ICOS* inducible T cell costimulator, *GLUT* glucose transporter, *HKs* hexokinases, *TK1* thymidine kinase 1, *dCK* deoxycytidine kinase, *dGK* deoxyguanosine kinase, *CTLA-4* cytotoxic T-lymphocyte-associated protein 4, *PD-1* programmed cell death receptor 1. **Nuclear imaging probes**: *mAb* monoclonal antibody, *Mb* minibody, *cDb* cys-diabody, *DFO* deferoxamine, *IL-2* interleukin-2, *FDG* fluorodeoxyglucose, *FLT* fluorothymidine, *FAC* fluoroarabinofuranosyl-cytosine, *CFA* clofarabine, *AraG* arabinofuranosyl guanine, *IFNγ* interferon-γ.

Biomarker imaging developmental stage assigned as "Clinical" indicates endogenous targets that are currently under clinical evaluation

[a]Metabolic pathways: overall levels of the associated biomarkers and their activity are upregulated during T cell activation and proliferation

tin domains [40], cysteine knots [41, 42], and adnectins [43] that have shown utility as both cancer and immune imaging agents. Obtaining clinical approval for radiolabeled antibodies, piggybacking off antibodies already approved for therapy, may however be easier than for new entities such as engineered proteins. Overall, the choice of vector, chelate, and radiometal requires careful consideration for optimal imaging and has been widely reviewed [27, 44].

2.2.2 Intracellular Metabolic Pathways

An alternative approach for imaging immune cells is to target endogenous intracellular metabolic pathways that are upregulated during specific functional states. Glycolysis [45] and DNA synthesis [46] typically increase during immune activation in order to fulfil the bioenergetic demands for growth and expansion. Small molecules are particularly well suited to probing intracellular metabolic pathways, and development of such radiotracers has benefited from high-throughput screening of existing small molecule chemical libraries. Depending on their lipophilicity, charge, molecular weight, and stability, small molecules (typically <500 Da) are able to passively or actively cross biological barriers and undergo rapid clearance [25]. Although they can be developed to bind to surface markers, their utility has mostly been explored for probing enzymatic/metabolic activity. A major advantage of this strategy is signal amplification, which results from the enzyme being able to act on several substrate molecules that subsequently become trapped intracellularly. The size of these probes makes them suited for radiolabeling with smaller radioisotopes such as ^{11}C ($t_{1/2}$ = 20 min) and ^{18}F ($t_{1/2}$ = 110 min) that are unlikely to alter their pharmacokinetics and targeting properties. Advantageously, small molecule probes can be radiolabeled at much higher specific activities than biologics; thus pico- to femtomole levels per gram of tissue are sufficient for imaging. At such low doses, any biological or pharmacological effects in vivo are highly unlikely though this can be confirmed with toxicity studies [47].

The most well-established metabolic PET tracer, [^{18}F]FDG, is a glucose analogue that has been used to probe the glycolytic pathway. [^{18}F]FDG is taken up by glucose transporters (GLUTs), and subsequently phosphorylated by hexokinase I, becoming trapped intracellularly. Since the majority of cancers exhibit increased glucose consumption to meet their metabolic needs (known as the Warburg effect), [^{18}F] FDG has become the gold standard for detection and staging of most cancers and for monitoring response to therapy [48]. Glycolysis is also upregulated in both innate and adaptive immune cells during immune activation and proliferation [49], leading to [^{18}F]FDG being assessed for immune activation in a number of indications including inflammation [50]

and transplant rejection [49] and for evaluating response to immune checkpoint blockade [51, 52]. Although it has shown some promise in these applications, the nonspecific nature of [^{18}F]FDG results in high rates of false-positive signals and has motivated the immune imaging field to evaluate other metabolic pathways and complimentary probes that are more specific for immune responses. These newer small molecule metabolic tracers have been used to probe T cell activation and will be discussed in more depth later on in this chapter and are summarized in Table 2.1.

2.2.3 Secreted Biomarkers

Much of the communication and signaling between cells is mediated by small proteins secreted by tissues and immune cells called cytokines [53]. Cytokines produced by immune cells along with other secreted effector molecules can reflect their functional state. Cytokines like interleukin (IL)-6, IL-10, and transforming growth factor-beta (TGF-β), for example, are considered immunosuppressive, and high serum levels of these are correlated with poor prognosis in cancer. Conversely pro-inflammatory cytokines such as IL-2 and interferon (IFN)-γ are associated with favorable prognosis [54]. Recent advances in immune-monitoring methods have made it possible to use peripheral blood to characterize the patient's immune profile. Despite the ease of sampling, cytokine concentrations in the blood do not always sensitively reflect the concentrations within a tumor microenvironment or at the site of immunopathology. This has motivated the development of imaging probes targeted to candidate secreted immune biomarkers [55–57]. Lymphocyte-associated secreted biomarkers imaged to date are summarized in Table 2.1. Possible dilution of imaging signal due to biomarker secretion is a potential concern for this class of biomarker; additionally cytokines can be produced by a wide distribution of immune and endo-epithelial cells.

2.2.4 Strengths and Limitations Compared to Ex Vivo Labeling Approaches

The major advantage of endogenous biomarker targeting strategies is that the isolation and ex vivo manipulation of cells, which can compromise cellular functionality, are bypassed. In contrast, ex vivo direct labeling first requires isolation of immune cells from a subject, these cells are then tagged with a radioactive molecule before reintroduction of the labeled cells back into the subject for cell tracking and imaging. This strategy was one of the earliest methods to track immune cells in vivo and is an established clinical nuclear imaging protocol specifically used for visualizing autologous white blood cells for detection of inflammatory foci [58]. To date multiple preclinical and clinical studies have utilized this approach to track adoptively transferred immune subsets and therapies in vivo [59–61]. Though relatively simple and generalizable to most cell types, a major limitation of this approach is low temporal resolution where the radiolabel is not uniformly passed on to daughter cells during proliferation. Lymphocytes can be sensitive to lipophilic chelates used [62] and to Auger electrons emitted from commonly used isotopes in direct labeling like indium-111 (^{111}In, $t_{1/2}$ = 2.8 days), which can negatively impact cells at a genetic or functional level [63, 64]. It therefore becomes important to characterize the overall health and functionality of lymphocytes labeled in this manner such as assessment of viability, proliferative capacity, and cytokine production [60].

Indirect labeling also involves isolation of cells so that a foreign reporter gene can be introduced using electroporation, transfection, or viral transduction, leading to the translation of a functional protein that is normally absent. Modified cells can subsequently be imaged with a corresponding radiotracer that can be metabolized by an artificially expressed intracellular protein or be specifically bound by an artificially expressed cell surface receptor [65, 66]. The advantage of this approach is overall low background tracer accumulation in other tissues lacking expression of the reporter gene and sustained reporter gene expression in subsequent generations of daughter cells allowing for longitudinal monitoring of immune cells in vivo. The reporter gene approach has dominated the imaging of adoptive T cell therapies which already require ex vivo manipulation, genetic engineering, and expansion during production [67, 68]. The most widely characterized PET reporter gene is the herpes simplex virus type 1 thymidine kinase (HSV1-tk) enzyme and its optimized mutant sr39tk [69, 70]. The clinical utility of HSV1-tk and its corresponding PET tracer 9-(4-[^{18}F]fluoro-3-(hydroxymethyl) butyl) guanine ([^{18}F]FHBG) for imaging T cell trafficking was shown in a landmark study reporting the first reporter gene imaging of adoptive T cells in patients with recurrent high-grade glioblastoma [71]. A number of challenges lie in the use of reporter genes including the phenomenon of promoter silencing, squelching, and potential negative impacts on cellular functionality. With viral genes there is an added risk of insertional oncogenesis [72], while expression of a foreign protein such as HSV1-tk can trigger immune responses [73] and has prompted the development of several humanized PET reporters [74–76]. Though most reporter systems used have been constitutive, inducible systems where reporter gene expression can be linked to certain biological responses such as immune activation have the potential to impart greater specificity and functional insights [77]. Despite the enormous potential of this approach, ex vivo handling of primary cells is not always feasible, and endogenous targeting remains the most widely used strategy for noninvasive imaging studies.

Biomarker identification and probe development have greatly aided the molecular imaging field to ensure specific and sensitive interrogation of immune cells. A principal drawback of this approach is the potential overlap in the expression of cell surface targets or metabolic demands of the target immune cell with other cells or tissues, resulting in binding or uptake of the imaging agent at non-intended sites which can confound interpretation of the signals. A further challenge is that the expression of surface markers can be very dynamic, for example, activation markers are switched on at different timepoints post-stimulation and can have varying temporal windows of expression. Identifying the appropriate imaging timepoint for a disease or therapy model can therefore be challenging. Additionally, many candidate antibodies used in immunoPET were originally developed as therapeutic agents and possess strong agonist or antagonistic functions. Although imaging doses are significantly lower than therapeutic doses, the protein dose injected (μg to mg quantities in preclinical and clinical imaging studies, respectively), may nevertheless have unwanted biological consequences on the immune cells depending on the target and probe selected [78]. Furthermore, the sensitivity for detecting the immune cell of interest and the overall image quality can be impacted by the presence of antigen sinks (tissues that also exhibit high target expression, e.g., spleen and lymph nodes) that may compete for the tracer and reduce its availability for binding to the target immune cell at sites of interest.

The prognostic value of endogenous immune biomarkers can vary depending on the disease and therapy regimens involved and therefore require careful characterization to fully establish how imaging may guide clinical decisions. Lastly, there are certain lymphocyte subsets such as regulatory T cells or functional states such as T cell exhaustion for which unique biomarkers have not been yet been characterized. Imaging these populations thus becomes challenging unless they are first isolated and specifically tagged ex vivo. The isolation and ex vivo labeling of cells in direct and indirect labeling methods can overcome some of the problems in specificity that targeting endogenous markers face. In the following section, we will discuss examples of these approaches that have allowed the detection of lymphocyte responses in preclinical and clinical settings and evaluate the utility of these imaging agents in the context of cancer and immunopathology.

2.3 Imaging T Cell Responses

2.3.1 Overview of T Cell Biology

T lymphocytes or T cells are by far the most abundant lymphocyte. In isolated peripheral blood mononuclear cells (PBMCs), T cells represent the most abundant cell type (40–70% of total cells). They are undoubtedly a primary focus in the molecular imaging field because of their dominant roles in driving anti-cancer responses and immunopathology and due to the growth in T cell-based therapies. T cells can be distinguished from other lymphocytes by the presence of T cell receptors (TCRs) on their cell surface which possess unique antigen specificity. T cells originally derive from the bone marrow and complete their maturation in the thymus where they differentiate into distinct subsets such as helper and cytotoxic T cells [79]. Carefully selected mature T cells egress from the thymus and can recirculate between blood, secondary lymphoid organs (SLOs), and lymph, potentially for many years. SLOs, including the spleen and lymph nodes, represent specialized sites where naïve T cells encounter their specific antigen and become activated [80]. Once activated, T cells expand rapidly, eventually creating potent effector mechanisms for eliminating microbes and aberrant cells. In the following sections, endogenous markers of these T cell responses and associated PET probes that have been developed will be discussed.

2.3.2 T Cell Activation and Proliferation

Initiated within SLOs, T cell activation is a critical event in protective immunity, where activated APCs having encountered pathogens or their products present foreign antigens to naïve T cells through the formation of an immune synapse [81]. The detection of early markers of T-cell activation at LNs, can act as indicators of an effective immune response. Our understanding of the molecular dynamics of this crucial interaction has benefited considerably from flow cytometry analyses and in vivo intravital microscopy of lymphoid compartments. Optimal T cell activation requires two distinct signaling events. Firstly, the TCR must bind and recognize its cognate antigen, presented on the major histocompatibility complex (MHC) located on target cells (MHC class I) or APCs (MHC class II). Here the co-receptors CD4 expressed on helper T cells and CD8 on cytotoxic T cells work to stabilize the MHC-TCR complex. TCR engagement alone is insufficient to induce cytokine production or sustain proliferation and can lead to apoptosis or anergy (an unresponsive state) [82]. The second required signal, known as costimulation, is antigen-independent and involves T cell costimulatory molecules such as CD28, binding to their respective ligands on activated APCs [83]. This dual event ensures optimal TCR signaling, high levels of IL-2 production, clonal expansion, and eventually differentiation of the naïve population into effector and memory cells [77]. Upon in vivo expansion, antigen-specific T cells are able to leave the LNs via the efferent lymphatic vessels or vasculature and migrate to sites of inflammation, eventually extravasating into tissues and organs to carry out effector function [84].

While CD28 is the most well-characterized costimulatory molecule, other "positive" costimulatory receptors that also drive activation have since been identified, many belonging to the tumor necrosis factor receptor (TNFR) superfamily including CD40, OX40 (CD134), GITR, and 4-1BB (CD137) [85]. In contrast to CD28 which is constitutively expressed on naïve T cells, expression of these costimulatory receptors is induced following T cell activation (within hours to days of antigen recognition) [86]. The low expression of these receptors on naïve cells and increased abundance on activated cells have made them attractive biomarkers for imaging T cell activation. Importantly, while costimulation provides protective immunity in response to infection, cancer, or cancer IOT, in the context of an innocuous agent, grafted organ, or self-organ, it can drive allergy, rejection, and autoimmunity, respectively. Thus, imaging activation in these contexts can provide novel insights into mechanisms of immune dysfunction underlying these conditions.

2.3.2.1 Targeting Cell Surface Lineage Markers

The last decade has seen the evaluation of several immunoPET agents to visualize T cell activation and expansion in vivo. Constitutively expressed lineage identifying T cell surface markers imaged to date include CD3 [87, 88], CD4 [89], and CD8 [90, 91]. Although not specific for activation, these markers are able to capture the expansion of T cells downstream of activation, and homing of effector T cells to specific sites.

CD3-targeted immunoPET approaches to visualize tumor infiltrating T cells have been evaluated in murine models of colorectal [87] and bladder cancer [88]. Larimer et al. reported a murine CD3-specific antibody radiolabeled with zirconium-89 (^{89}Zr) via bioconjugation with the chelate deferoxamine (DFO). Anti-mouse [^{89}Zr] Zr-DFO-anti-CD3-mAb was able to clearly visualize tumor-infiltrating lymphocytes (TILs) in a murine colon carcinoma model in response to anti-cytotoxic T lymphocyte-associated protein 4 (CTLA-4) therapy [87]. The tracer exhibited high uptake in tumors, prior to any anatomic changes, which correlated with greater therapeutic response at later timepoints, highlighting the potential clinical utility of this strategy to predict response to immune checkpoint blockade (ICB). Pektor et al. reported a human CD3-targeted immunoPET approach for imaging disease progression in a humanized mouse model of graft versus host disease (GVHD), a major complication of allogeneic hematopoietic cell transplantation (HCT) in which donor T cells are primarily activated upon interaction with host tissue, undergoing dramatic expansion and eventually mediating destruction of key tissues such as skin, liver, and the gastrointestinal tract [92]. Anti-human [^{89}Zr] Zr-DFO-CD3-mAb was able to clearly visualize kinetics of T cell migration from the SLOs to the liver over 10 days post-transplantation and was able to resolve the spread of disease within distinct parts of the target organ. The radiotracer was also able to detect response to treatment using immunosuppressive regulatory T cells (Tregs) that resulted in overall reduction in the liver PET signal. The advantage of targeting CD3, a pan T cell marker which forms part of the TCR complex, is its ability to report on the global T cell population. A potential caveat of this approach is that the CD3/TCR complex can be downregulated during T cell activation which could be confounding with the possibility of underestimating T cell number at sites of inflammation [93].

In the cancer immunity cycle, Chen and Mellman conceptually outline the steps necessary for an effective anti-tumor immune response. Briefly, the cycle describes the initiation of the endogenous anti-cancer immune response with the release of antigens by cancer cells that are processed by APCs and presented to T cells that then become primed to carry out effector functions. They traffic to the tumor eventually culminating in the destruction of tumor cells by cytotoxic T cells [6]. The presence of cytotoxic T cells (CTLs) in tumor biopsies, that have natural reactivity to autologous tumor antigens, are strongly associated with favorable outcomes, and are shown to be predictive of overall survival in a range of cancers [3, 94–96]. CD8, a transmembrane glycoprotein, is a marker for CTLs which exists as a disulfide-linked dimer of an α- and β-chain or two α-chains and serves as a co-receptor for the TCR. The importance of CD8+ CTLs in cancer and viral clearance has motivated the development of several CD8-targeted engineered antibody fragments with enhanced immunoPET characteristics (rapid clearance, abolished Fc interactions) to date. Tavaré et al. reported the feasibility of engineering minibodies from two different anti-murine CD8 depleting antibody clones (2.43 and YTS169.4.2.1). Minibodies, like intact antibodies, are bivalent and undergo hepatobiliary excretion but are more rapidly cleared more rapidly due to their smaller size making it feasible to image within 4 h post-administration. The fragments generated were subsequently radiolabeled with copper-64 ($t_{1/2}$ = 12.7 h), retained their antigen specificity, and demonstrated specific binding to CD8+ T cells in the thymus, spleen, and LNs of immunocompetent mice. Advantageously, removing part of the Fc region from the parental antibodies also abolished original Fc effector functions and CD8+ T cell-depleting capabilities in vivo [90]. Smaller CD8-targeted cys-diabodies evaluated by

the same group also retain target-specific binding but undergo renal clearance [85, 88]. [^{89}Zr] Zr-malDFO-169cDb, a cys-diabody (cDb) probe site-specifically modified with maleimide-DFO and radiolabeled with zirconium-89, has been evaluated extensively in cancer IOT models [91]. The probe was used to image systemic expansion of CD8+ T cells in lymphoid tissues and tumors in three mechanistically distinct syngeneic, murine models of immunotherapy. In the murine CT26 colorectal xenograft tumor model treated with anti-PD-L1 therapy, the probe showed increased tumor uptake in responders versus non-responders. Transverse PET/CT images revealed that the uptake pattern of the probe was diffuse throughout the tumor for responders indicating the presence of intratumoral CD8+ T cells, further confirmed by flow cytometry [91]. In contrast, the PET signal detected in the non-responders was restricted to the peripheral rim of the tumor (Fig. 2.1a). Ultimately the minibody (Mb) format was chosen for clinical translation likely due to superior binding and higher overall uptake in to target tissues compared to the cys-diabody [39]. The human CD8-targeted probe Df-IAB22M2C has been deemed safe in patients following an initial phase I study (NCT03107663) with acceptable dosimetry and was able to penetrate the blood-brain barrier (BBB), making it compatible for brain imaging. The tracer showed specific accumulation in CD8+ T cell-rich tissues such as the spleen and LNs and furthermore was able to delineate T cells within the tumor microenvironment [97]. A phase II study is currently underway in patients with advanced or metastatic solid tumors including melanoma and head and neck cancer (NCT03802123). These studies will be able to address the utility of Df-IAB22M2C for detecting CD8+ TIL density pre- and post-immunotherapy and thereby its ability to monitor response to therapy. Additionally, the correlation of Df-IAB22M2C PET signal with CD8+ T cell immunohistochemistry (IHC) will be assessed.

While CD8+ T cells have attracted much attention as effectors of cytotoxicity, the CD4+ T helper cells play a vital role in amplifying CTL response in cancer IOT, infection, inflammatory diseases and promoting humoral immunity

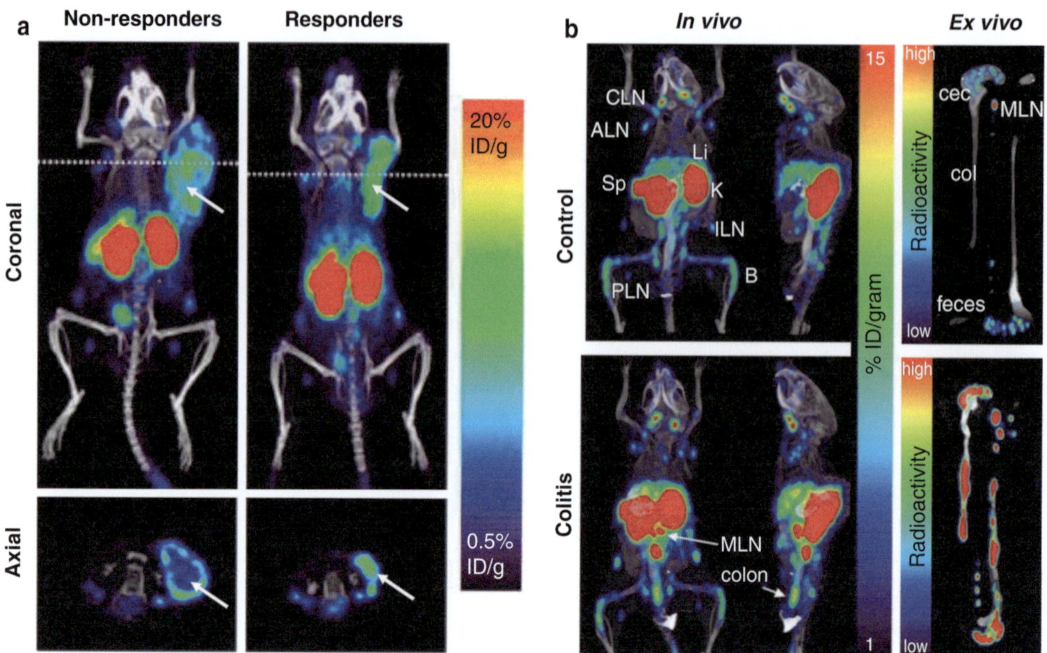

Fig. 2.1 ImmunoPET of constitutively expressed T cell lineage markers. (**a**) Representative anti-CD8 immunoPET-CT images of [^{89}Zr]Zr-malDFO-169cDb in Balb/c mice bearing subcutaneous CT26 colorectal tumors treated with anti-PD-L1 immunotherapy. ImmunoPET images were acquired 22 h post-tracer injection in responding (tumor <8 mm average diameter) and non-responding mice (tumor >8 mm average diameter). The tumor in the coronal and axial views is indicated with a white arrow (adapted from Tavaré et al. Cancer Research, 2016 [91]). Axial views show that the uptake pattern of the probe is diffuse throughout the tumor for the responder indicating the presence of intratumoral CD8$^+$ T cells, while in non-responders the PET signal is restricted to the tumor periphery. (**b**) Representative anti-CD4 immunoPET/CT (coronal and sagittal) images of control (top) and colitic (bottom) mice acquired with 2 µg of [^{89}Zr]Zr-malDFO-GK1.5 cDb. Images were acquired 20 h post-injection of probe and are displayed as 25 mm maximum-intensity projections (MIPs). Organs of interest are axillary LN (ALN), bone (B), cervical LN (CLN), inguinal LN (ILN), kidney (K), liver (Li), popliteal LN (PLN), mesenteric LN (MLN), and spleen (Sp). After in vivo PET/CT scans, mice were euthanized, and the colon, ceca, and MLNs were dissected and laid out for ex vivo PET-CT. Tissues from colitic mice showed higher probe accumulation versus control mice (adapted from Freise et al. Journal of Nuclear Medicine, 2018 [89])

[98–100]. CD4$^+$ helper T cells are an abundant target and account for approximately two-thirds of the total T cell population, while CD8$^+$ T cells account for the remaining. The safety and feasibility of CD4-specific scintigraphy has previously been evaluated in rheumatoid arthritis (RA) patients using [^{99m}Tc]Tc-HYNIC-CD4-Fab, which showed increased uptake in 68% of clinically effected joints [101]. In parallel to CD8-specific antibody fragments, CD4-specific engineered fragments have also been evaluated for PET. [^{89}Zr]Zr-malDFO-GK1.5cDb, a murine CD4 specific cys-diabody, was successfully able to visualize CD4$^+$ T cells in preclinical models of hematopoietic stem cell transplantation [102] and colitis, a major form of IBD marked by chronic inflammation of the large intestine [89]. In the colitis model, [^{89}Zr]Zr-malDFO-GK1.5cDb was able to detect elevated numbers of CD4$^+$ T cells in the colon, mesenteric lymph node, and ceca of colitic mice relative to control mice (Fig. 2.1b). PET imaging of CD4$^+$ T cells would obviate the need for patients to undergo colonoscopy and biopsy which are invasive procedures that can result in iatrogenic complications. Evaluation of the biological effects of [^{89}Zr]Zr-malDFO-GK1.5 cDb revealed that high concentrations of the probe (an excess of 25 nM in vitro and 40 µg in mice) could have perturbative effects. Specifically, a decrease in T cell proliferation and cytokine production was observed in vitro, and a transient decrease in CD4 expression (depletion) in thymus, spleen, LNs, and blood was observed in vivo. These effects were significantly reduced by lowering the dose of the probe [103].

2.3.2.2 Targeting Cell Surface Activation Markers

Despite the relative success of targeting T cell lineage identifying markers, this approach fails to directly report on the activated component that has been highlighted as a critical determinant of T cell response in IOT efficacy or disease pathogenesis. Probing activated T cells rather than the total immune infiltrate could provide a more sensitive and earlier indication of overall T cell response since activation precedes infiltration to effector sites and cytotoxic functions. We now understand that there are situations where detection of lineage markers fails to reveal significant changes in the T cell population pre- and post-cancer immunotherapy despite the occurrence of immune induction resulting in positive outcomes [55, 104]. Imaging activation would potentially be able to report on T cell efficacy more accurately in these scenarios. Some activation markers however can be skewed to certain subpopulations of T cells or be stimuli specific, which may limit their broader utility, and their temporal window of expression must also be considered. An expression profile that is narrow or highly dynamic makes it more challenging to accurately schedule imaging timepoints to capture the response.

The increased production of interleukin-2 (IL-2), a 15.5 kDa cytokine, during T cell activation is accompanied by the elevated expression of CD25, the alpha chain of the trimeric IL-2 receptor (IL-2RA). CD25 has a long history as a biomarker for T cell activation and its expression is advantageously sustained during activation. CD25 has been imaged with radiolabeled anti-CD25 antibodies [105] and radiolabeled IL-2 [106, 107]. The latter has been extensively evaluated in animal models and in patients for a variety of pathologies including IBD [108], atherosclerosis [109], and diabetes [110–112]. Type I diabetes is an autoimmune disease mediated

by autoreactive T cells that carry out the selective destruction of insulin-producing β-cells found in the islets of Langerhans in the pancreas. Crucially by the time of clinical diagnosis, >80% of β-cell mass may have already been damaged due to cytotoxic T cell activity [113]; thus early detection of islet-infiltrating activated lymphocytes is critically needed for early prediction and intervention. Iodine-123 (^{123}I) ($t_{1/2}$ = 13.2 h) [110, 111] and iodine-125 (^{125}I) ($t_{1/2}$ = 59.5 days) [112] labeled IL-2 have been evaluated in multiple rodent diabetes models and were able to detect the elevated levels of activated lymphocytes in the pancreas of diabetic and prediabetic mice, resulting in a higher pancreatic radioactive signal versus in healthy controls.

Concerns about the potential adverse effects of radioactive iodine and the limited availability of iodine-123 eventually motivated the development of IL-2 labeled with technetium-99m (^{99m}Tc, $t_{1/2}$ = 6 h) [114]. [^{99m}Tc]Tc-HYNIC-IL-2 for SPECT imaging of IL-2RA was evaluated in a phase I safety study on five metastatic melanoma patients receiving ICB therapy [115]. The protocol involved a scan prior to treatment initiation and at 12 weeks after anti-CTLA-4 or anti-PD-1 treatment. [^{99m}Tc]Tc-HYNIC-IL-2 was able to discriminate between true tumor progression and pseudoprogression, although only three of the patients were able to complete the pre- and posttreatment scans and in this small cohort. Overall the imaging agent was deemed to be safe with one patient experiencing grade 1 pruritus and grade 1 pain which was attributed to radiotracer bioactivity. More recently, ^{18}F-labeled IL-2 was developed for improved sensitivity and spatial resolution in CD25 imaging [107, 116]. PET images of N-(4-[^{18}F]fluorobenzoyl)-interleukin-2 ([^{18}F]FB-IL-2) in lung tumor-bearing mice showed elevated PET signal in the cohorts that were irradiated alone or in combination with immunization (a 10- and 27-fold increase, respectively), versus untreated controls [107]. [^{18}F]FB-IL-2 is currently being evaluated in the clinic in metastatic melanoma patients receiving ICB therapy (NCT02922283). CD25 is also broadly upregulated on other activated immune cell subsets including B cells and DC cells. Its expression on hematological cancer cells could be confounding for imaging anti-cancer immune responses [117].

Using a CD25-targeted approach to image immune activation may be further complicated by the fact that it is also present on Tregs (defined as CD4[+], CD25[+], FOXP3[+]) that are involved in immunosuppression. Recently a ^{18}F-labeled mutant version of IL-2 ([^{18}F]FB-IL-2v) was developed with the motivation of reducing immune-related toxicity [118]. The probe only binds to the beta and gamma subunits of the IL-2 receptor (and not to CD25, the alpha subunit) and retains specific binding to the IL-2R on activated human PBMCs. An added advantage of the mutant imaging agent would be that it would no longer bind to CD25 on the Treg population.

More recently the focus has shifted to imaging earlier markers of T cell activation with immunoPET such as CD69, which is upregulated rapidly within 2–4 h of TCR/CD3 engagement [119]. Expressed on both CD4 and CD8 populations, CD69 acts as a costimulatory molecule and plays a pivotal role in the preservation of tissue resident memory T cells that are critical for pathogen control at barrier sites [120] and as a metabolic gatekeeper highly expressed on TILs, helping to sustain their metabolic needs in the hypoxic environment [120]. Motivated by its important role in T cell activation, Tako et al. have developed a murine CD69-specific immunoPET agent ([^{64}Cu]Cu-NODAGA-CD69-mAb) [121]. The tracer was evaluated in a murine colon adenocarcinoma and melanoma tumor model treated with anti-PD-L1 and anti-LAG-3 therapy and was able to distinguish responders from non-responders within 3 days of treatment initiation. The early onset dynamics and narrow window of expression (CD69 levels were shown to return to baseline within 7 days post-initial treatment within this particular model) may make it more challenging to accurately time the imaging to capture the response that is prognostic of therapy response. Elevated CD69 expression has been documented in patients with RA [122] and MS [123] and in renal transplant rejection [124] though the utility of CD69 imaging in these indications is yet to be evaluated. CD69 expression can also overlap with other immune cells (inducible on B cells, NK cells, and myeloid cells and is constitutively expressed on human monocytes and platelets) [119].

OX40 (CD134) is a potent costimulatory molecule which becomes highly expressed on antigen-experienced effector T cells [85]. OX40 signaling conveys prosurvival signals to T conventional cells by binds to the ligand OX40L, preferentially expressed on APCs. This results in the downstream formation of a TCR-independent signaling complex and activation of the NF-κB pathway, triggering the production of cytokines such as IL-2 and interferon-γ (IFN-γ) which promote the survival, proliferation, and activation of T cells [125]. Humanized OX40 agonist mAbs are currently under evaluation in the clinic for therapy of liquid and solid tumors [125, 126]. Our group recently reported the noninvasive visualization of murine OX40 to image local and systemic responses in a paradigm changing IOT approach involving intratumoral administration of a clinically relevant immune stimulant, CpG oligodeoxynucleotides. This approach demonstrates the same potency of a 100-fold equivalent dose administered systemically [4]. [^{64}Cu]Cu-DOTA-OX40-mAb was able to clearly visualize local T cell activation, specifically within the CpG-treated tumor and the tumor-draining lymph node (TDLN) in a dual A20 murine lymphoma model, at day 2 post-therapy initiation (Fig. 2.2) [104]. Although OX40 is considered an early activation marker, its expression on T cells was shown to be sustained even 9 days post-stimulation. Systemic T cell activation was visualized at the later timepoint in CpG-treated mice; elevated PET signal was observed in the spleen, an organ involved in the priming of T cells prior to their deployment throughout the body for antigen surveillance, as well as in the distal untreated TDLNs. Moreover, incorporating multiple OX40 PET signals from the tumor, TDLN, and spleen taken from the early imaging timepoint (2 days posttreatment initiation), prior to divergence in tumor size between treated and control groups, was highly predictive of overall therapeutic response at day 9 ($R^2 = 0.674$) and outperformed the predictive value of anatomical and cytokine measurements. Although OX40 has been reported on both CD8+ and CD4+ T cells, it is often more skewed toward the latter [127, 128]. This strategy may therefore be better suited for IOTs where the magnitude of the CD4 response is reflective of treatment success or mainly CD4-driven pathologies where upregulation of OX40 has been implicated in disease pathogenesis such as GVHD [129], MS [130], and IBD [131] in addition to organ transplant rejection [132, 133].

The inducible T cell costimulatory receptor (ICOS or CD278) and its endogenous ligand ICOSL expressed on APCs are also currently under evaluation as potential targets for cancer immunotherapy [134, 135]. Like OX40, ICOS acts as a positive costimulatory molecule and binds to the ICOSL. ICOS signaling promotes T cell survival and production of both Th1 (IFNγ) and Th2 (IL-4, IL-10) cytokines in response to bacterial, viral, and parasitic infections [136]. Moreover, binding of ICOS to ICOSL leads to increase in CD40L expression on CD4 T cells which binds to CD40 on B cells, crucial for immunoglobulin class switching, production of antibodies, and formation of memory B cells [137]. Compared to OX40, ICOS has the added advantage of being highly upregulated on both activated CD4+ and CD8+ T cell subsets. The extent of circulating ICOS+ T cells has been correlated to improved survival in melanoma patients receiving ICB therapy, indicating its utility as an early marker of response [138]. Our group has recently developed an immunoPET agent ([^{89}Zr]Zr-DFO-ICOS-mAb) with

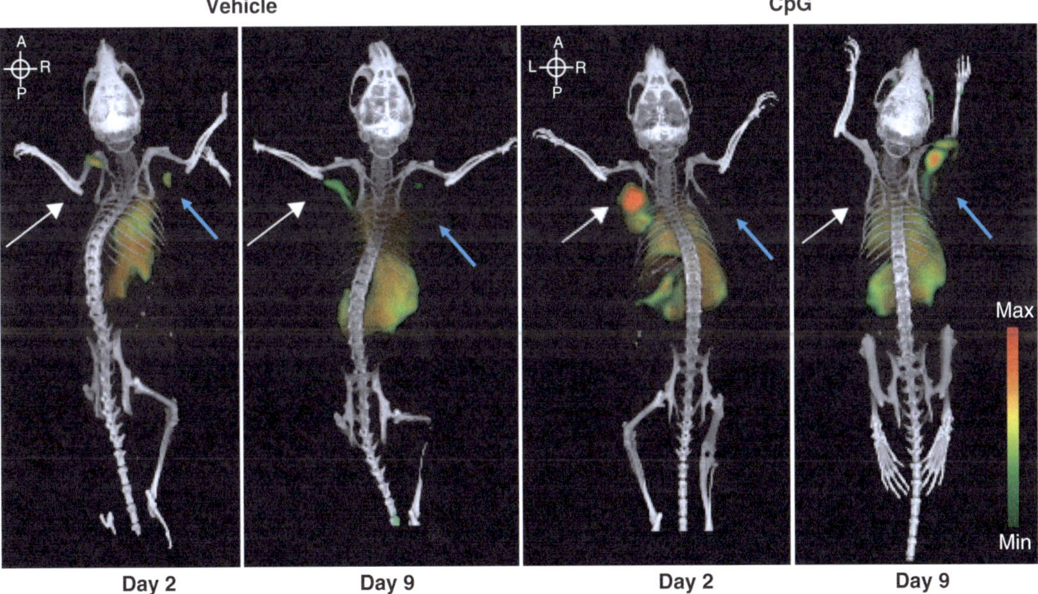

Fig. 2.2 ImmunoPET of a T cell activation marker OX40, in an intratumoral CpG vaccine model. OX40-immunoPET captures the spatiotemporal dynamics of activated T cells following intratumoral administration of CpG in a dual subcutaneous A20 lymphoma tumor model. Images were acquired 24 h post-injection of [^{64}Cu] Cu-DOTA-OX40-mAb. Volume rendered technique (VRT) PET-CT images of representative vehicle-treated and CpG-treated mice on days 2 and 9 after vaccination. White arrows indicate the vehicle (left panel)- or CpG (right panel)-treated tumor, and blue arrows indicate the distal untreated tumor. The OX40-PET signal is elevated in the tumor and tumor-draining lymph node (TDLN) of CpG-treated tumors (right panel, day 2, white arrow) not seen in the vehicle-treated mice (left panel, day 2, white arrow). The localized signal observed in the CpG-treated tumor at the early timepoint is no longer observed by day 9 by which time the tumor has shrunk (right panel, day 9, white arrow). Instead at day 9, an elevated OX40-PET signal is now observed in the distal untreated tumor and TDLN in the CpG-treated mouse indicating a systemic immune response at the later timepoint (right panel, day 9, blue arrow). Scale bar: maximum (Max) = red; minimum (Min) = green. (Adapted from Alam et al. Journal of Clinical Investigation, 2018 [104])

specificity for murine ICOS, which was able to visualize T cell activation in response to intratumoral anti PD-1 and STING agonist therapy in a Lewis lung carcinoma model [128]. Induction of ICOS expression was highly dependent on the therapy; while the STING agonist induced high levels of ICOS expression, PD-1 therapy alone failed to do so. Higher frequencies of ICOS$^+$ T cells in the TDLN and the spleen were confirmed using flow cytometry in STING agonist-treated cohorts. [^{89}Zr]Zr-DFO-ICOS-mAb PET revealed significant increases in PET signal in the tumor, TDLN, and spleen of STING-treated mice versus PD-1-treated and control groups at both early and late treatment timepoints. PET signal in the tumor and TDLN were identified as the strongest response predictors and integration of the early ICOS immunoPET signal from both regions strongly correlated with late therapeutic response ($R^2 = 0.768$) [128].

2.3.2.3 Targeting Intracellular Metabolic Pathways

The activation of T cells significantly increases their metabolic demands over the resting state in order to sustain clonal expansion, differentiation of the naïve population into effector and memory cells and to support effector functions [139]. Undifferentiated naïve T cells rely on oxidative phosphorylation for energy production; however upon TCR engagement, activated T cells become highly anabolic and switch to glycolysis [140]. Consequently glucose analog [^{18}F] FDG has been widely evaluated to probe inflammation in patients with RA [141], atherosclerotic plaques [142], GVHD [143], and infection [144]. However, glycolysis can be upregulated across multiple immune cell types and is reportedly higher in innate immune cells than T cells [145]. The high rates of glycolysis shared by cancer cells and immune cells can also give rise to false positives and make it challenging for [^{18}F]FDG to distinguish the two when colocalized, for example, at TDLNs where there may be LN metastasis and immune activation [146, 147].

In pursuit of more immune-specific imaging agents, alternate metabolic pathways have been evaluated (Table 2.1). While most tissues predominantly utilize de novo DNA synthesis, lymphoid organs and rapidly proliferating tissues rely on salvage pathways [139]. The nucleotide salvage pathway is involved in the production of precursors for DNA synthesis and primarily utilizes deoxyribonucleosides derived from degraded DNA or nutrients. These enter cells from the extracellular space via nucleoside transporters and are subsequently phosphorylated by four key enzymes to produce nucleotides: deoxycytidine kinase (dCK), deoxyguanosine kinase (dGK), and thymidine kinase (TK) 1 and 2 [148]. The PET tracer, 3′-deoxy-3′[^{18}F]-fluorothymidine ([^{18}F]FLT), a substrate for TK1, has been widely used for in vivo assessment of tumor proliferation in response to therapy since TK1 activity is closely correlated with the S-phase of DNA synthesis [149–151]. [^{18}F]FLT has also been clinically evaluated to detect proliferation of activated lymphocytes in response to IOT [152–154]. Aarntzen et al. demonstrated that [^{18}F]FLT was able to visualize immune activation following intranodal DC vaccination in melanoma patients with lymph node metastases [152]. Elevated [^{18}F] FLT signal was detected specifically in vaccinated LNs that received tumor antigen-loaded DCs and not in LNs that were injected with saline or DCs not loaded with antigen. Unlike [^{18}F]FDG, the [^{18}F]FLT PET was able to delineate lymphocyte activation in vaccinated LNs and its uptake correlated with antigen-specific T and B cell proliferative responses measured in peripheral blood. Ultimately due to the overlap in tracer uptake by both tumor and immune cells, many studies using [^{18}F]FDG and [^{18}F]FLT have focused on changes in the PET signal within major lymphoid compartments such as bone marrow and spleen post-ICB, instead of directly focusing on tumor sites where distinguishing the tumor and immune compartments could be challenging [152, 155].

The deoxynucleoside kinase enzymes, deoxycytidine kinase (dCK) and deoxyguanosine kinase(dGK), located in the cytosol and mitochondria, respectively, are also upregulated during lymphocyte activation and proliferation. The current toolbox of PET probes includes several candidates that were inspired by nucleoside analogues used in cancer therapy that are targeted to dCK and dGK. Radu and colleagues have developed a series of dCK-specific probes including [^{18}F]-2-fluoro-D-(arabinofuranosyl) cytosine ([^{18}F]FAC), an analog of deoxycytidine [156–158]. [^{18}F]FAC shows specific dCK-mediated retention in lymphoid organs and has been evaluated in numerous models of immune cell expansion. [^{18}F]FAC uptake in proliferating CD8$^+$ T cells isolated from TDLNs exceeded that of other immune cells, while effector CD8$^+$ T cells isolated from the spleen of mice with onco-retrovirus-induced sarcomas showed a fourfold higher accumulation of the tracer versus naïve CD8$^+$ T cells [156, 157]. Interestingly, in subsequent studies using a tritiated version of the probe, it was shown that tracer accumulation in TILs was significantly reduced versus in T cells isolated from TDLNs (approximately by twofold). This was attributed to environment-specific alterations in metabolism and proliferation, altering the sensitivity of the probe [145]. One of the major caveats of [^{18}F]FAC is its rapid deamination in vivo catalyzed by cytidine deaminase, which led to the evaluation of alternative analogs with unnatural L-chirality (L-[^{18}F]FAC and L-[^{18}F]FMAC). These candidates were successfully resistant to deamination while still acting as substrates for dCK which lacks enantioselectivity. The most recent iteration of the dCK-targeted probes [^{18}F]-clofarabine ([^{18}F]-CFA) has greater stability in humans compared to [^{18}F]FAC and is therefore more suited for clinical applications [159]. To date [^{18}F]CFA has been evaluated as a cancer imaging agent for patient stratification in dCK-dependent cytotoxic therapies (e.g., gemcitabine and clofarabine) [159] and also as an immune imaging agent [160]. [^{18}F]CFA was used to evaluate the immune response in glioblastoma (GBM) patients that received a tumor-lysate pulsed DC vaccination in combination with anti-PD-1 mAb therapy [160]. Post-treatment [^{18}F] CFA-PET scans indicated elevated signal in peripheral lymph nodes and within the tumor. The authors demonstrated that advanced MRI techniques could be used in conjunction with [^{18}F]CFA-PET to distinguish immune infiltration from tumor progression. Importantly, [^{18}F]CFA is unable to cross the BBB in healthy subjects [161]; thus evaluation in intracranial malignancies would require adequate disruption of the BBB [162].

Arabinofuranosyl guanine (AraG), a nucleoside analog of deoxyguanosine, is predominantly a substrate for dGK but also for dCK [163, 164]. Nelarabine, a water-soluble prodrug of AraG, is approved to treat patients with refractory or relapsed T cell acute lymphoblastic leukemia and T cell lymphoblastic lymphoma [165]. AraG's preferential accumulation in proliferating T cells inspired the synthesis of PET radiotracer 2′-deoxy-2′-[^{18}F]fluoro-9-β-D-arabinofuranosylguanine ([^{18}F]F-AraG) [166] which showed 19-fold higher uptake in activated versus resting human T cells in vitro [167]. To date [^{18}F]F-AraG has successfully been able to detect T cell activation and homing in murine models of GvHD [167], RA [168], and colon adenocarcinoma (MC38) treated with anti-PD-1 therapy [169]. In MC38 tumor-bearing mice, [^{18}F]F-AraG showed significant enhancement of intratumoral and TDLN signal in responders versus non-responders within 48 h of anti-PD-1 treatment (Fig. 2.3). In vitro, using a tritiated version of the radiotracer, Levi et al. characterized its uptake and retention in a broad range of immune subsets and demonstrated the highest uptake in activated human CD8$^+$ T cells, approximately threefold higher than in activated human CD4$^+$ cells. Evaluation of its potential toxicity confirmed that [^{18}F]F-AraG did not compromise the viability of stimulated PBMCs exposed to the tracer for 96 h in vitro [169]. In healthy volunteers, [^{18}F]F-AraG exhibits hepatobiliary and renal clearance and an overall favorable biodistribution with low background in the thorax and the gastrointestinal tract [167]. The radiotracer is currently being evaluated in multiple cancer immunotherapy clinical trials including head and neck cancer patients to monitor response to anti-PD-1 treatment (NCT03129061). The tracer is also being evaluated in suspected GVHD patients as a method for early disease detection (NCT03367962) and in HIV patients to detect residual immune activation in a cohort treated with antiretroviral therapy (ART) (NCT03684655). Though accumulation of [^{18}F]F-AraG in stimulated versus resting T cells is striking, and has been attributed to increased expression of equilibrative nucleoside transporters and dGK expression during activation, these endogenous markers can also become elevated in certain cancers and other immune cells such as macrophages and DCs [169].

2.3.3 T Cell Cytotoxicity

Biomarkers specifically associated with T cell effector functions represent later stages of activation and can be imaged to probe functionally effective cells directly engaged in T cell cytotoxicity. One of the major effector functions of CD8$^+$ T cells is their ability to kill infected or aberrant

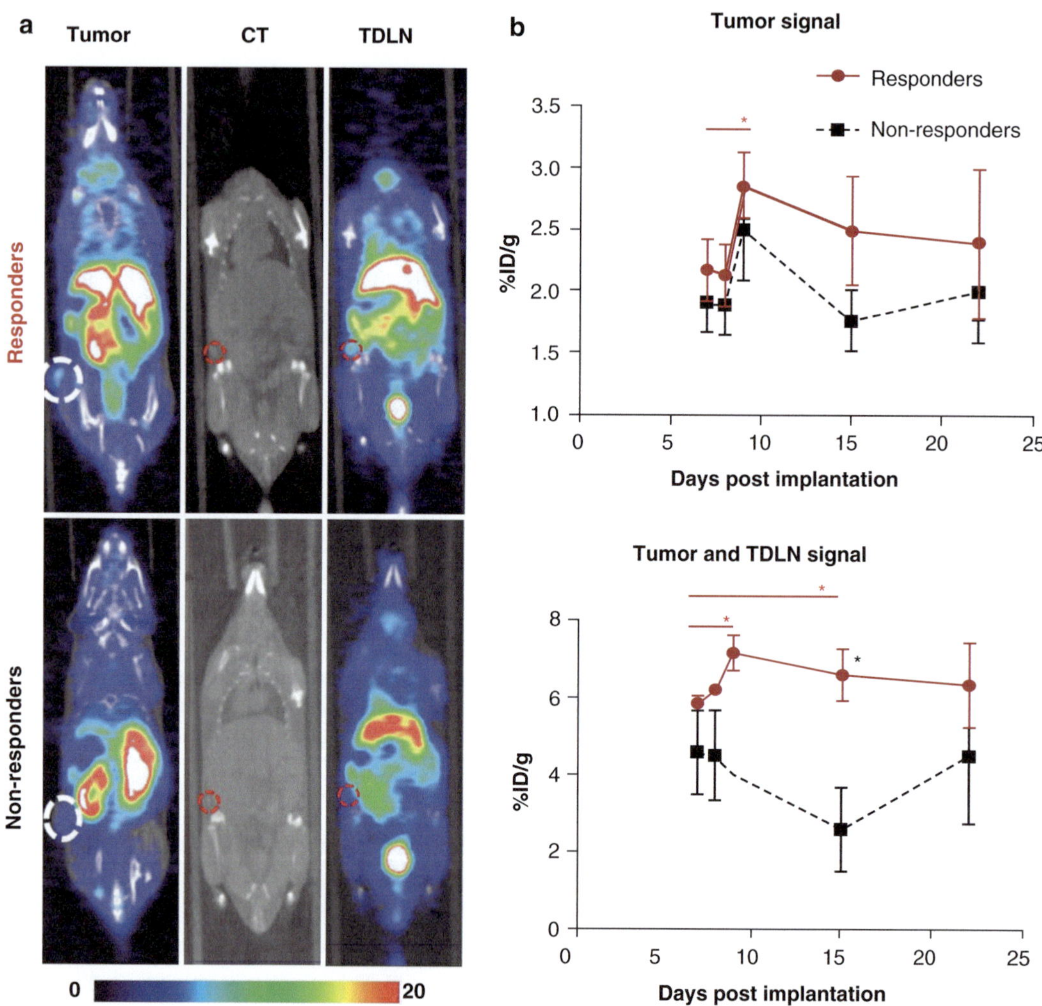

Fig. 2.3 PET imaging of metabolic pathways for visualization of T cell activation. (**a**) [^{18}F]F-AraG imaging of MC38 colon adenocarcinoma tumor-bearing mice receiving anti-PD-1 treatment. PET-CT images were acquired 48 h post-anti-PD-1 treatment. Higher [^{18}F]F-AraG signal in the tumor (white circles) and tumor-draining lymph nodes (red) was noted in the responding mice compared to non-responding mice. Tumor-draining lymph nodes (TDLN) are indicated in the CT and PET images. (**b**) At day 9 post-tumor implantation, the intratumoral signal in the responders was significantly increased over the pretreatment scan (day 7 post-tumor implantation). On days 9 and 15, the combined PET signal (intratumoral and intranodal) in the responders was significantly increased over the pretreatment scan and significantly higher than in non-responders. The combination [^{18}F]F-AraG signal in the responders was 6.587 ± 0.6874 versus 2.604 ± 1.083 in non-responders on day 15 post-tumor implantation. The bars represent standard deviation, *p < 0.05. (Adapted from Levi et al. Cancer Research, 2019 [169])

cells through the release of cytolytic mediators perforin and granzyme B [170]. The latter, a serine protease, is considered a classic effector of CTLs and NK cells. Upon release by CTLs, granzyme B can enter targeted cells through poreforming perforin and activate caspases, thereby triggering apoptosis. Larimer et al. recently reported the development of a PET tracer, a peptide probe ([68Ga]Ga-NOTA-GZP), that enables direct visualization of CTL activity by targeting secreted granzyme B [171]. The authors hypothesize that detection of the cytotoxic event may be more sensitive for predicting response to IOT than probing total immune infiltrate. [^{68}Ga]Ga-NOTA-GZP has high affinity for murine granzyme B and has been evaluated in preclinical cancer IOT models [55, 171]. Combination treatment with anti-CTLA-4 and anti-PD-1 in a murine colorectal CT26 tumor model was shown to induce a four-fold increase in granzyme B levels in treated versus untreated tumors without significant changes in overall CD3 and CD8 expression [55]. [^{68}Ga]Ga-NOTA-GZP PET on day 14 post-therapy initiation was able to distinguish responders from non-responders with significant differences in their tumor-to-blood (TBR) ratios derived from PET image analysis (Fig. 2.4). TBR ratios for responders, non-responders, and vehicle-treated mice were 1.90 ± 0.55, 0.89 ± 0.19, and 0.95 ± 0.20, respectively. Notably, the probe is unable to enter cells and thus only capable of detecting granzyme B that is secreted into the extracellular matrix. This may lead to higher specificity for probing cytotoxicity given that the target is produced at high levels constitutively in granules of T cells and is secreted only upon immune activation. Whether the peptide tracer exerts any inhibitory impact on the enzymatic activity of granzyme B is yet to be reported. The potential clinical utility of imaging granzyme B was highlighted in the same study, where IHC staining of melanoma biopsy samples obtained from patients receiving anti-PD-1 confirmed elevated detection of the target in responders. High infiltration of CTLs expressing granzyme B, as well as the location of TILs within the tumor bed, is associated with a positive clinical outcome in several cancers, including lung [96], colorectal [94], and ovarian cancer [95]. The authors have developed a human granzyme B-specific probe which is a candidate for clinical translation. These findings highlight the potential of granzyme B as an appropriate imaging biomarker of active cytotoxic response with predictive value for cancer therapy. Granzyme B-PET could potentially be expanded to the diagnosis and management of Crohn's disease, a major form of IBD, since higher granzyme B levels have been documented in gut mucosa of Crohn's patients [172, 173]. It is worth noting that NK cells and B cells are also capable of secreting granzyme B [174].

Interferon-γ (IFN-γ) is a soluble cytokine, produced and secreted by activated type 1 (Th1)-skewed CD4$^+$ and cytotoxic CD8$^+$ T cells. IFN-γ plays a critical role in T cell effector functions and is able to control tumor growth through multiple mechanisms including the induction of tumor cell cycle arrest, apoptosis, and activation of APCs. These properties recently motivated the development of an immunoPET agent, a murine IFN-γ-specific monoclonal antibody ([^{89}Zr]Zr-DFO-IFNγ-mAb) which was able to detect localized anti-tumor T cell response in spontaneous salivary and orthotopic neu$^+$ mammary tumors upon vaccination with HER2/neu DNA [56]. A caveat of imaging secreted biomarkers is the possibility of signal dilution. However, Gibson et al. were able to demonstrate that in response to treatment, [^{89}Zr]Zr-DFO-IFNγ-mAb was sequestered and clearly visualized within key tissues such as tumor and spleen, likely binding to receptor-bound IFN-γ. An advantage of this strategy is that while imaging lineage surface markers can result in high background in all SLOs and create a sink effect, this is avoided with IFN-γ imaging which is more specific to CTL activity.

2.3.4 T Cell Inhibition and Control

Just as positive costimulatory molecules drive immune activation, negative coinhibitory molecules exist on the T cell surface to downregulate T cell responses. Two such molecules are

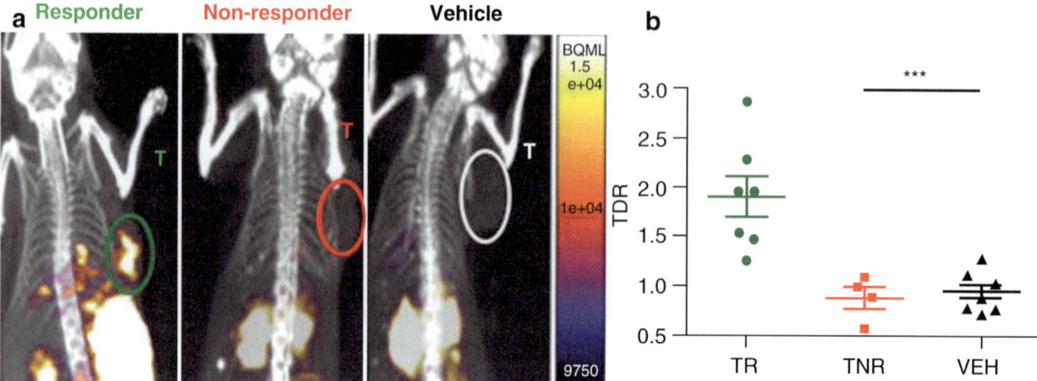

Fig. 2.4 PET imaging of granzyme B, a biomarker for T cell cytotoxicity. (**a**) Representative granzyme B PET-CT images of CT26 tumor-bearing mice that received combination therapy (anti-PD-1 and anti-CTLA-4) or vehicle. Mice were imaged with [^{68}Ga]Ga-NOTA-GZP peptide, 12 days post-inoculation (prior to any treatment-induced tumor shrinkage). Granzyme B PET imaging was able to differentiate treated responders from treated non-responders and vehicle-treated mice. Treated responders exhibited the highest PET tumor signal (T) which subsequently regressed, while tumors of treated non-responders increased in tumor size and showed low probe uptake. (**b**) Scatter plots of tumor-to-blood ratios (TBR) of individual mice within each group. The means of each group are represented by bars ± standard error mean, ***$p < 0.001$. *TR* treated responders, *TNR* treated non-responders, *VEH* vehicle-treated. (Adapted from Larimer et al., Cancer Research, 2017 [55])

the programmed cell death receptor 1 (PD-1) and cytotoxic T lymphocyte-associated protein 4 (CTLA-4). Inducibly expressed upon T cell activation, they subsequently bind to their respective ligands programmed cell death ligand 1 (PD-L1) and B7 family members (B7.1, B7.2), causing a negative feedback loop which downregulates T cell activation. A careful balance between the engagement of stimulatory and inhibitory receptors is critical for maintaining peripheral tolerance under physiological conditions and preventing overstimulation and autoimmunity. However, sustained expression of these molecules and engagement of these pathways, known as immune checkpoints, are observed in cancer and chronic infections and collectively outcompete or interrupt signaling via CD28, preventing T cells from progressing to their active effector states [175, 176]. Multiple mechanisms contribute to an overall immunosuppressive TME including upregulation of PD-L1 on tumor and myeloid-derived suppressor cells which engage PD-1 on T cells [177]. The interaction of PD-1 with PD-L1 promotes apoptosis of antigen-specific effector T cell while supporting proliferation of immunosuppressive Tregs [74]. Imbalanced immune checkpoint pathways and overexpression of these coinhibitory molecules result in dysfunctional T cell states such as exhaustion which can occur from chronic antigen-mediated TCR stimulation as observed in cancer and chronic viral infections [178]. Exhausted T cells lack effector cytokine function and fail to mount effective immune responses. Another type of dysfunction, anergy, describes T cells that become tolerant to specific antigens and occurs as a result of TCR activation in the absence of costimulatory signals, or in the presence of high levels of coinhibitory signaling, rendering the cells functionally inactive.

Immune checkpoint blockade (ICB) has emerged as a powerful arm of cancer immunotherapy which can disrupt immune checkpoint pathways and release the brakes they exert on the immune system. Currently there are four US Food and Drug Administration (FDA)-approved monoclonal antibody therapies that directly target the checkpoint markers on T cells: nivolumab, pembrolizumab and cemiplimab (all anti-PD-1) [179–181], and ipilimumab (anti-CTLA-4)

[182]. Despite durable responses in certain indications such as advanced melanoma and lung cancer, overall response rates have varied greatly with only a minority of patients responding and show long-term survival benefits. A cross-sectional analysis of US cancer patients eligible for ICB therapy for registered indications, estimated a response rate of 12.46% in 2018 [183]. This may be due to variable expression of the targets in malignant lesions or variability in antibody pharmacodynamics and pharmacokinetics between patients. Additionally, immune-related adverse events such as colitis and dermatitis are a significant complication of ICB. Nuclear imaging of these checkpoint molecules therefore has the potential to aid patient stratification, selecting for patients with confirmed expression of the targets at the tumor, reduce costs and side effects associated with ineffective therapy, and provide measurable biomarkers to predict early therapeutic response [184].

Preclinical studies have highlighted the utility of imaging PD-1 and CTLA-4 for visualization of TILs in humanized mouse models and predicting responders to ICB. Natarajan et al. demonstrated the feasibility of using both ^{64}Cu- and ^{89}Zr-labeled pembrolizumab to visualize PD-1 expression in vivo using humanized NSG mice. Both radiolabeled versions were able to visualize human PBMCs homing to the spleen and human melanoma xenografts [185] (Fig. 2.5a). The feasibility of imaging CTLA-4 on T cells has similarly been demonstrated in murine [186] and humanized mouse models [187, 188]. Ehlerding et al. compared ^{64}Cu-labeled NOTA-ipilimumab and its F(ab')$_2$ format to visualize T cell homing to the salivary glands of human PBMC-injected NSG mice that developed GVHD [188]. Imaging with [^{64}Cu]Cu-NOTA-ipilimumab-F(ab')$_2$ led to higher salivary gland-to-blood ratios at earlier timepoints due to faster clearance versus the full antibody format ([^{64}Cu]Cu-NOTA-ipilimumab). ImmunoPET of immune checkpoints molecules could potentially be used to also image T cell dysfunction. Key signatures

of an exhausted T cell phenotype include increased expression of multiple cell surface markers such as CTLA-4, PD-1, TIM-3, and LAG-3 in addition to reduced IL-2 and IFN-γ production [189]. Gibson et al. demonstrated the feasibility of confirming T cell dysfunction using [^{89}Zr]Zr-DFO-IFNγ-mAb, in a murine model of induced exhaustion [56].

Landmark study by Bensch et al. recently demonstrated the utility of immune checkpoint imaging for patient treatment stratification and as a companion diagnostic potentially superior to IHC [190]. In this first-in-human imaging study with [^{89}Zr]Zr-atezolizumab, the safety and feasibility of imaging PD-L1 and its potential to predict response to anti-PD-L1 therapy in 22 patients with 3 different tumor types was evaluated. [^{89}Zr]Zr-atezolizumab-PET performed at baseline showed high uptake in lymphoid tissues and high, heterogeneous intratumoral and intralesional uptake that correlated with PD-L1 IHC. Importantly lesions with highest baseline maximum standardized uptake value (SUVmax) showed greatest therapeutic response to anti-PD-L1 therapy. Overall, clinical responses were better correlated with the pretreatment PET signal than with IHC or RNA sequencing-based predictive biomarkers. Similarly a first-in-human study using [^{89}Zr]Zr-DFO-nivolumab (anti-PD-1), to monitor non-small cell lung cancer (NSCLC) patients eligible for nivolumab therapy (Fig. 2.5b), also demonstrated that pretreatment uptake of the imaging agent was higher in responding lesions and also more predictive than IHC [191]. [^{89}Zr]Zr-DFO-nivolumab uptake was significantly higher in patients whose tumor biopsies showed aggregates of PD-1-positive TILs versus in lesions where such cells were absent (median SUV$_{peak}$ 7.0 vs. 2.7, $p = 0.03$, Mann–Whitney U-test). The safety and utility of [^{89}Zr]Zr-pembrolizumab is currently under evaluation in NSCLC and melanoma patients, and results are pending (NCT03065764, NCT02760225). The same trial also reported the characterization of a PD-L1-targeted adnectin probe ([^{18}F]F-BMS-986192), which exhibited high uptake in NSCLC lesions which correlated with PD-L1 expression as determined by IHC [191].

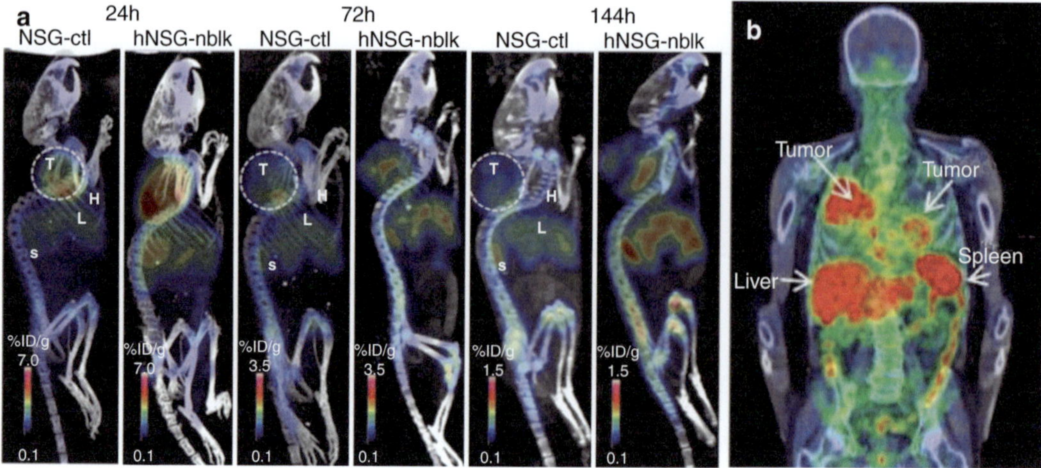

Fig. 2.5 Preclinical and clinical PET imaging of immune checkpoint molecule PD-1. (**a**) Representative PET-CT images of human PD-1 at 24, 72, and 144 h post-injection of [^{89}Zr]Zr-DFO-pembrolizumab in A375 melanoma tumor-bearing NSG control mice (NSG-ctl) and NSG mice injected with human PBMCs (hNSG-nblk). *L* liver, *H* heart, *T* tumor, and *S* spleen are indicated. The tumor-to-muscle ratios (TMR) of hNSG-nblk were significantly higher compared to the NSG-ctl group (adapted from Natarajan et al. Molecular Imaging and Biology, 2017 [185]). (**b**) PD-1 imaging in a patient with ^{89}Zr-labeled nivolumab. PET-CT image acquired 162 h post-injection, demonstrates heterogeneous tracer uptake within and between the two tumors in the lung and mediastinal lymph nodes (adapted from Niemeijer et al., Nature Communications, 2018 [191])

Though tracer uptake did not correlate with response to nivolumab treatment in this small cohort, nonetheless the study demonstrates the feasibility of using smaller engineered protein scaffolds to image and quantify expression of immune targets [192]. A phase 2 trial with [^{89}Zr]Zr-ipilimumab in metastatic melanoma patients is also currently underway with the aim of monitoring CTLA-4 expression in tumor lesions at the start of ipilimumab therapy and following the second therapeutic dose (NCT03313323) [193]. Studies like these will be crucial for obtaining a macroscopic view of target expression, understanding the correlation between radiotracer uptake with therapeutic response, in addition to the association between "on-target off-tumor" binding and toxicity.

While most ICB therapy and imaging have focused on immuno-oncology applications, PD-1, CTLA-4, and other checkpoints are also highly implicated in mediating pathogen persistence in infectious diseases such as malaria and HIV [194]. Targeting these pathways in infection has shown some therapeutic benefits although imaging studies in relevant preclinical models have yet to be reported [194, 195].

2.4 Imaging B Cell Responses

2.4.1 Overview of B Cell Biology

B lymphocytes or B cells constitute 5–25% of total lymphocytes in humans and play a critical role in the adaptive immune response, acting as both APCs and precursors for antibody-producing plasma cells. Early maturation and development of B cells from precursors of the B cell lineage is a well-characterized sequence of programmed steps that takes place in the bone marrow (Fig. 2.6). Here, hematopoietic stem cells mature into pro-B cells, then pre-B cells, and finally immature B cells which leave the bone marrow and travel via the blood to reside in the lymph nodes and spleen. It is within these peripheral lymphoid organs that antigen-dependent B cell maturation and activation occur [196].

B cell responses are classified as T cell-dependent or T cell-independent. In the latter scenario, B cells undergo activation by directly binding to non-protein antigen epitopes such as microbial polysaccharides, resulting in a transient, medium affinity immune response [197].

In contrast, B cell activation in response to protein antigens involves interaction with T cells and results in stronger, robust responses with long-lasting memory [137]. In the T cell-dependent activation, naïve B cells bind to foreign antigens through cell surface immunoglobulins that are also known as the B cell antigen receptor (BCR). The antigen is subsequently internalized along with the BCR and degraded by enzymes within the cell for eventual presentation on surface MHC II molecules to CD4+ T helper cells. Recognition of the antigen by the TCR along with costimulation triggers a signaling cascade which leads to B cell activation, proliferation, and eventual differentiation into plasma and antigen-specific memory B cells (Fig. 2.6) [137, 198].

Plasma cells are responsible for the production and secretion of millions of high affinity antibodies with the exact antigen specificity as their original BCR [137]. Antibodies (immunoglobulins) are glycoproteins that are highly specific to their corresponding antigen. In humans they are classified into five isotypes according to their heavy chains (IgA, IgD, IgE, IgM, and IgG) and fulfil distinct biological functions [137]. IgG represents 75% of antibody found in circulating blood and is composed of four subclasses, IgG1 to IgG4, named in order of their decreasing abundance in serum [199]. Antibodies mediate the clearance of invading pathogens using a variety of mechanisms. In addition to directly binding and neutralizing invading pathogens or toxins, antibodies can coat a pathogen in a process known as opsonization and facilitate phagocytosis by macrophages. Alternatively, by binding to antigens on the surface of a target cell, antibodies can recruit via their Fc region, NK cells, and eosinophils among others for antibody-dependent cell-mediated cytotoxicity (ADCC). Lastly, pathogen-bound antibodies can recruit complement resulting in the lysis of the target cell [200]. Memory B cells formed through T cell-dependent activation constitute approximately 40% of total B cells in adult humans and can persist for decades within SLOs, providing protective immunity against recurring pathogens. Upon encountering low doses of a previously encountered antigen, they undergo rapid proliferation and differentiation to antibody-producing plasma cells [201].

Given their highly specialized roles in immune surveillance and health, dysfunctional B cell responses can have grave consequences and are implicated in the development of chronic autoimmune disorders, such as multiple sclerosis [202], RA [203], and systemic lupus erythematosus [204]. Traditionally considered to be primarily T cell mediated, advances in immunobiology have dramatically reshaped the way autoimmune diseases are viewed today. Though

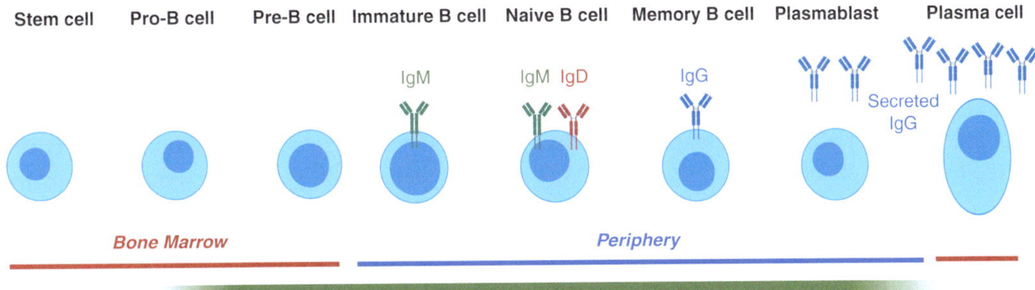

Fig. 2.6 Expression of B cell lineage-specific markers CD19 and CD20 at different stages of B cell development in the bone marrow (red line) and in the peripheral lymphoid organs (blue line). CD19, a pan-B cell surface marker, is expressed across a broader range of B cell subsets than CD20 including pro-B cells, pre-B cells, and antibody-secreting plasmablasts. The surface density of CD19 and CD20 is highly regulated throughout B cell development. (Created with BioRender.com)

incompletely understood, central to the pathophysiology of many of these diseases is the loss of peripheral B cell tolerance through autoantigen presentation, production of autoantibodies, and secretion of inflammatory cytokines [196, 205]. These insights have provided the rationale for B cell modulation and depletion as a potential therapeutic strategy in the management of autoimmune disorders [206]. B cell imaging offers a noninvasive method for accurate diagnosis of these heterogeneous diseases, identification of patients who are most likely to benefit from B cell-targeted therapies, and monitoring of associated therapeutic responses. Despite their central role in autoimmunity, fewer nuclear imaging approaches for in vivo tracking of B cells have been reported compared to that of T cells, focusing largely on two lineage cell surface markers, CD19 and CD20.

2.4.1.1 Targeting Cell Surface Lineage Markers

CD20 is a membrane-associated non-glycosylated phosphoprotein that is acquired relatively late in maturation, at the pre-B cell stage. Its expression is maintained through most of B cell development up until memory B cell formation and is ultimately lost on terminally differentiated plasma cells (Fig. 2.6). Rituximab, a chimeric IgG1 targeting CD20, was the first monoclonal antibody to be approved for oncology patients, specifically for B cell malignancies due to its potent B cell depletion capabilities attributed primarily to ADCC [207]. The nuclear imaging field has naturally embraced this FDA-approved and widely evaluated monoclonal antibody to monitor B cell responses in vivo. Rituximab is also approved for the treatment of rheumatoid arthritis (RA), a chronic inflammatory disease affecting the joints, which can lead to cartilage injury, bone erosion and symptoms of chronic pain, swelling, joint stiffness, and deformity [208]. While T cells are a major component of RA pathology, B cells play a role in the development of the disease through APC functions and production of autoantibodies [209]. B cell depletion with rituximab has been shown to ameliorate the disease in 50–60% of patients, suggesting that non-responders rep-

resent a different pathogenic subset of the disease. [^{89}Zr]Zr-rituximab PET has been evaluated for multiple indications in the clinic, including RA and orbital inflammatory disease with some promising results [210–212]. In a study by Bruijnen et al., 20 RA patients receiving rituximab treatment were also imaged with [^{89}Zr]Zr-rituximab at the start of treatment [210]. Responders showed significantly higher tracer uptake in their hand joints (Fig. 2.7a) than non-responders with median target-to-background ratios of 6.2 vs. 3.1 respectively, demonstrating the feasibility of using [^{89}Zr]Zr-rituximab PET to predict clinical response [210].

Multiple sclerosis (MS) is a chronic autoimmune disorder affecting the CNS, where B cell involvement has been dissected extensively [213, 214]. MS is characterized by immune-driven destruction of myelin, axonal degeneration, and white matter plaque formation principally observed in the spinal cord, optic nerve, and brain stem, resulting in disrupted neuronal signaling and neurological disability [215]. The presence of B cells, plasma cells, and excess autoantibodies have long been documented in lesions and in the cerebrospinal fluid of MS patients, providing strong evidence of the role of B cells in MS pathophysiology [215–217]. Depletion of B cells has been evaluated as therapeutic strategy in relapsing-remitting MS using rituximab as well as newer CD20-targeting mAb therapies with superior biologic properties such as reduced internalization and immunogenicity [218]. These have shown some benefit in a subset of patients by reducing relapse rates and delaying disability progression [219, 220]. Clinical tools to monitor the efficacy of these therapies are however limited. Pathological confirmation of B cell involvement in MS patients is complicated by the invasive nature of biops and location of affected tissues, further highlighting the potential utility of noninvasive B cell imaging. Preclinical studies have attempted to understand immune dysfunction in MS with the widely used experimental autoimmune encephalomyelitis (EAE) animal model, where demyelination is induced through the administration of myelin oligodendrocyte glycoprotein fragment in complete Freund's adjuvant along with pertussis toxin. James et al. specifically induced EAE in humanized transgenic mice with B cells expressing the human CD20 cell surface protein, to evaluate the feasibility of using [^{64}Cu] Cu-rituximab to assess B cell biodistribution in diseased mice [78]. [^{64}Cu]Cu-rituximab PET was able to clearly delineate increased B cell infiltration into the spinal cord and several regions of the brain of EAE versus control mice (Fig. 2.7b). Importantly this study highlighted some key challenges of using rituximab for B cell imaging. First, the requirement of adequate BBB disruption for the full-sized antibody to access B cell clusters in the CNS. Second, the therapeutic potency of rituximab leading to significant B cell depletion even at low doses of the antibody (3 μg), greatly limiting the amount of tracer that can be administered and reducing the overall sensitivity of the imaging approach [78].

Another caveat of rituximab, a type I anti-CD20 mAb, is that upon binding to CD20, internalization of the antigen (Ag) occurs more rapidly than with type II anti-CD20 mAbs [221, 222]. Cell surface retention of the mAb/Ag complex is favorable in the therapeutic context as it allows time for

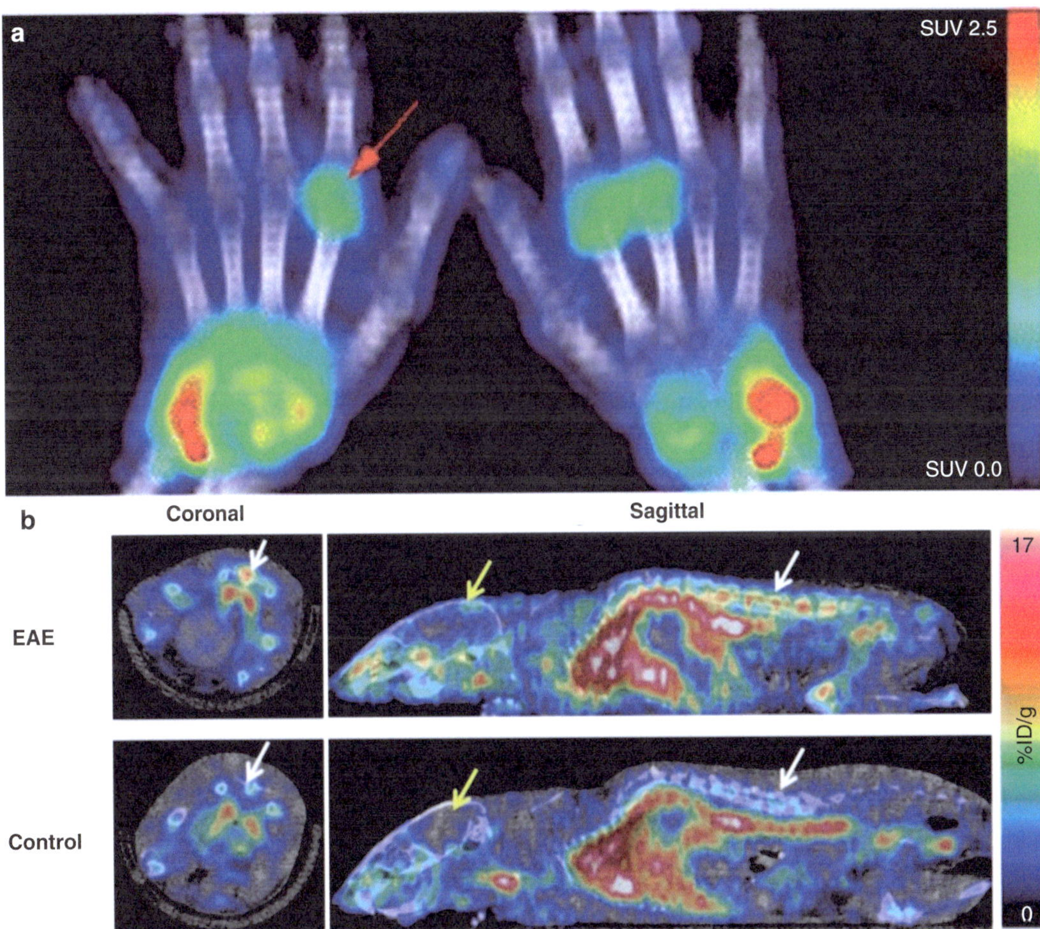

Fig. 2.7 ImmunoPET of B cell responses using CD20-targeted rituximab. (**a**) PET/CT image of the wrists and hands of a rheumatoid arthritis patient injected with [^{89}Zr] Zr-rituximab indicates enhanced signal in multiple joints, (red arrow). PET-positive joints typically correspond with clinical signs of arthritis. *SUV* standardized uptake value (adapted from Bruijnen et al. Arthritis Research and Therapy, 2016 [210]). (**b**) Representative PET/CT images of an EAE mouse (a preclinical model of multiple sclerosis) and a control naive mouse, 1 h post-injection of [^{64}Cu] Cu-rituximab. Elevated PET signals are observed in the brain (yellow arrow) and spinal cord (white arrow) of the EAE mouse, corresponding with increased B cell infiltration in these regions (adapted from James et al., Journal of Nuclear Medicine, 2017 [78])

optimal recruitment of immune cells for phagocytosis and ADCC [222] but is also preferable for imaging particularly when using conventionally labeled iodine-124 tracers. Upon internalization, and catabolism, degradation can release the radioactive iodine which readily diffuses out of the cell, thereby decreasing signal to background ratios [223]. Zettlitz et al. evaluated [124]I-labeled cys-minibody and cys-diabody antibody fragments based on humanized type II anti-CD20 mAb, obinutuzumab, for immunoPET imaging of mice bearing human CD20+ tumors [224]. The radioiodinated obinutuzumab fragments were compared to similarly labeled rituximab cys-minibody and cys-diabody fragments. Iodinated obinutuzumab fragments were superior to the respective rituximab fragments and showed higher accumulation in tumors, higher target-to-blood ratios, and consequently higher contrast images. Moreover [89]Zr-labeled obinutuzumab fragments showed slightly higher tumor uptake and retention than [124]I-labeled obinutuzumab fragments due to the residualizing nature of the zirconium-89 [224]. Collectively the results show that compared to rituximab, humanized obinutuzumab fragments show superior imaging characteristics, probably due to slower internalization, and warrant wider evaluation in preclinical models and in the clinic. This also demonstrates the merits of considering vector internalization when pairing with a diagnostic radionuclide.

As previously mentioned, smaller antibody fragments such as camelid single-domain antibodies (sdAbs), are currently under active evaluation in oncological applications specifically for radioimmunotherapy [225] and imaging [226]. Also known as VHH or nanobodies, these smaller entities are favored for their rapid pharmacokinetics, improved stability, solubility, and low immunogenicity. Motivated by the need to overcome the slow clearance and resultant off-target toxicities of full-length mAbs [227], CD20-specific sdAbs for radioimmunotherapy of CD20+ lymphomas were generated by Krasniqi et al. [228]. In the same study, the lead human CD20-specific sdAbs were radiolabeled for SPECT and PET imaging and evaluated in two different models: (1)

immunocompetent mice bearing human CD20-positive murine melanoma tumors or (2) human lymphoma-bearing immunocompromised SCID mice. [68Ga]Ga-NOTA-CD20 sdAbs showed rapid renal clearance and tumor uptake values of up to 2.2% ± 0.2% versus 0.2% ± 0.01% for a similarly radiolabeled control sdAb, confirming their specificity and illustrating the feasibility of imaging immune cells with sdAbs together with short-lived PET isotopes [228, 229].

CD19, a type I transmembrane glycoprotein, acts as a critical co-receptor for BCR signal transduction and plays a role in immunoglobulin-induced activation of B cells [230, 231]. In humans, CD19 is the most ubiquitous B cell lineage marker that is expressed on almost all phases of B cell development with the exception of terminally differentiated plasma cells (Fig. 2.6). CD19 expression is induced as early as the pro-B cell stage, and its expression is sustained all the way up to early plasma cells [137]. The surface density of CD19 is highly regulated throughout cell development and is threefold higher in mature versus immature B cells [230]. Due to its broader expression on B cell subsets relative to CD20, the potential advantages of CD19 over CD20 as a diagnostic and therapeutic target for B cell malignancies have been widely discussed [230, 232, 233], and newer CD19-targeted therapies such as inebilizumab are being actively pursued [234, 235]. CD19 also does not appear to be internalized and is potentially a more specific biomarker for B cells than CD20 (the latter is also expressed on a small subset of human T cells) [236]. For these reasons, anti-CD19 imaging probes could potentially capture B cell involvement in autoimmune diseases more accurately and specifically than CD20-targeted imaging.

Recently Stevens et al. reported the utility of a murine CD19-specific immunoPET probe for monitoring B cell infiltration into the CNS of EAE mice [237]. [64Cu]Cu-DOTA-CD19-mAb PET/CT images acquired 19 h post-tracer administration showed significantly higher tracer accumulation in the brain and spinal cord of EAE mice, compared to control mice. Ex vivo analyses of these CNS tissues using autoradiography and IHC revealed that the higher PET signals corresponded with increased B cell infiltration, implicated in EAE pathology. Interestingly the spleen and bone marrow of EAE mice showed a dramatic reduction in tracer-associated signal compared to control mice, reflecting a possible egress of B cells out of these lymphoid tissues ultimately trafficking to the CNS. This observation is in agreement with findings from a longitudinal ex vivo flow cytometric analysis of murine EAE tissues [238]. Further assessment of CD19 immunoPET probes will need to rule out any possible toxicities to B cells and has motivated the evaluation of mAb formats with Fc regions that are mutated or antibody fragments lacking this region altogether. Currently, human CD19-specific immunoPET probes are being actively evaluated in humanized mouse models. Collectively, these pre-clinical studies will lay the groundwork for future clinical evaluation of CD19-targeted tracers for imaging B cell responses.

2.5 Imaging Natural Killer (NK) Cell Responses

2.5.1 Overview of NK Cell Biology

Natural killer (NK) cells are classified as innate lymphoid cells (ILCs) which derive from the common lymphoid progenitors in the bone marrow but lack genetically rearranged antigen receptors [239]. Rather, NK cells have germline-encoded activating and inhibitory receptors that interact with the environment. NK cells are distinguished from other innate lymphoid cells by their dependence on interleukin 15 (IL-15) for development and intrinsic cytotoxic ability [240]. NK cells can kill target cells without the need for prior sensitization but can develop memory of previous antigen exposure [241]. NK cells constitute 5–15% of circulating lymphocytes [242] and are considered an important bridge between the innate and adaptive immune system. In particular, they play a vital role in the immunosurveillance of tumors and can kill aberrant cells via the perforin/granzyme B pathway or via the secretion of cytokines and chemokines that modulate other immune cells [243].

NK cells were the first described members of the expanding ILC family. The most recent ILC classification consists of five subsets: NK cells, ILC1s, ILC2s, ILC3s, and LTi cells [244]. These subsets are classified by the transcription factors that regulate their development and function and the cytokines they produce [245]. Although they have different developmental pathways, both NK cells and group 1 ILCs depend on the transcription factor Tbet, which turns on the expression of T-bet target genes such as IFN-γ and NKp46 [246]. Notably, many of the markers associated with NK cells such CD56 are also expressed on other ILCs such as ILC1; however, NK cells are the most prevalent ILC in the tumor microenvironment, varying from non-detectable to greater than 20% of lymphocytes depending on the tumor type [247]. Typically, in humans, immune cells that are CD3⁻CD56⁺ are reported as NK cells although more markers are necessary to delineate NK cells from rarer ILC subclasses such as ILC1.

The most prevalent model of NK cell development is a linear progression from CD34⁺ hematopoietic progenitors to NK cells that express CD16 and killer immunoglobulin-like receptors (KIR). While this model is easy to follow, recent findings indicate that a variety of precursor populations can develop into distinct subsets of mature NK cells [248]. In humans, NK cells are thought to progress from CD56^{bright} to CD56^{dim} cells that upregulate CD16 and KIR [249]. CD56 (also known as neural cell adhesion molecule, or NCAM) is the archetypal phenotypic marker of NK cells but can also be expressed by alpha beta T cells, gamma delta T cells, dendritic cells, monocytes, neurons, glia, and skeletal muscles [250]. A more specific class of receptors for NK cells are the natural cytotoxicity receptors (NCRs). NCRs are activation receptors expressed on human NK cells (along with rare innate lymphoid subsets) and include NKp30, NKp44, NKp46, and NKp80. While NKp44 is upregulated on activated NK cells, the other receptors are constitutively expressed. NK cells can also express inhibitory receptors such as PD-1, TIGIT, and LAG-3. A simplified model of NK cell receptor expression is shown in Fig. 2.8. Vivier et al. provide a thorough review of ILC development and phenotypic marker expression [244].

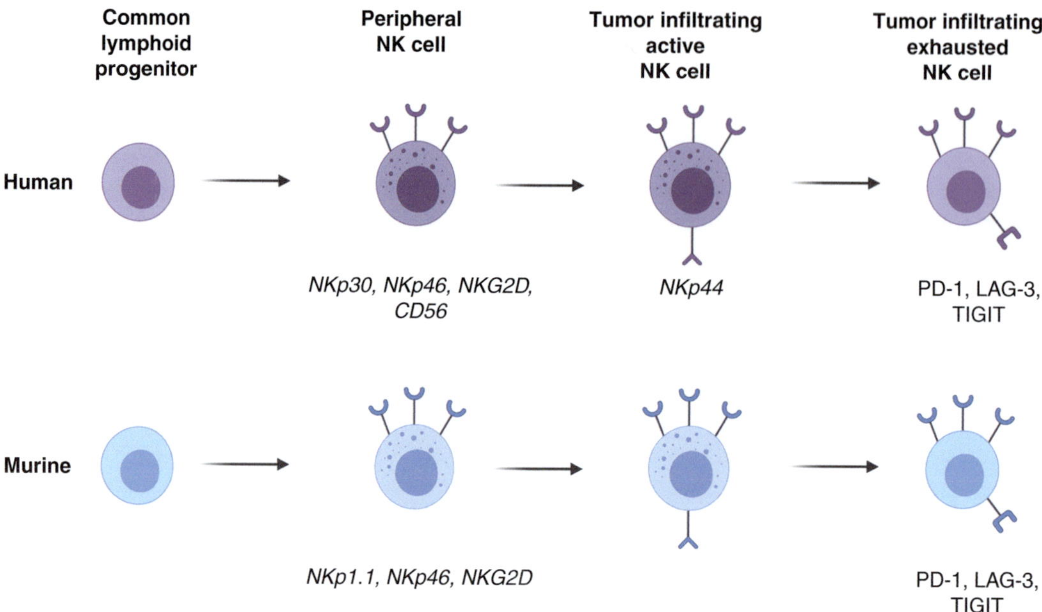

Fig. 2.8 Human and murine natural killer (NK) cells express different markers based on their functional state. NK cells interact with their environment through inhibitory and activation receptors, and the overall activity of NK cells is dictated by co-stimulation of these signals. While expression of certain NK receptors such as NKp46 remains unchanged during activation, others such as NKp44 are upregulated on human NK cells. Murine and human NK cells differ substantially in receptor expression. A candidate cell surface marker that would allow adequate visualization of murine tumor-infiltrating, active NK cell is yet to be proposed. Inhibitory receptors are elevated on exhausted NK cells and are emerging therapeutic targets. To date, nuclear imaging probes for only NKp30, NKp46, and CD56 have been reported and were evaluated in preclinical models. (Image created with BioRender.com)

2.5.1.1 Emergence of NK Cell Therapies

NK cells are essential mediators in specific therapeutic approaches including chimeric antigen receptor (CAR) NK cells and monoclonal antibody-mediated direct activation, as well as indirect activation of NK cells via ADCC [251]. Early studies investigated NK-92 cells and primary NK cells activated ex vivo with IL-2. NK-92 is an immortal, IL-2 dependent NK cell line established in 1992 from the peripheral blood of a 50-year-old male patient with non-Hodgkin's lymphoma, collected at the time of diagnosis [252]. To date, NK-92 has been engineered to express a number of different CARs to target CD19 or CD20 (anti-B cell malignancies), CD38 (anti-myeloma), or human epidermal growth factor receptor 2 (anti-epithelial cancers) [253]. CAR NK cells are an example of adoptive cell therapy where NK cells are genetically modified to target a specific tumor antigen, expanded ex vivo, and then injected into patients. CAR NK cells generated from cord blood have been evaluated in phase I and II trials and delivered promising results, with 7 of 11 patients having complete remission in CD19-positive cancers [254]. In contrast to first-generation CAR T cells, there were no substantial toxic effects, and the manufacturing of CAR NK cells is comparatively simpler. While CAR T cells have to be generated from individual patients, CAR NK cells can be generated from banked cord blood, eliminating the need to produce a unique CAR product for each patient. Another promising strategy is activating endogenous NK cells through the administration of small molecules or antibodies. The most established NK cell-mediated therapy involves the use of antibodies targeting cell surface antigens on tumor cells for ADCC [255]. The Fc domain of antibodies is recognized by the FcγRIII (CD16a) receptor on NK cells, resulting in the activation of potent cytotoxic processes. While these therapies have existed for decades, recent strategies have enhanced ADCC through the engineering of the Fc region of antibodies or through inhibition of endocytosis of targeted antigens [256]. There are currently 574 NK cell therapies in phase I/II clinical trials (the majority for oncology) and a multitude in preclinical development, fueling the demand for accurate immunomonitoring of NK cells [257].

2.5.1.2 Candidate Endogenous Targets for NK Cell Imaging

While the development of NK immunotherapies has exploded, therapeutic monitoring remains a challenge. There is a noticeable lack of imaging probes for adequate monitoring of NK cell therapies compared to T cells [258]. To date CAR NK cells have been labeled ex vivo with [^{111}In] In-oxine or [^{89}Zr]Zr-oxine in both murine [259] and primate models [260], much like previously discussed CAR T cells. However, imaging agents for direct visualization of endogenous NK cells are lacking. Differences in NK cell receptor expression between preclinical animal models and human NK cells are driving factors behind this shortage and render preclinical evaluation of potential approaches for NK cell imaging in the clinic challenging. Many human recep-

tors considered promising imaging biomarkers for NK cells are not expressed on murine NK cells. To address this challenge, transgenic murine models that express human IL-15 have been generated which, via the injection of CD34^{+} HSCs, allow for the development of functional human NK cells, along with T cells and semi-functional B cells [261]. As this model has only recently become commercially available, imaging studies in this model have yet to be reported. Indeed, only one endogenous NK cell marker-targeted imaging probe has been reported to date in a preclinical SCID model [262]. Here, the human CD56 receptor was imaged with a ^{99m}Tc-radiolabeled antibody for imaging with a high-resolution portable mini-γ camera. The chelator S-HYNIC (succinimidyl-6-hydrazinonicotinate hydrochloride) was conjugated to an anti-human CD56 mAb, prior to radiolabeling. Since murine NK cells lack expression of CD56, human NK cells were injected into SCID mice either sub-cutaneously as flank xenografts or intravenously into tumor-bearing mice. This was followed by injection of the [^{99m}Tc]Tc-hCD56-mAb SPECT probe, which was able to visualize tumor-infiltrating NK cells in anaplastic thyroid cancer (ARO) xenografts (Fig. 2.9). Due to the half-life

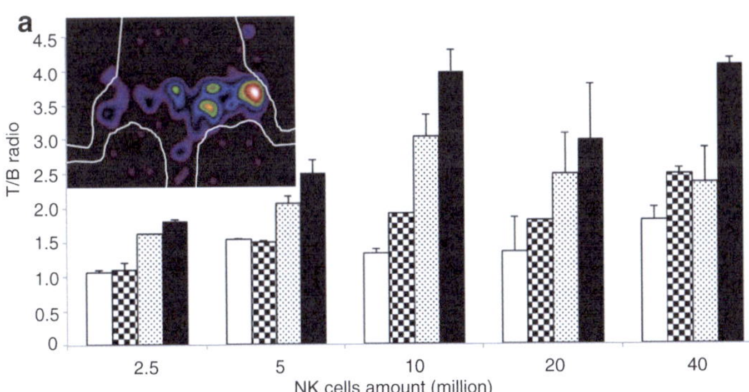
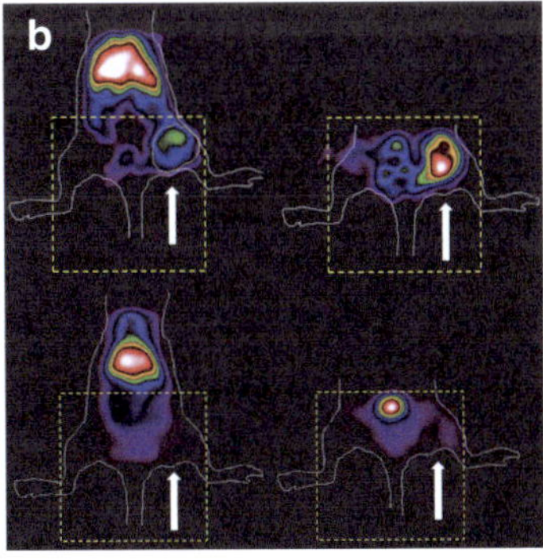

Fig. 2.9 In vivo imaging of human NK cells using [^{99m}Tc] Tc-hCD56-mAb. (a) Target-to-background (T/B) ratios calculated in mice injected with increasing numbers of CD56^{+} NK cells in the right thigh and with equivalent numbers of CD56^{-} control cells in the left thigh. Mice were imaged at 1 h (white bar), 3 h (squared bar), 6 h (dotted bar), and 24 h (black bar). Image of mouse injected with 10^{6} NK cells was acquired 24 h after injection of 5.5 MBq of radiolabeled mAb. (b) (Top) Total body (left) and lower body (right) scans of a mouse bearing an ARO xenograft (white arrow) in the right thigh. The animal intravenously received 10^{6} human NK cells and, after 24 h, 5.5 MBq of [^{99m}Tc]Tc-CD56-mAb. (Bottom) A negative control mouse bearing an ARO xenograft that intravenously received only radiolabeled antibody. Images were acquired 24 h after radiotracer injection. Each mouse is representative of a group of three mice (adapted from Galli et al., Journal of Nuclear Medicine, 2015 [262])

of ^{99m}Tc ($t_{1/2} = 6$ h), imaging was only conducted up to 24 h post-probe administration and demonstrated an optimal tumor-to-background ratio of 6.02 [262].

Although endogenous NK cell imaging is still in its infancy, efforts to develop further imaging agents are expected to grow as NK therapies mature. Choosing which aspect of NK cells to image is of paramount importance, and cell surface receptors are likely to be targeted in the first generation of nuclear imaging agents due to the specificity of these receptors and the availability of commercial antibodies. Ideally the imaging target should be expressed exclusively by the subset of NK cells of interest. A thorough genetic study showed that the most specific cell surface marker expressed by NK cells were *Klra8* (Ly49H) and *Ncr1* (NKp46) [263]. While Ly49H was expressed in only 50% of NK cells in C57BL/6 mice, it was not detectable in any other leukocyte population. Among the NCRs, activating ligands expressed by tumor and virally infected cells for NKp30 are the most widely known and include the tumor ligand B7-H6. Intense NKp30 immunohistochemistry staining has been shown to be a positive response indicator of survival in a variety of cancers, including acute myeloid leukemia and gastric and cervical cancer. NKp30 expression is also detected on tumor-infiltrating NK cells in human renal cell carcinoma (RCC) [264]. Our group has recently reported a ^{64}Cu- and ^{89}Zr-labeled mAb for specific imaging of the human NKp30 receptor in preclinical models [264, 265]. Other human NK cell targets include NKp44, NKp46, NKp80, and NKG2D as activating receptors, along with the killer cell immunoglobulin-like receptors (KIR). A major consideration is whether to image murine targets in immunocompetent murine models or human targets in humanized murine models. Murine NK cell targets include NK1.1 and NKp46 (Fig. 2.8). While NK1.1 is expressed primarily in C57BL/6 (B6) mice, NKp46 is expressed on NK cells in most mouse strains and shares 50–60% homology with human NKp46 [266]. NK cell numbers in the tumor milieu can vary greatly according to the tumor type; however they are typically quite low in the tumor microenvironment, necessitat-

ing the development of imaging probes with high specificity for NK cell targets with minimal background [267, 268]. NK cell imaging probes have the potential to aid the development of therapies that modulate the NK cell response and serve as early in vivo biomarkers of treatment response in clinical trials. Emerging therapies that require sensitive monitoring include mAbs that promote NK cell-mediated ADCC or bi- and tri-specific antibodies that directly target NK receptors. In contrast to biopsies or peripheral blood draws, noninvasive molecular imaging would provide a quantitative and much more accurate readout of whole-body NK cell response to therapy.

2.6 Priorities and Future Considerations

The last decade has experienced significant advancement in the characterization of lymphocyte biology and revealed their central roles in cancer immunity and immunopathology. This in turn has motivated the development of multiple imaging probes that are able to noninvasively capture their distinct behaviors in vivo. Targeting endogenous biomarkers of lymphocyte responses has been extremely useful where ex vivo labeling of cells is not feasible or desired. Nuclear imaging of immune cells has the potential to facilitate immunotherapy development, optimize therapy dose and scheduling, enable patient stratification, and elucidate the mechanisms of success or failure while also improving diagnosis and management of immunopathology such as type 1 diabetes, GVHD, and IBD. Significant advances in radiometal availability, chelate chemistry, and FDA-approved immune-modulating small molecules and biologics have boosted the development of lymphocyte imaging strategies, resulting in newer probes reaching clinical evaluation, with results of phase II trials for promising candidates such as the CD8-targeted Df-IAB22M2C and [^{18}F]F-AraG pending.

Despite significant advancements in the field, there is still a paucity of immune imaging agents that are clinically approved, and their potential to guide clinical management is yet to be realized.

There are several criteria that preclinical studies could fulfil in order to bridge this gap, for example, greater efforts to test the predictive capabilities of imaging probes, a critical step that is often omitted. Clearer demonstration of and how these imaging agents could be used to provide actionable insights into patient management is a requisite for rapid clinical translation and adoption. The hypothesis that imaging biomarkers of activation or cytotoxicity could provide more sensitive measurements of immune response, versus assaying constitutively expressed lineage markers is yet to be proved. Comparative studies of potential candidates demonstrating the value of one imaging agent over another in given models would help tailor their specific applications. The evaluation of possible immune modulating effects that the imaging probes could have, for example, inducing activation or depletion of certain subsets, is imperative especially in immunoPET studies targeting surface markers that play a key role in regulating immunity. The consequences of these perturbations will also be highly dependent on the scenario, for example, immune activation which is generally beneficial in immuno-oncology could be detrimental when imaging an immunopathological model. The likelihood of any biological impact is likely to be reduced through careful selection of antibody clones, generation of antibody fragments or engineered binders, and careful quality control. The search for more specific small molecule metabolic probes is ongoing and would be facilitated by the identification of metabolic signatures that are highly enriched in TILs but not utilized by the tumor. Additionally, while in vivo tracking of adoptive cell therapies has been dominated by ex vivo labeling and reporter genes, the evaluation of endogenous biomarker targeting approaches is also warranted for these therapies, which upon encountering their antigen, upregulate many of the targets discussed in this chapter.

A significant hurdle in the wider clinical application and serial imaging that is needed to monitor immune dynamics, is the high radiation dose associated with the use of longer-lived isotopes such as zirconium-89 and slower clearing agents such as intact antibodies. In addition to alternative faster clearing vectors, pre-targeted approaches whereby the vector and radiolabeled entity are injected separately are currently under active evaluation [269]. This approach may still allow the use of intact antibodies while minimizing radiation dose to healthy non-target tissues. Developments in PET instrumentation such as the whole-body PET EXPLORER system, with a reported 40-fold increased sensitivity, would dramatically reduce the radiation dose while generating dynamic images with high temporal and spatial resolution [270, 271]. Time-of-flight (ToF) PET has also significantly increased signal-to-noise ratios and improved visualization of low contrast lesions [272, 273]. By pushing the limits of sensitivity, one could envisage more rapid clinical evaluation of tracers with well-characterized PK like immunoPET agents, which currently take years to reach the clinic after initial preclinical evaluation. Further technological advances in PET scanner hardware will be key for improving the current molecular sensitivity in both preclinical and clinical research. Finally, artificial intelligence and machine learning approaches have the potential to facilitate the interpretation of large scan volumes and also parse out subtle systems level changes in tracer uptake, that may otherwise be missed by radiologists and nuclear medicine physicians.

It is important to highlight the utility of immune imaging approaches against a backdrop of other complimentary tools such as blood biomarker analysis and "omic" technologies such as RNA sequencing to improve the accuracy and frequency of immune monitoring and to potentially aid in the identification of novel imaging biomarkers. Multiplexed technologies such as flow cytometry, mass cytometry, and co-detection by indexing (CODEX) have made it possible to analyze several immune markers in parallel to facilitate understanding of the complex interplay between different immune populations and affected tissues. Although this chapter has focused on lymphocytes, myeloid cells are important contributors of the overall immune response [274]. As their roles in cancer and inflammatory disorders have become clearer and specific biomarkers for these populations have been identified, we have observed a growth in nuclear imaging probes for these cells [36, 275, 276]. Furthermore, simultaneous multi-isotope imaging would allow for the noninvasive visualization of multiple immune subsets in tandem to better capture the full complexity of immune responses. Efforts to develop PET detectors for multi-isotope imaging are currently underway and would be paradigm changing [277, 278].

2.7　Conclusion

The need for imaging immune responses is a critical priority for both preclinical research and clinical management of patients. Nuclear imaging approaches have the potential to allow noninvasive, systems level monitoring of early events and accurate prediction of therapeutic response in cancer immunotherapy and immunopathology. The sensitivity, translatability, and quantitative capabilities of PET make it an ideal modality to capture the complex spatiotemporal dynamics of immune cell responses, with the potential to change how therapies are applied and assessed for overall improved patient outcomes [25]. Targeting endogenous biomarkers of immune cell response negates the need for ex vivo manipulations that can perturb cell behavior. The success of this approach will be further boosted by identification of superior immune-specific biomarkers, continued advances in probe development, protein engineering, as well as the utilization of superior preclinical models that appropriately recapitulate clinical scenarios. With many promising first-in-human results for these targeted radiotracers on the horizon, it is anticipated that these approaches will play a major role in the clinic in years to come.

Acknowledgments We thank Drs. Federico Simonetta, Carmel T. Chan, Weiyu Chen and Nusrat S. Alam for valuable discussions and for reviewing the manuscript. Additionally we are grateful to Jim Strommer and Judy Schwimmer for their support with figures. We would also like to acknowledge funding support from the Ben and Catherine Ivy Foundation, Canary Foundation and National Cancer Institute (R01 CA201719-05). Finally, we are thankful to our colleagues in the imaging community that contributed to the development and translation of the strategies discussed in this chapter. This work is dedicated to the memory of my father Dr. Mohammed Shamsul Alam, my aunt Dr Dilara Huq and our mentor Professor Sanjiv Sam Gambhir; for their deep commitment to humanity, tireless efforts to serve others and above all for their passion and wonder for science and medicine.

Review Criteria: We have intentionally chosen to highlight studies that have been reported within the last decade with an emphasis on those that have been clinically evaluated or demonstrate strong translational potential. Pubmed was searched for relevant publications up until June 2020. ClinicalTrials.gov was queried for trials pertaining to the probes discussed. We chose to focus on endogenous imaging biomarkers, specifically associated with lymphocytes, rather than general markers associated with the inflammatory response that are upregulated on vasculature and stroma. We recognize that there are many valuable studies in the field that were not within the scope of this discussion and have cited references for readers who are interested in those areas.

Conflicts of Interest Dr Gambhir was the founder and equity holder of CellSight Inc. that develops and translates strategies for imaging cell trafficking/transplantation.

References

1. Iwasaki A, Medzhitov R. Control of adaptive immunity by the innate immune system. Nat Immunol. 2015;16(4):343–53. https://doi.org/10.1038/ni.3123.
2. Marshall JS, Warrington R, Watson W, Kim HL. An introduction to immunology and immunopathology. Allergy Asthma Clin Immunol. 2018;14(Suppl 2):49. https://doi.org/10.1186/s13223-018-0278-1.
3. Tumeh PC, Harview CL, Yearley JH, Shintaku IP, Taylor EJ, Robert L, et al. PD-1 blockade induces responses by inhibiting adaptive immune resistance. Nature. 2014;515(7528):568–71. https://doi.org/10.1038/nature13954.
4. Sagiv-Barfi I, Czerwinski DK, Levy S, Alam IS, Mayer AT, Gambhir SS, et al. Eradication of spontaneous malignancy by local immunotherapy. Sci Transl Med. 2018;10(426):eaan4488. https://doi.org/10.1126/scitranslmed.aan4488.
5. Benmebarek MR, Karches CH, Cadilha BL, Lesch S, Endres S, Kobold S. Killing mechanisms of chimeric antigen receptor (CAR) T cells. Int J Mol Sci. 2019;20(6):1283. https://doi.org/10.3390/ijms20061283.
6. Chen DS, Mellman I. Oncology meets immunology: the cancer-immunity cycle. Immunity. 2013;39(1):1–10. https://doi.org/10.1016/j.immuni.2013.07.012.
7. Beer L, Hochmair M, Prosch H. Pitfalls in the radiological response assessment of immunotherapy. Memo. 2018;11(2):138–43. https://doi.org/10.1007/s12254-018-0389-x.

8. Aide N, Hicks RJ, Le Tourneau C, Lheureux S, Fanti S, Lopci E. FDG PET/CT for assessing tumour response to immunotherapy: report on the EANM symposium on immune modulation and recent review of the literature. Eur J Nucl Med Mol Imaging. 2019;46(1):238–50. https://doi.org/10.1007/s00259-018-4171-4.

9. Somarouthu B, Lee SI, Urban T, Sadow CA, Harris GJ, Kambadakone A. Immune-related tumour response assessment criteria: a comprehensive review. Br J Radiol. 2018;91(1084):20170457. https://doi.org/10.1259/bjr.20170457.

10. Borcoman E, Nandikolla A, Long G, Goel S, Le Tourneau C. Patterns of response and progression to immunotherapy. Am Soc Clin Oncol Educ Book. 2018;38:169–78. https://doi.org/10.1200/EDBK_200643.

11. Ventola CL. Cancer immunotherapy, Part 3: Challenges and future trends. P T. 2017;42(8):514–21.

12. Liu Z, Li Z. Molecular imaging in tracking tumor-specific cytotoxic T lymphocytes (CTLs). Theranostics. 2014;4(10):990–1001. https://doi.org/10.7150/thno.9268.

13. Wei W, Jiang D, Ehlerding EB, Luo Q, Cai W. Noninvasive PET imaging of T cells. Trends Cancer. 2018;4(5):359–73. https://doi.org/10.1016/j.trecan.2018.03.009.

14. Krekorian M, Fruhwirth GO, Srinivas M, Figdor CG, Heskamp S, Witney TH, et al. Imaging of T-cells and their responses during anti-cancer immunotherapy. Theranostics. 2019;9(25):7924–47. https://doi.org/10.7150/thno.37924.

15. Pugliese A. Autoreactive T cells in type 1 diabetes. J Clin Invest. 2017;127(8):2881–91. https://doi.org/10.1172/JCI94549.

16. Fletcher JM, Lalor SJ, Sweeney CM, Tubridy N, Mills KH. T cells in multiple sclerosis and experimental autoimmune encephalomyelitis. Clin Exp Immunol. 2010;162(1):1–11. https://doi.org/10.1111/j.1365-2249.2010.04143.x.

17. Maynard CL, Weaver CT. Intestinal effector T cells in health and disease. Immunity. 2009;31(3):389–400. https://doi.org/10.1016/j.immuni.2009.08.012.

18. Comte D, Karampetsou MP, Tsokos GC. T cells as a therapeutic target in SLE. Lupus. 2015;24(4–5):351–63. https://doi.org/10.1177/0961203314556139.

19. Ingulli E. Mechanism of cellular rejection in transplantation. Pediatr Nephrol. 2010;25(1):61–74. https://doi.org/10.1007/s00467-008-1020-x.

20. Ford ML. T cell cosignaling molecules in transplantation. Immunity. 2016;44(5):1020–33. https://doi.org/10.1016/j.immuni.2016.04.012.

21. Zeiser R, Blazar BR. Acute graft-versus-host disease - biologic process, prevention, and therapy. N Engl J Med. 2017;377(22):2167–79. https://doi.org/10.1056/NEJMra1609337.

22. Beilhack A, Schulz S, Baker J, Beilhack GF, Wieland CB, Herman EI, et al. In vivo analyses of early events in acute graft-versus-host disease reveal sequential infiltration of T-cell subsets. Blood. 2005;106(3):1113–22. https://doi.org/10.1182/blood-2005-02-0509.

23. Cazaux M, Grandjean CL, Lemaitre F, Garcia Z, Beck RJ, Milo I, et al. Single-cell imaging of CAR T cell activity in vivo reveals extensive functional and anatomical heterogeneity. J Exp Med. 2019;216(5):1038–49. https://doi.org/10.1084/jem.20182375.

24. Balagopalan L, Sherman E, Barr VA, Samelson LE. Imaging techniques for assaying lymphocyte activation in action. Nat Rev Immunol. 2011;11(1):21–33. https://doi.org/10.1038/nri2903.

25. James ML, Gambhir SS. A molecular imaging primer: modalities, imaging agents, and applications. Physiol Rev. 2012;92(2):897–965. https://doi.org/10.1152/physrev.00049.2010.

26. Mayer AT, Gambhir SS. The immunoimaging toolbox. J Nucl Med. 2018;59(8):1174–82. https://doi.org/10.2967/jnumed.116.185967.

27. Wei W, Rosenkrans ZT, Liu J, Huang G, Luo QY, Cai W. ImmunoPET: concept, design, and applications. Chem Rev. 2020;120(8):3787–851. https://doi.org/10.1021/acs.chemrev.9b00738.

28. Sharma SK, Chow A, Monette S, Vivier D, Pourat J, Edwards KJ, et al. Fc-mediated anomalous biodistribution of therapeutic antibodies in immunodeficient mouse models. Cancer Res. 2018;78(7):1820–32. https://doi.org/10.1158/0008-5472.CAN-17-1958.

29. Vivier D, Sharma SK, Adumeau P, Rodriguez C, Fung K, Zeglis BM. The impact of FcgammaRI binding on immuno-PET. J Nucl Med. 2019;60(8):1174–82. https://doi.org/10.2967/jnumed.118.223636.

30. Freise AC, Wu AM. In vivo imaging with antibodies and engineered fragments. Mol Immunol. 2015;67(2 Pt A):142–52. https://doi.org/10.1016/j.molimm.2015.04.001.

31. Fu R, Carroll L, Yahioglu G, Aboagye EO, Miller PW. Antibody fragment and affibody ImmunoPET imaging agents: radiolabelling strategies and applications. ChemMedChem. 2018;13(23):2466–78. https://doi.org/10.1002/cmdc.201800624.

32. Rashidian M, Keliher EJ, Bilate AM, Duarte JN, Wojtkiewicz GR, Jacobsen JT, et al. Noninvasive imaging of immune responses. Proc Natl Acad Sci U S A. 2015;112(19):6146–51. https://doi.org/10.1073/pnas.1502609112.

33. Iezzi ME, Policastro L, Werbajh S, Podhajcer O, Canziani GA. Single-domain antibodies and the promise of modular targeting in cancer imaging and treatment. Front Immunol. 2018;9:273. https://doi.org/10.3389/fimmu.2018.00273.

34. Chakravarty R, Goel S, Cai W. Nanobody: the "magic bullet" for molecular imaging? Theranostics. 2014;4(4):386–98. https://doi.org/10.7150/thno.8006.

35. Van Elssen C, Rashidian M, Vrbanac V, Wucherpfennig KW, Habre ZE, Sticht J, et al. Noninvasive imaging of human immune responses in a human xenograft model of graft-versus-host disease. J Nucl Med. 2017;58(6):1003–8. https://doi.org/10.2967/jnumed.116.186007.

36. Rashidian M, LaFleur MW, Verschoor VL, Dongre A, Zhang Y, Nguyen TH, et al. Immuno-PET identifies the myeloid compartment as a key contributor to the outcome of the antitumor response under PD-1 blockade. Proc Natl Acad Sci U S A. 2019;116(34):16971–80. https://doi.org/10.1073/pnas.1905005116.

37. Rashidian M, Ingram JR, Dougan M, Dongre A, Whang KA, LeGall C, et al. Predicting the response to CTLA-4 blockade by longitudinal noninvasive monitoring of CD8 T cells. J Exp Med. 2017;214(8):2243–55. https://doi.org/10.1084/jem.20161950.

38. Schneider DW, Heitner T, Alicke B, Light DR, McLean K, Satozawa N, et al. In vivo biodistribution, PET imaging, and tumor accumulation of 86Y- and 111In-antimindin/RG-1, engineered antibody fragments in LNCaP tumor-bearing nude mice. J Nucl Med. 2009;50(3):435–43. https://doi.org/10.2967/jnumed.108.055608.

39. Carter LM, Poty S, Sharma SK, Lewis JS. Preclinical optimization of antibody-based radiopharmaceuticals for cancer imaging and radionuclide therapy-model, vector, and radionuclide selection. J Labelled Comp Radiopharm. 2018;61(9):611–35. https://doi.org/10.1002/jlcr.3612.

40. Natarajan A, Hackel BJ, Gambhir SS. A novel engineered anti-CD20 tracer enables early time PET imaging in a humanized transgenic mouse model of B-cell non-Hodgkins lymphoma. Clin Cancer Res. 2013;19(24):6820–9. https://doi.org/10.1158/1078-0432.CCR-13-0626.

41. Ackerman SE, Currier NV, Bergen JM, Cochran JR. Cystine-knot peptides: emerging tools for cancer imaging and therapy. Expert Rev Proteomics. 2014;11(5):561–72. https://doi.org/10.1586/14789450.2014.932251.

42. Kimura RH, Wang L, Shen B, Huo L, Tummers W, Filipp FV, et al. Evaluation of integrin alphavbeta6 cystine knot PET tracers to detect cancer and idiopathic pulmonary fibrosis. Nat Commun. 2019;10(1):4673. https://doi.org/10.1038/s41467-019-11863-w.

43. Donnelly DJ, Smith RA, Morin P, Lipovsek D, Gokemeijer J, Cohen D, et al. Synthesis and biologic evaluation of a novel (18)F-labeled adnectin as a PET radioligand for imaging PD-L1 expression. J Nucl Med. 2018;59(3):529–35. https://doi.org/10.2967/jnumed.117.199596.

44. Wu AM. Engineered antibodies for molecular imaging of cancer. Methods. 2014;65(1):139–47. https://doi.org/10.1016/j.ymeth.2013.09.015.

45. Menk AV, Scharping NE, Moreci RS, Zeng X, Guy C, Salvatore S, et al. Early TCR signaling induces rapid aerobic glycolysis enabling distinct acute T cell effector functions. Cell Rep. 2018;22(6):1509–21. https://doi.org/10.1016/j.celrep.2018.01.040.

46. Fairbanks LD, Bofill M, Ruckemann K, Simmonds HA. Importance of ribonucleotide availability to proliferating T-lymphocytes from healthy humans. Disproportionate expansion of pyrimidine pools and contrasting effects of de novo synthesis inhibitors. J Biol Chem. 1995;270(50):29682–9.

47. Cherry SR, Gambhir SS. Use of positron emission tomography in animal research. ILAR J. 2001;42(3):219–32. https://doi.org/10.1093/ilar.42.3.219.

48. Endo K, Oriuchi N, Higuchi T, Iida Y, Hanaoka H, Miyakubo M, et al. PET and PET/CT using 18F-FDG in the diagnosis and management of cancer patients. Int J Clin Oncol. 2006;11(4):286–96. https://doi.org/10.1007/s10147-006-0595-0.

49. Daly KP, Dearling JL, Seto T, Dunning P, Fahey F, Packard AB, et al. Use of [18F]FDG positron emission tomography to monitor the development of cardiac allograft rejection. Transplantation. 2015;99(9):e132–9. https://doi.org/10.1097/TP.0000000000000618.

50. Vaidyanathan S, Patel CN, Scarsbrook AF, Chowdhury FU. FDG PET/CT in infection and inflammation—current and emerging clinical applications. Clin Radiol. 2015;70(7):787–800. https://doi.org/10.1016/j.crad.2015.03.010.

51. Wong ANM, McArthur GA, Hofman MS, Hicks RJ. The advantages and challenges of using FDG PET/CT for response assessment in melanoma in the era of targeted agents and immunotherapy. Eur J Nucl Med Mol Imaging. 2017;44(Suppl 1):67–77. https://doi.org/10.1007/s00259-017-3691-7.

52. Takada K, Toyokawa G, Yoneshima Y, Tanaka K, Okamoto I, Shimokawa M, et al. (18)F-FDG uptake in PET/CT is a potential predictive biomarker of response to anti-PD-1 antibody therapy in non-small cell lung cancer. Sci Rep. 2019;9(1):13362. https://doi.org/10.1038/s41598-019-50079-2.

53. Turner MD, Nedjai B, Hurst T, Pennington DJ. Cytokines and chemokines: at the crossroads of cell signalling and inflammatory disease. Biochim Biophys Acta. 2014;1843(11):2563–82. https://doi.org/10.1016/j.bbamcr.2014.05.014.

54. Lippitz BE. Cytokine patterns in patients with cancer: a systematic review. Lancet Oncol. 2013;14(6):e218–28. https://doi.org/10.1016/S1470-2045(12)70582-X.

55. Larimer BM, Wehrenberg-Klee E, Dubois F, Mehta A, Kalomeris T, Flaherty K, et al. Granzyme B PET imaging as a predictive biomarker of immunotherapy response. Cancer Res. 2017;77(9):2318–27. https://doi.org/10.1158/0008-5472.CAN-16-3346.

56. Gibson HM, McKnight BN, Malysa A, Dyson G, Wiesend WN, McCarthy CE, et al. IFNgamma PET imaging as a predictive tool for monitoring response to tumor immunotherapy. Cancer Res. 2018;78(19):5706–17. https://doi.org/10.1158/0008-5472.CAN-18-0253.

57. Beckford-Vera DR, Gonzalez-Junca A, Janneck JS, Huynh TL, Blecha JE, Seo Y, et al. PET/CT imaging of human TNFalpha using [(89)Zr]Certolizumab pegol in a transgenic preclinical model of rheumatoid arthritis. Mol Imaging Biol. 2020;22(1):105–14. https://doi.org/10.1007/s11307-019-01363-0.

58. Signore A, Jamar F, Israel O, Buscombe J, Martin-Comin J, Lazzeri E. Clinical indications, image acquisition and data interpretation for white blood cells and anti-granulocyte monoclonal antibody scin-

tigraphy: an EANM procedural guideline. Eur J Nucl Med Mol Imaging. 2018;45(10):1816–31. https://doi.org/10.1007/s00259-018-4052-x.

59. Sato N, Wu H, Asiedu KO, Szajek LP, Griffiths GL, Choyke PL. (89)Zr-oxine complex PET cell imaging in monitoring cell-based therapies. Radiology. 2015;275(2):490–500. https://doi.org/10.1148/radiol.15142849.

60. Man F, Lim L, Volpe A, Gabizon A, Shmeeda H, Draper B, et al. In vivo PET tracking of (89)Zr-labeled Vgamma9Vdelta2 T cells to mouse xenograft breast tumors activated with liposomal alendronate. Mol Ther. 2019;27(1):219–29. https://doi.org/10.1016/j.ymthe.2018.10.006.

61. Fisher B, Packard BS, Read EJ, Carrasquillo JA, Carter CS, Topalian SL, et al. Tumor localization of adoptively transferred indium-111 labeled tumor infiltrating lymphocytes in patients with metastatic melanoma. J Clin Oncol. 1989;7(2):250–61. https://doi.org/10.1200/JCO.1989.7.2.250.

62. Kassis AI, Adelstein SJ. Chemotoxicity of indium-111 oxine in mammalian cells. J Nucl Med. 1985;26(2):187–90.

63. Signore A, Beales P, Sensi M, Zuccarini O, Pozzilli P. Labelling of lymphocytes with indium 111 oxine: effect on cell surface phenotype and antibody-dependent cellular cytotoxicity. Immunol Lett. 1983;6(3):151–4.

64. Sahu SK, Kassis AI, Makrigiorgos GM, Baranowska-Kortylewicz J, Adelstein SJ. The effects of indium-111 decay on pBR322 DNA. Radiat Res. 1995;141(2):193–8.

65. Acton PD, Zhou R. Imaging reporter genes for cell tracking with PET and SPECT. Q J Nucl Med Mol Imaging. 2005;49(4):349–60.

66. MacLaren DC, Gambhir SS, Satyamurthy N, Barrio JR, Sharfstein S, Toyokuni T, et al. Repetitive, non-invasive imaging of the dopamine D2 receptor as a reporter gene in living animals. Gene Ther. 1999;6(5):785–91. https://doi.org/10.1038/sj.gt.3300877.

67. Lee JT, Moroz MA, Ponomarev V. Imaging T cell dynamics and function using PET and human nuclear reporter genes. Methods Mol Biol. 1790;2018:165–80. https://doi.org/10.1007/978-1-4939-7860-1_13.

68. Minn I, Rowe SP, Pomper MG. Enhancing CAR T-cell therapy through cellular imaging and radiotherapy. Lancet Oncol. 2019;20(8):e443–e51. https://doi.org/10.1016/S1470-2045(19)30461-9.

69. Gambhir SS, Bauer E, Black ME, Liang Q, Kokoris MS, Barrio JR, et al. A mutant herpes simplex virus type 1 thymidine kinase reporter gene shows improved sensitivity for imaging reporter gene expression with positron emission tomography. Proc Natl Acad Sci U S A. 2000;97(6):2785–90. https://doi.org/10.1073/pnas.97.6.2785.

70. Yaghoubi SS, Gambhir SS. PET imaging of herpes simplex virus type 1 thymidine kinase (HSV1-tk) or mutant HSV1-sr39tk reporter gene expression in mice and humans using [18F]FHBG. Nat Protoc. 2006;1(6):3069–75. https://doi.org/10.1038/nprot.2006.459.

71. Keu KV, Witney TH, Yaghoubi S, Rosenberg J, Kurien A, Magnusson R, et al. Reporter gene imaging of targeted T cell immunotherapy in recurrent glioma. Sci Transl Med. 2017;9(373):eaag2196. https://doi.org/10.1126/scitranslmed.aag2196.

72. Blumenthal M, Skelton D, Pepper KA, Jahn T, Methangkool E, Kohn DB. Effective suicide gene therapy for leukemia in a model of insertional oncogenesis in mice. Mol Ther. 2007;15(1):183–92. https://doi.org/10.1038/sj.mt.6300015.

73. Berger C, Flowers ME, Warren EH, Riddell SR. Analysis of transgene-specific immune responses that limit the in vivo persistence of adoptively transferred HSV-TK-modified donor T cells after allogeneic hematopoietic cell transplantation. Blood. 2006;107(6):2294–302. https://doi.org/10.1182/blood-2005-08-3503.

74. Campbell DO, Yaghoubi SS, Su Y, Lee JT, Auerbach MS, Herschman H, et al. Structure-guided engineering of human thymidine kinase 2 as a positron emission tomography reporter gene for enhanced phosphorylation of non-natural thymidine analog reporter probe. J Biol Chem. 2012;287(1):446–54. https://doi.org/10.1074/jbc.M111.314666.

75. Minn I, Huss DJ, Ahn HH, Chinn TM, Park A, Jones J, et al. Imaging CAR T cell therapy with PSMA-targeted positron emission tomography. Sci Adv. 2019;5(7):eaaw5096. https://doi.org/10.1126/sciadv.aaw5096.

76. Sharif-Paghaleh E, Sunassee K, Tavare R, Ratnasothy K, Koers A, Ali N, et al. In vivo SPECT reporter gene imaging of regulatory T cells. PLoS One. 2011;6(10):e25857. https://doi.org/10.1371/journal.pone.0025857.

77. Ponomarev V, Doubrovin M, Lyddane C, Beresten T, Balatoni J, Bornman W, et al. Imaging TCR-dependent NFAT-mediated T-cell activation with positron emission tomography in vivo. Neoplasia. 2001;3(6):480–8. https://doi.org/10.1038/sj.neo.7900204.

78. James ML, Hoehne A, Mayer AT, Lechtenberg K, Moreno M, Gowrishankar G, et al. Imaging B cells in a mouse model of multiple sclerosis using (64)cu-rituximab PET. J Nucl Med. 2017;58(11):1845–51. https://doi.org/10.2967/jnumed.117.189597.

79. Kumar BV, Connors TJ, Farber DL. Human T cell development, localization, and function throughout life. Immunity. 2018;48(2):202–13. https://doi.org/10.1016/j.immuni.2018.01.007.

80. Hughes CE, Benson RA, Bedaj M, Maffia P. Antigen-presenting cells and antigen presentation in tertiary lymphoid organs. Front Immunol. 2016;7:481. https://doi.org/10.3389/fimmu.2016.00481.

81. Bogle G, Dunbar PR. T cell responses in lymph nodes. Wiley Interdiscip Rev Syst Biol Med. 2010;2(1):107–16. https://doi.org/10.1002/wsbm.47.

82. Zheng Y, Delgoffe GM, Meyer CF, Chan W, Powell JD. Anergic T cells are metabolically anergic. J Immunol. 2009;183(10):6095–101. https://doi.org/10.4049/jimmunol.0803510.

83. June CH, Ledbetter JA, Linsley PS, Thompson CB. Role of the CD28 receptor in T-cell activation. Immunol Today. 1990;11(6):211–6. https://doi.org/10.1016/0167-5699(90)90085-n.

84. Masopust D, Schenkel JM. The integration of T cell migration, differentiation and function. Nat Rev Immunol. 2013;13(5):309–20. https://doi.org/10.1038/nri3442.

85. Watts TH. TNF/TNFR family members in costimulation of T cell responses. Annu Rev Immunol. 2005;23:23–68. https://doi.org/10.1146/annurev.immunol.23.021704.115839.

86. Croft M. The role of TNF superfamily members in T-cell function and diseases. Nat Rev Immunol. 2009;9(4):271–85. https://doi.org/10.1038/nri2526.

87. Larimer BM, Wehrenberg-Klee E, Caraballo A, Mahmood U. Quantitative CD3 PET imaging predicts tumor growth response to anti-CTLA-4 therapy. J Nucl Med. 2016;57(10):1607–11. https://doi.org/10.2967/jnumed.116.173930.

88. Beckford Vera DR, Smith CC, Bixby LM, Glatt DM, Dunn SS, Saito R, et al. Immuno-PET imaging of tumor-infiltrating lymphocytes using zirconium-89 radiolabeled anti-CD3 antibody in immune-competent mice bearing syngeneic tumors. PLoS One. 2018;13(3):e0193832. https://doi.org/10.1371/journal.pone.0193832.

89. Freise AC, Zettlitz KA, Salazar FB, Tavare R, Tsai WK, Chatziioannou AF, et al. Immuno-PET in inflammatory bowel disease: imaging CD4-positive T cells in a murine model of colitis. J Nucl Med. 2018;59(6):980–5. https://doi.org/10.2967/jnumed.117.199075.

90. Tavare R, McCracken MN, Zettlitz KA, Knowles SM, Salazar FB, Olafsen T, et al. Engineered antibody fragments for immuno-PET imaging of endogenous CD8+ T cells in vivo. Proc Natl Acad Sci U S A. 2014;111(3):1108–13. https://doi.org/10.1073/pnas.1316922111.

91. Tavare R, Escuin-Ordinas H, Mok S, McCracken MN, Zettlitz KA, Salazar FB, et al. An effective immuno-PET imaging method to monitor CD8-dependent responses to immunotherapy. Cancer Res. 2016;76(1):73–82. https://doi.org/10.1158/0008-5472.CAN-15-1707.

92. Pektor S, Schloder J, Klasen B, Bausbacher N, Wagner DC, Schreckenberger M, et al. Using immuno-PET imaging to monitor kinetics of T cell-mediated inflammation and treatment efficiency in a humanized mouse model for GvHD. Eur J Nucl Med Mol Imaging. 2019; https://doi.org/10.1007/s00259-019-04507-0.

93. San Jose E, Borroto A, Niedergang F, Alcover A, Alarcon B. Triggering the TCR complex causes the downregulation of nonengaged receptors by a signal transduction-dependent mechanism. Immunity. 2000;12(2):161–70. https://doi.org/10.1016/s1074-7613(00)80169-7.

94. Galon J, Costes A, Sanchez-Cabo F, Kirilovsky A, Mlecnik B, Lagorce-Pages C, et al. Type, density, and location of immune cells within human colorectal tumors predict clinical outcome. Science. 2006;313(5795):1960–4. https://doi.org/10.1126/science.1129139.

95. Zhang L, Conejo-Garcia JR, Katsaros D, Gimotty PA, Massobrio M, Regnani G, et al. Intratumoral T cells, recurrence, and survival in epithelial ovarian cancer. N Engl J Med. 2003;348(3):203–13. https://doi.org/10.1056/NEJMoa020177.

96. Al-Shibli KI, Donnem T, Al-Saad S, Persson M, Bremnes RM, Busund LT. Prognostic effect of epithelial and stromal lymphocyte infiltration in non-small cell lung cancer. Clin Cancer Res. 2008;14(16):5220–7. https://doi.org/10.1158/1078-0432.CCR-08-0133.

97. Pandit-Taskar N, Postow M, O'Donoghue J, Harding J, Ziolkowska M, Lyashchenko S, et al. First in human phase I imaging study with 89Zr-IAB22M2C anti CD8 minibody in patients with solid tumors. J Nucl Med. 2018;59

98. Spitzer MH, Carmi Y, Reticker-Flynn NE, Kwek SS, Madhireddy D, Martins MM, et al. Systemic immunity is required for effective cancer immunotherapy. Cell. 2017;168(3):487–502.e15. https://doi.org/10.1016/j.cell.2016.12.022.

99. Bhattacharyya M, Madden P, Henning N, Gregory S, Aid M, Martinot AJ, et al. Regulation of CD4 T cells and their effects on immunopathological inflammation following viral infection. Immunology. 2017;152(2):328–43. https://doi.org/10.1111/imm.12771.

100. Borst J, Ahrends T, Babala N, Melief CJM, Kastenmuller W. CD4(+) T cell help in cancer immunology and immunotherapy. Nat Rev Immunol. 2018;18(10):635–47. https://doi.org/10.1038/s41577-018-0044-0.

101. Steinhoff K, Pierer M, Siegert J, Pigla U, Laub R, Hesse S, et al. Visualizing inflammation activity in rheumatoid arthritis with Tc-99 m anti-CD4-mAb fragment scintigraphy. Nucl Med Biol. 2014;41(4):350–4. https://doi.org/10.1016/j.nucmedbio.2013.12.018.

102. Tavare R, McCracken MN, Zettlitz KA, Salazar FB, Olafsen T, Witte ON, et al. Immuno-PET of murine T cell reconstitution postadoptive stem cell transplantation using anti-CD4 and anti-CD8 Cys-diabodies. J Nucl Med. 2015;56(8):1258–64. https://doi.org/10.2967/jnumed.114.153338.

103. Freise AC, Zettlitz KA, Salazar FB, Lu X, Tavare R, Wu AM. ImmunoPET imaging of murine CD4(+) T cells using anti-CD4 Cys-diabody: effects of protein dose on T cell function and imaging. Mol Imaging Biol. 2017;19(4):599–609. https://doi.org/10.1007/s11307-016-1032-z.

104. Alam IS, Mayer AT, Sagiv-Barfi I, Wang K, Vermesh O, Czerwinski DK, et al. Imaging activated T cells predicts response to cancer vaccines. J Clin Invest. 2018;128(6):2569–80. https://doi.org/10.1172/JCI98509.

105. Dancey G, Violet J, Malaroda A, Green AJ, Sharma SK, Francis R, et al. A phase I clinical trial of CHT-

25 a 131I-labeled chimeric anti-CD25 antibody showing efficacy in patients with refractory lymphoma. Clin Cancer Res. 2009;15(24):7701–10. https://doi.org/10.1158/1078-0432.CCR-09-1421.

106. Glaudemans AW, Bonanno E, Galli F, Zeebregts CJ, de Vries EF, Koole M, et al. In vivo and in vitro evidence that (9)(9)mTc-HYNIC-interleukin-2 is able to detect T lymphocytes in vulnerable atherosclerotic plaques of the carotid artery. Eur J Nucl Med Mol Imaging. 2014;41(9):1710–9. https://doi.org/10.1007/s00259-014-2764-0.

107. Hartimath SV, Draghiciu O, van de Wall S, Manuelli V, Dierckx RA, Nijman HW, et al. Noninvasive monitoring of cancer therapy induced activated T cells using [(18)F]FB-IL-2 PET imaging. Oncoimmunology. 2017;6(1):e1248014. https://doi.org/10.1080/2162402X.2016.1248014.

108. Signore A, Chianelli M, Annovazzi A, Bonanno E, Spagnoli LG, Pozzilli P, et al. 123I-interleukin-2 scintigraphy for in vivo assessment of intestinal mononuclear cell infiltration in Crohn's disease. J Nucl Med. 2000;41(2):242–9.

109. Hubalewska-Dydejczyk A, Stompor T, Kalembkiewicz M, Krzanowski M, Mikolajczak R, Sowa-Staszczak A, et al. Identification of inflamed atherosclerotic plaque using 123 I-labeled interleukin-2 scintigraphy in high-risk peritoneal dialysis patients: a pilot study. Perit Dial Int. 2009;29(5):568–74.

110. Signore A, Parman A, Pozzilli P, Andreani D, Beverley PC. Detection of activated lymphocytes in endocrine pancreas of BB/W rats by injection of 123I-interleukin-2: an early sign of type 1 diabetes. Lancet. 1987;2(8558):537–40. https://doi.org/10.1016/s0140-6736(87)92925-4.

111. Signore A, Chianelli M, Ferretti E, Toscano A, Britton KE, Andreani D, et al. New approach for in vivo detection of insulitis in type I diabetes: activated lymphocyte targeting with 123I-labelled interleukin 2. Eur J Endocrinol. 1994;131(4):431–7. https://doi.org/10.1530/eje.0.1310431.

112. Rolandsson O, Stigbrand T, Riklundahlstrom K, Eary J, Greenbaum C. Accumulation of (125) iodine labeled interleukin-2 in the pancreas of NOD mice. J Autoimmun. 2001;17(4):281–7. https://doi.org/10.1006/jaut.2001.0555.

113. Klinke DJ II. Extent of beta cell destruction is important but insufficient to predict the onset of type 1 diabetes mellitus. PLoS One. 2008;3(1):e1374. https://doi.org/10.1371/journal.pone.0001374.

114. Chianelli M, Mather SJ, Grossman A, Sobnak R, Fritzberg A, Britton KE, et al. 99mTc-interleukin 2 scintigraphy in normal subjects and in patients with autoimmune thyroid diseases: a feasibility study. Eur J Nucl Med Mol Imaging. 2008;35(12):2286–93. https://doi.org/10.1007/s00259-008-0837-7.

115. Markovic SN, Galli F, Suman VJ, Nevala WK, Paulsen AM, Hung JC, et al. Non-invasive visualization of tumor infiltrating lymphocytes in patients with metastatic melanoma undergoing immune checkpoint inhibitor therapy: a pilot study. Oncotarget. 2018;9(54):30268–78. https://doi.org/10.18632/oncotarget.25666.

116. Di Gialleonardo V, Signore A, Glaudemans AW, Dierckx RA, De Vries EF. N-(4-18F-fluorobenzoyl) interleukin-2 for PET of human-activated T lymphocytes. J Nucl Med. 2012;53(5):679–86. https://doi.org/10.2967/jnumed.111.091306.

117. Flynn MJ, Hartley JA. The emerging role of anti-CD25 directed therapies as both immune modulators and targeted agents in cancer. Br J Haematol. 2017;179(1):20–35. https://doi.org/10.1111/bjh.14770.

118. Hartimath SV, Manuelli V, Zijlma R, Signore A, Nayak TK, Freimoser-Grundschober A, et al. Pharmacokinetic properties of radiolabeled mutant Interleukin-2v: a PET imaging study. Oncotarget. 2018;9(6):7162–74. https://doi.org/10.18632/oncotarget.23852.

119. Gonzalez-Amaro R, Cortes JR, Sanchez-Madrid F, Martin P. Is CD69 an effective brake to control inflammatory diseases? Trends Mol Med. 2013;19(10):625–32. https://doi.org/10.1016/j.molmed.2013.07.006.

120. Cibrian D, Sanchez-Madrid F. CD69: from activation marker to metabolic gatekeeper. Eur J Immunol. 2017;47(6):946–53. https://doi.org/10.1002/eji.201646837.

121. Bredi Tako PK, Maurer A, Kneilling M, Pichler B, Sonanini D. ImmunoPET of the early activation antigen CD69 enables response prediction of cancer immunotherapies. Montreal, Canada: World Molecular Imaging Congress; 2019.

122. Afeltra A, Galeazzi M, Ferri GM, Amoroso A, De Pita O, Porzio F, et al. Expression of CD69 antigen on synovial fluid T cells in patients with rheumatoid arthritis and other chronic synovitis. Ann Rheum Dis. 1993;52(6):457–60. https://doi.org/10.1136/ard.52.6.457.

123. Perrella O, Carrieri PB, De Mercato R, Buscaino GA. Markers of activated T lymphocytes and T cell receptor gamma/delta+ in patients with multiple sclerosis. Eur Neurol. 1993;33(2):152–5. https://doi.org/10.1159/000116923.

124. Posselt AM, Vincenti F, Bedolli M, Lantz M, Roberts JP, Hirose R. CD69 expression on peripheral CD8 T cells correlates with acute rejection in renal transplant recipients. Transplantation. 2003;76(1):190–5. https://doi.org/10.1097/01.TP.0000073614.29680.A8.

125. Weinberg AD, Morris NP, Kovacsovics-Bankowski M, Urba WJ, Curti BD. Science gone translational: the OX40 agonist story. Immunol Rev. 2011;244(1):218–31. https://doi.org/10.1111/j.1600-065X.2011.01069.x.

126. Peng W, Williams LJ, Xu C, Melendez B, McKenzie JA, Chen Y, et al. Anti-OX40 antibody directly enhances the function of tumor-reactive CD8(+) T

cells and synergizes with PI3Kbeta inhibition in PTEN loss melanoma. Clin Cancer Res. 2019;25(21):6406–16. https://doi.org/10.1158/1078-0432.CCR-19-1259.

127. Gramaglia I, Weinberg AD, Lemon M, Croft M. Ox-40 ligand: a potent costimulatory molecule for sustaining primary CD4 T cell responses. J Immunol. 1998;161(12):6510–7.

128. Xiao Z, Mayer AT, Nobashi TW, Gambhir SS. ICOS is an indicator of T cell-mediated response to cancer immunotherapy. Cancer Res. 2020; https://doi.org/10.1158/0008-5472.CAN-19-3265.

129. Blazar BR, Sharpe AH, Chen AI, Panoskaltsis-Mortari A, Lees C, Akiba H, et al. Ligation of OX40 (CD134) regulates graft-versus-host disease (GVHD) and graft rejection in allogeneic bone marrow transplant recipients. Blood. 2003;101(9):3741–8. https://doi.org/10.1182/blood-2002-10-3048.

130. Carboni S, Aboul-Enein F, Waltzinger C, Killeen N, Lassmann H, Pena-Rossi C. CD134 plays a crucial role in the pathogenesis of EAE and is upregulated in the CNS of patients with multiple sclerosis. J Neuroimmunol. 2003;145(1–2):1–11.

131. Mahmood T, Yang PC. OX40L-OX40 interactions: a possible target for gastrointestinal autoimmune diseases. N Am J Med Sci. 2012;4(11):533–6. https://doi.org/10.4103/1947-2714.103311.

132. Kinnear G, Wood KJ, Fallah-Arani F, Jones ND. A diametric role for OX40 in the response of effector/memory CD4+ T cells and regulatory T cells to alloantigen. J Immunol. 2013;191(3):1465–75. https://doi.org/10.4049/jimmunol.1300553.

133. Demirci G, Li XC. Novel roles of OX40 in the allograft response. Curr Opin Organ Transplant. 2008;13(1):26–30. https://doi.org/10.1097/MOT.0b013e3282f3def3.

134. Amatore F, Gorvel L, Olive D. Inducible Co-Stimulator (ICOS) as a potential therapeutic target for anti-cancer therapy. Expert Opin Ther Targets. 2018;22(4):343–51. https://doi.org/10.1080/14728222.2018.1444753.

135. Marinelli O, Nabissi M, Morelli MB, Torquati L, Amantini C, Santoni G. ICOS-L as a potential therapeutic target for cancer immunotherapy. Curr Protein Pept Sci. 2018;19(11):1107–13. https://doi.org/10.2174/1389203719666180608093913.

136. Wikenheiser DJ, Stumhofer JS. ICOS co-stimulation: friend or foe? Front Immunol. 2016;7:304. https://doi.org/10.3389/fimmu.2016.00304.

137. Parham P. The immune system. 4th ed. Oxford, UK: Garland Science, Taylor & Francis Group, LLC; 2015.

138. Di Giacomo AM, Calabro L, Danielli R, Fonsatti E, Bertocci E, Pesce I, et al. Long-term survival and immunological parameters in metastatic melanoma patients who responded to ipilimumab 10 mg/kg within an expanded access programme. Cancer Immunol Immunother. 2013;62(6):1021–8. https://doi.org/10.1007/s00262-013-1418-6.

139. Quemeneur L, Beloeil L, Michallet MC, Angelov G, Tomkowiak M, Revillard JP, et al. Restriction of de novo nucleotide biosynthesis interferes with clonal expansion and differentiation into effector and memory CD8 T cells. J Immunol. 2004;173(8):4945–52. https://doi.org/10.4049/jimmunol.173.8.4945.

140. Buck MD, O'Sullivan D, Pearce EL. T cell metabolism drives immunity. J Exp Med. 2015;212(9):1345–60. https://doi.org/10.1084/jem.20151159.

141. Elzinga EH, van der Laken CJ, Comans EF, Lammertsma AA, Dijkmans BA, Voskuyl AE. 2-Deoxy-2-[F-18]fluoro-D-glucose joint uptake on positron emission tomography images: rheumatoid arthritis versus osteoarthritis. Mol Imaging Biol. 2007;9(6):357–60. https://doi.org/10.1007/s11307-007-0113-4.

142. Rudd JH, Myers KS, Bansilal S, Machac J, Pinto CA, Tong C, et al. Atherosclerosis inflammation imaging with 18F-FDG PET: carotid, iliac, and femoral uptake reproducibility, quantification methods, and recommendations. J Nucl Med. 2008;49(6):871–8. https://doi.org/10.2967/jnumed.107.050294.

143. Stelljes M, Hermann S, Albring J, Kohler G, Loffler M, Franzius C, et al. Clinical molecular imaging in intestinal graft-versus-host disease: mapping of disease activity, prediction, and monitoring of treatment efficiency by positron emission tomography. Blood. 2008;111(5):2909–18. https://doi.org/10.1182/blood-2007-10-119164.

144. Basu S, Chryssikos T, Moghadam-Kia S, Zhuang H, Torigian DA, Alavi A. Positron emission tomography as a diagnostic tool in infection: present role and future possibilities. Semin Nucl Med. 2009;39(1):36–51. https://doi.org/10.1053/j.semnuclmed.2008.08.004.

145. Nair-Gill E, Wiltzius SM, Wei XX, Cheng D, Riedinger M, Radu CG, et al. PET probes for distinct metabolic pathways have different cell specificities during immune responses in mice. J Clin Invest. 2010;120(6):2005–15. https://doi.org/10.1172/JCI41250.

146. Chang JM, Lee HJ, Goo JM, Lee HY, Lee JJ, Chung JK, et al. False positive and false negative FDG-PET scans in various thoracic diseases. Korean J Radiol. 2006;7(1):57–69. https://doi.org/10.3348/kjr.2006.7.1.57.

147. Tumeh PC, Radu CG, Ribas A. PET imaging of cancer immunotherapy. J Nucl Med. 2008;49(6):865–8. https://doi.org/10.2967/jnumed.108.051342.

148. Arner ES, Eriksson S. Mammalian deoxyribonucleoside kinases. Pharmacol Ther. 1995;67(2):155–86.

149. Chen W, Cloughesy T, Kamdar N, Satyamurthy N, Bergsneider M, Liau L, et al. Imaging proliferation in brain tumors with 18F-FLT PET: comparison with 18F-FDG. J Nucl Med. 2005;46(6):945–52.

150. Shields AF, Grierson JR, Dohmen BM, Machulla HJ, Stayanoff JC, Lawhorn-Crews JM, et al. Imaging proliferation in vivo with [F-18]FLT and positron emission tomography. Nat Med. 1998;4(11):1334–6. https://doi.org/10.1038/3337.

151. Hoeben BA, Troost EG, Span PN, van Herpen CM, Bussink J, Oyen WJ, et al. 18F-FLT PET during

radiotherapy or chemoradiotherapy in head and neck squamous cell carcinoma is an early predictor of outcome. J Nucl Med. 2013;54(4):532–40. https://doi.org/10.2967/jnumed.112.105999.

152. Aarntzen EH, Srinivas M, De Wilt JH, Jacobs JF, Lesterhuis WJ, Windhorst AD, et al. Early identification of antigen-specific immune responses in vivo by [18F]-labeled 3′-fluoro-3′-deoxy-thymidine ([18F]FLT) PET imaging. Proc Natl Acad Sci U S A. 2011;108(45):18396–9. https://doi.org/10.1073/pnas.1113045108.

153. Scarpelli M, Zahm C, Perlman S, McNeel DG, Jeraj R, Liu G. FLT PET/CT imaging of metastatic prostate cancer patients treated with pTVG-HP DNA vaccine and pembrolizumab. J Immunother Cancer. 2019;7(1):23. https://doi.org/10.1186/s40425-019-0516-1.

154. Ribas A, Benz MR, Allen-Auerbach MS, Radu C, Chmielowski B, Seja E, et al. Imaging of CTLA4 blockade-induced cell replication with (18)F-FLT PET in patients with advanced melanoma treated with tremelimumab. J Nucl Med. 2010;51(3):340–6. https://doi.org/10.2967/jnumed.109.070946.

155. Schwenck JSB, Fiz F, Sonanini D, Forschner A, Eigentler T, Weide B, Martella M, Gonzalez-Menendez I, Campi C, Sambuceti G, Seith F, Quintanilla-Martinez L, Garbe C, Pfannenberg C, Röcken M, la Fougere C, Pichler BJ, Kneilling M. Cancer immunotherapy is accompanied by distinct metabolic patterns in primary and secondary lymphoid organs observed by non-invasive in vivo 18F-FDG-PET. Theranostics. 2019; https://doi.org/10.7150/thno.35989.

156. Radu CG, Shu CJ, Nair-Gill E, Shelly SM, Barrio JR, Satyamurthy N, et al. Molecular imaging of lymphoid organs and immune activation by positron emission tomography with a new [18F]-labeled 2′-deoxycytidine analog. Nat Med. 2008;14(7):783–8. https://doi.org/10.1038/nm1724.

157. Shu CJ, Campbell DO, Lee JT, Tran AQ, Wengrod JC, Witte ON, et al. Novel PET probes specific for deoxycytidine kinase. J Nucl Med. 2010;51(7):1092–8. https://doi.org/10.2967/jnumed.109.073361.

158. Schwarzenberg J, Radu CG, Benz M, Fueger B, Tran AQ, Phelps ME, et al. Human biodistribution and radiation dosimetry of novel PET probes targeting the deoxyribonucleoside salvage pathway. Eur J Nucl Med Mol Imaging. 2011;38(4):711–21. https://doi.org/10.1007/s00259-010-1666-z.

159. Kim W, Le TM, Wei L, Poddar S, Bazzy J, Wang X, et al. [18F]CFA as a clinically translatable probe for PET imaging of deoxycytidine kinase activity. Proc Natl Acad Sci U S A. 2016;113(15):4027–32. https://doi.org/10.1073/pnas.1524212113.

160. Antonios JP, Soto H, Everson RG, Moughon DL, Wang AC, Orpilla J, et al. Detection of immune responses after immunotherapy in glioblastoma using PET and MRI. Proc Natl Acad Sci U S A. 2017;114(38):10220–5. https://doi.org/10.1073/pnas.1706689114.

161. Chen BY, Ghezzi C, Villegas B, Quon A, Radu CG, Witte ON, et al. (18)F-FAC PET visualizes brain-infiltrating leukocytes in a mouse model of multiple sclerosis. J Nucl Med. 2019; https://doi.org/10.2967/jnumed.119.229351.

162. Sarkaria JN, Hu LS, Parney IF, Pafundi DH, Brinkmann DH, Laack NN, et al. Is the blood-brain barrier really disrupted in all glioblastomas? A critical assessment of existing clinical data. Neuro Oncol. 2018;20(2):184–91. https://doi.org/10.1093/neuonc/nox175.

163. Zhu C, Johansson M, Permert J, Karlsson A. Enhanced cytotoxicity of nucleoside analogs by overexpression of mitochondrial deoxyguanosine kinase in cancer cell lines. J Biol Chem. 1998;273(24):14707–11.

164. Rodriguez CO Jr, Mitchell BS, Ayres M, Eriksson S, Gandhi V. Arabinosylguanine is phosphorylated by both cytoplasmic deoxycytidine kinase and mitochondrial deoxyguanosine kinase. Cancer Res. 2002;62(11):3100–5.

165. Roecker AM, Stockert A, Kisor DF. Nelarabine in the treatment of refractory T-cell malignancies. Clin Med Insights Oncol. 2010;4:133–41. https://doi.org/10.4137/CMO.S4364.

166. Namavari M, Chang YF, Kusler B, Yaghoubi S, Mitchell BS, Gambhir SS. Synthesis of 2′-deoxy-2′-[18F]fluoro-9-beta-D-arabinofuranosylguanine: a novel agent for imaging T-cell activation with PET. Mol Imaging Biol. 2011;13(5):812–8. https://doi.org/10.1007/s11307-010-0414-x.

167. Ronald JA, Kim BS, Gowrishankar G, Namavari M, Alam IS, D'Souza A, et al. A PET imaging strategy to visualize activated T cells in acute graft-versus-host disease elicited by allogeneic hematopoietic cell transplant. Cancer Res. 2017;77(11):2893–902. https://doi.org/10.1158/0008-5472.CAN-16-2953.

168. Franc BL, Goth S, MacKenzie J, Li X, Blecha J, Lam T, et al. In vivo PET imaging of the activated immune environment in a small animal model of inflammatory arthritis. Mol Imaging. 2017;16:1536012117712638. https://doi.org/10.1177/1536012117712638.

169. Levi J, Lam T, Goth SR, Yaghoubi S, Bates J, Ren G, et al. Imaging of activated T cells as an early predictor of immune response to anti-PD-1 therapy. Cancer Res. 2019;https://doi.org/10.1158/0008-5472.CAN-19-0267.

170. Voskoboinik I, Whisstock JC, Trapani JA. Perforin and granzymes: function, dysfunction and human pathology. Nat Rev Immunol. 2015;15(6):388–400. https://doi.org/10.1038/nri3839.

171. Larimer BM, Bloch E, Nesti S, Austin EE, Wehrenberg-Klee E, Boland G, et al. The effectiveness of checkpoint inhibitor combinations and administration timing can be measured by granzyme B PET imaging. Clin Cancer Res. 2019;25(4):1196–205. https://doi.org/10.1158/1078-0432.CCR-18-2407.

172. Cupi ML, Sarra M, Marafini I, Monteleone I, Franze E, Ortenzi A, et al. Plasma cells in the mucosa of

patients with inflammatory bowel disease produce granzyme B and possess cytotoxic activities. J Immunol. 2014;192(12):6083–91. https://doi.org/10.4049/jimmunol.1302238.

173. Boschetti G, Nancey S, Moussata D, Cotte E, Francois Y, Flourie B, et al. Enrichment of circulating and mucosal cytotoxic CD8+ T cells is associated with postoperative endoscopic recurrence in patients with Crohn's disease. J Crohns Colitis. 2016;10(3):338–45. https://doi.org/10.1093/ecco-jcc/jjv211.

174. Hagn M, Sontheimer K, Dahlke K, Brueggemann S, Kaltenmeier C, Beyer T, et al. Human B cells differentiate into granzyme B-secreting cytotoxic B lymphocytes upon incomplete T-cell help. Immunol Cell Biol. 2012;90(4):457–67. https://doi.org/10.1038/icb.2011.64.

175. Hui E, Cheung J, Zhu J, Su X, Taylor MJ, Wallweber HA, et al. T cell costimulatory receptor CD28 is a primary target for PD-1-mediated inhibition. Science. 2017;355(6332):1428–33. https://doi.org/10.1126/science.aaf1292.

176. Rudd CE, Taylor A, Schneider H. CD28 and CTLA-4 coreceptor expression and signal transduction. Immunol Rev. 2009;229(1):12–26. https://doi.org/10.1111/j.1600-065X.2009.00770.x.

177. Lu C, Redd PS, Lee JR, Savage N, Liu K. The expression profiles and regulation of PD-L1 in tumor-induced myeloid-derived suppressor cells. Oncoimmunology. 2016;5(12):e1247135. https://doi.org/10.1080/2162402X.2016.1247135.

178. Blank CU, Haining WN, Held W, Hogan PG, Kallies A, Lugli E, et al. Defining 'T cell exhaustion'. Nat Rev Immunol. 2019;19(11):665–74. https://doi.org/10.1038/s41577-019-0221-9.

179. Weber JS, D'Angelo SP, Minor D, Hodi FS, Gutzmer R, Neyns B, et al. Nivolumab versus chemotherapy in patients with advanced melanoma who progressed after anti-CTLA-4 treatment (CheckMate 037): a randomised, controlled, open-label, phase 3 trial. Lancet Oncol. 2015;16(4):375–84. https://doi.org/10.1016/S1470-2045(15)70076-8.

180. Robert C, Schachter J, Long GV, Arance A, Grob JJ, Mortier L, et al. Pembrolizumab versus ipilimumab in advanced melanoma. N Engl J Med. 2015;372(26):2521–32. https://doi.org/10.1056/NEJMoa1503093.

181. Migden MR, Rischin D, Schmults CD, Guminski A, Hauschild A, Lewis KD, et al. PD-1 blockade with cemiplimab in advanced cutaneous squamous-cell carcinoma. N Engl J Med. 2018;379(4):341–51. https://doi.org/10.1056/NEJMoa1805131.

182. Hodi FS, O'Day SJ, McDermott DF, Weber RW, Sosman JA, Haanen JB, et al. Improved survival with ipilimumab in patients with metastatic melanoma. N Engl J Med. 2010;363(8):711–23. https://doi.org/10.1056/NEJMoa1003466.

183. Haslam A, Prasad V. Estimation of the percentage of US patients with cancer who are eligible for and respond to checkpoint inhibitor immunotherapy drugs. JAMA Netw Open. 2019;2(5):e192535. https://doi.org/10.1001/jamanetworkopen.2019.2535.

184. van de Donk PP, Kist de Ruijter L, Lub-de Hooge MN, Brouwers AH, van der Wekken AJ, Oosting SF, et al. Molecular imaging biomarkers for immune checkpoint inhibitor therapy. Theranostics. 2020;10(4):1708–18. https://doi.org/10.7150/thno.38339.

185. Natarajan A, Mayer AT, Reeves RE, Nagamine CM, Gambhir SS. Development of novel ImmunoPET tracers to image human PD-1 checkpoint expression on tumor-infiltrating lymphocytes in a humanized mouse model. Mol Imaging Biol. 2017;19(6):903–14. https://doi.org/10.1007/s11307-017-1060-3.

186. Higashikawa K, Yagi K, Watanabe K, Kamino S, Ueda M, Hiromura M, et al. 64Cu-DOTA-anti-CTLA-4 mAb enabled PET visualization of CTLA-4 on the T-cell infiltrating tumor tissues. PLoS One. 2014;9(11):e109866. https://doi.org/10.1371/journal.pone.0109866.

187. Ehlerding EB, England CG, Majewski RL, Valdovinos HF, Jiang D, Liu G, et al. ImmunoPET imaging of CTLA-4 expression in mouse models of non-small cell lung cancer. Mol Pharm. 2017;14(5):1782–9. https://doi.org/10.1021/acs.molpharmaceut.7b00056.

188. Ehlerding EB, Lee HJ, Jiang D, Ferreira CA, Zahm CD, Huang P, et al. Antibody and fragment-based PET imaging of CTLA-4+ T-cells in humanized mouse models. Am J Cancer Res. 2019;9(1):53–63.

189. Wherry EJ, Kurachi M. Molecular and cellular insights into T cell exhaustion. Nat Rev Immunol. 2015;15(8):486–99. https://doi.org/10.1038/nri3862.

190. Bensch F, van der Veen EL, Lub-de Hooge MN, Jorritsma-Smit A, Boellaard R, Kok IC, et al. (89) Zr-atezolizumab imaging as a non-invasive approach to assess clinical response to PD-L1 blockade in cancer. Nat Med. 2018;24(12):1852–8. https://doi.org/10.1038/s41591-018-0255-8.

191. Niemeijer AN, Leung D, Huisman MC, Bahce I, Hoekstra OS, van Dongen G, et al. Whole body PD-1 and PD-L1 positron emission tomography in patients with non-small-cell lung cancer. Nat Commun. 2018;9(1):4664. https://doi.org/10.1038/s41467-018-07131-y.

192. Huisman M, Niemeijer AL, Windhorst B, Schuit R, Leung D, Hayes W, et al. Quantification of PD-L1 expression with [(18)F]BMS-986192 PET/CT in patients with advanced stage non-small-cell lung cancer. J Nucl Med. 2020; https://doi.org/10.2967/jnumed.119.240895.

193. McKnight BN, Viola-Villegas NT. (89) Zr-ImmunoPET companion diagnostics and their impact in clinical drug development. J Labelled Comp Radiopharm. 2018;61(9):727–38. https://doi.org/10.1002/jlcr.3605.

194. Wykes MN, Lewin SR. Immune checkpoint blockade in infectious diseases. Nat Rev Immunol. 2018;18(2):91–104. https://doi.org/10.1038/nri.2017.112.

195. Boyer Z, Palmer S. Targeting immune checkpoint molecules to eliminate latent HIV. Front Immunol. 2018;9:2339. https://doi.org/10.3389/fimmu.2018.02339.

196. Carter RH. B cells in health and disease. Mayo Clin Proc. 2006;81(3):377–84. https://doi.org/10.4065/81.3.377.

197. Vos Q, Lees A, Wu ZQ, Snapper CM, Mond JJ. B-cell activation by T-cell-independent type 2 antigens as an integral part of the humoral immune response to pathogenic microorganisms. Immunol Rev. 2000;176:154–70. https://doi.org/10.1034/j.1600-065x.2000.00607.x.

198. Parker DC. T cell-dependent B cell activation. Annu Rev Immunol. 1993;11:331–60. https://doi.org/10.1146/annurev.iy.11.040193.001555.

199. Vidarsson G, Dekkers G, Rispens T. IgG subclasses and allotypes: from structure to effector functions. Front Immunol. 2014;5:520. https://doi.org/10.3389/fimmu.2014.00520.

200. Heyman B. Regulation of antibody responses via antibodies, complement, and Fc receptors. Annu Rev Immunol. 2000;18:709–37. https://doi.org/10.1146/annurev.immunol.18.1.709.

201. Seifert M, Kuppers R. Human memory B cells. Leukemia. 2016;30(12):2283–92. https://doi.org/10.1038/leu.2016.226.

202. Hausser-Kinzel S, Weber MS. The role of B cells and antibodies in multiple sclerosis, neuromyelitis optica, and related disorders. Front Immunol. 2019;10:201. https://doi.org/10.3389/fimmu.2019.00201.

203. O'Neill SK, Shlomchik MJ, Glant TT, Cao Y, Doodes PD, Finnegan A. Antigen-specific B cells are required as APCs and autoantibody-producing cells for induction of severe autoimmune arthritis. J Immunol. 2005;174(6):3781–8. https://doi.org/10.4049/jimmunol.174.6.3781.

204. Karrar S, Cunninghame Graham DS. Abnormal B cell development in systemic lupus erythematosus: what the genetics tell us. Arthritis Rheumatol. 2018;70(4):496–507. https://doi.org/10.1002/art.40396.

205. Hampe CS. B cell in autoimmune diseases. Scientifica (Cairo). 2012; https://doi.org/10.6064/2012/215308.

206. Browning JL. B cells move to centre stage: novel opportunities for autoimmune disease treatment. Nat Rev Drug Discov. 2006;5(7):564–76. https://doi.org/10.1038/nrd2085.

207. Grillo-Lopez AJ, White CA, Varns C, Shen D, Wei A, McClure A, et al. Overview of the clinical development of rituximab: first monoclonal antibody approved for the treatment of lymphoma. Semin Oncol. 1999;26(5 Suppl 14):66–73.

208. Mok CC. Rituximab for the treatment of rheumatoid arthritis: an update. Drug Des Devel Ther. 2013;8:87–100. https://doi.org/10.2147/DDDT.S41645.

209. Marston B, Palanichamy A, Anolik JH. B cells in the pathogenesis and treatment of rheumatoid arthritis. Curr Opin Rheumatol. 2010;22(3):307–15. https://doi.org/10.1097/BOR.0b013e3283369cb8.

210. Bruijnen S, Tsang ASM, Raterman H, Ramwadhdoebe T, Vugts D, van Dongen G, et al. B-cell imaging with zirconium-89 labelled rituximab PET-CT at baseline is associated with therapeutic response 24 weeks after initiation of rituximab treatment in rheumatoid arthritis patients. Arthritis Res Ther. 2016;18(1):266. https://doi.org/10.1186/s13075-016-1166-z.

211. Jauw YW, Zijlstra JM, de Jong D, Vugts DJ, Zweegman S, Hoekstra OS, et al. Performance of 89Zr-labeled-rituximab-PET as an imaging biomarker to assess CD20 targeting: a pilot study in patients with relapsed/refractory diffuse large B cell lymphoma. PLoS One. 2017;12(1):e0169828. https://doi.org/10.1371/journal.pone.0169828.

212. Laban KG, Kalmann R, Leguit RJ, de Keizer B. Zirconium-89-labelled rituximab PET-CT in orbital inflammatory disease. EJNMMI Res. 2019;9(1):69. https://doi.org/10.1186/s13550-019-0530-9.

213. Disanto G, Morahan JM, Barnett MH, Giovannoni G, Ramagopalan SV. The evidence for a role of B cells in multiple sclerosis. Neurology. 2012;78(11):823–32. https://doi.org/10.1212/WNL.0b013e318249f6f0.

214. Greenfield AL, Hauser SL. B-cell therapy for multiple sclerosis: entering an era. Ann Neurol. 2018;83(1):13–26. https://doi.org/10.1002/ana.25119.

215. Arneth BM. Impact of B cells to the pathophysiology of multiple sclerosis. J Neuroinflammation. 2019;16(1):128. https://doi.org/10.1186/s12974-019-1517-1.

216. Lucchinetti C, Bruck W, Parisi J, Scheithauer B, Rodriguez M, Lassmann H. Heterogeneity of multiple sclerosis lesions: implications for the pathogenesis of demyelination. Ann Neurol. 2000;47(6):707–17. https://doi.org/10.1002/1531-8249(200006)47:6<707::aid-ana3>3.0.co;2-q.

217. Colombo M, Dono M, Gazzola P, Roncella S, Valetto A, Chiorazzi N, et al. Accumulation of clonally related B lymphocytes in the cerebrospinal fluid of multiple sclerosis patients. J Immunol. 2000;164(5):2782–9. https://doi.org/10.4049/jimmunol.164.5.2782.

218. Gasperi C, Stuve O, Hemmer B. B cell-directed therapies in multiple sclerosis. Neurodegener Dis Manag. 2016;6(1):37–47. https://doi.org/10.2217/nmt.15.67.

219. Castillo-Trivino T, Braithwaite D, Bacchetti P, Waubant E. Rituximab in relapsing and progressive forms of multiple sclerosis: a systematic review. PLoS One. 2013;8(7):e66308. https://doi.org/10.1371/journal.pone.0066308.

220. Salzer J, Svenningsson R, Alping P, Novakova L, Bjorck A, Fink K, et al. Rituximab in multiple sclerosis: a retrospective observational study on safety and efficacy. Neurology. 2016;87(20):2074–81. https://doi.org/10.1212/WNL.0000000000003331.

221. Beers SA, Chan CH, James S, French RR, Attfield KE, Brennan CM, et al. Type II (tositumomab) anti-CD20 monoclonal antibody out performs type I (rituximab-like) reagents in B-cell depletion regardless of complement activation. Blood. 2008;112(10):4170–7. https://doi.org/10.1182/blood-2008-04-149161.

222. Beers SA, French RR, Chan HT, Lim SH, Jarrett TC, Vidal RM, et al. Antigenic modulation limits the efficacy of anti-CD20 antibodies: implications for antibody selection. Blood. 2010;115(25):5191–201. https://doi.org/10.1182/blood-2010-01-263533.

223. Shih LB, Thorpe SR, Griffiths GL, Diril H, Ong GL, Hansen HJ, et al. The processing and fate of antibodies and their radiolabels bound to the surface of tumor cells in vitro: a comparison of nine radiolabels. J Nucl Med. 1994;35(5):899–908.

224. Zettlitz KA, Tavare R, Knowles SM, Steward KK, Timmerman JM, Wu AM. ImmunoPET of malignant and normal B cells with (89)Zr- and (124)I-labeled obinutuzumab antibody fragments reveals differential CD20 internalization in vivo. Clin Cancer Res. 2017;23(23):7242–52. https://doi.org/10.1158/1078-0432.CCR-17-0855.

225. Witzig TE. Efficacy and safety of 90Y ibritumomab tiuxetan (Zevalin) radioimmunotherapy for non-Hodgkin's lymphoma. Semin Oncol. 2003;30(6 Suppl 17):11–6. https://doi.org/10.1053/j.seminoncol.2003.10.007.

226. Keyaerts M, Xavier C, Heemskerk J, Devoogdt N, Everaert H, Ackaert C, et al. Phase I study of 68Ga-HER2-nanobody for PET/CT assessment of HER2 expression in breast carcinoma. J Nucl Med. 2016;57(1):27–33. https://doi.org/10.2967/jnumed.115.162024.

227. Witzig TE, White CA, Gordon LI, Wiseman GA, Emmanouilides C, Murray JL, et al. Safety of yttrium-90 ibritumomab tiuxetan radioimmunotherapy for relapsed low-grade, follicular, or transformed non-Hodgkin's lymphoma. J Clin Oncol. 2003;21(7):1263–70. https://doi.org/10.1200/JCO.2003.08.043.

228. Krasniqi A, D'Huyvetter M, Xavier C, Van der Jeught K, Muyldermans S, Van Der Heyden J, et al. Theranostic radiolabeled anti-CD20 sdAb for targeted radionuclide therapy of non-Hodgkin lymphoma. Mol Cancer Ther. 2017;16(12):2828–39. https://doi.org/10.1158/1535-7163.MCT-17-0554.

229. Movahedi K, Schoonooghe S, Laoui D, Houbracken I, Waelput W, Breckpot K, et al. Nanobody-based targeting of the macrophage mannose receptor for effective in vivo imaging of tumor-associated macrophages. Cancer Res. 2012;72(16):4165–77. https://doi.org/10.1158/0008-5472.CAN-11-2994.

230. Wang K, Wei G, Liu D. CD19: a biomarker for B cell development, lymphoma diagnosis and therapy. Exp Hematol Oncol. 2012;1(1):36. https://doi.org/10.1186/2162-3619-1-36.

231. Forsthuber TG, Cimbora DM, Ratchford JN, Katz E, Stuve O. B cell-based therapies in CNS autoimmunity: differentiating CD19 and CD20 as therapeutic targets. Ther Adv Neurol Disord. 2018;11:1756286418761697. https://doi.org/10.1177/1756286418761697.

232. Kalos M, Levine BL, Porter DL, Katz S, Grupp SA, Bagg A, et al. T cells with chimeric antigen receptors have potent antitumor effects and can establish memory in patients with advanced leukemia. Sci Transl Med. 2011;3(95):95ra73. https://doi.org/10.1126/scitranslmed.3002842.

233. Maude SL, Teachey DT, Porter DL, Grupp SA. CD19-targeted chimeric antigen receptor T-cell therapy for acute lymphoblastic leukemia. Blood. 2015;125(26):4017–23. https://doi.org/10.1182/blood-2014-12-580068.

234. Agius MA, Klodowska-Duda G, Maciejowski M, Potemkowski A, Li J, Patra K, et al. Safety and tolerability of inebilizumab (MEDI-551), an anti-CD19 monoclonal antibody, in patients with relapsing forms of multiple sclerosis: results from a phase 1 randomised, placebo-controlled, escalating intravenous and subcutaneous dose study. Mult Scler. 2019;25(2):235–45. https://doi.org/10.1177/1352458517740641.

235. Cree BAC, Bennett JL, Kim HJ, Weinshenker BG, Pittock SJ, Wingerchuk DM, et al. Inebilizumab for the treatment of neuromyelitis optica spectrum disorder (N-MOmentum): a double-blind, randomised placebo-controlled phase 2/3 trial. Lancet. 2019;394(10206):1352–63. https://doi.org/10.1016/S0140-6736(19)31817-3.

236. Schuh E, Berer K, Mulazzani M, Feil K, Meinl I, Lahm H, et al. Features of human CD3+CD20+ T cells. J Immunol. 2016;197(4):1111–7. https://doi.org/10.4049/jimmunol.1600089.

237. Stevens M, Cropper H, Jackson I, Chaney A, Lechtenberg K, Buckwalter M, James ML. Radiolabeling and pre-clinical evaluation of a first-in-class CD19 PET tracer for imaging B cells in multiple sclerosis. Reston, VA: Society of Nuclear Medicine and Molecular Imaging; 2019.

238. Barthelmes J, Tafferner N, Kurz J, de Bruin N, Parnham MJ, Geisslinger G, et al. Induction of experimental autoimmune encephalomyelitis in mice and evaluation of the disease-dependent distribution of immune cells in various tissues. J Vis Exp. 2016;(111):53933. https://doi.org/10.3791/53933.

239. Kim S, Poursine-Laurent J, Truscott SM, Lybarger L, Song YJ, Yang L, et al. Licensing of natural killer cells by host major histocompatibility complex

class I molecules. Nature. 2005;436(7051):709–13. https://doi.org/10.1038/nature03847.

240. Ali AK, Nandagopal N, Lee SH. IL-15-PI3K-AKT-mTOR: a critical pathway in the life journey of natural killer cells. Front Immunol. 2015;6:355. https://doi.org/10.3389/fimmu.2015.00355.

241. Geary CD, Sun JC. Memory responses of natural killer cells. Semin Immunol. 2017;31:11–9. https://doi.org/10.1016/j.smim.2017.08.012.

242. Terren I, Orrantia A, Mikelez-Alonso I, Vitalle J, Zenarruzabeitia O, Borrego F. NK cell-based immunotherapy in renal cell carcinoma. Cancers (Basel). 2020;12(2):316. https://doi.org/10.3390/cancers12020316.

243. Habif G, Crinier A, Andre P, Vivier E, Narni-Mancinelli E. Targeting natural killer cells in solid tumors. Cell Mol Immunol. 2019;16(5):415–22. https://doi.org/10.1038/s41423-019-0224-2.

244. Vivier E, Artis D, Colonna M, Diefenbach A, Di Santo JP, Eberl G, et al. Innate lymphoid cells: 10 years on. Cell. 2018;174(5):1054–66. https://doi.org/10.1016/j.cell.2018.07.017.

245. Spits H, Artis D, Colonna M, Diefenbach A, Di Santo JP, Eberl G, et al. Innate lymphoid cells—a proposal for uniform nomenclature. Nat Rev Immunol. 2013;13(2):145–9. https://doi.org/10.1038/nri3365.

246. Constantinides MG, McDonald BD, Verhoef PA, Bendelac A. A committed precursor to innate lymphoid cells. Nature. 2014;508(7496):397–401. https://doi.org/10.1038/nature13047.

247. Simoni Y, Fehlings M, Kloverpris HN, McGovern N, Koo SL, Loh CY, et al. Human innate lymphoid cell subsets possess tissue-type based heterogeneity in phenotype and frequency. Immunity. 2017;46(1):148–61. https://doi.org/10.1016/j.immuni.2016.11.005.

248. Cichocki F, Grzywacz B, Miller JS. Human NK cell development: one road or many? Front Immunol. 2019;10:2078. https://doi.org/10.3389/fimmu.2019.02078.

249. Chan A, Hong DL, Atzberger A, Kollnberger S, Filer AD, Buckley CD, et al. CD56bright human NK cells differentiate into CD56dim cells: role of contact with peripheral fibroblasts. J Immunol. 2007;179(1):89–94. https://doi.org/10.4049/jimmunol.179.1.89.

250. Van Acker HH, Capsomidis A, Smits EL, Van Tendeloo VF. CD56 in the immune system: more than a marker for cytotoxicity? Front Immunol. 2017;8:892. https://doi.org/10.3389/fimmu.2017.00892.

251. Minetto P, Guolo F, Pesce S, Greppi M, Obino V, Ferretti E, et al. Harnessing NK cells for cancer treatment. Front Immunol. 2019;10:2836. https://doi.org/10.3389/fimmu.2019.02836.

252. Gong JH, Maki G, Klingemann HG. Characterization of a human cell line (NK-92) with phenotypical and functional characteristics of activated natural killer cells. Leukemia. 1994;8(4):652–8.

253. Suck G, Odendahl M, Nowakowska P, Seidl C, Wels WS, Klingemann HG, et al. NK-92: an 'off-the-shelf therapeutic' for adoptive natural killer cell-based cancer immunotherapy. Cancer Immunol Immunother. 2016;65(4):485–92. https://doi.org/10.1007/s00262-015-1761-x.

254. Liu E, Marin D, Banerjee P, Macapinlac HA, Thompson P, Basar R, et al. Use of CAR-transduced natural killer cells in CD19-positive lymphoid tumors. N Engl J Med. 2020;382(6):545–53. https://doi.org/10.1056/NEJMoa1910607.

255. Wang W, Erbe AK, Hank JA, Morris ZS, Sondel PM. NK cell-mediated antibody-dependent cellular cytotoxicity in cancer immunotherapy. Front Immunol. 2015;6:368. https://doi.org/10.3389/fimmu.2015.00368.

256. Chew HY, De Lima PO, Gonzalez Cruz JL, Banushi B, Echejoh G, Hu L, et al. Endocytosis inhibition in humans to improve responses to ADCC-mediating antibodies. Cell. 2020;180(5):895–914.e27. https://doi.org/10.1016/j.cell.2020.02.019.

257. Tang J, Pearce L, O'Donnell-Tormey J, Hubbard-Lucey VM. Trends in the global immuno-oncology landscape. Nat Rev Drug Discov. 2018;17(12):922. https://doi.org/10.1038/nrd.2018.202.

258. Shapovalova M, Pyper SR, Moriarity BS, LeBeau AM. The molecular imaging of natural killer cells. Mol Imaging. 2018;17:1536012118794816. https://doi.org/10.1177/1536012118794816.

259. Marincola FM, Drucker BJ, Keeling CA, Siao DY, Starnes HF Jr, Goodwin DA, et al. The in vivo distribution of human peripheral blood lymphocytes and lymphokine-activated killer cells adoptively transferred in human pancreatic cancer-bearing nude mice. Surgery. 1989;105(1):79–85.

260. Sato N, Stringaris K, Davidson-Moncada JK, Reger R, Adler SS, Dunbar C, et al. In vivo tracking of adoptively transferred natural killer cells in rhesus macaques using (89)zirconium-oxine cell labeling and PET imaging. Clin Cancer Res. 2020; https://doi.org/10.1158/1078-0432.CCR-19-2897.

261. Katano I, Nishime C, Ito R, Kamisako T, Mizusawa T, Ka Y, et al. Long-term maintenance of peripheral blood derived human NK cells in a novel human IL-15-transgenic NOG mouse. Sci Rep. 2017;7(1):17230. https://doi.org/10.1038/s41598-017-17442-7.

262. Galli F, Rapisarda AS, Stabile H, Malviya G, Manni I, Bonanno E, et al. In vivo imaging of natural killer cell trafficking in tumors. J Nucl Med. 2015;56(10):1575–80. https://doi.org/10.2967/jnumed.114.152918.

263. Bezman NA, Kim CC, Sun JC, Min-Oo G, Hendricks DW, Kamimura Y, et al. Molecular definition of the identity and activation of natural killer cells. Nat Immunol. 2012;13(10):1000–9. https://doi.org/10.1038/ni.2395.

264. Shaffer T, Gambhir SS, Aalipour A, Schurch C. PET imaging of the natural killer cell activation receptor

NKp30. J Nucl Med. 2020; https://doi.org/10.2967/jnumed.119.233163.

265. Shaffer TAA, Gambhir SS. PET imaging of activation and inhibition natural killer cell receptors. Montreal, Canada: World Molecular Imaging Congress; 2019.

266. Carlyle JR, Mesci A, Ljutic B, Belanger S, Tai LH, Rousselle E, et al. Molecular and genetic basis for strain-dependent NK1.1 alloreactivity of mouse NK cells. J Immunol. 2006;176(12):7511–24. https://doi.org/10.4049/jimmunol.176.12.7511.

267. Schleypen JS, Baur N, Kammerer R, Nelson PJ, Rohrmann K, Grone EF, et al. Cytotoxic markers and frequency predict functional capacity of natural killer cells infiltrating renal cell carcinoma. Clin Cancer Res. 2006;12(3 Pt 1):718–25. https://doi.org/10.1158/1078-0432.CCR-05-0857.

268. Lavin Y, Kobayashi S, Leader A, Amir ED, Elefant N, Bigenwald C, et al. Innate immune landscape in early lung adenocarcinoma by paired single-cell analyses. Cell. 2017;169(4):750–65.e17. https://doi.org/10.1016/j.cell.2017.04.014.

269. Altai M, Membreno R, Cook B, Tolmachev V, Zeglis BM. Pretargeted imaging and therapy. J Nucl Med. 2017;58(10):1553–9. https://doi.org/10.2967/jnumed.117.189944.

270. Cherry SR, Jones T, Karp JS, Qi J, Moses WW, Badawi RD. Total-body PET: maximizing sensitivity to create new opportunities for clinical research and patient care. J Nucl Med. 2018;59(1):3–12. https://doi.org/10.2967/jnumed.116.184028.

271. Badawi RD, Shi H, Hu P, Chen S, Xu T, Price PM, et al. First human imaging studies with the EXPLORER total-body PET scanner. J Nucl Med. 2019;60(3):299–303. https://doi.org/10.2967/jnumed.119.226498.

272. Vandenberghe S, Mikhaylova E, D'Hoe E, Mollet P, Karp JS. Recent developments in time-of-flight PET. EJNMMI Phys. 2016;3(1):3. https://doi.org/10.1186/s40658-016-0138-3.

273. Conti M, Bendriem B. The new opportunities for high time resolution clinical TOF PET. Clin Transl Imaging. 2019;7(2):139–47.

274. Vacchelli E, Vitale I, Eggermont A, Fridman WH, Fucikova J, Cremer I, et al. Trial watch: Dendritic cell-based interventions for cancer therapy. Oncoimmunology. 2013;2(10):e25771. https://doi.org/10.4161/onci.25771.

275. Liu Q, Johnson EM, Lam RK, Wang Q, Bo Ye H, Wilson EN, et al. Peripheral TREM1 responses to brain and intestinal immunogens amplify stroke severity. Nat Immunol. 2019;20(8):1023–34. https://doi.org/10.1038/s41590-019-0421-2.

276. Nigam S, McCarl L, Kumar R, Edinger RS, Kurland BF, Anderson CJ, et al. Preclinical ImmunoPET imaging of glioblastoma-infiltrating myeloid cells using zirconium-89 labeled anti-CD11b antibody. Mol Imaging Biol. 2019; https://doi.org/10.1007/s11307-019-01427-1.

277. Andreyev A, Celler A. Dual-isotope PET using positron-gamma emitters. Phys Med Biol. 2011;56(14):4539–56. https://doi.org/10.1088/0031-9155/56/14/020.

278. Fukuchi T, Okauchi T, Shigeta M, Yamamoto S, Watanabe Y, Enomoto S. Positron emission tomography with additional gamma-ray detectors for multiple-tracer imaging. Med Phys. 2017;44(6):2257–66. https://doi.org/10.1002/mp.12149.

279. Vera DRB, Smith CC, Bixby LM, Glatt DM, Dunn SS, Saito R, et al. Immuno-PET imaging of tumor-infiltrating lymphocytes using zirconium-89 radiolabeled anti-CD3 antibody in immune-competent mice bearing syngeneic tumors. PLoS One. 2018;13(3):e0193832. https://doi.org/10.1371/journal.pone.0193832.

280. Seo JW, Tavare R, Mahakian LM, Silvestrini MT, Tam S, Ingham ES, et al. CD8(+) T-cell density imaging with Cu-64-labeled Cys-diabody informs immunotherapy protocols. Clin Cancer Res. 2018;24(20):4976–87. https://doi.org/10.1158/1078-0432.Ccr-18-0261.

281. Olafsen T, Torgov M, Zhang GG, Romero J, Zampila C, Marchioni F, et al. Pet imaging of cytotoxic human T cells using an 89Zr-labeled anti-CD8 minibody. J Immunother Cancer. 2015;3(Suppl 2):P388. https://doi.org/10.1186/2051-1426-3-S2-P388.

282. Mayer KE, Mall S, Yusufi N, Gosmann D, Steiger K, Russelli L, et al. T-cell functionality testing is highly relevant to developing novel immuno-tracers monitoring T cells in the context of immunotherapies and revealed CD7 as an attractive target. Theranostics. 2018;8(21):6070–87. https://doi.org/10.7150/thno.27275.

283. Hettich M, Braun F, Bartholoma MD, Schirmbeck R, Niedermann G. High-resolution PET imaging with therapeutic antibody-based PD-1/PD-L1 checkpoint tracers. Theranostics. 2016;6(10):1629–40. https://doi.org/10.7150/thno.15253.

284. England CG, Ehlerding EB, Hernandez R, Rekoske BT, Graves SA, Sun H, et al. Preclinical pharmacokinetics and biodistribution studies of 89Zr-labeled pembrolizumab. J Nucl Med. 2017;58(1):162–8. https://doi.org/10.2967/jnumed.116.177857.

285. England CG, Jiang D, Ehlerding EB, Rekoske BT, Ellison PA, Hernandez R, et al. (89)Zr-labeled nivolumab for imaging of T-cell infiltration in a humanized murine model of lung cancer. Eur J Nucl Med Mol Imaging. 2018;45(1):110–20. https://doi.org/10.1007/s00259-017-3803-4.

286. Higashikawa K, Yagi K, Watanabe K, Kamino S, Ueda M, Hiromura M, et al. Cu-64-DOTA-anti-CTLA-4 mAb enabled PET visualization of CTLA-4 on the T-cell infiltrating tumor tissues. PLoS One. 2014;9(11):e109866. https://doi.org/10.1371/journal.pone.0109866.

287. Muylle K, Flamen P, Vugts DJ, Guiot T, Ghanem G, Meuleman N, et al. Tumour targeting and radiation

dose of radioimmunotherapy with (90)Y-rituximab in CD20+ B-cell lymphoma as predicted by (89)Zr-rituximab immuno-PET: impact of preloading with unlabelled rituximab. Eur J Nucl Med Mol Imaging. 2015;42(8):1304–14. https://doi.org/10.1007/s00259-015-3025-6.

288. Natarajan A, Gambhir SS. Radiation dosimetry study of [(89)Zr]rituximab tracer for clinical transla-tion of B cell NHL imaging using positron emission tomography. Mol Imaging Biol. 2015;17(4):539–47. https://doi.org/10.1007/s11307-014-0810-8.

289. Olafsen T, Betting D, Kenanova VE, Salazar FB, Clarke P, Said J, et al. Recombinant anti-CD20 anti-body fragments for small-animal PET imaging of B-cell lymphomas. J Nucl Med. 2009;50(9):1500–8. https://doi.org/10.2967/jnumed.108.060426.

Áron Roxin and François Bénard

Contents

3.1   Introduction

Cancer immunotherapy (CIT) encompasses a broad range of strategies that involves the action of immune cells or antibodies, each with the common goal of specific tumor cell eradication that spares healthy tissues and imposes minimal systemic toxicity. The topic of CIT has been extensively reviewed since 2015 [1–13]. Some investigations have focused on CIT methods that involve the use of natural killer (NK) cell [14–19], macrophages [20], tumor-reactive T cells [21–28] (more specifically $\gamma\delta$-T cells [29–31] or chimeric antigen receptor (CAR) T cells [32–59]), interferon therapy [60], immune checkpoint blockade (ICB) therapy [61–64], and combined immune therapies [65, 66]. Other reports and reviews have focused on describing the biological mechanisms involved during T cell activation [9, 67–86], have suggested refinements for optimal CIT [87, 88], and have highlighted challenges that hinder current CIT cfforts [89–95]. CIT research strives to develop safe and effective ICB therapy, radioimmunotherapy (i.e., antibodies conjugated to radioisotopes emitting ionizing radiation, α-particles, or β-particles), and adop-

Á. Roxin
Molecular Oncology, British Columbia Cancer Agency Research Centre, Vancouver, BC, Canada
e-mail: aroxin@bccrc.ca

F. Bénard (✉)
Molecular Oncology, British Columbia Cancer Agency Research Centre, Vancouver, BC, Canada

Department of Radiology, University of British Columbia, Vancouver, BC, Canada
e-mail: fbenard@bccrc.ca

© Springer Nature Switzerland AG 2022
S. Harsini et al. (eds.), *Nuclear Medicine and Immunology*,
https://doi.org/10.1007/978-3-030-81261-4_3

tive cell therapy (ACT). Generally, ACT involves the use of ex vivo expanded tumor-infiltrating lymphocytes (TILs), cytolytic T lymphocytes (CTLs), or genetically modified T cells from peripheral blood. While ICB therapy allows the patient's immune response to attack tumor cells avoiding detection, ACT introduces immune cells with modified T cell receptors (TCR) or CARs that can confer tumor homing and anti-tumor activity. Moreover, contemporary CIT employing adoptively transferred (AT) T cells is moving toward achieving personalization, wherein a patient's own immune cells would be used for treatment regime selection, as the treatment itself or the means of monitoring treatment outcomes. There is, therefore, a fueling need to track the location and function of immune cells that are a part of CIT. Ideally, functional immune cells would be monitored by noninvasive means over the long-term course of the chosen therapy with negligible toxicity to healthy tissues. Being able to understand the biodistribution, kinetics, interactions, and fates of immune cells would aid in establishing patient risk stratifications [96] and may guide future interventions. The accurate monitoring of activated T cells can also serve applications beyond CIT, specifically for those involving autoimmune disorders and organ transplantations.

CIT generally presents major challenges for treatment monitoring [97–104]. The outcomes of conventional chemotherapeutic drugs and radiation therapy are routinely monitored by 2-[^{18}F] FDG PET by means of imaging metabolically active regions as a proxy for assessing tumor progression and function. The signal intensity recorded from primary tumors or metastatic regions is then used to calculate tumor burden and to subsequently inform the outcomes of the selected therapy. Treatment assessments have been improved with a refined version of the Response Evaluation Criteria in Solid Tumours (RECIST), namely, RECIST version 1.1 that has established additional guidelines pertaining to detection of new lesions, lymph node invasion, and tumor burden assessment criteria [105]. Yet,

CIT that involves leukocyte recruitment, invasion, and expansion at tumor sites may result in inflammation that can give rise to increased tumor volumes (pseudo-progression) as an expected part of successful immunotherapy [106]. This poses a challenge for serial CIT monitoring with 2-[^{18}F]FDG, and in fact, there are currently few definite methods of accurately predicting clinical outcomes of CIT [107]. The immune-related response criteria (irRC) incorporate guidelines that are better suited according to expected results of CIT and were demonstrated to provide more accurate treatment assessments compared to RECIST 1.1 during clinical CIT evaluations [108]. The accurate monitoring of immune cells, particularly activated T cells (e.g., CTLs and TILs), to tumors and lymphoid tissues would therefore aid in predicting therapeutic response and understanding the complex mechanisms governing anti-tumor response and off-target toxicity.

Previous reviews have summarized reports describing the use of PET and SPECT imaging [97, 109–130], MRI [131–136], and nanoparticles [137–141] for tracking immune cells, with some focusing on clinical cell tracking studies [95, 142–144]. Several reviews have also highlighted the use of immune cell tracking as a means for assessing CIT [106, 107, 145–162] or specifically as a part of a theranostic approach [96], wherein molecular diagnostic agents also served as therapeutics. This chapter will focus on summarizing reports that have employed radio-imaging methods to monitor activated T cells in the contexts of preclinical and clinical cancer investigations. These have been categorized according to methods that involve directly labeling T cells ex vivo prior to infusion (direct labeling) and those that labeled T cells in vivo (indirect labeling) for T cell tracking studies (Fig. 3.1). The latter section is described with relatively more breadth, as it includes the use of transduced T cells expressing reporter genes, tracers preferentially uptaken by proliferating T cells, and also targeting agents specific to endogenous or engineered T cell markers.

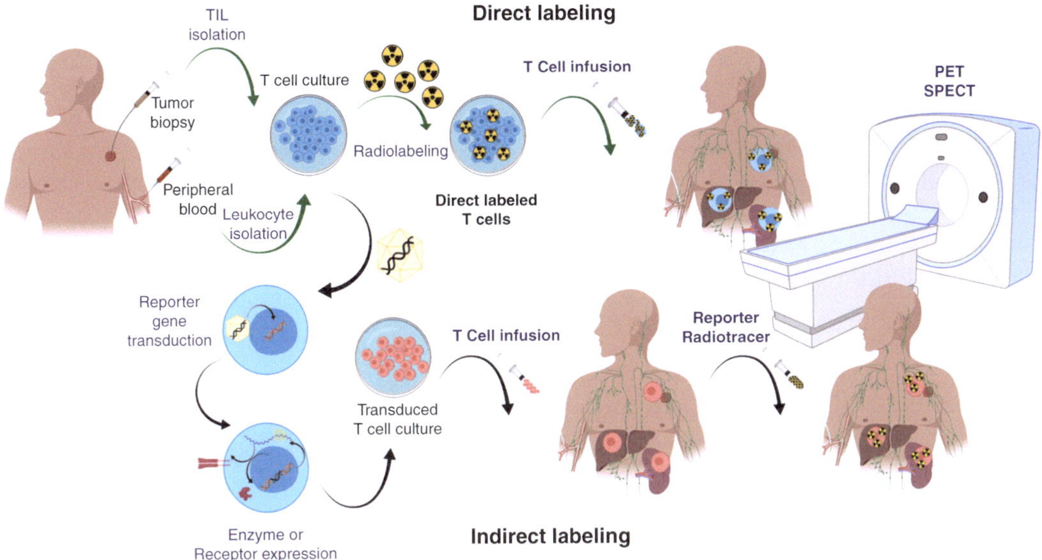

Fig. 3.1 Representation of direct labeling (top) and indirect labeling (bottom) strategies employed for tracking activated T cells in vivo. (Created with BioRender.com)

3.2 Direct Labeling

Immune cells that are isolated from patient's peripheral blood or from tumor biopsies/resections that are subsequently modified and expanded for ACT regimes can also be monitored in vivo after applying radioisotope labels. Several reports have described the direct radiolabeling of cancer cells [163], non-immune cells for imaging non-malignant disease [164, 165], immune cells other than T cells (e.g., natural killer (NK) cells, dendritic cells (DC), neutrophils, and monocytes) for imaging cancer [166–171] and non-malignant disease [172–183], and T cells for applications other than cancer imaging [165, 184–187]. Moreover, many reports have described the direct labeling of immune cells with non-radioactive contrast agents for in vivo MRI [188–197], CT [198], and fluorescence [199, 200] imaging. The scope of this section is, therefore, limited to the direct radiolabeling and subsequent in vivo tracking of activated T cells in preclinical and clinical cancer investigations.

TILs have been clinically evaluated as imaging agents with the ability to home to primary tumors and their metastatic loci. For example, a report by Fisher et al. described clinical studies with autologous TILs from six patients with metastatic melanoma undergoing cyclophosphamide therapy, wherein TILs were isolated from resected tumors or lymph nodes [201]. The TILs were cultured, directly labeled by [^{111}In]oxine incubation, purified, and reinjected (~750 µCi/10^{10} cells) into circulation along with administrations of IL-2 (every 8 h) to investigate the tumor- and metastasis-targeting ability of the [^{111}In]oxine-TILs. While the TILs were either predominantly leu 2 positive cytotoxic T cells (four patients) or leu 3 positive helper T cells (two patients), accumulation of [^{111}In]oxine-TILs was observed in tumors of five of six patients at 3–40 tumor-to-background contrasts. Moreover, the labeling treatments did not reduce TIL viability, while side effects were attributed to IL-2 administrations only. In addition to tumor localization, gamma camera images revealed uptake of [^{111}In]oxine-TILs in the lungs, liver, and spleen within 2 h of injection, but clearance from the lungs after 24 h. A follow-up clinical study by Griffith et al. involved 24 patients with metastatic melanoma undergoing cyclophosphamide therapy [202]. Specifically, this report investigated the use of [^{111}In]oxine-labeled autologous TILs for 19 patients and [^{111}In]oxine-labeled peripheral blood lymphocytes (PBLs; mixture of T cells, B cells, NK cells, and monocytes) coinjected for 5 patients along with non-labeled TILs as tumor-targeting agents. After T cell activation with IL-2 (30,000 or 100,000 U/kg infusions every 8 h), gamma camera images and biopsies revealed higher tumor accumulation of [^{111}In]oxine-TILs (0.0049%ID/g) in tumor tissues as compared to [^{111}In]oxine-PBLs (0.001%ID/g) with approximately three times higher mean tumor-to-background contrasts for labeled TILs compared to PBLs. Moreover, gamma camera images detected [^{111}In]oxine-TILs in tumors of 13 of the 18 patient scans, versus 1 of 4 patients who received [^{111}In]oxine-PBLs. Using gamma camera imaging and biopsy analyses, Pockaj et al. conducted a subsequent evaluation of [^{111}In] oxine-TIL tumor localization using TILs derived from resected tumors of 38 metastatic melanoma patients [203]. Gamma camera images identified the uptake of IL-2-activated [^{111}In]oxine-TILs in metastatic loci for 21 of 26 patients who received cyclophosphamide (25 mg/kg) prior to TIL infusion, compared to only observing [^{111}In]oxine-TIL uptake in lung metastases for 5 of 12 patients in the control group. These early reports highlighted the potential of ex vivo radiolabeled TILs as imaging agents with specificity to clinical presentations of advanced melanoma.

Preclinical research conducted by Wallace et al. was designed to investigate the mechanisms of TIL-mediated tumor regression using [^{125}I]-labeled PKH95, capable of lipid membrane partitioning [204]. [^{125}I]PKH95 was used to directly label TILs (CD3$^+$, CD4$^-$, and CD8$^+$) which were subsequently monitored in vivo to examine the relationships between [^{125}I]PKH95-TIL dynamics and treatment outcomes. While TIL-based ACT reduced the number of MCA-207 lung metastases in C57BL/6 mice, tumor uptake of [^{125}I]PKH95-TILs was <1%ID/g, while healthy lung tissue uptake ranged from 10 to 20%ID/g. Since their labeling techniques did not affect TIL viability and deiodination was stated to be unlikely, it was concluded that tumor uptake was potentially passive and not determined by TIL-mediated tumor homing for this metastatic murine tumor model as expected. This preclinical study suggested that the observed accumulation patterns were likely not representative of those expected for human patients and reflect the need for establishing animal models that mimic clinical outcome more accurately.

T cells may be directly labeled by a choice of various radioisotopes, but it is not obvious which strategy allows modified cells to retain their desired functions. Research from Botti et al. compared the ovarian tumor localization and cytotoxicity of CTL directly labeled by either [^{111}In]oxine, [^{99m}Tc]D,L-hexamethylpropylene amine oxime ([^{99m}Tc]HMPAO), or 2-[^{18}F]FDG [205]. This was in conjunction with a pre-targeting strategy using heterobifunctional mAb, MOvl8/anti-CD3 (biMAb OC/TR), that displays specificity for folate-binding protein (FBP) expressed by IGROV1 ovarian carcinomas and the CD3$^+$ T cell receptor of TILs. The labeling efficiency (using 2.5×10^8 T lymphocytes) was highest for the [^{111}In]oxine (68%) and 2-[^{18}F] FDG (64%) methods compared to using [^{99m}Tc] HMPAO (31%), while neither method significantly reduced CTL viability. Yet, each labeling approach reduced CTL cytotoxicity and long-term proliferation and resulted in poor therapeutic specificity to IGROV1 cells compared to the FBP-negative MeWo human melanoma controls. These investigations also found that loss of cytotoxicity could be mitigated by reducing the specific activity of directly labeled CTLs from 26 MBq/10^8 cells to 0.7 MBq/10^8 cells, wherein more cells (1.4×10^9) were incubated with the same amount of [^{111}In]oxine (55.5 MBq). These studies were instrumental in further optimizing CTL labeling methods and for identifying additional challenges involved with tumor-specific immunotherapy.

Inspired to develop methods for translatable longitudinal monitoring of autologous CTL ACT, Pittet et al. evaluated the use of [^{111}In]oxine-CTLs for SPECT-CT imaging [206]. This multimodal imaging approach enabled high-sensitivity tracking of radioisotope via SPECT while providing anatomical details via CT for accurately assessing in vivo tracer localization. Cell lines that either expressed (HA$^+$CT44) or showed negligible expression (HA$^-$CT26) of the HA$_{512-520}$

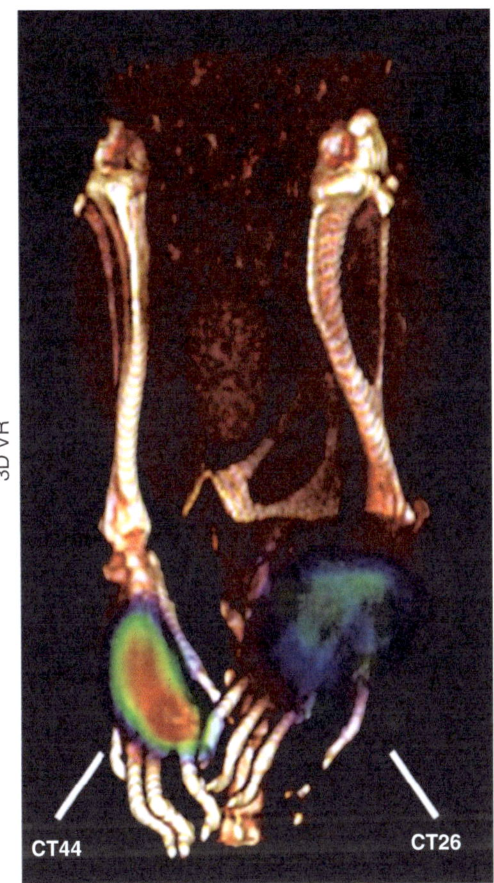

Fig. 3.2 SPECT-CT image showing [^{111}In]oxine-CTL localization in a Thy1.1 BALB/c mouse bearing a HA$_{512-520}$ peptide-expressing HA$^+$CT44 (left) foot pad tumor and a HA$^-$CT26 control tumor (right). (Adapted from Pittet et al., Proceedings of the National Academy of Sciences, 2007 [206])

tumors. These studies identified HA as a potential biomarker for clinical ACT and described methods for monitoring HA-specific CTL in vivo activity.

A combined PET-MRI approach was employed by Agger et al. to enable in vivo tracking of transgenic CD8$^+$ T cells modified to target an ovalbumin peptide (OVA$_{257-264}$, SIINFEKL) expressed by subcutaneous B16-OVA melanoma tumors in C57BL/6 mice [207]. Analogous to the aforementioned SPECT-CT methods of Pittet et al., the use of PET provides sensitive detection of tracers undergoing positron decay, while MRI defines anatomical features for accurate assessments of in vivo tracer localization. The PET tracer, [^{124}I]deoxyuridine ([^{124}I]dU), was incubated with OVA-targeting T cells ([^{124}I]IdU-OVA T cells) and were injected into mice with B16-OVA tumors. PET and MRI were then performed 5 days after [^{124}I]IdU-OVA T cell injection on sacrificed mice, which showed higher uptake of [^{124}I]IdU-OVA T cells in tumors and in 2 mm tumor margins compared to contralateral healthy control volumes. Ex vivo γ-counting experiments performed on sacrificed mice with contralateral B16-OVA and B16-F10 (control) tumors revealed higher activity per gram of tissue from OVA$^+$ tumors compared to controls. These studies identified OVA as a potential biomarker for tumor-specific ACT and validated in vivo targeting with a murine melanoma model. Further investigations may continue exploring the use of this targeting strategy for assessing modified T cell accumulation in human melanoma tumors using additional direct-labeling approaches.

peptide were used to develop foot pad tumors in Thy1.1 BALB/c mice (Fig. 3.2). Extracted CTLs were then harvested and T cell receptors (TCRs) were modified to enable targeting to HA. The [^{111}In]oxine-CTLs were then injected into lymphodepleted mice (pretreated with 300 rad irradiation) with the described tumors and were monitored in vivo by SPECT-CT for 5 days. Results showed that HA-targeting CTLs first localized in the lungs and HA$^+$CT44 tumors (2 h post injection (p.i.)) and then accumulated in the tumors, liver, and spleen after 24 h. Significantly less activity was detected in HA$^-$CT26 control

While the clinical relevance of biomarkers chosen for targeting by T cells is of great importance, injection routes also influence in vivo accumulation patterns of T cells within ACT regimes. A report from Maher's group investigated the in vivo fate of adoptively transferred T cells with CARs that targeted either MUC1 (HOX) or ErbB proteins (T1E-28z), with each co-expressing 4$\alpha\beta$ (to induce expansion with IL-4 stimulation) [208]. CAR T cells were passively loaded with [^{111}In]tropolone and monitored by SPECT-CT in beige SCID mice (Fig. 3.3). Following intravenous (i.v.) injection of [^{111}In]

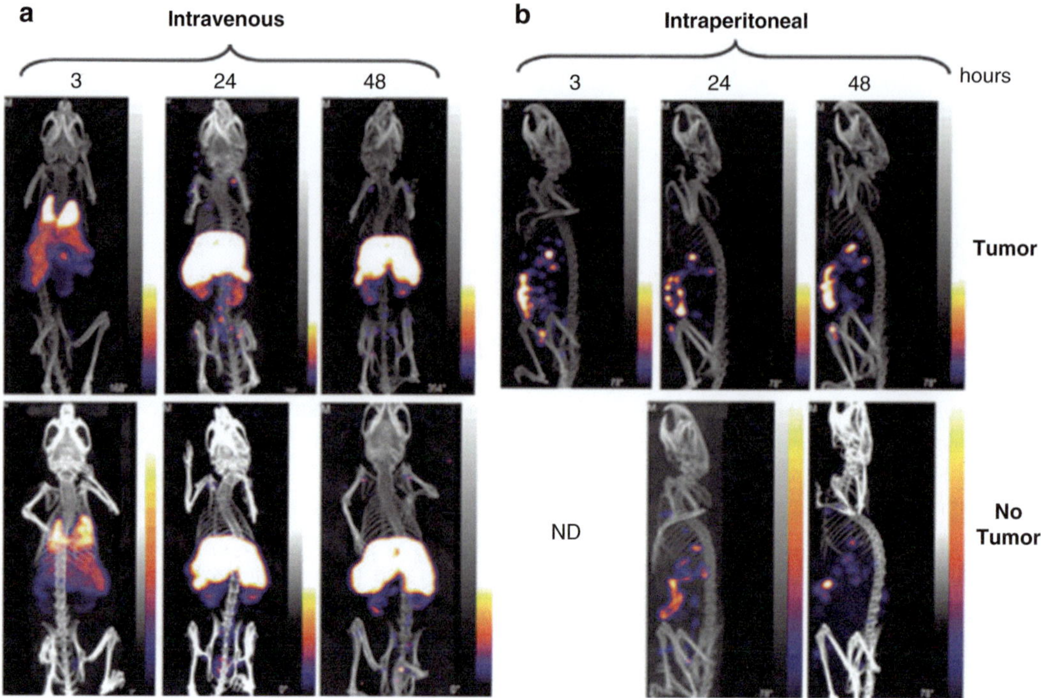

Fig. 3.3 SPECT-CT images showing accumulation of passively loaded [^{111}In]tropolone-HOX$^+$4αβ$^+$ CAR T cells in hMUC1$^+$MDA-MB-435 tumor-bearing beige SCID mice (top panels) or tumor-free mice (bottom panels) after (**a**) i.v. or (**b**) i.p. injections at the indicated timepoints p.i. (Adapted from Parente-Pereira et al., Journal of clinical immunology, 2011 [208])

tropolone-HOX$^+$4αβ$^+$ CAR T cells, SPECT observed trafficking to the lungs (residing for 3 h) and then to the liver, spleen, and LNs (axillary, retroperitoneal, and popliteal lymph) in mice with hMUC1$^+$MDA-MB-435 breast cancer tumors (expressing firefly luciferase, ffLuc). This was in contrast to [^{111}In]tropolone-HOX$^+$4αβ$^+$ CAR T cells that were injected intraperitoneally (i.p.), which resulted in limiting CAR T cell localization to the peritoneal cavity over the 48 h investigation. [^{111}In]tropolone-T1E-28z$^+$4αβ$^+$ CAR T cells injected i.v. also successfully migrated to subcutaneous ErbB$^+$ HN3 SC (head and neck) tumors and lymphoid organs, yet, cells injected subcutaneously beside these tumors remained localized over 96 h with no systemic absorption. Although minimal tumor infiltration was observed while targeting MUC1 and ErbB, this report found differential localization patterns of CAR T cells depending on administration route. These findings are vital for optimizing ACT protocols aimed for clinical translation.

Multiple imaging modalities may be coupled to provide information regarding the dynamics of injected T cells. Yet, these complex labeling strategies must be optimized to ensure that modifications do not disrupt the tumor-targeting ability or viability of AT T cells. Studies by Bhatnagar et al. evaluated the in vitro behavior of CD19-specific CAR T cells that were transduced to express EGFP and ffLuc (for BLI) and also loaded with super paramagnetic iron oxide-[^{64}Cu]DOTA-nanoparticles ([^{64}Cu]DOTA-SPION) to enable sensitive tracking via PET imaging [209]. [^{64}Cu]DOTA-SPION CAR T cells where evaluated for target specificity using CD19$^+$ NALM-6 B cell lymphoma cells compared to EL-4 control cells. Chromium release assays showed dose-dependent lysis of CD19$^+$ NALM-6 B cell, and microscopy revealed subsequent apoptosis, while control cells were minimally affected. The methods allowed the modified CAR T cells to remain viable and functional toward CD19[+] tumor cells, and future studies were planned to evaluate the construct in vivo with coupled PET, MRI, and BLI. The described use of nanoparticles (NPs) also illustrated the convergence of nanotechnology and CIT, an approach with great potential for theranostic CIT.

A more recent example of direct T cell labeling comes from a report by Man et al. that employed $[^{89}Zr]Zr(oxinate)_4$ for labeling Vγ9Vδ2 T cells for tracking TILs to MDA-MB-231 hNIS-GFP breast cancer tumors in NSG mice by PET imaging [210]. Tumor-bearing mice were injected with $[^{89}Zr]$Vγ9Vδ2 T cells alone, with free alendronate (aminobisphosphonate drug for induction of isopentenyl pyrophosphate (IPP) and subsequent Vγ9Vδ2 T cell activation) or liposomal alendronate formulations (PLA) (also labeled with $[^{111}In]In(oxinate)_3$ for SPECT imaging of $[^{111}In]$PLA). PET imaging showed substantial $[^{89}Zr]$Vγ9Vδ2 T accumulation in the spleen and liver of all animal groups. Yet, PET images taken at 48 h post-coinjection of $[^{89}Zr]$Vγ9Vδ2 T with PLA revealed significantly higher tumor uptake (~0.6%ID/g) compared to the other groups, while SPECT imaging demonstrated passive tumor uptake of $[^{111}In]$PLA by EPR. Ex vivo biodistribution studies (performed 7 days post-Vγ9Vδ2 T cell injection) confirmed the enhanced tumor uptake offered by PLA compared to controls, while anti-CD3 IHC confirmed the presence Vγ9Vδ2 T cells in the tumor and liver. This technique enabled the selective activation, tumor migration, and sensitive detection of γδ-T cells. Future efforts may continue to refine alendronate delivery methods to further enhance γδ-T activation and tumor accumulation.

The described direct labeling approaches offer some powerful advantages. Firstly, because cell labeling is performed ex vivo, many aspects of labeling (i.e., cell concentrations, tracer molar activities (A_m), buffer conditions, incubation methods, etc.) can be explored and optimized with relative ease prior to administration. Within the same context, labeling stability, cell viability, and biomarker-targeting specificity may be eval-

uated and confirmed in vitro. Moreover, directly labeled T cells can be purified prior to in vivo administration. These inherent aspects of the direct labeling approach confer the ability to create pure products with high stability and specificity. Yet, the greatest hindrance to this approach is the continuous dilution of the signal as the labeled cells proliferate and concomitantly share the loaded tracers with their respective daughter cells. While direct labeling offers great potential for tracking AT T cells, there is a notable trend showing growing use of alternate cell tracking strategies, namely, the multitude of indirect labeling methods.

3.3   Indirect Labeling

Indirect cell labeling, in the context of activated T cell imaging, refers to the use of tracers with high specificity for cell surface receptors of T cell or the use of tracers that are preferentially uptaken and trapped within targeted T cells. Because tracers can be administered multiple times, this approach allows longitudinal cell tracking without being as limited by tracer dilution resulting from cell division of labeled cells. This approach is more diverse compared to direct labeling strategies and encompasses the broad use of reporter genes, biomarker-targeting antibodies and analogues, and substrates that are preferentially uptaken by proliferating T cells.

3.3.1   Reporter Genes

A now mainstream method for indirect labeling involves genetic modifications of autologous immune cells by viral or nonviral transduction of reporter genes. Such reporter genes are subsequently transcribed and translated by the modified cells to either present unique targets or to produce enzymes for the metabolic trapping of radiotracers. The use of reporter genes for cell imaging and tracking has been previously reviewed [211–215]. Several studies therein have shown the use of PET and SPECT tracers applied for tracking reporter genes expressed by transduced tumors [216–233], non-cancerous and non-immune cells [234–236], and immune cells other than T cells for imaging cancer [237, 238] or other conditions [239–242]. This section will summarize the use of reporter genes and their respective tracers aimed to track transduced activated T cells in preclinical or clinical cancer investigations. Specifically, tracers specific for reporter gene systems including thymidine kinase (TK), sodium-iodine symporter (NIS), human norepinephrine transporter (hNET), and genetically modified TCRs will be described in this section.

3.3.1.1 Thymadine Kinase Reporter Gene Tracers

FIAU

The thymadine kinase (TK) reporter gene strategy involves the uptake of thymidine-based tracers and site-specific phosphorylation by TK, which results in trapping of the metabolite within TK-expressing cells [213]. Ideally, nonspecific tracer uptake would be quickly cleared from off-target sites to enhance the contrast of tracers trapped in targeted cells. In a 2001 report from Ponomarev et al., the herpes simplex virus 1 thymidine kinase (HSV1-TK) and GFP (TKGFP) dual reporter system was coupled with nuclear factor of activated T cells (NFAT) transcription factor and incorporated into human Jurkat cells via recombinant retroviral transduction to specifically identify activated T cells [243]. This elegant strategy involved the in vivo activation of T cell receptors (TCR) using anti-CD3 and anti-CD28 mAbs, followed by the TCR-dependent NFAT-mediated activation of endogenous T cells. Once activated, PET imaging was achieved by identifying TK-mediated tracer trapping using 2′-fluoro-2′-deoxy-1-β-D-arabinofuranosyl-5-iodouracil ([^{124}I]FIAU) in *nu/nu* mouse models with palpable Jurkat cell infiltrates. Tracer trapping in Jurkat cells was validated by antibody controls, and the accumulation of activated T cells was confirmed by anti-CD69 flow cytometry. These evaluations demonstrated the feasibility of using the described *TKGFP-NAFT* gene

reporter system and [^{124}I]FIAU for identifying activated T cells in vivo.

Studies by Koehne et al. demonstrated the ability of FIAU to track activated T cells transduced with *HSV1-TK* and human low-affinity nerve growth factor receptor (*LNGFR*), NIT$^+$ CTL, specific for Epstein-Barr virus-induced B lymphoblastoid cell line (EBV-BLCL) that expressed T cells' restricting HLA allele [244]. T cell imaging was accomplished using the tracers [^{131}I]FIAU and [^{124}I]FIAU for imaging by scintigraphy and PET, respectively. The NIT$^+$ CTLs were initially labeled ex vivo with either [^{131}I] FIAU or [^{111}In]oxine (control) or labeled with [^{131}I]FIAU in vivo. Scintigraphy showed higher accumulation of [^{131}I]FIAU-NIT$^+$ CTLs in autologous tumors compared to allogeneic (mismatched HLA allele-expressing) tumors (~7×), spleen (~2.5×), liver (~12×), and skeletal muscle (~57×) that was also higher compared to the accumulation of [^{111}In]oxine-NIT$^+$ CTLs in the respect tissues. In vivo labeling of NIT$^+$ CTLs with [^{124}I]FIAU (recorded 4 h after tracer injection) at 1, 8, and 15 days after CLT infusion provided PET images showing tracer accumulation in EBV$^+$ BLCL tumors, while radiation dose calculations (2, 8, and 16 days after CTL infusion) showed stable accumulation of tracer at each tumor and in the spleen (decreasing from 8 to 16 days after CTL infusion). In vitro toxicity studies were performed in a subsequent report by Zanzonico et al. that evaluated [^{131}I]FIAU following 2 h in vitro incubations with NIT$^+$ T cells [245]. These calculations found the maximum tolerated dose (MTD) of ~800 cGy to cell nuclei. These reports demonstrated the in vivo targeting specificity of FIAU-based tracers and revealed that the described labeling methods resulted in radiation dose that would not disrupt T cell function.

FHBG

The TK-mediated imaging strategy has been expanded with the use of other tracers that are structurally similar to FIAU. For example, a study by Dubey et al. involved harvesting tumor-targeting T cells from primary splenic lymphocytes that

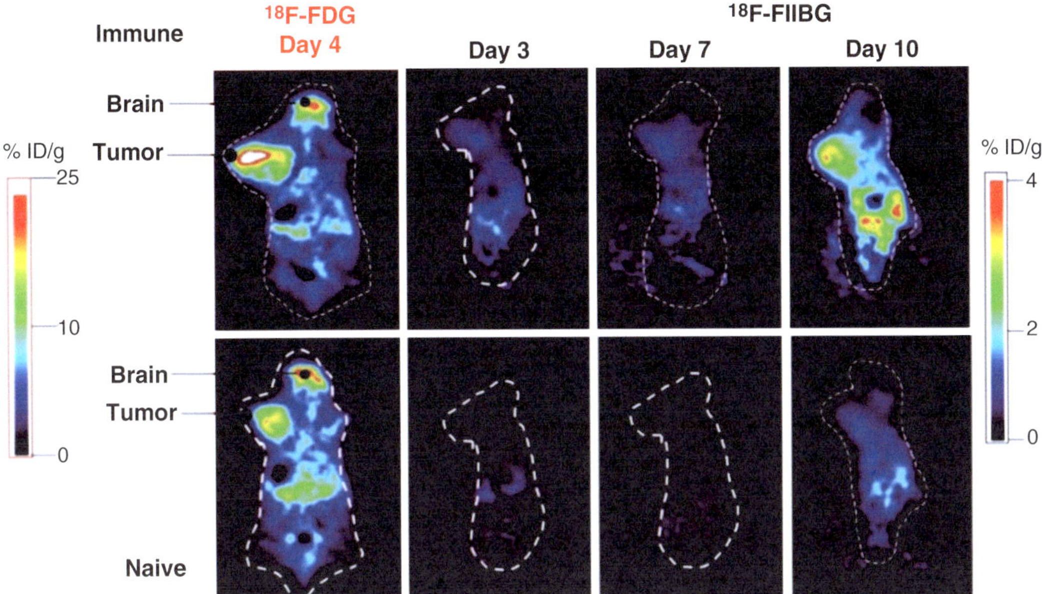

Fig. 3.4 PET images showing uptake of [18F]FHBG in M-MSV/M-MuLV-induced tumors by transduced tumor-targeting T cells (top panels) and naïve T cells (bottom panels), as compared to 2-[18F]FDG (left red panels). (Adapted from Dubey et al., Proceedings of the National Academy of Sciences, 2003 [246])

rejected tumors induced by Moloney murine sarcoma/leukemia virus (M-MSV/M-MuLV) [246]. These T cells were then transduced with the *HSV1-sr39TK* (a mutant variant of *HSV1-TK* with reduced immunogenicity) and *GFP* reporter genes after stimulation by α-CD3 and α-CD28. Flow cytometry confirmed *GFP* transduction, while the HSV1-sr39TK specific tracer, 9-[4-[18F]fluoro-3-(hydroxymethyl)butyl]guanine ([18F]FHBG), was evaluated for tracking AT T cells by PET imaging in immunodeficient mice displaying M-MSV/M-MuLV-induced tumors. PET imaging revealed higher uptake of activated T cells throughout virus-induced tumors compared to naïve T cells (Fig. 3.4). These results were recapitulated by autoradiography using the 14C-labeled 1-(2′-deoxy-2′-fluoro-β-D-arabinofuranosyl)-5-iodouracil ([14C]FIAU) that also recognized the sr39TK reporter. Su et al. continued to refine methods for quantifying AT (activated via α-CD3 and α-CD28 stimulation) T cells transduced with *GFP* and mouse stem cell virus (MSCV)-*sr39TK* reporter genes by PET imaging [247]. Among their PET studies, AT T cells were labeled with [18F]FHBG ex vivo and subcutaneously injected into C57BL/6 mouse with N2A-TK

cells to generate dose-activity standard curves, while unmodified N2A glioma controls without TK expression did not induce tracer trapping. In separate animal experiments, varying numbers of *sr39TK*-transduced T cells were injected into EL4 lymphoma tumors that were subsequently labeled with [18F]FHBG in vivo. Then, dose-activity regressions found that ~10⁶ [18F]FHBG-ATCs were accurately observed within 0.1 mL volumes, which corresponded to ~0.2%ID/g of EL4 tumor uptake. This report detailed quantification methods that can be readily applied to future studies with the goal of enhancing cell detection limits, especially pertaining to detecting minute T cell accumulation in small tumors and LNs.

In a following set of studies reported by Shu et al., bone marrow chimeric mice were developed with reconstituted hematopoietic stem cells that were transduced with the trifusion reporter gene (*hrl-egfp-tk*) that incorporated sr39TK for tracer trapping [248]. This allowed multimodal cell tracking involving GPF-enabled flow cytometry for confirming transduction, in vivo and ex vivo luciferase-based BLI, and [18F]FHBG-enabled monitoring with PET. BLI showed reconstituted lymphoid (CD4+, CD8+, and B220+) cells in the thymus and spleen and myeloid (CD11b+) cells in the bone marrow. PET imaging revealed accumulation of [^{18}F]FHBG in M-MSV/M-MuLV-induced rhabdomyosarcoma tumors and in tumor-draining lymph nodes (TDLNs). Immunosuppression with dexamethasone resulted in partial suppression of CD4+ and CD8+ T cells, which reduced tracer accumulation in TDLNs, but surprisingly still allowed tumor infiltration and expansion of reconstituted T cells. A subsequent report by Shu et al. used [^{18}F]FHBG to investigate early correlates of PET imaging and various CIT regimes [249]. T cells containing TCR specific for an epitope of gp100 (an unmutated melanoma/melanocyte-associated antigen) of B16-F10 melanoma tumors were retrovirally transduced ex vivo with the *sr39TK* reporter gene and monitored by PET using [^{18}F]FHBG in mouse models. This revealed significant T cell accumulation in the spleen and in axillary, brachial, and cervical lymph nodes 3 days post-infusion in mice receiving full combined immunotherapy (T cell adoptive therapy, lymphodepletion, DC vaccination, and systemic IL-2 injection) compared to controls receiving incomplete immunotherapy regimes. The tracer also accumulated in B16-F10 tumors, but this uptake was similar for mice experiencing tumor regression (full combined immunotherapy) and control animals showing tumor progression. Thus, while tumor uptake of [^{18}F]FHBG did not correlate with successful anti-tumor response to immunotherapy, the high uptake of the tracer in secondary lymphoid organs served as a proxy measure that indicated subsequent treatment efficacy.

The *HSV1-sr39TK* reporter gene and corresponding tracer, [^{18}F]FHBG, was further used to evaluate the in vivo localization patterns of naïve T cells (from OT-1 mouse splenocytes) as compared with memory CD8+ T cells (from C57BL/6 mice immunized by irradiated OVA-expressing E.G7 thymoma cells), each transduced to express GFP and sr39TK [250]. PET imaging studies performed by Su et al. revealed E.G7 tumor accumulation of memory T cells with no accumulation in EL4 control tumors at 1 day post injection. PET also identified the

migration of memory T cells to the lungs and to the cervical and mediastinal LNs after 8 days. Conversely, PET imaging did not detect naïve T cell accumulation in E.G7 or EL4 control tumors during the 10 day longitudinal evaluations with [^{18}F]FHBG. This report validated the tumor-targeting properties of transduced memory T cells using the sr39TK/[^{18}F]FHBG reporter system and highlighted the feasibility for longitudinal monitoring by PET.

A clinical study reported by Yaghoubi et al. evaluated the specificity of [^{18}F]FHBG for PET imaging of autologous CD8+ CTLs, transduced with *HSV1-TK* and *interleukin-13 zetakine* (therapeutic gene for tumor targeting), harvested from peripheral blood mononuclear cells (PBMCs) of a patient diagnosed with grade III/IV glioblastoma multiforme [251]. After a 5-week course of CTL therapy (total of 10^9 CTLs), PET imaging displayed two to three times higher activity at the tumor resection site and also in a tumor of the corpus callosum. In addition, there was no indication of toxicity from [^{18}F]FHBG exposure during the trial. More recently, Keu et al. infused either autologous or allogeneic engineered CTLs transduced to express the IL-13 zetakine chimeric antigen receptor (CAR) and HSV1-TK to evaluate the specificity of [^{18}F]FHBG-enabled PET for seven patients (involving IL-2 activation of CTLs for five patients) with recurrent high-grade gliomas [252]. Possibly as a result of blood-brain barrier (BBB) disruption, pre-CTL infusion imaging showed significant nonspecific tracer retention in gliomas and in healthy brain tissue. While specific tracer uptake was observed for all patients, PET imaging showed highly variable distribution and retention of [^{18}F]FHBG in tumors and in different brain regions, depending on techniques employed for CLT infusion and the sites of gliomas and resection beds. Aside from one patient developing a rash (successfully treated with 25 mg diphenhydramine) after [^{18}F]FHBG injection but prior to CLT infusion, none of the patients showed major responses to either the PET tracer or to the CLTs. These evaluations demonstrate the applicability of the TK/FHBG reporter system and suggest potential for successful clinical translation.

FEAU

In addition to FIAU and FHBG, another thymidine derivative, that is, 2′-fluoro-2′-deoxy-1-β-D-arabinofuranosyl-5-ethyluracil (FEAU), has been employed for cell tracking studies with the described TK reporter gene strategy. For example, a report by Dobrenkov et al. described the use of human T lymphocytes, transduced to express the click beetle red luciferase (and/or GFP), TK, and CAR specific for human prostate specific membrane antigen (hPSMA) [253]. This strategy enabled in vivo targeting of RM1 murine prostate carcinoma tumors (transduced to express hPSMA and *Renilla* luciferase) and PET imaging using 2′-[^{18}F]-fluoro-2′-deoxy-1-β-D-arabinofuranosyl-5-ethyluracil ([^{18}F]FEAU). The in vivo BLI signals from transduced CAR T cells (targeting hPSMA or carcinoembryonic antigen (hCEA, control)) were surprisingly inversely correlated with tumor BLI intensities. Yet, PET imaging with [^{18}F]FEAU 3 days after CAR T lymphocyte infusion revealed approximately one-fold higher activity of the tracer in animals infused with hPSMA-targeting CAR T cells (with tumor-to-background ratios ranging from 1.74 to 2.47) compared to control CAR T cells. A subsequent report by Dotti et al. used repeated PET imaging to investigate the localization of [^{18}F]FEAU in two rhesus macaques injected with T cells retrovirally transduced to express *HSV1-rs39tk* and *LNGFR* [254]. PET imaging (at 90 min, 24 h and 7 days post-T cell infusions) revealed consistent tracer localization in cervical and axillary LNs, thymus, and parotid glands and in sites of minor inflammation but surprisingly low accumulation in the lungs. More recently, a report by Najjar et al. investigated the sensitivity of [^{18}F]FEAU-enabled PET and BLI for detecting CD19-specific CAR T cells (co-stimulated by CD19, CD64, CD86, CD137L, and IL-15) expressing ffLuc and HSV1-TK (modified with nonviral Sleeping Beauty (SB) transposon/transposase) in *NOD.Cg-Prkdc^{scid}Il2rg^{tm1wjl}/SzJ* mice [255]. BLI signals corresponded to PET images that detected 3.75 × 10^6 ex vivo [^{18}F]FEAU-labeled CAR T cells subcutaneously injected into mice, while 7.5 × 10^6 subcutaneously injected CAR T cells were detected 2 h following subsequent in vivo labeling with [^{18}F]FEAU (Fig. 3.5). These animal studies, including the use of non-human primates, demonstrated the use of the TK/FEAU reporter system with AT T cells modified to detect different tumor biomarkers. The more recent study also presents the sensitivity offered by PET imaging for accurately detecting in vivo labeled CAR T cells. Together, these results may help guide future studies with the goal of translating the use of FEAU for human patients.

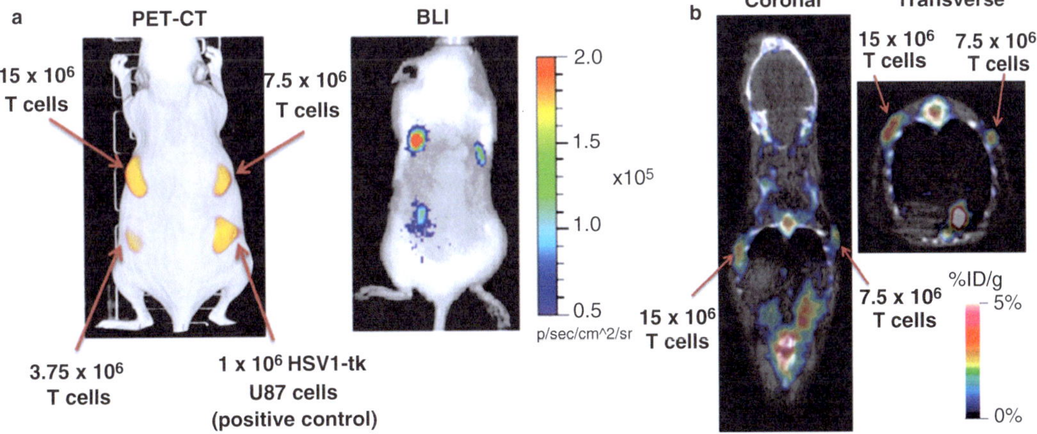

Fig. 3.5 Images showing (**a**) subcutaneously injected CD19-specific CAR T cells labeled ex vivo with [^{18}F]FEAU visualized by PET-CT (left panel) and BLI (right panel) and (**b**) PET-CT of subcutaneously injected CD19-specific CAR T cells scanned 2 h post-intravenous injection of [^{18}F]FEAU in *NOD.Cg-Prkdc^{scid}Il2rg^{tm1wjl}/SzJ* mice. (Adapted from Najjar et al., Mol Imaging Biol, 2016 [255])

3.3.1.2 T Cell Receptor Targeting

Recent strategies have directed reporter genes to become expressed by modified TCRs. For example, Vedvyas et al. developed genetically engineered T cells with a CAR that co-expressed the single-chain variable fragment (R6.5 scFv) of the known R6.5 antibody, with specificity for the tumor biomarker intercellular adhesion molecule 1 (ICAM-1; CD54), and somatostatin receptor 2 (SSTR2) for allowing longitudinal PET tracking with [^{68}Ga]gallium-labeled (DOTA^0-Phe^1-Tyr^3) octreotide ([^{68}Ga]DOTATOC) [256]. Non-obese diabetic (NOD)/LtSz-Prkdc^{scid} Il2rg^{tm1Wjl}/J (NSG) mice were inoculated with FLuc$^+$GFP$^+$ 8505C anaplastic thyroid carcinoma cells which developed into lung tumors and liver metastases that were detected by BLI. SSTR2-R6.5 scFv CAR T cells (2–3 × 10^6) were injected at either days 7 and 10 (SR1–4 group) or days 13 and 15 (SR5–9 group) post-inoculation, and CAR T cells dynamics were monitored with [^{68}Ga]DOTATOC on days 10, 16, 20, 23, and 27. PET imaging and BLI showed a biphasic anti-tumor response for SR1–4 mice (responders), which corresponded to the infiltration, expansion, and contraction of CAR T cells, while SR5–9 mice showed continued tumor growth regardless of increasing CAR T cell proliferation. In a following study, Park et al. developed T cells with a CAR that mimicked the I domain (G128–G311; F292A) of lymphocyte function-associated antigen (LFA-1), with specific binding (K_D = ~20 μM) to ICAM-1/CD54, and incorporated SSTR2 linked to the N-terminus of the I domain with porcine teschovirus-1 2 A (P2A) [257]. This enabled [^{18}F] NOTA-octreotide (OCT)-based PET imaging to evaluate in vivo anti-tumor activity of SSTR2-F292A CAR T cells. BLI revealed that systemic injection of FLuc$^+$GFP$^+$ 8505C cells in NOD/NSG mice resulted in tumors in the lungs and liver. Mice were then treated with SSTR2-F292A CAR T cells (~1–3 × 10^6) 8 days after xenograft inoculation. [^{18}F]NOTAOCT was administered on days 8, 15, 18, 22, 25, 29, 32, and 81 (post-tumor inoculation) to monitor the distribution, kinetics, and anti-tumor activity of SSTR2-F292A CAR T cells via PET imaging (correlated with BLI). Imaging results revealed the progressive elimination of lung tumors that

coincided with the expansion and contraction of infiltrating CAR T cells, as indicated by the surge and rebound of IFN-γ, IL-6, and CXCL10 levels in the blood. These studies provided a strategy for using anti-tumor CAR T cells with the SSTR2 reporter gene for longitudinal PET monitoring of CAR T cell therapy.

Using a strategy similar to the aforementioned studies, Mall et al. developed CD8$^+$ central memory T cells (T$_{CM}$) transduced to express the genetically engineered TCR, TCR2.5D6, as a reporter that allows tracking via PET imaging using the complimentary tracer, [^{89}Zr]aTCRmu-F(ab′)$_2$ [258]. This system was evaluated in vivo using NSG and BRG mice bearing GFP$^+$ML2-B7 myeloid sarcoma tumors, along with injections of hIL-15 producing NSO cells for supplementing T$_{CM}$ activation. Among these studies, PET imaging revealed differential patterns of TILs (confirmed ex vivo by anti-CD3 IHC) either at the periphery of larger tumors or homogeneously distributed within smaller tumors, depending on the phase of tumor rejection by TILs. In a following report from Yusufi et al., PET imaging with [^{89}Zr]aTCRmu-F(ab′)$_2$ and complimentary BLI detected the accumulation of TILs in GFP$^+$ML2-B7 tumors after injection of 3 × 10^6 and 1.5 × 10^6 iRFP$^+$TCR2.5D6-transgenic T$_{CM}$ but not in contralateral GFP$^+$ML2-B15 control tumors or in mice injected with non-transduced T$_{CM}$ [259] (Fig. 3.6). TILs were subsequently confirmed ex vivo by IHC for γH2AX, cleaved caspase-3 and CD3, and flow cytometry for hCD3 and hCD45. A spot-assay further showed that this PET imaging approach with [^{89}Zr] aTCRmu-F(ab′)$_2$ detected a minimum of 10^4 subcutaneously injected iRFP$^+$TCR2.5D6-transgenic T$_{CM}$ cells in NSG mice.

More recently, Krebs et al. employed CAR T cells expressing the reporter gene, DOTA antibody reporter 1 (*DAbR1*), that was developed from the scFv of the anti-lanthanoid-DOTA antibody, 2D12.5/G54C, which is specific for lanthanoid-(S)-2-(4-acrylamidobenzyl)-DOTA (AABD) chelate complexes [261]. PET (with [^{86}Y]AABD) and SPECT (with [^{177}Lu]AABD) imaging detected in vivo labeled DAbR1-CAR T cells homing to U373.eGFP glioma tumors in IcrTac:ICR-Prkdc^{scid} (ICR-SCID) mice. Both

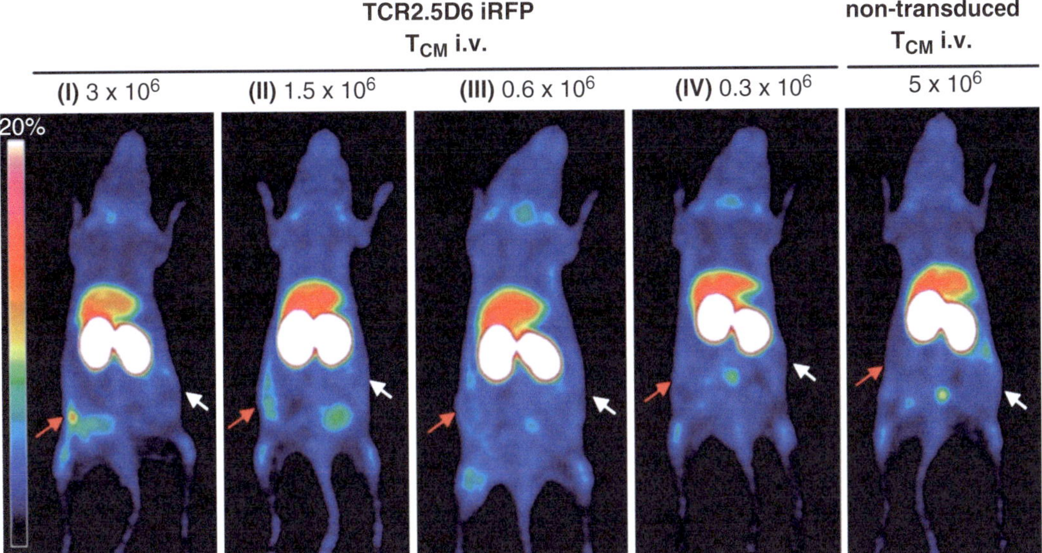

Fig. 3.6 PET images showing accumulation of [^{89}Zr] aTCRmu-F(ab′)$_2$ in NSG mice with GFP$^+$ML2-B7 tumors (red arrows) after injection of (I) 3×10^6 and (II) 1.5×10^6 iRFP$^+$TCR2.5D6-transgenic T$_{CM}$ but not in contralateral GFP$^+$ML2-B15 control tumors (white arrows) or in mice injected with non-transduced T$_{CM}$ (right panel). (Adapted from Yusufi et al., Theranostics, 2017 [260])

PET and SPECT also revealed uptake of adoptively transferred CD19-targeting DAbR1-CAR T in ffLuc$^+$GFP$^+$ NALM-6 B cell precursor leukemia tumors in NOD/SCID/IL-2Rg-null mice that was confirmed by ex vivo anti-CD3 IHC for TILs. The mean absorbed doses to T cells were then calculated, and it was suggested that [^{86}Y] AABD (20 cGy) likely did not affect T cell function, while [^{177}Lu]AABD (1.1 Gy/MBq) may eradicate clustered T cells. This elegant system shows potential to track and deliver therapeutic (β- or α-emitting) radionuclides to TILs, yet dosimetry must be optimized to preclude undesired toxicity to non-tumor tissues. This latter report illustrates the convergence of TCR targeting and theranostics, a strategy that certainly holds great potential for activated T cell tracking and site-specific radioimmunotherapy.

3.3.1.3 hNIS Reporter Gene Tracer: [^{99m}Tc]TcO$_4^-$

The cell surface protein, sodium-potassium symporter (NIS), functions to concentrate iodide in the thyroid gland, and clinical imaging investigations with [^{131}I]iodide identified NIS in other healthy tissues including the salivary glands and the stomach [262]. A recent report by Emami-Shahri et al. described the development of CAR T cells, by retroviral transduction with a tricistronic vector for stoichiometric co-expression of *P28ζ* (for PSMA targeting), *4αβ* (chimeric IL-4 receptor), and *hNIS* as a reporter gene, for cell tracking via [^{99m}Tc]pertechnetate ([^{99m}Tc]TcO$_4^-$)-enabled SPECT imaging [126]. Varying numbers of 4P28ζN CAR T were subcutaneously injected into NSG mice, and i.v. injected [^{99m}Tc]TcO$_4^-$ allowed detection by SPECT-CT with a limit of 1.5×10^4 cells. PC3-LN3 prostate cancer cells were transduced to co-express ffLuc, tdTomato-RFP, and PSMA (PLP tumor cells), and in vivo PSMA targeting of 4P28ζN CAR T (10^6 cells) was compared to PL control tumor cells (without PSMA) and 4PTrN CAR T control cells at 7 days (low tumor burden group, LTBG) or 14 days (high tumor burden group, HTBG) after tumor cell inoculations. BLI revealed PLP tumor regression for the LTBG post-4P28ζN CAR T administration, while 4PTrN CAR T-treated mice exhibited continued tumor growth. Tumors as well as the stomach, thyroid and salivary glands were clearly visible by SPECT at 1 h p.i. of [^{99m}Tc]TcO$_4^-$ (blockable with coinjection of NaClO$_4^-$). While the AT cell dose was not sufficient to alleviate tumors from the HTBG, ex vivo IHC of resected tumors confirmed the presence of CD3$^+$ TILs in 4P28ζN CAR T cell-treated PLP tumors, but not in PL tumors or tumors treated with 4PTrN CAR T cells. These studies demonstrated successful PSMA-targeting, anti-tumor therapy by AT CAR T cells and illustrated an elegant study design for monitoring tumor progression and CAR T cell migration.

3.3.1.4 hNET Reporter Gene Tracer: MIBG

The [^{123}I]-labeled norepinephrine derivative, metaiodobenzylguanidine ([^{123}I]MIBG), has been extensively employed as a clinical SPECT tracer for detecting and monitoring neuroblastomas, while [^{131}I]MIBG has been evaluated for *β*-therapy [263]. In addition to these clinical applications, MIBG has been evaluated as a potential tracer for tracking T cells transduced to express the human norepinephrine transporter (*hNET*) reporter gene. For example, Moroz et al. developed cell lines transduced to express *GFP* and *hNET* reporter gene to evaluate the in vitro uptake of ^{123}I- or ^{124}I-labeled hNET-specific tracer, metaiodobenzylguanidine (MIBG) [264]. Cell uptake experiments showed almost 50-fold higher distribution volumes (V_d) of [^{124}I]MIBG in transduced Jurkat cells (T cell line) compared to wild-type Jurkat cells, owing to the ~30-fold higher influx rate of MIBG in transduced cells. Subsequent in vivo evaluations compared SPECT ([^{123}I]MIBG) to PET ([^{124}I]MIBG) using *hNET*-expressing C6 glioma tumors in mouse models and found better contrast by PET, potentially due to the lower specific activity of [^{124}I]MIBG. A report by Doubrovin et al. also evaluated the use of [^{123}I]MIBG and [^{124}I]MIBG for SPECT and PET imaging (respectively) for tracking EBV-specific CTLs transduced to express GFP and hNET in mouse models with EBV-transformed B cell lymphomas (EBV-BLCL) [265]. Imaging data revealed accumulation of both MIBG tracers

in tumors at 4 h post-injection, even with injections of 10^4 transduced CTLs, which was comparable to the sensitivity provided by HSV1-TK-transduced CTLs evaluated by the reporter gene PET tracer, [^{124}I]FIAU, in this report. Moreover, all tracers were able to detect EBV$^+$ tumors at 28 days post-i.v. infusion of transduced CTLs by SPECT and PET imaging. These studies illustrated in vivo T cell labeling, tumor specificity of labeled T cells, and high-sensitivity imaging of labeled T cells. Yet, the perfuse expression of endogenous hNET may pose a challenge for this reporter gene/tracer strategy.

3.3.2 Deoxyribonucleotide Salvage Pathway Reporters

The deoxyribonucleotide salvage pathway has been explored as a means for in vivo labeling activated T cells using various radiolabeled derivatives of cytosine, adenine, thymidine, guanine, and uracil. Similarly to 2-[^{18}F]FDG, successful targeting and imaging are governed by enhanced tracer uptake by metabolically active cells. The goal of this strategy is to achieve preferential tracer uptake by proliferating T cells that display enhanced deoxyribonucleotide salvage pathway activity, whereas most other cells rely on de novo DNA synthesis [266].

3.3.2.1 FAC

A report from Radu et al. introduced 1-(2′-deoxy-2′-[^{18}F]fluoroarabinofuranosyl) cytosine ([^{18}F]FAC) as a PET tracer capable of specific uptake in proliferating T cells [266]. In vivo PET experiments comparing lymphoid organ uptake of [^{18}F]FAC to [^{18}F]fluoro-3′-deoxythymidine ([^{18}F]FLT) and 1-(2-deoxy-2-[^{18}F]-β-arabino-furanosyl)-5-methyluracil ([^{18}F]FMAU) showed higher uptake of [^{18}F]FAC in the spleen (~1-fold) and thymus (~1.5-fold). PET imaging also revealed elevated uptake of [^{18}F]FAC in U87 GBM tumors (~1.9 %ID/g) in the spleen and thymus 15 days after anti-tumor challenging with Moloney murine sarcoma and leukemia virus complex (MSV/MuLV). PET studies further showed [^{18}F]FAC activity in the thymus and lymph nodes of *B6. MRL-Faslpr/J* mice displaying systemic autoimmunity, which was later reduced upon treatment with the immunosuppressant drug, dexamethasone. A following report by Nair-Gill et al. demonstrated the preferential uptake of [^{18}F]FAC in the GI tract and in CD8$^+$ T cells of the spleen and thymus and in tumor-draining lymph nodes of immunocompetent C57BL/6 mice challenged with MSV/MuLV [111]. This was in contrast to the significantly lower tracer uptake observed in lymphoid organs of CB17$^{SCID/SCID}$ immune-defective mice with deficient T and B cells that were also challenged with MSV/MuLV. While non-metastatic rhabdomyosarcoma tumor uptake of [^{18}F]FAC was relatively low compared to the uptake of 2-[^{18}F]FDG, this was attributed to low deoxycytidine kinase (dCK) activity and, thus, minor activation of the deoxyribonucleotide salvage pathway in these animal models.

A comparison report by Schwarzenberg et al. investigated the targeting specificity of [^{18}F]FAC, [^{18}F]L-FAC, and a 5-position methylated derivative, 2′-deoxy-2′-[^{18}F]-fluoro-5-methyl-β-L--arabinofuranosylcytosine ([^{18}F]L-FMAC) [267]. The goal of these studies was to evaluate tracer uptake in regions of enhanced dCK activity in nine healthy human volunteers (three volunteers per tracer) with the long-term goal of identifying if these PET tracers may help stratify patients undergoing chemotherapy with nucleoside analogue prodrugs (e.g., cladribine, clofarabine, cytarabine, decitabine, and gemcitabine). PET imaging results showed higher tracer uptake of [^{18}F]FAC in the spleen and lower retention in bone marrow. This was explained to be indicative of CDA-catalyzed deamination (to [^{18}F]FAU), while the higher liver uptake of L-enantiomer tracers was proposed to be related to differential transport and "washout" of [^{18}F]L-FAC and [^{18}F]L-FMAC by hepatocytes. PET-CT imaging further evaluated [^{18}F]L-FMAC with one patient with ovarian cancer and found tracer localization in a gastric metastatic lesion, potentially due to increased dCK activity.

A more recent report by Antonios et al. evaluated the use of [^{18}F]FAC-enabled PET-CT and also MRI for identifying orthotopic malignant GL261 murine gliomas in syngeneic immuno-competent mice subjected to DC vaccination (with DCVax-L) and/or ICB therapy (with the PD-1 mAb, pembrolizumab) [268]. In vivo labeling of proliferating T cells with [^{18}F]FAC provided PET images (1 h p.i.) showing significant activity in gliomas of mice treated with DCVax-L (with and without pembrolizumab) and also in cervical and axillary LNs of mice treated with DCVax-L and pembrolizumab. These studies concluded that [^{18}F]FAC activity correlated with activated TILs and with upregulated dCK activity of proliferating T lymphocyte. Furthermore, the validated study design may be translated to investigating clinical outcomes of combination CITs.

3.3.2.2 CFA

The prodrug, clofarabine (Clolar), is a nucleic acid synthesis inhibitor with approval for the treatment of recurrent pediatric acute lymphoid leukemia and has been modified to explore its utility as an activated T cell tracer. An initial report by Shu et al. found that the [^{18}F]-labeled derivative, 2-chloro-2′-deoxy-2′-[^{18}F]fluoro-9-β-D-arabinofuranosyl-adenine ([^{18}F]CFA), provided PET images that displayed unexpectedly low tracer uptake in lymphoid structures (spleen, thymus, and marrow) in immunocompetent C57BL/6J mice [269]. Yet, a more recent report by Kim et al. demonstrated that in vivo targeting of [^{18}F]CFA to activated T cells is cytidine deaminase (CDA)-mediated and specific for cells displaying enhanced deoxyribonucleoside salvage via upregulation of deoxycytosine kinase (dCK) [270]. These studies were performed using NSG mice and also in a first-in-human trial. PET imaging showed specific accumulation of [^{18}F]CFA in CEM-CDA leukemia tumors (blockable with CDA inhibitor, DI-82) compared to CEM-EYFP control tumors. The first-in-human PET images of [^{18}F]CFA with a healthy volunteer showed tracer accumulation in the liver, spleen, bone marrow, LNs, kidneys, and bladder (Fig. 3.7a). In comparison, the tracer notably localized in a skull bone lesion of a patient with paraganglioma (Fig. 3.7b) and did not accumulate in lumbar spine vertebrae previously irradiated to treat regional tumors (Fig. 3.7c). These results reflect

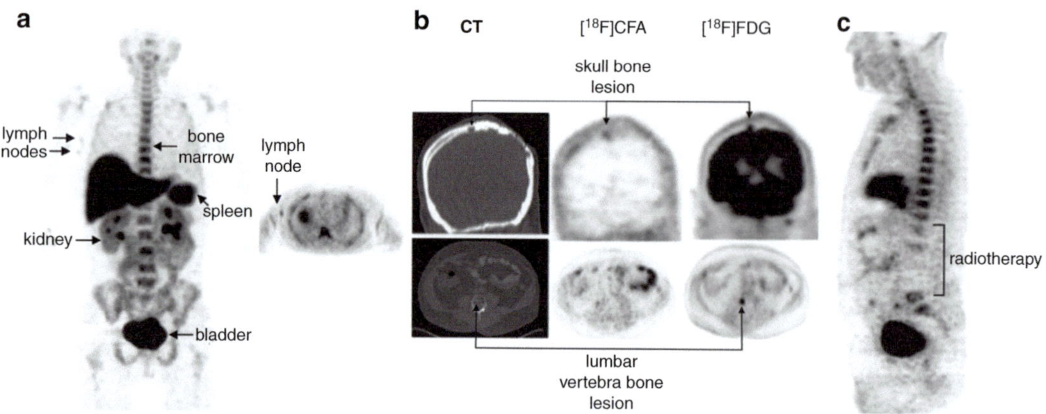

Fig. 3.7 PET images showing accumulation of [^{18}F]CFA in (**a**) a healthy volunteer, (**b**) a patient with paraganglioma, and (**c**) a patient post-radiotherapy. (Adapted from Kim et al., Proc Natl Acad Sci USA, 2016 [270])

the expected uptake of [^{18}F]CFA in major lymphoid structures and its applicability for clinical cancer imaging.

3.3.2.3 AraG

The guanine derivative, 9-β-D-arabinofuranosylguanine (AraG), can be uptaken by activated T cells displaying upregulated mitochondrial deoxyguanosine kinase (dGK) activity, phosphorylated and trapped within, making this nucleoside a useful T cell imaging agent [271]. A report by Namavari et al. described the synthesis of the dCK-specific PET tracer, 2′-deoxy-2′-[^{18}F]fluoro-9-β-D-arabinofuranosylguanine ([^{18}F] F-AraG), and investigated its uptake in activated primary thymocytes [272]. Cell studies showed significant tracer uptake in T cells activated with IL-2 (1.4-fold increase) and co-activated with phorbol myristate acetate (PMA) and ionomycin (4.7-fold increase) compared to inactivated thymocytes. Successful [^{18}F]fluoride ion radiolabeling via nucleophilic substitution of the triflate precursor gave acceptable decay-corrected radiochemical yields (7–10%, n = 10) and molar activities (A_m, 0.8–1.3 Ci/μmol) for [^{18}F]F-AraG—showing promise for PET imaging.

A recent report by Levi et al. described the use of [^{18}F]F-AraG as an activated T cell PET tracer for monitoring T cell response during anti-PD-1 ICB therapy [273]. In vivo evaluations with Balb/C mice confirmed the localization of [^{18}F] F-AraG to MSV-MuLV-induced rhabdomyosar-coma tumors via uptake and retention by CD8$^+$ and CD4$^+$ TILs. In further animal experiments, B2 mice bearing MC38 colon carcinoma tumors were administered with anti-PD-1 mAb, RMP1–14 (7 × 5 mg/kg), or isotype control (2A3) and were longitudinally monitored by PET over 3 weeks using [^{18}F]F-AraG. Mice in the treatment group that responded to ICB therapy displayed significant elevation of tracer uptake in the tumor (9 days post-therapy) and also in TDNLs of responders at 9 and 15 days post-therapy, compared to non-responder animals. The latter observation was key for providing early indications of the desired ICB therapy response. [^{18}F]F-AraG (CellSight Technologies) is currently being evaluated in a phase 2 US clinical trial (NCT03217071) for monitoring response to combined radiation therapy and pembrolizumab ICB therapy with NSCLC patients.

3.3.2.4 FMAU

A report by McCracken et al. from Witte's group detailed the development of tumor models that express a mutant variant of dCK, hdCK3mut (3-amino acid active site substitution), in L1210-10K mouse leukemia cells lacking dCK activity and subsequent evaluations of 2′-deoxy-2′-[^{18}F]-fluoro-5-methyl-1-β-L-arabinofuranosyluracil ([^{18}F]L-FMAU) as a PET reporter [240]. PET imaging revealed the specificity of [^{18}F]L-FMAU to hdCK3mut expressed by transduced L1210-10K tumors in NSG mice, while significantly

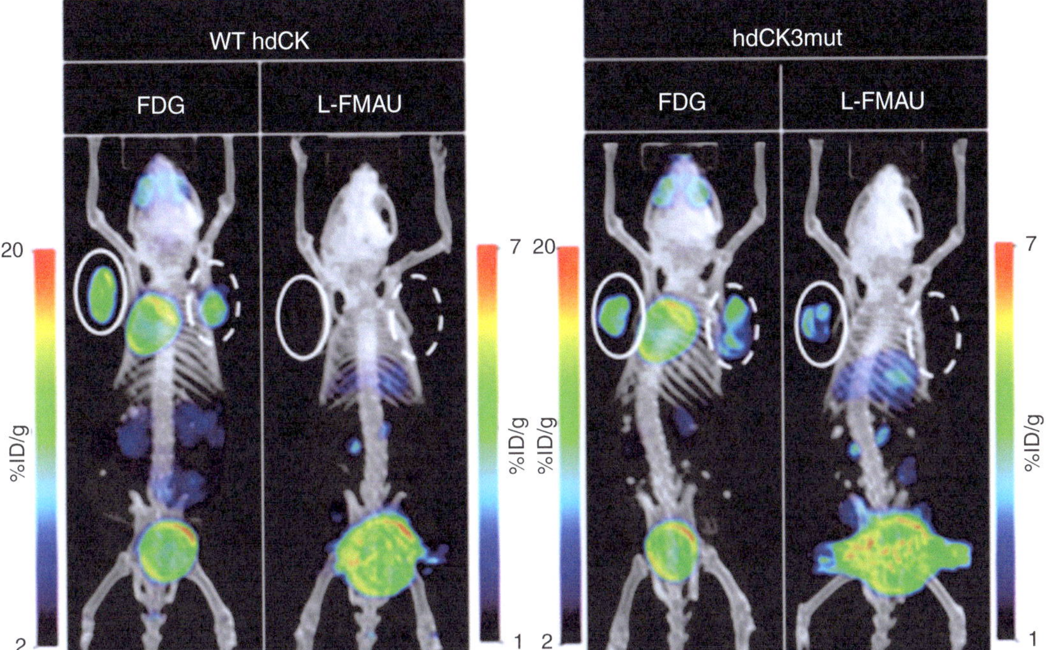

Fig. 3.8 PET-CT images of NGS mice bearing non-transduced L1210-10K control tumors (dotted lines) and contralateral L1210-10K tumors transduced (solid lines) to express either WT hdCK (left panels) or hdCK3mut (right panels). Mice were imaged using 2-[¹⁸F]FDG and [¹⁸F]L-FMAU. (Adapted from McCracken et al., Proc Natl Acad Sci USA, 2013 [240])

lower [¹⁸F]L-FMAU activity was observed in L1210-10K tumors expressing wild-type hdCK and non-transduced tumors (Fig. 3.8). While tumor uptake of 2-[¹⁸F]FDG was higher compared to [¹⁸F]L-FMAU under all conditions, 2-[¹⁸F]FDG did not display specificity toward transduced L1210-10K tumors since glucose metabolism was noted to be similar. A following report by McCracken et al. explored the use of [¹⁸F]L-FMAU as a PET tracer for detecting TILs transduced to express human deoxycytidine kinase triple mutant (hdCK3mut) and anti-melanoma T cell receptor, F5 (specific for melanoma antigen recognized by T cells 1, MART-1), in immune-deficient NSG mice models with human melanoma tumors [274]. PET imaging showed high tracer uptake in M202 (HLA-matched) tumors at 1 day and 8 days after injection of engineered TILs (expressing hdCK3mut and F5, but not hdCK3mut only) compared to IL-2-activated PBMNs. PET imaging with [¹⁸F]L-FMAU also revealed tracer specificity for M202 tumors over M207 (HLA-mismatched)

tumors in mice previously injected with hdCK3mut⁺F5⁺ TILs but displayed low tumor uptake in mice injected with T cells expressing only hdCK3mut. Thus, these studies validated F5-specific targeting and tracking of AT T cells with [¹⁸F]L-FMAU.

3.3.2.5 FLT

A clinical report from Ribas et al. described the use of PET imaging for detecting T cells with enhanced nucleoside transporter and TK1 activity using the cell replication reporter, 3′-deoxy-3′-[¹⁸F]-fluorothymidine ([¹⁸F]FLT) [275]. The tracer was evaluated with nine patients with advanced melanoma undergoing coinhibitory molecule cytotoxic T lymphocyte-associated antigen 4 (CTLA4) blockade therapy (disrupting CTLA4-CD80 and CTLA4-CD86 binding) with the anti-CTLA4 mAb, tremelimumab. PET imaging with [¹⁸F]FLT was performed prior to and 43–98 days post-tremelimumab treatments, along with 2-[¹⁸F]FDG PET imaging (within 2 weeks after [¹⁸F]FLT imaging) to monitor tumor progression. SUV measurements found increased [18F]FLT accumulation in the spleens in seven of nine patients, while spleen accumulation was reduced for two patients post-mAb therapy. While there was no apparent tracer uptake in tumors or draining lymph nodes, the authors highlighted that the differential spleen uptake may provide insights for improving patient stratification strategies for immune checkpoint blockade therapies.

Further clinical investigations by Aarntzen et al. evaluated the use of [18F]FLT for monitoring activated T and B cell response to intranodal DC vaccination (expressing gp100 and tyrosinase) for melanoma patients with lymph node metastasis [276]. Imaging studies revealed colocalization of [111In]oxine-SPIO-loaded DCs (SPECT imaging) and [18F]FLT signals (PET) in metastatic lymph nodes, while IHC confirmed the presence of CD4+ and CD8+ TILs following DC vaccinations. A recent clinical study by Scarpelli et al. evaluated [18F]FLT as a tracer for monitoring CIT response to pTVG-HP DNA vaccination and pembrolizumab ICB therapy for 17 patients with metastatic prostate cancer [277]. Enhanced tracer accumulation was observed in vaccine-draining LNs compared to non-draining LNs, as expected. Yet, higher tracer uptake by tumors and spleen was found to be indicative of a shorter progression-free survival, while baseline thyroid uptake predicted thyroid-associated pembrolizumab toxicity. Ex vivo immunofluorescence imaging of tumor biopsies further suggested that tracer uptake was, at least, partially mediated by expansion of proliferation CD8+ Ki67+ T cells. These clinical studies highlighted the in vivo dynamics of [18F] FLT and provided methods for investigating correlates of tracer uptake patterns and expected treatment outcomes.

3.3.3 Interleukins

Radiolabeled interleukins (ILs) have been explored as imaging agents for assessing relationships between immune cell recruitment/activation and tracer uptake in studies involving organ allografts

([123I]IL-2) [278], colitis-related inflammation ([99mTc]HYNIC-IL-2) [279, 280], diabetes-related infections ([131I]IL-8) [281], inflammation from cardiac plaque formation ([99mTc]HYNIC-IL-2) [282], CD28-mediated xenograft-induced inflammation (4-[18F]-fluorobenzoate-IL-2, [18F]FB-IL-2) [283], and animal models with subcutaneously injected activated T cells ([18F]FB-IL-2) [284]. This section summarizes the results from studies in which radiolabeled IL-2 has been evaluated in preclinical and clinical cancer investigations that examined tracer uptake by TILs.

A report by Signore et al. described the use of [99mTc]S-tetrahydrofurfurylacetyl(thio-2,3,5,6 tetrafluorophenyl)adipylglycylglycine ([99mTc] N_3S) conjugated to IL-2 ([99mTc]N_3S-IL-2), with specificity for CD25 (IL-2 receptor, IL-2R) of TILs, with the goal of aiding predictions of in vivo TIL response to IL-2 therapy for patients with advanced cutaneous melanoma [285]. All 30 patients with atypical pigmentary cutaneous lesions were administered with [99mTc]N_3S-IL-2 (111–185 MBq), and planer γ-camera imaging (1 h p.i.) detected significant tracer uptake ($\geq$1.1 target-to-background, T/B) in lesions confirmed as malignant melanoma (~71%, 15 of 21) or benign (~22%, 2 of 9). IHC analyses (for CD3, CD4, CD8, CD16, CD25) further revealed significant correlations between [99mTc]N_3S-IL-2 uptake and CD25 expression of TILs (~73%, 11 of 15) and also CD16 expression by NK cells in resected melanoma tumors, whereas tracer uptake by melanoma cells did not correlate with tumor CD25 expression. A following study from Loose et al. evaluated the biodistribution of [123I] IL-2 by SPECT imaging for 17 patients with squamous cell carcinoma of the head and neck (SSCHN) to assess the relationship between tracer distribution and CD28 expression of TILs from tumor resections or biopsies [286]. SPECT (following 300 mg oral KI to block thyroid uptake of 123I) revealed significant uptake of [123I] IL-2 (1.2 median T/B) in tumors for ~80% (14 of 17) of patients, and subsequent IHC (for CD3 and CD25) showed a positive correlations between tracer accumulation and CD28 expression by TILs, but not with CD28 expression by SSCHN tumor cells. A recent clinical pilot study

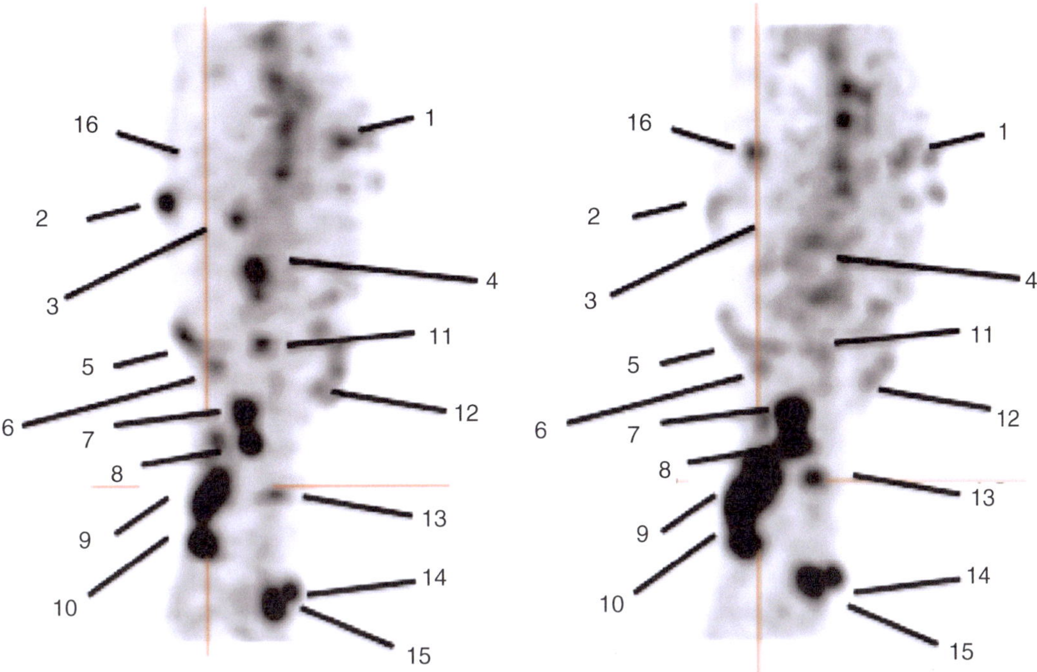

Fig. 3.9 Planar scintigraphy showing accumulation of [^{99m}Tc]HYNIC-IL-2 in metastatic lesions pre-therapy (left) and post-therapy (right) for patient no. 1. (Adapted from Markovic et al., Oncotarget, 2018 [287])

from Signore's group used [^{99m}Tc]HYNIC-IL-2 (with tricine as a co-ligand)-enabled SPECT-CT for assessing tracer uptake by TILs for patients with metastatic melanoma before (five patients) and 12 weeks after (three patients) undergoing ICB therapy with the anti-CTLA-4 mAb, ipilimumab (IPI, one patient), or anti-PD-1 mAb, pembrolizumab (PEMBRO, two patients) [287]. Imaging analyses found significant correlations (Spearman rank) between CT-assessed tumor burden and [^{99m}Tc]HYNIC-IL-2 uptake, both before and after (coefficients = 0.592 and 0.618, respectively) therapy, that suggested a proportional relationship between tumor size and TIL accumulation in tumors (Fig. 3.9). While some patients were excluded from post-therapy imaging studies, negative symptoms were attributed to expected side effects from the respective mAb therapies and not from [^{99m}Tc]HYNIC-IL-2.

In addition to exploring the use of [^{99m}Tc]- and [^{123}I]-labeled IL-2 for SPECT, [^{18}F]-labeling has also been applied to enable PET imaging of activated T cells in preclinical cancer imaging investigations. Specifically, Hartimath et al. evaluated [^{18}F]FB-IL-2 as a tracer for detecting differential activated T cell migration following immunization (SFVeE6,7) with and without irradiation (14 Gy) of TC-1 lung cancer tumors in C57BL/6 mice [121]. PET imaging showed distinct tracer accumulation in tumors with CD8$^+$ TILs (confirmed by anti-CD8 IHC) for both treatment groups, wherein higher tracer uptake was observed following combined therapy (9.1 ± 2.7 %ID/g) and radiation therapy (3.4 ± 0.7 %ID/g), compared to sham controls (0.34 ± 0.16 %ID/g). Interestingly, administration of the CXCR4 antagonist, Plerixafor (3 mg/kg daily × 6, i.p.), significantly reduced tracer accumulation in irradiated tumors. This revealed that CD8$^+$ T cell migration to tumors following irradiation is likely a CXCR4-mediated response. Further ex vivo biodistribution studies found that the described combined therapy enhanced activated T cell migration to the thymus, spleen, bone marrow, salivary gland, and lymph nodes, compared to other animal groups. Recently, mutant variants of IL-2, that is, IL-2v [288], and corresponding antibody conjugates (e.g., carcinoembryonic antigen (CEA)-specific mAb, cergutuzumab; CEA-IL-2v) have been explored as immunocytokines for CIT [289]. These reports suggest that radiolabeled IL-2 derivatives show promise as activated T cell imaging agents, therapeutics, and tracers for monitoring response to CIT.

3.3.4 Antibodies, Antibody Fragments, and Peptides

Antibodies and associated amino acid-based macromolecules (e.g., peptides, single-chain fragments (scFv), etc.) have been developed to display high specificity and binding affinity toward molecular targets overexpressed by hematological cancer cells and those expressed by tumors attempting to avoid immune system detection and clearance. Radiolabeled antibodies and analogues have been reported for tracking migrating B cells [271, 290], B cell lymphoma cells [291–296], activated macrophages [297–300], and T cells in healthy animals [301, 302] and in models of inflammation (e.g., colitis [303, 304] and arthritis [271]), infection [305], or hematopoietic stem cell (HSC) transplantation [306, 307]. Radiolabeled antibodies and corresponding analogues have also been employed to detect cancer cells expressing programmed death ligand 1 (PD-L1) [308–317] or cytotoxic T lymphocyte-associated protein 4 (CTLA-4) [318], both targets for ICB therapy. This section will focus on summarizing the use of PET and SPECT imaging for tracking activated T cells after in vivo labeling with radiolabeled antibodies and analogues specific for T cell markers that include programmed death 1 (PD-1), CTLA-4 (CD152), CD3, CD8, OX40 (CD134), modified TCRs, and granzyme B.

3.3.4.1 PD-1

PD-1 is expressed by T cells and may bind to cancer cells expressing the inhibitory ligand, PD-L1, which provides cancer cells a means of escaping detection and subsequent immune system eradication. Natarajan et al. developed a [^{64}Cu]DOTA-anti-mouse-PD-1 mAb conjugate and evaluated

in vivo PD-1 targeting specificity to PD-1$^+$ murine TILs in Foxp3$^+$.LuciDTR4 transgenic mice with B16–F10 murine melanoma tumors by PET-CT imaging [319]. PET imaging (from 1 to 48 h p.i.) (Fig. 3.10) and ex vivo biodistribution (48 h p.i.) studies revealed blockable tracer uptake in the tumor, spleen, and liver at 48 h p.i., while ex vivo BLI detected FoxP3$^+$CD4$^+$ Tregs in the tumor and spleen. The colocalization of PET and BLI signals suggested that uptake of [^{64}Cu]DOTA-anti-mouse-PD-1 was related to the PD-1 expression of Tregs that homed to and infiltrated tumors. Hettich et al. reported the conjugation of [^{64}Cu]S-2-(4-isothiocyanatobenzyl)-1,4,7-triazacyclononane-1,4,7-triacetic acid (p-SCN-Bn-NOTA) to an α-PD-1 mAb (RMP1–14) and the subsequent PET imaging of [^{64}Cu]NOTA-Bn- α-PD-1 in C57BL/6N mice with subcutaneous CD133-expressing B16-F10 murine melanoma tumors [320]. Mice were either healthy, displayed tumors but were not treated or had tumors that were treated with 2 × 12 Gy γ-irradiation and ICB therapy (with anti-CTLA-4 and anti-PD-L1 mAbs; 200 μg, i.p) once tumors reached 500 mm^3. The treated and untreated tumor-bearing mice displayed blockable PD-1$^+$ TIL-associated tracer uptake in the tumor and also higher (and blockable) uptake of the tracer in the spleen and LNs compared to healthy mice.

The humanized IgG4 anti-PD-1 mAb, pembrolizumab (Keytruda; Merck), selectively binds to PD-1 on activated T cells which disrupts binding with PD-L1 expressed by tumor cells attempting to evade immune system recognition and has been approved by the FDA for treating non-small cell lung cancer (NSCLC), renal cell cancer, and advanced melanoma. The [^{89}Zr]-labeled conjugate, [^{89}Zr]deferoxamine(Df)-pembrolizumab, was evaluated by PET imaging and in vivo biodistribution studies using mouse (female ICR (CD-1), SCID γ-(NSG), and NSG with human peripheral blood lymphocytes (hu-PBL-SCID)) and rat (Hsd: Sprague–Dawley) models by England et al. with the goal of extrapolating results to estimate radiation dosimetry for humans [321]. The 78.4 h half-life of [^{89}Zr]zirconium allowed longitudinal in vivo tracking of the

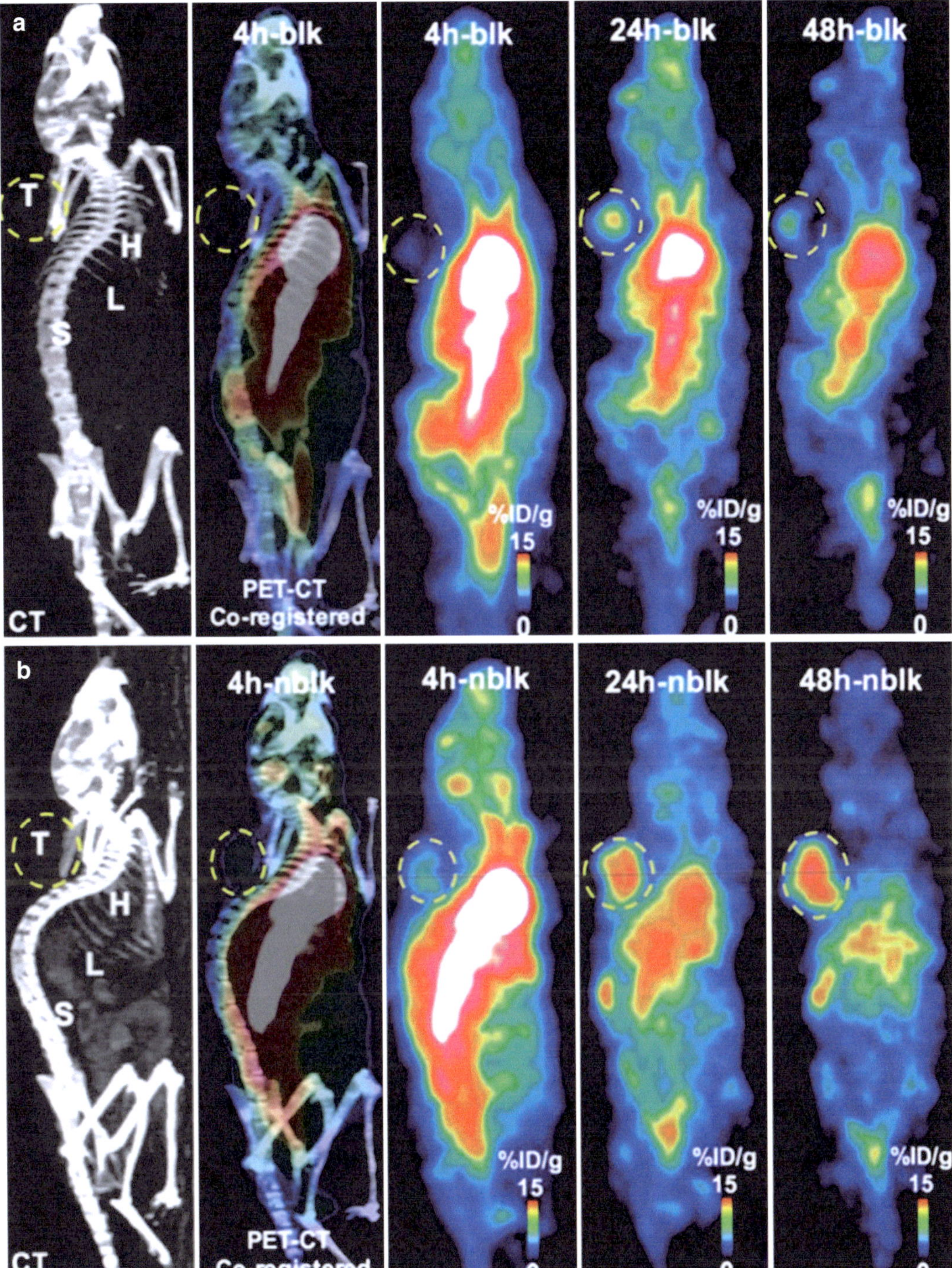

Fig. 3.10 Representative CT (left column), PET-CT (second from left column, 4 h p.i.), and PET images (4 h, 24 h and 48 h p.i.) showing accumulation of [^{64}Cu]DOTA-anti-mouse-PD-1 mAb in B16–F10 murine melanoma tumor-bearing Foxp3$^+$.LuciDTR4 transgenic mice (**a**) with and (**b**) without non-radioactive pembrolizumab blocking. (Adapted from Natarajan et al., Bioconjug Chem, 2015 [319])

conjugate and revealed tracer stability and retention in the blood (>10 %ID/g at 168 h p.i.) with clearance mostly via the liver (versus the spleen and kidneys) in CD-1 mice, while the tracer was cleared via the liver and spleen equally in Hsd rats. Also, hu-PBL-SCID mice displayed elevated tracer accumulation in the salivary glands (from T cell infiltration), liver, and kidneys but lower retention in the blood pool and spleen compared to SCID γ-(NSG) controls — resulting in higher estimated radiation doses for hu-PBL-SCID (1.246 mGy/MBq) mice compared to controls (0.838 mGy/MBq).

A report from Natarajan et al. described the use of PET imaging for tracking the tracers, [89Zr]benzyl-desferrioxamine (Df-Bz)-pembrolizumab and [64Cu]DOTA-pembrolizumab, to hPBMC (with huCD45[+] and hPD-1[+] lymphocytes) injected into NOD-scid IL-2Rγ[null] (hNSG) mice with A375 human melanoma tumors compared to control NSG mice without hPBMC engraftment [322]. PET imaging (1–144 h p.i. for [89Zr]mAb and 1–48 h p.i. for [64Cu]mAb) revealed blockable homing of both tracers to hPD-1[+] TILs in the tumor (~4 %ID/g and ~6.4 %ID/g, respectively) and significant clearance via the spleen and liver of hPBMC-engrafted mice compared to controls at 24 h p.i. Natarajan et al. further evaluated hPD-1 targeting of [64Cu]DOTA-pembrolizumab to hPD-1[+] 293T cells engrafted to NOD-scid IL-2Rγ[null] mice and hPBMC i.v. injected to NSG mice with subcutaneous A375 tumors to determine hPD-1 specificity and to calculate estimated human radiation dosimetry [323]. PET-CT revealed distinct and blockable tracer uptake in hPD-1 expressing 293T xenografts at 24 h and 48 h p.i., with significant initial retention in the heart, slow clearance from the liver, and gradual accumulation in the spleen. Mice with engrafted hPBMC displayed blockable hPD-1-specific tracer targeting to TILs in A375 tumors compared to controls, but with faster clearance from the heart, liver, and spleen compared to 293T engrafted mice. Human dosimetry estimates (OLINDA/EXM v 1.2 software from in vivo and ex vivo PET ROI's) further found the liver as dose-limiting, but calculations were still within acceptable limits.

England et al. synthesized a [89Zr]Df-labeled conjugate of the FDA-approved PD-1 specific mAb, nivolumab, and evaluated [89Zr]Df-nivolumab for tracking CD4[+]/CD8[+] TILs in NSG mice and human peripheral blood lymphocytes-severe combined immunodeficiency (PBL) mice, each bearing A549 lung cancer tumors [324]. PBL mice were used as a positive control, as they are known to experience chronic graft-versus-host disease (GvHD), and thus display enhanced T cell activation and infiltration in lacrimal and salivary glands. PET imaging (performed at 3 h, 6 h, 12 h, 24 h, 48 h, 72 h, and 168 h p.i.) revealed higher tracer uptake in the tumor (at 72 h and 168 h p.i.) and salivary glands (24–168 h p.i.) of PBL mice compared to NSG mice. Moreover, [89Zr]Df-nivolumab showed higher tumor (3–168 h p.i.) and salivary gland (6–168 h p.i.) uptake in PBL mice compared to the [89Zr]Df-IgG control. Ex vivo IHC (anti-hCD3 and anti-hPD-1 staining) confirmed the presence of TILs in the tumor, spleen, salivary glands, and lungs.

Doxorubicin-loaded liposomes were formulated (1,2-distearoyl-*sn*-glycero-3-phosphocholine (DSPC), cholesterol, 1,2-distearoyl-*sn*-glycero-3-phosphoethanol-amine (DSPE) conjugated to IRDye800CW (near-infrared (NIR) fluorescent dye, 0.1 mol%), DSPE conjugated to DOTA (2 mol%), and DSPE-PEG conjugated to the rat IgG2a PD-1 mAb (RMP1-14, 2.5 mol%)) and labeled with [64Cu]copper to evaluate PD-1-specific targeting and therapy in 4T1-fLuc (luciferase-expressing) mammary tumor-bearing female Balb/c mice [325]. In vivo fluorescence imaging and BLI showed 4T1-fLuc-specific accumulation of liposomes at 24 h p.i., while PET imaging revealed PD-1-specific localization of targeting liposomes in tumors. Significant tracer uptake was also noted for the spleen, liver, and kidneys in all groups. Moreover, PD-1 targeting doxorubicin-loaded liposomes significantly reduced tumors volumes (monitored for 15 days) and prolonged animal survival (up to 80 days) compared to control groups (under 50 days). This study highlights the immense multimodal potential of nanotechnology as it pertains to the specific detection of activated T cells, in vivo imaging with fluorophores/radioisotopes, and target-specific therapy with chemotherapeutics. Future studies, therefore, have multiple options for selecting from a host of targeting agents, contrasts, and drugs for site-specific theranostics.

3.3.4.2 Anti-CD152 (CTLA-4) mAb

CTLA-4 (CD152) is a transmembrane receptor that is upregulated by activated T cells and outcompetes the co-stimulatory protein, CD28, for binding with CD80 and CD86, and thus leads to T cell suppression [318]. CTLA-4 has been exploited as a target for ICB therapy, and therefore, agents specific for CTLA-4 have potential for in vivo labeling and tracking activated T cells. For example, Higashikawa et al. developed a [^{64}Cu]DOTA-labeled conjugate of an anti-mouse CTLA-4 (CD152) mAb (~4 DOTA/mAb) and evaluated anti-cytotoxic T lymphocyte-associated protein 4 (CTLA-4)-specific targeting of CT29 mouse colon tumors in BALB/c and BALB/c nude (*nu/nu*; thymus-deficient) mice by PET imaging [326]. PET imaging showed higher tumor retention of [^{64}Cu]DOTA-anti-CTLA-4 mAb (SUV$_{max}$ = 2.65 ± 0.01) compared to the nonspecific control conjugate ([^{64}Cu]DOTA-IgG, SUV$_{max}$ = 2.06 ± 0.32) at 48 h p.i. (Fig. 3.11) (but not at 24 h p.i.). Furthermore, in vitro assays for the expression of T cell markers from normal colon cells, cultured CT29 cells, and CT29 tumors from BALB/c and BALB/c nude control mice linked tracer uptake in CT29 tumors with CD4, CD8, Foxp3, FR4, CD69, CD154, and

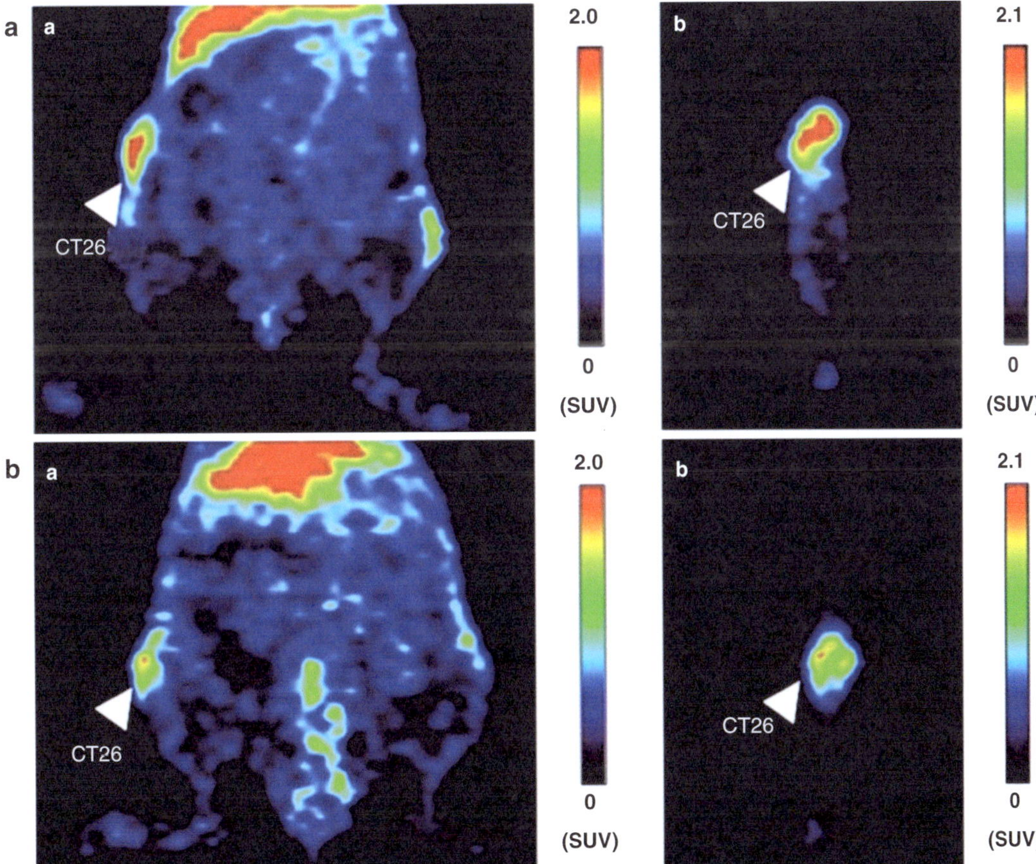

Fig. 3.11 PET images showing accumulation of (**a**) [^{64}Cu]DOTA-anti-CTLA-4 mAb and the (**b**) [^{64}Cu]DOTA-IgG control ((a) coronal and (b) sagittal views) in CT26 tumor-bearing BALB/c mice. (Adapted from Higashikawa et al., PLoS One, 2014 [327])

CD25 that was likely expressed by Tregs and activated TILs. As CTLA-4 ICB therapy becomes more mainstream, additional mAbs may be introduced that would also serve as ligands capable of activated T cell tracking. Such tracers would be useful for stratifying patients into potential responder/non-responder groups for subsequent anti-CTLA-4 therapy, for monitoring anti-CTLA-4 treatment outcomes, and/or for deciding treatment interventions.

3.3.4.3 Anti-CD3 mAb

The CD3 receptor has been routinely stained by IHC to confirm the presence of T cells, and therefore, presents a useful target for labeling and tracking T cells in vivo. For example, Malviya et al. synthesized a [99mTc]HYNIC-labeled conjugate of the CD3-specific mAb, visilizumab, and evaluated the ability of [99mTc]HYNIC-visilizumab to track TILs [328]. Specifically, these investigations involved the inoculation of HuT78 human lymphoma cells in athymic nude BALB/c *nu/nu* mice and in SCID mice reconstituted with hPBMCs (8×10^6) following NK cell and monocyte depletion (3 Gy whole-body ^{137}Cs irradiation). Gamma-camera imaging (6 h and 24 h p.i.) detected [99mTc]HYNIC-visilizumab uptake in HuT78 ($5–20 \times 10^6$) cells subcutaneously injected in the legs of BALB/c *nu/nu* mice and also showed enhanced tracer uptake in HuT78 (2×10^7) cells compared to contralateral CD3$^-$ TPC1 (2×10^7) control cells. Scintigraphic imaging (15–180 min p.i.) and ex vivo anti-CD3 IHC suggested that i.v. injected [99mTc]HYNIC-visilizumab bound to circulating CD3$^+$ T cells and subsequently tracked accumulation to the spleen, liver, and GI tract in SCID mice, while the [99mTc]HYNIC-IgG2 control conjugate remained largely in circulation after 3 h p.i. These investigations demonstrated a CD3-targeting strategy for tracking T cells and may be further applied to patient stratification regimes for predicting responders of visilizumab therapy.

The use of anti-CD3 mAb conjugates was also explored by Larimer et al., who reported a PET imaging strategy wherein a [89Zr]Df-Bz-anti-CD3 conjugate was employed to assess female BALB/c mice with CT29 tumors as responders or non-responders to anti-CTLA-4 therapy with a murine anti-CTLA-4 mAb (3×200 ng i.p.) compared to untreated (saline-injected) mice [329]. Mice that showed reduced tumor volumes at 17 days post-CTLA-4 treatment (responders) provided PET images (injected 11 days post-treatment and scanned on day 14) showing higher tumor-to-liver (known to contain CD3$^+$ T cells) ratios compared to non-responder mice (Fig. 3.12). This method illustrated the use of PET imaging for assessing CD3-based imaging of TILs as a correlate of anti-CTLA-4 immunotherapy response. More recently, Beckford Vera et al. used PET imaging, ex vivo biodistribution studies, and flow cytometry to evaluate the [89Zr]DFO-anti-CD3 mAb conjugate for detecting activated CD3$^+$ TILs in C57BL/6J mice with BBN975 syngeneic bladder tumors compared to the isotype control tracer, [89Zr]DFO-IgG2b [330]. PET imaging of healthy and tumor-bearing mice at 72 h p.i. showed [89Zr]DFO-anti-CD3 mAb accumulation in the thymus, spleen, LNs (cervical, axillary, and inguinal), and tumors. While ex vivo biodistribution revealed similar tumor uptake of [89Zr]DFO-IgG2b ($9.99 \pm 1.81\%$ID/g) compared to [89Zr]DFO-anti-CD3 mAb ($7.20 \pm 4.79\%$ID/g), this was likely nonspecific, as significant isotype control tracer remained in circulation ($8.3 \pm 0.37\%$ID/g versus $0.5 \pm 0.05\%$ID/g for anti-CD3 conjugate) at 72 h p.i. Flow cytometry performed on resected tumors found increases in total CD8$^+$ T$_{CM}$ (CD14$^-$NK1.1$^-$ CD44$^+$ and CD62L$^+$) and CD8$^+$ effector memory T cells (CD14$^-$NK1.1$^-$ CD44$^+$ and CD62L$^-$) with reduced CD4$^+$ T cells in response to anti-CD3 mAb injections. As this shift in TIL populations has been correlated with immunotherapy response, it was suggested that anti-CD3 mAbs may also serve as potential immune system modulators.

3.3.4.4 Anti-CD8 mAb

The CD8 receptor of T cells presents a useful target for in vivo labeling and cell tracking. Tavaré et al. generated the [89Zr]malDFO-labeled anti-CD8 cys-diabody (dimer of scFv) conjugate, [89Zr]malDFO-169 cDb, and employed PET imaging (at 22 h p.i.) to determine its use for assessing outcomes of AT T cell therapy (MHC-

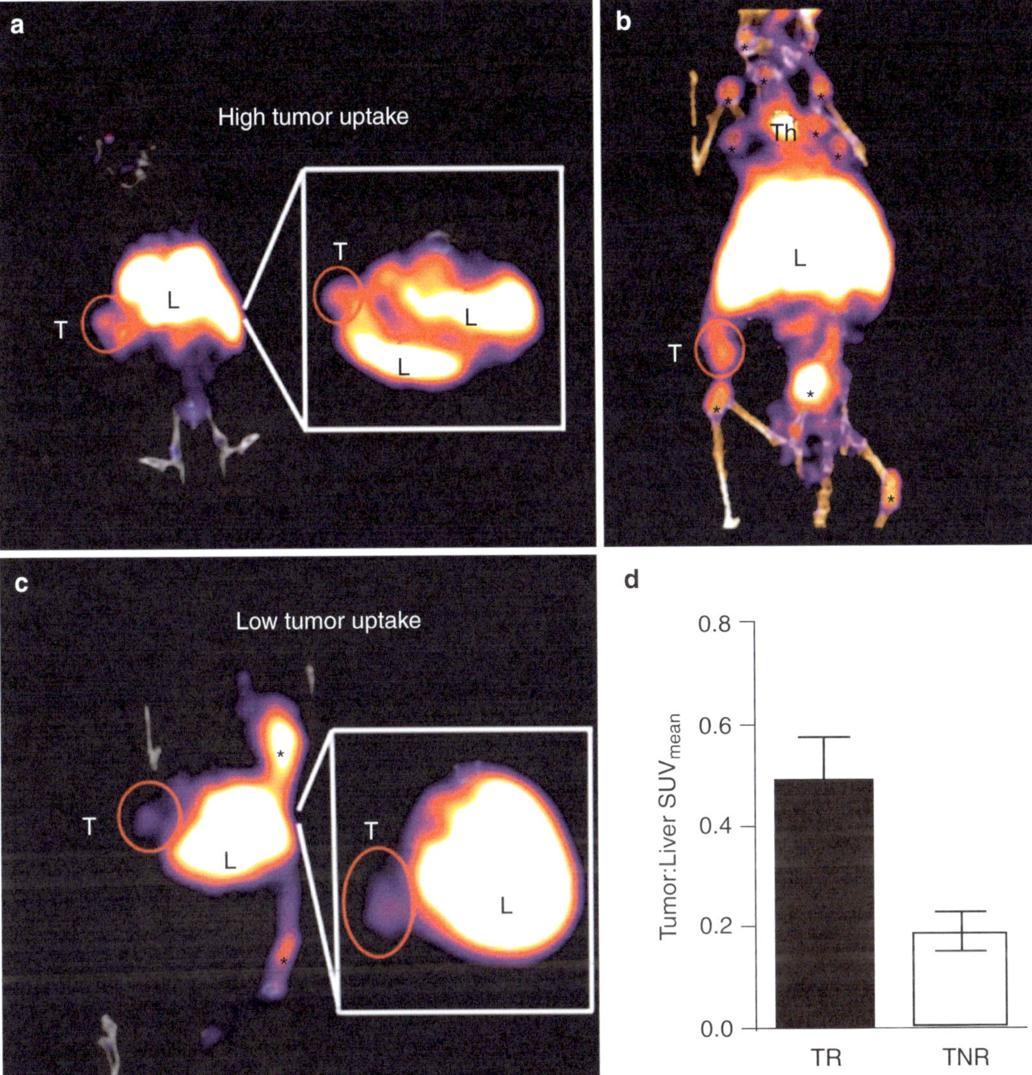

Fig. 3.12 PET-CT images showing the accumulation of [⁸⁹Zr]Df-Bz-anti-CD3 in CT29 tumor-bearing female BALB/c mice designated as responders (**a** and **c**) or non-responders (**b**) to murine anti-CTLA-4 mAb therapy with (**d**) tumor:liver SUV measurements. *L* liver, *Th* thymus, *T* tumor, *TR* treatment responders, *TNR* treatment non-responders. (Adapted from Larimer et al., J Nucl Med, 2016 [329])

I-restricted TCR specific for OVA), anti-CD137 mAb (clone 3H3) agonistic immunotherapy, and anti-PD-L1 mAb (clone 10F.9G2) ICB [331]. C57BL/6 mice, following BM transplantation and vaccination with OVA$_{257-264}$ peptide-pulsed DCs, with contralateral EL4-Ova and EL4 tumors were injected with OVA-targeting T cells (activated in vivo with supplemented IL-2) and [⁸⁹Zr] malDFO-169 cDb. PET imaging and ex vivo biodistribution revealed blockable tracer uptake in

EL4-Ova tumors and the axillary LN beside EL4-Ova tumors. Balb/c mice with CT29 tumors that were treated with anti-CD137 mAb therapy also exhibited blockable tracer uptake in tumors that corresponded to CD8$^+$ TILs stained by IHC, whereas untreated mice showed tracer uptake at the periphery of tumors due to resident CD8$^+$ T cells and non-specific tracer retention due to EPR. Similarly, CT29 tumor-bearing Balb/c mice that responded to anti-PD-L1 mAb therapy displayed higher tracer uptake in the tumor and had greater CD45+CD8+ TILs compared to non-responders and untreated mice. The summary of these results suggested that anti-CD8 PET imaging may be employed to stratify candidates for immunotherapy based on expected CD8+ TIL recruitment.

Rashidian et al. evaluated a 20-kDa PEGylated anti-CD8 single-binding domain fragment (VHH-X118) labeled with [89Zr]Df to evaluate the use of PET imaging for assessing responders and non-responders to anti-CTLA-4 immunotherapy in C57BL/6 mice with either B16 melanoma, mesenchymal PB3, or epithelial PB2 breast cancer tumors [332]. PET imaging revealed that mice treated with GVAX (granulocyte-macrophage colony-stimulating factor (GM-CSF)-secreting whole-cell melanoma vaccine) and anti-CTLA-4 mAb (7 days after inoculation) that exhibited a strong response to therapy also displayed homogenous tracer distribution in tumors. Moreover, PET imaging showed homogeneous activity in PB2 tumors from mice that responded to anti-CTLA-4 mAb therapy compared to untreated controls, while heterogeneous patterns of activity were observed in PB3 tumors that progressed similarly to respective control mice. By monitoring the presence of CD8+ TILs and their level of homogeneity in tumors, this report highlighted methods that can be applied to PET imaging analysis to help predict response to anti-CTLA-4 mAb therapy.

3.3.4.5 OX40 (CD134)

In addition to CD152, CD3 and CD8, other cell surface receptors displayed by activated T cells may be targeted for in vivo labeling and cell tracking studies. For example, Alam et al. described the synthesis and in vivo evaluation of a [64Cu]DOTA-labeled mAb conjugate ([64Cu]DOTA-AbOX40) with specificity for the cell surface receptor, OX40 (CD135), expressed by antigen-specific activated T cells [333]. Specifically, [64Cu]DOTA-AbOX40-enabled PET imaging was used to monitor tumor response to in situ vaccination with 50 µg CpG (ssDNA with unmethylated cytosine-guanine) in dual contra-lateral A20 lymphoma tumor-bearing BALB/c mice. PET imaging was performed 24 h after tracer injection and showed that CpG vaccination initially enhanced tracer uptake in treated tumors (2 days p.i.), but this became nonsignificant compared to control tumors at 9 days p.i. due to the reduced volumes of treated tumors (observable 7–9 days p.i.) that coincided with enhanced CD3+ T cell recruitment. Greater tracer uptake was also observed in TDLNs associated with treated tumors and in the enlarged spleens of vaccinated mice compared to control mice. These investigations highlighted the use of an OX40/CD134-specific PET tracer that allowed tracking of activated T cells and shows promise for stratifying patient cohorts.

3.3.4.6 T Cell Receptor Targeting

Antibodies can be generated to display binding specificity toward TCRs as a means of labeling and tracking activated T cells in vivo. For example, Matsui et al. reported the development [64Cu]DOTA-anti-Thy1.2 mAb PET tracer for tracking tERK-I (epitope: QYIHSANVL)-activated AT DUC18 CD8+ TCR transgenic T cells (Thy1.2) with specificity for CMS5 fibrosarcoma tumors in BALB/c-Thy1.1 mice [334]. Eight days after CMS5 tumor cell (3 × 10^6) inoculation, mice were i.v. injected with 4 × 10^7 ex vivo-activated Thy1.2 cells, and PET imaging was performed (12 h p.i.) after 14 days, 7 days, or 4 days of Thy1.2 cell infusions. PET imaging revealed higher tracer uptake in tumors of mice injected with Thy1.2 cells 4 days prior to imaging (1.97 %ID/g) compared to mice injected 7 days prior (0.71 %ID/g, only residual tumors remained near inoculation sites), while tumors were not detected in the final group. These results demonstrate that signal intensity was inversely correlated with tumor size, as the CMS5-targeting transgenic T cells displayed both tumor homing and anti-tumor activity. The tracer also showed Thy1.2 cell accumulation in the spleen and in the inguinal, brachial, and axial lymph nodes for all groups, each with higher activity compared to saline-injected control mice.

3.3.4.7 Granzyme B

Granzyme B is a serine-protease that is expressed by activated CD8[+] T cells and NK cells and has been implicated to mediate anti-tumor response by CTLs [335]. Larimer et al. developed a [^{68}Ga]NOTA-labeled conjugate of the granzyme B-specific peptide (βA-GG-**IEFD**-OH; GZP) and evaluated CTL-associated detection of granzyme B in CT26 tumor-bearing BALB/c mice by PET imaging. Specifically, 14 days after tumor cell inoculation, mice that were treated with anti-PD-L1 therapy, combined anti-PD-L1 and anti-CTLA-4 therapy or vehicle, were i.v. injected with [^{68}Ga]NOTA-BZP and monitored by PET at 1 h p.i. Images were processed to employ tumor-to-blood ratios (TBR) as a proxy measure of differential granzyme B retention in tumors. This showed enhanced granzyme B presence in mice that underwent combined therapy (TBR = 1.83 ± 0.18) and monotherapy (TBR = 1.29 ± 0.12), compared to untreated (TBR = 0.96 ± 0.11) control mice. Moreover, mice that responded to therapy showed higher tumor uptake of [^{68}Ga]NOTA-BZP compared to mice that did not display tumor regression. In vitro investigations suggested that granzyme B content was CD8-independent and was released by CTL within tumor cells. This trend was also observed with human melanoma biopsy samples that showed a positive correlation between granzyme B content and tumor regression post-ICB therapy. Thus, granzyme B may serve as a useful biomarker for future clinical investigations, whereby tumor uptake of granzyme B-specific tracers may predict therapeutic response for patients undergoing ICB therapy.

3.4 Conclusions

This chapter has presented summaries of reports that have employed a wide array of strategies for labeling and monitoring activated T cells within the context of preclinical and clinical cancer investigations. The overarching goal of this chapter was to highlight the key results of each study in order to provide readers with a host of options for accomplishing efficient T cell labeling and methods for assessing in vivo migration by PET, SPECT, or planar γ-camera imaging. The convergence of nanotechnology with CIT particularly broadens the range of strategies available for multimodal imaging and for the development of agents with theranostic capability. While each labeling strategy is accompanied by inherent advantages that can be capitalized, challenges have also been identified that must be mitigated. Briefly, ex vivo direct labeling of T cells provides a convenient means for optimizing labeling efficiency, labeling stability, cell viability and targeting specificity prior to in vivo administration. Indirect labeling methods include the use of reporter genes, metabolic targeting approaches, and high-affinity targeting ligands. While indirect in vivo labeling may be relatively more prone to nonspecific tracer uptake by healthy tissues, these strategies are not significantly hindered by the dilution of tracers upon cell proliferation and allows for convenient serial administration of tracers for longitudinal cell tracking.

CIT, particularly the use of radioimmunotherapy, ICB, and ATC therapy, holds promise for effective and safe cancer treatment. Yet, the high cost of most CIT and challenges related to patient stratification presents clinicians with significant hurdles. The complex nature of CIT that encompasses a range of dynamic interactions between immune cells and cancer cells, thus, demands a clear understanding of how immune cell functions and migration patterns relate to treatment effectiveness. The use of combined CITs further elevates the level of complexity of these cellular interactions. The goal of T cell tracking investigations, therefore, is to provide accurate insights for linking migration patterns of activated T cells to clinical therapeutic outcomes. For example, treatment costs may be significantly reduced if image-guided screenings could distinguish patients as likely responders for the selected CIT regimes. Moreover, accurate assessments during the course of CIT would distinguish patients that display expected responses from those requiring treatment interventions. As the safety, feasibility, and merits of immune cell tracking continue to become evaluated in clinical settings, results of these studies should inspire preclinical efforts to provide solutions to address challenges. This reciprocal relationship between clinical evaluations and preclinical discoveries could lead to the development of optimized tracers, labeling methods, treatment protocols, and assessment criteria for maximizing the benefits of CIT.Conflicts of InterestThe authors report no conflict of interest with the material presented in this study. Dr. François Bénard is co-founder, director, and shareholder of Alpha-9 Theranostics, a radiopharmaceutical company. No other potential conflicts of interest relevant to this article exist.

References

1. Miller JF, Sadelain M. The journey from discoveries in fundamental immunology to cancer immunotherapy. Cancer Cell. 2015;27(4):439–49. https://doi.org/10.1016/j.ccell.2015.03.007.

2. Ayed AO, Chang LJ, Moreb JS. Immunotherapy for multiple myeloma: current status and future directions. Crit Rev Oncol Hematol. 2015;96(3):399–412. https://doi.org/10.1016/j.critrevonc.2015.06.006.

3. Littman DR. Releasing the brakes on cancer immunotherapy. Cell. 2015;162(6):1186–90. https://doi.org/10.1016/j.cell.2015.08.038.

4. Sharma P, Allison JP. Immune checkpoint targeting in cancer therapy: toward combination strategies with curative potential. Cell. 2015;161(2):205–14. https://doi.org/10.1016/j.cell.2015.03.030.

5. Palucka AK, Coussens LM. The basis of oncoimmunology. Cell. 2016;164(6):1233–47. https://doi.org/10.1016/j.cell.2016.01.049.

6. Emens LA, Ascierto PA, Darcy PK, Demaria S, Eggermont AMM, Redmond WL, et al. Cancer immunotherapy: opportunities and challenges in the rapidly evolving clinical landscape. Eur J Cancer. 2017;81:116–29. https://doi.org/10.1016/j.ejca.2017.01.035.

7. Jung SH, Lee HJ, Vo MC, Kim HJ, Lee JJ. Immunotherapy for the treatment of multiple myeloma. Crit Rev Oncol Hematol. 2017;111:87–93. https://doi.org/10.1016/j.critrevonc.2017.01.011.

8. Rasche L, Weinhold N, Morgan GJ, van Rhee F, Davies FE. Immunologic approaches for the treatment of multiple myeloma. Cancer Treat Rev. 2017;55:190–9. https://doi.org/10.1016/j.ctrv.2017.03.010.

9. Franchina DG, Dostert C, Brenner D. Reactive oxygen species: involvement in T cell signaling and metabolism. Trends Immunol. 2018;39(6):489–502. https://doi.org/10.1016/j.it.2018.01.005.

10. Spitzer MH, Carmi Y, Reticker-Flynn NE, Kwek SS, Madhireddy D, Martins MM, et al. Systemic immunity is required for effective cancer immunotherapy. Cell. 2017;168(3):487–502.e15. https://doi.org/10.1016/j.cell.2016.12.022.

11. Madden DL. From a patient advocate's perspective: does cancer immunotherapy represent a paradigm shift? Curr Oncol Rep. 2018;20(1):8. https://doi.org/10.1007/s11912-018-0662-5.

12. Tang J, Shalabi A, Hubbard-Lucey VM. Comprehensive analysis of the clinical immuno-oncology landscape. Ann Oncol. 2018;29(1):84–91. https://doi.org/10.1093/annonc/mdx755.

13. Danhof S, Hudecek M, Smith EL. CARs and other T cell therapies for MM: the clinical experience. Best Pract Res Clin Haematol. 2018;31(2):147–57. https://doi.org/10.1016/j.beha.2018.03.002.

14. Suck G, Koh MBC. Emerging natural killer cell immunotherapies: large-scale ex vivo production of highly potent anticancer effectors. Hematol Oncol Stem Cell Ther. 2010;3(3):135–42.

15. Granzin M, Soltenborn S, Muller S, Kollet J, Berg M, Cerwenka A, et al. Fully automated expansion and activation of clinical-grade natural killer cells for adoptive immunotherapy. Cytotherapy. 2015;17(5):621–32. https://doi.org/10.1016/j.jcyt.2015.03.611.

16. Fang F, Xiao W, Tian Z. NK cell-based immunotherapy for cancer. Semin Immunol. 2017;31:37–54. https://doi.org/10.1016/j.smim.2017.07.009.

17. Malmberg KJ, Carlsten M, Bjorklund A, Sohlberg E, Bryceson YT, Ljunggren HG. Natural killer cell-mediated immunosurveillance of human cancer. Semin Immunol. 2017;31:20–9. https://doi.org/10.1016/j.smim.2017.08.002.

18. Lin C, Zhang J. Reformation in chimeric antigen receptor based cancer immunotherapy: redirecting natural killer cell. Biochim Biophys Acta Rev Cancer. 2018;1869(2):200–15. https://doi.org/10.1016/j.bbcan.2018.01.005.

19. Daher M, Rezvani K. Next generation natural killer cells for cancer immunotherapy: the promise of genetic engineering. Curr Opin Immunol. 2018;51:146–53. https://doi.org/10.1016/j.coi.2018.03.013.

20. Andón FT, Digifico E, Maeda A, Erreni M, Mantovani A, Alonso MJ, et al., editors. Targeting tumor associated macrophages: the new challenge for nanomedicine, Seminars in immunology. Amsterdam: Elsevier; 2017.

21. Dudley ME, Wunderlich JR, Robbins PF, Yang JC, Hwu P, Schwartzentruber DJ, et al. Cancer regression and autoimmunity in patients after clonal repopulation with antitumor lymphocytes. Science. 2002;298(5594):850–4.

22. Park TS, Rosenberg SA, Morgan RA. Treating cancer with genetically engineered T cells. Trends Biotechnol. 2011;29(11):550–7. https://doi.org/10.1016/j.tibtech.2011.04.009.

23. Wang M, Yin B, Wang HY, Wang R-F. Current advances in T-cell-based cancer immunotherapy. Immunotherapy. 2014;6(12):1265–78.

24. Parkhurst MR, Yang JC, Langan RC, Dudley ME, Nathan DA, Feldman SA, et al. T cells targeting carcinoembryonic antigen can mediate regression of metastatic colorectal cancer but induce severe transient colitis. Mol Ther. 2011;19(3):620–6. https://doi.org/10.1038/mt.2010.272.

25. Wu CY, Rupp LJ, Roybal KT, Lim WA. Synthetic biology approaches to engineer T cells. Curr Opin Immunol. 2015;35:123–30. https://doi.org/10.1016/j.coi.2015.06.015.

26. Klebanoff CA, Restifo NP. Customizing functionality and payload delivery for receptor-engineered T cells. Cell. 2016;167(2):304–6. https://doi.org/10.1016/j.cell.2016.09.033.

27. Johnson LA, June CH. Driving gene-engineered T cell immunotherapy of cancer. Cell Res. 2017;27(1):38–58. https://doi.org/10.1038/cr.2016.154.

28. Yee C. Adoptive T cell therapy: points to consider. Curr Opin Immunol. 2018;51:197–203. https://doi.org/10.1016/j.coi.2018.04.007.

29. Tyler CJ, Doherty DG, Moser B, Eberl M. Human Vgamma9/Vdelta2 T cells: innate adaptors of the immune system. Cell Immunol. 2015;296(1):10–21. https://doi.org/10.1016/j.cellimm.2015.01.008.

30. Chitadze G, Oberg H-H, Wesch D, Kabelitz D. The ambiguous role of γδ T lymphocytes in antitumor immunity. Trends Immunol. 2017;38(9):668–78.

31. Kabelitz D. Human γδ T cells: from a neglected lymphocyte population to cellular immunotherapy: a personal reflection of 30 years of γδ T cell research. Clin Immunol. 2016;100(172):90–7.

32. Allegra A, Innao V, Gerace D, Vaddinelli D, Musolino C. Adoptive immunotherapy for hematological malignancies: current status and new insights in chimeric antigen receptor T cells. Blood Cells Mol Dis. 2016;62:49–63. https://doi.org/10.1016/j.bcmd.2016.11.001.

33. Blidner AG, Marino KV, Rabinovich GA. Driving CARs into sweet roads: targeting glycosylated antigens in cancer. Immunity. 2016;44(6):1248–50. https://doi.org/10.1016/j.immuni.2016.06.010.

34. Brown CE, Adusumilli PS. Next frontiers in CAR T-cell therapy. Mol Ther Oncolytics. 2016;3:16028. https://doi.org/10.1038/mto.2016.28.

35. Fesnak A, Lin C, Siegel DL, Maus MV. CAR-T cell therapies from the transfusion medicine perspective. Transfus Med Rev. 2016;30(3):139–45. https://doi.org/10.1016/j.tmrv.2016.03.001.

36. Gad AZ, El-Naggar S, Ahmed N. Realism and pragmatism in developing an effective chimeric antigen receptor T-cell product for solid cancers. Cytotherapy. 2016;18(11):1382–92. https://doi.org/10.1016/j.jcyt.2016.07.004.

37. Geyer MB, Brentjens RJ. Review: Current clinical applications of chimeric antigen receptor (CAR) modified T cells. Cytotherapy. 2016;18(11):1393–409. https://doi.org/10.1016/j.jcyt.2016.07.003.

38. Gill S, Maus MV, Porter DL. Chimeric antigen receptor T cell therapy: 25 years in the making. Blood Rev. 2016;30(3):157–67. https://doi.org/10.1016/j.blre.2015.10.003.

39. Newick K, Moon E, Albelda SM. Chimeric antigen receptor T-cell therapy for solid tumors. Mol Ther Oncolytics. 2016;3:16006. https://doi.org/10.1038/mto.2016.6.

40. Sadelain M. Chimeric antigen receptors: driving immunology towards synthetic biology. Curr Opin Immunol. 2016;41:68–76. https://doi.org/10.1016/j.coi.2016.06.004.

41. Smith AJ, Oertle J, Warren D, Prato D. Chimeric antigen receptor (CAR) T cell therapy for malignant cancers: summary and perspective. J Cell Immunother. 2016;2(2):59–68. https://doi.org/10.1016/j.jocit.2016.08.001.

42. Wang X, Riviere I. Clinical manufacturing of CAR T cells: foundation of a promising therapy. Mol Ther Oncolytics. 2016;3:16015. https://doi.org/10.1038/mto.2016.15.

43. Bollino D, Webb TJ. Chimeric antigen receptor-engineered natural killer and natural killer T cells for cancer immunotherapy. Transl Res. 2017;187:32–43. https://doi.org/10.1016/j.trsl.2017.06.003.

44. Chang ZL, Chen YY. CARs: synthetic immunoreceptors for cancer therapy and beyond. Trends Mol Med. 2017;23(5):430–50. https://doi.org/10.1016/j.molmed.2017.03.002.

45. de Wilde S, Guchelaar HJ, Zandvliet ML, Meij P. Understanding clinical development of chimeric antigen receptor T cell therapies. Cytotherapy. 2017;19(6):703–9. https://doi.org/10.1016/j.jcyt.2017.03.070.

46. Frey N. The what, when and how of CAR T cell therapy for ALL. Best Pract Res Clin Haematol. 2017;30(3):275–81. https://doi.org/10.1016/j.beha.2017.07.009.

47. Han S, Latchoumanin O, Wu G, Zhou G, Hebbard L, George J, et al. Recent clinical trials utilizing chimeric antigen receptor T cells therapies against solid tumors. Cancer Lett. 2017;390:188–200. https://doi.org/10.1016/j.canlet.2016.12.037.

48. Jaspers JE, Brentjens RJ. Development of CAR T cells designed to improve antitumor efficacy and safety. Pharmacol Ther. 2017;178:83–91. https://doi.org/10.1016/j.pharmthera.2017.03.012.

49. Lim WA, June CH. The principles of engineering immune cells to treat cancer. Cell. 2017;168(4):724–40. https://doi.org/10.1016/j.cell.2017.01.016.

50. Riviere I, Sadelain M. Chimeric antigen receptors: a cell and gene therapy perspective. Mol Ther. 2017;25(5):1117–24. https://doi.org/10.1016/j.ymthe.2017.03.034.

51. Kenderian SS, Porter DL, Gill S. Chimeric antigen receptor T cells and hematopoietic cell transplantation: how not to put the CART before the horse.

Biol Blood Marrow Transplant. 2017;23(2):235–46. https://doi.org/10.1016/j.bbmt.2016.09.002.

52. Zheng PP, Kros JM, Li J. Approved CAR T cell therapies: ice bucket challenges on glaring safety risks and long-term impacts. Drug Discov Today. 2018;23(6):1175–82. https://doi.org/10.1016/j.drudis.2018.02.012.

53. Si W, Li C, Wei P. Synthetic immunology: T-cell engineering and adoptive immunotherapy. Synth Syst Biotechnol. 2018;3(3):179–85. https://doi.org/10.1016/j.synbio.2018.08.001.

54. Siddiqi HF, Staser KW, Nambudiri VE. Research techniques made simple: CAR T-cell therapy. J Invest Dermatol. 2018;138(12):2501–4.e1. https://doi.org/10.1016/j.jid.2018.09.002.

55. Ramello MC, Haura EB, Abate-Daga D. CAR-T cells and combination therapies: what's next in the immunotherapy revolution? Pharmacol Res. 2018;129:194–203. https://doi.org/10.1016/j.phrs.2017.11.035.

56. Grupp S. Beginning the CAR T cell therapy revolution in the US and EU. Curr Res Transl Med. 2018;66(2):62–4. https://doi.org/10.1016/j.retram.2018.03.004.

57. Halim L, Ajina A, Maher J. Pre-clinical development of chimeric antigen receptor T-cell immunotherapy: implications of design for efficacy and safety. Best Pract Res Clin Haematol. 2018;31(2):117–25. https://doi.org/10.1016/j.beha.2018.04.002.

58. Calmels B, Mfarrej B, Chabannon C. From clinical proof-of-concept to commercialization of CAR T cells. Drug Discov Today. 2018;23(4):758–62. https://doi.org/10.1016/j.drudis.2018.01.024.

59. Chen N, Li X, Chintala NK, Tano ZE, Adusumilli PS. Driving CARs on the uneven road of antigen heterogeneity in solid tumors. Curr Opin Immunol. 2018;51:103–10. https://doi.org/10.1016/j.coi.2018.03.002.

60. Minn AJ, Wherry EJ. Combination cancer therapies with immune checkpoint blockade: convergence on interferon signaling. Cell. 2016;165(2):272–5. https://doi.org/10.1016/j.cell.2016.03.031.

61. Gibney GT, Weiner LM, Atkins MB. Predictive biomarkers for checkpoint inhibitor-based immunotherapy. Lancet Oncol. 2016;17(12):e542–e51. https://doi.org/10.1016/s1470-2045(16)30406-5.

62. Gay F, D'Agostino M, Giaccone L, Genuardi M, Festuccia M, Boccadoro M, et al. Immuno-oncologic approaches: CAR-T cells and checkpoint inhibitors. Clin Lymphoma Myeloma Leuk. 2017;17(8):471–8. https://doi.org/10.1016/j.clml.2017.06.014.

63. Shao J, Xu Q, Su S, Meng F, Zou Z, Chen F, et al. Engineered cells for costimulatory enhancement combined with IL-21 enhance the generation of PD-1-disrupted CTLs for adoptive immunotherapy. Cell Immunol. 2017;320:38–45. https://doi.org/10.1016/j.cellimm.2017.09.003.

64. Jacobson CA, Armand P. Immunotherapy in aggressive B-cell lymphomas. Best Pract Res Clin Haematol. 2018;31(3):299–305. https://doi.org/10.1016/j.beha.2018.07.015.

65. Roybal KT, Rupp LJ, Morsut L, Walker WJ, McNally KA, Park JS, et al. Precision tumor recognition by T cells with combinatorial antigen-sensing circuits. Cell. 2016;164(4):770–9. https://doi.org/10.1016/j.cell.2016.01.011.

66. Themeli M, Sadelain M. Combinatorial antigen targeting: ideal T-cell sensing and anti-tumor response. Trends Mol Med. 2016;22(4):271–3. https://doi.org/10.1016/j.molmed.2016.02.009.

67. Biggs MJ, Milone MC, Santos LC, Gondarenko A, Wind SJ. High-resolution imaging of the immunological synapse and T-cell receptor microclustering through microfabricated substrates. J R Soc Interface. 2011;8(63):1462–71. https://doi.org/10.1098/rsif.2011.0025.

68. Illingworth JJ, Anton van der Merwe P. Dissecting T-cell activation with high-resolution live-cell microscopy. Immunology. 2012;135(3):198–206. https://doi.org/10.1111/j.1365-2567.2011.03537.x.

69. Neve-Oz Y, Razvag Y, Sajman J, Sherman E. Mechanisms of localized activation of the T cell antigen receptor inside clusters. Biochim Biophys Acta. 2015;1853(4):810–21. https://doi.org/10.1016/j.bbamcr.2014.09.025.

70. Chang CH, Qiu J, O'Sullivan D, Buck MD, Noguchi T, Curtis JD, et al. Metabolic competition in the tumor microenvironment is a driver of cancer progression. Cell. 2015;162(6):1229–41. https://doi.org/10.1016/j.cell.2015.08.016.

71. Zitvogel L, Ayyoub M, Routy B, Kroemer G. Microbiome and anticancer immunosurveillance. Cell. 2016;165(2):276–87. https://doi.org/10.1016/j.cell.2016.03.001.

72. Hu KH, Butte MJ. T cell activation requires force generation. J Cell Biol. 2016;213(5):535–42. https://doi.org/10.1083/jcb.201511053.

73. Le Borgne M, Raju S, Zinselmeyer BH, Le VT, Li J, Wang Y, et al. Real-time analysis of calcium signals during the early phase of T cell activation using a genetically encoded calcium biosensor. J Immunol. 2016;196(4):1471–9.

74. Sathappan A, van Panhuys N. Advances in in vivo imaging techniques for the visualization and quantification of DC-T cell interactions. J Immunobiol. 2017;2:2. https://doi.org/10.4172/2476-1966.1000125.

75. Stein JV, Gonzalez SF. Dynamic intravital imaging of cell-cell interactions in the lymph node. J Allergy Clin Immunol. 2017;139(1):12–20.

76. Beaurepaire E, Pavone FS, So PTC, Gavgiotaki E, Filippidis G, Zerva I, et al. Nonlinear microscopy as diagnostic tool for the discrimination of activated T cells. Adv Microsc Imaging. 2017; https://doi.org/10.1117/12.2282895.

77. Andrejeva G, Rathmell JC. Similarities and distinctions of cancer and immune metabolism in inflam-

mation and tumors. Cell Metab. 2017;26(1):49–70. https://doi.org/10.1016/j.cmet.2017.06.004.

78. Mukherjee M, Mace EM, Carisey AF, Ahmed N, Orange JS. Quantitative imaging approaches to study the CAR immunological synapse. Mol Ther. 2017;25(8):1757–68. https://doi.org/10.1016/j.ymthe.2017.06.003.

79. Beckermann KE, Dudzinski SO, Rathmell JC. Dysfunctional T cell metabolism in the tumor microenvironment. Cytokine Growth Factor Rev. 2017;35:7–14. https://doi.org/10.1016/j.cytogfr.2017.04.003.

80. Dugnani E, Pasquale V, Bordignon C, Canu A, Piemonti L, Monti P. Integrating T cell metabolism in cancer immunotherapy. Cancer Lett. 2017;411:12–8. https://doi.org/10.1016/j.canlet.2017.09.039.

81. Ho P-C, Kaech SM. Reenergizing T cell anti-tumor immunity by harnessing immunometabolic checkpoints and machineries. Curr Opin Immunol. 2017;46:38–44.

82. Kishton RJ, Sukumar M, Restifo NP. Metabolic regulation of T cell longevity and function in tumor immunotherapy. Cell Metab. 2017;26(1):94–109. https://doi.org/10.1016/j.cmet.2017.06.016.

83. Hardaway JC, Prince E, Arepally A, Katz SC. Regional infusion of chimeric antigen receptor T cells to overcome barriers for solid tumor immunotherapy. J Vasc Intervent Radiol. 2018;29(7):1017–21.e1.

84. Xiong W, Chen Y, Kang X, Chen Z, Zheng P, Hsu YH, et al. Immunological synapse predicts effectiveness of chimeric antigen receptor cells. Mol Ther. 2018;26(4):963–75. https://doi.org/10.1016/j.ymthe.2018.01.020.

85. Zhang L, Romero P. Metabolic control of CD8+ T cell fate decisions and antitumor immunity. Trends Mol Med. 2018;24(1):30–48.

86. Moogk D, Natarajan A, Krogsgaard M. T cell receptor signal transduction: affinity, force and conformational change. Curr Opin Chem Eng. 2018;19:43–50. https://doi.org/10.1016/j.coche.2017.12.007.

87. Sukumar M, Kishton RJ, Restifo NP. Metabolic reprograming of anti-tumor immunity. Curr Opin Immunol. 2017;46:14–22.

88. Yang QY, Yang JD, Wang YS. Current strategies to improve the safety of chimeric antigen receptor (CAR) modified T cells. Immunol Lett. 2017;190:201–5. https://doi.org/10.1016/j.imlet.2017.08.018.

89. Wolchok JD, Hoos A, O'Day S, Weber JS, Hamid O, Lebbe C, et al. Guidelines for the evaluation of immune therapy activity in solid tumors: immune-related response criteria. Clin Cancer Res. 2009;15(23):7412–20. https://doi.org/10.1158/1078-0432.CCR-09-1624.

90. Bonifant CL, Jackson HJ, Brentjens RJ, Curran KJ. Toxicity and management in CAR T-cell therapy. Mol Ther Oncolytics. 2016;3:16011. https://doi.org/10.1038/mto.2016.11.

91. Pitt JM, Vetizou M, Daillere R, Roberti MP, Yamazaki T, Routy B, et al. Resistance mechanisms to immune-checkpoint blockade in cancer: tumor-intrinsic and -extrinsic factors. Immunity. 2016;44(6):1255–69. https://doi.org/10.1016/j.immuni.2016.06.001.

92. Frey N. Cytokine release syndrome: who is at risk and how to treat. Best Pract Res Clin Haematol. 2017;30(4):336–40. https://doi.org/10.1016/j.beha.2017.09.002.

93. Kim S, Moon EK. Development of novel avenues to overcome challenges facing CAR T cells. Transl Res. 2017;187:22–31. https://doi.org/10.1016/j.trsl.2017.05.009.

94. Perales MA, Kebriaei P, Kean LS, Sadelain M. Building a safer and faster CAR: seatbelts, airbags, and CRISPR. Biol Blood Marrow Transplant. 2018;24(1):27–31. https://doi.org/10.1016/j.bbmt.2017.10.017.

95. Gauthier J, Yakoub-Agha I. Chimeric antigen-receptor T-cell therapy for hematological malignancies and solid tumors: clinical data to date, current limitations and perspectives. Curr Res Transl Med. 2017;65(3):93–102. https://doi.org/10.1016/j.retram.2017.08.003.

96. Bailly C, Clery PF, Faivre-Chauvet A, Bourgeois M, Guerard F, Haddad F, et al. Immuno-PET for clinical theranostic approaches. Int J Mol Sci. 2016;18(1):57. https://doi.org/10.3390/ijms18010057.

97. Wu C, Ma G, Li J, Zheng K, Dang Y, Shi X, et al. In vivo cell tracking via (1)(8)F-fluorodeoxyglucose labeling: a review of the preclinical and clinical applications in cell-based diagnosis and therapy. Clin Imaging. 2013;37(1):28–36. https://doi.org/10.1016/j.clinimag.2012.02.023.

98. Tirumani SH, Ramaiya NH, Keraliya A, Bailey ND, Ott PA, Hodi FS, et al. Radiographic profiling of immune-related adverse events in advanced melanoma patients treated with ipilimumab. Cancer Immunol Res. 2015;3(10):1185–92.

99. Kong BY, Menzies AM, Saunders CA, Liniker E, Ramanujam S, Guminski A, et al. Residual FDG-PET metabolic activity in metastatic melanoma patients with prolonged response to anti-PD-1 therapy. Pigment Cell Melanoma Res. 2016;29(5):572–7. https://doi.org/10.1111/pcmr.12503.

100. Cottereau AS, Becker S, Broussais F, Casasnovas O, Kanoun S, Roques M, et al. Prognostic value of baseline total metabolic tumor volume (TMTV0) measured on FDG-PET/CT in patients with peripheral T-cell lymphoma (PTCL). Ann Oncol. 2016;27(4):719–24. https://doi.org/10.1093/annonc/mdw011.

101. Cho SY, Lipson EJ, Im HJ, Rowe SP, Gonzalez EM, Blackford A, et al. Prediction of response to immune checkpoint inhibitor therapy using early-time-point (18)F-FDG PET/CT imaging in patients with advanced melanoma. J Nucl Med. 2017;58(9):1421–8. https://doi.org/10.2967/jnumed.116.188839.

102. Shah NN, Nagle SJ, Torigian DA, Farwell MD, Hwang WT, Frey N, et al. Early positron emission tomography/computed tomography as a predictor of response after CTL019 chimeric antigen receptor-T-cell therapy in B-cell non-Hodgkin lymphomas. Cytotherapy. 2018;20(12):1415–8. https://doi.org/10.1016/j.jcyt.2018.10.003.

103. Mekki A, Dercle L, Lichtenstein P, Marabelle A, Michot J-M, Lambotte O, et al. Detection of immune-related adverse events by medical imaging in patients treated with anti-programmed cell death 1. Eur J Cancer. 2018;96:91–104.

104. Wang J, Hu Y, Yang S, Wei G, Zhao X, Wu W, et al. Role of fluorodeoxyglucose positron emission tomography/computed tomography in predicting the adverse effects of chimeric antigen receptor T cell therapy in patients with non-Hodgkin lymphoma. Biol Blood Marrow Transplant. 2019;25(6):1092–8. https://doi.org/10.1016/j.bbmt.2019.02.008.

105. Eisenhauer EA, Therasse P, Bogaerts J, Schwartz LH, Sargent D, Ford R, et al. New response evaluation criteria in solid tumours: revised RECIST guideline (version 1.1). Eur J Cancer. 2009;45(2):228–47.

106. Bauckneht M, Piva R, Sambuceti G, Grossi F, Morbelli S. Evaluation of response to immune checkpoint inhibitors: is there a role for positron emission tomography? World J Radiol. 2017;9(2):27–33. https://doi.org/10.4329/wjr.v9.i2.27.

107. Evangelista L, de Jong M, Del Vecchio S, Cai W. The new era of cancer immunotherapy: what can molecular imaging do to help? Clin Transl Imaging. 2017;5(4):299–301. https://doi.org/10.1007/s40336-017-0241-z.

108. Hodi FS, Hwu WJ, Kefford R, Weber JS, Daud A, Hamid O, et al. Evaluation of immune-related response criteria and RECIST v1.1 in patients with advanced melanoma treated with pembrolizumab. J Clin Oncol. 2016;34(13):1510–7. https://doi.org/10.1200/JCO.2015.64.0391.

109. Hildebrandt IJ, Gambhir SS. Molecular imaging applications for immunology. Clin Immunol. 2004;111(2):210–24. https://doi.org/10.1016/j.clim.2003.12.018.

110. Skitzki JJ, Muhitch JB, Evans SS. Tracking the elusive lymphocyte: methods of detection during adoptive immunotherapy. Immunol Investig. 2007;36(5–6):807–27. https://doi.org/10.1080/08820130701712867.

111. Nair-Gill E, Wiltzius SM, Wei XX, Cheng D, Riedinger M, Radu CG, et al. PET probes for distinct metabolic pathways have different cell specificities during immune responses in mice. J Clin Invest. 2010;120(6):2005–15. https://doi.org/10.1172/JCI41250.

112. Srinivas M, Aarntzen EH, Bulte JW, Oyen WJ, Heerschap A, de Vries IJ, et al. Imaging of cellular therapies. Adv Drug Deliv Rev. 2010;62(11):1080–93. https://doi.org/10.1016/j.addr.2010.08.009.

113. Kircher MF, Gambhir SS, Grimm J. Noninvasive cell-tracking methods. Nat Rev Clin Oncol. 2011;8(11):677–88. https://doi.org/10.1038/nrclinonc.2011.141.

114. Ottobrini L, Martelli C, Trabattoni DL, Clerici M, Lucignani G. In vivo imaging of immune cell trafficking in cancer. Eur J Nucl Med Mol Imaging. 2011;38(5):949–68. https://doi.org/10.1007/s00259-010-1687-7.

115. Youn H, Hong KJ. In vivo non invasive molecular imaging for immune cell tracking in small animals. Immune Netw. 2012;12(6):223–9. https://doi.org/10.4110/in.2012.12.6.223.

116. Leech JM, Sharif-Paghaleh E, Maher J, Livieratos L, Lechler RI, Mullen GE, et al. Whole-body imaging of adoptively transferred T cells using magnetic resonance imaging, single photon emission computed tomography and positron emission tomography techniques, with a focus on regulatory T cells. Clin Exp Immunol. 2013;172(2):169–77. https://doi.org/10.1111/cei.12087.

117. Srinivas M, Melero I, Kaempgen E, Figdor CG, de Vries IJ. Cell tracking using multimodal imaging. Contrast Media Mol Imaging. 2013;8(6):432–8. https://doi.org/10.1002/cmmi.1561.

118. Liu Z, Li Z. Molecular imaging in tracking tumor-specific cytotoxic T lymphocytes (CTLs). Theranostics. 2014;4(10):990.

119. Neri D. Imaging T cells in vivo. J Nucl Med. 2015;56(8):1135–6. https://doi.org/10.2967/jnumed.115.159533.

120. Lee HW, Gangadaran P, Kalimuthu S, Ahn BC. Advances in molecular imaging strategies for in vivo tracking of immune cells. Biomed Res Int. 2016;2016:1946585. https://doi.org/10.1155/2016/1946585.

121. Hartimath SV, Draghiciu O, van de Wall S, Manuelli V, Dierckx RA, Nijman HW, et al. Noninvasive monitoring of cancer therapy induced activated T cells using [(18)F]FB-IL-2 PET imaging. Oncoimmunology. 2017;6(1):e1248014. https://doi.org/10.1080/2162402X.2016.1248014.

122. Du Y, Jin Y, Sun W, Fang J, Zheng J, Tian J. Advances in molecular imaging of immune checkpoint targets in malignancies: current and future prospect. Eur Radiol. 2019;29(8):4294–302. https://doi.org/10.1007/s00330-018-5814-3.

123. Wei W, Jiang D, Ehlerding EB, Luo Q, Cai W. Noninvasive PET imaging of T cells. Trends Cancer. 2018;4(5):359–73. https://doi.org/10.1016/j.trecan.2018.03.009.

124. Zeelen C, Paus C, Draper D, Heskamp S, Signore A, Galli F, et al. In-vivo imaging of tumor-infiltrating immune cells: implications for cancer immunotherapy. Q J Nucl Med Mol Imaging. 2018;62(1):56–77. https://doi.org/10.23736/S1824-4785.17.03052-7.

125. Mayer AT, Gambhir SS. The immunoimaging toolbox. J Nucl Med. 2018;59(8):1174–82. https://doi.org/10.2967/jnumed.116.185967.

126. Emami-Shahri N, Foster J, Kashani R, Gazinska P, Cook C, Sosabowski J, et al. Clinically compliant spatial and temporal imaging of chimeric antigen

receptor T-cells. Nat Commun. 2018;9(1):1081. https://doi.org/10.1038/s41467-018-03524-1.

127. Adams CL, Rush CM, Smith KM, Garside P. Tracking antigen-specific lymphocytes in vivo. In: D'Ambrosio D, Sinigaglia F, editors. Cell migration in inflammation and immunity: methods and protocols. Totowa, NJ: Humana Press; 2003. p. 133–46.

128. Diken M, Pektor S, Miederer M. Harnessing the potential of noninvasive in vivo preclinical imaging of the immune system: challenges and prospects. Nanomedicine. 2016;11(20):2711–22.

129. Hong H, Yang Y, Zhang Y, Cai W. Non-invasive cell tracking in cancer and cancer therapy. Curr Top Med Chem. 2010;10(12):1237–48.

130. Singh A, Radu C, Ribas A. PET imaging of the immune system: immune monitoring at the whole body level. Q J Nucl Med Mol Imaging. 2010;54(3):281–90.

131. Bulte JW. In vivo MRI cell tracking: clinical studies. AJR Am J Roentgenol. 2009;193(2):314–25. https://doi.org/10.2214/AJR.09.3107.

132. Himmelreich U, Dresselaers T. Cell labeling and tracking for experimental models using magnetic resonance imaging. Methods. 2009;48(2):112–24. https://doi.org/10.1016/j.ymeth.2009.03.020.

133. Ahrens ET, Bulte JW. Tracking immune cells in vivo using magnetic resonance imaging. Nat Rev Immunol. 2013;13(10):755–63. https://doi.org/10.1038/nri3531.

134. Seth A, Park HS, Hong KS. Current perspective on in vivo molecular imaging of immune cells. Molecules. 2017;22(6):881. https://doi.org/10.3390/molecules22060881.

135. Chapelin F, Capitini CM, Ahrens ET. Fluorine-19 MRI for detection and quantification of immune cell therapy for cancer. J Immunother Cancer. 2018;6(1):105.

136. Beckmann N, Cannet C, Babin AL, Blé FX, Zurbruegg S, Kneuer R, et al. In vivo visualization of macrophage infiltration and activity in inflammation using magnetic resonance imaging. Wiley Interdiscip Rev Nanomed Nanobiotechnol. 2009;1(3):272–98.

137. Wang Y, Xu C, Ow H. Commercial nanoparticles for stem cell labeling and tracking. Theranostics. 2013;3(8):544–60. https://doi.org/10.7150/thno.5634.

138. Weissleder R, Nahrendorf M, Pittet MJ. Imaging macrophages with nanoparticles. Nat Mater. 2014;13(2):125–38. https://doi.org/10.1038/nmat3780.

139. Meir R, Popovtzer R. Cell tracking using gold nanoparticles and computed tomography imaging. Wiley Interdiscip Rev Nanomed Nanobiotechnol. 2018;10(2):28544497. https://doi.org/10.1002/wnan.1480.

140. Meir R, Motiei M, Popovtzer R. Gold nanoparticles for in vivo cell tracking. Nanomedicine. 2014;9(13):2059–69.

141. Zanganeh S, Spitler R, Hutter G, Ho JQ, Pauliah M, Mahmoudi M. Tumor-associated macrophages, nanomedicine and imaging: the axis of success in the future of cancer immunotherapy. Immunotherapy. 2017;9(10):819–35.

142. Thanarajasingam G, Bennani-Baiti N, Thompson CA. PET-CT in staging, response evaluation, and surveillance of lymphoma. Curr Treat Options Oncol. 2016;17(5):24. https://doi.org/10.1007/s11864-016-0399-z.

143. Gambhir SS. Imaging of T cells in patients with recurrent glioblastoma. Transl Cancer Res. 2017;6(S7):S1291–S2.

144. Karls S, Shah H, Jacene H. PET/CT for lymphoma post-therapy response assessment in other lymphomas, response assessment for autologous stem cell transplant, and lymphoma follow-up. Semin Nucl Med. 2018;48(1):37–49. https://doi.org/10.1053/j.semnuclmed.2017.09.004.

145. Shah K. Current advances in molecular imaging of gene and cell therapy for cancer. Cancer Biol Ther. 2005;4(5):518–23. https://doi.org/10.4161/cbt.4.5.1706.

146. Lucignani G, Ottobrini L, Martelli C, Rescigno M, Clerici M. Molecular imaging of cell-mediated cancer immunotherapy. Trends Biotechnol. 2006;24(9):410–8. https://doi.org/10.1016/j.tibtech.2006.07.003.

147. Tumeh PC, Radu CG, Ribas A. PET imaging of cancer immunotherapy. J Nucl Med. 2008;49(6):865–8. https://doi.org/10.2967/jnumed.108.051342.

148. Lazovic J, Jensen MC, Ferkassian E, Aguilar B, Raubitschek A, Jacobs RE. Imaging immune response in vivo: cytolytic action of genetically altered T cells directed to glioblastoma multiforme. Clin Cancer Res. 2008;14(12):3832–9. https://doi.org/10.1158/1078-0432.CCR-07-5067.

149. Akins EJ, Dubey P. Noninvasive imaging of cell-mediated therapy for treatment of cancer. J Nucl Med. 2008;49(Suppl 2):180S–95S. https://doi.org/10.2967/jnumed.107.045971.

150. Ponomarev V. Nuclear imaging of cancer cell therapies. J Nucl Med. 2009;50(7):1013–6. https://doi.org/10.2967/jnumed.109.064055.

151. Liu G, Swierczewska M, Niu G, Zhang X, Chen X. Molecular imaging of cell-based cancer immunotherapy. Mol BioSyst. 2011;7(4):993–1003. https://doi.org/10.1039/c0mb00198h.

152. Kurtz DM, Gambhir SS. Tracking cellular and immune therapies in cancer. Adv Cancer Res. 2014;124:257–96.

153. McCracken MN, Tavaré R, Witte ON, Wu A. Advances in PET detection of the antitumor T cell response. Adv Immunol. 2016;131:187–231.

154. Ehlerding EB, England CG, McNeel DG, Cai W. Molecular imaging of immunotherapy targets in cancer. J Nucl Med. 2016;57(10):1487–92. https://doi.org/10.2967/jnumed.116.177493.

155. Haris M, Bagga P, Hariharan H, McGettigan-Croce B, Johnson LA, Reddy R. Molecular imaging biomarkers for cell-based immunotherapies. J Transl

Med. 2017;15(1):140. https://doi.org/10.1186/s12967-017-1240-6.

156. Kurozumi S, Fujii T, Matsumoto H, Inoue K, Kurosumi M, Horiguchi J, et al. Significance of evaluating tumor-infiltrating lymphocytes (TILs) and programmed cell death-ligand 1 (PD-L1) expression in breast cancer. Med Mol Morphol. 2017;50(4):185–94. https://doi.org/10.1007/s00795-017-0170-y.

157. Ponomarev V. Advancing immune and cell-based therapies through imaging. Mol Imaging Biol. 2017;19(3):379–84. https://doi.org/10.1007/s11307-017-1069-7.

158. Fruhwirth GO, Kneilling M, de Vries IJM, Weigelin B, Srinivas M, Aarntzen E. The potential of in vivo imaging for optimization of molecular and cellular anti-cancer immunotherapies. Mol Imaging Biol. 2018;20(5):696–704. https://doi.org/10.1007/s11307-018-1254-3.

159. Marciscano AE, Thorek DLJ. Role of noninvasive molecular imaging in determining response. Adv Radiat Oncol. 2018;3(4):534–47. https://doi.org/10.1016/j.adro.2018.07.006.

160. Shields AF, Jacobs PM, Sznol M, Graham MM, Germain RN, Lum LG, et al. Immune modulation therapy and imaging: workshop report. J Nucl Med. 2018;59(3):410–7. https://doi.org/10.2967/jnumed.117.195610.

161. van der Veen EL, Bensch F, Glaudemans A, Lub-de Hooge MN, de Vries EGE. Molecular imaging to enlighten cancer immunotherapies and underlying involved processes. Cancer Treat Rev. 2018;70:232–44. https://doi.org/10.1016/j.ctrv.2018.09.007.

162. Wang Q, Ornstein M, Kaufman HL. Imaging the immune response to monitor tumor immunotherapy. Expert Rev Vaccines. 2009;8(10):1427–37.

163. Bier G, Hoffmann V, Kloth C, Othman AE, Eigentler T, Garbe C, et al. CT imaging of bone and bone marrow infiltration in malignant melanoma—challenges and limitations for clinical staging in comparison to 18FDG-PET/CT. Eur J Radiol. 2016;85(4):732–8. https://doi.org/10.1016/j.ejrad.2016.01.012.

164. Gholamrezanezhad A, Mirpour S, Ardekani JM, Bagheri M, Alimoghadam K, Yarmand S, et al. Cytotoxicity of 111In-oxine on mesenchymal stem cells: a time-dependent adverse effect. Nucl Med Commun. 2009;30(3):210–6.

165. Adonai N, Nguyen KN, Walsh J, Iyer M, Toyokuni T, Phelps ME, et al. Ex vivo cell labeling with 64Cu–pyruvaldehyde-bis (N4-methylthiosemicarbazone) for imaging cell trafficking in mice with positron-emission tomography. Proc Natl Acad Sci U S A. 2002;99(5):3030–5.

166. Paik J-Y, Lee K-H, Byun S-S, Choe Y, Kim B-T. Use of insulin to improve [18F] fluorodeoxyglucose labelling and retention for in vivo positron emission tomography imaging of monocyte trafficking. Nucl Med Commun. 2002;23(6):551–7.

167. Ridolfi R, Riccobon A, Galassi R, Giorgetti G, Petrini M, Fiammenghi L, et al. Evaluation of in vivo labelled dendritic cell migration in cancer patients. J Transl Med. 2004;2(1):27.

168. Meller B, Frohn C, Brand JM, Lauer I, Schelper LF, von Hof K, et al. Monitoring of a new approach of immunotherapy with allogenic (111)In-labelled NK cells in patients with renal cell carcinoma. Eur J Nucl Med Mol Imaging. 2004;31(3):403–7. https://doi.org/10.1007/s00259-003-1398-4.

169. Meier R, Piert M, Piontek G, Rudelius M, Oostendorp RA, Senekowitsch-Schmidtke R, et al. Tracking of [18F] FDG-labeled natural killer cells to HER2/neu-positive tumors. Nucl Med Biol. 2008;35(5):579–88.

170. Melder RJ, Brownell AL, Shoup TM, Brownell GL, Jain RK. Imaging of activated natural killer cells in mice by positron emission tomography: preferential uptake in tumors. Cancer Res. 1993;53(24):5867–71.

171. Melder RJ, Elmaleh D, Brownell AL, Brownell GL, Jain RK. A method for labeling cells for positron emission tomography (PET) studies. J Immunol Methods. 1994;175(1):79–87.

172. Allan R, Sladen G, Bassingham S, Lazarus C, Clarke S, Fogelman I. Comparison of simultaneous 99m Tc-HMPAO and 111 In oxine labelled white cell scans in the assessment of inflammatory bowel disease. Eur J Nucl Med. 1993;20(3):195–200.

173. Blocklet D, Toungouz M, Kiss R, Lambermont M, Velu T, Duriau D, et al. 111 In-oxine and 99m Tc-HMPAO labelling of antigen-loaded dendritic cells: in vivo imaging and influence on motility and actin content. Eur J Nucl Med Mol Imaging. 2003;30(3):440–7.

174. Quillien V, Moisan A, Carsin A, Lesimple T, Lefeuvre C, Adamski H, et al. Biodistribution of radiolabelled human dendritic cells injected by various routes. Eur J Nucl Med Mol Imaging. 2005;32(7):731–41. https://doi.org/10.1007/s00259-005-1825-9.

175. Bhargava KK, Gupta RK, Nichols KJ, Palestro CJ. In vitro human leukocyte labeling with 64Cu: an intraindividual comparison with 111In-oxine and 18F-FDG. Nucl Med Biol. 2009;36(5):545–9.

176. de Vries EF, Roca M, Jamar F, Israel O, Signore A. Guidelines for the labelling of leucocytes with (99m) Tc-HMPAO. Inflammation/Infection Taskgroup of the European Association of Nuclear Medicine. Eur J Nucl Med Mol Imaging. 2010;37(4):842–8. https://doi.org/10.1007/s00259-010-1394-4.

177. Roca M, de Vries EF, Jamar F, Israel O, Signore A. Guidelines for the labelling of leucocytes with (111)In-oxine. Inflammation/Infection Taskgroup of the European Association of Nuclear Medicine. Eur J Nucl Med Mol Imaging. 2010;37(4):835–41. https://doi.org/10.1007/s00259-010-1393-5.

178. McAfee J, Samin A. In-111 labeled leukocytes: a review of problems in image interpretation. Radiology. 1985;155(1):221–9.

179. Müller C, Zielinski C, Linkesch W, Ludwig H, Sinzinger H. In vivo tracing of indium-111 oxine-labeled human peripheral blood mononuclear cells

in patients with lymphatic malignancies. J Nucl Med. 1989;30(6):1005–11.

180. Olasz EB, Lang L, Seidel J, Green MV, Eckelman WC, Katz SI. Fluorine-18 labeled mouse bone marrow-derived dendritic cells can be detected in vivo by high resolution projection imaging. J Immunol Methods. 2002;260(1–2):137–48.

181. Read EJ, Keenan AM, Carter CS, Yolles PS, Davey RJ. In vivo traffic of indium-111-oxine labeled human lymphocytes collected by automated apheresis. J Nucl Med. 1990;31(6):999–1006.

182. Segal A, Arnot R, Thakur M, Lavender J. Indium-111-labelled leucocytes for localisation of abscesses. Lancet. 1976;308(7994):1056–8.

183. Thakur ML, Seifert CL, Madsen MT, McKenney SM, Desai AG, Park CH, editors. Neutrophil labeling: problems and pitfalls, Seminars in nuclear medicine. Amsterdam: Elsevier; 1984.

184. Hughes DK. Nuclear medicine and infection detection: the relative effectiveness of imaging with 111In-oxine-, 99mTc-HMPAO-, and 99mTc-stannous fluoride colloid-labeled leukocytes and with 67Ga-citrate. J Nucl Med Technol. 2003;31(4):196–201.

185. Ulker O, Genc S, Ates H, Durak H, Atabey N. 99mTc-HMPAO labelling inhibits cell motility and cell proliferation and induces apoptosis of NC-NC cells. Mutat Res. 2007;631(2):69–76. https://doi.org/10.1016/j.mrgentox.2006.12.009.

186. Eriksson O, Sadeghi A, Carlsson B, Eich T, Lundgren T, Nilsson B, et al. Distribution of adoptively transferred porcine T-lymphoblasts tracked by (18)F-2-fluoro-2-deoxy-D-glucose and position emission tomography. Nucl Med Biol. 2011;38(6):827–33. https://doi.org/10.1016/j.nucmedbio.2011.02.011.

187. Bhatnagar P, Li Z, Choi Y, Guo J, Li F, Lee DY, et al. Imaging of genetically engineered T cells by PET using gold nanoparticles complexed to Copper-64. Integr Biol (Camb). 2013;5(1):231–8. https://doi.org/10.1039/c2ib20093g.

188. de Vries IJ, Lesterhuis WJ, Barentsz JO, Verdijk P, van Krieken JH, Boerman OC, et al. Magnetic resonance tracking of dendritic cells in melanoma patients for monitoring of cellular therapy. Nat Biotechnol. 2005;23(11):1407–13. https://doi.org/10.1038/nbt1154.

189. Srinivas M, Morel PA, Ernst LA, Laidlaw DH, Ahrens ET. Fluorine-19 MRI for visualization and quantification of cell migration in a diabetes model. Magn Reson Med. 2007;58(4):725–34.

190. Smirnov P, Poirier-Quinot M, Wilhelm C, Lavergne E, Ginefri JC, Combadiere B, et al. In vivo single cell detection of tumor-infiltrating lymphocytes with a clinical 1.5 Tesla MRI system. Magn Reson Med. 2008;60(6):1292–7. https://doi.org/10.1002/mrm.21812.

191. Srinivas M, Turner MS, Janjic JM, Morel PA, Laidlaw DH, Ahrens ET. In vivo cytometry of antigen-specific t cells using 19F MRI. Magn Reson Med. 2009;62(3):747–53.

192. Arbab AS, Janic B, Jafari-Khouzani K, Iskander AS, Kumar S, Varma NR, et al. Differentiation of glioma and radiation injury in rats using in vitro produce magnetically labeled cytotoxic T-cells and MRI. PLoS One. 2010;5(2):e9365. https://doi.org/10.1371/journal.pone.0009365.

193. Bannas P, Graumann O, Balcerak P, Peldschus K, Kaul MG, Hohenberg H, et al. Quantitative magnetic resonance imaging of enzyme activity on the cell surface: in vitro and in vivo monitoring of ADP-ribosyltransferase 2 on T cells. Mol Imaging. 2010;9(4):211–22. https://doi.org/10.2310/7290.2010.00017.

194. Liu L, Ye Q, Wu Y, Hsieh WY, Chen CL, Shen HH, et al. Tracking T-cells in vivo with a new nano-sized MRI contrast agent. Nanomedicine. 2012;8(8):1345–54. https://doi.org/10.1016/j.nano.2012.02.017.

195. Bouchlaka MN, Ludwig KD, Gordon JW, Kutz MP, Bednarz BP, Fain SB, et al. (19)F-MRI for monitoring human NK cells in vivo. Oncoimmunology. 2016;5(5):e1143996. https://doi.org/10.1080/2162402X.2016.1143996.

196. Gonzales C, Yoshihara HA, Dilek N, Leignadier J, Irving M, Mieville P, et al. In-vivo detection and tracking of T cells in various organs in a melanoma tumor model by 19F-fluorine MRS/MRI. PLoS One. 2016;11(10):e0164557. https://doi.org/10.1371/journal.pone.0164557.

197. Daldrup-Link HE, Meier R, Rudelius M, Piontek G, Piert M, Metz S, et al. In vivo tracking of genetically engineered, anti-HER2/neu directed natural killer cells to HER2/neu positive mammary tumors with magnetic resonance imaging. Eur Radiol. 2005;15(1):4–13.

198. Meir R, Shamalov K, Betzer O, Motiei M, Horovitz-Fried M, Yehuda R, et al. Nanomedicine for cancer immunotherapy: tracking cancer-specific T-cells in vivo with gold nanoparticles and CT imaging. ACS Nano. 2015;9(6):6363–72.

199. Deguine J, Breart B, Lemaître F, Di Santo JP, Bousso P. Intravital imaging reveals distinct dynamics for natural killer and CD8+ T cells during tumor regression. Immunity. 2010;33(4):632–44.

200. Xu W-L, Li S-l, Ming W, Wen J-y, Jie H, Zhang H-z, et al. Tracking in vivo migration and distribution of antigen-specific cytotoxic T lymphocytes by 5,6-carboxyfluorescein diacetate succinimidyl ester staining during cancer immunotherapy. Chin Med J. 2013;126(16):3019–25.

201. Fisher B, Packard BS, Read EJ, Carrasquillo JA, Carter CS, Topalian SL, et al. Tumor localization of adoptively transferred indium-111 labeled tumor infiltrating lymphocytes in patients with metastatic melanoma. J Clin Oncol. 1989;7(2):250–61.

202. Griffith KD, Read EJ, Carrasquillo JA, Carter CS, Yang JC, Fisher B, et al. In vivo distribution of adoptively transferred indium-111-labeled tumor infiltrating lymphocytes and peripheral blood lymphocytes in patients with metastatic melanoma. J Natl Cancer Inst. 1989;81(22):1709–17.

203. Pockaj BA, Sherry RM, Wei JP, Yannelli JR, Carter CS, Leitman SF, et al. Localization of 111Indium-labeled tumor infiltrating lymphocytes to tumor in patients receiving adoptive immunotherapy. Augmentation with cyclophosphamide and correlation with response. Cancer. 1994;73(6):1731–7.

204. Wallace PK, Palmer LD, Perry-Lalley D, Bolton ES, Alexander RB, Horan PK, et al. Mechanisms of adoptive immunotherapy: improved methods for in vivo tracking of tumor-infiltrating lymphocytes and lymphokine-activated killer cells. Cancer Res. 1993;53(10):2358–67.

205. Botti C, Negri DR, Seregni E, Ramakrishna V, Arienti F, Maffioli L, et al. Comparison of three different methods for radiolabelling human activated T lymphocytes. Eur J Nucl Med. 1997;24(5):497–504.

206. Pittet MJ, Grimm J, Berger CR, Tamura T, Wojtkiewicz G, Nahrendorf M, et al. In vivo imaging of T cell delivery to tumors after adoptive transfer therapy. Proc Natl Acad Sci U S A. 2007;104(30):12457–61.

207. Agger R, Petersen MS, Petersen CC, Hansen SB, Stødkilde-Jørgensen H, Skands U, et al. T cell homing to tumors detected by 3D-coordinated positron emission tomography and magnetic resonance imaging. J Immunother. 2007;30(1):29–39.

208. Parente-Pereira AC, Burnet J, Ellison D, Foster J, Davies DM, van der Stegen S, et al. Trafficking of CAR-engineered human T cells following regional or systemic adoptive transfer in SCID beige mice. J Clin Immunol. 2011;31(4):710–8.

209. Bhatnagar P, Alauddin M, Bankson JA, Kirui D, Seifi P, Huls H, et al. Tumor lysing genetically engineered T cells loaded with multi-modal imaging agents. Sci Rep. 2014;4:4502.

210. Man F, Lim L, Volpe A, Gabizon A, Shmeeda H, Draper B, et al. In vivo PET tracking of (89)Zr-labeled Vgamma9Vdelta2 T cells to mouse xenograft breast tumors activated with liposomal alendronate. Mol Ther. 2019;27(1):219–29. https://doi.org/10.1016/j.ymthe.2018.10.006.

211. Herschman HR. PET reporter genes for noninvasive imaging of gene therapy, cell tracking and transgenic analysis. Crit Rev Oncol Hematol. 2004;51(3):191–204. https://doi.org/10.1016/j.critrevonc.2004.04.006.

212. Serganova I, Ponomarev V, Blasberg R. Human reporter genes: potential use in clinical studies. Nucl Med Biol. 2007;34(7):791–807. https://doi.org/10.1016/j.nucmedbio.2007.05.009.

213. Yaghoubi SS, Campbell DO, Radu CG, Czernin J. Positron emission tomography reporter genes and reporter probes: gene and cell therapy applications. Theranostics. 2012;2(4):374.

214. Brader P, Serganova I, Blasberg RG. Noninvasive molecular imaging using reporter genes. J Nucl Med. 2013;54(2):167–72. https://doi.org/10.2967/jnumed.111.099788.

215. Herschman HR. Noninvasive imaging of reporter gene expression in living subjects. Adv Cancer Res. 2004;92:30–80.

216. Gambhir SS, Bauer E, Black ME, Liang Q, Kokoris MS, Barrio JR, et al. A mutant herpes simplex virus type 1 thymidine kinase reporter gene shows improved sensitivity for imaging reporter gene expression with positron emission tomography. Proc Natl Acad Sci U S A. 2000;97(6):2785–90.

217. Doubrovin M, Ponomarev V, Beresten T, Balatoni J, Bornmann W, Finn R, et al. Imaging transcriptional regulation of p53-dependent genes with positron emission tomography in vivo. Proc Natl Acad Sci U S A. 2001;98(16):9300–5.

218. Jacobs A, Tjuvajev JG, Dubrovin M, Akhurst T, Balatoni J, Beattie B, et al. Positron emission tomography-based imaging of transgene expression mediated by replication-conditional, oncolytic herpes simplex virus type 1 mutant vectors in vivo. Cancer Res. 2001;61(7):2983–95.

219. Liang Q, Gotts J, Satyamurthy N, Barrio J, Phelps ME, Gambhir SS, et al. Noninvasive, repetitive, quantitative measurement of gene expression from a bicistronic message by positron emission tomography, following gene transfer with adenovirus. Mol Ther. 2002;6(1):73–82.

220. Tjuvajev JG, Doubrovin M, Akhurst T, Cai S, Balatoni J, Alauddin MM, et al. Comparison of radiolabeled nucleoside probes (FIAU, FHBG, and FHPG) for PET imaging of HSV1-tk gene expression. J Nucl Med. 2002;43(8):1072–83.

221. Min JJ, Iyer M, Gambhir SS. Comparison of [18F]FHBG and [14C]FIAU for imaging of HSV1-tk reporter gene expression: adenoviral infection vs stable transfection. Eur J Nucl Med Mol Imaging. 2003;30(11):1547–60. https://doi.org/10.1007/s00259-003-1238-6.

222. Ponomarev V, Doubrovin M, Serganova I, Vider J, Shavrin A, Beresten T, et al. A novel triple-modality reporter gene for whole-body fluorescent, bioluminescent, and nuclear noninvasive imaging. Eur J Nucl Med Mol Imaging. 2004;31(5):740–51.

223. Ponomarev V, Doubrovin M, Shavrin A, Serganova I, Beresten T, Ageyeva L, et al. A human-derived reporter gene for noninvasive imaging in humans: mitochondrial thymidine kinase type 2. J Nucl Med. 2007;48(5):819–26. https://doi.org/10.2967/jnumed.106.036962.

224. Niu G, Gaut AW, Ponto LLB, Hichwa RD, Madsen MT, Graham MM, et al. Multimodality noninvasive imaging of gene transfer using the human sodium iodide symporter. J Nucl Med. 2004;45(3):445–9.

225. Ray P, De A, Min J-J, Tsien RY, Gambhir SS. Imaging tri-fusion multimodality reporter gene expression in living subjects. Cancer Res. 2004;64(4):1323–30.

226. Chin FT, Namavari M, Levi J, Subbarayan M, Ray P, Chen X, et al. Semiautomated radiosynthesis and biological evaluation of [18F]FEAU: a novel PET imaging agent for HSV1-tk/sr39tk reporter gene expression. Mol Imaging Biol. 2008;10(2):82–91. https://doi.org/10.1007/s11307-007-0122-3.

227. Cho SY, Ravasi L, Szajek LP, Seidel J, Green MV, Fine HA, et al. Evaluation of 76Br-FBAU as a PET reporter probe for HSV1-tk gene expression imaging

using mouse models of human glioma. J Nucl Med. 2005;46(11):1923–30.

228. Yaghoubi SS, Barrio JR, Namavari M, Satyamurthy N, Phelps ME, Herschman HR, et al. Imaging progress of herpes simplex virus type 1 thymidine kinase suicide gene therapy in living subjects with positron emission tomography. Cancer Gene Ther. 2005;12(3):329.

229. Soghomonyan S, Hajitou A, Rangel R, Trepel M, Pasqualini R, Arap W, et al. Molecular PET imaging of HSV1-tk reporter gene expression using [18F] FEAU. Nat Protoc. 2007;2(2):416–23. https://doi.org/10.1038/nprot.2007.49.

230. Barton KN, Stricker H, Brown SL, Elshaikh M, Aref I, Lu M, et al. Phase I study of noninvasive imaging of adenovirus-mediated gene expression in the human prostate. Mol Ther. 2008;16(10):1761–9. https://doi.org/10.1038/mt.2008.172.

231. Miyagawa T, Gogiberidze G, Serganova I, Cai S, Balatoni JA, Thaler HT, et al. Imaging of HSV-tk Reporter gene expression: comparison between [18F]FEAU, [18F]FFEAU, and other imaging probes. J Nucl Med. 2008;49(4):637–48. https://doi.org/10.2967/jnumed.107.046227.

232. Chan P-C, Wu C-Y, Chang W-Y, Chang W-T, Alauddin M, Liu R-S, et al. Evaluation of F-18-labeled 5-iodocytidine (18F-FIAC) as a new potential positron emission tomography probe for herpes simplex virus type 1 thymidine kinase imaging. Nucl Med Biol. 2011;38(7):987–95.

233. Niers JM, Chen JW, Lewandrowski G, Kerami M, Garanger E, Wojtkiewicz G, et al. Single reporter for targeted multimodal in vivo imaging. J Am Chem Soc. 2012;134(11):5149–56. https://doi.org/10.1021/ja209868g.

234. Lee WW, Moon DH, Park SY, Jin J, Kim SJ, Lee H. Imaging of adenovirus-mediated expression of human sodium iodide symporter gene by 99mTcO4 scintigraphy in mice. Nucl Med Biol. 2004;31(1):31–40.

235. Bettegowda C, Foss CA, Cheong I, Wang Y, Diaz L, Agrawal N, et al. Imaging bacterial infections with radiolabeled 1-(2′-deoxy-2′-fluoro-β-D-arabinofuranosyl)-5-iodouracil. Proc Natl Acad Sci U S A. 2005;102(4):1145–50.

236. Sun H, Mangner TJ, Collins JM, Muzik O, Douglas K, Shields AF. Imaging DNA synthesis in vivo with 18F-FMAU and PET. J Nucl Med. 2005;46(2):292–6.

237. Le LQ, Kabarowski JH, Wong S, Nguyen K, Gambhir SS, Witte ON. Positron emission tomography imaging analysis of G2A as a negative modifier of lymphoid leukemogenesis initiated by the BCR-ABL oncogene. Cancer Cell. 2002;1(4):381–91.

238. Park J-J, Lee T-S, Son J-J, Chun K-S, Song I-H, Park Y-S, et al. Comparison of cell-labeling methods with 124I-FIAU and 64Cu-PTSM for cell tracking using chronic myelogenous leukemia cells expressing HSV1-tk and firefly luciferase. Cancer Biother Radiopharm. 2012;27(10):719–28.

239. Mayer-Kuckuk P, Doubrovin M, Bidaut L, Budak-Alpdogan T, Cai S, Hubbard V, et al. Molecular imaging reveals skeletal engraftment sites of transplanted bone marrow cells. Cell Transplant. 2006;15(1):75–82.

240. McCracken MN, Gschweng EH, Nair-Gill E, McLaughlin J, Cooper AR, Riedinger M, et al. Long-term in vivo monitoring of mouse and human hematopoietic stem cell engraftment with a human positron emission tomography reporter gene. Proc Natl Acad Sci U S A. 2013;110(5):1857–62. https://doi.org/10.1073/pnas.1221840110.

241. Lee HW, Yoon SY, Singh TD, Choi YJ, Lee HJ, Park JY, et al. Tracking of dendritic cell migration into lymph nodes using molecular imaging with sodium iodide symporter and enhanced firefly luciferase genes. Sci Rep. 2015;5:9865. https://doi.org/10.1038/srep09865.

242. Lee SB, Lee HW, Lee H, Jeon YH, Lee SW, Ahn BC, et al. Tracking dendritic cell migration into lymph nodes by using a novel PET probe (18)F-tetrafluoroborate for sodium/iodide symporter. EJNMMI Res. 2017;7(1):32. https://doi.org/10.1186/s13550-017-0280-5.

243. Ponomarev V, Doubrovin M, Lyddane C, Beresten T, Balatoni J, Bornman W, et al. Imaging TCR-dependent NFAT-mediated T-cell activation with positron emission tomography in vivo. Neoplasia (New York, NY). 2001;3(6):480.

244. Koehne G, Doubrovin M, Doubrovina E, Zanzonico P, Gallardo HF, Ivanova A, et al. Serial in vivo imaging of the targeted migration of human HSV-TK-transduced antigen-specific lymphocytes. Nat Biotechnol. 2003;21(4):405.

245. Zanzonico P, Koehne G, Gallardo HF, Doubrovin M, Doubrovina E, Finn R, et al. [131I]FIAU labeling of genetically transduced, tumor-reactive lymphocytes: cell-level dosimetry and dose-dependent toxicity. Eur J Nucl Med Mol Imaging. 2006;33(9):988–97. https://doi.org/10.1007/s00259-005-0057-3.

246. Dubey P, Su H, Adonai N, Du S, Rosato A, Braun J, et al. Quantitative imaging of the T cell antitumor response by positron-emission tomography. Proc Natl Acad Sci U S A. 2003;100(3):1232–7.

247. Su H, Forbes A, Gambhir SS, Braun J. Quantitation of cell number by a positron emission tomography reporter gene strategy. Mol Imaging Biol. 2004;6(3):139–48.

248. Shu CJ, Guo S, Kim YJ, Shelly SM, Nijagal A, Ray P, et al. Visualization of a primary anti-tumor immune response by positron emission tomography. Proc Natl Acad Sci U S A. 2005;102(48):17412–7.

249. Shu CJ, Radu CG, Shelly SM, Vo DD, Prins R, Ribas A, et al. Quantitative PET reporter gene imaging of CD8+ T cells specific for a melanoma-expressed self-antigen. Int Immunol. 2009;21(2):155–65. https://doi.org/10.1093/intimm/dxn133.

250. Su H, Chang DS, Gambhir SS, Braun J. Monitoring the antitumor response of naive and memory CD8 T cells in RAG1−/− mice by positron-emission tomography. J Immunol. 2006;176(7):4459–67. https://doi.org/10.4049/jimmunol.176.7.4459.

251. Yaghoubi SS, Jensen MC, Satyamurthy N, Budhiraja S, Paik D, Czernin J, et al. Noninvasive detection of therapeutic cytolytic T cells with 18 F–FHBG PET in a patient with glioma. Nat Rev Clin Oncol. 2009;6(1):53.

252. Keu KV, Witney TH, Yaghoubi S, Rosenberg J, Kurien A, Magnusson R, et al. Reporter gene imaging of targeted T cell immunotherapy in recurrent glioma. Sci Transl Med. 2017;9(373):eaag2196.

253. Dobrenkov K, Olszewska M, Likar Y, Shenker L, Gunset G, Cai S, et al. Monitoring the efficacy of adoptively transferred prostate cancer-targeted human T lymphocytes with PET and bioluminescence imaging. J Nucl Med. 2008;49(7):1162–70. https://doi.org/10.2967/jnumed.107.047324.

254. Dotti G, Tian M, Savoldo B, Najjar A, Cooper LJ, Jackson J, et al. Repetitive noninvasive monitoring of HSV1-tk-expressing T cells intravenously infused into nonhuman primates using positron emission tomography and computed tomography with 18F-FEAU. Mol Imaging. 2009;8(4):230–7.

255. Najjar AM, Manuri PR, Olivares S, Flores L II, Mi T, Huls H, et al. Imaging of sleeping beauty-modified CD19-specific T cells expressing HSV1-thymidine kinase by positron emission tomography. Mol Imaging Biol. 2016;18(6):838–48. https://doi.org/10.1007/s11307-016-0971-8.

256. Vedvyas Y, Shevlin E, Zaman M, Min IM, Amor-Coarasa A, Park S, et al. Longitudinal PET imaging demonstrates biphasic CAR T cell responses in survivors. JCI Insight. 2016;1(19):e90064. https://doi.org/10.1172/jci.insight.90064.

257. Park S, Shevlin E, Vedvyas Y, Zaman M, Park S, Hsu YS, et al. Micromolar affinity CAR T cells to ICAM-1 achieves rapid tumor elimination while avoiding systemic toxicity. Sci Rep. 2017;7(1):14366. https://doi.org/10.1038/s41598-017-14749-3.

258. Mall S, Yusufi N, Wagner R, Klar R, Bianchi H, Steiger K, et al. Immuno-PET imaging of engineered human T cells in tumors. Cancer Res. 2016;76(14):4113–23. https://doi.org/10.1158/0008-5472.CAN-15-2784.

259. Yusufi N, Mall S, Bianchi HO, Steiger K, Reder S, Klar R, et al. In-depth characterization of a TCR-specific tracer for sensitive detection of tumor-directed transgenic T cells by immuno-PET. Theranostics. 2017;7(9):2402–16. https://doi.org/10.7150/thno.17994.

260. Yusufi N, Mall S, de Oliveira Bianchi H, Steiger K, Reder S, Klar R, et al. In-depth characterization of a TCR-specific tracer for sensitive detection of tumor-directed transgenic T cells by immuno-PET. Theranostics. 2017;7(9):2402.

261. Krebs S, Ahad A, Carter LM, Eyquem J, Brand C, Bell M, et al. Antibody with infinite affinity for in vivo tracking of genetically engineered lymphocytes. J Nucl Med. 2018;59(12):1894–900. https://doi.org/10.2967/jnumed.118.208041.

262. Bruno R, Giannasio P, Ronga G, Baudin E, Travagli J, Russo D, et al. Sodium iodide symporter expression and radioiodine distribution in extrathyroidal tissues. J Endocrinol Investig. 2004;27(11):1010–4.

263. Sharp SE, Trout AT, Weiss BD, Gelfand MJ. MIBG in neuroblastoma diagnostic imaging and therapy. Radiographics. 2016;36(1):258–78.

264. Moroz MA, Serganova I, Zanzonico P, Ageyeva L, Beresten T, Dyomina E, et al. Imaging hNET reporter gene expression with 124I-MIBG. J Nucl Med. 2007;48(5):827–36.

265. Doubrovin MM, Doubrovina ES, Zanzonico P, Sadelain M, Larson SM, O'Reilly RJ. In vivo imaging and quantitation of adoptively transferred human antigen-specific T cells transduced to express a human norepinephrine transporter gene. Cancer Res. 2007;67(24):11959–69. https://doi.org/10.1158/0008-5472.CAN-07-1250.

266. Radu CG, Shu CJ, Nair-Gill E, Shelly SM, Barrio JR, Satyamurthy N, et al. Molecular imaging of lymphoid organs and immune activation by positron emission tomography with a new [18F]-labeled 2′-deoxycytidine analog. Nat Med. 2008;14(7):783–8. https://doi.org/10.1038/nm1724.

267. Schwarzenberg J, Radu CG, Benz M, Fueger B, Tran AQ, Phelps ME, et al. Human biodistribution and radiation dosimetry of novel PET probes targeting the deoxyribonucleoside salvage pathway. Eur J Nucl Med Mol Imaging. 2011;38(4):711–21. https://doi.org/10.1007/s00259-010-1666-z.

268. Antonios JP, Soto H, Everson RG, Moughon DL, Wang AC, Orpilla J, et al. Detection of immune responses after immunotherapy in glioblastoma using PET and MRI. Proc Natl Acad Sci U S A. 2017;114(38):10220–5. https://doi.org/10.1073/pnas.1706689114.

269. Shu CJ, Campbell DO, Lee JT, Tran AQ, Wengrod JC, Witte ON, et al. Novel PET probes specific for deoxycytidine kinase. J Nucl Med. 2010;51(7):1092–8. https://doi.org/10.2967/jnumed.109.073361.

270. Kim W, Le TM, Wei L, Poddar S, Bazzy J, Wang X, et al. [18F]CFA as a clinically translatable probe for PET imaging of deoxycytidine kinase activity. Proc Natl Acad Sci U S A. 2016;113(15):4027–32. https://doi.org/10.1073/pnas.1524212113.

271. Franc BL, Goth S, MacKenzie J, Li X, Blecha J, Lam T, et al. In vivo PET imaging of the activated immune environment in a small animal model of inflammatory arthritis. Mol Imaging. 2017;16:1536012117712638. https://doi.org/10.1177/1536012117712638.

272. Namavari M, Chang YF, Kusler B, Yaghoubi S, Mitchell BS, Gambhir SS. Synthesis of 2′-deoxy-2′-[18F]fluoro-9-beta-D-arabinofuranosylguanine: a novel agent for imaging T-cell activation with PET. Mol Imaging Biol. 2011;13(5):812–8. https://doi.org/10.1007/s11307-010-0414-x.

273. Levi J, Lam T, Goth SR, Yaghoubi S, Bates J, Ren G, et al. Imaging of activated T cells as an early predictor of immune response to anti-PD-1 therapy. Cancer Res. 2019;79(13):3455–65.

274. McCracken MN, Vatakis DN, Dixit D, McLaughlin J, Zack JA, Witte ON. Noninvasive detection of

tumor-infiltrating T cells by PET reporter imaging. J Clin Invest. 2015;125(5):1815–26.

275. Ribas A, Benz MR, Allen-Auerbach MS, Radu C, Chmielowski B, Seja E, et al. Imaging of CTLA4 blockade-induced cell replication with (18)F-FLT PET in patients with advanced melanoma treated with tremelimumab. J Nucl Med. 2010;51(3):340–6. https://doi.org/10.2967/jnumed.109.070946.

276. Aarntzen EH, Srinivas M, De Wilt JH, Jacobs JF, Lesterhuis WJ, Windhorst AD, et al. Early identification of antigen-specific immune responses in vivo by [18F]-labeled 3′-fluoro-3′-deoxy-thymidine ([18F] FLT) PET imaging. Proc Natl Acad Sci U S A. 2011;108(45):18396–9.

277. Scarpelli M, Zahm C, Perlman S, McNeel DG, Jeraj R, Liu G. FLT PET/CT imaging of metastatic prostate cancer patients treated with pTVG-HP DNA vaccine and pembrolizumab. J Immunother Cancer. 2019;7(1):23.

278. Abbs IC, Pratt JR, Dallman MJ, Sacks SH. Analysis of activated T cell infiltrates in rat renal allografts by gamma camera imaging after injection of 123iodine-interleukin 2. Transpl Immunol. 1993;1(1):45–51.

279. Annovazzi A, Biancone L, Caviglia R, Chianelli M, Capriotti G, Mather SJ, et al. 99mTc-interleukin-2 and (99m)Tc-HMPAO granulocyte scintigraphy in patients with inactive Crohn's disease. Eur J Nucl Med Mol Imaging. 2003;30(3):374–82. https://doi.org/10.1007/s00259-002-1069-x.

280. Annovazzi A, D'Alessandria C, Bonanno E, Mather SJ, Cornelissen B, van de Wiele C, et al. Synthesis of 99mTc-HYNIC-interleukin-12, a new specific radiopharmaceutical for imaging T lymphocytes. Eur J Nucl Med Mol Imaging. 2006;33(4):474–82. https://doi.org/10.1007/s00259-005-0001-6.

281. Gross MD, Shapiro B, Fig LM, Steventon R, Skinner RW, Hay RV. Imaging of human infection with 131I-labeled recombinant human interleukin-8. J Nucl Med. 2001;42(11):1656–9.

282. Glaudemans AW, Bonanno E, Galli F, Zeebregts CJ, de Vries EF, Koole M, et al. In vivo and in vitro evidence that (9)(9)mTc-HYNIC-interleukin-2 is able to detect T lymphocytes in vulnerable atherosclerotic plaques of the carotid artery. Eur J Nucl Med Mol Imaging. 2014;41(9):1710–9. https://doi.org/10.1007/s00259-014-2764-0.

283. Di Gialleonardo V, Signore A, Willemsen AT, Sijbesma JW, Dierckx RA, de Vries EF. Pharmacokinetic modelling of N-(4-[(18)F]fluorobenzoyl)interleukin-2 binding to activated lymphocytes in an xenograft model of inflammation. Eur J Nucl Med Mol Imaging. 2012;39(10):1551–60. https://doi.org/10.1007/s00259-012-2176-y.

284. Di Gialleonardo V, Signore A, Glaudemans AW, Dierckx RA, De Vries EF. N-(4-18F-fluorobenzoyl) interleukin-2 for PET of human-activated T lymphocytes. J Nucl Med. 2012;53(5):679–86. https://doi.org/10.2967/jnumed.111.091306.

285. Signore A, Annovazzi A, Barone R, Bonanno E, D'Alessandria C, Chianelli M, et al. 99mTc-interleukin-2 scintigraphy as a potential tool for evaluating tumor-infiltrating lymphocytes in melanoma lesions: a validation study. J Nucl Med. 2004;45(10):1647–52.

286. Loose D, Signore A, Staelens L, Bulcke KV, Vermeersch H, Dierckx RA, et al. (123)I-Interleukin-2 uptake in squamous cell carcinoma of the head and neck carcinoma. Eur J Nucl Med Mol Imaging. 2008;35(2):281–6. https://doi.org/10.1007/s00259-007-0609-9.

287. Markovic SN, Galli F, Suman VJ, Nevala WK, Paulsen AM, Hung JC, et al. Non-invasive visualization of tumor infiltrating lymphocytes in patients with metastatic melanoma undergoing immune checkpoint inhibitor therapy: a pilot study. Oncotarget. 2018;9(54):30268.

288. Hartimath SV, Manuelli V, Zijlma R, Signore A, Nayak TK, Freimoser-Grundschober A, et al. Pharmacokinetic properties of radiolabeled mutant Interleukin-2v: a PET imaging study. Oncotarget. 2018;9(6):7162.

289. Klein C, Waldhauer I, Nicolini VG, Freimoser-Grundschober A, Nayak T, Vugts DJ, et al. Cergutuzumab amunaleukin (CEA-IL2v), a CEA-targeted IL-2 variant-based immunocytokine for combination cancer immunotherapy: overcoming limitations of aldesleukin and conventional IL-2-based immunocytokines. Oncoimmunology. 2017;6(3):e1277306. https://doi.org/10.1080/2162402X.2016.1277306.

290. Walther M, Gebhardt P, Grosse-Gehling P, Wurbach L, Irmler I, Preusche S, et al. Implementation of 89Zr production and in vivo imaging of B-cells in mice with 89Zr-labeled anti-B-cell antibodies by small animal PET/CT. Appl Radiat Isot. 2011;69(6):852–7. https://doi.org/10.1016/j.apradiso.2011.02.040.

291. Olafsen T, Sirk SJ, Betting DJ, Kenanova VE, Bauer KB, Ladno W, et al. ImmunoPET imaging of B-cell lymphoma using 124I-anti-CD20 scFv dimers (diabodies). Protein Eng Des Sel. 2010;23(4):243–9.

292. Olafsen T, Betting D, Kenanova VE, Salazar FB, Clarke P, Said J, et al. Recombinant anti-CD20 antibody fragments for small-animal PET imaging of B-cell lymphomas. J Nucl Med. 2009;50(9):1500–8.

293. Natarajan A, Gambhir SS. Radiation dosimetry study of [(89)Zr]rituximab tracer for clinical translation of B cell NHL imaging using positron emission tomography. Mol Imaging Biol. 2015;17(4):539–47. https://doi.org/10.1007/s11307-014-0810-8.

294. Natarajan A, Habte F, Gambhir SS. Development of a novel long-lived immunoPET tracer for monitoring lymphoma therapy in a humanized transgenic mouse model. Bioconjug Chem. 2012;23(6):1221–9. https://doi.org/10.1021/bc300039r.

295. Natarajan A, Hackel BJ, Gambhir SS. A novel engineered anti-CD20 tracer enables early time PET imaging in a humanized transgenic mouse model of B-cell non-Hodgkins lymphoma. Clin Cancer Res. 2013;19(24):6820–9.

296. Zettlitz KA, Tavaré R, Knowles SM, Steward KK, Timmerman JM, Wu AM. ImmunoPET of malignant and normal B cells with 89Zr-and 124I-labeled obinutuzumab antibody fragments reveals differential CD20 internalization in vivo. Clin Cancer Res. 2017;23(23):7242–52.

297. Rashidian M, Keliher EJ, Bilate AM, Duarte JN, Wojtkiewicz GR, Jacobsen JT, et al. Noninvasive imaging of immune responses. Proc Natl Acad Sci U S A. 2015;112(19):6146–51.

298. Movahedi K, Schoonooghe S, Laoui D, Houbracken I, Waelput W, Breckpot K, et al. Nanobody-based targeting of the macrophage mannose receptor for effective in vivo imaging of tumor-associated macrophages. Cancer Res. 2012;72(16):4165–77. https://doi.org/10.1158/0008-5472.CAN-11-2994.

299. Blykers A, Schoonooghe S, Xavier C, D'Hoe K, Laoui D, D'Huyvetter M, et al. PET imaging of macrophage mannose receptor-expressing macrophages in tumor stroma using 18F-radiolabeled camelid single-domain antibody fragments. J Nucl Med. 2015;56(8):1265–71. https://doi.org/10.2967/jnumed.115.156828.

300. Seo JH, Jeon YH, Lee YJ, Yoon GS, Won DI, Ha JH, et al. Trafficking macrophage migration using reporter gene imaging with human sodium iodide symporter in animal models of inflammation. J Nucl Med. 2010;51(10):1637–43. https://doi.org/10.2967/jnumed.110.077891.

301. Freise AC, Zettlitz KA, Salazar FB, Lu X, Tavare R, Wu AM. ImmunoPET imaging of murine CD4(+) T cells using anti-CD4 Cys-Diabody: effects of protein dose on T cell function and imaging. Mol Imaging Biol. 2017;19(4):599–609. https://doi.org/10.1007/s11307-016-1032-z.

302. Tavare R, McCracken MN, Zettlitz KA, Knowles SM, Salazar FB, Olafsen T, et al. Engineered antibody fragments for immuno-PET imaging of endogenous CD8+ T cells in vivo. Proc Natl Acad Sci U S A. 2014;111(3):1108–13. https://doi.org/10.1073/pnas.1316922111.

303. Kanwar B, Gao DW, Hwang AB, Grenert JP, Williams SP, Franc B, et al. In vivo imaging of mucosal CD4+ T cells using single photon emission computed tomography in a murine model of colitis. J Immunol Methods. 2008;329(1–2):21–30. https://doi.org/10.1016/j.jim.2007.09.008.

304. Freise AC, Zettlitz KA, Salazar FB, Tavare R, Tsai WK, Chatziioannou AF, et al. Immuno-PET in inflammatory bowel disease: imaging CD4-positive T cells in a murine model of colitis. J Nucl Med. 2018;59(6):980–5. https://doi.org/10.2967/jnumed.117.199075.

305. Di Mascio M, Srinivasula S, Kim I, Duralde G, St Claire A, DeGrange P, et al. Total body CD4+ T cell dynamics in treated and untreated SIV infection revealed by in vivo imaging. JCI Insight. 2018;3(13):e97880. https://doi.org/10.1172/jci.insight.97880.

306. Ronald JA, Kim BS, Gowrishankar G, Namavari M, Alam IS, D'Souza A, et al. A PET imaging strategy to visualize activated T cells in acute graft-versus-host disease elicited by allogenic hematopoietic cell transplant. Cancer Res. 2017;77(11):2893–902. https://doi.org/10.1158/0008-5472.CAN-16-2953.

307. Tavare R, McCracken MN, Zettlitz KA, Salazar FB, Olafsen T, Witte ON, et al. Immuno-PET of murine T cell reconstitution postadoptive stem cell transplantation using anti-CD4 and anti-CD8 Cys-Diabodies. J Nucl Med. 2015;56(8):1258–64. https://doi.org/10.2967/jnumed.114.153338.

308. Heskamp S, Hobo W, Molkenboer-Kuenen JD, Olive D, Oyen WJ, Dolstra H, et al. Noninvasive imaging of tumor PD-L1 expression using radiolabeled anti-PD-L1 antibodies. Cancer Res. 2015;75(14):2928–36. https://doi.org/10.1158/0008-5472.CAN-14-3477.

309. Maute RL, Gordon SR, Mayer AT, McCracken MN, Natarajan A, Ring NG, et al. Engineering high-affinity PD-1 variants for optimized immunotherapy and immuno-PET imaging. Proc Natl Acad Sci U S A. 2015;112(47):E6506–14. https://doi.org/10.1073/pnas.1519623112.

310. Chatterjee S, Lesniak WG, Gabrielson M, Lisok A, Wharram B, Sysa-Shah P, et al. A humanized antibody for imaging immune checkpoint ligand PD-L1 expression in tumors. Oncotarget. 2016;7(9):10215.

311. Lesniak WG, Chatterjee S, Gabrielson M, Lisok A, Wharram B, Pomper MG, et al. PD-L1 detection in tumors using [(64)Cu]Atezolizumab with PET. Bioconjug Chem. 2016;27(9):2103–10. https://doi.org/10.1021/acs.bioconjchem.6b00348.

312. Josefsson A, Nedrow JR, Park S, Banerjee SR, Rittenbach A, Jammes F, et al. Imaging, biodistribution, and dosimetry of radionuclide-labeled PD-L1 antibody in an immunocompetent mouse model of breast cancer. Cancer Res. 2016;76(2):472–9. https://doi.org/10.1158/0008-5472.CAN-15-2141.

313. Mayer AT, Natarajan A, Gordon SR, Maute RL, McCracken MN, Ring AM, et al. Practical immuno-PET radiotracer design considerations for human immune checkpoint imaging. J Nucl Med. 2017;58(4):538–46. https://doi.org/10.2967/jnumed.116.177659.

314. Nedrow JR, Josefsson A, Park S, Ranka S, Roy S, Sgouros G. Imaging of programmed cell death ligand 1: impact of protein concentration on distribution of anti-PD-L1 SPECT agents in an immunocompetent murine model of melanoma. J Nucl Med. 2017;58(10):1560–6. https://doi.org/10.2967/jnumed.117.193268.

315. Chatterjee S, Lesniak WG, Nimmagadda S. Noninvasive imaging of immune checkpoint ligand PD-L1 in tumors and metastases for guiding immunotherapy. Mol Imaging. 2017;16:1536012117718459.

316. Kikuchi M, Clump DA, Srivastava RM, Sun L, Zeng D, Diaz-Perez JA, et al. Preclinical immunoPET/CT imaging using Zr-89-labeled anti-PD-L1 monoclonal antibody for assessing radiation-induced PD-L1

upregulation in head and neck cancer and melanoma. Oncoimmunology. 2017;6(7):e1329071.

317. Truillet C, Oh HLJ, Yeo SP, Lee CY, Huynh LT, Wei J, et al. Imaging PD-L1 expression with ImmunoPET. Bioconjug Chem. 2018;29(1):96–103. https://doi.org/10.1021/acs.bioconjchem.7b00631.

318. Ehlerding EB, England CG, Majewski RL, Valdovinos HF, Jiang D, Liu G, et al. ImmunoPET imaging of CTLA-4 expression in mouse models of non-small cell lung cancer. Mol Pharm. 2017;14(5):1782–9. https://doi.org/10.1021/acs.molpharmaceut.7b00056.

319. Natarajan A, Mayer AT, Xu L, Reeves RE, Gano J, Gambhir SS. Novel radiotracer for ImmunoPET imaging of PD-1 checkpoint expression on tumor infiltrating lymphocytes. Bioconjug Chem. 2015;26(10):2062–9. https://doi.org/10.1021/acs.bioconjchem.5b00318.

320. Hettich M, Braun F, Bartholoma MD, Schirmbeck R, Niedermann G. High-resolution PET imaging with therapeutic antibody-based PD-1/PD-L1 checkpoint tracers. Theranostics. 2016;6(10):1629–40. https://doi.org/10.7150/thno.15253.

321. England CG, Ehlerding EB, Hernandez R, Rekoske BT, Graves SA, Sun H, et al. Preclinical pharmacokinetics and biodistribution studies of 89Zr-labeled pembrolizumab. J Nucl Med. 2017;58(1):162–8. https://doi.org/10.2967/jnumed.116.177857.

322. Natarajan A, Mayer AT, Reeves RE, Nagamine CM, Gambhir SS. Development of novel ImmunoPET tracers to image human PD-1 checkpoint expression on tumor-infiltrating lymphocytes in a humanized mouse model. Mol Imaging Biol. 2017;19(6):903–14. https://doi.org/10.1007/s11307-017-1060-3.

323. Natarajan A, Patel CB, Habte F, Gambhir SS. Dosimetry prediction for clinical translation of (64)Cu-pembrolizumab ImmunoPET targeting human PD-1 expression. Sci Rep. 2018;8(1):633. https://doi.org/10.1038/s41598-017-19123-x.

324. England CG, Jiang D, Ehlerding EB, Rekoske BT, Ellison PA, Hernandez R, et al. (89)Zr-labeled nivolumab for imaging of T-cell infiltration in a humanized murine model of lung cancer. Eur J Nucl Med Mol Imaging. 2018;45(1):110–20. https://doi.org/10.1007/s00259-017-3803-4.

325. Du Y, Liang X, Li Y, Sun T, Jin Z, Xue H, et al. Nuclear and fluorescent labeled PD-1-liposome-DOX-(64)Cu/IRDye800CW allows improved breast tumor targeted imaging and therapy. Mol Pharm. 2017;14(11):3978–86. https://doi.org/10.1021/acs.molpharmaceut.7b00649.

326. Higashikawa K, Yagi K, Watanabe K, Kamino S, Ueda M, Hiromura M, et al. 64Cu-DOTA-anti-CTLA-4 mAb enabled PET visualization of CTLA-4 on the T-cell infiltrating tumor tissues. PLoS One. 2014;9(11):e109866. https://doi.org/10.1371/journal.pone.0109866.

327. Higashikawa K, Yagi K, Watanabe K, Kamino S, Ueda M, Hiromura M, et al. 64 Cu-DOTA-anti-CTLA-4 mAb enabled PET visualization of CTLA-4 on the T-cell infiltrating tumor tissues. PLoS One. 2014;9(11):e109866.

328. Malviya G, D'Alessandria C, Bonanno E, Vexler V, Massari R, Trotta C, et al. Radiolabeled humanized anti-CD3 monoclonal antibody visilizumab for imaging human T-lymphocytes. J Nucl Med. 2009;50(10):1683–91.

329. Larimer BM, Wehrenberg-Klee E, Caraballo A, Mahmood U. Quantitative CD3 PET imaging predicts tumor growth response to anti-CTLA-4 therapy. J Nucl Med. 2016;57(10):1607–11. https://doi.org/10.2967/jnumed.116.173930.

330. Beckford Vera DR, Smith CC, Bixby LM, Glatt DM, Dunn SS, Saito R, et al. Immuno-PET imaging of tumor-infiltrating lymphocytes using zirconium-89 radiolabeled anti-CD3 antibody in immune-competent mice bearing syngeneic tumors. PLoS One. 2018;13(3):e0193832. https://doi.org/10.1371/journal.pone.0193832.

331. Tavare R, Escuin-Ordinas H, Mok S, McCracken MN, Zettlitz KA, Salazar FB, et al. An effective Immuno-PET imaging method to monitor CD8-dependent responses to immunotherapy. Cancer Res. 2016;76(1):73–82. https://doi.org/10.1158/0008-5472.CAN-15-1707.

332. Rashidian M, Ingram JR, Dougan M, Dongre A, Whang KA, LeGall C, et al. Predicting the response to CTLA-4 blockade by longitudinal non-invasive monitoring of CD8 T cells. J Exp Med. 2017;214(8):2243–55. https://doi.org/10.1084/jem.20161950.

333. Alam IS, Mayer AT, Sagiv-Barfi I, Wang K, Vermesh O, Czerwinski DK, et al. Imaging activated T cells predicts response to cancer vaccines. J Clin Investig. 2018;128(6):2569–80.

334. Matsui K, Wang Z, McCarthy TJ, Allen PM, Reichert DE. Quantitation and visualization of tumor-specific T cells in the secondary lymphoid organs during and after tumor elimination by PET. Nucl Med Biol. 2004;31(8):1021–31. https://doi.org/10.1016/j.nucmedbio.2004.06.002.

335. Larimer BM, Wehrenberg-Klee E, Dubois F, Mehta A, Kalomeris T, Flaherty K, et al. Granzyme B PET imaging as a predictive biomarker of immunotherapy response. Cancer Res. 2017;77(9):2318 27. https://doi.org/10.1158/0008-5472.CAN-16-3346.

Gallium Imaging of Infection and Inflammation

4

Mariza Vorster and Mike Sathekge

Contents

4.1   Introduction

Infection is still a significant contributor to global mortality and morbidity, with tuberculosis, acquired immunodeficiency syndrome (AIDS), and malaria, responsible for around half of infection-related deaths [1, 2]. Inflammation

M. Vorster (✉) · M. Sathekge
Department of Nuclear Medicine, Steve Biko Academic Hospital, University of Pretoria, Pretoria, South Africa
e-mail: marizavorster@up.ac.za; mike.sathekge@up.ac.za

© Springer Nature Switzerland AG 2022
S. Harsini et al. (eds.), *Nuclear Medicine and Immunology*,
https://doi.org/10.1007/978-3-030-81261-4_4

represents the host's response to dangerous stimuli and may therefore accompany any pathogen invasion or occur in the absence of any pathogen as sterile inflammation. The latter forms a crucial component of many systemic and debilitating conditions, such as auto-immune conditions, arthritis, cardiovascular disease, respiratory conditions, and diabetes [3, 4]. The accurate distinction between these two different, but often overlapping, conditions remains an important clinical need in order to accurately guide medical management.

As such, positron emission tomography/computed tomography (PET/CT) provides an attractive diagnostic tool that is able to image the whole body, combining morphological and functional imaging, and that is ideally suited to disease detection at an early stage. This is especially true in an era of improved access to PET/CT imaging. Considering the cost and the logistics related to cyclotron-produced PET tracers, a generator-based PET tracer is a sensible choice. Germanium-68/gallium-68 generators are ideal in that they provide nearly year-long tracer availability, on an as-needed basis with the possibility of at least two generator elutions per day providing doses for at least two patients per eluate [5, 6].

Gallium (in the form of [^{67}Ga]Ga-citrate) has traditionally provided nuclear physicians with a versatile tool for use over a broad spectrum of clinical applications that included indications related to infection and inflammation (e.g., tuberculosis, sarcoidosis, skeletal infections). The mechanism of action is generally accepted to be related to its similarities to iron and its binding to transferrin, ferritin, and lactoferrin [7]. It stands to reason that gallium-68 would be as useful as gallium-67 with the added PET/CT advantages of improved image resolution, improved sensitivity and quantification possibilities, dynamic imaging possibilities, and versatile compounding options. Gallium-68 can be linked via several chelators (i.e., DOTA, NOTA, NODAGA, TRAP) to antibodies, receptors on white blood cells, selectins, integrins, chemokines, folate receptors, antimicrobial proteins, peptides, and siderophores [8].

Some of the potential additional advantages of using gallium-68-based tracers over the more widely used 2-[^{18}F]fluoro-2-deoxy-D-glucose (2-[^{18}F]FDG) include improved specificity, improved distinction between infection and inflammation, and improved biodistribution in areas such as the brain and heart. Advantages over the more traditional single-photon emission computed tomography (SPECT) infection tracers include the absence of contact with infectious material, improved logistics, improved imaging characteristics, and possibly fewer false negatives in the settings of immune-suppression, spinal and chronic infections [9–11].

This chapter aims to summarize some of the most prominent work done with gallium, in particular gallium-68-based PET tracers in the settings of infection and inflammation.

4.2 Infection Imaging

Infection is regarded as an important cause of morbidity and mortality worldwide. It is therefore crucial to obtain an accurate and timeous diagnosis in order to appropriately manage the condition. Conventional diagnostic modalities are often time-consuming and/or invasive, and it may not always be practical to await the results of blood cultures or obtain tissue for histology. On the other hand, empirical treatment may have significant side effects, may contribute to antibiotic resistance or result in allergic reactions, and might ultimately end up being suboptimal or entirely inappropriate.

Whole-body imaging provides a "one-stop" noninvasive diagnostic study and might be especially valuable in cases where the site of the infection is unknown. Gallium is a dark gray trivalent transition metal, solid at room temperature but liquid at normal body temperature. The most common forms used in nuclear medicine are the cyclotron-produced gallium-67, used in the form of [^{67}Ga]Ga-citrate for SPECT imaging, and the generator-produced gallium-68, for PET imaging.

[^{67}Ga]Ga-citrate acts within the body as an iron analog and for the first 16–20 h is primarily in its free form with high blood pool activity and renal excretion. After 20 h, it becomes bound to transferrin and lactoferrin, where it acts as an iron analog, and later, excretion takes place via the gastrointestinal tract. Imaging is performed at 24 and 48 h in order to provide the best target to background ratio. The advent of SPECT/CT allows for more precise localization of uptake and better clarification between physiological and pathological activity and has extended the role of [^{67}Ga]Ga-citrate in the sites without labeled leukocytes or funding for 2-[^{18}F]FDG PET (Fig. 4.1 demonstrates the expected biodistribution of [^{67}Ga]Ga-citrate and [^{68}Ga]Ga-citrate) [7, 12].

In order to image infection, specific and unique elements of the offending invasive organism have to be targeted, and this remains challenging. Some of the most frequently implemented infection-specific approaches so far have included targeting of the bacterial wall, passive and active internalization, several extracellular and membrane-bound receptors and enzymes, intracellular proteins and enzymes, DNA synthesis and translation, antimicrobials, and antimicrobial peptides [13].

Gallium-68 provides versatile labeling options with the following tracers often used in infection imaging: [^{68}Ga]Ga-NOTA-UBI, [^{68}Ga]Ga-chloride, ^{68}Ga-labeled siderophores, [^{68}Ga]Ga-apo-transferrin, [^{68}Ga]Ga-TF, [^{68}Ga]Ga-DOTAVAP-P1, [^{68}Ga]Ga-ciprofloxacin, and [^{68}Ga]Ga-citrate (Table 4.1).

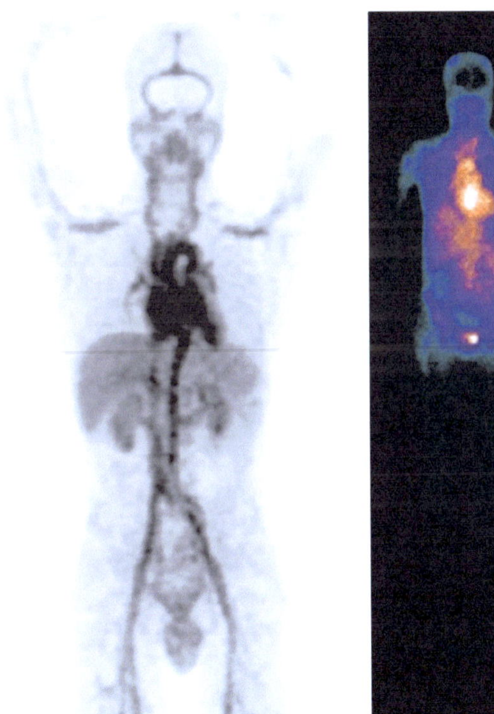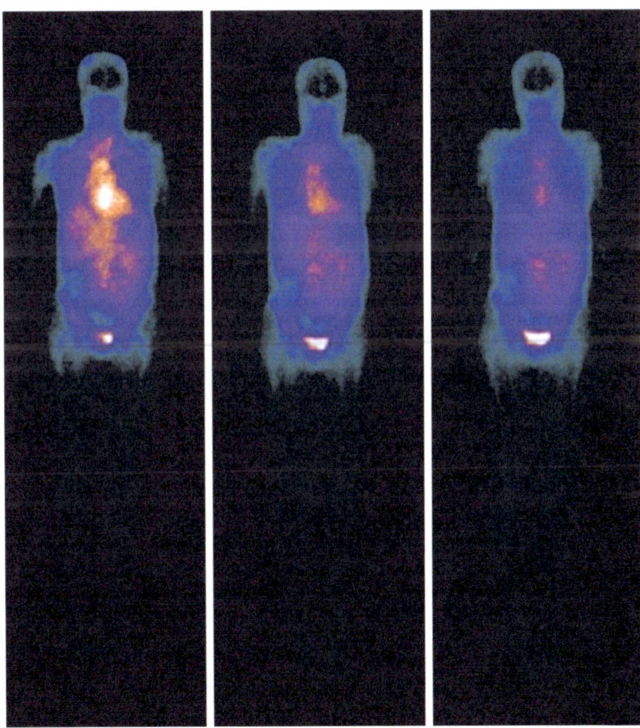

Fig. 4.1 A maximum intensity projection (MIP) image demonstrates the expected biodistribution of [^{68}Ga]Ga-citrate (left image). This image was acquired on a Siemens Biograph 40 PET/CT scanner at 60 min postinjection of 185 MBq of [^{68}Ga]Ga-citrate. The normal biodistribution includes high vascular activity and activity in the salivary glands, liver, spleen, and bone marrow. The series of images on the right demonstrates the biodistribution of [^{67}Ga]Ga-citrate at the following time points: 30, 60, and 120 min for comparison

Table 4.1 Gallium imaging in infection

Tracer	Target	Application	Setting	First author (year)
[^{67}Ga]Ga-citrate	Transferrin receptors, ferritin, lactoferrin	Musculoskeletal infection, TB, FUO	C	Palestro (1994, 1997)
[^{68}Ga]Ga-NOTA-UBI 29-41	Bacterial cell wall	Musculoskeletal infection vs. inflammation, TB	PC	Ebenhan (2014)
[^{68}Ga]Ga-DOTA-depsidomycin	Bacterial cell wall	Tuberculosis, *E. coli*	PC	Mokaleng (2014)
[^{68}Ga]Ga-ciprofloxacin	Bacterial DNA gyrase	Musculoskeletal infections	PC	Satpati (2015)
[^{68}Ga]Ga-TAFC/FOXE	Siderophores; iron transporters in bacteria and fungi	Aspergillosis	PC	Petrik (2010–2012)
[^{68}Ga]Ga-chloride	Transferrin receptors, ferritin, lactoferrin	Chlamydia genitourinary tract infections	PC	Nanni (2009)
[^{68}Ga]Ga-chloride/ apo-transferrin	Transferrin receptors, ferritin, lactoferrin	Musculoskeletal infection vs. inflammation	PC	Kumar (2011)
[^{68}Ga]Ga-citrate	Transferrin receptors, ferritin, lactoferrin	Inflammatory bowel disease	C	Rizzello (2009)
[^{68}Ga]Ga-citrate	Transferrin receptors, ferritin, lactoferrin	Musculoskeletal infections	C	Nanni (2010)
[^{68}Ga]Ga-citrate	Transferrin receptors, ferritin, lactoferrin	Tuberculosis	C	Vorster (2014)
[^{68}Ga]Ga-DOTAVAP-P1	Vascular adhesion protein-1 (VAP-1)	Infection vs. inflammation	C	Lankinen (2008)

TB tuberculosis, *FUO* fever of unknown origin, *PC* preclinical, *C* clinical

4.3 Preclinical Studies in Infection

One promising infection-specific agent that has emerged is probably [^{68}Ga]Ga-UBI, which followed from the development of the bacteria-specific peptide [^{99m}Tc]Tc-UBI. There has been particular interest in the development of new radiotracers based on antibiotic derivatives, the assessment of its biodistribution, and binding to the target bacteria, as reported on by Ebenhan et al. and in particular with the use of [^{68}Ga]Ga-NOTA-UBI-29-41 [14].

PET/CT imaging with [^{68}Ga]Ga-UBI in *Staphylococcus aureus*-infected rabbits demonstrated relatively increased tracer uptake in infected muscles when compared with healthy and inflamed muscles, which supports, at least in part, bacteria-specific binding. This also correlated well with the in vitro results that confirmed bacterial binding. Injection of healthy monkeys with [^{68}Ga]Ga-NOTA-UBI-29-41 demonstrated mainly rapid renal clearance and the absence of activity in target organs, such as the lungs, the musculoskeletal system, and the abdomen. Although these ^{68}Ga-labeled tracers offer many advantages in logistics and costs, it should be noted that the intensity of the uptake in infective lesions is notably less when compared to that of 2-[^{18}F]FDG (Fig. 4.2) [14].

Satpati et al. investigated two ^{68}Ga-labeled ciprofloxacin conjugates in vitro and in vivo with promising results. Increased tracer accumulation was noted in *Staphylococcus aureus* cells when compared to nonviable cells in vitro, and they reported discriminatory values between bacterial infection and inflammation in a rat model [15].

Mokaleng et al. reported on the use of [^{68}Ga]Ga-DOTA-depsidomycin in a proof-of-concept study in a mouse model. Tuberculosis (TB) was induced in the thigh muscle, and this demonstrated increased uptake with no uptake noted on the contralateral side. Uptake was also reported in infections with *Escherichia coli* (Fig. 4.3) [16].

Preclinical results in bone infection imaging have indicated that fewer false-positive results due to postsurgical inflammatory changes were noticed when using [^{68}Ga]Ga-chloride, that it is possible to differentiate between infection and inflammation as early as 7 days after the intervention when using [^{68}Ga]Ga-DOTAVAP-P1, and that detection of *Staphylococcus aureus* and other anaerobic infections is possible as early as 1 h after injection with [^{68}Ga]Ga-Transferrin [17].

Kumar et al. have reported on the potential use of [^{68}Ga]Ga-TF in the detection of *Staphylococcus aureus* infection and gram-negative organisms such as *Proteus mirabilis* with promising results [18].

The emergence of hybrid tracers with the added ability to image optically during procedures opens the door to exciting new imaging possibilities. This is especially attractive in the setting of infected implants for the intraoperative guidance and monitoring of procedures. Welling et al. recently reported on an antimicrobial peptide conjugated to a hybrid label containing both a radioisotope and a fluorescent dye, as [^{111}In]In-DTPA-Cy5-UBI29-41. They reported good target to background ratios and specific accumulation in bacterial infections. Other advantages include detailed imaging of the infective process at microscopic level and real-time feedback during surgery. This novel approach is likely to find its way to PET imaging as well [19].

4.3.1 Chlamydia

Gallium-67-citrate imaging was long used in the detection of various infectious diseases based on its similarities to iron and its metabolism. It was then noticed that [^{68}Ga]Ga-citrate/[^{68}Ga]Ga-chloride with its similar mechanism of uptake and better imaging characteristics could be applied similarly.

Nanni et al. investigated genital infections caused by *Chlamydia muridarum* in a mouse model where infected mice were imaged serially with [^{68}Ga]Ga-chloride PET for up to 19 days post-inoculation. They reported increased tracer accumulation in the infected mice when compared with the normal controls,

which was validated with cervical swabs and in vivo analysis. The authors concluded that the [^{68}Ga]Ga-chloride could be used for genital infection imaging, despite its inability to clearly distinguish between infection and sterile inflammatory changes and suggested that [^{68}Ga]Ga-citrate might be promising in this setting considering its higher stability [20].

4.3.2 Aspergillosis

Aspergillus fumigatus is one of the most common airborne fungi, easily eliminated in the immunocompetent host. However, infection with this pathogen in the immunocompromised individuals remains potentially fatal, and the diagnosis of aspergillosis with the use of conventional investigations remains suboptimal. Iron plays an essential role in the nutrition, survival, and virulence of the causative pathogen *A. fumigatus*. Many of its siderophores (which function as iron transporters in most bacteria and fungi) demonstrate an affinity for gallium-68 similar to that for iron.

The in vitro and in vivo potential of gallium-68 siderophores to diagnose invasive pulmonary aspergillosis have been investigated by a group from Innsbruck. Petrik et al. labeled two different siderophores from *A. fumigatus* (desferri-triacetylfusarinine C/TAFC and desferriferricrocin/FC) with gallium-68. They injected it into a group of immunosuppressed mice as well as into a healthy group and reported that the tracer uptake in the lungs depended on the severity of the infection and that no uptake was noted in the lungs of the control group and rapid accumulation was noted in mice with severe infection. They also reported that tracer accumulation was highly dependent on the iron load, which could be blocked by administering high amounts of siderophores or NaN$_3$. Petrik et al. have reported on the possibilities of various gallium-68 (and zirconium-89)-labeled siderophores in a series of publications making use of animal models. The most promising results have been reported with [^{68}Ga]Ga-TAFC and [^{68}Ga]Ga-FOXE in the detection of aspergillosis, as these tracers accumulate selectively in infective lung lesions and

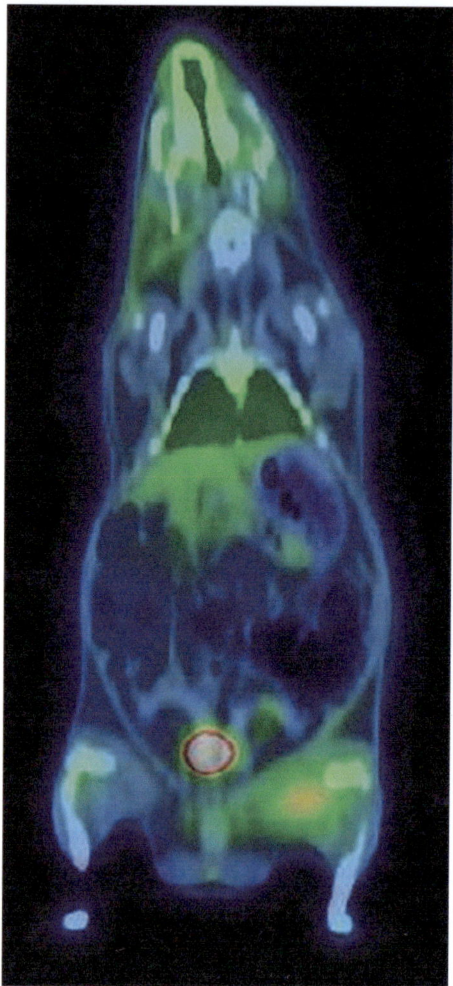

Fig. 4.2 [^{68}Ga]Ga-NOTA-UBI uptake in an induced tuberculosis infection of the left thigh in a guinea pig, demonstrating significantly increased uptake in the left-sided tuberculosis infection when compared to the right-sided control with turpentine-induced inflammation

correlate to both tracer intensity and infection severity [21–23].

4.3.3 Intra-abdominal Infections

[^{68}Ga]Ga-citrate PET imaging of intra-abdominal infections in an *S. aureus*-infected rat model demonstrated early increased tracer accumulation (at 5 min post-injection) with intense uptake noted between 30 min and 6 h at the site of infection. These findings were confirmed in a patient

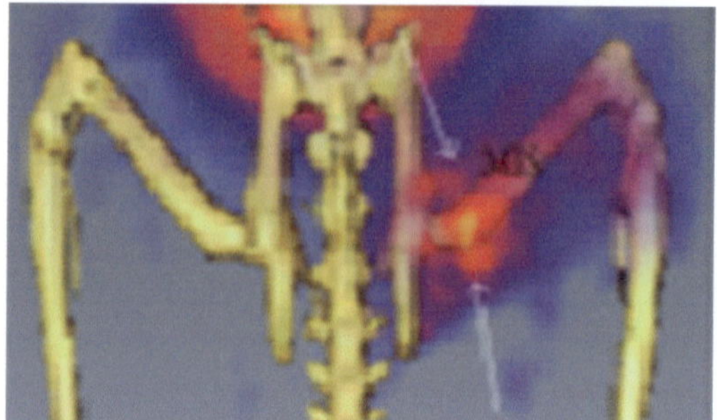

Fig. 4.3 Micro-PET imaging with [^{68}Ga]Ga-DOTA-depsidomycin demonstrates increased uptake in the left thigh muscle with induced tuberculosis infection

with postoperative intra-abdominal infection, which highlights the possible clinical application of [^{68}Ga]Ga-citrate in infection imaging [24].

4.4 Clinical Studies Using Infection Imaging

4.4.1 Osteomyelitis

The most well-known and validated application of [^{67}Ga]Ga-citrate is in the diagnosis of skeletal (and prosthetic) infections in combination with the use of [^{99m}Tc]Tc-methylene diphosphonate (MDP) imaging. Osteomyelitis is confirmed based on a relative increase in the intensity and/or extent of gallium-67 uptake when compared to the MDP scan. Vertebral osteomyelitis and discitis are two conditions where imaging with gallium-67 scintigraphy is still considered superior to other imaging techniques, such as white blood cell imaging [25, 26].

Considering gallium-67-citrate's good track record in the identification of infected limb prosthesis and osteomyelitis, it only makes sense that [^{68}Ga]Ga-citrate/chloride/transferrin would also perform well in the clinical setting of skeletal infections [27]. [^{68}Ga]Ga-DOTAVAP-P1 PET imaging has also been used in this setting [17].

Detection of infection with ^{68}Ga-labeled compounds has been best documented in the setting of osteomyelitis. In this clinical scenario, there is a need for a tracer with improved specificity when compared to 2-[^{18}F]FDG. Ideally, such a tracer should be able to distinguish accurately between infection and the inflammation associated with normal healing of bone or osteo-degenerative changes.

In a study by Nanni et al. (Fig. 4.4), 31 patients were evaluated for skeletal infections with [^{68}Ga] Ga-citrate PET/CT acquired at 60 min post-injection. Images demonstrated increased tracer accumulation in all patients with confirmed infection. The diagnostic indices were reported as follows: overall diagnostic accuracy of 90%, sensitivity of 100%, specificity of 76%, positive predictive value of 85%, and negative predictive value of 100%. Advantages of [^{68}Ga]Ga-citrate included favorable dosimetry, no contraindications before scanning, and the possibility of evaluating the therapeutic response [28].

4.4.2 Tuberculosis

Vorster et al. were the first to evaluate the use of [^{68}Ga]Ga-citrate in the imaging of patients with confirmed TB in a pilot study. All of the TB patients (some of whom were co-infected with human immunodeficiency virus) demonstrated abnormal tracer accumulation in the lungs, extra-pulmonary, or both (with a median maximum standardized uptake value of 3.71). [^{68}Ga] Ga-citrate accumulated in the pulmonary tuber-culous lesions noted on CT in almost half of the cases, whereas in the remainder of the cases, some of the lung lesions noted on CT were not [^{68}Ga]Ga-citrate avid, considered as consistent with nonactive tuberculous lesions. The majority of patients demonstrated extrapulmonary involvement, and affected sites included various lymph node groups, skeletal lesions, and the pleura, spleen, and gastrointestinal tract. The authors concluded that [^{68}Ga]Ga-citrate PET may provide a way of distinguishing active from inac-tive lesions for treatment response evaluation and that it appeared superior to CT in the detection of extrapulmonary involvement. Validation from larger trials is, however, still needed (Figs. 4.5 and 4.6) [29].

PET imaging with [^{68}Ga]Ga-NOTA-UBI has also been applied in this setting, and although ini-tial findings appeared promising in the detection and monitoring of TB, larger studies are needed to validate its potential use in these patients [30].

A case study of a patient with a central ner-vous system tuberculous granuloma demon-strated increased uptake of [^{68}Ga]Ga-citrate and [^{68}Ga]Ga-NOTA-RGD. This highlights the advantages of using a tracer that does not have uptake in the brain as part of its normal biodistri-bution (Fig. 4.7).

4.4.3 Fever of Unknown Origin (FUO)

Localization of abnormally increased activity of [^{67}Ga]Ga-citrate traditionally provided important clues with regard to the possible source of FUO. Possible sites of occult infection include infected cysts (renal or hepatic), abdominal or graft-related sepsis, and skeletal or joint infec-tion. When interpreting the findings of a gallium-67 study, it is important to compare the intensity of abnormal uptake to the liver, spleen, and bone/bone marrow or alternatively to the contralateral site or surrounding tissue [26].

In systemic infections, [^{67}Ga]Ga-citrate also offers significant advantages over labeled leuko-cytes, such as elimination of the need to handle potentially infected human blood and imaging patients with a relative leukopenia. However, in many places, 2-[^{18}F]FDG PET has replaced some of these indications. In some cases such as in sus-pected infected renal transplants, [^{67}Ga]Ga-citrate could still be used in combination with SPECT-CT, considering the absence of renal excretion after 24 h. This may result in a greater than 85% accuracy in a difficult group of patients who may have multiple comorbidities.

Immunocompromised patients (such as those infected with human immunodeficiency virus), or patients with an unidentified focus of infec-tion, could also potentially benefit from gallium-68 PET/CT imaging. Immunocompromised patients often suffer from (multiple) opportunis-tic infections, such as *Pneumocystis jirovecii* pneumonia, TB, chlamydia, aspergillosis, and candida in addition to the usual infections with *S.*

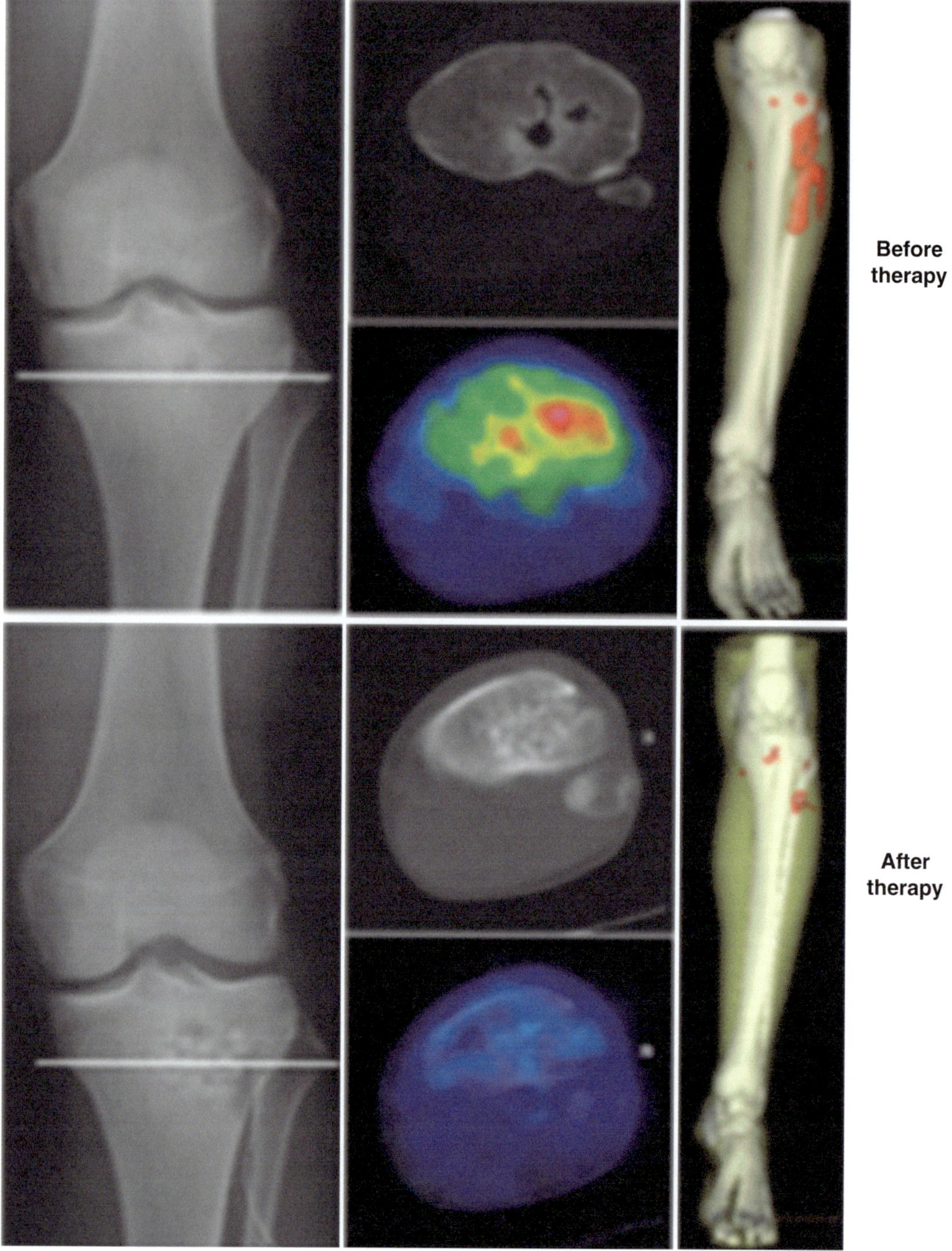

Fig. 4.4 A patient with osteomyelitis of the left fibula with a good treatment response on follow-up evaluation. (Adapted from Nanni et al. [28])

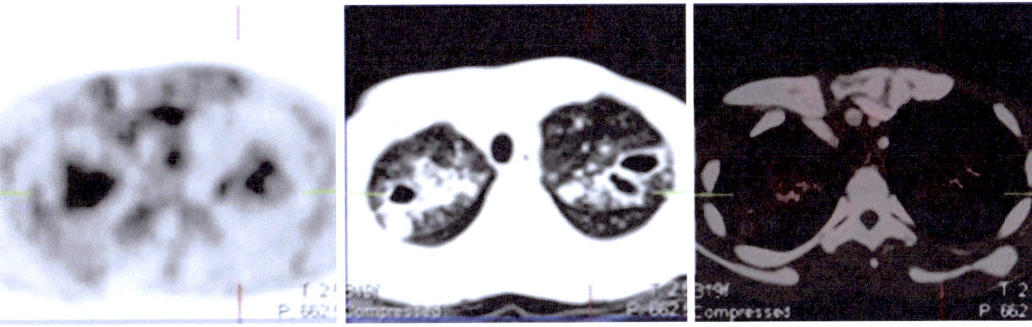

Fig. 4.5 A 44-year-old male smoker with right ventricular dilatation who presented with bilateral apical lung changes. Transverse [⁶⁸Ga]Ga-citrate PET, CT, and fused [⁶⁸Ga]Ga-citrate PET/CT images demonstrate increased tracer uptake in both apical lobes. Sputum cultures confirmed *Mycobacterium tuberculosis*

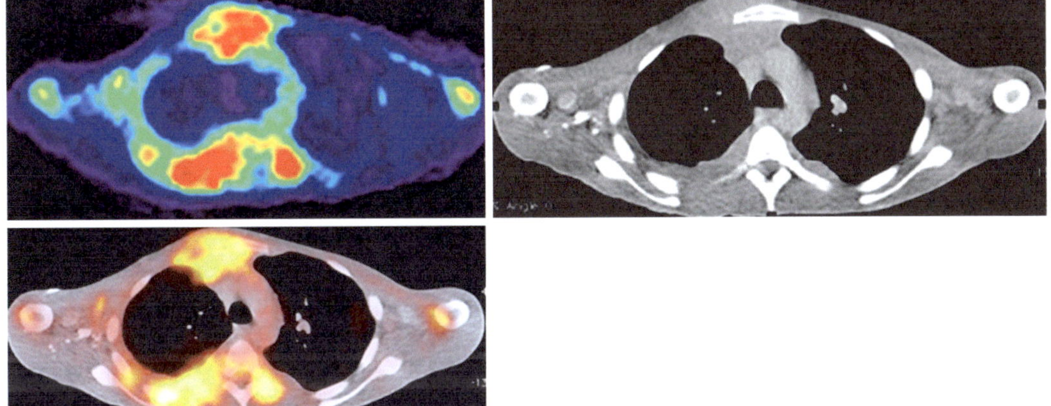

Fig. 4.6 A 28-year-old man with a large right-sided pleural effusion and *Mycobacterium tuberculosis* on pleural fluid analysis. Dual-time point imaging was performed at 60 and 120 min following intravenous administration of 224.59 MBq of [⁶⁸Ga]Ga-citrate and intravenous contrast. Intense tracer accumulation was noted in the anterior chest wall and posterior thickened pleura on the right side (SUVmax 1: 7.42; SUVmax 2: 7.17; decrease of 3.4%; hepatic SUVmax: 3.90)

aureus and other infective agents. Whole-body gallium-68-based PET imaging may direct further investigations or management in the same way as 2-[¹⁸F]FDG PET in the setting of fever of unknown origin [31].

4.5 Inflammation Imaging

The process of inflammation forms an integral part of the host's defense mechanism, and in acute inflammation, it represents the first response to harmful triggers such as trauma, chemical stimuli, and invasion by microorganisms. If left unchecked, inappropriate or prolonged inflammation may lead to unintended damage to normal cells and chronic inflammation. Inflammation may be associated with infection or not (sterile inflammation) and may be either localized or systemic [32]. Systemic inflammation underpins many debilitating diseases such as Alzheimer's disease, atherosclerosis, graft rejection, arthritis, diabetes, and autoimmune diseases and is often associated with the tumor microenvironment. Important role players in inflammation include macrophages, neutrophils, mitochondria, matrix metalloproteinase, various cytokines, leukotrienes, and chemokines released from inflammatory cells and the vascular endothe-

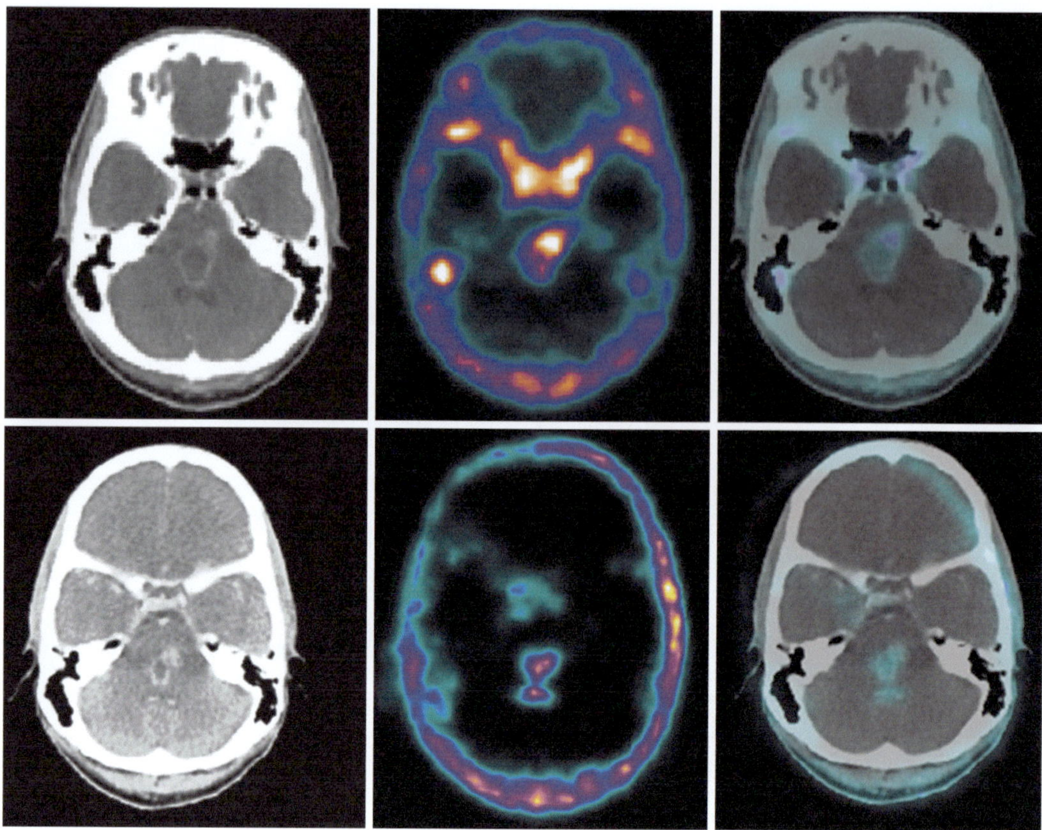

Fig. 4.7 PET/CT imaging with [68Ga]Ga-citrate on the top row demonstrate increased tracer accumulation in the tuberculous granuloma. The absence of normal tracer accumulation in the brain makes this an attractive agent for imaging suspected CNS infections. PET/CT imaging with [68Ga]Ga-RGD performed on the same patient on the bottom row demonstrates (slightly less intense) increased tracer accumulation in the tuberculous granuloma

lium [2, 3]. These aforementioned role players provide attractive targets for molecular imaging, thereby enabling insight into the underlying pathophysiology, early detection, identification of possible new therapeutic targets, evaluation of treatment response, and prognostication.

Gallium-68 PET/CT imaging can be used to image nonspecific inflammatory events, such as vasodilation or increased permeability (leading to an influx of macrophages and neutrophils), or used to target a specific aspect of inflammation (e.g., the somatostatin receptors on activated lymphocytes and macrophages), depending on what it is labeled to.

4.5.1 Nonspecific Inflammation Processes and Tracers

Vascular permeability increases significantly to allow a significant influx of macrophages and neutrophils with associated release of cytokines, chemokines, and leukotrienes from endothelial and inflammatory cells. [67Ga]Ga-citrate had long been used in this setting and could be substituted easily with [68Ga]Ga-citrate with its improved PET imaging capabilities and better logistics. Its mechanism of uptake also includes binding to transferrin receptors, ferritin, and lactoferrin [33].

4.5.2 Specific Inflammatory Processes and Tracers

The following brief discussion on some of the major role players during the process of inflammation (and potential imaging targets) is by no means exhaustive, and a complete list together with the different inflammatory pathways falls outside the scope of this chapter.

- **Somatostatin receptors** present an attractive target on activated lymphocytes and macrophages and have been imaged in the settings of sarcoidosis, pulmonary fibrosis, coronary artery disease, and vulnerable plaques. Somatostatin receptor 2A (SSTR2A) appears to be the dominant receptor subtype and may also play a role in T-cell regulation [34].
- **Formyl peptide R (FPR)** is a G protein-coupled receptor expressed on neutrophils, which is responsible for the migration cascade taking place during inflammation. Three FPRs have been identified in humans (FPR1–3), and these have been implicated in wound repair and angiogenesis besides their role in the regulation of innate immune responses [35].
- **Cyclo-oxygenase-2 (COX-2)** is an inducible enzyme that is responsible for the conversion of arachidonic acid into prostaglandins, expressed at elevated levels at sites of inflammation and malignant transformation, and is normally absent in most epithelial cells. It plays an important role in the inflammatory process and as such presents an interesting imaging and therapeutic target which can be inhibited by the COX enzyme inhibitor celecoxib. Preclinical studies have been performed making use of COX-2-targeted fluorine-18/crbon-11 PET imaging with promising results, which could be possibly extended to labeling with gallium-68 [36].
- **Interleukin-2 (IL-2)** is synthesized and secreted by activated T lymphocytes (especially cluster of differentiation (CD)4$^+$ and CD8$^+$ T helper 1 lymphocytes). IL-2 is present in degenerative diseases, graft failure, tumor inflammation, autoimmune diseases, celiac disease, vulnerable plaques, and insulin resistance [4].
- **Tumor necrosis factor-alpha (TNF-α)** is a cytokine involved in cell apoptosis and organ dysfunction, which increases the transport of white blood cells to the inflammation sites early in the process. In the late phase, the TNF-α level decreases and may cause the apoptosis of inflammatory cells in order to limit further unnecessary inflammation. TNF-α is an important role player in acute immune response to infection, injury, and autoimmune and chronic inflammatory disorders [37].
- **Integrin αvb3**: Overexpression of this integrin is found on the endothelial cells of neovasculature, cancer cells, and macrophages. RGD peptides containing the Arg-Gly-Asp amino-acid sequence are specific ligands for the αvb3 integrin and represent angiogenesis during chronic inflammation. [^{68}Ga]Ga-DOTA/NOTA-RGD PET has been applied to the imaging of cardiovascular pathologies such as atherosclerosis, vulnerable plaques, myocarditis, post-myocardial infarction inflammation, and cerebral infarction [38].
- **Vascular adhesion protein 1 (VAP-1)** is an endothelial adhesion protein stored in intracellular granules and translocated onto the luminal surface of endothelial cells at sites of inflammation upon stimulation. The stimulation causes leukocyte migration, especially CD8$^+$ T lymphocytes, from the blood into the non-lymphoid inflammatory foci [39]. Both [^{68}Ga]Ga-DOTA-VAP-1 and [^{68}Ga]Ga-DOTA-VAP-PEG-P2 have been used to target this vascular adhesion protein in order to distinguish inflammation from malignant processes (Fig. 4.8) [41].
- **The mitochondria** are a rich endogenous source of damage-associated molecular-pattern molecules (DAMPs). There is increasing evidence that mitochondria play a central role in innate immune activation leading to regulation of the adaptive immune response, and there is growing evidence that mitochondrial DNA is released in the setting of tissue injury.

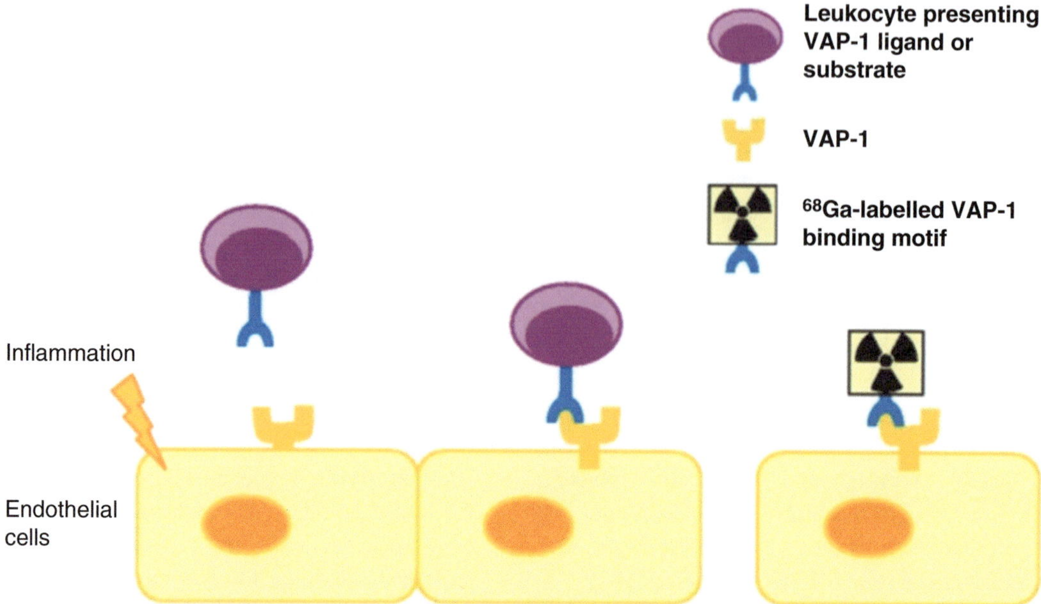

Fig. 4.8 Imaging inflammation with [^{68}Ga]Ga-VAP-1 in vivo. (Adapted from Roivainen et al., Eur J Nucl Med Mol Imaging (2012) [40])

It may also play a key role in the pathogenesis of autoimmune diseases such as systemic lupus erythematosus (SLE) and rheumatoid arthritis (RA) [42].

4.5.3 Tumor-Related Inflammation

Inflammatory cells and mediators are present in the microenvironment of almost all tumors. Tumor-associated macrophages (TAMS or TIMS) represent interesting targets for both imaging and therapy, and depletion of these cells has been shown to enhance the therapeutic effect of chemotherapy in some cancers [17, 18].

4.6 PET Imaging of Inflammation

Inflammation imaging with the help of ^{68}Ga-based tracers has been successfully used to image various types of pathologies as they occur in the central nervous system, cardiovascular system, respiratory system, and gastrointestinal system. Table 4.2 presents a summary of inflammation

scans performed with ^{68}Ga-based PET/CT in various preclinical and clinical settings.

4.6.1 Central Nervous System

4.6.1.1 Preclinical

Alzheimer's disease remains an important diagnostic and therapeutic problem characterized by the extracellular deposition of amyloid-β (Aβ) plaques. Several carbon-11- and fluorine-18-based PET tracers have been investigated to target these plaques. [^{68}Ga]Ga-DOTA-C3-BF is a novel ^{68}Ga-based benzofuran derivative which has demonstrated a high affinity for Aβ aggregates in the brain tissue of mice, with only low levels of uptake reported in the brains of normal mice with promising clinical translation possibilities [43].

4.6.1.2 Clinical

Angiogenesis with overexpression of integrin αvβ3 may follow an episode of cerebral ischemia during the recovery process and as such provides an ideal imaging target for [^{68}Ga]Ga-RGD. In a

Table 4.2 Gallium imaging in inflammation

Tracer	Target	Application	Setting	First author (year)
[^{67}Ga]Ga-citrate	Transferrin receptors, ferritin, lactoferrin	Sarcoidosis	C	Sobic-Saranovi (2013)
[^{68}Ga]Ga-DOTA-C3-BF	β-Amyloid (Aβ) plaques in the brain	Alzheimer's disease	PC	Watanabe (2014)
[^{68}Ga]Ga-NOTA/DOTA-RGD	Integrin αυβ3; angiogenesis	Cardiovascular (e.g., atherosclerosis, vulnerable plaque, myocarditis, post-MI inflammation) Cerebral infarction	PC PC C	Haukkala (2009) Caforio (2013) Eo (2013) Choi (2013)
[^{68}Ga]Ga-DOTATATE/TOC/NOC	Somatostatin receptor expression	Vulnerable plaque Sarcoidosis Pulmonary fibrosis Coronary artery disease	PC C C	Caforio (2013) Soydal l (2015) Ambrosini (2010) Rominger (2010)
[^{68}Ga]Ga-Fucoidan	P-selectin	Vulnerable plaques	PC	Lee (2014)
[^{68}Ga]Ga-DOTA-E-[c(RGDfk)]$_2$	Integrin expression; extracellular matrix remodeling	Myocardial remodeling	PC	Kiugel (2014)
[^{68}Ga]Ga-MPO-platelets/streptokinase	Platelet/plasminogen detection	Thrombus detection	PC	Jalilian (2008)
[^{68}Ga]Ga-DOTAVAP-P1	Vascular adhesion protein-1	Inflammation vs. malignancy	PC	Autio (2010)
[^{68}Ga]Ga-DOTAVAP-PEG-P2	Vascular adhesion protein-1	Inflammation vs. malignancy	PC	Silvola (2010)
[^{68}Ga]Ga-DOTA-PEG-FA	Folate receptors on macrophages	Post-medical implant inflammation	PC	Zhou (2013)
[^{68}Ga]Ga-citrate/[^{68}Ga]Ga-chloride	Transferrin receptors, ferritin, lactoferrin	Pulmonary fibrosis IBD Vulnerable plaque	C C PC	Vorster (2014) Rizzello (2009) Silvola (2010)
[^{68}Ga]Ga-DOTA-Siglec-9	Vascular adhesion protein-1; sialic acid-binding immunoglobulin-like lectin-9	Synovitis/arthritis	PC	Virtanen (2015)
[^{68}Ga]Ga-Anti-CD163 Ab	CD 163 Hb scavenger receptor on monocytes and macrophages	Inflammatory conditions, such as arthritis	PC	Eichendorff (2014)

IBD inflammatory bowel disease, *PC* preclinical, *C* clinical

first-in-human study, the uptake of [^{68}Ga]Ga-RGD was evaluated in a group of children with cerebral infarcts due to Moyamoya disease. Choi et al. reported significantly increased tracer accumulation in these infarcts, which appeared most intense shortly after the clinical event. It follows that [^{68}Ga]Ga-RGD PET/CT may be used in the detection and follow-up of cerebral (and other) infarcts and may provide important information with regard to disease detection, possible therapeutic target evaluation, treatment response evaluation, and prognostication [44].

4.6.2 Cardiovascular System

Cardiovascular diseases remain an important cause of morbidity and mortality, and the following inflammatory conditions have been evaluated with ^{68}Ga-based tracers: atherosclerosis, the vulnerable plaque, myocarditis, post-myocardial infarct inflammation, post-medical device implantation, and platelet and thrombus imaging. The majority of the aforementioned research was evaluated at the preclinical level and has frequently made use of ^{68}Ga]Ga-NOTA-RGD and ^{68}Ga]Ga-DOTATATE [45, 46].

[68]Ga-based tracers applied in the setting of cardiovascular pathology may add advantages over 2-^{18}F]FDG with its variable physiological uptake in the myocardium and interpretation difficulties [9]. The normal biodistribution of ^{68}Ga]Ga-RGD consists of renal excretion with significant tracer accumulation in the lungs, liver, spleen, and bowel.

It is further anticipated that the combination of complementary imaging modalities, such as PET/magnetic resonance imaging (MRI), will lead to hybrid imaging systems with improved sensitivity to provide powerful imaging tools for the spectrum of cardiovascular pathologies that are currently not diagnosed optimally.

4.6.2.1 Atherosclerosis

The changes that occur in vessels affected by atherosclerosis is partly regulated by anb3 and anb5 integrins, which are also increased on CD-68[+] macrophages. Integrin anb3 mediates intercellular adhesion of all proteins in which RGD is exposed and is expressed in the necrotic core of atherosclerotic lesions and in the shoulder of advanced plaques. The presence of micro-vessel formation within the atherosclerotic vessel walls together with the migration of activated endothelial cells regulated in part by the anb3 and anb5 integrins lends itself in particular to imaging with ^{68}Ga]Ga-RGD peptides [45, 47].

In a preclinical study on a group of atherosclerotic mice, the feasibility of occlusive atherosclerotic imaging with ^{68}Ga]Ga-DOTA-RGD PET was investigated. Haukkala et al. demonstrated a statistically significantly higher tracer accumulation in atherosclerotic plaques when compared to normal vessels with a mean ratio of 1.4. This suggests the feasibility of imaging with this tracer, although its clinical translation has not yet been established [45].

PET imaging with ^{68}Ga]Ga-NOTA-RGD and ^{68}Ga]Ga-DOTATATE have shown the most promise in the setting of atherosclerosis, and the demonstration of increased expression of integrins such as anb3 and anb5 has generated novel imaging possibilities for both the diagnosis and treatment of atherosclerosis.

4.6.2.2 Vulnerable Plaque

These lesions frequently lead to cardiac events and are characterized by a lipid-rich core, a thin fibrous cap, and inflammatory infiltrates. Macrophages play an important role in the expression of SSTRs subtypes 1 and 2 and as such can be imaged with ^{68}Ga]Ga-DOTATATE. PET imaging with ^{68}Ga]Ga-NOTA-RGD has also been used for imaging of these culprit lesions.

There is a significant expression of P-selectin by the endothelium which overlies advanced active atherosclerotic plaques in contrast to the endothelium which overlies inactive fibrous plaques. This has led to the use of ^{68}Ga]Ga-fucoidan for the imaging of vulnerable plaques. Li et al. concluded that ^{68}Ga]Ga-fucoidan could potentially be used to detect vulnerable plaques in vivo [48].

[68]Ga]Ga-chloride PET has been used to target and image rupture-prone plaques in a mouse model consisting of LDLR$^{-/-}$ ApoB100/100 mice which were compared to a control group of normal mice. PET findings were quantified by drawing standardized regions of interest (ROIs) over the left ventricle, the aortic arch, and the brachiocephalic artery which were identified on CT angiography. Silvola et al. reported significantly increased ^{68}Ga]Ga-chloride activity (1.8 ± 0.2) in areas of atherosclerotic plaques (especially in macrophage-rich plaques) when compared to healthy vessels. Challenges to the clinical translation of this study include the high level of plasma activity combined with the slow clear-

ance and relatively short half-life of [^{68}Ga]Ga-chloride [47].

4.6.2.3 Post-myocardial Infarct Inflammation

Imaging targets in this setting are presented by the SSTR expression on macrophages, integrin expression, and angiogenesis, among other role players that are intricately involved in the processes of post-ischemic inflammation and myocarditis. PET imaging with [^{68}Ga]Ga-NOTA-RGD, [^{68}Ga]Ga-DOTA-E-[c(RGDfK)]2, [^{68}Ga]Ga-DOTAVAP-P1, and [^{68}Ga]Ga-DOTAVAP-PEG-P2 has been applied in this setting, and the use of [^{68}Ga]Ga-DOTATATE PET has also been suggested for the imaging of myocarditis [41, 45, 49].

In a preclinical study involving rats, [^{68}Ga]Ga-NOTA-RGD PET imaging was used to evaluate post-MI inflammation in order to monitor the efficacy of angiogenesis induction therapy with basic fibroblast growth factor. Eo et al. reported significantly higher accumulation of [^{68}Ga]Ga-NOTA-RGD in areas of infarction, which corresponded to the amount of macrophage accumulation and expression of vascular endothelial growth factor. Significantly higher tracer accumulation was noted in the fibroblast growth factor-injected group when compared with the control group. This suggests that [^{68}Ga]Ga-NOTA-RGD PET may be a valuable angiogenesis imaging modality in understanding the underlying pathophysiology and in monitoring treatment response [46].

Kiugel et al. made use of [^{68}Ga]Ga-DOTA-E-[c(RGDfK)]2 PET to image the integrin expression associated with extracellular matrix remodeling after MI. PET imaging of rats at days 4 and 7 post-infarction demonstrated significantly higher tracer uptake in the corresponding infarcted areas, which correlated with the amount of β3 integrin subunits present. The authors suggested the possibility of using this integrin-targeting tracer to monitor post-MI myocardial extracellular matrix remodeling [50].

PET imaging with [^{68}Ga]Ga-DOTAVAP-P1 has been used to differentiate inflammation from malignant processes in a rat model. Autio et al. reported that [^{68}Ga]Ga-DOTAVAP-P1 PET was "more inflammation-selective" than imaging with 2-[^{18}F]FDG or [^{11}C]C-choline. Improvements to the biochemical properties of [^{68}Ga]Ga-DOTAVAP-P1 have resulted in the development of [^{68}Ga]Ga-DOTAVAP-PEG-P2 which has a significantly longer metabolic half-life, slower renal excretion, a higher target to background ratio, and radiochemical purity of more than 95% [41].

James Thackeray et al. compared the use of [^{68}Ga]Ga-citrate and [^{68}Ga]Ga-DOTATATE in a mouse model to evaluate post-infarct inflammation imaging. This was done with the view to guide and possibly facilitate improved therapy and healing. Unfortunately, the gallium images demonstrated high blood pool activity with nonspecific cardiac accumulation, which may pose a significant limitation to its clinical translation [51].

4.6.2.4 Post-medical Device Implantation

Imaging and quantification of macrophage accumulation in this setting may result in interesting insights and novel prevention strategies as these cells play an important role in the inflammatory response and in many of the complications that may occur following the implantation of a medical device. PET imaging with [^{68}Ga]Ga-DOTA-PEG-FA targets the folic acid receptors on macrophages and has been used in animals to detect acute inflammation post-implantation of a medical device. Zhou et al. suggested the clinical application of this macrophage-specific PET probe for the detection of inflammatory responses following various implants such as surgical mesh, degradable implants, soft tissue encapsulated cell implants, implantable sensors, and temporomandibular and other joint implants [52].

4.6.2.5 Platelet and Thrombus Imaging

PET imaging with [^{68}Ga]Ga-MPO-platelets and [^{68}Ga]Ga-streptokinase have been used to evaluate platelet behavior in thrombosis. Thrombus imaging may find clinical translation in stroke management and may also increase understanding of the underlying pathophysiologic processes in cardiovascular disease.

Clinical

In one of the few studies carried out in humans, a German group retrospectively evaluated the use of [^{68}Ga]Ga-DOTATATE in imaging of the coronary arteries in 70 consecutive oncology patients. Tracer accumulation was assessed in the left anterior descending artery and correlated with vascular calcium burden and other cardiac risk factors. Rominger et al. reported a significant correlation between increased [^{68}Ga] Ga-DOTATATE accumulation and the presence of vessel wall calcifications. In addition, a significant correlation between increased uptake in the left anterior descending and the presence of prior cardiovascular events was discovered. The authors suggested that [^{68}Ga]Ga-DOTATATE PET/CT could be useful in the imaging of coronary artery plaques [53].

Constantin Lapa et al. suggested that [^{68}Ga] Ga-DOTATOC PET/CT may evolve as a potential predictor of cardiac remodeling. They reported on [^{68}Ga]Ga-DOTATOC PET/CT findings in 12 patients (6 patients with active myocarditis and 6 patients with subacute MI), which they also compared to MRI. Imaging patterns on the two modalities showed high overall concordance and were closely related to structural changes and macrophage concentrations in vivo [49].

4.6.3 Respiratory System

Gallium-67 imaging has traditionally played an important role in the imaging of granulomatous diseases such as tuberculosis and sarcoidosis [7, 12]. Pulmonary infection imaging with [^{67}Ga] Ga-citrate is advantageous in light of the limited physiological uptake present in the thorax. In the past, [^{67}Ga]Ga-citrate was used to look for the cause of respiratory symptoms in patients infected with HIV and a low CD4 lymphocyte count. Differentiation was especially needed between *Pneumocystis jiroveci* (previously known as pneumocystis carinii) pneumonia and

Kaposi's sarcoma, the former demonstrating intense uptake, while the latter would be negative. More recent developments with regard to antiretroviral drugs and chest CT have both resulted in [^{67}Ga]Ga-citrate no longer being used in this clinical context. TB presented an ideal clinical condition for imaging with [^{67}Ga] Ga-citrate as chronic TB produces a large lymphocytic infiltration, which is very iron-rich and, as a consequence, very [^{67}Ga]Ga-citrate avid [54].

The distinction between infective, inflammatory, and malignant processes becomes especially important in the immune-compromised patient, in particular in patients co-infected with HIV and TB and where many of these conditions may coexist. It is now well known that 2-[^{18}F]FDG is unable to distinguish between tuberculosis and malignant processes and ^{68}Ga-based tracers may play a role in these settings [55].

Sarcoidosis is an incompletely understood, multisystemic, chronic auto-inflammatory disease in which a lymphocytic inflammatory infiltration, non-caseating granulomas, and, oftentimes, fibrosis are seen histologically. The skin and respiratory and cardiovascular systems are frequently involved; however, any organ in the body may be involved, including the central nervous system. Historically, [^{67}Ga]Ga-citrate SPECT imaging has played an important role in evaluating the disease extent as well as the treatment response. A recent review reported that despite the use of serum anti-converting enzyme and 2-[^{18}F]FDG, [^{67}Ga]Ga-citrate still has a role in identifying sites of active sarcoid, especially in neuro-sarcoidosis where extra-cranial sites of involvement could be identified [56]. [^{67}Ga] Ga-citrate has proven useful in identifying sites of active sarcoid and also could be used semi-quantitatively to assess the degree of inflammation and response to treatment. A semi-quantitative grading system comparing lung uptake with the liver and heart has proven to be robust in those patients who have diffuse lung involvement and seems to indicate a poorer prognosis [12]. It follows therefore that gallium-68 PET/CT with its superior spatial resolution, more favorable dosimetry, and improved quantification possibilities should be used in this setting [57]. Today, 2-[^{18}F]FDG has replaced this indication in many centers with its better image quality and logistics. However, the cost of 2-[^{18}F]FDG is higher, and there is little evidence that this changes patient outcomes or management in most patients with sarcoidosis.

Following on the initial work of Kwekkeboom et al. with SSTR scintigraphy, Soydal et al. reported image findings with [^{68}Ga]Ga-DOTATATE in patients with sarcoidosis. Disease activity on PET/CT was analyzed in combination with lung function tests and angiotensin-converting enzyme levels [58].

In a small series of patients with histologically confirmed pulmonary fibrosis that were imaged with both [^{68}Ga]Ga-citrate and 2-[^{18}F]FDG PET/CT, it was observed that patients had a distinct absence of [^{68}Ga]Ga-citrate accumulation in areas of fibrosis, which was in contrast to the increased tracer accumulation noted on 2-[^{18}F]FDG in the corresponding areas. The authors suggested that unnecessary invasive procedures could potentially be avoided in patients with absent uptake on [^{68}Ga]Ga-citrate PET/CT and that such patients could potentially rather be followed up and a watch-and-wait strategy employed (Fig. 4.9). The use of [^{68}Ga]Ga-DOTA-NOC PET/CT was also evaluated in a small series of patients with various forms of pulmonary fibrosis with promising results [59].

4.6.4 Gastrointestinal Tract (GIT)

Detection of pathology in the gastrointestinal tract is difficult with 2-[^{18}F]FDG due to its variable normal biodistribution, which may also be altered by certain medications, such as metformin. There is therefore a need for more suitable PET alternatives. Good clinical evidence remains lacking at this point with only a few reports available for GIT applications with gallium-68 imaging.

[^{67}Ga]Ga-citrate had been previously applied in the setting of inflammatory bowel disease, and therefore this translation to [^{68}Ga]Ga-citrate is not necessarily unexpected. In one of the first examples thereof, Rizzello et al. shared an image of a patient with inflammatory bowel disease in their article on the synthesis and quality control of [^{68}Ga]Ga-citrate. The image demonstrated increased tracer accumulation in the affected descending bowel, which suggested possible novel applications for [^{68}Ga]Ga-citrate in the imaging of inflammatory bowel disease as well as in the imaging of post-surgical abdominal infections. Nanni et al. and other groups have also since confirmed the value of this application [24].

Imaging of sulfonylurea receptor-1 to determine the β-cell mass of the pancreas with the use of [^{68}Ga]Ga-NODAPA-NCS-glibenclamide may be valuable in patients with type 1 diabetes mellitus who require transplants.

4.6.5 Inflammatory Joint Diseases

Imaging targets in the setting of inflammatory joint diseases such as arthritis and synovitis include VAP-1 and the CD163 receptor. VAP-1 is an adhesion molecule that moves from its intracellular sources to the endothelial surface during inflammation [60], and the CD163 receptor is a hemoglobin scavenger receptor exclusively expressed on monocytes and tissue macrophages, which may provide important diagnostic and prognostic information [61]. Available imaging tools to target these aforementioned molecules include [^{68}Ga]Ga-DOTA-siglec-9 and [^{68}Ga]Ga-anti-CD163-antibody conjugate. [^{68}Ga]Ga-siglec-9 (sialic acid binding immunoglobulin-like lectin-9) is a leukocyte ligand of VAP-1 that may be used for the detection of vascular inflammation (and malignant tumors).

In the preclinical setting, rabbits with synovial inflammation have been imaged with [^{68}Ga]Ga-siglec-9, compared to 2-[^{18}F]FDG. The authors reported that [^{68}Ga]Ga-DOTA-siglec-9 PET imaging detected VAP-1-positive vasculature in rabbits with mild synovitis in a way that was comparable to 2-[^{18}F]FDG, suggesting a potential role in the imaging of synovial inflammation in patients with rheumatic diseases [62]. Virtanen et al. also reported on [^{68}Ga]Ga-DOTA-

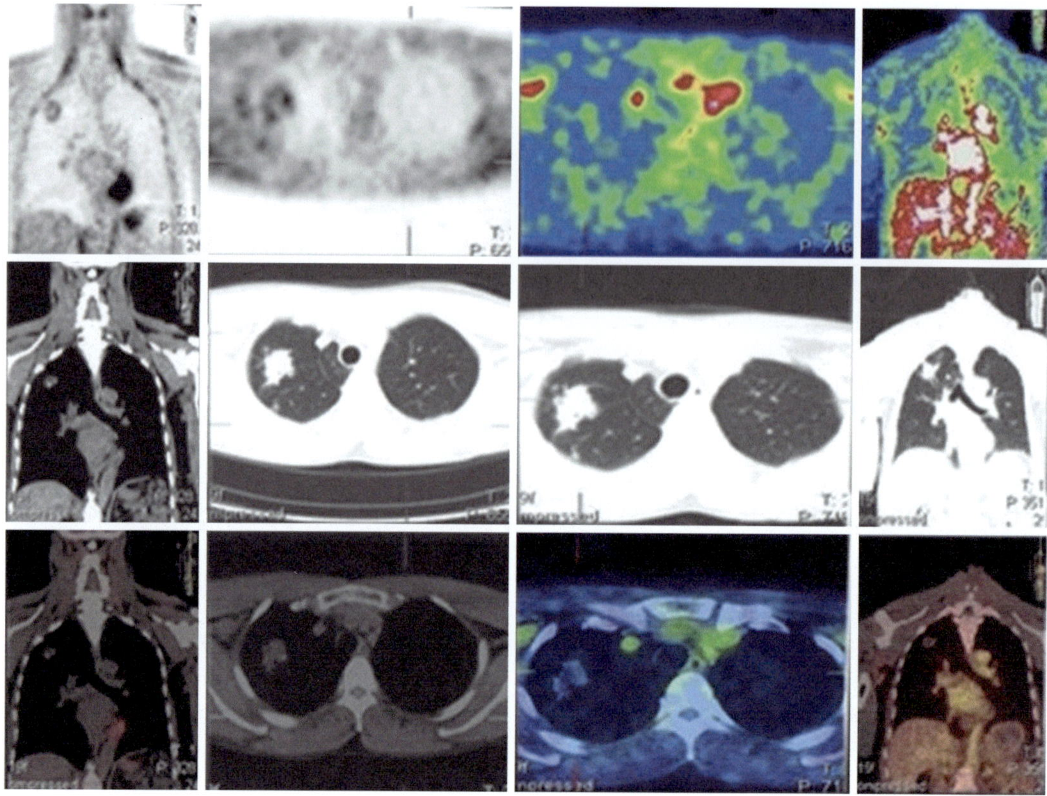

Fig. 4.9 A 49-year-old male presented with a right upper lobe mass, which was discovered incidentally following a routine chest X-ray. He had a long-standing smoking history (greater than 20 years) and worked in a coal mine for 17 years. He was completely asymptomatic and had no other comorbidities. The pretest probability combined with the suspicious CT features was highly suggestive of a malignant process. Two PET/CT scans were performed within a week of one another, one with [68Ga]Ga-citrate and the other with 2-[18F]FDG for comparison. The 2-[18F] FDG images (on the left) clearly demonstrate uptake, whereas there is no demonstrable uptake on the [68Ga] Ga-citrate images (right). Histology confirmed the presence of fibrosis. (Adapted from Vorster et al., Current Pharmaceutical Design, 2018, Vol. 24 [27])

siglec-9 as a novel imaging tool for the detection of synovitis [63].

Eichendorff et al. made use of a rat model to report on the biodistribution and PET imaging of a [68Ga]Ga-anti-CD163-antibody conjugate and concluded that it could be used in the imaging of macrophages in inflammatory conditions [64].

4.7 Summary and Future Considerations

This chapter summarizes some of the highlights with regard to gallium imaging, especially gallium-68, as applied to PET imaging of infection and inflammation. These conditions, namely, infection and inflammation, remain important contributors to morbidity and mortality and encompass a broad spectrum of pathologies, the distinction and diagnosis of which is not always clear. There remains therefore a need for improved imaging modalities to direct patient management appropriately, evaluate treatment response, and prognosticate more accurately.

68Ga-based tracers provide all of the advantages of imaging with PET/CT or PET/MRI without the need for a nearby cyclotron and show promise in addressing the relatively poor record of infection and inflammation imaging. These advantages follow from the excellent track record established by gallium-67 infection and inflammation SPECT imaging. Several further important recent advances regarding PET/MRI, improved chelators, tracer delivery possibilities, and antimicrobial peptides that are conjugated to both a radioisotope and a fluorescent dye may further advance this field.

Despite the explosion in the development of new ^{68}Ga-labeled tracers, most of these have still only been evaluated in the preclinical settings. Imaging methodologies also remain non-standardized for now, so the possibility of performing a meta-analysis on the results of various groups remain for now elusive. There are also several interesting novel targets, such as COX-2, matrix metalloproteinase, TNF-α, and various cytokines, which have not yet been labeled with gallium-68.

The ^{68}Ga-based infection and inflammation tracers, which have been used in limited numbers of patients so far, are [^{68}Ga]Ga-NOTA-UBI29-41, [^{68}Ga]Ga-DOTATATE, [^{68}Ga]Ga-DOTA, and [^{68}Ga]Ga-citrate. These tracers have shown promising results in the imaging of various musculo-skeletal, respiratory, and cardiovascular inflammatory and infectious conditions. Another future development may include the possibility of therapeutic options following imaging diagnosis in a theranostic approach similar to that used in treating oncology patients.

References

1. MacNeil A, Glaziou P, Sismanidis C, Maloney S, Floyd K. Global epidemiology of tuberculosis and progress toward achieving global targets - 2017. MMWR Morb Mortal Wkly Rep. 2019;68:263–6.
2. Espinoza J. Malaria resurgence in the Americas: an underestimated threat. Pathogens. 2019;8:11–4.
3. Hotamisligil GS. Inflammation and metabolic disorders. Nature. 2006;444:860–7.
4. Coussens LM, Werb Z. Inflammation and cancer. Nature. 2002;420:860–7.
5. Decristoforo C. Gallium-68—a new opportunity for PET available from a long shelf-life generator - automation and applications. Curr Radiopharm. 2012;5:212–20.
6. Roesch F. Maturation of a key resource - the germanium-68/gallium-68 generator: development and new insights. Curr Radiopharm. 2012;5:202–11.
7. Tsuchiya Y, Nakao A, Komatsu T, Yamamoto M, Shimokata K. Relationship between gallium 67 citrate scanning and transferrin receptor expression in lung diseases. Chest. 1992;102:530–4.
8. Spang P, Herrmann C, Roesch F. Bifunctional Gallium-68 chelators—past, present, and future. Semin Nucl Med. 2016;46:373–94.
9. Vorster M, Maes A, Van deWiele C, Sathekge M. Gallium-68: a systematic review of its non-oncological applications. Nucl Med Commun. 2013;34:834–54.
10. Vorster M, Maes A, Van de Wiele C, Sathekge M. Gallium-68 PET—a powerful generator-based alternative to infection and inflammation imaging. Semin Nucl Med. 2016;46:436–47.
11. Velikyan I. Prospective of 68Ga radionuclide contribution to the development of imaging agents for infection and inflammation. Contrast Media Mol Imaging. 2018;2018:1–24.
12. Siemsen JK, Grebe SF, Waxman AD. The use of gallium-67 in pulmonary disorders. Semin Nucl Med. 1978;8:235–49.
13. Auletta S, Varani M, Horvat R, Galli F, Signore A, Hess S. PET radiopharmaceuticals for specific bacteria imaging: a systematic review. JCM. 2019;8:197–25.
14. Ebenhan T, Chadwick N, Sathekge MM, Govender P, Govender T, Kruger HG, Marjanovic-Painter B, Zeevaart JR. Peptide synthesis, characterization and 68Ga-radiolabeling of NOTA-conjugated ubiquicidin fragments for prospective infection imaging with PET/CT. Nucl Med Biol. 2014;41:390–400.
15. Satpati D, Arjun C, Krishnamohan R, Samuel G, Banerjee S. 68Ga-labeled ciprofloxacin conjugates as radiotracers for targeting bacterial infection. Chem Biol Drug Des. 2015;87:680–6.
16. Mokaleng BB, Ebenhan T, Ramesh S, et al. Synthesis, 68Ga-radiolabeling, and preliminary in vivo assessment of a depsipeptide-derived compound as a potential PET/CT infection imaging agent. Biomed Res Int. 2015;2015:1–12.
17. Lankinen P, Mäkinen TJ, Pöyhönen TA, Virsu P, Salomäki S, Hakanen AJ, Jalkanen S, Aro HT, Roivainen A. 68Ga-DOTAVAP-P1 PET imaging capable of demonstrating the phase of inflammation in healing bones and the progress of infection in osteomyelitic bones. Eur J Nucl Med Mol Imaging. 2007;35:352–64.
18. Kumar V, Boddeti DK, Evans SG, Roesch F, Howman-Giles R. Potential use of 68Ga-apo-transferrin as a PET imaging agent for detecting Staphylococcus aureus infection. Nucl Med Biol. 2011;38:393–8.
19. Welling MM, Bunschoten A, Kuil J, Nelissen RGHH, Beekman FJ, Buckle T, van Leeuwen FWB. Development of a hybrid tracer for SPECT and optical imaging of bacterial infections. Bioconjug Chem. 2015;26:839–49.
20. Nanni C, Marangoni A, Quarta C, et al. Small animal PET for the evaluation of an animal model of genital infection. Clin Physiol Funct Imaging. 2009;29:187–92.

21. Petrik M, Haas H, Dobrozemsky G, Lass-Florl C, Helbok A, Blatzer M, Dietrich H, Decristoforo C. 68Ga-siderophores for PET imaging of invasive pulmonary aspergillosis: proof of principle. J Nucl Med. 2010;51:639–45.

22. Petrik M, Franssen GM, Haas H, Laverman P, Hörtnagl C, Schrettl M, Helbok A, Lass-Flörl C, Decristoforo C. Preclinical evaluation of two 68Ga-siderophores as potential radiopharmaceuticals for Aspergillus fumigatus infection imaging. Eur J Nucl Med Mol Imaging. 2012;39:1175–83.

23. Petrik M, Haas H, Laverman P, Schrettl M, Franssen GM, Blatzer M, Decristoforo C. 68Ga-Triacetylfusarinine C and 68Ga-ferrioxamine E for Aspergillus infection imaging: uptake specificity in various microorganisms. Mol Imaging Biol. 2013;16:102–8.

24. Rizzello A, Di Pierro D, Lodi F, et al. Synthesis and quality control of 68Ga citrate for routine clinical PET. Nucl Med Commun. 2009;30:542–5.

25. Palestro CJ, Torres MA. Radionuclide imaging in orthopedic infections. Semin Nucl Med. 1997;27:334–45.

26. Palestro CJ. The current role of gallium imaging in infection. Semin Nucl Med. 1994;24:128–41.

27. Vorster M, Buscombe J, Saad Z, Sathekge M. Past and future of Ga-citrate for infection and inflammation imaging. Curr Pharm Des. 2018;24:787–94.

28. Nanni C, Errani C, Boriani L, et al. 68Ga-citrate PET/CT for evaluating patients with infections of the bone: preliminary results. J Nucl Med. 2010;51:1932–6.

29. Vorster M, Maes A, Jacobs A, Malefahlo S, Pottel H, Van de Wiele C, Sathekge MM. Evaluating the possible role of 68Ga-citrate PET/CT in the characterization of indeterminate lung lesions. Ann Nucl Med. 2014;20:303–8.

30. Mukherjee A, Bhatt J, Shinto A, Korde A, Kumar M, Kamaleshwaran K, Joseph J, Sarma HD, Dash A. 68Ga-NOTA-ubiquicidin fragment for PET imaging of infection: from bench to bedside. J Pharm Biomed Anal. 2018;159:245–51.

31. Besson FL, Chaumet-Riffaud P, Playe M, Noel N, Lambotte O, Goujard C, Prigent A, Durand E. Contribution of 18F-FDG PET in the diagnostic assessment of fever of unknown origin (FUO): a stratification-based meta-analysis. Eur J Nucl Med Mol Imaging. 2016;43(10):1887–95.

32. Chen C-J, Kono H, Golenbock D, Reed G, Akira S, Rock KL. Identification of a key pathway required for the sterile inflammatory response triggered by dying cells. Nat Med. 2007;13:851–6.

33. Tsan M-F. Mechanism of gallium-67 accumulation in inflammatory lesions. J Nucl Med. 1985;26:88–92.

34. Elliott DE, Li J, Blum AM, Metwali A, Patel YC, Weinstock JV. SSTR2A is the dominant somatostatin receptor subtype expressed by inflammatory cells, is widely expressed and directly regulates T cell IFN-gamma release. Eur J Immunol. 1999;29:2454–63.

35. Prevete N, Liotti F, Marone G, Melillo RM, de Paulis A. Formyl peptide receptors at the interface of inflammation, angiogenesis and tumor growth. Pharmacol Res. 2015;102:184–91.

36. Uddin MJ, Crews BC, Ghebreselasie K, Huda I, Kingsley PJ, Ansari MS, Tantawy MN, Reese J, Marnett LJ. Fluorinated COX-2 inhibitors as agents in PET imaging of inflammation and cancer. Cancer Prev Res. 2011;4:1536–45.

37. Bradley JR. TNF-mediated inflammatory disease. J Pathol. 2008;214:149–60.

38. Hodivala-Dilke K. αvβ3 integrin and angiogenesis: a moody integrin in a changing environment. Curr Opin Cell Biol. 2008;20:514–9.

39. Jalkanen S, Salmi M. VAP-1 and CD73, endothelial cell surface enzymes in leukocyte extravasation. Arterioscler Thromb Vasc Biol. 2008;28:18–26.

40. Roivainen A, Jalkanen S, Nanni C. Gallium-labelled peptides for imaging of inflammation. Eur J Nucl Med Mol Imaging. 2012;39:68–77.

41. Autio A, Henttinen T, Sipilä HJ, Jalkanen S, Roivainen A. Mini-PEG spacering of VAP-1-targeting 68 Ga-DOTAVAP-P1 peptide improves PET imaging of inflammation. EJNMMI Res. 2011;1:1–7.

42. Brennan TV, Rendell VR, Yang Y. Innate immune activation by tissue injury and cell death in the setting of hematopoietic stem cell transplantation. Front Immunol. 2015;6:1813–9.

43. Watanabe H, Ono M, Iikuni S, Yoshimura M, Matsumura K, Kimura H, Saji H. A 68Ga complex based on benzofuran scaffold for the detection of β-amyloid plaques. Bioorg Med Chem Lett. 2014;24:4834–7.

44. Choi H, Phi JH, Paeng JC, Kim S-K, Lee Y-S, Jeong JM, Chung J-K, Lee DS, Wang K-C. Imaging of integrin α(v)β(3) expression using 68Ga-RGD positron emission tomography in pediatric cerebral infarct. Mol Imaging. 2013;12:213–7.

45. Haukkala J, Laitinen I, Luoto P, et al. 68Ga-DOTA-RGD peptide: biodistribution and binding into atherosclerotic plaques in mice. Eur J Nucl Med Mol Imaging. 2009;36:2058–67.

46. Eo JS, Paeng JC, Lee S, Lee Y-S, Jeong JM, Kang KW, Chung J-K, Lee DS. Angiogenesis imaging in myocardial infarction using 68Ga-NOTA-RGD PET. Coron Artery Dis. 2013;24:303–11.

47. Silvola JM, Laitinen I, Sipilä HJ, Laine VJO, Leppänen P, Ylä-Herttuala S, Knuuti J, Roivainen A. Uptake of 68 gallium in atherosclerotic plaques in LDLR−/− ApoB 100/100 mice. EJNMMI Res. 2011;1:1–8.

48. Li X, Bauer W, Israel I, Kreissl MC, et al. Targeting P-selectin by gallium-68–labeled fucoidan positron emission tomography for noninvasive characterization of vulnerable plaques: correlation with in vivo. Am Heart Assoc. 2014; https://doi.org/10.1161/ATVBAHA.114.303485/-/DC1.

49. Lapa C, Reiter T, Li X, Werner RA, Samnick S, Jahns R, Buck AK, Ertl G, Bauer WR. Imaging of myocardial inflammation with somatostatin receptor based PET/CT—a comparison to cardiac MRI. Int J Cardiol. 2015;194:44–9.

50. Kiugel M, Dijkgraaf I, Kytö V, et al. Dimeric [68Ga]DOTA-RGD peptide targeting αvβ3 integrin reveals extracellular matrix alterations after myocardial infarction. Mol Imaging Biol. 2014;16:793–801.
51. Thackeray JT, Bankstahl JP, Wang Y, Korf-Klingebiel M, Walte A, Wittneben A, Wollert KC, Bengel FM. Targeting post-infarct inflammation by PET imaging: comparison of 68Ga-citrate and 68Ga-DOTATATE with 18F-FDG in a mouse model. Eur J Nucl Med Mol Imaging. 2014;42:317–27.
52. Zhou J, Hao G, Weng H, Tsai Y-T, Baker DW, Sun X, Tang L. In vivo evaluation of medical device-associated inflammation using a macrophage-specific positron emission tomography (PET) imaging probe. Bioorg Med Chem Lett. 2013;23:2044–7.
53. Rominger A, Saam T, Vogl E, et al. In vivo imaging of macrophage activity in the coronary arteries using 68Ga-DOTATATE PET/CT: correlation with coronary calcium burden and risk factors. J Nucl Med. 2010;51:193–7.
54. Bekerman C, Bitran J. Gallium-67 scanning in the clinical evaluation of human immunodeficiency virus infection: indications and limitations. Semin Nucl Med. 1988;18:273–86.
55. Sathekge MM, Maes A, Pottel H, Stoltz A, Van de Wiele C. Dual time-point FDG PET-CT for differentiating benign from malignant solitary pulmonary nodules in a TB endemic area. S Afr Med J. 2010;100:598–601.
56. Allard AB, Buscombe J, Kidd DP. The role of gallium (Ga-67) scintigraphy in the diagnosis of sarcoidosis. MRI. 2014;03:99–107.
57. Sobic-Saranovic D, Artiko V, Obradovic V. FDG PET imaging in sarcoidosis. Semin Nucl Med. 2013;43:404–11.
58. Soydal C, Kucuk ON, Ozkan E, Metin KK. Ga-68 DOTATATE accumulation in sarcoidosis. Int J Nucl Med Res. 2015;2:1–4.
59. Ambrosini V, Zompatori M, De Luca F, et al. 68Ga-DOTANOC PET/CT allows somatostatin receptor imaging in idiopathic pulmonary fibrosis: preliminary results. J Nucl Med. 2010;51:1950–5.
60. Jensen SB, Käkelä M, Jødal L, Moisio O, Alstrup AKO, Jalkanen S, Roivainen A. Exploring the radiosynthesis and in vitro characteristics of [68Ga] Ga-DOTA-Siglec-9. J Label Compd Radiopharm. 2017;60:439–49.
61. Buechler C, Ritter M, Orsó E, Langmann T, Klucken J, Schmitz G. Regulation of scavenger receptor CD163 expression in human monocytes and macrophages by pro- and antiinflammatory stimuli. J Leukoc Biol. 2000;67:97–103.
62. Virtanen H, Silvola JMU, Autio A, et al. Comparison of 68Ga-DOTA-Siglec-9 and 18F-Fluorodeoxyribose-Siglec-9: inflammation imaging and radiation dosimetry. Contrast Media Mol Imaging. 2017;2017:1–10.
63. Virtanen H, Autio A, Siitonen R, et al. 68Ga-DOTA-Siglec-9 – a new imaging tool to detect synovitis. Arthritis Res Ther. 2015;17:308.
64. Eichendorff S, Svendsen P, Bender D, Keiding S, Christensen EI, Deleuran B, Moestrup SK. Biodistribution and PET imaging of a novel [68Ga]-anti-CD163-antibody conjugate in rats with collagen-induced arthritis and in controls. Mol Imaging Biol. 2014;17:87–93.

¹¹¹Indium-Labeled Leukocyte Imaging of Infection and Inflammation

Sara K. Meibom, Ilan Y. Benador-Shen, and Gustavo A. Mercier

Contents

S. K. Meibom (✉) · G. A. Mercier
Department of Radiology, Boston University, Boston, MA, USA
e-mail: sara.meibom@bmc.org; Gustavo.Mercier@bmc.org

I. Y. Benador-Shen
Department of Radiology and Biomedical Imaging, University of California, San Francisco, CA, USA
e-mail: ilan.benador@uscf.edu

© Springer Nature Switzerland AG 2022
S. Harsini et al. (eds.), *Nuclear Medicine and Immunology*,
https://doi.org/10.1007/978-3-030-81261-4_5

5.1 Introduction

Infection and inflammation still represent significant clinical problems despite advances in microbiology, the molecular biology of the immune system, and therapy [1]. Infection remains one of the top ten causes of mortality worldwide [2]. Worldwide, malaria, tuberculosis, and acquired immunodeficiency syndrome (AIDS) cause 50%

of all the lethal cases of infection resulting in 5 million deaths and 300 million illnesses per year [3]. The emergence of multidrug-resistant bacteria also presents threats to patients, and delays in diagnosis are life-threatening. Early and accurate detection of sources of infection in the body is critical for tissue sampling and helps clinicians identify microorganisms and choose effective antimicrobials.

The clinical workup for infection includes physical examination, blood tests such as white blood cell count and levels of C-reactive protein, and analysis of aspirated fluid from sites of suspected infection. Although aspirates of infected tissues and fluids are ideal for diagnosis and selection of antimicrobial therapy, this requires knowledge of the site or source of infection that is suitable for sampling. Unfortunately, it is common for patients to show features of infection while the source or primary site remains unknown. The imaging of infection and inflammation fills the important medical need of locating the source of infection to help guide treatment. There are multiple imaging modalities that detect features of inflammation and infection in humans. Regional imaging methods that assess for a morphologic abnormality use cross-sectional imaging such as ultrasonography, computed tomography (CT), and magnetic resonance imaging (MRI) scans [4]. These imaging modalities help to locate abscesses for aspiration or drainage. However, these conventional imaging techniques rely on structural changes that occur in a later stage of infection and that can also be seen in sterile inflammation. For nearly half a century, scintigraphic imaging has been used to locate infections. A distinct advantage of nuclear medicine imaging is its ability to detect infection in an early phase before a morphologic change such as abscess formation has occurred at the site of infection [5, 6]. Whole body imaging is also easier to do with scintigraphy and is important in cases of fever of unknown origin (FUO) where locating an occult source is critical for adequate management [7].

Scintigraphy of infection and inflammation is possible using a variety of radiopharmaceuticals such as gallium-67 (^{67}Ga) citrate, radiolabeled antibodies and antibiotics, and radiolabeled leukocytes [8]. [^{67}Ga]Ga-citrate was the first scintigraphic imaging agent able to detect infection and inflammation. However, this agent suffered from lack of specificity due to binding to neoplasms and reduced sensitivity due to background activity in the liver, spleen, and gut. Although still useful in selected situations, [^{67}Ga]Ga-citrate has been replaced by [^{111}In]In-oxine or [^{99m}Tc]Tc-HMPAO-labeled leukocytes. Recently, 2-[^{18}F]fluoro-2-deoxy-D-glucose (2-[^{18}F]FDG) has also been used for infection and inflammation imaging with particular success in the diagnosis of spine osteomyelitis and FUO. [^{67}Ga]Ga-citrate is now reserved for diagnosis of suspected spine osteomyelitis when 2-[^{18}F]FDG is not available.

[^{68}Ga]Ga-citrate, radiolabeled leukocytes, and 2-[^{18}F]FDG cannot discriminate between infection and inflammation [9]. Despite this, they remain useful in clinical practice. Scintigraphy with radiolabeled leukocytes is still clinically relevant even with the availability of MRI and 2-[^{18}F]FDG PET/CT imaging [4]. This is particularly true given the development of hybrid gamma imaging equipment to parallel PET/CT equipment such as single-photon emission computed tomography (SPECT)/CT. These hybrid scanners allow fusion of cell tracking scintigraphy with anatomic imaging [10].

This chapter will focus on the clinical applications of leukocyte scintigraphy in the detection of infection in joint prosthesis and cardiovascular devices such as vascular grafts, endocarditis, and diabetic infections in adult patients. We also discuss their application in the workup of FUO origin in the adult, appendicitis, inflammatory bowel disease, and rheumatoid arthritis.

5.2 Inflammation

Inflammation is an immune response to invasion by a microbe or to an injury from a physical, chemical, or immunologic agent or from radiation. This results in local swelling, heat, and redness and sometimes causes pain. Inflammation can be acute or chronic depending on the duration of inflammation from the time of injury. Acute inflammation lasts for a short time (8–10 days) with chronic inflammation lasting weeks to years [11]. The pathology of inflammation involves multiple cell types of the immune system (monocytes, macrophages, leukocytes and neutrophils, eosinophils, B and T lymphocytes, natural killer (NK) cells, mast cells). These immune cells can act via phagocytosis and can secrete chemical signals that modulate the process of inflammation such as cytokines. Cytokines produced by macrophages, T and B lymphocytes, and mast cells include interferons, lymphokines, chemokines, and interleukins. These bind to cell surface receptors on macrophages, leukocytes, and granulocytes and steer the immune response. The release of cytokines results in an inflammatory migration cascade that is supported by enzymes on the surface of endothelial cells and leukocytes that lead to arteriolar and capillary vasodilation with increased vascular permeability and subsequent leukocyte and protein-rich fluid extravasation [11, 12]. The result is an exudate that can be purulent if leukocyte-rich or hemorrhagic when rich in red blood cells. Part of this process includes the migration, margination, and subsequent emigration of leukocytes as a response to the chemotactic factors [11]. These exudates are the hallmark of acute inflammation. The exudate may evolve into an abscess or the formation of granulation tissue which involves fibrin deposition, macrophage involvement, angiogenesis, and fibrosis with subsequent scar formation. Alternatively, acute inflammation may heal with restitution of normal tissue. Acute inflammation may also evolve into chronic inflammation where a proliferative response is the key feature instead of an exudative response. In chronic inflammation, there is a decrease in the number of polymorphonuclear cells over time and subsequent infiltration of mononuclear cells consisting of macrophages, lymphocytes, plasma cells, and fibroblasts. The proliferative response is fibroblastic and vascular [13].

Since inflammation is a response to an insult, it may be seen in settings where there is no invading microbe responsible for the infection. In this case, the process is sterile. For effective treatment, it is important to determine if the inflammation is due to infection or a sterile response. Leukocytes are unable to discriminate between these two scenarios. Hence, the clinical context is important in interpreting labeled leukocyte scans.

5.3 Radiolabeled Leukocytes

McAfee and Thakur discovered that the lipid-soluble ^{111}Indium-oxine ([^{111}In]In-oxine) was the most efficient agent in labeling leukocytes in human abscesses [14]. They described a technique for the radiolabeling of leukocytes with [^{111}In]In-oxine that remains in use to this day. [^{111}In]In-oxine is a neutral lipophilic complex that diffuses rapidly across the cell membrane into the cell. Within the cell, indium-111 associates with the cytoplasm and oxine exits the cell [15]. [^{111}In]In-oxine-labeled leukocytes have higher specificity than [^{67}Ga]Ga-citrate in imaging infection, and this makes it a better imaging agent. For example, [^{111}In]In-oxine-labeled leukocyte was found to have a specificity of 97% versus 64% for [^{67}Ga]Ga-citrate in the detection of abscesses [16]. Other benefits of [^{111}In]In-oxine-labeled leukocytes over [^{67}Ga]Ga-citrate include a more consistent biodistribution in the spleen, liver, and bone marrow and the absence of radiotracer accumulation in the gastrointestinal or genitourinary tract. Studies in the 1980s and early 1990s reported sensitivities of 38–100%, specificities of 15–100%, and accuracies of 60–96% for [^{111}In]In-oxine-labeled leukocyte scans for infection [17–20]. At the same time, [^{111}In]In-oxine-labeled leukocytes became the agent of choice for evaluation of patients with FUO, osteomyelitis, and prosthetic graft infections and were considered for the evaluation of inflammatory bowel disease (IBD) [21]. Four decades later, [^{111}In]In-oxine is still regarded as the gold standard for leukocyte labeling for infection imaging in routine clinical practice [5, 11]. Increasing focal accumulation of [^{111}In]In-oxine-labeled leukocytes over time is highly specific for infection [22] with a sensitivity for infection that is comparable to anatomic imaging modalities [23].

Rather than reporting sensitivity and specificity in evaluating the diagnostic performance of leukocyte scans, Lewis et al. evaluated the clinical utility of this imaging modality in cases of diagnostic uncertainty over a 7-year period [24]. A clinically useful scan was defined as one that definitely or possibly contributed to subsequent clinical management decisions made for the patient. This definition acknowledged that both positive and negative scans can benefit the patient. Lewis et al. reviewed 136 cases of suspected infection from 2005 to 2011 and found that 30% of scans were positive (defined as focal, non-physiologic increased uptake subsequently found to be a site of injection) and 62% were ultimately determined to have an infection. [^{111}In] In-oxine-labeled leukocyte scans were found to be most helpful for indications of osteomyelitis (79% clinical utility), vascular access infection (67% clinical utility), and FUO (34% clinical utility) [24]. Scans positive for vascular graft infection failed to contribute to clinical management when surgeons had opted not to operate and instead treated the patient with a prolonged course of antibiotics. Given findings such as those of Lewis et al., it is not surprising that leukocyte scintigraphy is still the gold standard for infection imaging.

The labeling of leukocytes requires strict sterile conditions and safeguards in place to guarantee that autologous cells are injected after radiolabeling ex vivo. In addition, personnel working with blood products must be protected against exposure to blood-borne pathogens. In the United States, the recently codified USP825 law specifies requirements for preparation, compounding, dispensing, and repackaging of radiopharmaceuticals [25]. The USP797 law specifies requirements for sterile handling of cell preparations to use in clinical imaging [26]. The regulations are complex but include the use of clean rooms and laminar flood hoods within a hot lab to avoid the risk of contaminating blood products meant for injection into a patient.

Cell labeling is done ex vivo after collecting 25–50 ml of whole blood [27]. Gravity sedimentation is used to remove the red blood cells. Centrifugation removes platelets and allows the collection of a blood fraction rich in leukocytes that is suitable for radiolabeling.

It is not necessary to separate out the neutrophils since it does not affect the concentration of radiolabeled cells in abscesses, and no difference in sensitivity has been found in studies using populations containing mixed cells [28]. Usually

[^{111}In]In-oxine-labeled "mixed" leukocytes are adequate for localizing the source of sepsis obviating the need to label pure granulocytes except in a few conditions such as intravascular sepsis (to avoid unintentional labeling of platelets and erythrocytes in the blood pool) and in patient with neutropenia. When using mixed leukocytes, about 60–70% of the radioactivity is bound to the granulocytes [29].

The presence of any [^{111}In]In-transferrin, with its higher stability constant, can decrease the labeling efficiency so the leukocytes need to be washed to remove natural plasma nutrients. Oxine is a bacteriostatic chelating agent. Though oxine is toxic in very high amounts, the safety factor is high because the amount of oxine needed for labeling is minute, less than 150 μg [30]. Oxine forms a 3:1 complex with indium-111 resulting in a neutral lipophilic complex that readily crosses the cell membrane. Once intracellular, the complex disassociates and the indium-111 binds to nuclear and cytoplasmic proteins where it remains bound for 24 h. The oxine leaves the cell via diffusion.

In addition to [^{111}In]In-oxine-labeled leukocytes, it is now possible to label leukocytes with [^{99m}Tc]Tc-hexamethylpropyleneamine oxime ([^{99m}Tc]Tc-HMPAO) [31, 32]. [^{99m}Tc]Tc-HMPAO is lipophilic, and labeling of leukocytes with this agent follows a process similar to labeling with [^{111}In]In-oxine. [^{99m}Tc]Tc-pertechnetate is eluted from a technetium-99m/molybdenum-99 (^{99m}Tc/^{99}Mo) generator and must be used within 30 min for cell labeling. [^{99m}Tc]Tc-HMPAO is retained inside cells by binding to proteins and cell organelles. [^{111}In]In-oxine-labeled leukocytes are washed with plasma, but [^{99m}Tc] Tc-HMPAO-labeled cells are washed with saline. Washing with plasma is thought to keep the cells under more physiologic conditions, but there is little scientific evidence to support one medium over the other [33]. Labeling requires a minimum of 2×10^8 total cells, corresponding to approximated 5000 cells/mm^3 using the standard 60 mL collection. Some studies showed that the leukocytes had preserved physiologic functions of chemotaxis, migration, and bactericidal activity [34], while others have reported a 50% decrease in chemotaxis and migration [35]. For this reason, it is prudent to test the labeled cells for viability and function using such methods as dye exclusion test. Injection of the [^{99m}Tc]Tc-HMPAO-labeled leukocytes into the patient should be performed within 1 h of labeling. Radiation damage to the leukocytes occurs, but the risk of lymphoid malignancy associated with administration of [^{99m}Tc]Tc-HMPAO-labeled leukocytes is negligible since the labeled leukocytes cannot divide and are then removed by phagocytosis and apoptosis.

It is possible to label individual populations of leukocytes, but the labeling of mixed cell populations is more common in clinical practice. The overall labeling efficiency is high, 95%, but the labeling reflects the distribution of leukocyte subtypes. Hence, 80% of the radioactivity is associated with neutrophils and 15% with lymphocytes. Due to imperfect cell separation by centrifugation, 5% of the labeling is to red blood cells [36, 37]. Due to neutrophil predominance, this mode of imaging is particularly useful for the detection of infection and inflammatory processes that are dominated by the chemotaxis of neutrophils, such as acute bacterial infections. Chronic bacterial infections, where macrophage accumulation is the significant immunological response, are frequently false negative in leukocyte scintigraphy. A common example is tuberculosis. For these infections, [^{67}Ga]Ga-citrate scintigraphy or 2-[^{18}F]FDG PET imaging is preferred. These modalities do not depend on the chemotaxis of neutrophils to detect infection [38, 39].

The main benefit to radiolabeling with [^{99m}Tc]Tc-HMPAO is that technetium-99m is readily available from generators, while indium-111 is produced in a cyclotron [29]. Advantages of using [^{111}In]In-oxine to label leukocytes include higher labeling efficiency, lower efflux of radiolabeled leukocytes, and lower cost compared to [^{99m}Tc]Tc-HMPAO. In addition, due to the breakdown of HMPAO linker, [^{99m}Tc]Tc-HMPAO-labeled leukocytes show activity in the gastrointestinal tract and some excretion in the genitourinary tract that reduces the sensitivity of this tracer for detection of infection in the abdomen and pelvis. Dual-isotope imaging that combines radiopharmaceuticals labeled with two different radioisotopes for simultaneous imaging is possible with [^{111}In]In-oxine-labeled leukocytes. This ^{111}In-based agent is combined with a ^{99m}Tc-labeled agent such as [^{99m}Tc]Tc-sulfur colloid for bone marrow imaging to generate a simultaneous scan that improves the accuracy of the leukocyte scan.

The major disadvantage of [^{111}In]In-oxine-labeled leukocyte is its poor dosimetry. Significant organ radiation doses limit the total dose injected to the patient. Hence, image quality with ^{111}In-leukocyte is inferior to [^{99m}Tc]Tc-HMPAO leukocyte because it is count poor. The low count rates of ^{111}In-leukocyte make SPECT imaging impractical, although not impossible. Imaging time must be increased when compared to [^{99m}Tc]Tc-HMPAO to compensate for the low count rate. Prolonged scan times lead to greater motion artifacts.

The dose-limiting organ for both [^{111}In]In-oxine-labeled leukocytes and [^{99m}Tc]Tc-HMPAO-labeled leukocytes is the spleen. In an adult given a dose of 10–18.5 MBq of [^{111}In]In-oxine-labeled leukocytes, the spleen receives a radiation dose of 55–101.75 mGy, and the effective dose equivalent to the body is 5.9–10.915 mSv. In an adult given a dose of 185–370 MBq of [^{99m}Tc]Tc-HMPAO-labeled leukocytes, the spleen receives a dose of 27.75–55.5 mGy, and the effective dose equivalent to the body is 2.035–4.07 mSv. The higher activity of [^{99m}Tc]Tc-HMPAO-labeled leukocytes improves image quality, while at the same time radiation exposure is half that seen with [^{111}In]In-oxine-labeled leukocytes. The smaller body size of a child relative to the size of the liver and spleen and the resultant difference in pediatric S factors result in higher doses to non-target tissues relative to a dose in the adult. The radiation dose to the spleen in children can therefore be quite high and is higher in cases with splenic hyperfunction or enlargement [40]. In children given a dose of 3.7–7.4 MBq/kg, the dose-limiting organ is also the spleen which receives a dose of 0.48 mGy/MBq, with an effective dose equivalent to the body of 0.034 mSv/MBq [29, 37].

5.4 Normal Distribution and Kinetics of Radiolabeled Leukocytes

The leukocyte pool is composed of 59% neutrophils, 34% lymphocytes, 4% monocytes, 3% eosinophils, and 0.5% basophils. Neutrophils originate in the bone marrow and have a life cycle of 2 weeks with a survival time of 2–3 days in circulation. Neutrophils migrate in the bloodstream to sites of inflammation via chemotaxis. Under the influence of lactoferrin, leukocytes adhere to the vascular endothelium [41]. Chemotactic factors activate leukocytes, and within 30 min they begin to migrate into the perivascular space [41]. Several hours later monocytes migrate with overall less than 1% of circulating monocytes entering the site of inflammation. Up to 10% of the neutrophils in circulation accumulate in the sites of inflammation. Bacteria are phagocytized by neutrophils and trapped in cytoplasmic vacuole where they are destroyed by enzymes [41].

[^{111}In]In-oxine-labeled leukocytes are more stable in vivo than [^{99m}Tc]Tc-HMPAO-labeled ones. The biologic half-life in blood of [^{99m}Tc]Tc-HMPAO-labeled leukocytes is 4 h, shorter than the 6 h of [^{111}In]In-oxine-labeled leukocytes. Immediately after the injection of radiolabeled leukocytes, about 60% of the activity accumulates in the liver, spleen, and bone marrow [42]. Marginating labeled granulocytes equilibrate into the spleen over 30 min after injection. There is some margination into the liver, but equilibrium occurs sooner, within about 5 min, due to the large amount of hepatic blood flow. The splenic activity should always be higher than liver activity with both labeling agents. A reversal of this pattern may indicate liver damage. First-pass transit through the lungs is similar with both [^{111}In]In-oxine- and [^{99m}Tc]Tc-HMPAO-labeled leukocytes. Transient margination of labeled leukocytes into the lungs is seen shortly after injection. This is illustrated in Fig. 5.1 for [^{99m}Tc]Tc-HMPAO-labeled leukocytes. The lung activity starts to fade 3–5 h after injection and is eliminated by 18–24 h under normal conditions [29, 37]. The prolongation of the uptake in the lungs

would indicate a quality control issue resulting in damaged cells. The margination into the lungs is less with [^{111}In]In-oxine-labeled leukocytes than with [^{99m}Tc]Tc-HMPAO-labeled leukocytes, but it is clinically significant for both agents. It hinders the early detection of lung infections. The bone marrow uptake is prominent very early after injection due to bone marrow margination. In the steady-state, when no further clearance is seen from the blood, the final uptake of [^{111}In]In-oxine-labeled leukocytes by the liver is 20%, the spleen is 25%, and the bone marrow is 30%. The distribution for [^{99m}Tc]Tc-HMPAO-labeled leukocytes is similar. There is very little clearance of [^{111}In]In-oxine-labeled leukocytes in the urine [29], but free [^{99m}Tc]Tc-pertechnetate and [^{111}In]In-oxine are excreted in the urine. There is no excretion of [^{111}In]In-oxine-labeled leukocytes in the feces, as illustrated in Fig. 5.2. The lack of bowel activity when imaging with ^{111}In-leukocyte is useful when evaluating abdominal infections, including inflammatory bowel disease or appendicitis. [^{99m}Tc]Tc-HMPAO-labeled leukocytes lose their labeling starting 2–3 h after labeling due to the instability of the linker. This leads to the visualization of activity in the bowel 3 h after injection of [^{99m}Tc]Tc-HMPAO leukocyte, since the radioisotope is excreted in the feces. This together with the excretion of [^{99m}Tc]Tc-HMPAO by the hepatobiliary system into the bowel can interfere with the localization of abdominal and perihepatic abscesses.

Early uptake of labeled leukocytes depends on the severity of the inflammatory reaction and the chelate employed to label the cells [43]. In clinical practice, there is a 24 h delay in imaging with [^{111}In]In-oxine-labeled leukocytes in order to achieve maximal sensitivity [44] even though it is possible to detect infection as early as 30 min after injection. [^{99m}Tc]Tc-HMPAO-labeled leukocytes localize more rapidly. Therefore, 1-h post-injection imaging in adults (30 min post-injection in children) can be done before hepatobiliary excretion and gut activity occur. Numerous studies have shown localization in infectious sites with imaging 30 min post-injection, although it is common in clinical practice to obtain 3 h and sometimes 18 or 24 h delayed

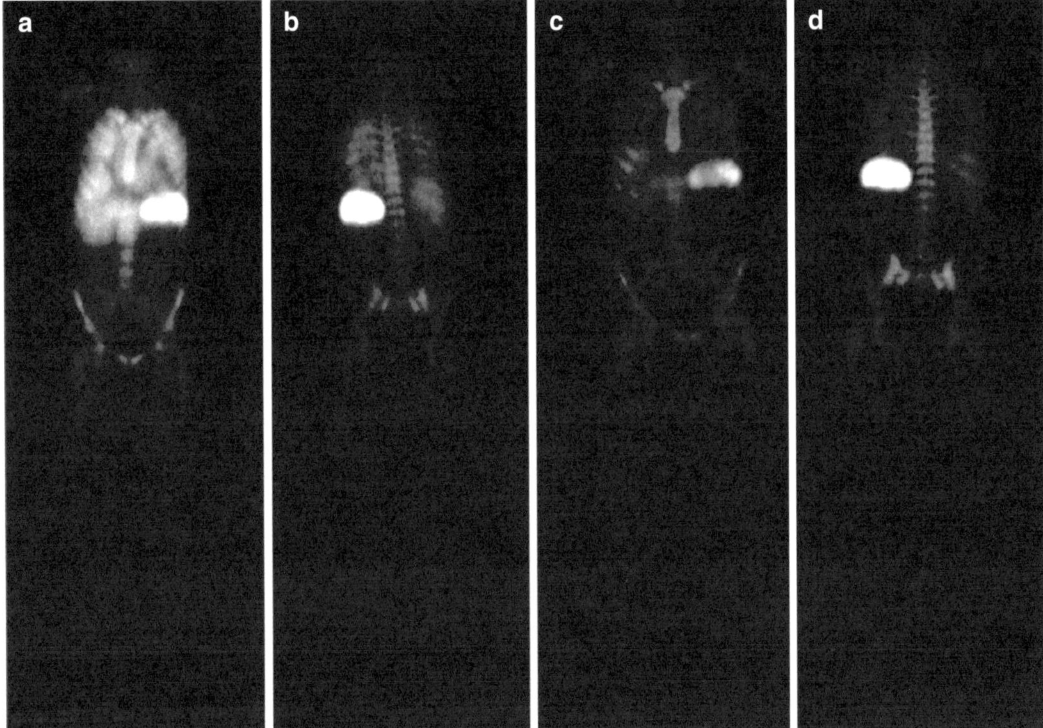

Fig. 5.1 Normal [^{99m}Tc]Tc-HMPAO-labeled leukocyte whole body scintigraphy. At 2.5 h post-injection: (**a**) is an anterior image, (**b**) is a posterior image with normal distribution to the spleen, bone marrow, and liver and transient physiologic residence of labeled leukocytes in the lungs. At 4 h post-injection: (**c**) is an anterior image, (**d**) is a posterior image with expected washout from lungs and continued activity in the spleen (greatest activity), liver, and bone marrow. Early images are performed as early as 1 h before potentially interfering physiologic bowel activity appears on delayed images. In this case, there is no gastrointestinal activity on early or delayed images

images [41]. This delayed imaging adds sensitivity. Larikka et al. showed that delayed imaging with [^{99m}Tc]Tc-HMPAO-labeled leukocytes was superior to early 2–4 h imaging [45]. The performance metrics of early imaging, 50% sensitivity, 90% specificity, and 95% negative predictive value (NPV), improved with 24 h delayed imaging to 83%, 100%, and 100%, respectively. The positive predictive value (PPV) also increased to 100% in this study. Since [^{111}In]In-oxine-labeled leukocytes are most suitable for delayed imaging, this agent shows higher target-to-background activity than [^{99m}Tc]Tc-HMPAO labeled leukocytes. This is particularly useful in the evaluation of abdominal and pelvic infections [46] because the gut activity is seen in delayed views with [^{99m}Tc]Tc-HMPAO-labeled leukocytes due to excretion. The target-to-background ratio for [^{99m}Tc]Tc-HMPAO-labeled leukocytes is one-third that of [^{111}In]In-oxine-labeled leukocytes in *Escherichia coli* abscesses when using blood pool or normal tissue as background [47].

5.5 Pathological Distribution of Radiolabeled Leukocytes

The uptake of radiolabeled leukocytes in pathology is due to cellular migration triggered by chemotaxis. Given the kinetics, optimal imaging is around 24 h after the injection of radiolabeled leukocytes [45, 48]. Pathologic uptake consistent with infection shows progressively increased activity over time in a distribution inconsistent with the normal distribution described above. Foci of initial accumulation that decrease or fail to increase in delayed imaging are considered negative for infection. This analysis can be done

Fig. 5.2 Normal [^{111}In] In-oxine-labeled leukocyte whole body scan. (**a**) is the anterior view and (**b**) is the posterior view. Both views are acquired 24 h after injection. The most intense uptake is seen in the spleen followed by the liver and bone marrow. There is no physiologic bowel and lung activity with this tracer. There is a small expected focus of activity from the tracer at the injection site in the right arm

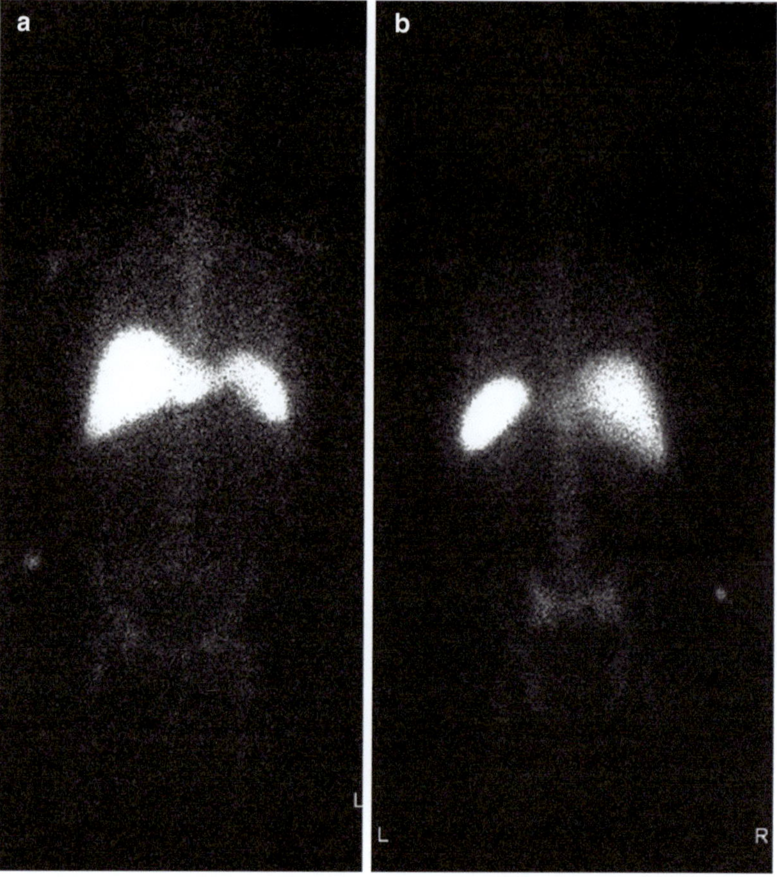

by visual inspection of properly normalized images, but semi-quantitative analysis has also been shown to be useful [49, 50].

There are reports of noninfectious uptake by radiolabeled leukocytes. Examples include metastatic disease to the bone and sources of inflammation such as colostomy drains. In addition, it is possible to swallow phlegm containing radiolabeled leukocytes from sinusitis or lung infection that lead to the detection of activity in the gut [21].

In theory, mixed radiolabeled leukocyte imaging, as performed in routine clinical practice, should be better at detecting acute than chronic infection given that the neutrophil fraction represents the largest number of labeled leukocytes. Moreover, a biofilm may develop with time around the site of infection that hinders infiltration by leukocytes. This should further reduce the sensitivity of leukocyte scintigraphy for the

detection of chronic low-grade infections. Although an initial study by Sfakianakis et al. was consistent with this theoretical expectation [51], subsequent investigators challenged their findings on the basis of technical problems with their labeling method and lower than the recommended dose of radioisotope [52]. In a retrospective study by Datz and Thorne, there was no statistical difference in performance when imaging acute versus chronic infection with [^{111}In] In-oxine-labeled leukocytes [52]. In that study, there was a 90% sensitivity for the detection of infection of 0–14 days duration versus 86% sensitivity for those lasting 15 days or longer. Al-Sheikh et al. reported findings consistent with Datz and Thorne's work [53]. They found no difference in the sensitivity between [^{67}Ga]Ga-citrate and [^{111}In]In-oxine leukocyte imaging for subacute or chronic bone infections. Explanations for the larger than unexpected sensitivity of

[¹¹¹In]In-oxine-labeled leukocytes in the detection of chronic infection include the presence of a large number of labeled granulocytes even when the dominant cells in these infections are mononuclear cells [54]. Merkel et al. also proposed that the large numbers of lymphocytes obtained by gravity sedimentation might be the reason for the high sensitivity of [¹¹¹In]In-oxine-labeled leukocytes in chronic infection [55].

5.6   Clinical Applications

5.6.1   Clinical Guidelines

Guidelines for imaging infection and inflammation are offered by the American College of Radiology (ACR), the Society of Nuclear Medicine and Molecular Imaging (SNMMI), and the European Association of Nuclear Medicine (EANM), among others. ACR provides clinical appropriateness criteria [56] and practice parameters [57]. In the former, the document defines a clinical scenario, and different imaging modalities are graded by a committee of experts on how clinically appropriate they are and their degree of radiation exposure. In the latter, the document summarizes potential applications and discusses technical issues regarding imaging such as optimal parameters and training expected for those supervising and reading the studies. The SNMMI and EANM have traditionally defined practice standards analogous to the ACR practice parameters but more recently have defined appropriateness criteria like the ACR. The SNMMI labels both documents as "clinical guidelines" [58], and the EANM simply calls them "guidelines" [59]. The EANM has published guidelines for the diagnosis of musculoskeletal infections and endocarditis and cardiovascular implantable electronic device infections among others, in addition to tracer-specific practice guidelines [60]. The SNMMI has published procedure standards that are largely tracer specific [61] and does not have developed appropriateness criteria for infection or inflammation imaging. The ACR practice parameter for the performance of scintigraphy in infection and inflammation [57] was

revised in 2018, and the document includes a discussion of radiolabeled leukocyte imaging. The ACR appropriateness criteria for diagnostic imaging studies include a large number of clinical scenarios stratified by the organ system [56]. Examples relevant to infection or inflammation imaging include documents "suspected osteomyelitis of the foot in patients with diabetes mellitus" and "suspected infective endocarditis" [62]. The applications we discuss in this chapter fall within these guidelines. However, we note that in general, the ACR favors anatomic imaging such as radiography or MRI over scintigraphy in the workup of osteomyelitis, soft tissue infection, and joint prosthesis infection [63]. We note when evidence supports leukocyte imaging in disagreement with the guidelines.

5.6.2   Fever of Unknown Origin (FUO)

Fever of unknown origin is defined as a febrile illness with the following features: "(1) temperature equal to or greater than 38.3 °C (101 °F) on at least two occasions; (2) duration of illness equal to or greater than 3 weeks or multiple febrile episodes in equal to or greater than 3 weeks; (3) not immunocompromised (defined as neutropenia for at least 1 week in the 3 months before the start of the fever; known HIV infection; known hypogammaglobinemia or use of 10 mg prednisone or equivalent for at least 2 weeks in the 3 months before the start of fever); and (4) uncertain diagnosis despite thorough history-taking, physical examination, and the following investigations: erythrocyte sedimentation rate (ESR) or C-reactive protein (CRP), hemoglobin, platelet count, leukocyte count and differentiation, electrolytes, creatinine, total serum protein, protein electrophoresis, alkaline phosphatase, aspartate aminotransferase, alanine aminotransferase, lactate dehydrogenase, creatinine kinase, ferritin, antinuclear antibodies, rheumatoid factor, microscopic urinalysis, three blood cultures, urine culture, chest x-ray, abdominal ultrasonography and tuberculin skin test or interferon gamma release assay" [64]. Studies of the etiology of FUO point to four main causes: infection, noninfectious inflammatory diseases, neoplasms, and miscellaneous causes. As the leading etiology, infections are responsible for one-third of all cases, and these include occult abscesses, endocarditis, tuberculosis, and urinary tract infections. However, noninfectious causes of FUO are more prevalent in elderly patients [65].

Leukocyte scintigraphy is sensitive and specific for detecting infection or inflammation in FUO. [^{111}In]In-oxine-labeled leukocytes have a role in detecting the source of fever of unknown origin in patients who have undergone non-localizing evaluation with other imaging modalities [8]. Published data found that the sensitivity of [^{111}In]In-oxine-labeled leukocytes in fever of unknown origin is 80% with somewhat higher specificity [66]. A negative test virtually excludes infectious or inflammatory causes with an NPV of 94% [7, 67]. Hence, it is not surprising that for more than two decades, the agent of choice for the workup of FUO has been labeled leukocytes imaging. However, recent literature supports 2-[^{18}F]FDG PET/CT as a first-line imaging modality for FUO [64, 68].

2-[^{18}F]FDG PET was originally employed as a tumor agent but was noted to accumulate at sites of infection because leukocytes exhibited high glucose uptake and utilization. 2-[^{18}F]FDG uptake in inflammation peaks at 60 min and then stabilizes or decreases. It is a convenient modality because there is no need to harvest and label cells. The main drawback off 2-[^{18}F]FDG PET is its lack of specificity since it also localizes in malignancies and sites of trauma, in addition to infection and inflammation [4]. Leukocyte scintigraphy is a useful adjunct because it has high specificity for infection. A meta-analysis of 42 studies with 2058 patients found that 2-[^{18}F]FDG PET/CT is 86% sensitive and 52% specific in detecting infections in FUO [68]. In comparison, leukocyte scintigraphy had a summed sensitivity of 33% and specificity of 83%. 2-[^{18}F]FDG PET/CT was successful in locating the source of infection in about 60% of patients, while leukocyte scintigraphy was only successful in 20% of the cases. It is noteworthy that the success of 2-[^{18}F]FDG PET/CT was largely due to the detection of

neoplastic causes of FUO than detection of infectious causes. In the absence of localizing signs and symptoms, Kouijzer recommends 2-[^{18}F]FDG PET/CT [64] to help determine which additional diagnostic tests should be done. The implication is that 2-[^{18}F]FDG PET/CT may be a good initial imaging modality, but it needs support from either tissue sampling or leukocyte scintigraphy to discriminate between neoplasm and infection. The specificity of leukocyte imaging, particularly when combined with SPECT/CT, is important in such situation as illustrated in Fig. 5.3 where an abscess accumulates labeled leukocytes, but there is no accumulation in the adjacent liposarcoma.

5.6.3 Infective Endocarditis and Cardiac Electronic Devices

The modified Duke criteria remain the gold standard for the diagnosis of infective endocarditis (IE) in native and prosthetic valves [69]. This criterion relies on physical exam findings, blood cultures positive for organisms consistent with IE, and imaging evidence, largely from echocardiography. Because of the protean syndromic presentations of IE, there are ongoing efforts to improve early diagnosis that allows for early and effective treatment to reduce mortality and morbidity. This drive for early diagnosis with improved imaging is most relevant to the widespread use of prosthetic valves [70]. Scintigraphic modalities to assist in the diagnosis of IE include leukocyte imaging and 2-[^{18}F]FDG PET/CT [71]. SPECT/CT when using labeled leukocytes is crucial in the detection of endocarditis and implantable cardiac devices since it affects treatment decisions [72]. In the setting of IE, these modalities complement each other due to differences in sensitivity and specificity. In a case series of 131 patients with suspected infectious endocarditis, leucocytes SPECT/CT was more specific for detecting foci of infection than 2-[^{18}F]FDG PET/CT, but 2-[^{18}F]FDG PET/CT was faster and had superior spatial resolution [73]. Indeed, a major disadvantage of leukocyte imaging is the limited

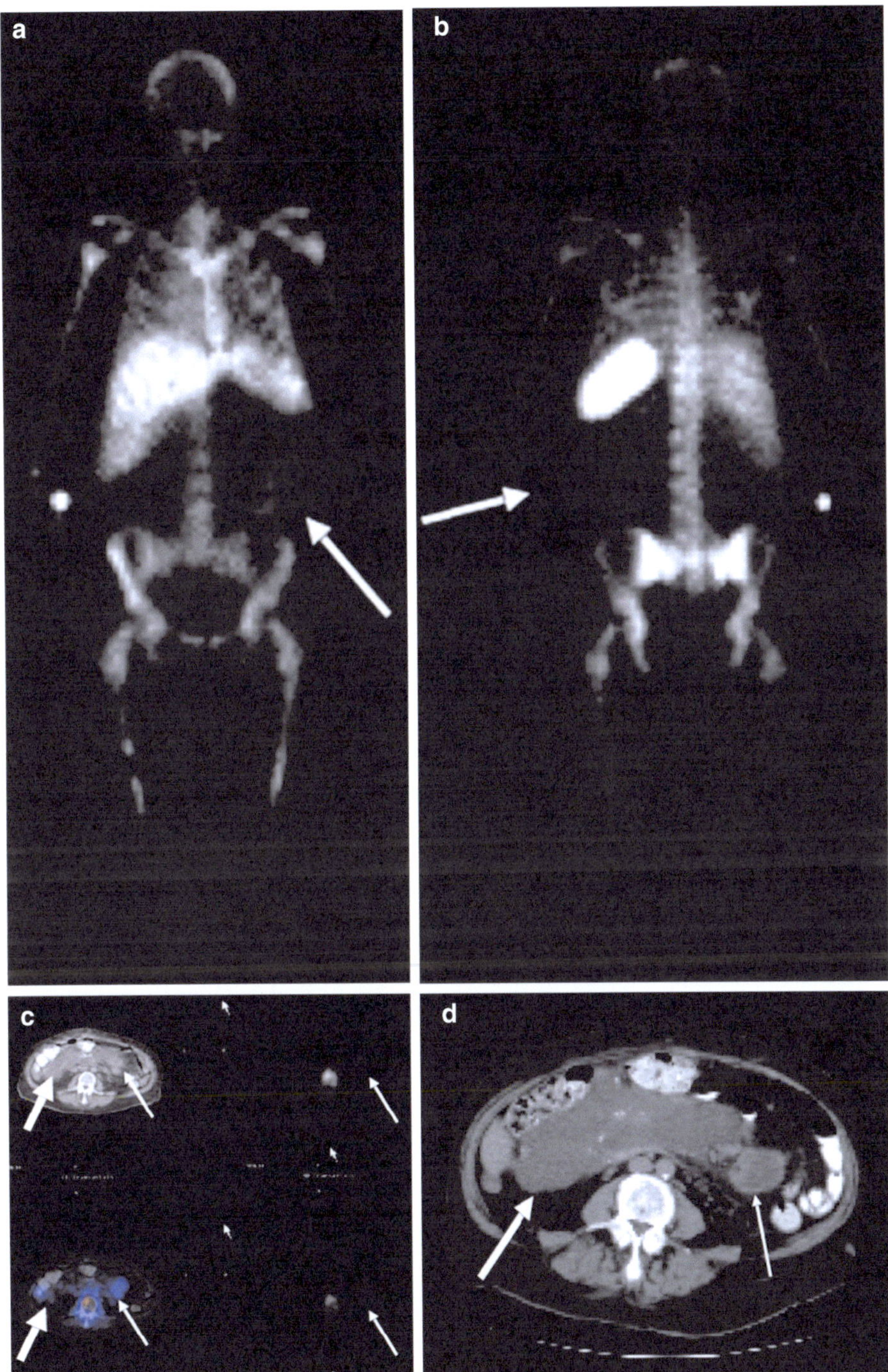

Fig. 5.3 [^{99m}Tc]Tc-HMPAO-labeled leukocyte scan with SPECT/CT. Middle-age male with fever several days after CT-guided biopsy of liposarcoma of the abdomen to assess for infection. Whole body planar images acquired 2.5 h after injection (**a** is anterior, **b** is posterior) show a focus of activity seen in the left mid-abdomen. (**c**) is of a SPECT/CT scan (top left is axial low-dose CT scan of mid-abdomen, top and bottom right are adjacent axial slices of attenuation corrected SPECT scan, bottom left is fused axial slice of CT and SPECT scans), where there is focal leukocyte accumulation (thin arrow, abscess) separate from the liposarcoma (thick arrow, tumor). No leukocyte accumulation is seen in the tumor. (**d**) is a contrast-enhanced CT scan showing enhancing collection consistent with an abscess at the site of leukocyte accumulation

spatial resolution of gamma photon imaging. Studies suggest that valvular vegetations need to be at least 5 mm in size for detection with [^{111}In] In-oxine-labeled leukocytes [74]. Moreover, false-negative results may occur with fungal infections [75]. Despite these limitations, the European Society of Cardiology guidelines recommends 2-[^{18}F]FDG PET/CT scan or labeled leukocyte scans for cases of possible or highly suspicious IE [76].

Recent work by Calais et al. provides additional support for the use of scintigraphy in the setting of cardiac-related infection [77]. Calais and coworkers studied 48 consecutive patients (50% female, 60% with prosthetic heart valve, 38% with staphylococcus) with inconclusive echocardiography and suspected infection of a cardiovascular implantable electronic device (CIED) with [^{99m}Tc]Tc-HMPAO leukocyte SPECT/CT scans at 4 and 24 h and 2-[^{18}F]FDG PET/CT scans. The final diagnosis was based on pathological and clinical modified Duke-Li criteria after a 3-month follow-up, positive culture from the device, or clinically evident pocket infection. The study demonstrated that [^{99m}Tc]Tc-HMPAO leukocyte scans were highly specific for infection and 2-[^{18}F]FDG PET/CT was highly sensitive for the diagnosis of chronic CIED infection. The [^{99m}Tc]Tc-HMPAO leukocyte study was instrumental in excluding infection by reducing the number of cases to less than half of those initially suspected.

5.6.4 Vascular Graft Infection

Vascular graft infection (VGI) is a late complication that occurs several months after implantation and generally requires removal of the graft for adequate treatment [78]. It is an uncommon complication but carries high morbidity and mortality. The earlier the diagnosis of vascular graft infection is made, the better the functional outcome [79]. The incidence of vascular graft infection ranges from 0.6% to 5% [80]. The presenting symptoms include fever, chills, redness and swelling around superficial grafts, or pain or pulsatile mass in the location of deeper grafts.

Infections are most commonly bacterial involving *Staphylococcus aureus* [80]. Discriminating between infection and postoperative changes is challenging using traditional anatomic imaging [80, 81].

In the evaluation of imaging modalities for the diagnosis of infected vascular graft, the meta-analysis by Reinders et al. is noteworthy [82]. In this meta-analysis, the literature from January 1997 to October 2017 was reviewed, and from 4259 articles, 14 were considered suitable for analysis and generation of pooled data and statistics. Inclusion criteria included details of study design, number of participants ($\geq$5 human adults with suspected VGI of any type), and endpoints (sensitivity, specificity, positive predictive value, negative predictive value, with biochemical or microbiological confirmation). Both prospective and retrospective observational cohort studies were included. The authors noted that studies failed to report the age of the graft or if the patient had received antibiotics by the time imaging was performed. Table 5.1 is a summary of the pooled sensitivities and specificities reported by imaging modality and illustrates the superior sensitivity and specificity of leukocyte imaging, particularly when combined with SPECT/CT. The meta-analysis also evaluated post-test probabilities as a proxy for true positives in imaging. In this metric, labeled leukocyte SPECT/CT was identified as having the highest rate of true imaging positive findings while keeping the lowest rate of false-negative imaging findings. 2-[^{18}F]FDG PET and PET/CT imaging had only slightly worse performance in this proxy metric. Given that radiolabeling of leukocytes is not readily available, 2-[^{18}F]FDG PET/CT was considered a favorable alternative to leukocyte imaging. The meta-analysis recognized that interpretation of 2-[^{18}F]FDG PET/CT findings was dependent on reader expertise and that patterns of vascular graft activity that have the highest association with infection are not well defined. In spite of these limitations, the meta-analysis concluded that CT angiography alone for the diagnosis of vascular graft infection is obsolete.

The American Heart Association also recommends [^{111}In]In-oxine-labeled leukocyte imaging

Table 5.1 Performance of imaging modalities in diagnosis of vascular graft infection adapted from *Reinders Folmer* et al. [82]

Modality	Sensitivity	Specificity	Comment
CT angiography	0.67 (0.57–0.75)[a]	0.63 (0.48–0.76)	4 studies
2-[^{18}F]FDG PET	0.94 (0.88–0.98)	0.70 (0.59–0.79)	4 studies
2-[^{18}F]FDG PET/CT	0.95 (0.87–0.99)	0.80 (0.69–0.89)	5 studies
Leukocyte scintigraphy	0.90 (0.85–0.94)	0.88 (0.81–1.94)	[^{111}In]In-oxine leukocytes: 3 studies [^{99m}Tc]Tc-HMPAO leukocytes: 5 studies
Leukocyte SPECT/CT	0.99 (0.92–1.00)	0.82 (0.57–0.96)	Either low-dose CT or contrast-enhanced CT: 3 studies

[a]95% confidence intervals in parentheses

to assist in the diagnosis of extra-cavitary (i.e., largely groin and lower extremity) vascular graft infection [83]. Surprisingly, the recommendation is limited to when ultrasound, CT angiography, or MRI studies are inconclusive [83]. This class IIb recommendation is based on a reported relatively high specificity (87%) and modest sensitivity (67–73%) of [^{111}In]In-oxine-labeled leukocyte imaging in detecting vascular graft infection that neglects the more recent meta-analysis results outlined above. For this reason, the recommendation most likely will be revised in the future. Figure 5.4 illustrates significant background to uptake contrast ratio in a patient with left femoral arterial bypass graft using [^{111}In]In-oxine-labeled leukocyte imaging in correlation with CT scan.

5.6.5 Joint Prosthesis Infection

Joint replacements are common. There are more than one million total joint arthroplasties performed annually worldwide, and this number is projected to be nearly four million by the year 2030 [84, 85]. Despite advances in arthroplasties, complications like aseptic and septic loosening are still common. By 10 years post-implantation, 50% of prostheses show evidence of loosening on radiographs and 30% need revision [86]. Aseptic loosening and septic loosening often present with very similar clinical and histopathological findings making it difficult to discriminate between the two etiologies [86]. CT and MRI scans are limited by metal artifacts from the

implanted hardware and suffer from poor sensitivity and specificity in the detection of infected prostheses [87]. [^{111}In]In-oxine-labeled leukocyte imaging with concurrent [^{99m}Tc]Tc-sulfur colloid scans, the dual-isotope scan, remains the gold standard imaging modality to discriminate between septic and aseptic prosthetic loosening [88]. A meta-analysis of the literature between January 1980 and December 2008 identified 44 prospective cohort and retrospective case-control studies with 1634 total patients [89]. The highest diagnostic accuracy of 95% for bone and joint infections was observed with dual-isotope scans. The principle behind dual-isotope imaging is that both [^{99m}Tc]Tc-sulfur colloid and [^{111}In]In-oxine-labeled leukocytes migrate to the bone marrow, but due to chemotaxis induced by infection and the replacement of the infected bone marrow by pus, [^{111}In]In-oxine-labeled leukocytes will still accumulate at the site of infection and [^{99m}Tc]Tc-sulfur colloid will not. This results in an incongruent imaging pattern for the distribution of activity that is characteristic of infection and is illustrated in Fig. 5.5.

The addition of 2-[^{18}F]FDG PET imaging in infection may challenge the dual-isotope scan as the preferred imaging modality for infected prostheses in the future. Several studies have been published comparing the diagnostic performance of 2-[^{18}F]FDG PET to leukocyte scans with various, and occasionally contradictory, results [38, 90–92]. The joint EANM/SNMMI guidelines for the use of 2-[^{18}F]FDG in inflammation and infection reported sensitivity of 95% and specificity of

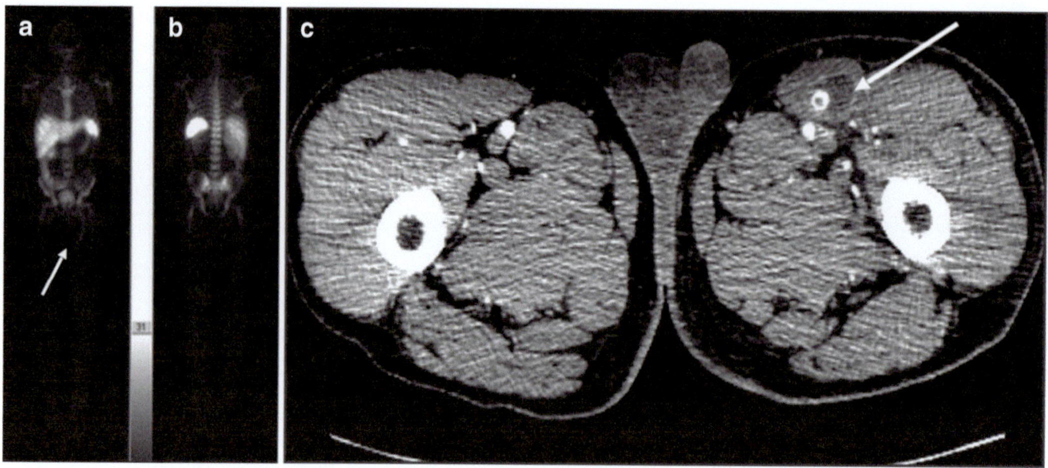

Fig. 5.4 [⁹⁹ᵐTc]Tc-HMPAO-labeled leukocyte scan. Middle-aged man with left groin pain and fever. Whole body leukocyte scan at 24 h, **a** is the anterior view and **b** is the posterior view. Notice physiologic bowel and bladder activity. There is abnormal linear activity medial to the left femur that corresponds to uptake in the vascular graft infection (arrow). (**c**) shows a small collection around a left femoral artery graft that correlates with leukocyte scan findings

98% for knee and hip PJI [93]. A report by the EANM applied a multidisciplinary review of the literature from the fields of nuclear medicine, radiology, orthopedics, infectious disease, and microbiology to provide evidence-based uniform statements regarding the diagnosis of prosthetic joint infection [94]. This consensus paper made key recommendations using the Oxford Centre for Evidence Based Medicine rankings (summarized in Table 5.2). In this ranking system, Level 1 represents the highest level of evidence, and Level 5 represents the lowest [95]. The EANM concludes that there is good evidence for the use of scintigraphy in evaluating PJI.

Planar scintigraphic imaging is enhanced with tomography such as SPECT. SPECT/CT scanners allow for hybrid imaging where it is possible to use the CT scan for lesion localization and attenuation correction of the scintigraphy. However, the metal in the prostheses may generate artifacts both on the CT and on the CT-corrected SPECT scan. For these reasons, it is important to review CT (attenuation corrected) and non-CT-corrected SPECT scans when performing hybrid scans. Hybrid scanners with diagnostic CT are capable of "metal suppression" CT imaging. However, this technique results in high radiation exposure because it relies on a high-energy X-ray photon flux to "burn" through the metal. The development of dual-beam CT imaging provides for a different approach to eliminate metal artifacts on CT, but this type of CT scan is not available in hybrid mode [99]. Joint infection imaging is one potential clinical application for a future generation of hybrid scanners.

5.6.6 Diabetic Infections

Peripheral neuropathy and peripheral vascular disease are complications of long-standing diabetes that contribute to foot wounds. These soft tissue infections frequently evolve to diabetic foot osteomyelitis (DFO) by means of direct extension. It results in an increased incidence of amputations in diabetics and in increased mortality [100, 101]. The early diagnosis of DFO is difficult. Foot ulcers may or may not be infected, and there may be soft tissue infection without reaching the bone or bone marrow. Diabetics suffer from Charcot neuro-osteoarthropathy with bone changes that may mimic osteomyelitis in morphologic imaging. Multiple imaging modalities are available to assist in the diagnosis of DFO,

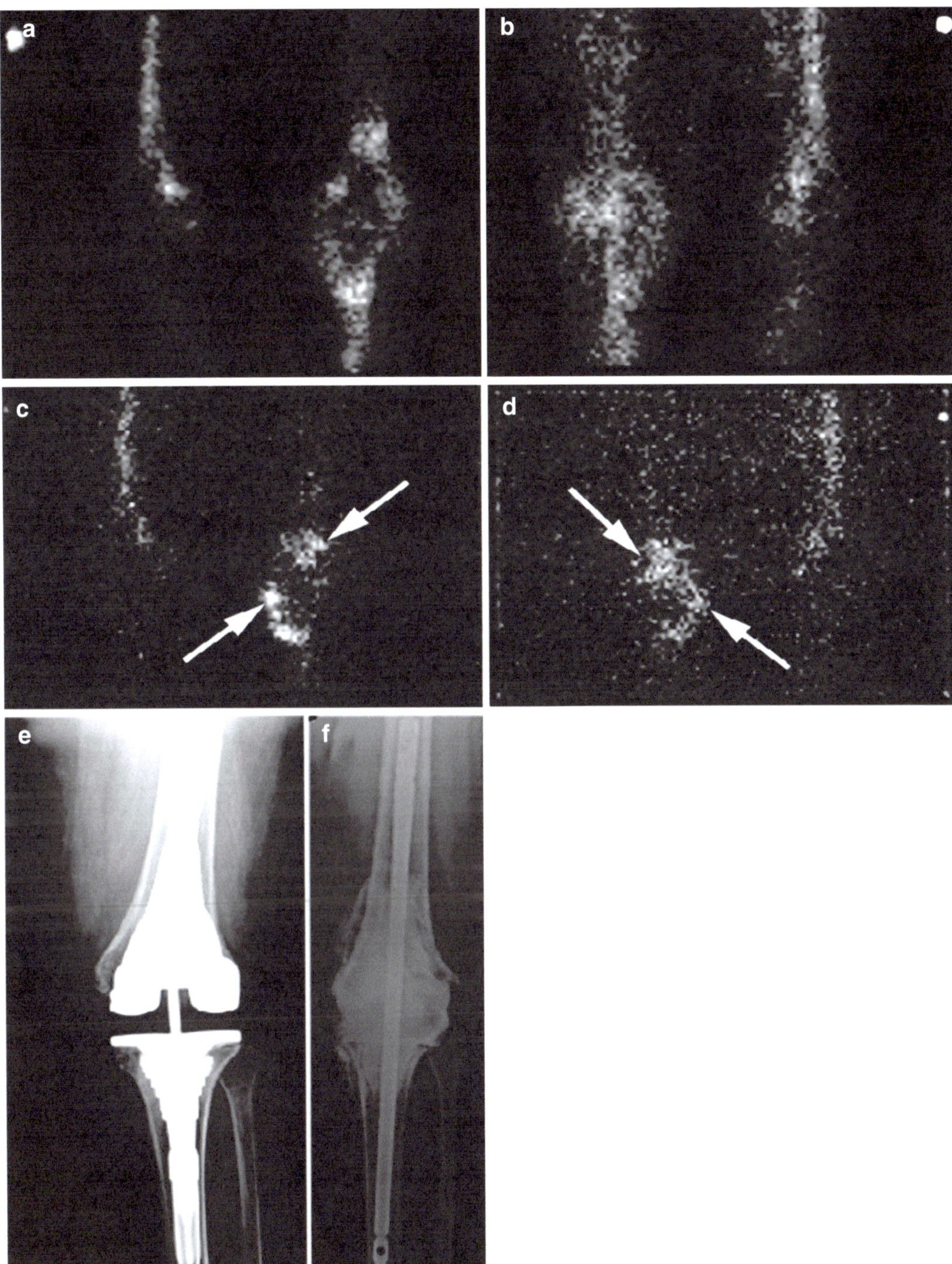

Fig. 5.5 [^{111}In]In-oxine-labeled leukocyte scan with [^{99m}Tc]Tc-sulfur colloid bone marrow planar dual-isotope imaging to assess for a prosthetic knee infection. Image **a** (anterior) and image **b** (posterior) view of [^{99m}Tc]Tc-sulfur colloid bone marrow imaging of both knees, with a right dot marker identifying the right side of the patient. Image **c** (anterior) and image **d** (posterior) demonstrate corresponding [^{111}In]In-oxine-labeled leukocyte scans, showing incongruent accumulation of labeled leukocytes (arrows), particularly in the medial left knee. Photopenia is due to metallic left knee prosthesis as seen on the X-ray of the left total knee prosthesis (**e**) on the left. This immunocompromised patient had developed a draining sinus in the left knee that grew *Bacteroides fragilis*. The prosthesis was removed and replaced with an antibiotic spacer and a transfixing rod as shown on the right side in image **f**

Table 5.2 Highlights of the European Association of Nuclear Medicine multidisciplinary review of imaging of prosthetic joint infections [94]

Statement	Level of evidence	Comment
In the case of negative leukocyte scintigraphy, the probability of prosthetic joint infection is low	2	
2-[^{18}F]FDG PET in patients with suspected prosthetic joint infection has higher sensitivity but lower specificity than leukocyte scintigraphy or anti-granulocyte antibody scintigraphy	2	
Anti-granulocyte scintigraphy is a good alternative to leukocyte scintigraphy, with similar sensitivity and specificity	2	Similar results for [^{99m}Tc] Tc-besilesomab versus ^{99m}Tc-labeled leukocytes [96] Overall sensitivity of 83% and specificity of 79–80% of anti-granulocyte antibodies in prosthetic joint [97, 98]
Hybrid SPECT/CT imaging can improve localization of infection (and diagnostic accuracy)	2	Current interpretation of leukocyte scans is based on planar images, but SPECT/CT would theoretically increase diagnostic accuracy since SPECT/CT is well established to do so with other pathologies
Dual-isotope imaging increases diagnostic accuracy for prosthetic joint infection	2	
Semiquantitative analysis of leukocyte accumulation over time in leukocyte scan increases diagnostic accuracy for prosthetic joint infection	3	

including CT, MRI, and scintigraphy as dominant imaging modalities after initial investigation with radiography.

Current guidelines from the ACR recommend imaging for patients with at least soft tissue swelling and favor MRI over scintigraphy [102]. The evidence that follows is inconsistent with this recommendation, particularly in light of advances in hybrid imaging. Indeed, a normal delayed phase bone scan excludes osteomyelitis and is a valuable exam for patients without evidence of Charcot neuro-osteoarthropathy in radiography and a low clinical suspicion of osteomyelitis. [^{111}In]In-oxine-labeled leukocyte scintigraphy has a sensitivity of at least 89% and specificity of at least 79% for DFO [103]. In a study of 459 patients, dual-isotope SPECT/CT using [^{111}In]In-oxine-labeled leukocyte and [^{99m}Tc]Tc-methylene diphosphonate was more accurate than planar scintigraphy, CT, and MRI in diagnosing diabetic foot osteomyelitis [104].

A meta-analysis by Lauri et al. reviewed the literature up to August 2016 to identify a total of 27 articles and 2 abstracts out of 6649 publications that met inclusion criteria [6]. Included studies were either prospective or retrospective in design. Table 5.3 shows a summary of the performance metrics. When the 95% confidence intervals are considered, there is a significant similarity in the performance of all four modalities with possibly 2-[^{18}F]FDG PET/CT and [^{99m}Tc]Tc-HMPAO leukocyte imaging having a slight edge in specificity. Group data like this makes it difficult to support the ACR recommendation.

In a meta-analysis of 50 original papers and 7 reviews that described the imaging of the diabetic foot and examined a total of 2889 lesions, Capriotti et al. concluded that, in contrast to bone scans which had poor specificity (particularly in noninfected neuropathic-related fractures in Charcot joints), radiolabeled leukocytes were not taken up in uninfected bone [105]. Their sensitivity, specificity, and accuracy in the detection of osteomyelitis for diabetic feet were 86%, 74.4%, and 77%, respectively, for ^{111}In-oxine-labeled leukocytes and were 85.8%, 84.5%, and 85.9%, respectively, with [^{99m}Tc]Tc-HMPAO-labeled

Table 5.3 Diagnostic performance of [¹¹¹In]In-oxine versus [⁹⁹ᵐTc]Tc-HMPAO-labeled leukocyte scans in infected joint prostheses

Agent	Sensitivity	Specificity	Diagnostic odds ratio	Positive likelihood ratio	Negative likelihood ratio	Comment
[¹¹¹In]n-Oxine leukocytes	92% (72–98)[a]	75% (66–82)	34 (6.9–165.7)	3.6 (1.9–6.7)	0.1 (0.03–0.4)	9 studies, 206 patients
[⁹⁹ᵐTc]Tc-HMPAO leukocytes	91% (86–94)	92% (78–98)	118 (30–459)	12 (3.7–36.3)	0.1 (0.06–0.16)	10 studies, 406 patients
2-[¹⁸F]FDG	89% (68–97)	92% (85–96)	95 (18–504)	11 (4.7–25.0)	0.11 (0.03–0.4)	6 studies, 254 patients
MRI	93% (82–97)	75% (63–84)	37 (11.3–121.3)	3.66 (2.1–6.4)	0.10 (0.04–0.26)	13 studies, 421 patients

[a]95% confidence intervals in parenthesis

leukocytes. The better specificity and accuracy with [⁹⁹ᵐTc]Tc-HMPAO-labeled leukocytes were thought likely to be related to better spatial resolution and anatomical landmarks. Though MRI had a higher sensitivity of 90.1%, it suffered from lower specificity of 73.9% and lower accuracy of 80.5%.

Medical treatment for diabetic foot osteomyelitis, though effective, carries a risk of relapse of up to 30%. Vouillarmet et al. evaluated the role of SPECT/CT in detecting relapse in this group of patients. They showed that a negative leukocyte SPECT/CT effectively rules out relapse [106]. Although [⁹⁹ᵐTc]Tc-MDP three-phase scintigraphy was sensitive in detecting relapse, its specificity and the subsequent positive predictive value were poor (15%). However, the addition of [⁹⁹ᵐTc]Tc-HMPAO-labeled leukocyte SPECT/CT had significantly improved specificity (92%) without sacrificing high sensitivity. The end result was an improved positive predictive value to 72%, with an unchanged negative predictive value of 100%.

5.6.7 Appendicitis

Appendicitis classically presents with diffuse mid-abdominal pain, loss of appetite, and nausea, followed by localization of pain to the right lower quadrant, guarding, and elevated leukocyte count [107]. However, almost half of the patients have an atypical presentation. Delay in diagnosis and surgical intervention puts patients at risk for perforation, which can lead to abscess formation, peritonitis, sepsis, and even death [108]. On the other hand, unnecessary laparotomy can lead to morbid consequences as well. [⁹⁹ᵐTc]Tc-HMPAO-labeled leukocyte scan has been shown to be a highly sensitive and accurate, noninvasive, diagnostic test for appendicitis. Importantly, it carries a high negative predictive value that makes it a useful test to exclude appendicitis in cases with equivocal presentation or inconclusive anatomic imaging such as CT or ultrasound. The ACR currently classifies leukocyte scans as "usually not appropriate" for suspected appendicitis [109]. Albiston reviewed 32 prospective studies from 1987 to 2001 comparing the performance of [⁹⁹ᵐTc]Tc-HMPAO leukocyte scans with CT and ultrasound imaging. Although most of the experience was with anatomic imaging, the sensitivities, specificities, and accuracies of the three modalities were similar, ranging from 80% to 100% [110]. Two contemporaneous prospective studies [111, 112] reached similar conclusions. In light of these findings, we believe the ACR recommendation should be qualified and leukocyte imaging is considered an option for inconclusive anatomic imaging of suspected appendicitis.

5.6.8 Inflammatory Bowel Disease

Inflammatory bowel disease (IBD) is a chronic, idiopathic, granulomatous inflammatory condition that results from a defective immune system and damages the integrity of the gut epithelium. IBD is not considered an infection. The two major types of IBD are Crohn's disease (CD) and ulcerative colitis (UC). Both are relapsing-remitting diseases. Ulcerative colitis begins at the rectum and progresses in a contiguous retrograde fashion to involve the rest of the large bowel. It involves all three layers of the bowel wall. CD involves discontinuous segments of the bowel, large and small, and may only involve the mucosa and submucosal layers. The gold standard for diagnosis is endoscopy, which is invasive. However, the diagnosis can be suggested from fluoroscopic, CT, or MRI imaging. These exams require bowel preparation that is particularly demanding for patients [113]. Endoscopy and fluoroscopy are limited in that they cannot detect deep intestinal wall involvement or extra-intestinal extension of disease. CT and MRI are useful adjuncts to address these limitations, but results can be inconclusive in the setting of relapsing disease where discriminating between residual from old inflammation and new injury from a flare-up of disease is important.

A systematic review of 55 articles concluded that radiolabeled leukocyte imaging is a useful tool in the detection of active IBD, but prospective multicenter studies are still lacking [113]. [^{111}In]In-oxine-labeled leukocytes have been shown to be sensitive and specific for the detection of active inflammation of the intestine [114]. However, poor image quality and limited availability have hampered its acceptance in this clinical scenario. [^{99m}Tc]Tc-HMPAO leukocyte scintigraphy has acceptable dosimetry (fourfold less than CT imaging [115]) and superior image resolution and provides results within 4 h of injection. Combined published data for [^{99m}Tc] Tc-HMPAO-labeled leukocyte imaging shows sensitivity of 95–100%, specificity of 85–100%, and accuracy of 92–100%, to detect, localize, and assess for inflammatory bowel disease [115]. A specific example is a study by Charron et al. where [^{99m}Tc]Tc-HMPAO-labeled leukocyte scans were shown to be useful in detecting active IBD with a sensitivity of 90%, specificity of 97%, positive predictive value of 97%, negative predictive value of 93%, and overall accuracy of 93% in 215 patients [116]. Inflammation on a [^{99m}Tc] Tc-HMPAO-labeled leukocyte study appears as a bowel-shaped region of uptake that is persistent on delayed imaging. [^{99m}Tc]Tc-HMPAO-labeled leukocyte scintigraphy can evaluate the entire bowel and assess if a stricture is actively inflamed [115]. SPECT, and particularly SPECT/CT, imaging helps to determine if the inflammation is in the large or small bowel or outside the intestines. SPECT imaging allows for one-to-one correlation with CT or MR anatomic imaging. Software fusion of SPECT imaging with CT was shown to be superior to side by side correlation resulting in higher diagnostic confidence [10]. For these reasons, Stathaki and coworkers suggested that leukocyte scintigraphy can be considered a reference method to determine the extent of inflammation in situations where colonoscopy could not be completed or when radiographic imaging is negative [115]. In spite of these benefits, CT imaging remains as a "usually appropriate" imaging modality for Crohn's disease under current guidelines from ACR, while [^{99m}Tc] Tc-HMPAO-labeled leukocyte scintigraphy is considered "usually not appropriate" [62].

Although [^{99m}Tc]Tc-HMPAO-labeled leukocyte is useful in detecting active inflammation in IBD, it is unable to detect complications such as strictures, fistulas, or pre-stenotic dilation. These findings are detected by CT or MRI imaging and may be the reason for the choice in the ACR guidelines. SPECT/CT presents a unique opportunity to detect active inflammation and its complications by combining [^{99m}Tc]Tc-HMPAO-labeled leukocyte imaging with contrast enhanced CT scans. This hybrid imaging modality should correct common problems with [^{99m}Tc]Tc-HMPAO-labeled leukocyte scans such as pinpointing the site of localization of tracer and discriminating extravasation of tracer due to bleeding from localization as a consequence of inflammation. However, there have been no studies to support the clinical use of such hybrid imaging, thus far.

5.6.9 Rheumatoid Arthritis

There is limited experience with leukocyte imaging in rheumatoid arthritis. This chronic inflammatory joint condition has flare-ups that may be detectable by leukocyte imaging.

Uno et al. evaluated the association between [111In]In-oxine-labeled leukocyte scans of wrist and knee joints in 33 patients with the flare-up of rheumatoid arthritis [117]. No uptake was seen in joints that had neither pain nor swelling consistent with significant specificity of the imaging for active inflammation. The authors suggested that imaging may be valuable in monitoring disease activity. Gaál et al. reached a similar conclusion using [99mTc]Tc-HMPAO-labeled leukocytes [118]. Pilot work by Al-Janabi et al. found that clinical response to steroid injections in joints of rheumatoid arthritis patients correlated with a 50–80% decrease in [99mTc]Tc-HMPAO-labeled leukocyte uptake [119].

5.7 Improvements in Leukocyte Scans

Leukocyte imaging could be improved by selective labeling of specific white cell populations that play different roles in the process of inflammation. However, this strategy has not been pursued. It is also of interest to avoid the risks associated with ex vivo labeling and subsequent reinjection of autologous cells by labeling in vivo. This can be accomplished by injecting radiopharmaceutical that targets leukocytes in vivo. Antibody or antibody fragments have been used in this strategy [88]. Two products are currently available: besilesomab, a whole murine immunoglobulin (Ig)G anti-NCA-95 antibody, and sulesomab, a Fab′ fragment anti-NCA-90 [75]. Neither are approved for clinical use in the United States as of 2019, but they are available in Europe. While both bind neutrophils with very high specificity and affinity (dissociation constant in nanomolar range), they exhibit important differences in biodistribution. Besilesomab, a whole antibody, shows intense uptake in bone marrow, greater uptake in the spleen than in the liver, and only slight kidney uptake 4 h post injection. After 24 h, nonspecific uptake is seen in the gastrointestinal tract as a result of radiolabel instability. Sulesomab shows intense uptake in the kidneys due to renal excretion, and liver uptake is greater than the spleen in the first 4 h

post-injection. Its bone marrow uptake is much lower compared to besilesomab. Nonspecific gastrointestinal uptake is seen as early as 4 h due to the faster breakdown of this tracer. These antibodies are accepted as fast and sensitive for the evaluation of osteomyelitis, diabetic foot infection, bone prosthetic infections, fever of unknown origin, vascular graft infection, prosthetic heart valve infection, and inflammatory bowel disease [96–98, 105, 120–123]. However, they have not replaced leukocyte scintigraphy. For instance, as a murine antibody, besilesomab can induce human anti-mouse antibodies in humans, and this limits its use in clinical practice. Sulesomab does not suffer this limitation, but in Europe, it is only approved for peripheral musculoskeletal infections.

Significant improvements in leukocyte clinical imaging have been achieved with the introduction of hybrid scanners such as SPECT/CT. The review by Erba and Israel provides numerous examples [10]. This is particularly true if the imaging can be coupled with quantitative analysis to supplement visual inspection and help with reproducibility of results across multiple viewers. Semi-quantitative analysis has been shown to be useful by several authors [49, 50].

The addition of SPECT/CT to planar whole body imaging increases the sensitivity and specificity of the scans for the detection of infection [3]. CT imaging for lesion localization and attenuation correction improves SPECT imaging and allows accurate localization of findings to guide tissue sampling and therapy. Ingui et al. reported that SPECT/CT added value to diagnoses of infection with [111In]In-oxine-labeled leukocytes by increasing reader confidence to 71% in nearly half of cases [124]. Similar improvements have been reported with [67Ga]Ga-citrate imaging [125]. Djekidel et al. have also shown that SPECT/CT increases sensitivity [126]. This is seen without loss of specificity. As an example, the work of Heib et al. showed that for soft tissue infection, the sensitivity and specificity of planar imaging for infection increased from 78% and 96% to 81% and 100%, respectively, with the addition of SPECT, and to 94% and 100%, respectively, with the addition of SPECT/CT. A similar trend was seen for osteomyelitis [127]. The ability to locate the site of uptake is most crucial in endocarditis, implantable cardiac device infection, vascular graft infection, and diabetic foot infection, because it can affect treatment decisions [72]. For instance, in diabetic foot infection, it is critical to discriminate between infection confined to the soft tissues versus the bone because the length of antibiotic treatment is significantly longer when there is osteomyelitis and not just myositis. SPECT/CT imaging helps to discriminate atypical physiologic uptake or benign inflammation from pathologic uptake in leukocyte imaging [21]. Examples included gut uptake due to swallowed cells from sinusitis or lung infections, inflammation around devices like colostomy drains, or uptake in accessory spleens. The value of SPECT is illustrated in Figs. 5.6 and 5.7. In Fig. 5.6, a dual-isotope scan combining [^{99m}Tc]Tc-methylene diphosphonate and [^{111}In] In-oxine-labeled leukocytes is able to discriminate between osteomyelitis and underlying myositis/cellulitis in a below the knee amputation stump. Confirmation of the location of the abnormal leukocyte uptake could have been achieved with SPECT or SPECT/CT imaging, as was done in Fig. 5.7 where a persistent infection at the site of the fracture is confirmed using [^{111}In]In-oxine-

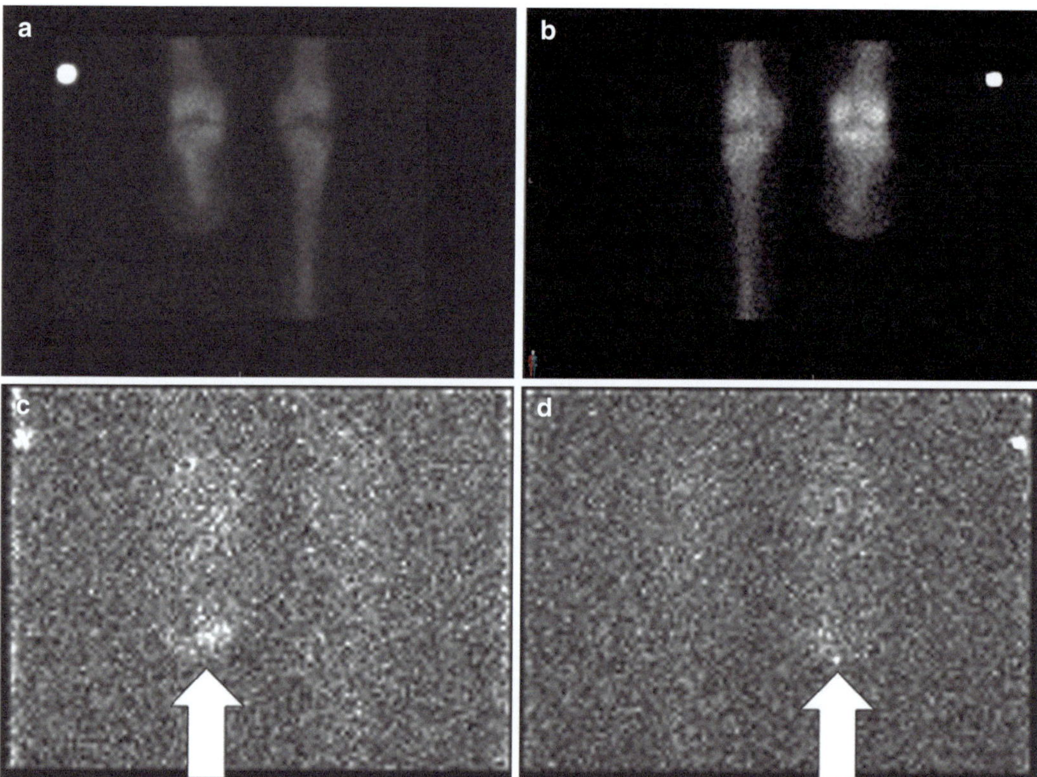

Fig. 5.6 [^{111}In]In-oxine labeled leukocyte with [^{99m}Tc] Tc-methylene diphosphonate (MDP) bone planar dual isotope scans. **a** (anterior) and **b** (posterior) planar views of a bone scan ([^{99m}Tc]Tc-MDP) 3 h after injection with a bright dot marker identifying the right side of the patient. **c** (anterior) and **d** (posterior) views of the [^{111}In]In-oxine labeled leukocyte scan imaged 24 h after injection. Simultaneous imaging of both isotopes is achieved with a multichannel analyzer to discriminate different emission energy peaks. The bone scan agent is injected the day after leukocyte injection for imaging on the day of bone tracer injection. The bone scan shows a below-knee amputation on the right side but is otherwise normal. Leukocyte scan shows accumulation in the soft tissue on the edge of the right lower extremity stump (arrow). The combination of findings excludes osteomyelitis and confirms infection or inflammation limited to the soft tissues at the end of the stump. Notice that the background activity is high in the leukocyte scan because the injected dose is significantly less than the bone scan dose. After all, poor dosimetry with [^{111}In]In-oxine labeled leukocytes requires a lower dose to reduce radiation exposure

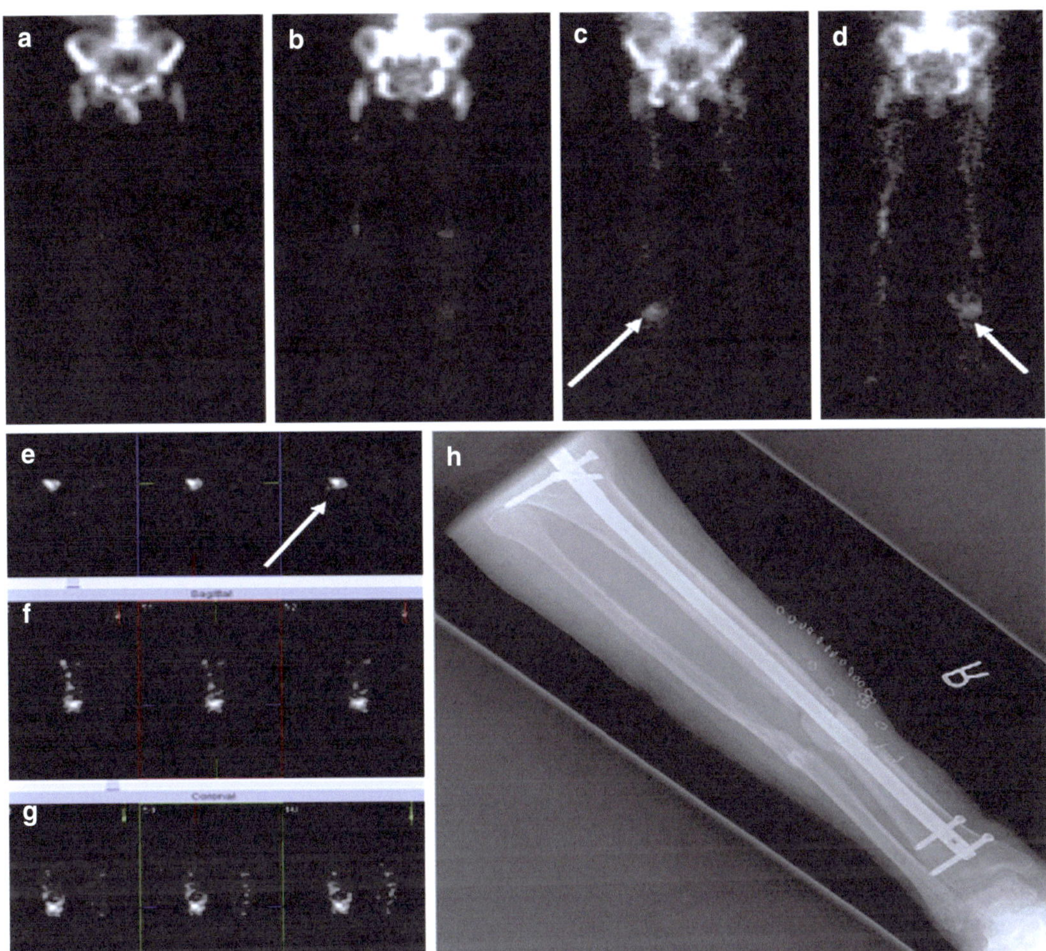

Fig. 5.7 [¹¹¹In]In-oxine labeled leukocyte scan, dual isotope technique. The exam was to evaluate for infection in a fracture, s/p rod and screw fixation s/p debridement, and insertion of a cement plug containing antibiotics. Images **a** (anterior) and **b** (posterior) are planar images of a [⁹⁹ᵐTc]Tc-sulfur colloid bone marrow scan, and images **c** (anterior) and **d** (posterior) are views of [¹¹¹In]In-oxine labeled leukocyte scans. The white arrow points to the site of incongruent uptake on the leukocyte scan where there is no corresponding uptake on the bone marrow scan. Images **e**, **f**, and **g** show axial, sagittal, and coronal SPECT slices (respectively) of [¹¹¹In]In-oxin-labeled leukocyte SPECT scan, demonstrating uptake within the bone consistent with osteomyelitis, resulting in fracture non-union. Image **h** shows the radiograph of the fracture non-union. Sagittal and coronal slices of [¹¹¹In]In-oxine labeled leukocyte SPECT scan demonstrated uptake within the bone and not the overlying soft tissues. **h** is a corresponding radiograph showing a rod transfixing a fracture that had been debrided and unsuccessfully treated with a cement plug containing antibiotics. Infection persists at the fracture site

labeled leukocytes and SPECT imaging. However, in the case of the stump infection, the additional tomographic scan was considered unnecessary. This was not the case for the intra-abdominal abscess in Fig. 5.3. In this case, SPECT/CT imaging was critical to provide convincing evidence that abdominal activity was related to an abscess that had been incorrectly characterized as a tumor on a CT scan prior to scintigraphic imaging.

Given that image quality and resolution are better with PET than with SPECT, there has been interest in labeling leukocytes for PET/CT imaging. Rini et al. compared 2-[¹⁸F]FDG-labeled leukocyte PET imaging to [¹¹¹In]In-oxine-labeled leukocyte scintigraphy. They reported similar leukocyte viability and similar performance with sensitivity (87% vs. 73%), specificity (82% vs. 86%), and accuracy (84% vs. 81%) [128]. A meta-analysis by Meyer et al. on the diagnostic accuracy of 2-[^{18}F]FDG-labeled leukocyte PET and PET/CT imaging showed that the benefit of this modality was the detection of faint uptake in the brain and myocardium [129]. Since the gastrointestinal and genitourinary tracts do not take up 2-[^{18}F]FDG-labeled leukocytes, this imaging modality is suitable for the detection of intra-abdominal and renal infections in addition to cardiac and cerebral infections. One drawback of radiolabeling with 2-[^{18}F]FDG is the much shorter half-life of fluorine-18 (1.8 h), which precludes the delayed imaging that is known to improve the accuracy of leukocyte imaging. It has been suggested that leukocytes be labeled with copper-64 because its half-life is 12.7 h, allowing for delayed imaging at 18–24 h after injection [4].

## 5.8	Conclusion

Radiolabeled leukocytes are still considered the gold standard for imaging of most infections [130]. They are a useful clinical tool supported by the multiple studies described in this chapter. [^{111}In]In-oxine-labeled leucocyte imaging is a significant improvement over [^{67}Ga]Ga-citrate imaging for infection and inflammation. The leukocyte scans are more reliable, show more consistent biodistribution, and are more specific for the detection of infection with less uptake in healing wounds, malignancy, and traumatic bone injury. With [^{99m}Tc]Tc-HMPAO-labeled leukocytes, results are often available within 4 h as opposed to 24 or 48 h with [^{111}In]In-oxine-labeled leukocytes and [^{67}Ga]Ga-citrate, respectively. The major drawback of leukocyte scans is the laborious process of in vitro cell labeling and the inability to harvest enough cells in patients with severe leukopenia or inconsistent red cell sedimentation as is the case with those suffering from sickle cell disease [131].

[^{99m}Tc]Tc-HMPAO-labeled leukocyte is an improvement over [^{111}In]In-oxine-labeled leuko-cyte not only because it yields results faster but also because it has lower radiation dose and better imaging properties. For these reasons, it is the agent of choice in children. It is also convenient because indium-111 is cyclotron produced and not always available [108]. The drawback of [^{99m}Tc]Tc-HMPAO-labeled leukocyte scans is the accumulation in the gastrointestinal and genitourinary tract starting 2–3 h after injection [132]. Therefore, [^{111}In]In-oxine-labeled leukocytes are preferred for the evaluation of infection of the kidneys, bladder, gallbladder, abdomen, and intestines [8].

Leukocyte scans supplement the use of 2-[^{18}F]FDG PET/CT imaging in the evaluation of fever of unknown origin and vertebral osteomyelitis. For these applications, 2-[^{18}F]FDG PET/CT has emerged as a first-line modality because it is highly sensitive, and in the setting of fever of unknown origin, it can detect malignancies like lymphoma that often present with fever. However, 2-[^{18}F]FDG imaging of infection and inflammation suffers from low specificity, and leukocyte scans can improve the specificity for the detection of infection. This is most useful when aspiration is difficult or when it is necessary to initiate therapy before waiting for culture results.

Leukocytes scans, particularly combined with SPECT/CT imaging, have a clinical role in the evaluation of infected grafts, cardiac devices, and endocarditis. The scans remain a useful tool in the evaluation of suspected infection in joint prostheses given that these prostheses generate significant artifacts in MRI and CT imaging. For evaluation of diabetic foot infection, leukocytes remain a gold standard even though in clinical practice, MRI has replaced this application due to its widespread availability, delivery of faster results, and ability to guide surgical interventions. MRI is a sensitive imaging modality, but like is the case with PET/CT imaging, leukocyte imaging provides specificity. Many of the drawbacks of leukocyte imaging in this setting are likely to be overcome with SPECT/CT of dual-isotope scans. However, comparison of these imaging strategies remains to be done. Leukocyte scans can help in the evaluation of appendicitis when CT scans and ultrasounds are equivocal.

The use of [^{99m}Tc]Tc-HMPAO-labeled leukocytes allows for the detection of hyperemia in a radionuclide angiogram and early detection of bowel inflammation. Localization is also possible with SPECT/CT imaging. Detecting active flare-ups in inflammatory bowel disease is another similar application that remains under-utilized. In this setting, 2-[^{18}F]FDG PET/CT scans detect active inflammation and assist MRI and CT in discriminating the bowel segment relevant to the patient's symptoms and a target for intervention. Leukocyte scan with SPECT/CT is an alternative when the goal is to improve on the sensitivity of the anatomic imaging modalities. We believe there is enough evidence to recommend radiolabeled leukocyte imaging when CT and MRI scans are inconclusive. We encourage the ACR to reconsider its position and generate new recommendations that are in line with new evidence and the recommendations from sister medical societies.

References

1. Institute for Health Metrics and Evaluation (IHME). Global burden of disease study 2017 [Internet]. 2019 [cited 2019 Jul 28]. Available from: http://ghdx.healthdata.org/gbd-results-tool.
2. WHO. Global health estimates 2016: deaths by cause, age, sex, by country and by region [Internet]. Health statistics and information systems. 2018 [cited 2019 Sep 19]. Available from: https://www.who.int/healthinfo/global_burden_disease/estimates/en/.
3. Velikyan I. Prospective of 68Ga radionuclide contribution to the development of imaging agents for infection and inflammation. Contrast Media Mol Imaging. 2018;2018:9713691.
4. Ady J, Fong Y. Imaging for infection: from visualization of inflammation to visualization of microbes. Surg Infect. 2014;15(6):700–7.
5. Salmanoglu E, Kim S, Thakur ML. Currently available radiopharmaceuticals for imaging infection and the holy grail. Semin Nucl Med. 2018;48(2):86–99.
6. Lauri C, Tamminga M, Glaudemans AWJM, Juárez Orozco LE, Erba PA, Jutte PC, et al. Detection of osteomyelitis in the diabetic foot by imaging techniques: a systematic review and meta-analysis comparing MRI, white blood cell scintigraphy, and FDG-PET. Diabetes Care. 2017;40(8):1111–20.
7. Kjaer A, Lebech A-M. Diagnostic value of (111) In-granulocyte scintigraphy in patients with fever of unknown origin. J Nucl Med. 2002;43(2):140–4.
8. Censullo A, Vijayan T. Using nuclear medicine imaging wisely in diagnosing infectious diseases. Open Forum Infect Dis. 2017;4(1):ofx011.
9. Wing VW, van Sonnenberg E, Kipper S, Bieberstein MP. Indium-111-labeled leukocyte localization in hematomas: a pitfall in abscess detection. Radiology. 1984;152(1):173–6.
10. Erba PA, Israel O. SPECT/CT in infection and inflammation. Clin Transl Imaging. 2014;2(6):519–35.
11. Goldsmith SJ, Vallabhajosula S. Clinically proven radiopharmaceuticals for infection imaging: mechanisms and applications. Semin Nucl Med. 2009;39(1):2–10.
12. Jalkanen S, Salmi M. VAP-1 and CD73, endothelial cell surface enzymes in leukocyte extravasation. Arterioscler Thromb Vasc Biol. 2008;28(1):18–26.
13. Wilhelm DL. Pathology, vol. 1. 7th ed. St Louis: The CV Mosby Company; 1977. p. 25–89.
14. McAfee JG, Thakur ML. Survey of radioactive agents for in vitro labeling of phagocytic leukocytes. I. Soluble agents. J Nucl Med. 1976;17(6):480–7.
15. Thakur ML, Segal AW, Louis L, Welch MJ, Hopkins J, Peters TJ. Indium-111-labeled cellular blood components: mechanism of labeling and intracellular location in human neutrophils. J Nucl Med. 1977;18(10):1022–6.
16. McDougall IR, Goodwin DA. Gallium scan v indium 111-labeled oxyquinoline WBC scan. Arch Intern Med. 1982;142(7):1407–8.
17. Glithero PR, Grigoris P, Harding LK, Hesslewood SR, McMinn DJ. White cell scans and infected joint replacements. Failure to detect chronic infection. J Bone Joint Surg Br. 1993;75(3):371–4.
18. Pring DJ, Henderson RG, Rivett AG, Krausz T, Coombs RR, Lavender JP. Autologous granulocyte scanning of painful prosthetic joints. J Bone Joint Surg Br. 1986;68(4):647–52.
19. Pring DJ, Henderson RG, Keshavarzian A, Rivett AG, Krausz T, Coombs RR, et al. Indium-granulocyte scanning in the painful prosthetic joint. AJR Am J Roentgenol. 1986;147(1):167–72.
20. Wukich DK, Abreu SH, Callaghan JJ, Van Nostrand D, Savory CG, Eggli DF, et al. Diagnosis of infection by preoperative scintigraphy with indium-labeled white blood cells. J Bone Joint Surg Am. 1987;69(9):1353–60.
21. Froelich JW, Swanson D. Imaging of inflammatory processes with labeled cells. Semin Nucl Med. 1984;14(2):128–40.
22. Datz F, Luers P, Baker W, Christian P. Improved detection of upper abdominal abscesses by combination of 99mTc sulfur colloid and 111In leukocyte scanning. Am J Roentgenol. 1985;144(2):319–23.
23. Knochel JQ, Koehler PR, Lee TG, Welch DM. Diagnosis of abdominal abscesses with computed tomography, ultrasound, and 111In leukocyte scans. Radiology. 1980;137(2):425–32.
24. Lewis SS, Cox GM, Stout JE. Clinical utility of indium 111-labeled white blood cell scintigraphy

for evaluation of suspected infection. Open Forum Infect Dis. 2014;1(2):ofu089.

25. USP. USP General Chapter <825> Radiopharmaceuticals—preparation, compounding, dispensing, and repackaging I USP [Internet]. USP General Chapter <825> Radiopharmaceuticals—preparation, compounding, dispensing, and repackaging I USP. 2019 [cited 2019 Jul 28]. Available from: https://www.usp.org/chemical-medicines/general-chapter-825.

26. USP. General Chapter <797> Pharmaceutical compounding—sterile preparations I USP [Internet]. General Chapter <797> Pharmaceutical compounding—sterile preparations I USP. 2019 [cited 2019 Jul 28]. Available from: https://www.usp.org/compounding/general-chapter-797.

27. Steffel FG, Rao SA. Rapid and simple methods for labeling white blood cells and platelets with indium-111-oxine. J Nucl Med Technol. 1987;15(2):61–5.

28. Datz FL, Bedont RA, Baker WJ, Alazraki NP, Taylor A. No difference in sensitivity for occult infection between tropolone- and oxine-labeled indium-111 leukocytes. J Nucl Med. 1985;26(5):469–73.

29. Roca M, de Vries EFJ, Jamar F, Israel O, Signore A. Guidelines for the labelling of leucocytes with (111)In-oxine. Inflammation/Infection Taskgroup of the European Association of Nuclear Medicine. Eur J Nucl Med Mol Imaging. 2010;37(4):835–41.

30. Thakur ML, Coleman RE, Welch MJ. Indium-111-labeled leukocytes for the localization of abscesses: preparation, analysis, tissue distribution, and comparison with gallium-67 citrate in dogs. J Lab Clin Med. 1977;89(1):217–28.

31. SNMMI. Society of Nuclear Medicine Procedure Guideline for 99mTc-Exametazime (HMPAO)-labeled leukocyte scintigraphy for suspected infection/inflammation [Internet]. 2004 [cited 2019 Sep 20]. Available from: http://snmmi.files.cms-plus.com/docs/HMPAO_v3.pdf.

32. SNMMI. Society of Nuclear Medicine Procedure Guideline for 111In-leukocyte scintigraphy for suspected infection/inflammation [Internet]. 2004 [cited 2019 Sep 20]. Available from: http://snmmi.files.cms-plus.com/docs/Leukocyte_v3.pdf.

33. de Vries EFJ, Roca M, Jamar F, Israel O, Signore A. Guidelines for the labelling of leucocytes with 99mTc-HMPAO. Eur J Nucl Med Mol Imaging. 2010;37(4):842–8.

34. Zakhireh B, Thakur ML, Malech HL, Cohen MS, Gottschalk A, Root RK. Indium-111-labeled human polymorphonuclear leukocytes: viability, random migration, chemotaxis, bactericidal capacity, and ultrastructure. J Nucl Med. 1979;20(7):741–7.

35. Segal AW, Deteix P, Garcia R, Tooth P, Zanelli GD, Allison AC. Indium-111 labeling of leukocytes: a detrimental effect on neutrophil and lymphocyte function and an improved method of cell labelling. J Nucl Med. 1978;19:11. Available from: https://www.osti.gov/biblio/6203551.

36. Thakur ML, Coleman RE, Mayhall CG, Welch MJ. Preparation and evaluation of 111In-labeled leukocytes as an abscess imaging agent in dogs. Radiology. 1976;119(3):731.

37. de Vries EFJ, Roca M, Jamar F, Israel O, Signore A. Guidelines for the labelling of leucocytes with (99m)Tc-HMPAO. Inflammation/Infection Taskgroup of the European Association of Nuclear Medicine. Eur J Nucl Med Mol Imaging. 2010;37(4):842–8.

38. Love C, Palestro CJ. Radionuclide imaging of infection. J Nucl Med Technol. 2004;32(2):47–57.

39. Love C, Tomas MB, Tronco GG, Palestro CJ. FDG PET of infection and inflammation. Radiographics. 2005;25(5):1357–68.

40. Gainey MA, Siegel JA, Smergel EM, Jara BJ. Indium-111-labeled white blood cells: dosimetry in children. J Nucl Med. 1988;29(5):689–94.

41. Datz FL. Indium-111-labeled leukocytes for the detection of infection: current status. Semin Nucl Med. 1994;24(2):92–109.

42. Thakur ML, Lavender JP, Arnot RN, Silvester DJ, Segal AW. Indium-111-labeled autologous leukocytes in man. J Nucl Med. 1977;18(10):1014–21.

43. Datz FL, Jacobs J, Baker W, Landrum W, Alazraki N, Taylor A. Decreased sensitivity of early imaging with In-111 oxine-labeled leukocytes in detection of occult infection: concise communication. J Nucl Med. 1984;25(3):303–6.

44. Peters AM, Saverymuttu SH, Reavy HJ, Danpure HJ, Osman S, Lavender JP. Imaging of inflammation with indium-111 tropolonate labeled leukocytes. J Nucl Med. 1983;24(1):39–44.

45. Larikka MJ, Ahonen AK, Junila JA, Niemelä O, Hämäläinen MM, Syrjälä HP. Extended combined 99mTc-white blood cell and bone imaging improves the diagnostic accuracy in the detection of hip replacement infections. Eur J Nucl Med. 2001;28(3):288–93.

46. Peters AM. The utility of [99mTc]HMPAO-leukocytes for imaging infection. Semin Nucl Med. 1994;24(2):110–27.

47. Mcafee J, Subramanian GA, Gagne G, Schneider RF, Zapf-Longo C. 99mTc-HM-PAO for leukocyte labeling—experimental comparison with 111In oxine in dogs. Eur J Nucl Med. 1987;13:353–7.

48. Glaudemans AWJM, Israel O, Slart RHJA. Pitfalls and limitations of radionuclide and hybrid imaging in infection and inflammation. Semin Nucl Med. 2015;45(6):500–12.

49. Glaudemans AWJM, de Vries EFJ, Vermeulen LEM, Slart RHJA, Dierckx RAJO, Signore A. A large retrospective single-centre study to define the best image acquisition protocols and interpretation criteria for white blood cell scintigraphy with 99mTc-HMPAO-labelled leucocytes in musculoskeletal infections. Eur J Nucl Med Mol Imaging. 2013;40(11):1760–9.

50. Erba PA, Glaudemans AWJM, Veltman NC, Sollini M, Pacilio M, Galli F, et al. Image acquisition and interpretation criteria for 99mTc-HMPAO-

labelled white blood cell scintigraphy: results of a multicentre study. Eur J Nucl Med Mol Imaging. 2014;41(4):615–23.

51. Sfakianakis GN, Al-Sheikh W, Heal A, Rodman G, Zeppa R, Serafini A. Comparisons of scintigraphy with In-111 leukocytes and Ga-67 in the diagnosis of occult sepsis. J Nucl Med. 1982;23(7):618–26.

52. Datz F, Thorne D. Effect of chronicity of infection on the sensitivity of the In-111-labeled leukocyte scan. Am J Roentgenol. 1986;147(4):809–12.

53. Al-Sheikh W, Sfakianakis GN, Mnaymneh W, Hourani M, Heal A, Duncan RC, et al. Subacute and chronic bone infections: diagnosis using In-111, Ga-67 and Tc-99m MDP bone scintigraphy, and radiography. Radiology. 1985;155(2):501–6.

54. Robbins SL, Ramzi SC, Robbins SL, Cotran RS. Pathologic basis of disease. 2nd ed. Philadelphia: W.B. Saunders; 1979. p. 82–4.

55. Merkel KD, Brown ML, Dewanjee MK, Fitzgerald RH. Comparison of indium-labeled-leukocyte imaging with sequential technetium-gallium scanning in the diagnosis of low-grade musculoskeletal sepsis. A prospective study. J Bone Joint Surg Am. 1985;67(3):465–76.

56. ACR Appropriateness Criteria® [Internet]. [cited 2019 Dec 20]. Available from: https://www.acr.org/Clinical-Resources/ACR-Appropriateness-Criteria.

57. Practice Parameters and Technical Standards | American College of Radiology [Internet]. [cited 2019 Dec 20]. Available from: https://www.acr.org/Clinical-Resources/Practice-Parameters-and-Technical-Standards.

58. Clinical guidelines—SNMMI [Internet]. [cited 2019 Dec 20]. Available from: http://www.snmmi.org/ClinicalPractice/content.aspx?ItemNumber=10817&navItemNumber=10786.

59. Guidelines [Internet]. EANM. 2016 [cited 2019 Dec 20]. Available from: https://www.eanm.org/publications/guidelines/.

60. Inflammation/infection [Internet]. EANM. 2016 [cited 2019 Dec 20]. Available from: https://www.eanm.org/publications/guidelines/inflammationinfection/.

61. Procedure standards—SNMMI [Internet]. [cited 2019 Dec 20]. Available from: http://www.snmmi.org/ClinicalPractice/content.aspx?ItemNumber=6414#InfecInflamm.

62. Appropriateness criteria [Internet]. [cited 2019 Dec 20]. Available from: https://acsearch.acr.org/list.

63. ACR Appropriateness Criteria. Suspected osteomyelitis, septic arthritis, or soft tissue infection (excluding spine and diabetic foot) [Internet]. ACR.org. 2016 [cited 2019 Sep 19]. Available from: https://acsearch.acr.org/docs/3094201/Narrative/.

64. Kouijzer IJE, Mulders-Manders CM, Bleeker-Rovers CP, Oyen WJG. Fever of unknown origin: the value of FDG-PET/CT. Semin Nucl Med. 2018;48(2):100–7.

65. Unger M, Karanikas G, Kerschbaumer A, Winkler S, Aletaha D. Fever of unknown origin (FUO) revised. Wien Klin Wochenschr. 2016;128(21–22):796–801.

66. Syrjälä MT, Valtonen V, Liewendahl K, Myllylä G. Diagnostic significance of indium-111 granulocyte scintigraphy in febrile patients. J Nucl Med. 1987;28(2):155–60.

67. Seshadri N, Solanki C, Balan K. Utility of 111In-labelled leucocyte scintigraphy in patients with fever of unknown origin in an era of changing disease spectrum and investigational techniques. Nucl Med Commun. 2008;29(3):277–82.

68. Takeuchi M, Dahabreh IJ, Nihashi T, Iwata M, Varghese GM, Terasawa T. Nuclear imaging for classic fever of unknown origin: meta-analysis. J Nucl Med. 2016;57(12):1913–9.

69. Li JS, Sexton DJ, Mick N, Nettles R, Fowler VG, Ryan T, et al. Proposed modifications to the Duke criteria for the diagnosis of infective endocarditis. Clin Infect Dis. 2000;30(4):633–8.

70. Musso M, Petrosillo N. Nuclear medicine in diagnosis of prosthetic valve endocarditis: an update [Internet]. BioMed Res Int. 2015 [cited 2019 Jun 20]. Available from: https://www.hindawi.com/journals/bmri/2015/127325/.

71. Kestler M, Muñoz P, Rodríguez-Créixems M, Rotger A, Jimenez-Requena F, Mari A, et al. Role of (18) F-FDG PET in patients with infectious endocarditis. J Nucl Med. 2014;55(7):1093–8.

72. Schillaci O. Hybrid imaging systems in the diagnosis of osteomyelitis and prosthetic joint infection. Q J Nucl Med Mol Imaging. 2009;53(1):95–104.

73. Bruun NE, Habib G, Thuny F, Sogaard P. Cardiac imaging in infectious endocarditis. Eur Heart J. 2014;35(10):624–32.

74. Erba PA, Conti U, Lazzeri E, Sollini M, Doria R, De Tommasi SM, et al. Added value of 99mTc-HMPAO-labeled leukocyte SPECT/CT in the characterization and management of patients with infectious endocarditis. J Nucl Med. 2012;53(8):1235–43.

75. Signore A, Jamar F, Israel O, Buscombe J, Martin-Comin J, Lazzeri E. Clinical indications, image acquisition and data interpretation for white blood cells and anti-granulocyte monoclonal antibody scintigraphy: an EANM procedural guideline. Eur J Nucl Med Mol Imaging. 2018;45(10):1816–31.

76. Habib G, Lancellotti P, Antunes MJ, Bongiorni MG, Casalta J-P, Del Zotti F, et al. 2015 ESC guidelines for the management of infective endocarditis The Task Force for the Management of Infective Endocarditis of the European Society of Cardiology (ESC) Endorsed by: European Association for Cardio-Thoracic Surgery (EACTS), the European Association of Nuclear Medicine (EANM). Eur Heart J. 2015;36(44):3075–128.

77. Jérémie C, Aziza T, Nathalie G, Cédric L, Khadija B, Besma M, et al. Diagnostic impact of 18F-fluorodeoxyglucose positron emission tomography/computed tomography and white blood cell SPECT/computed tomography in patients with suspected cardiac implantable electronic device chronic infection. Circ Cardiovasc Imaging. 2019;12(7):e007188.

78. Keidar Z, Nitecki S. FDG-PET in prosthetic graft infections. Semin Nucl Med. 2013;43(5):396–402.

79. Perera GB, Fujitani RM, Kubaska SM. Aortic graft infection: update on management and treatment options. Vasc Endovasc Surg. 2006;40(1):1–10.

80. Bruggink JLM, Slart RHJA, Pol JA, Reijnen MMPJ, Zeebregts CJ. Current role of imaging in diagnosing aortic graft infections. Semin Vasc Surg. 2011;24(4):182–90.

81. Shahidi S, Eskil A, Lundof E, Klaerke A, Jensen BS. Detection of abdominal aortic graft infection: comparison of magnetic resonance imaging and indium-labeled white blood cell scanning. Ann Vasc Surg. 2007;21(5):586–92.

82. Reinders Folmer EI, Von Meijenfeldt GCI, Van der Laan MJ, Glaudemans AWJM, Slart RHJA, Saleem BR, et al. Diagnostic imaging in vascular graft infection: a systematic review and meta-analysis. Eur J Vasc Endovasc Surg. 2018;56(5):719–29.

83. Wilson Walter R, Bower Thomas C, Creager Mark A, Sepideh A-H, O'Gara Patrick T, Lockhart Peter B, et al. Vascular graft infections, mycotic aneurysms, and endovascular infections: a scientific statement from the American Heart Association. Circulation. 2016;134(20):e412–60.

84. Etkin CD, Springer BD. The American Joint Replacement Registry—the first 5 years. Arthroplast Today. 2017;3(2):67–9.

85. Kurtz S. Projections of primary and revision hip and knee arthroplasty in the United States from 2005 to 2030. J Bone Joint Surg Am. 2007;89(4):780.

86. Love C, Tomas MB, Marwin SE, Pugliese PV, Palestro CJ. Role of nuclear medicine in diagnosis of the infected joint replacement. Radiographics. 2001;21(5):1229–38.

87. Gratz S, Behr T, Reize P, Pfestroff A, Kampen W, Höffken H. (99m)Tc-Fab′ fragments (sulesomab) for imaging septically loosened total knee arthroplasty. J Int Med Res. 2009;37(1):54–67.

88. Gemmel F, Van den Wyngaert H, Love C, Welling MM, Gemmel P, Palestro CJ. Prosthetic joint infections: radionuclide state-of-the-art imaging. Eur J Nucl Med Mol Imaging. 2012;39(5):892–909.

89. van der Bruggen W, Bleeker-Rovers CP, Boerman OC, Gotthardt M, Oyen WJG. PET and SPECT in osteomyelitis and prosthetic bone and joint infections: a systematic review. Semin Nucl Med. 2010;40(1):3–15.

90. Basu S, Kwee TC, Saboury B, Garino JP, Nelson CL, Zhuang H, et al. FDG-PET for diagnosing infection in hip and knee prostheses: prospective study in 221 prostheses and subgroup comparison with combined 111In-labeled leukocyte/99mTc-sulfur colloid bone marrow imaging in 88 prostheses. Clin Nucl Med. 2014;39(7):609–15.

91. Jin H, Yuan L, Li C, Kan Y, Hao R, Yang J. Diagnostic performance of FDG PET or PET/CT in prosthetic infection after arthroplasty: a meta-analysis. Q J Nucl Med Mol Imaging. 2014;58(1):85–93.

92. Pill SG, Parvizi J, Tang PH, Garino JP, Nelson C, Zhuang H, et al. Comparison of fluorodeoxyglucose positron emission tomography and 111Indium–white blood cell imaging in the diagnosis of periprosthetic infection of the hip. J Arthroplasty. 2006;21(6 Suppl):91–7.

93. Jamar F, Buscombe J, Chiti A, Christian PE, Delbeke D, Donohoe KJ, et al. EANM/SNMMI guideline for 18F-FDG use in inflammation and infection. J Nucl Med. 2013;54(4):647–58.

94. Signore A, Sconfienza LM, Borens O, Glaudemans AWJM, Cassar-Pullicino V, Trampuz A, et al. Consensus document for the diagnosis of prosthetic joint infections: a joint paper by the EANM, EBJIS, and ESR (with ESCMID endorsement). Eur J Nucl Med Mol Imaging. 2019;46(4):971–88.

95. Howick J, Chalmers I, Glasziou P, Greenhalgh T, Heneghan C, Liberati A, et al. The Oxford 2011 levels of evidence [Internet]. Oxford Centre for Evidence-Based Medicine; 2011. Available from: http://www.cebm.net/index.aspx?o=5653.

96. Richter WS, Ivancevic V, Meller J, Lang O, Le Guludec D, Szilvazi I, et al. 99mTc-besilesomab (Scintimun) in peripheral osteomyelitis: comparison with 99mTc-labelled white blood cells. Eur J Nucl Med Mol Imaging. 2011;38(5):899–910.

97. Pakos EE, Trikalinos TA, Fotopoulos AD, Ioannidis JPA. Prosthesis infection: diagnosis after total joint arthroplasty with antigranulocyte scintigraphy with 99mTc-labeled monoclonal antibodies—a meta-analysis. Radiology. 2007;242(1):101–8.

98. Xing D, Ma X, Ma J, Wang J, Chen Y, Yang Y. Use of anti-granulocyte scintigraphy with 99mTc-labeled monoclonal antibodies for the diagnosis of periprosthetic infection in patients after total joint arthroplasty: a diagnostic meta-analysis. PLoS One. 2013;8(7):e69857.

99. Katsura M, Sato J, Akahane M, Kunimatsu A, Abe O. Current and novel techniques for metal artifact reduction at CT: practical guide for radiologists. Radiographics. 2018;38(2):450–61.

100. Armstrong DG, Wrobel J, Robbins JM. Guest Editorial: Are diabetes-related wounds and amputations worse than cancer? Int Wound J. 2007;4(4):286–7.

101. Ertugrul BM, Oncul O, Tulek N, Willke A, Sacar S, Tunccan OG, et al. A prospective, multi-center study: factors related to the management of diabetic foot infections. Eur J Clin Microbiol Infect Dis. 2012;31(9):2345–52.

102. ACR. ACR appropriateness criteria. Suspected osteomyelitis of the foot in patients with diabetes mellitus [Internet]. 2019 [cited 2019 Sep 20]. Available from: https://acsearch.acr.org/docs/69340/Narrative/.

103. Malhotra R, Chan CS-Y, Nather A. Osteomyelitis in the diabetic foot. Diabet Foot Ankle [Internet]. 2014 30 [cited 2019 May 10];5. Available from: https://www.ncbi.nlm.nih.gov/pmc/articles/PMC4119293/.

104. Heiba S, Kolker D, Ong L, Sharma S, Travis A, Teodorescu V, et al. Dual-isotope SPECT/CT impact on hospitalized patients with suspected diabetic foot infection: saving limbs, lives, and resources. Nucl Med Commun. 2013;34(9):877–84.

105. Capriotti G, Chianelli M, Signore A. Nuclear medicine imaging of diabetic foot infection: results of meta-analysis. Nucl Med Commun. 2006;27(10):757–64.

106. Vouillarmet J, Morelec I, Thivolet C. Assessing diabetic foot osteomyelitis remission with white blood cell SPECT/CT imaging. Diabet Med. 2014;31(9):1093–9.

107. Sarosi GJ, Turnage R. Appendicitis. In: Feldman M, Tschumy WJ, Friedman L, Sleisenger M, editors. Sleisenger and Fordtran's gastrointestinal and liver disease. 7th ed. Philadelphia, PA: W.B. Saunders; 2002. p. 2089–99.

108. Aydın F, Kın Cengiz A, Güngör F. Tc-99m labeled HMPAO white blood cell scintigraphy in pediatric patients. Mol Imaging Radionucl Ther. 2012;21(1):13–8.

109. ACR. ACR appropriateness criteria: right lower quadrant pain—suspected appendicitis [Internet]. 2010 [cited 2019 Sep 25]. Available from: http://www.emergencyultrasoundteaching.com/assets/articles/Appy_2011_Rosen_J_Am_Coll_Radiol.pdf.

110. Albiston E. The role of radiological imaging in the diagnosis of acute appendicitis. Can J Gastroenterol. 2002;16(7):451–63.

111. Cheng K-S, Shiau Y-C, Lin C-C, Lee C-C, Kao A. Comparison between technetium-99m hexamethylpropyleneamineoxide labeled white blood cell abdomen scan and abdominal sonography to detect appendicitis in female patients with an atypical clinical presentation. Hepatogastroenterology. 2003;50(49):136–9.

112. Sun S-S, Wu H-S, Wang J-J, Ho S-T, Kao A. Comparison between technetium 99m hexamethylpropyleneamine oxide labeled white blood cell abdominal scan and abdominal sonography to detect appendicitis in adult patients with atypical clinical presentation. Abdom Imaging. 2002;27(6):734–8.

113. Caobelli F, Evangelista L, Quartuccio N, Familiari D, Altini C, Castello A, et al. Role of molecular imaging in the management of patients affected by inflammatory bowel disease: state-of-the-art. World J Radiol. 2016;8(10):829–45.

114. Zhang J, Li L-F, Zhu Y-J, Qiu H, Xu Q, Yang J, et al. Diagnostic performance of 18F-FDG-PET versus scintigraphy in patients with inflammatory bowel disease: a meta-analysis of prospective literature. Nucl Med Commun. 2014;35(12):1233–46.

115. Stathaki MI, Koukouraki SI, Karkavitsas NS, Koutroubakis IE. Role of scintigraphy in inflammatory bowel disease. World J Gastroenterol. 2009;15(22):2693–700.

116. Charron M, Di Lorenzo C, Kocoshis S. Are 99mTc leukocyte scintigraphy and SBFT studies useful in children suspected of having inflammatory bowel disease? Am J Gastroenterol. 2000;5(95):1208–12.

117. Uno K, Matsui N, Nohira K, Suguro T, Kitakata Y, Uchiyama G, et al. Indium-111 leukocyte imaging in patients with rheumatoid arthritis. J Nucl Med. 1986;27(3):339–44.

118. Gaál J, Mézes A, Síró B, Varga J, Galuska L, Jánoky G, et al. 99mTc-HMPAO labelled leukocyte scintigraphy in patients with rheumatoid arthritis: a comparison with disease activity. Nucl Med Commun. 2002;23(1):39.

119. Al-Janabi MA, Jones AKP, Solanki K, Sobnack R, Bomanji J, Al-Nahhas AA, et al. 99Tcm-labelled leucocyte imaging in active rheumatoid arthritis. Nucl Med Commun. 1988;9(12):987.

120. Becker W, Bair J, Behr T, Repp R, Streckenbach H, Beck H, et al. Detection of soft-tissue infections and osteomyelitis using a technetium-99m-labeled antigranulocyte monoclonal antibody fragment. J Nucl Med. 1994;35(9):1436–43.

121. Gratz S, Braun HG, Behr TM, Meller J, Herrmann A, Conrad M, et al. Photopenia in chronic vertebral osteomyelitis with technetium-99m-antigranulocyte antibody (BW 250/183). J Nucl Med. 1997;38(2):211–6.

122. Gratz S, Schipper ML, Dorner J, Höffken H, Becker W, Kaiser JW, et al. LeukoScan for imaging infection in different clinical settings: a retrospective evaluation and extended review of the literature. Clin Nucl Med. 2003;28(4):267–76.

123. Papos M, Nagy F, Narai G, Rajtar M, Szantai G, Lang J, et al. Anti-granulocyte immunoscintigraphy and [99mTc]hexamethylpropyleneamine-oxime-labeled leukocyte scintigraphy in inflammatory bowel disease. Dig Dis Sci. 1996;41(2):412–20.

124. Ingui CJ, Shah NP, Oates ME. Infection scintigraphy: added value of single-photon emission computed tomography/computed tomography fusion compared with traditional analysis. J Comput Assist Tomogr. 2007;31(3):375–80.

125. Bar-Shalom R, Yefremov N, Guralnik L, Keidar Z, Engel A, Nitecki S, et al. SPECT/CT using 67Ga and 111In-labeled leukocyte scintigraphy for diagnosis of infection. J Nucl Med. 2006;47(4):587–94.

126. Djekidel M, Brown RKJ, Piert M. Benefits of hybrid SPECT/CT for (111)In-oxine- and Tc-99m-hexamethylpropylene amine oxime-labeled leukocyte imaging. Clin Nucl Med. 2011;36(7):e50–6.

127. Heiba S, Rangaswamy B, Kolker D, Kostakoglu L, Machac J. The diagnostic confidence of SPECT & SPECT/CT in Indium-111 leukocyte scintigraphy. J Nucl Med. 2007;48(Suppl 2):63P.

128. Rini JN, Bhargava KK, Tronco GG, Singer C, Caprioli R, Marwin SE, et al. PET with FDG-labeled leukocytes versus scintigraphy with 111In-oxine-labeled leukocytes for detection of infection. Radiology. 2006;238(3):978–87.

129. Meyer M, Testart N, Jreige M, Kamani C, Moshebah M, Muoio B, et al. Diagnostic performance of PET or PET/CT using 18F-FDG labeled white blood

cells in infectious diseases: a systematic review and a bivariate meta-analysis. Diagnostics (Basel). 2019;9(2):60. Available from: https://www.ncbi.nlm.nih.gov/pmc/articles/PMC6627172/.

130. Love C, Palestro CJ. Radionuclide imaging of infection. J Nucl Med Technol. 2004;32(2):12.

131. Palestro CJ. The current role of gallium imaging in infection. Semin Nucl Med. 1994;24(2):128–41.

132. Ballinger JR, Gnanasegaran G. Radiolabelled leukocytes for imaging inflammation: how radiochemistry affects clinical use. Q J Nucl Med Mol Imaging. 2005;49(4):308–18.

[^{99m}Tc]Tc-HMPAO-Labeled Leukocyte Imaging of Infection and Inflammation

6

Joanna E. Kusmirek and Scott B. Perlman

Contents

J. E. Kusmirek · S. B. Perlman (✉)
Department of Radiology, University of Wisconsin
School of Medicine and Public Health,
Madison, WI, USA
e-mail: JKusmirek@uwhealth.org;
SPerlman@uwhealth.org

© Springer Nature Switzerland AG 2022
S. Harsini et al. (eds.), *Nuclear Medicine and Immunology*,
https://doi.org/10.1007/978-3-030-81261-4_6

6.1 Introduction

Identification of infection and/or inflammation in a patient can be difficult. The clinical findings in a patient with a suspected infection may not be localized, and anatomic imaging modalities such as CT can be negative. The technetium-99m (^{99m}Tc)-labeled white blood cell (^{99m}Tc-WBC) exam provides an important method of examining the entire body to identify a source of the infection. In other cases, such as a complicated skeletal fracture or a vascular graft, this physiologic procedure can add important information as to whether an infection is present. This chapter will review the technical and clinical uses of the ^{99m}Tc-labeled leukocyte technique for the identification of inflammation and infection.

6.2 Leukocyte Labeling Procedure

Labeled leukocytes play an important role in the identification of infection, especially when the anatomic imaging modalities such as computed tomography (CT) are negative. This technique is a sensitive way of identifying the focus of infection. The procedure has been used since it was discovered that the patient's blood could be separated into its components, and the neutrophils could be labeled with a radioactive marker in such a way that the WBC chemotaxis would not be affected. Therefore, the labeled cells move toward the infection site the same as native unlabeled leukocytes. The first real labeling of leukocytes for clinical utility used [^{111}In]In-oxine, which enters the cells due to its lipophilicity and remains bound to cyto-

plasmic components. The leukocytes retained their function and have been used in the identification of infection with reasonably good accuracy. However, the indium-111 (^{111}In)-labeled cell method had a number of limitations, including a less-than-optimal dosimetry (longer half-life of 2.8 days and unfavorable radionuclide decay scheme) and the lower count rate making SPECT imaging difficult, limited availability of the indium-111 because it is a cyclotron product, and the expense of the radionuclide. Thus, there was a need to develop a better method of cell labeling for infection identification. This led to the development of the technetium labeling method using the readily available technetium-99m which can be obtained at a significantly lower cost due to its availability from the molybdenum/technetium generator which is present in many nuclear medicine departments. Furthermore, the higher photon flux allows single photon emission computed tomography (SPECT) imaging to be performed when needed to help localize the abnormal activity.

One of the earliest reports on the technetium-99m method of cell labeling used only 10–20 mL of blood. The diluted heparinized blood was centrifuged to separate out into three liquid layers, with lymphocytes present in the interface between the top two layers and the leukocytes between the second and bottom layers. The leukocytes could be moved into another tube, and the red blood cells (RBCs) removed by lysis when sterile water was added. These leukocytes could then be labeled with 740–1110 MBq (20–30 mCi) of [^{99m}Tc]Tc-O$_4$ after being incubated with a solution containing sodium pyrophosphate and stannous chloride. The labeling efficiency was approximately 81% and was stable [1].

More recently, this technique has been improved to involve the labeling of the leukocytes with [^{99m}Tc]Tc-HMPAO (hexamethylpropyleneamine oxime). The labeling technique involves the use of [^{99m}Tc]Tc-HMPAO, which was originally developed as a lipophilic brain imaging agent by Amersham International. The [^{99m}Tc]Tc-HMPAO is retained within the cell. Proposed mechanisms are conversion of the lipophilic complex into a hydrophilic one by reducing agents and binding of the [^{99m}Tc]Tc-HMPAO to nondiffusible proteins and organelles [2]. A thorough discussion of the [^{99m}Tc]Tc-HMPAO-labeling technique has been published, and a very brief summary follows:

1. Add 51 mL of blood to 9 mL of acid-citrate-dextrose (ACD) solution and mix gently.
   (a) >2 × 10^8 leukocytes are required for a good labeling efficiency.
2. Centrifuge 15 mL of this solution at 2000 *g* for 10 min.
   (a) The cell-free plasma and pellet are separated.
3. Add 10% 2-hydroxyethyl starch (HES) to 45 mL of the blood-ACD solution and allow the erythrocytes to sediment.
4. Collect the leukocyte-rich plasma and centrifuge at 150 *g* for 5 min.
5. Remove the platelet-rich plasma.
6. Gently resuspend the mixed leukocytes in 1 mL of fresh cell-free plasma.
7. Add 1 mL of 750–1000 MBq of [^{99m}Tc]Tc-HMPAO to the mixed leukocyte suspension, and incubate for 10 min at room temperature.
8. Add >3 mL of cell-free plasma and centrifuge at 150 *g* for 5 min.
9. Remove the supernatant containing the unbound [^{99m}Tc]Tc-HMPAO.
10. Measure the amount of radioactivity in the supernatant and in the pellet to calculate the labeling efficiency.
11. Gently resuspend the labeled mixed leukocyte pellet in 3–5 mL of cell-free plasma.
12. The appropriate quality control measures should be performed, and the patient's dose can be drawn from this cell suspension [2].

Peters and coworkers used this agent to label leukocytes in six patients with suspected or known inflammatory diseases and determined that 78% of the cell-bound activity was present on granulocytes when a mixed leukocyte suspension was labeled (mean efficiency of 47%) [3]. This represented a significant advance in labeled cell imaging as a technetium-labeled agent had better imaging characteristics and lower patient radiation exposure.

6.3 Biodistribution

The biodistribution of the ^{99m}Tc-leukocytes differs a little from ^{111}In-leukocytes on the early images. There is excretion of the unbound [^{99m}Tc]Tc-HMPAO into the gallbladder and gastrointestinal (GI) tract, so most protocols recommend early imaging at around 2 h to evaluate the abdomen as well as delayed images at around 4–8 h and if needed at 24 h postinjection. An abdominal focus of infection will often be seen on the early images, prior to significant gastrointestinal excretion, thus normal physiologic GI excretion can be separated from an intra-abdominal abscess. Furthermore, the higher photon flux of the larger dose of technetium-99m compared to indium-111 allows the addition of high-quality SPECT/CT to the planar images, thus providing the benefit of early localization of an area of abscess/infection. These advantages, combined with the lower cost and lower radiation exposure, are a major reason that when possible, the [^{99m}Tc]Tc-WBC technique is preferable to ^{111}In-WBC. Another difference in the biodistribution of the [^{99m}Tc]Tc-HMPAO-labeled cells is the appearance of early bone marrow activity, which decreases over an approximate 3-h time period [4]. Other normal areas of ^{99m}Tc-WBC accumulation include the liver, kidneys, spleen, and lungs. The activity seen in the lungs on early imaging clears by 4 h and thus should not be seen on the delayed images. This is due to the fact that the ^{99m}Tc-WBC spends more time in contact with the pulmonary endothelium than the systemic vascular endothelium for a number of reasons including prolonged pulmonary transit due to cell trauma during the labeling process (Figs. 6.1 and 6.2) [5].

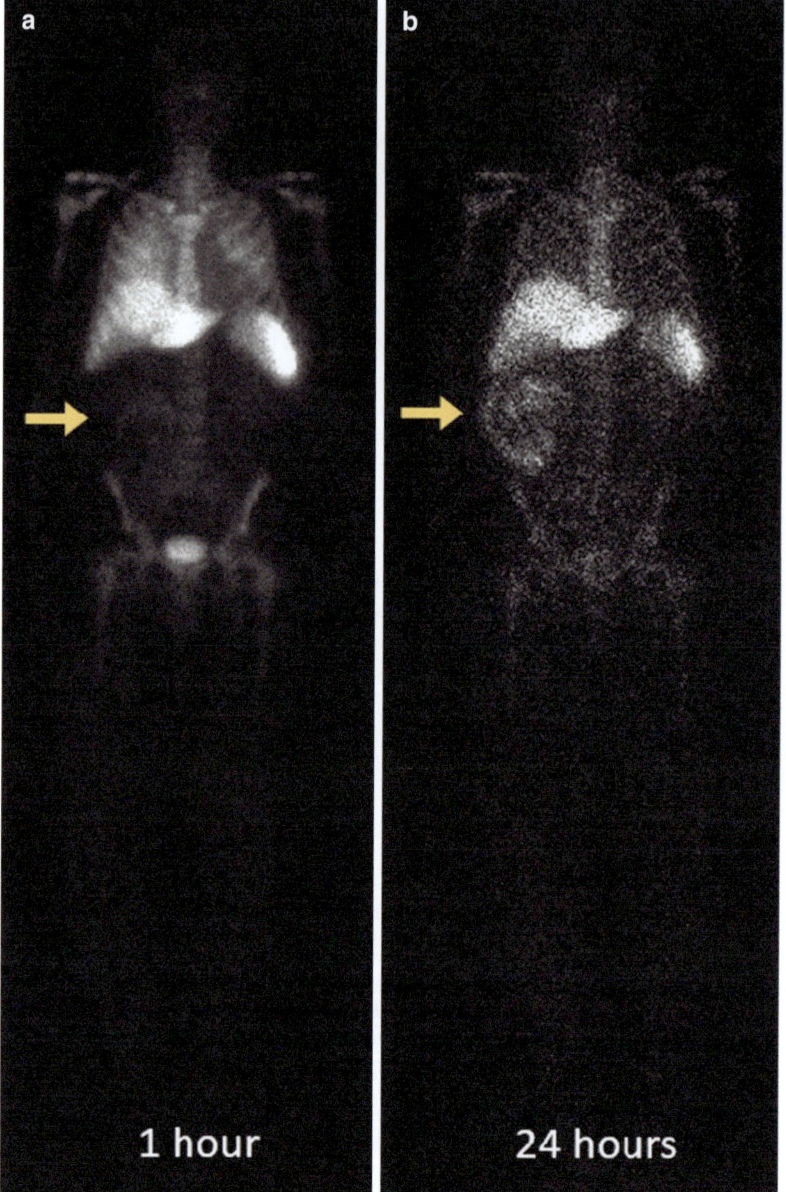

Fig. 6.1 A 64-year-old man with bacteremia. This exam was to look for infection. Note images at about 1 h after injection of labeled [^{99m}Tc]Tc-HMPAO WBCs show minimal small bowel activity (**a**, arrow), but images at 24 h show significant physiologic small bowel activity (**b**). The exam is negative for an infection source

6.4   Comparison of ^{99m}Tc-WBC with ^{111}In-WBC Scintigraphy

There are several benefits of using the ^{99m}Tc-WBC method over the ^{111}In-WBC method. Advantages of the [^{99m}Tc]Tc-HMPAO-labeled leukocytes include a higher photon flux allowing for high-quality SPECT/CT imaging, very important for being able to localize an infection site for possible biopsy and/or drainage, and ready availability as the molybdenum/technetium generator is in widespread use and readily available to most nuclear medicine departments. The time to a positive examination might also be an important concern. The [^{99m}Tc]Tc-HMPAO-WBC technique may be positive as early as a few

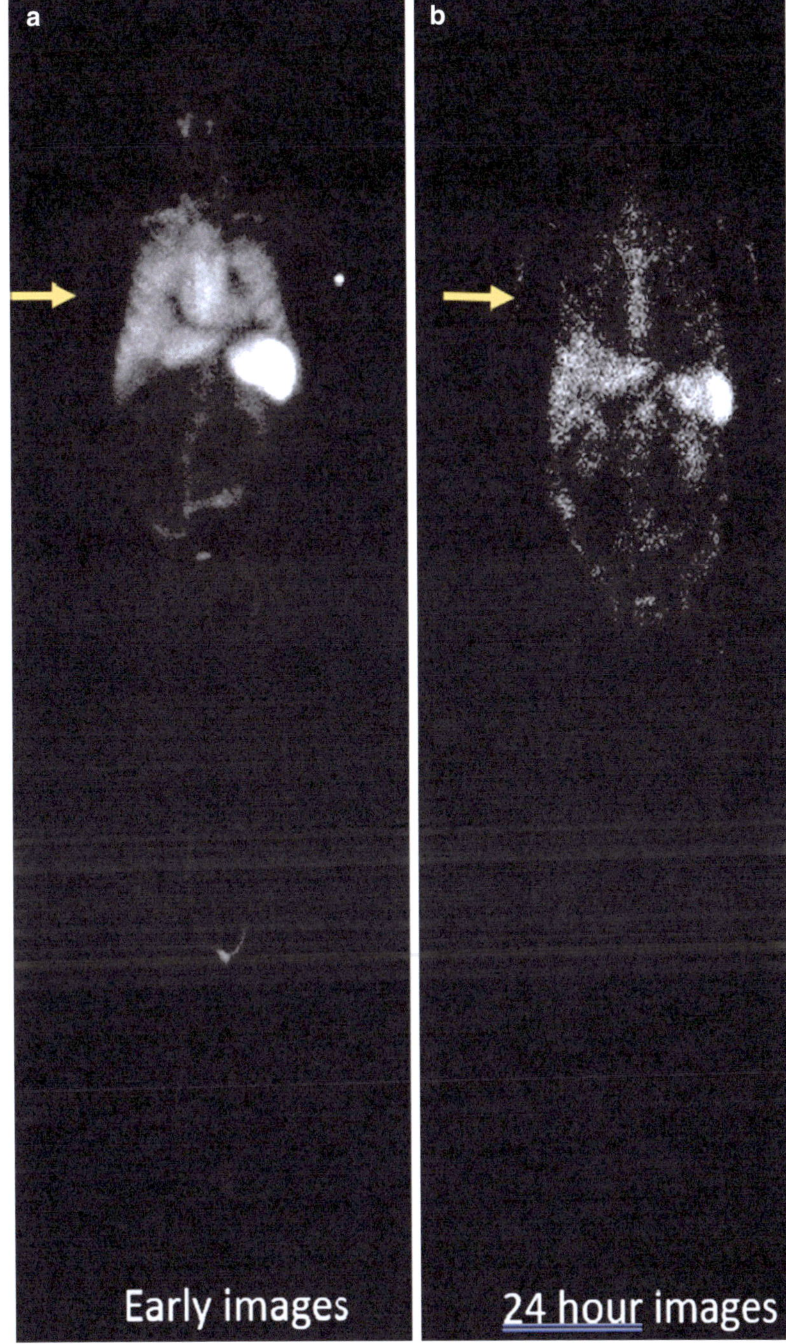

Fig. 6.2 A 68-year-old man with an exam performed to look for a source of infection. 1039.7 MBq of [^{99m}Tc]Tc-HMPAO-labeled leukocytes injected. Note the increased uptake in the lungs on the early images (**a**) which clears on the 24-h images (**b**), indicating normal biodistribution

hours after injection. As noted earlier, images are usually acquired both at 2 h and at 4–8 h with delayed imaging at 24 h after injection if needed. Images at 2 h will often localize an abscess, allowing an earlier intervention, instead of waiting for the 24-h images. Early images should be free of the excreted gastrointestinal activity, so an early focal area of uptake is suspicious for an infection/abscess. Imaging as early as 0.5 h after injection has been shown to have a sensitivity of

88% which increased to 95% at 2 h and 96% at 4 h, [6], so it would seem that imaging at the 2-h time point might be the most advantageous with repeat imaging around 4–8 h later and again at 24 h if needed. The 2-h imaging time point is early enough to avoid problems in interpretation from nonspecific gastrointestinal activity, with additional later imaging for maximal sensitivity.

The difference in distribution between ^{99m}Tc-WBC and ^{111}In-labeled WBC was described in the preceding paragraph, and the dosimetry is discussed in the following section.

6.5 Dosimetry

A very important consideration for every type of medical imaging is patient radiation exposure (Table 6.1). The recommended dose of the labeled leukocytes is 259–925 MBq (7–25 mCi), with an effective dose per administered activity of 7.5 µSv/MBq (28 mrem/mCi), the critical organ being the spleen receiving 88 µGy/ MBq (327 mrad/mCi) (US Food and Drug Administration (FDA) package insert, Jubilant DraxImage Inc., Quebec, Canada, revised 8/2017). This is in comparison to the $[^{111}$In] In-oxyquinoline (oxine)-labeled WBC, where the recommended dose is 10–20 MBq (0.3–0.5 mCi), giving an effective dose equivalent of 0.59 mSv/ MBq (2.2 rem/mCi) and the critical organ, the spleen, receiving 5.5 mGy/MBq (20 rad/mCi) (Society of Nuclear Medicine (SNM) Procedure Guideline for ^{111}In-leukocyte Scintigraphy for Suspected Infection/Inflammation, Version 3.0, approved June 2, 2004). Therefore, one must carefully consider which agent to use in each specific case, and if they are equal in accuracy, it

would be wise to choose the agent with the lower patient radiation exposure.

6.6 Infection/Inflammation Evaluation-General Considerations

The Society of Nuclear Medicine and Molecular Imaging (SNMMI) guidelines recommend ^{99m}Tc-WBC imaging for the detection of suspected sites of acute inflammation/infection in a febrile patient to detect the site of inflammation as a cause of abdominal pain or in patients with granulocytosis and/or positive blood cultures. Additionally, the study can be used to detect and determine the extent of inflammatory or ischemic bowel disease as well as to detect and follow up musculoskeletal infection, such as septic arthritis and osteomyelitis [7].

The European Association of Nuclear Medicine (EANM) guidelines [2] state that $[^{99m}$Tc]Tc-HMPAO-labeled WBC scintigraphy may be used to detect and localize any occult site of infection and to determine the extent of the process in various disorders, including:

- Osteomyelitis of the appendicular skeleton
- Infected joint and vascular prosthesis
- Diabetic foot
- Fever of unknown origin
- Postoperative abscesses
- Lung infections
- Endocarditis
- Inflammatory bowel disease
- Neurological infections
- Infected central venous catheters or other devices

Table 6.1 Radiation dosimetry for the ^{99m}Tc and ^{111}In-labeled leukocyte radiopharmaceuticals

	Dose	Critical organ: spleen	Effective dose
$[^{99m}$Tc]Tc-HMPAO WBCs			
FDA Package Insert 8/2017	259–925 MBq (7–25 mCi)	88 µGy/MBq (327 mrad/ mCi)	7.5 µSv/MBq (28 mrem/ mCi)
$[^{111}$In]In-oxine WBCs			
SNM Practice Guideline 6/2/2004	10–20 MBq (0.3–0.5 mCi)	5.5 mGy/MBq (20 rad/ mCi)	0.59 mSv/MBq (2.2 rem/ mCi)

Technetium-99m labeling enables higher-resolution images (compared to ^{111}In-labeled WBC). The imaging can be performed shortly after injection; however, the short half-life of technetium-99m limits delayed imaging beyond 24 h. In addition, technetium-99m has favorable characteristics for SPECT and SPECT/CT imaging.

^{99m}Tc-labeled WBC distribution can be quite variable in a healthy individual. Technetium is excreted by the kidneys and hepatobiliary system [8]. Therefore, in addition to the uptake in the spleen, liver, and bone marrow, normal distribution includes various degree of the radiotracer activity in the urinary tract, bowel, and gallbladder. This can be a potential cause for false-positive results in the evaluation of liver abscess; however, there should be focally increased uptake between 1- and 4-h imaging [9]. In some cases, imaging with [^{111}In]In-oxine may be preferred. In addition, assessment of renal and splenic abscesses may be limited. On the other hand, ^{99m}Tc-labeled WBC scintigraphy is preferred for suspected soft tissue infection/sepsis [9]

6.7   Inflammatory Bowel Disease

The determination of the activity of inflammatory bowel disease (IBD) can be a diagnostic challenge. Anatomic modalities can accurately identify areas of abnormal bowel, but it can often be very difficult to determine if the abnormal bowel is due to scar from inactive old disease or active inflammation. Endoscopy during an active flare of disease might lead to perforation, and the sites of active disease might not be apparent from an endoscope due to inflammation that is predominantly below the superficial layers of the bowel mucosa. A noninvasive technique that can accurately determine active disease in both the small and large bowel would be a great benefit to patient care and may be especially useful in patients unable to tolerate adequate bowel preparation for the colonoscopy as this radiopharmaceutical technique does not require bowel preparation. New drugs to treat active disease are effective but are expensive and carry several side effects. Therefore, it is important to determine if a flare in symptoms is secondary to active disease or other causes such as scarring so that drug treatment can be used most effectively. Activity indexes or blood and stool tests are indirect methods of determining disease activity. A direct method of determining disease activity would be a great advancement in the care of these patients.

The [^{99m}Tc]Tc-HMPAO-labeled leukocyte technique is a relatively simple technique for the evaluation of bowel inflammation. Early imaging needs to be performed in order to avoid the confusion of normal activity in the bowel from physiologic biliary excretion. Imaging is typically performed at 1 and 3 h after injection of the labeled leukocytes, with inflamed bowel often seen at 1 h and increasing on the 3-h image.

Various rating scales have been used to evaluate the bowel for inflammation as determined by the labeled cells. One simple rating scale uses a 4-grade semiquantitative scale as follows: 0 = no activity, 1 = detectable but minor activity, 2 = activity between 1 and 3, and 3 = strikingly intense activity. The presence of inflammation was judged as equal to or greater than grade 1 [10]. A more detailed scale calculated a scintigraphic index (SI), where the abdomen was divided into five zones that roughly represented the ascending colon, transverse colon, descending colon, sigmoid colon/rectum, and the small bowel. Activity in each zone was graded as 1 = activity less than bone activity, 2 = activity greater than bone activity, 3 = activity greater than liver activity, and 4 = activity greater than spleen activity. The SI was the sum of the degree of activity in each zone plus the number of zones affected, with an SI greater than 2 indicating active disease [11].

The labeled WBC technique has proven to be very useful in identifying abnormal bowel in patients with inflammatory bowel disease. A sensitivity of 97% has been reported in assessing colonic inflammation compared with colonoscopy. The leukocyte scan showed a similar degree of inflammation in the terminal ileum in 17 of 19 patients when visualized either endoscopically or surgically. The WBC scan did not show any false-positive findings in the terminal ileum in 83 control patients [12]. A review paper by Stathaki and coworkers reported that [^{99m}Tc]Tc-HMPAO-labeled leukocytes had a sensitivity of 95–100% and a specificity of 85–100% and an accuracy of 92–100% when used for the detection, localization, and assessment of disease activity in patients with inflammatory bowel disease [13].

Patients with a flare of disease would benefit from an exam that is noninvasive as colonoscopy during a flare might lead to an increased risk of complications. Twenty patients who were hospitalized with severe exacerbations of ulcerative colitis were studied with Tc-WBC 45 and 120 min after injection of the labeled cells, and rectosigmoidoscopy was performed within 24 h of scintigraphy [14]. The 45-min image was used for the visual grading as the later image may have nonspecific bowel accumulation. They reported that all patients had pathologic uptake in the rectosigmoid (100% sensitivity), with ten patients

having disease involving the left side of the colon, and pancolitis in the other patients.

One potential advantage of the molecular imaging technique over direct colonoscopy would be the identification of submucosal disease that might not be seen at direct visual endoscopy. Indeed, it has been reported that when the Crohn's Disease Activity Index, blood tests, and C-reactive protein were examined in patients with Crohn's disease and compared to [^{99m}Tc]Tc-HMPAO-labeled leukocytes, 70% of patients (14/20) did not show congruent results. Their conclusion was that [^{99m}Tc]Tc-HMPAO-labeled leukocyte scintigraphy could be important for determining inflammatory activity in Crohn's disease even in the absence of clinical symptoms (Fig. 6.3) [11].

The labeled WBC technique has been reported to be very useful in the evaluation of the small bowel in patients with Crohn's disease. The test had a sensitivity for macroscopically evident small bowel inflammation of 0.85 and a specific-

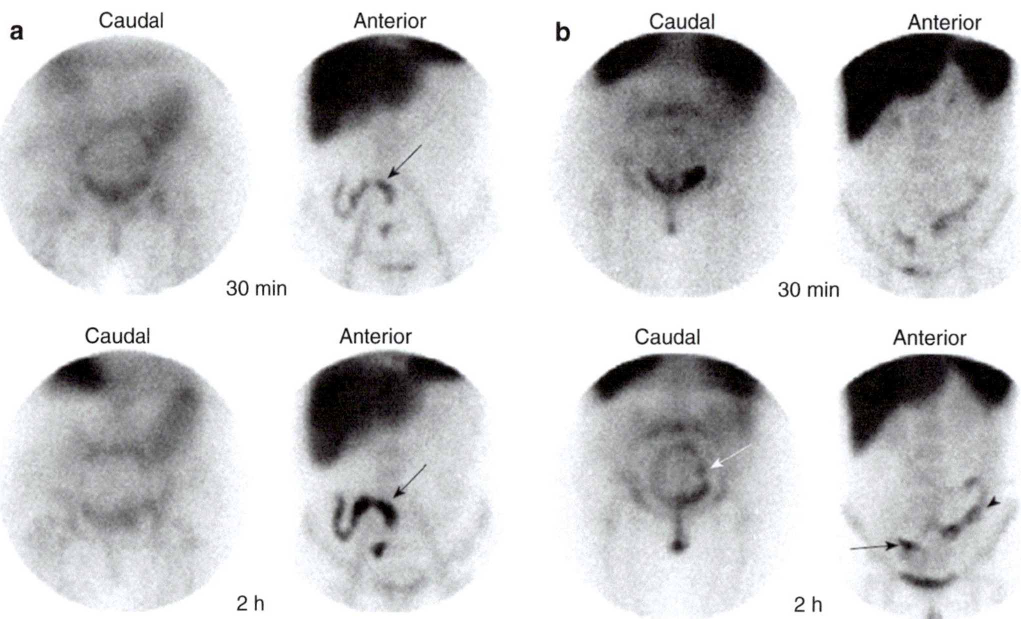

Fig. 6.3 (**a**) Images obtained 30 min and 2 h postinjection of [^{99m}Tc]Tc-HMPAO-labeled leukocytes in the caudal and anterior views in a 54-year-old female. The arrows indicate the region of the intestine affected by the inflammation. (**b**) Images obtained 30 min and 2 h postinjection of [^{99m}Tc]Tc-HMPAO-labeled leukocytes in the caudal and anterior views in a 24-year-old female. The arrows indicate [^{99m}Tc]Tc-HMPAO-labeled leukocyte uptake in the terminal ileum, descending colon, and rectosigmoid. The black arrows indicate terminal ileum; the arrowhead indicates descending colon; the white arrow indicates rectosigmoid. (Adapted from Mota et al., World Journal of Gastroenterology, 2010) [11]

ity of 0.81 and further detected inflammatory lesions not known before laparotomy in 34% (16 of 47). Uptake was also seen in fistulas and abscesses [10].

This imaging technique is especially useful in children in whom bowel preparation is a challenge to obtain for an adequate direct colonoscopy exam. The ^{99m}Tc-WBC technique has been investigated in children suspected of having inflammatory bowel disease and has been reported to demonstrate different patterns of uptake in Crohn's disease versus ulcerative colitis, with the pattern being continuous bowel uptake in ulcerative colitis (4/4 true-positive results) and discontinuous uptake in Crohn's disease (14/15 true-positive) [15].

The addition of SPECT to the planar images represents an improvement in localization of the abnormal bowel segments in some patients. In a 2016 review of molecular imaging in the management of patients with inflammatory bowel disease, the role of SPECT imaging in these techniques was discussed. This review concluded that planar and SPECT had comparable diagnostic accuracies, but SPECT provided a more detailed visualization of inflammatory bowel disease lesions in critical sites, such as the terminal ileum, pelvic floor, and rectum, which can be obscured by overlying background activity [16].

The ^{99m}Tc-WBC technique has been reported to be able to predict therapy response within 1 week after beginning treatment in patients with ulcerative colitis. Using a 4-point grading scale based on the counts in each colon segment on the SPECT image and comparing this to the count obtained in the lumbar spine bone marrow and converting this ratio into a severity score (normal = 0; and grades 1–3 indicating mild, moderate, and severe disease, respectively), the investigators found that the responders had a decrease in the scintigraphic activity score of >50%, and 10/14 nonresponders had an activity score increase of >10%, 2 had unchanged scores, and 2 patients had a decrease in their activity scores but had a residual mean segmental WBC SPECT uptake

ratio of >1.5 when the bowel activity was compared to the bone marrow [17].

One of the main disadvantages of the labeled WBC technique is the need to follow all the necessary precautions when handling a patient's blood, labeling the cells, and readministering these labeled cells in a patient, which takes about 2.5–3 h. A technique that does not require the labeling of cells would simplify the evaluation of a patient with inflammatory bowel disease. The ^{99m}Tc-LeukoScan represented a less complex technique. ^{99m}Tc-LeukoScan is an antigranulocyte murine monoclonal antibody fragment which has been used to image inflammation and infection. This agent was used to image 22 patients with inflammatory bowel disease and was compared to [⁹⁹ᵐTc]Tc-HMPAO-labeled leukocytes. The ^{99m}Tc-LeukoScan was seen to be taken up into most cases of IBD; however, normal bowel was also seen at 4 h. The [⁹⁹ᵐTc] Tc-HMPAO-labeled leukocyte technique was reported to be superior to the ^{99m}Tc-LeukoScan method for the identification of IBD [18]. In another report of six patients with clinically active inflammatory bowel disease and increased uptake on [⁹⁹ᵐTc]Tc-HMPAO leukocyte images, the LeukoScan was not found to be helpful and was inferior to [⁹⁹ᵐTc]Tc-HMPAO-labeled leukocytes in identifying active IBD found by colonoscopy [19].

In summary, the [⁹⁹ᵐTc]Tc-HMPAO-labeled leukocyte scan is a very good method of evaluating the bowel in patients with IBD. The molecular technique is accurate for identifying bowel inflammation, is relatively noninvasive, and might be able to identify submucosal disease that is not apparent on endoscopy. Newer techniques are being studied, including 2-[¹⁸F]fluoro-2-deoxy-D-glucose (2-[¹⁸F]FDG) positron emission tomography (PET)/CT and 2-[¹⁸F]FDG PET/ magnetic resonance imaging (MRI) of patients with IBD. These methods have the advantage of not requiring the labeling of the patient's cells, plus the diagnostic CT or MRI to help localize the abnormal 2-[¹⁸F]FDG signal. Studies are underway to determine the accuracy of these newer molecular techniques.

6.8　Musculoskeletal Infections

6.8.1　Peripheral Bone Infections

Peripheral bone infections (PBI) including osteitis and osteomyelitis have an incidence of less than 2% per year [20] but are more prevalent after trauma or surgery and in immunocompromised patients. The disease is associated with high morbidity and requires prolonged therapy, often surgical, but still has a high recurrence rate. The early diagnosis is difficult to establish, with diagnostic criteria, including physical exam and history, laboratory data, imaging studies, and bone biopsy (the gold standard). In general, radiographs are used as the first imaging modality in suspected musculoskeletal infection, with additional imaging including CT, MRI, PET/CT, and nuclear scintigraphy. Per SNMMI procedure guidelines [7], [^{99m}Tc]Tc-HMPAO-labeled WBC scan can be used for detection and follow-up of musculoskeletal infections, such as septic arthritis and osteomyelitis. Similarly, European guidelines state that this modality can be used to detect, to localize, and to determine the extent of the infection in osteomyelitis of the appendicular skeleton as well as joints [2]. Typically, the imaging is performed 1 and 4 h after labeled WBC injection. Extremities can be imaged at 2–6 h. Dual-time point WBC scintigraphy protocol with imaging at 3–4 h and 20–24 h after injection has been reported as highly accurate with a sensitivity of 85.1%, a specificity of 97.1%, a diagnostic accuracy of 94.5%, a positive predictive value of 88.8%, and a negative predictive value of 95.9% [21]. In this study, semiquantitative analysis was also used with the reference being the contralateral soft tissue or contralateral bone marrow. This semiquantitative analysis was used when visual analysis was inconclusive and improved the accuracy of interpretation.

6.8.2　Neuropathic Joint Versus Osteomyelitis

The neuropathic (Charcot) joint is associated with diabetes mellitus and most often affects the foot. The typical locations are tarsal and metatarsal (Lisfranc) joints (~60% of cases), the metatarsophalangeal joints (~30%), and the tibiotalar joint (~10%) [22]. Repetitive stress, injuries, and fractures, with incomplete healing, lead to extensive joints destruction, instability, and gross deformity [23]. Labeled leukocyte imaging is the radionuclide gold standard for diagnosing diabetic pedal osteomyelitis and differentiating this from soft tissue infection (Figs. 6.4, 6.5, and 6.6). The sensitivity and specificity of planar ^{99m}Tc-labeled leukocyte imaging range from 86% to 93% and from 80% to 98%, respectively [24]. SPECT/CT improves the accuracy of WBC-labeled scintigraphy in the evaluation of diabetic foot infection [25, 26]. Vouillarmet et al. reported the sensitivity, specificity, positive predictive value, and negative predictive value of SPECT/CT for foot osteomyelitis using SPECT/CT of 100%, 91.5%, 71.5%, and 100%, respectively. In addition to the detection and evaluation of the disease extent, SPECT/CT can help in guiding therapy [27, 28].

6.8.2.1 Combined WBC-Marrow Imaging

White blood cells do not accumulate in the cortex of normal bones. However, WBCs are present in the hematopoietically active (red) marrow. The distribution of active and inactive (fatty) marrow is variable. In young children, essentially all the marrow is hematopoietically active and becomes gradually replaced by fatty marrow with aging. Systemic diseases alter marrow distribution, causing generalized expansion (e.g., anemias) or fatty replacement (e.g., starvation). Insults and pathologic processes can cause focal changes with decreased (e.g., radiation therapy) or increased marrow activity (e.g., trauma) [29]. In addition, there is a wide range of variation between individuals [30]. Therefore, adding bone marrow imaging with sulfur colloid can greatly help in the assessment of suspected abnormal WBC accumulation. To avoid false-positive results in areas of expanded marrow, comparison with [^{99m}Tc]Tc-sulfur colloid images should be made. Labeled WBC accumulation in the uninfected Charcot joint is related to the pres-

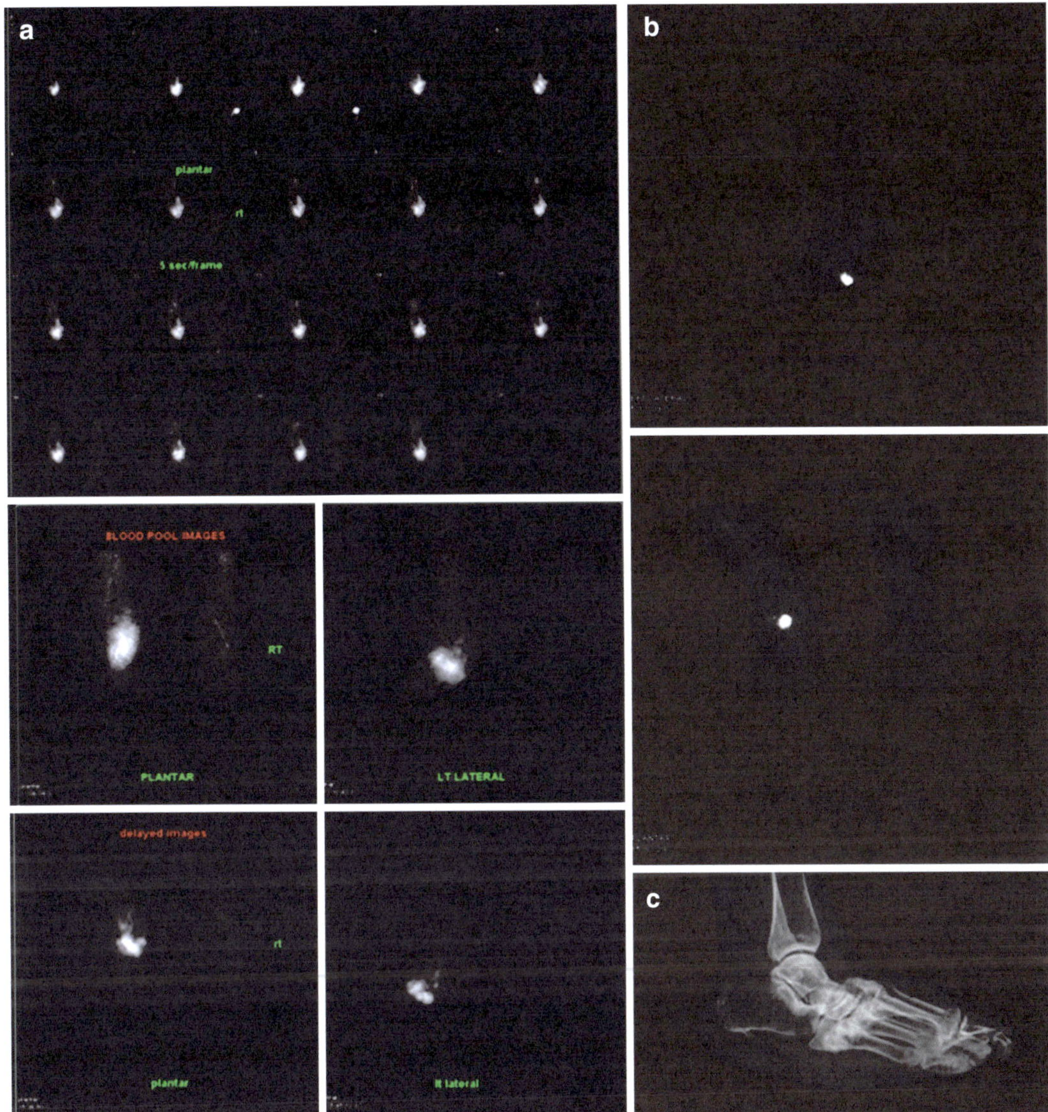

Fig. 6.4 Osteomyelitis. A 65-year-old female with diabetes presented with foot swelling. Three-phase bone scan (**a**) demonstrated intense focal uptake seen on all three phases suspicious for osteomyelitis versus Charcot joint. [⁹⁹ᵐTc]Tc-HMPAO-labeled WBC scan (**b**) shows focal uptake located in the subcutaneous tissue on the plantar surface of the left midfoot that extends to the lateral aspect of cuboid bone when correlated with radiographs (**c**). Findings are consistent with a soft tissue abscess and cuboid bone osteomyelitis

ence of hematopoietically active marrow. Sulfur colloid localizes in areas of noninfected marrow. Osteomyelitis stimulates the uptake of WBC and suppresses the uptake of sulfur colloid. The study is positive for infection when there is increased uptake on the labeled WBC image without corresponding activity on the sulfur colloid scan (images are spatially incongruent) (Fig. 6.7) [8]. Any other pattern is considered negative. Typically, these two scans are performed 2–3 days apart. The accuracy of a combined WBC/sulfur colloid exam is approximately 90% [22]. The WBC can be labeled with indium-111 or technetium-99 m. If ⁹⁹ᵐTc-labeled WBC is used, WBC imaging and marrow imaging should be carried out at least 48 h, and preferably 72 h,

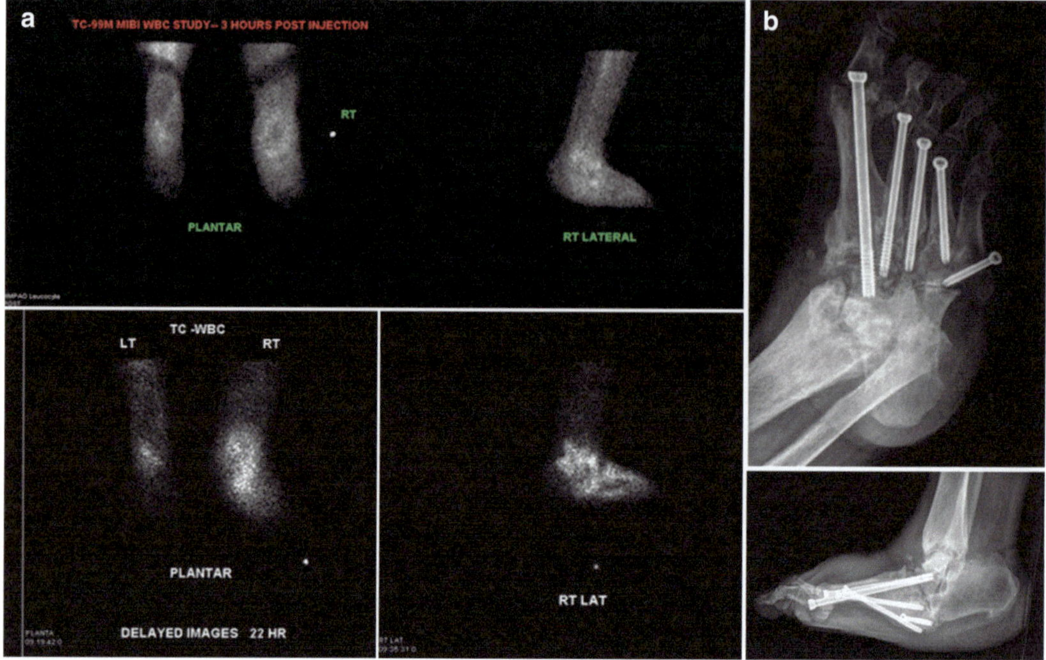

Fig. 6.5 Charcot foot. A 53-year-old female complaining of right foot pain and swelling for 3 days, labs notable for leukocytosis and elevated inflammatory markers. [^{99m}Tc] Tc-HMPAO-labeled WBC scan (**a**) shows asymmetric diffusely increased uptake in the right foot that involves the ankle, tarsal, and metatarsal regions with no evidence of focal area of increased uptake. These results were consistent with the known right Charcot foot as seen on the accompanying radiographs (**b**)

apart [22]. Importantly, improper preparation of sulfur colloid or preparation of more than 2 h old can cause artifacts [31].

6.8.3 Postoperative/Prosthesis Infections

Aseptic prosthesis loosening and infection can present with similar symptoms and may be difficult to differentiate clinically. Elevation of inflammatory markers is nonspecific in the postoperative period and can persist for months. Imaging with CT and MR is often limited due to postsurgical changes and metal-related artifacts. Therefore, scintigraphic imaging plays an important role in the evaluation of these patients. Images' interpretation may be challenging because WBCs are commonly seen around the prosthesis. This can be explained by the presence of active marrow around joint prosthesis due to displacement during surgery. In addition, there may be con-

version of fatty marrow into hematopoietically active marrow secondary to inflammation as a consequence of aseptic loosening. Therefore, combined WBC-marrow imaging should be performed. If there is no uptake on the WBC exam, marrow imaging is not indicated. If there is activity on the WBC image with corresponding marrow activity, the study is negative for infection keeping in mind that sulfur colloid images become photopenic about 1 week after infection [24]; therefore, acute infections may not demonstrate the typical pattern, and image should be interpreted with caution. If there is activity on the WBC image without corresponding activity on the marrow scan (spatial incongruence), the study is considered positive for infection. The abnormality is most often located within or adjacent to the joint space. The intensity of periprosthetic-labeled WBC activity should not be considered [22]. Per joint guidelines by the European Association of Nuclear Medicine, European Bone and Joint Infection Society, European

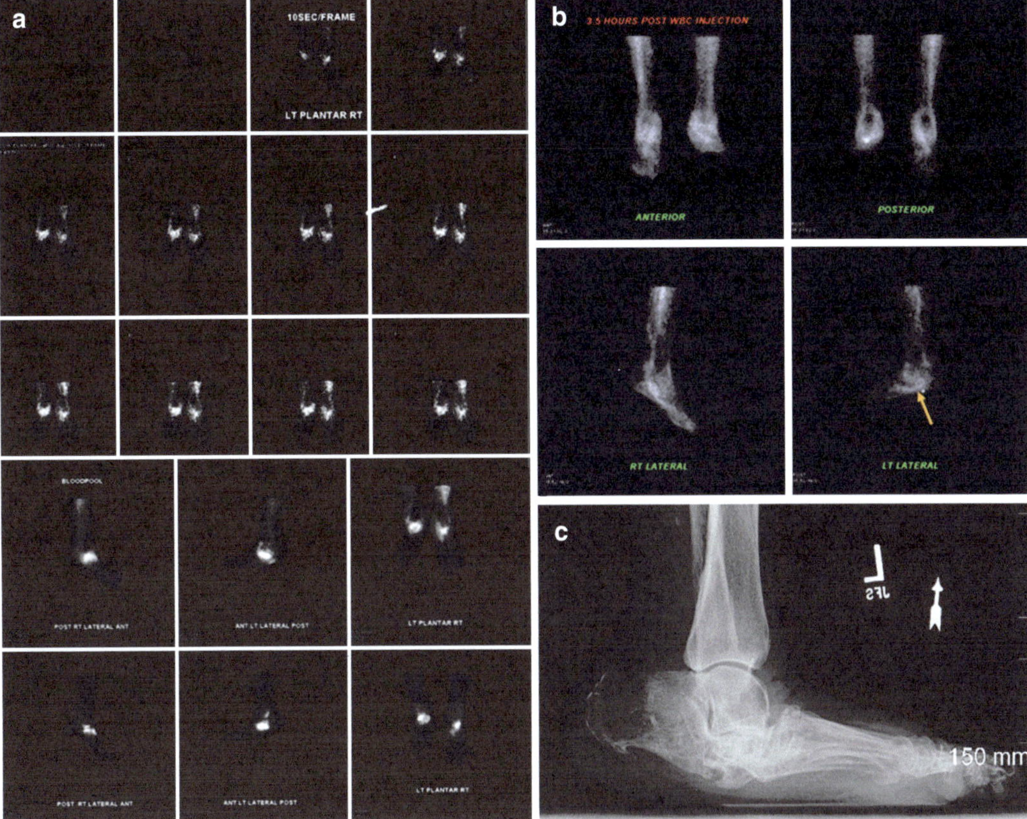

Fig. 6.6 Soft tissue abscess without osteomyelitis. A 65-year-old female with a history of diabetic foot ulcer. Radiographs (**c**) were consistent with neuropathic arthropathy. In addition, cuboid osteomyelitis was questioned. Three-phase bone scan (**a**) shows increased radiotracer uptake in the midfoot on all three phases, which can be seen in the setting of Charcot arthropathy or osteomyelitis. [⁹⁹ᵐTc]Tc-HMPAO-labeled WBC scan (**b**) shows superficial intense focal uptake within the skin and subcutaneous tissue on the plantar surface of the left midfoot consistent with a soft tissue abscess; however, no osseous uptake was seen, excluding osteomyelitis

Society of Radiology, and European Society of Microbiology and Infectious Diseases, choosing between three-phase bone scan and WBC scintigraphy should be based on pretest probability of infection (fractures, recent surgery, osteosynthesis, highly positive serological tests)—level of evidence 5 (expert opinion) [20]. This is justified by high sensitivity but low specificity of the three-phase bone scan, especially after recent surgery/fracture or in the setting of metallic hardware in situ. In these cases, WBC scintigraphy is considered the preferred nuclear medicine imaging technique (level of evidence 2). In addition, the guidelines state that hybrid SPECT-CT WBC imaging can be performed for the exact localization of infection sites (level of evidence 2). WBC scan has higher sensitivity and specificity than anti-granulocyte antibodies (AGA) scan, 2-[¹⁸F] FDG PET, and MRI and is preferred when available and indicated for the patient (Fig. 6.8). WBC scan can not only differentiate aseptic loosening and pseudoarthrosis from infection but also provide information about the extent of the disease process and treatment monitoring.

An additional consideration for early postoperative imaging is soft tissue infection. SPECT/ CT can be helpful to exclude concomitant osteomyelitis. Noninfected surgical wounds typically do not accumulate leukocytes. However, granulating wounds can demonstrate WBC accumulation. Specifically, WBC scan can show focal activity associated with ostomies and skin grafts

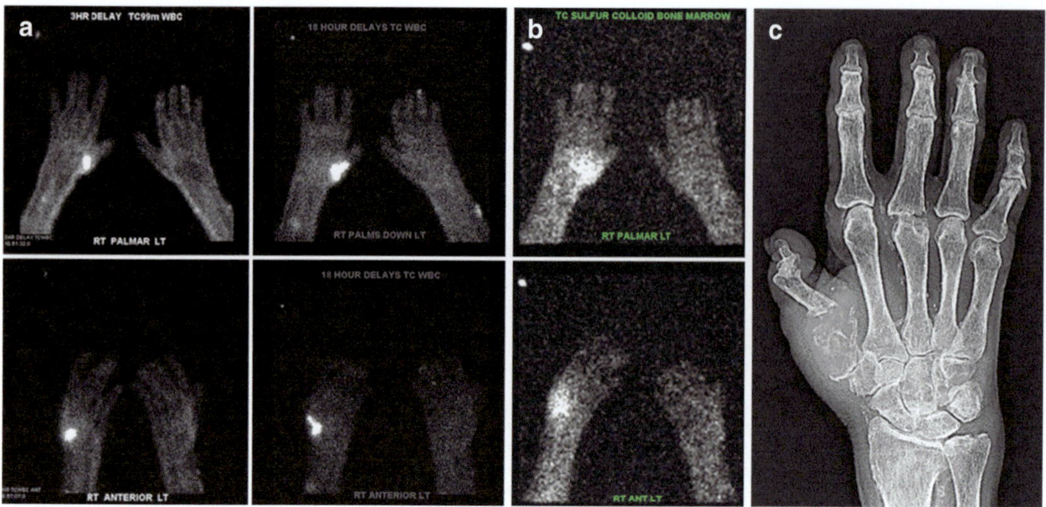

Fig. 6.7 Osteomyelitis. A 55-year-old male with hand pain. [⁹⁹ᵐTc]Tc-HMPAO-labeled WBC scan (**a**) shows focal uptake at the right first metacarpal region, most likely within the bone and adjacent soft tissue, which correlates with the area of osseous destruction identified on the radiograph (**c**). Superficial foci of mild radiotracer uptake at the left fourth distal finger, ulnar aspect of the left forearm, and along the midline of the right forearm correlated with sites of skin wounds noted on physical exam. Sulfur colloid scan (**b**) showed a more diffuse but lesser degree of uptake consistent with reactive bone marrow. The abnormal uptake on WBC scan was much more intense and focal; thus, the diagnosis of osteomyelitis of the right first metacarpal bone was made. This was confirmed on the subsequent biopsy

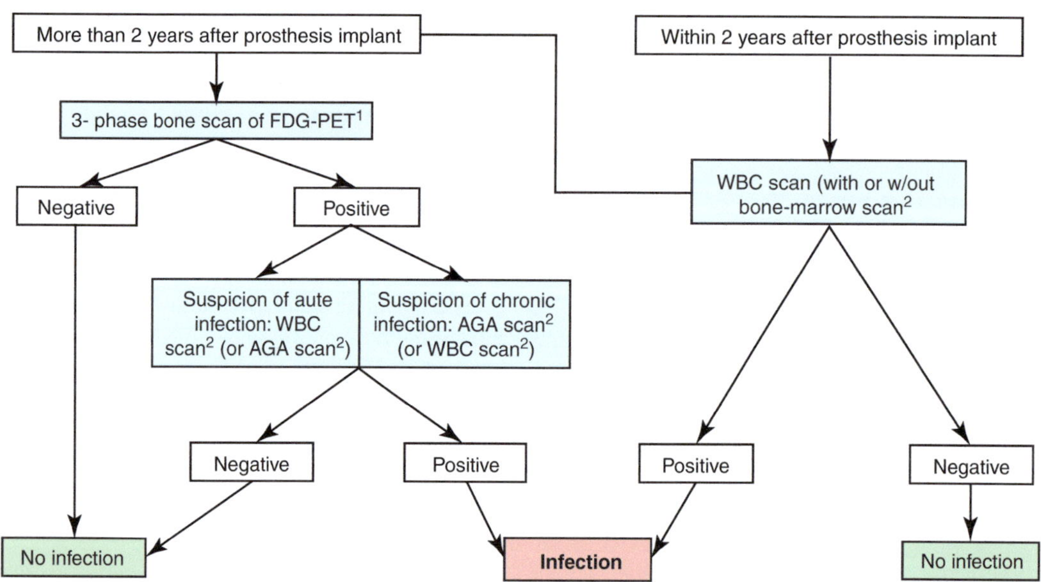

Fig. 6.8 Diagnostic flowchart for prosthetic joint infection when nuclear medicine procedures are considered. Initial stratification is based on time after implant (more or less than 2 years). This is particularly true for hip and shoulder prostheses, but knee prosthesis may require up to 5 years post-implant to reduce physiological inflammation. Some differences may also depend on the type of prosthesis (cemented or not), with cemented prostheses having a shorter post-implant time for physiological inflammatory reaction. (Adapted from Signore et al., Eur J Nucl Med Mol Imaging (2019) [32])

[33]. In addition, central venous lines and other catheters (dialysis, spinal) can show increased WBC accumulation [32].

6.8.4 Spondylodiscitis

Spondylodiscitis typically spreads hematogenously, less often via direct inoculation (e.g., procedures). Spine infection may present on WBC scan as areas of increased or decreased activity compared with normal bone marrow [34]. Approximately 50% of cases present as areas of nonspecifically decreased activity [35]. In the presence of photopenic or "cold" defects, several entities should be in the differential, including osteomyelitis, neoplasm, postradiation changes, congenital deformities, compression fracture, and other postsurgical/post-traumatic changes. Overall, labeled leukocyte imaging is not preferred for diagnosing spine infections. Bone scintigraphy is used for screening, and gallium-67 imaging improves the specificity and may detect infection sooner [36]; however, 2-[^{18}F]FDG PET/CT is the test of choice [24].

6.8.5 Chronic Infection/CMRO

In general, [99mTc]Tc-HMPAO is sensitive for the detection of acute osteomyelitis or exacerbated chronic osteomyelitis [36]. Chronic walled-off abscesses or low-grade infections, particularly in bone, have less [99mTc]Tc-granulocyte accumulation and are more likely not to be visualized [7, 37]. Chronic recurrent multifocal osteomyelitis (CRMO), or chronic nonbacterial osteomyelitis (CNO), is a rare disease in children that manifests as recurrent flares of inflammatory bone pain with or without a fever [38, 39]. SAPHO (synovitis, acne, pustulosis, hyperostosis, osteitis) syndrome is the adult equivalent of CRMO. CRMO is typically evaluated using [99mTc]Tc-methylene diphosphonate (MDP), which shows increased osteoblastic activity and can identify sites of asymptomatic disease [40]. [99mTc]Tc-HMPAO-labeled WBC scan can aid in the diagnosis of

chronic recurrent multifocal osteomyelitis [41]. The final diagnosis of CRMO requires correlation of clinical findings, laboratory data, imaging, and pathology results.

6.8.5.1 SPECT and SPECT/CT

The addition of SPECT to planar [99mTc] Tc-HMPAO-WBC images results in better contrast, helps to localize the abnormal uptake and differentiate soft tissue infection from osteomyelitis, and improves the assessment of the disease extent [42, 43]. However, despite this improvement, SPECT does not provide the exact location of WBC accumulation. SPECT/CT improves accuracy in the detection of osteomyelitis and can be performed for the exact localization of the infection site [32]. In addition, SPECT/CT improves reader confidence compared to planar imaging with SPECT [44]. The study by Erdman et al. concluded that 99mTc-WBC SPECT/CT imaging has value in prognostication in diabetic foot infection [26]. In a study by Filippi et al., SPECT/CT demonstrated significant change or contribution to the final diagnosis in 10 of 28 patients (35.7%) [43]. Overall, SPECT-CT can improve both sensitivity and specificity compared to planar scintigraphy or SPECT alone. Diagnostic accuracy of SPECT/CT imaging in diabetic foot osteomyelitis may be similar to MRI. The study by La Fontaine et al. reported sensitivity, specificity, positive predictive value, and negative predictive value for SPECT/CT of 89%, 35%, 74%, and 60%, respectively, whereas for MRI, the sensitivity, specificity, positive predictive value, and negative predictive value were 87%, 37%, 74%, and 58%, respectively [45]. However, further research is required for comparison between SPET/CT and MR for specific indications in musculoskeletal imaging [46].

SPECT and SPECT/CT can be helpful not only in the evaluation of musculoskeletal pathology because in many instances, the exact location of the lesion is desired. This is a piece of crucial information in many clinical scenarios including the evaluation of unknown sources of infection and can lead to a change in the patient's management (Fig. 6.9).

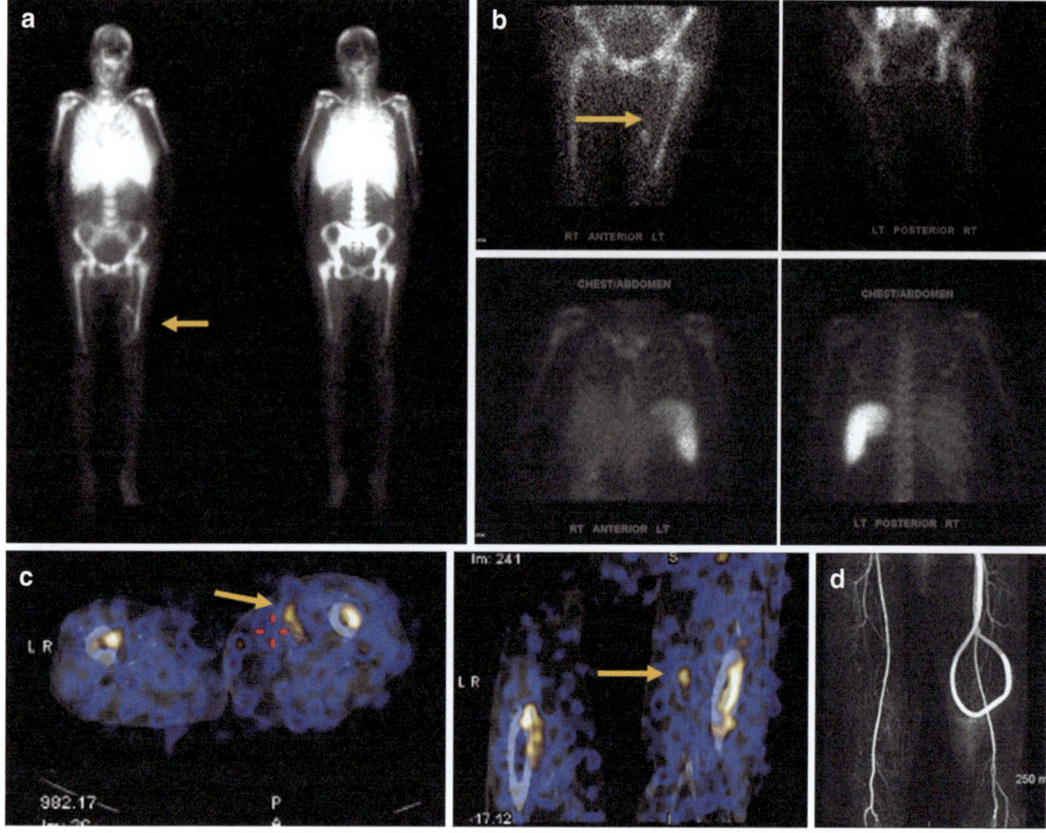

Fig. 6.9 A 50-year-old female with end-stage renal disease on hemodialysis via left thigh fistula and methicillin-resistant *Staphylococcus aureus* (MRSA)-positive blood culture. Whole-body 4-h (**a**) and delayed 17-h (**b**) planar [99mTc]Tc-HMPAO-labeled WBC images show a deep focus of increased uptake within the left medial mid-thigh, in the subcutaneous tissue, medial to the left femur (arrow). SPECT/CT images (**c**) and correlation with magnetic resonance angiography (MRA) (**d**) localize this focus near the top of the vascular fistula loop consistent with vascular graft infection

6.9 Fever of Unknown Origin (FUO)

Fever of unknown origin (FUO) is defined as the following: (1) temperature greater than 38.3 °C (101 °F) on several occasions, (2) more than 3 weeks' duration of illness, and (3) failure to reach a diagnosis despite initial investigation in an immunocompetent patient [47, 48]. Despite multiple available diagnostic tests, FUO still remains challenging. Both [99mTc]Tc-HMPAO-WBC scan and 2-[18F]FDG PET can be used in FUO. A high pretest probability for infection favors the WBC scan over PET/CT as a first study (Fig. 6.10) [49].

6.10 Cardiovascular Infections

6.10.1 Infectious Endocarditis (IE)

Infectious endocarditis (IE) is a life-threatening disease, establishing a diagnosis of which is often challenging. The diagnosis is established with modified Duke criteria which include pathological, clinical, and echocardiographic findings [50]. [99mTc]Tc-HMPAO-WBC scan can help in the diagnosis of infectious endocarditis. The study is considered positive if there is an accumulation of WBC in the cardiac region on early images, progressive on delayed images. Stable or decreasing accumulation is equivocal [49].

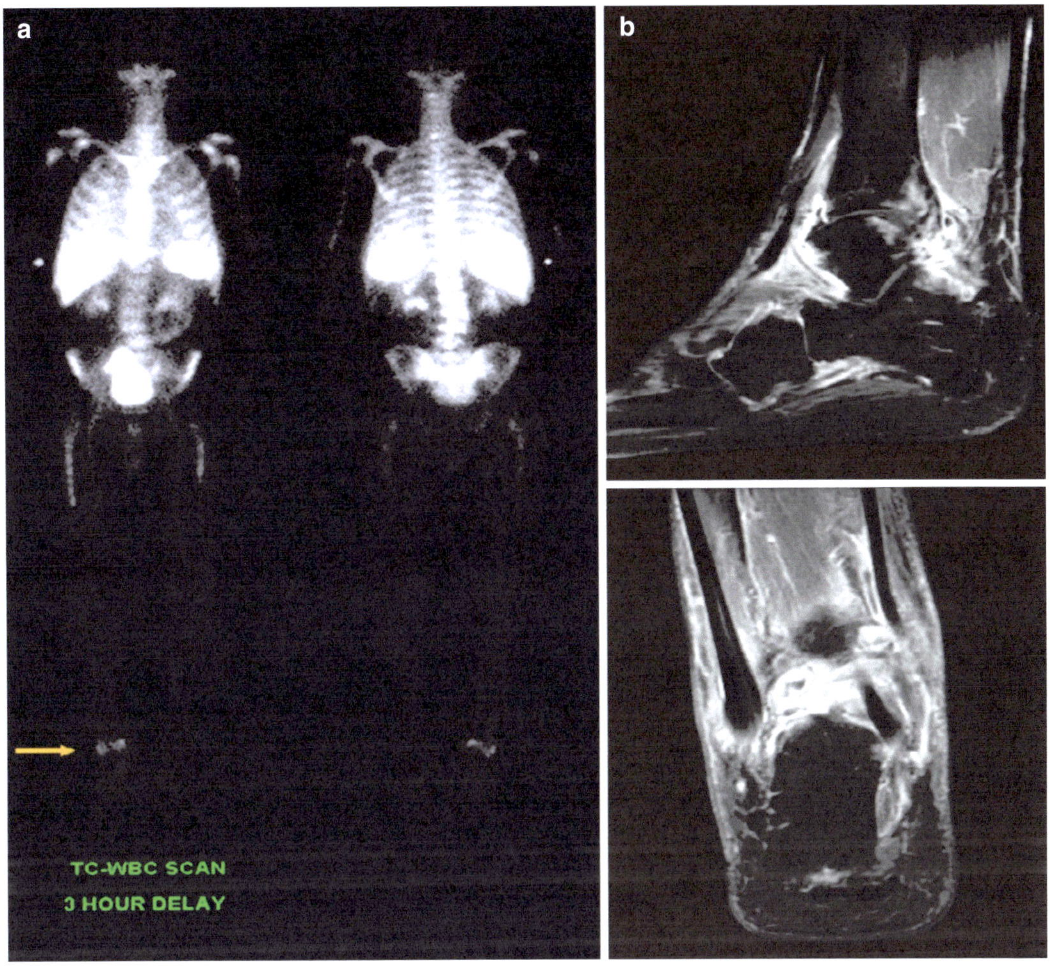

Fig. 6.10 A 62-year-old male admitted to the hospital with a group G Streptococcus bacteremia of unknown source, migratory arthralgias, and myalgias. [^{99m}Tc] Tc-HMPAO-labeled WBC scan was done to evaluate for a source of infection. Whole-body images (**a**) show focally increased radiotracer uptake in the region of the right ankle suspicious for infectious arthritis. Ankle MRI (**b**) shows severe synovitis/tenosynovitis. The final diagnosis was septic arthritis

Importantly, isotope decay has to be taken into account in order to have the same statistics in both images. Total body scans are performed to detect possible septic embolisms [51]. SPECT/CT should be obtained and both CT-attenuated and non-attenuation corrected (NAC) images should be reviewed to avoid false-positive results due to metallic artifacts in prosthetic valves [49]. The study by Erba et al. showed a sensitivity of 90%, specificity of 100%, and a negative predictive value of 94% [52]. This study showed that [^{99m}Tc]Tc-HMPAO-WBC scan was most valuable in patients with "possible IE" by Duke criteria, when there is a high level of clinical suspicion but negative or indeterminate echocardiographic findings. Almost half of the patients with a positive study had extracardiac uptake indicative of septic emboli. Another study by Holcman et al. reported 90% accuracy, 93% sensitivity, 88% specificity, 96% negative predictive value (NPV), and 81% positive predictive value (PPV) for [^{99m}Tc]Tc-HMPAO WBC compared to 60% accuracy, 93% sensitivity, 42% specificity, 92% NPV, and 46% PPV for transthoracic echocardiography (TTE) [31]. The addition of the WBC scan reduced the number of misdiagnosed IE classified in the "possible IE" category by modified Duke criteria by 27%. The study was most helpful in the differentiation of infectious and sterile echocardiographic lesions. In a study by Hyafil et al., the addition of the WBC scan resulted in a change in management in 12 out of 42 patients with prosthetic valve endocarditis (29%) [53]. Radiolabeled WBC SPECT/CT is more specific for the detection of prosthetic valve IE and infectious foci than 2-[^{18}F]FDG PET/CT. In the study by Rouzet et al., the reported sensitivity, specificity, PPV, NPV, and accuracy for 2-[^{18}F]FDG PET in prosthetic valve endocarditis were 93%, 71%, 68%, 94%, and 80%, respectively, and for WBC-labeled scintigraphy were 64%, 100%, 100%, 81%, and 86%, respectively [54]. Therefore, scintigraphy is preferred when higher specificity is required. Disadvantages of scintigraphy with radiolabeled WBC include the longer duration of the procedure in comparison with PET/CT, lower spatial resolution, and the requirement of blood handling for radiopharmaceutical preparation. European Society of Cardiology 2015 modified criteria included molecular imaging in the guidelines in the setting of the suspicion of endocarditis on a prosthetic valve [55]. Abnormal activity around the prosthetic valve detected by radiolabeled leukocyte SPECT/CT or 2-[^{18}F]FDG PET/CT (only if the prosthesis was implanted for more than 3 months) is considered a major criterion. Identification of recent embolic events or infectious aneurysms by imaging only is considered a minor criterion [56].

6.10.2 Mycotic Aneurysm

Mycotic aneurysm is an aortic aneurysm due to infection. This is a life-threatening complication of endocarditis or other bacteremia/sepsis. The diagnosis is challenging with variable clinical presentations, nonspecific laboratory abnormalities, and blood or tissue culture being positive in only approximately 50–75% of the cases [57]. Mycotic aneurysm can be difficult to differentiate on CT or MR from noninfectious aneurysm, and WBC scan can be useful in establishing the diagnosis as well as detecting additional sites of the disease; however, typically, indium-111 is used (Fig. 6.11).

6.10.3 Vascular Graft Infection

[^{99m}Tc]Tc-HMPAO-WBC imaging can be used for detecting, localizing, and defining the extent of graft infection (Fig. 6.12). The study by Fiorani et al. reported sensitivity of 100%, specificity of 94.4%, PPV of 90%, and NPV of 100% for aortic graft infection [58]. However, evaluation in the early postoperative period is limited since noninfected vascular grafts and shunts can show increased uptake due to bleeding or inflammation secondary to the procedure [59]. The study by Erba et al. concluded that WBC scintigraphy with SPECT/CT can be used in patients with late infections and inconclusive findings on ultrasound and CT [60]. False-positive results can be seen especially in the early postoperative period and may be related to hemorrhage, hematomas, graft thrombosis, pseudoaneurysms, and graft endothelialization (typically the first 1–2 weeks post-procedure) [33].

6.10.4 Cardiovascular Implantable Electronic Device (CIED) Infection

Cardiovascular implantable electronic device (CIED) infections are associated with significant morbidity and mortality. Often, they pose a diagnostic challenge due to variable clinical presentation, and cardiac imaging is commonly utilized. [^{99m}Tc]Tc-HMPAO-WBC scintigraphy can help detect infection associated with CIEDs, especially if SPECT/CT technique is utilized [61]. In a study by Erba et al., the specificity of SPECT/CT for detection and localization of CIED infection was 94%. Of note, no false-positive results were found. In a septic patient during a febrile episode, the scan excluded device-associated

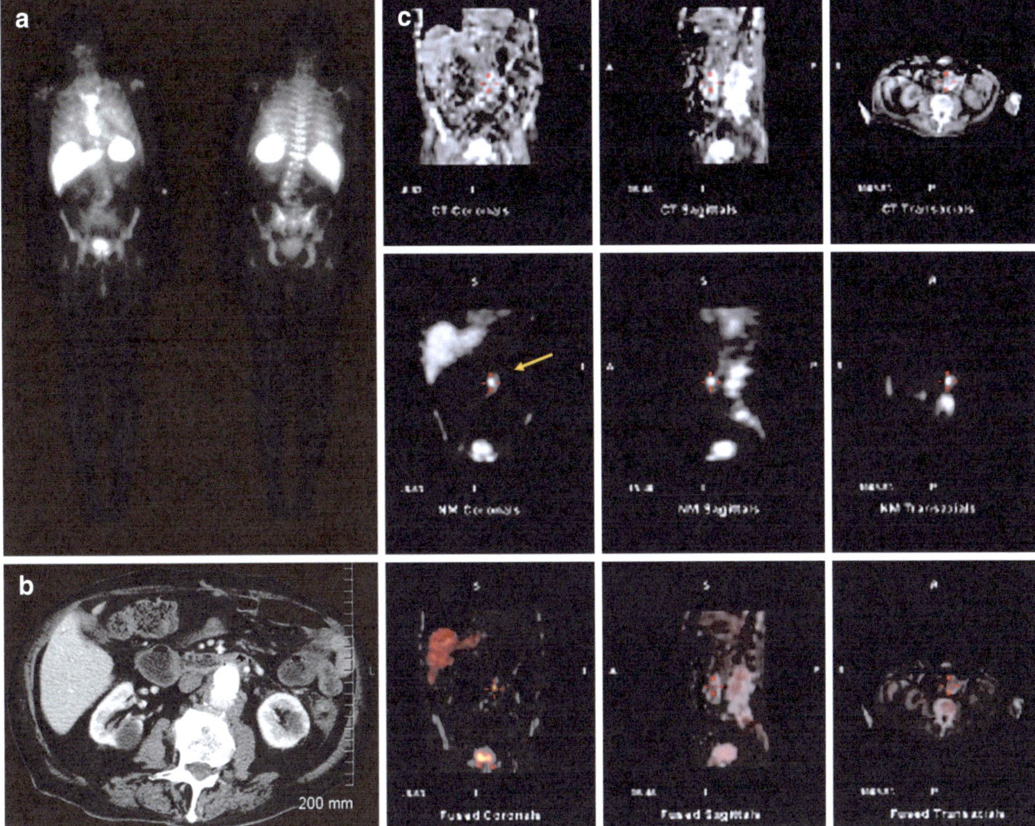

Fig. 6.11 An 85-year-old male with a history of prior aortic aneurysm repair; current concern for infection, suspected colitis. [^{99m}Tc]Tc-HMPAO-labeled WBC planar images show no obvious abnormality (**a**); however, there is a focus of abnormal tracer accumulation on SPECT images (**c**). Fused SPECT/CT images allow localizing this to the aortic graft, consistent with infection. Diagnostic CT image (**b**) shows an abnormality in the infrarenal aorta

infection with a 95% negative predictive value [62]. Based on available data, both WBC SPECT/CT and 2-[^{18}F]FDG PET/CT studies might play an additional role in the diagnosis of CIED infection; however, they are not incorporated in the 2015 European Society of Cardiology guidelines [56]. A study by Hitzel et al. evaluated ^{99m}Tc-leukocyte SPECT/CT in patients with suspected left ventricular assist device (LVAD) infections and concluded that this modality is accurate and allows to evaluate the extent of the disease [63]. Litzler et al. evaluated 13 patients with suspected LVAD infection and concluded that SPECT/CT led to an increase in diagnostic accuracy for the diagnosis of LVAD-related infection [64].

6.11 Pulmonary Infections

6.11.1 Interpretation

Diffuse lung activity on early (1-h) images is considered normal if this clears on delayed (4-h) images. Persistent diffuse uptake is nonspecific and may indicate infection or inflammation with a broad differential. Atypical lung infections and opportunistic infections, like *Pneumocystis jiroveci* as well as sepsis, can present with diffuse uptake. Diffuse lung injury of various etiologies can have this appearance, including drug- and radiation-related lung injury, acute respiratory distress syndrome (ARDS), eosino-

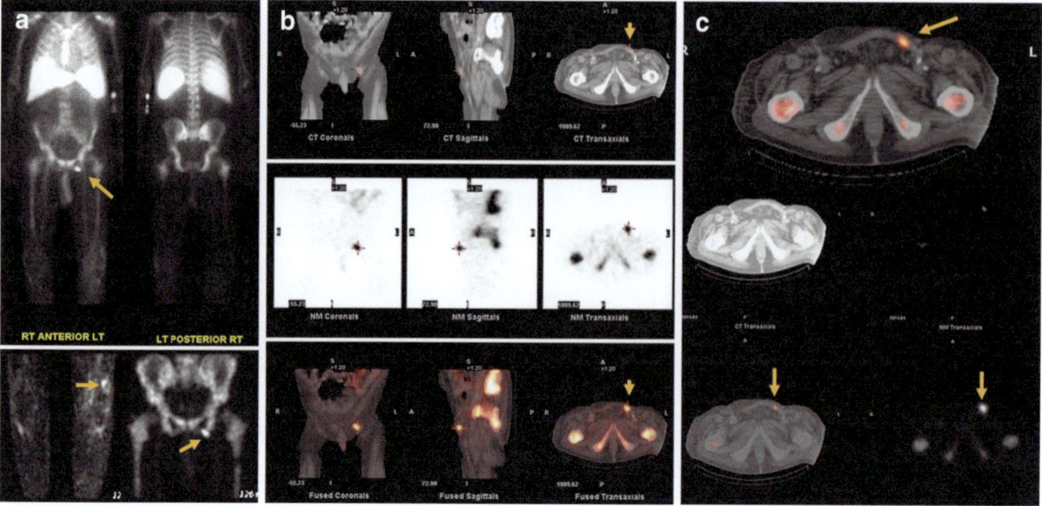

Fig. 6.12 A 78-year-old male with prior femoral-femoral and bilateral femoral-popliteal bypasses, currently with fever and septic left knee joint. [^{99m}Tc]Tc-HMPAO-labeled WBC planar images (**a**) show intense focal WBC accumulation in the left anterior pelvis. SPECT/CT images (**b** and **c**) localize this focus to the left segment of the femoral-femoral bypass, consistent with infected graft. In addition, there is increased radiotracer uptake in the left knee reflecting postoperative inflammation

philic syndromes, graft versus host disease, etc. Focal uptake on delayed images can be lobar/segmental or in nonanatomic distribution. Segmental and lobar uptake suggest pneumonia [65]. If nonanatomic distribution of uptake is seen, the images and tracer delivery/preparation should be closely scrutinized for possible technical errors.

6.12 Imaging pitfalls

6.12.1 Pitfalls in Lung Imaging

1. Even 4–6 h after injection, diffuse lung activity may be seen, particularly in patients with heart or renal failure. This may obscure focal lung infections [7].
2. Swallowed WBCs from an upper respiratory infection can cause a false-positive exam for GI disease.

6.12.2 Pitfalls Elsewhere in the Body

- Active bleeding and hematomas can present as focal WBC accumulation.
- Inflammation around neoplasms such as lymphomas may mimic an abscess.
- Focal collections of inflamed peritoneal fluid or sites of focal bowel inflammation can be mistaken for an abscess.
- Lymph node uptake can cause false-positive results [66].
- Postsurgical/postprocedural (ostomies, skin grafts, and central venous catheters) changes can lead to false-positive results [32] (Figs. 6.13 and 6.14).
- Antibiotic therapy can cause false-negative results.

6.13 Other Considerations

6.13.1 Tumors

Rarely, some tumors (e.g., melanoma, lymphoma) will also accumulate labeled leukocytes [66].

6.13.2 Eosinophilic Syndromes

[^{99m}Tc]Tc-HMPAO predominantly labels neutrophils; however, it also has an affinity to

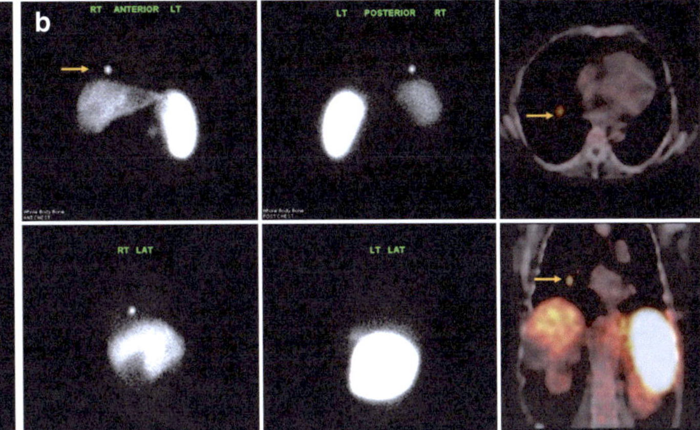

Fig. 6.13 A 50-year-old male with status post liver transplant with bilomas with persistent fever and bacteremia. [⁹⁹ᵐTc]Tc-HMPAO-labeled WBC scan was performed including whole-body planar images (**a**) and spot images of the lower chest and abdomen (**b**) 1 h after injection, and additional axial SPECT/CT images of the lower chest and abdomen were obtained approximately 4 h after injection. There is a small focus of radiotracer uptake in the posterior right middle lobe or right lower lung on early images. This persists on delayed SPECT images; however, there is no correlate on low-dose CT scan. This likely represents a small focus of labeled thrombus formation (a technical artifact). There is a somewhat heterogeneous appearance of the uptake in the liver with areas of decreased radiotracer uptake within regions of prior abscess with drainage

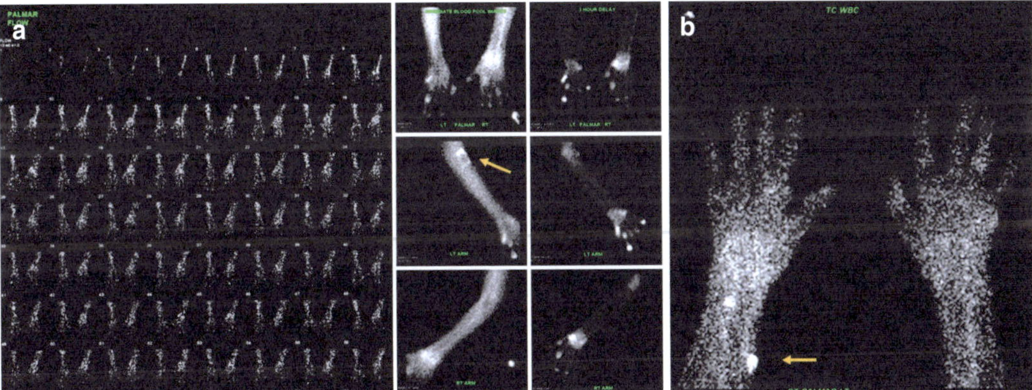

Fig. 6.14 An 87-year-old female with right wrist pain. Three-phase bone scan (**a**) shows mildly increased arterial flow to the region of the right wrist, with corresponding moderately increased radiotracer activity in the same region on blood pool and delayed images. This is nonspecific and a WBC scan was recommended for further evaluation. There is also moderate to intense radiotracer uptake of the joints of bilateral hands including the left fourth metacarpal-phalangeal and proximal metacarpal bone/joint and right fifth proximal metacarpal bone/joint region likely due to degenerative changes. [⁹⁹ᵐTc]Tc-HMPAO-labeled WBC scan (**b**) shows two punctate areas of radiotracer activity overlying the distal right forearm, related to the injection site and radiotracer within the intravenous catheter tubing (arrow). No scintigraphic evidence of the infectious etiology of arthritis

eosinophils, which may cause false positivity in disorders with eosinophilic infiltration [67].

6.13.3 Graft Versus Host Disease (GVHD)

Leukocyte scintigraphy can be used to evaluate gastrointestinal graft versus host disease (GVHD) [68]. This can manifest as uptake in the bowel or lungs. There are also reports indicating the utility of this method in cutaneous GVHD [69].

6.13.4 Treatment Monitoring

^{99m}Tc-labeled neutrophils can be used to quantify lung neutrophil inflammation in chronic obstructive pulmonary disease (COPD) in order to evaluate the efficacy of therapy [67].

6.14 Pediatric Population

In general, ^{99m}Tc-labeling is preferred over indium-111 in the pediatric population due to lower radiation dose and superior resolution [68]. In children, three-phase bone scintigraphy with [^{99m}Tc]Tc-MDP has lower specificity in the evaluation of osteomyelitis compared to adults. [^{99m}Tc]Tc-HMPAO can be especially helpful for children younger than 6 months as at this age, the sensitivity of [^{99m}Tc]Tc-MDP is low [69]. WBC imaging can be a valuable tool in postoperative settings [70]. For fever of unknown origin, negative study during a febrile episode can exclude infection. Koranda et al. reported two cases of successfully detected infection (necrotizing enterocolitis and osteomyelitis) in premature low birth weight infants using small blood sample volumes [71]. In addition to typical indications such as musculoskeletal infections and fever of unknown origin, [^{99m}Tc]Tc-HMPAO-WBC scintigraphy has high accuracy in the evaluation of suspected appendicitis [68, 72] and for the evaluation of IBD in children [73, 74]. In a study by Caobelli et al., reported sensitivity was 93.7%, specificity 86.1%, and negative predictive value

96.4%. In addition, scintigraphy was able to correctly recognize relapses and remissions, as well as to assess the extent and grade of the activity of the disease [75].

6.15 Future Directions

As mentioned before, the WBC labeling technique is time-consuming and requires handling of patient's blood. Anti-granulocyte monoclonal antibodies have been developed, including whole murine IgG anti-NCA-95 antibody ([^{99m}Tc]Tc-Besilesomab, Scintimun®) and a Fab fragment anti-NCA-90 (sulesomab, [^{99m}Tc]Tc-LeukoScan®). Besilesomab may induce the production of human anti-mouse antibodies (HAMA) that must be checked before performing the study and limits its use to one single administration in life. Sulesomab does not induce HAMA production and is licensed in Europe for peripheral musculoskeletal infections [49]. ^{99m}Tc-labeled antibiotics can be used for specific indications. For example, [^{99m}Tc]Tc-ciprofloxacin (Infecton®) can be used in suspected infections caused by gram-positive, gram-negative, and anaerobic bacteria [76]. Other antibiotics, such as cephalosporins and fluoroquinolones, antifungals, and other antimicrobial peptides, for example [^{99m}Tc]Tc-ubiquicidin (UBI), have also been investigated [77].

References

1. Farid NA, White SM, Heck LL, Van Hove ED. Tc-99m labeled leukocytes: preparation and use in identification of abscess and tissue rejection. Radiology. 1983;148(3):827–31. https://doi.org/10.1148/radiology.148.3.6308712.
2. de Vries EF, Roca M, Jamar F, Israel O, Signore A. Guidelines for the labelling of leucocytes with (99m)Tc-HMPAO. Inflammation/Infection Taskgroup of the European Association of Nuclear Medicine. Eur J Nucl Med Mol Imaging. 2010;37(4):842–8. https://doi.org/10.1007/s00259-010-1394-4.
3. Peters AM, Danpure HJ, Osman S, Hawker RJ, Henderson BL, Hodgson HJ, et al. Clinical experience with 99mTc-hexamethylpropylene-amineoxime for labelling leucocytes and imaging inflammation. Lancet. 1986;2(8513):946–9.

4. Connolly CM, Donohoe KJ. Nuclear medicine imaging of infection. Semin Roentgenol. 2017;52(2):114–9. https://doi.org/10.1053/j.ro.2016.07.001.

5. Love C, Palestro CJ. Altered biodistribution and incidental findings on gallium and labeled leukocyte/bone marrow scans. Semin Nucl Med. 2010;40(4):271–82. https://doi.org/10.1053/j.semnuclmed.2010.03.004.

6. Lantto EH, Lantto TJ, Vorne M. Fast diagnosis of abdominal infections and inflammations with technetium-99m-HMPAO labeled leukocytes. J Nucl Med. 1991;32(11):2029–34.

7. Palestro C, Brown M, Forstrom LA, Green BS, Truman HS, McAfee JG et al. Society of Nuclear Medicine Procedure Guideline for 99mTc-Exametazime (HMPAO)-labeled leukocyte scintigraphy for suspected infection/inflammation; 2019.

8. Palestro CJ. Radionuclide imaging of musculoskeletal infection: a review. J Nucl Med. 2016;57(9):1406–12. https://doi.org/10.2967/jnumed.115.157297.

9. Hughes DK. Nuclear medicine and infection detection: the relative effectiveness of imaging with 111In-oxine-, 99mTc-HMPAO-, and 99mTc-stannous fluoride colloid-labeled leukocytes and with 67Ga-citrate. J Nucl Med Technol. 2003;31(4):196–201; quiz 3–4.

10. Almer S, Granerus G, Strom M, Olaison G, Bonnet J, Lemann M, et al. Leukocyte scintigraphy compared to intraoperative small bowel enteroscopy and laparotomy findings in Crohn's disease. Inflamm Bowel Dis. 2007;13(2):164–74. https://doi.org/10.1002/ibd.20001.

11. Mota LG, Coelho LG, Simal CJ, Ferrari ML, Toledo C, Martin-Comin J, et al. Leukocyte-technetium-99m uptake in Crohn's disease: does it show subclinical disease? World J Gastroenterol. 2010;16(3):365–71. https://doi.org/10.3748/wjg.v16.i3.365.

12. Charron M, Del Rosario F, Kocoshis S. Assessment of terminal ileal and colonic inflammation in Crohn's disease with 99mTc-WBC. Acta Paediatr. 1999;88(2):193–8.

13. Stathaki MI, Koukouraki SI, Karkavitsas NS, Koutroubakis IE. Role of scintigraphy in inflammatory bowel disease. World J Gastroenterol. 2009;15(22):2693–700. https://doi.org/10.3748/wjg.15.2693.

14. Bennink R, Peeters M, D'Haens G, Rutgeerts P, Mortelmans L. Tc-99m HMPAO white blood cell scintigraphy in the assessment of the extent and severity of an acute exacerbation of ulcerative colitis. Clin Nucl Med. 2001;26(2):99–104.

15. Alberini JL, Badran A, Freneaux E, Hadji S, Kalifa G, Devaux JY, et al. Technetium-99m HMPAO-labeled leukocyte imaging compared with endoscopy, ultrasonography, and contrast radiology in children with inflammatory bowel disease. J Pediatr Gastroenterol Nutr. 2001;32(3):278–86.

16. Caobelli F, Evangelista L, Quartuccio N, Familiari D, Altini C, Castello A, et al. Role of molecular imaging in the management of patients affected by inflammatory bowel disease: state-of-the-art. World J Radiol. 2016;8(10):829–45. https://doi.org/10.4329/wjr.v8.i10.829.

17. Bennink RJ, Peeters M, Rutgeerts P, Mortelmans L. Evaluation of early treatment response and predicting the need for colectomy in active ulcerative colitis with 99mTc-HMPAO white blood cell scintigraphy. J Nucl Med. 2004;45(10):1698–704.

18. Kerry JE, Marshall C, Griffiths PA, James MW, Scott BB. Comparison between Tc-HMPAO labelled white cells and Tc LeukoScan in the investigation of inflammatory bowel disease. Nucl Med Commun. 2005;26(3):245–51.

19. Stokkel MP, Reigman HE, Pauwels EK. Scintigraphic head-to-head comparison between 99mTc-WBCs and 99mTc-LeukoScan in the evaluation of inflammatory bowel disease: a pilot study. Eur J Nucl Med Mol Imaging. 2002;29(2):251–4.

20. Jutte P, Lazzeri E, Sconfienza LM, Cassar-Pullicino V, Trampuz A, Petrosillo N, et al. Diagnostic flowcharts in osteomyelitis, spondylodiscitis and prosthetic joint infection. Q J Nucl Med Mol Imaging. 2014;58(1):2–19.

21. Glaudemans AW, de Vries EF, Vermeulen LE, Slart RH, Dierckx RA, Signore A. A large retrospective single-centre study to define the best image acquisition protocols and interpretation criteria for white blood cell scintigraphy with (9)(9)mTc-HMPAO-labelled leucocytes in musculoskeletal infections. Eur J Nucl Med Mol Imaging. 2013;40(11):1760–9. https://doi.org/10.1007/s00259-013-2481-0.

22. Palestro CJ, Love C, Tronco GG, Tomas MB, Rini JN. Combined labeled leukocyte and technetium 99m sulfur colloid bone marrow imaging for diagnosing musculoskeletal infection. Radiographics. 2006;26(3):859–70. https://doi.org/10.1148/rg.263055139.

23. Love C, Palestro CJ. Radionuclide imaging of infection. J Nucl Med Technol. 2004;32(2):47–57; quiz 8–9.

24. Palestro CJ. Radionuclide imaging of osteomyelitis. Semin Nucl Med. 2015;45(1):32–46. https://doi.org/10.1053/j.semnuclmed.2014.07.005.

25. Filippi L, Uccioli L, Giurato L, Schillaci O. Diabetic foot infection: usefulness of SPECT/CT for 99mTc-HMPAO-labeled leukocyte imaging. J Nucl Med. 2009;50(7):1042–6. https://doi.org/10.2967/jnumed.108.059493.

26. Erdman WA, Buethe J, Bhore R, Ghayee HK, Thompson C, Maewal P, et al. Indexing severity of diabetic foot infection with 99mTc-WBC SPECT/CT hybrid imaging. Diabetes Care. 2012;35(9):1826–31. https://doi.org/10.2337/dc11-2425.

27. Vouillarmet J, Morelec I, Thivolet C. Assessing diabetic foot osteomyelitis remission with white blood cell SPECT/CT imaging. Diabet Med. 2014;31(9):1093–9. https://doi.org/10.1111/dme.12445.

28. Lazaga F, Van Asten SA, Nichols A, Bhavan K, La Fontaine J, Oz OK, et al. Hybrid imaging with 99mTc-WBC SPECT/CT to monitor the effect of therapy in diabetic foot osteomyelitis. Int Wound J. 2016;13(6):1158–60. https://doi.org/10.1111/iwj.12433.

29. Seabold JE, Ferlic RJ, Marsh JL, Nepola JV. Periarticular bone sites associated with traumatic injury: false-positive findings with In-111-labeled white blood cell and Tc-99m MDP scintigraphy. Radiology. 1993;186(3):845–9. https://doi.org/10.1148/radiology.186.3.8430197.

30. Compston JE. Bone marrow and bone: a functional unit. J Endocrinol. 2002;173(3):387–94.

31. Holcman K, Szot W, Rubis P, Lesniak-Sobelga A, Hlawaty M, Wisniowska-Smialek S, et al. 99mTc-HMPAO-labeled leukocyte SPECT/CT and transthoracic echocardiography diagnostic value in infective endocarditis. Int J Cardiovasc Imaging. 2019;35(4):749–58. https://doi.org/10.1007/s10554-018-1487-x.

32. Signore A, Sconfienza LM, Borens O, Glaudemans AW, Cassar-Pullicino V, Trampuz A, et al. Consensus document for the diagnosis of prosthetic joint infections: a joint paper by the EANM, EBJIS, and ESR (with ESCMID endorsement). Eur J Nucl Med Mol Imaging. 2019;46(4):971–88.

33. Palestro CJ, Love C, Tronco GG, Tomas MB. Role of radionuclide imaging in the diagnosis of postoperative infection. Radiographics. 2000;20(6):1649–60. https://doi.org/10.1148/radiographics.20.6.g00nv101649.

34. Palestro CJ, Torres MA. Radionuclide imaging in orthopedic infections. Semin Nucl Med. 1997;27(4):334–45.

35. Palestro CJ, Love C, Bhargava KK. Labeled leukocyte imaging: current status and future directions. Q J Nucl Med Mol Imaging. 2009;53(1):105–23.

36. Wolf G, Aigner RM, Schwarz T. Diagnosis of bone infection using 99m Tc-HMPAO labelled leukocytes. Nucl Med Commun. 2001;22(11):1201–6.

37. Chong A, Ha JM, Hong R, Kwon SY. Variations in findings on (18)F-FDG PET/CT, Tc-99m HDP bone scan and WBC scan in chronic multifocal osteomyelitis. Int J Rheum Dis. 2014;17(3):344–5. https://doi.org/10.1111/1756-185x.12205.

38. Wipff J, Adamsbaum C, Kahan A, Job-Deslandre C. Chronic recurrent multifocal osteomyelitis. Joint, Bone, Spine: Revue du Rhumatisme. 2011;78(6):555–60. https://doi.org/10.1016/j.jbspin.2011.02.010.

39. Ata Y, Inaba Y, Choe H, Kobayashi N, Machida J, Nakamura N, et al. Bone metabolism and inflammatory characteristics in 14 cases of chronic nonbacterial osteomyelitis. Pediatr Rheumatol Online J. 2017;15(1):56. https://doi.org/10.1186/s12969-017-0183-z.

40. Khanna G, Sato TS, Ferguson P. Imaging of chronic recurrent multifocal osteomyelitis. Radiographics. 2009;29(4):1159–77. https://doi.org/10.1148/rg.294085244.

41. Dailey TA, Berven MD, Vroman PJ. 99mTc-HMPAO-labeled WBC scan for the diagnosis of chronic recurrent multifocal osteomyelitis. J Nucl Med Technol. 2014;42(4):299–301. https://doi.org/10.2967/jnmt.114.138073.

42. Sanli Y, Ozkan ZG, Unal SN, Turkmen C, Kilicoglu O. The additional value of Tc 99m HMPAO white blood cell SPECT in the evaluation of bone and soft tissue infections. Mol Imaging Radionucl Ther. 2011;20(1):7–13. https://doi.org/10.4274/mirt.20.02.

43. Filippi L, Schillaci O. Usefulness of hybrid SPECT/CT in 99mTc-HMPAO-labeled leukocyte scintigraphy for bone and joint infections. J Nucl Med. 2006;47(12):1908–13.

44. Djekidel M, Brown RK, Piert M. Benefits of hybrid SPECT/CT for (111)In-oxine- and Tc-99m-hexamethylpropylene amine oxime-labeled leukocyte imaging. Clin Nucl Med. 2011;36(7):e50–6. https://doi.org/10.1097/RLU.0b013e31821738a0.

45. La JF, Bhavan K, Lam K, Van SA, Erdman W, Lavery LA, et al. Comparison between Tc-99m WBC SPECT/CT and MRI for the diagnosis of biopsy-proven diabetic foot osteomyelitis. Wounds. 2016;28(8):271–8.

46. Saha S, Burke C, Desai A, Vijayanathan S, Gnanasegaran G. SPECT-CT: applications in musculoskeletal radiology. Br J Radiol. 2013;86(1031):20120519. https://doi.org/10.1259/bjr.20120519.

47. Gaeta GB, Fusco FM, Nardiello S. Fever of unknown origin: a systematic review of the literature for 1995–2004. Nucl Med Commun. 2006;27(3):205–11.

48. Mulders-Manders C, Simon A, Bleeker-Rovers C. Fever of unknown origin. Clin Med (Lond). 2015;15(3):280–4. https://doi.org/10.7861/clinmedicine.15-3-280.

49. Signore A, Jamar F, Israel O, Buscombe J, Martin-Comin J, Lazzeri E. Clinical indications, image acquisition and data interpretation for white blood cells and anti-granulocyte monoclonal antibody scintigraphy: an EANM procedural guideline. Eur J Nucl Med Mol Imaging. 2018;45(10):1816–31. https://doi.org/10.1007/s00259-018-4052-x.

50. Baddour LM, Wilson WR, Bayer AS, Fowler VG, Tleyjeh IM, Rybak MJ, et al. Infective endocarditis in adults: diagnosis, antimicrobial therapy, and management of complications. Circulation. 2015;132(15):1435–86. https://doi.org/10.1161/CIR.0000000000000296.

51. Iung B, Erba PA, Petrosillo N, Lazzeri E. Common diagnostic flowcharts in infective endocarditis. Q J Nucl Med Mol Imaging. 2014;58(1):55–65.

52. Erba PA, Conti U, Lazzeri E, Sollini M, Doria R, De Tommasi SM, et al. Added value of 99mTc-HMPAO-labeled leukocyte SPECT/CT in the characterization and management of patients with infectious endocarditis. J Nucl Med. 2012;53(8):1235–43. https://doi.org/10.2967/jnumed.111.099424.

53. Hyafil F, Rouzet F, Lepage L, Benali K, Raffoul R, Duval X, et al. Role of radiolabelled leucocyte scintigraphy in patients with a suspicion of prosthetic valve endocarditis and inconclusive echocardiography. Eur Heart J Cardiovasc Imaging. 2013;14(6):586–94. https://doi.org/10.1093/ehjci/jet029.

54. Rouzet F, Chequer R, Benali K, Lepage L, Ghodbane W, Duval X, et al. Respective performance of 18F-FDG PET and radiolabeled leukocyte scintigraphy for the diagnosis of prosthetic valve endocarditis. J Nucl Med. 2014;55(12):1980–5. https://doi.org/10.2967/jnumed.114.141895.

55. Hyafil F, Rouzet F, Le Guludec D. Nuclear imaging for patients with a suspicion of infective endocarditis: be part of the team! J Nucl Cardiol. 2017;24(1):207–11. https://doi.org/10.1007/s12350-015-0369-z.

56. Habib G, Lancellotti P, Antunes MJ, Bongiorni MG, Casalta JP, Del Zotti F, et al. 2015 ESC Guidelines for the management of infective endocarditis: The Task Force for the Management of Infective Endocarditis of the European Society of Cardiology (ESC). Endorsed by: European Association for Cardio-Thoracic Surgery (EACTS), the European Association of Nuclear Medicine (EANM). Eur Heart J. 2015;36(44):3075–128. https://doi.org/10.1093/eurheartj/ehv319.

57. Sörelius K, di Summa PG. On the diagnosis of mycotic aortic aneurysms. Clin Med Insights Cardiol. 2018;12:1179546818759678. https://doi.org/10.1177/1179546818759678.

58. Fiorani P, Speziale F, Rizzo L, De Santis F, Massimi GJ, Taurino M, et al. Detection of aortic graft infection with leukocytes labeled with technetium 99m-hexametazime. J Vasc Surg. 1993;17(1):87–95; discussion 96.

59. Fujii T, Watanabe Y. Multidisciplinary treatment approach for prosthetic vascular graft infection in the thoracic aortic area. Ann Thorac Cardiovasc Surg. 2015;21(5):418–27. https://doi.org/10.5761/atcs.ra.15-00187.

60. Erba PA, Leo G, Sollini M, Tascini C, Boni R, Berchiolli RN, et al. Radiolabelled leucocyte scintigraphy versus conventional radiological imaging for the management of late, low-grade vascular prosthesis infections. Eur J Nucl Med Mol Imaging. 2014;41(2):357–68. https://doi.org/10.1007/s00259-013-2582-9.

61. Sarrazin J-F, Philippon F, Trottier M, Tessier M. Role of radionuclide imaging for diagnosis of device and prosthetic valve infections. World J Cardiol. 2016;8(9):534.

62. Erba PA, Sollini M, Conti U, Bandera F, Tascini C, De Tommasi SM, et al. Radiolabeled WBC scintigraphy in the diagnostic workup of patients with suspected device-related infections. JACC Cardiovasc Imaging. 2013;6(10):1075–86. https://doi.org/10.1016/j.jcmg.2013.08.001.

63. Hitzel A, Manrique A, Etienne M, Chastan M, Salles A, Edet-Sanson A, et al. 99mTc leukocyte SPECT/CT for diagnosis of left ventricular assist device (LVAD) infection. J Nucl Med. 2009;50(Suppl 2):1343.

64. Litzler P-Y, Manrique A, Etienne M, Salles A, Edet-Sanson A, Vera P, et al. Leukocyte SPECT/CT for detecting infection of left-ventricular-assist devices: preliminary results. J Nucl Med. 2010;51(7):1044–8. https://doi.org/10.2967/jnumed.109.070664.

65. Love C, Opoku-Agyemang P, Tomas M, Pugliese PV, Bhargava K, Palestro C. Pulmonary activity on labeled leukocyte images: physiologic, pathologic, and imaging correlation. Radiographics. 2002;22(6):1385–93.

66. Palestro CJ, Torres MA. Radionuclide imaging of nonosseous infection. Q J Nucl Med. 1999;43(1):46–60.

67. Tregay N, Begg M, Cahn A, Farahi N, Povey K, Madhavan S, et al. Use of autologous ⁹⁹ᵐTechnetium-labelled neutrophils to quantify lung neutrophil clearance in COPD. Thorax. 2019;74(7):659–66. https://doi.org/10.1136/thoraxjnl-2018-212509.

68. Aydin F, Kin Cengiz A, Gungor F. Tc-99m labeled HMPAO white blood cell scintigraphy in pediatric patients. Mol Imaging Radionucl Ther. 2012;21(1):13–8. https://doi.org/10.4274/Mirt.165.

69. Peters AM. The utility of [99mTc]HMPAO-leukocytes for imaging infection. Semin Nucl Med. 1994;24(2):110–27. https://doi.org/10.1016/S0001-2998(05)80226-0.

70. Elgazzar AH, Abdel-Dayem HM, Clark JD, Maxon HR III. Multimodality imaging of osteomyelitis. Eur J Nucl Med. 1995;22(9):1043–63.

71. Koranda P, Drymlová J, Malý T, Kantor L, Ptácek J, Myslivecek M. Tc-99m exametazime (HMPAO)-labeled leukocyte scintigraphy in premature infants: detection and localization of necrotic enterocolitis and osteomyelitis. Clin Nucl Med. 2011;36(6):e35–e6. https://doi.org/10.1097/RLU.0b013e3182173954.

72. Chang CC, Tsai CY, Lin CC, Jeng LB, Lee CC, Kao CH. Comparison between technetium-99m hexamethylpropyleneamineoxide labeled white blood cell abdomen scan and abdominal sonography to detect appendicitis in children with an atypical clinical presentation. Hepato-Gastroenterology. 2003;50(50):426–9.

73. Aydin F, Dincer D, Gungor F, Boz A, Akca S, Yildiz A, et al. Technetium-99m hexamethyl propylene amine oxime-labeled leukocyte scintigraphy at three different times in active ulcerative colitis: comparison with colonoscopy and clinico-biochemical parameters in the assessment of disease extension and severity. Ann Nucl Med. 2008;22(5):371–7. https://doi.org/10.1007/s12149-008-0131-6.

74. Grahnquist L, Chapman SC, Hvidsten S, Murphy MS. Evaluation of 99mTc-HMPAO leukocyte scintigraphy in the investigation of pediatric inflammatory bowel disease. J Pediatr. 2003;143(1):48–53. https://doi.org/10.1016/s0022-3476(03)00280-4.

75. Caobelli F, Panarotto MB, Andreoli F, Ravelli A, De Agostini A, Giubbini R. Is 99mTc-HMPAO granulocyte scan an alternative to endoscopy in pediatric chronic inflammatory bowel disease (IBD)? Eur J Pediatr. 2011;170(1):51–7. https://doi.org/10.1007/s00431-010-1269-5.

76. Auletta S, Galli F, Lauri C, Martinelli D, Santino I, Signore A. Imaging bacteria with radiolabelled quinolones, cephalosporins and siderophores for imaging infection: a systematic review. Clin Transl Imaging. 2016;4:229–52. https://doi.org/10.1007/s40336-016-0185-8.

77. Signore A, Lauri C, Auletta S, Anzola K, Galli F, Casali M, et al. Immuno-imaging to predict treatment response in infection, inflammation and oncology. J Clin Med. 2019;8(5):681. https://doi.org/10.3390/jcm8050681.

2-[^{18}F]FDG PET Imaging of Infection and Inflammation

7

Ryogo Minamimoto

Contents

7.1 Introduction

2-[^{18}F]fluoro-2-deoxy-D-glucose (2-[^{18}F]FDG) positron emission tomography (PET) has impacted the staging, restaging, and assessment of the therapeutic effect in a variety of malignancies. However, 2-[^{18}F]FDG uptake is not specific for malignancies,

R. Minamimoto (✉)
Division of Nuclear Medicine, Department of Radiology, National Center for Global Health and Medicine, Tokyo, Japan

© Springer Nature Switzerland AG 2022
S. Harsini et al. (eds.), *Nuclear Medicine and Immunology*,
https://doi.org/10.1007/978-3-030-81261-4_7

and nonmalignant lesions such as infection, inflammation, granulomatous diseases, and autoimmune diseases with increased glycolysis can be visualized with 2-[^{18}F]FDG PET. Currently, 2-[^{18}F]FDG PET provides outstanding performance for the diagnosis of several infectious and inflammatory diseases and monitoring of response to therapy. This chapter describes the roles and limitations of 2-[^{18}F]FDG PET and 2-[^{18}F]FDG PET/computed tomography (CT) in the field of infectious and inflammatory diseases and adds some valuable knowledge about 2-[^{18}F]FDG PET for the assessment of autoimmune diseases.

7.2 Mechanism of 2-[^{18}F]FDG Uptake in Malignant and Inflammatory Cells

2-[^{18}F]FDG is a glucose analog, which follows the same physiological processes as glucose, being taken up through cell surface glucose transporters and subsequently phosphorylated by the hexokinase enzyme to 2-[^{18}F]FDG-6 phosphate, which is not metabolized further and remains trapped inside the cell. The degree of cellular 2-[^{18}F]FDG uptake is related to the cellular metabolic rate and the number of glucose transporters [1–3]. Increased 2-[^{18}F]FDG uptake in tumors is generally due to an increased number of glucose transporters in malignant cells. 2-[^{18}F]FDG PET/CT has played an important role in staging, restaging, and evaluation of the therapeutic effect in a variety of malignancies.

Multiple mechanistic similarities in underlying metabolic pathways have been demonstrated between inflammatory and malignant cells [4, 5]. Inflammation can be broadly divided into three phases: (1) early vascular phase, (2) acute cellular phase, and (3) late cellular/healing phases. The earliest phase of inflammation shows tissue hyperemia, enhanced vascular permeability, and release of inflammatory mediators. The increase in tissue perfusion results in greater 2-[^{18}F]FDG delivery to the affected sites [6, 7]. The second stage is that of active cell recruitment, migration, and proliferation at the site of inflammation. In this stage, glycolytic pathways are enhanced

through the release of a multitude of cytokines, followed by upregulation of glucose transporter-1 (GLUT-1) and GLUT-3 and an increase in hexokinase activity [2, 4, 5, 8]. Hypoxia and toll-like-receptor activation are also influential factors that lead to the activation of this process [5]. Finally, in the transition from acute to chronic inflammation, the cellular environment changes from polymorphonuclear leukocytes to macrophages and monocytes along with tissue healing. However, a consistent shift in the balance toward cell glycolysis and away from anabolic pathways persists even during chronic inflammation [9, 10].

Neutrophils and the monocyte/macrophage family are cells involved in infection and inflammation that express high levels of GLUT-1 and GLUT-3 and show increased hexokinase activity. Macrophages, which are regarded as a substantial component of 2-[^{18}F]FDG uptake in tumors, are localized as peri-tumoral inflammatory cells [11]. A high degree of 2-[^{18}F]FDG uptake is seen in neutrophils during the acute phase of inflammation, whereas macrophages and polymorphonuclear leukocytes take up 2-[^{18}F]FDG during the chronic phase. A significant linear correlation between 2-[^{18}F]FDG uptake and inflammatory cells density was confirmed in both acute and chronic inflammation [12]. These observations explain the superior accuracy of 2-[^{18}F]FDG PET over traditional imaging techniques in chronic infection/inflammation.

Two major differences are present in the process of 2-[^{18}F]FDG uptake in tumor cells and inflammatory cells. First, glucose-6-phosphatase levels decrease in tumor cells but remain high in inflammatory cells, leading to washout of 2-[^{18}F]FDG from inflammatory cells. The other is the extremely increased GLUT levels in tumor cells compared to inflammatory cells [13]. However, differentiating a tumor from inflammation has always been a clinical challenge with 2-[^{18}F]FDG PET.

7.3 Tissue Infection

Infection of tissues can progress to an acute or chronic phase due to hematogenous spreading of pathogenic microorganisms or local contamination. Tissue infection usually presents with non-specific signs and symptoms, such that reaching an accurate diagnosis is difficult. Microorganism isolation with multiple sampling or histology of biopsies and imaging provides suggestive information that may hasten the process of diagnosis. When a 2-[¹⁸F]FDG PET scan is conducted for the evaluation of malignancy, tissue infection may show positive 2-[¹⁸F]FDG uptake that is generally regarded as a false-positive finding. Obviously, 2-[¹⁸F]FDG PET has a limitation for differentiating infection from malignant lesions. In general, the mediastinum, hilar, and cervical areas are among those frequently showing non-specific 2-[¹⁸F]FDG uptake, which can lead to inaccurate staging of malignancy.

Although nuclear medicine imaging has not been the first choice for diagnosis and has some limitations, increasing evidence has shown a role for 2-[¹⁸F]FDG PET in infectious diseases. 2-[¹⁸F]FDG PET is clinically useful for the detection of occult foci of infection in patients with sepsis of unknown origin and with fever of unknown origin (FUO). This is because underlying infectious and inflammatory disorders, such as osteomyelitis, infected vascular grafts, meta-static infectious disease, vasculitis, sarcoidosis, and inflammatory bowel disease (IBD), can be identified with 2-[¹⁸F]FDG PET/CT, which is superior to conventional clinical imaging modalities [14].

Recent reports have shown the utility of 2-[¹⁸F]FDG PET/CT for diagnosing, treating, and evaluating inflammatory diseases, strongly suggesting that 2-[¹⁸F]FDG would be useful in the diagnosis of FUO. 2-[¹⁸F]FDG PET may allow easier detection of lesion sites at an early stage, confirmation of pathological diagnosis with precise biopsy or operation, and identification of the etiological agent, which could lead to timely treatment of the underlying disease [15, 16]. The value of 2-[¹⁸F]FDG PET for the diagnosis of FUO is described in more detail in Chap. 8.

Diagnosis of postoperative tissue infection is difficult due to various clinical manifestations. Although 2-[¹⁸F]FDG may have the potential to indicate the postoperative focal infection site, persistent 2-[¹⁸F]FDG uptake in uninfected surgical incisions has been observed after at least several weeks, suggesting that evaluation of a residual tumor by 2-[¹⁸F]FDG PET after surgery is unreliable (Figs. 7.1, 7.2, and 7.3).

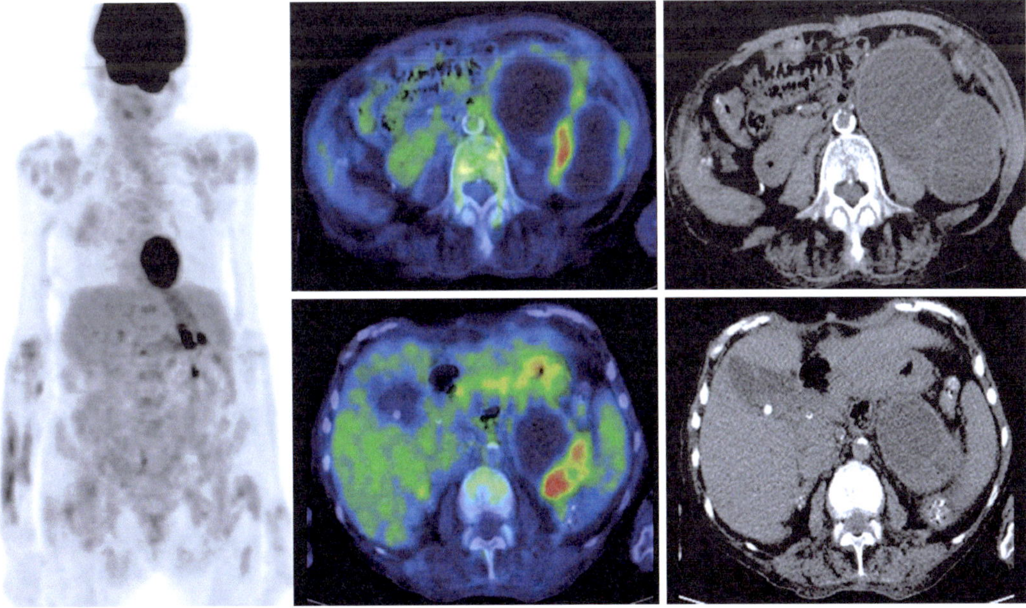

Fig. 7.1 Renal infection in polycystic kidney disease. Focal 2-[¹⁸F]FDG uptake is confirmed in the infectious site in the polycystic kidney

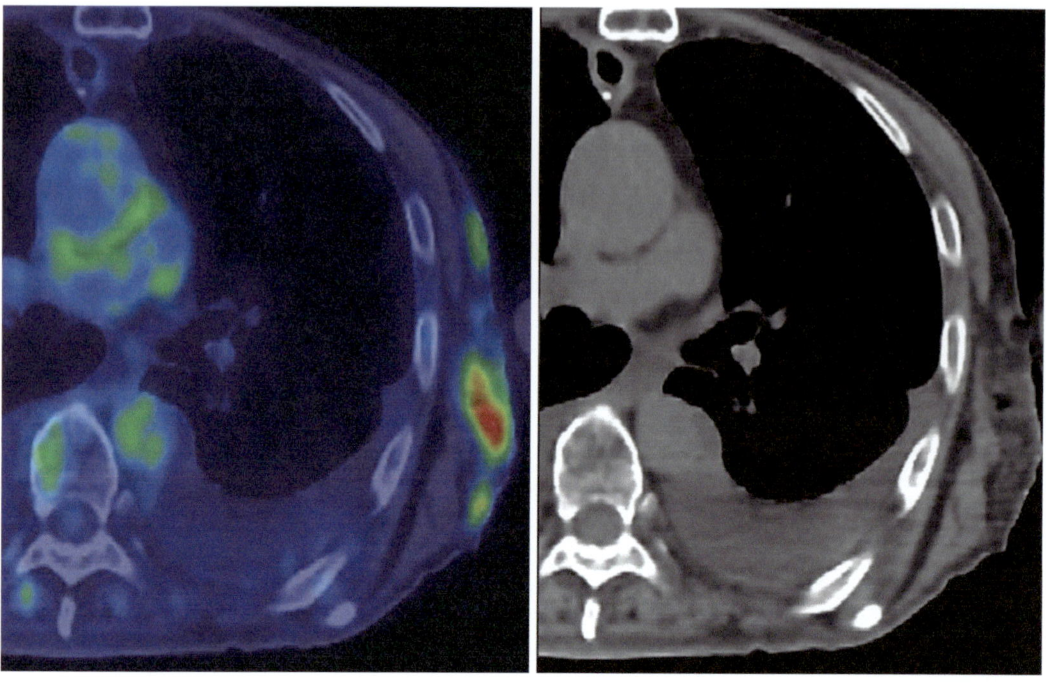

Fig. 7.2 Soft tissue infection (cellulitis) at left chest wall

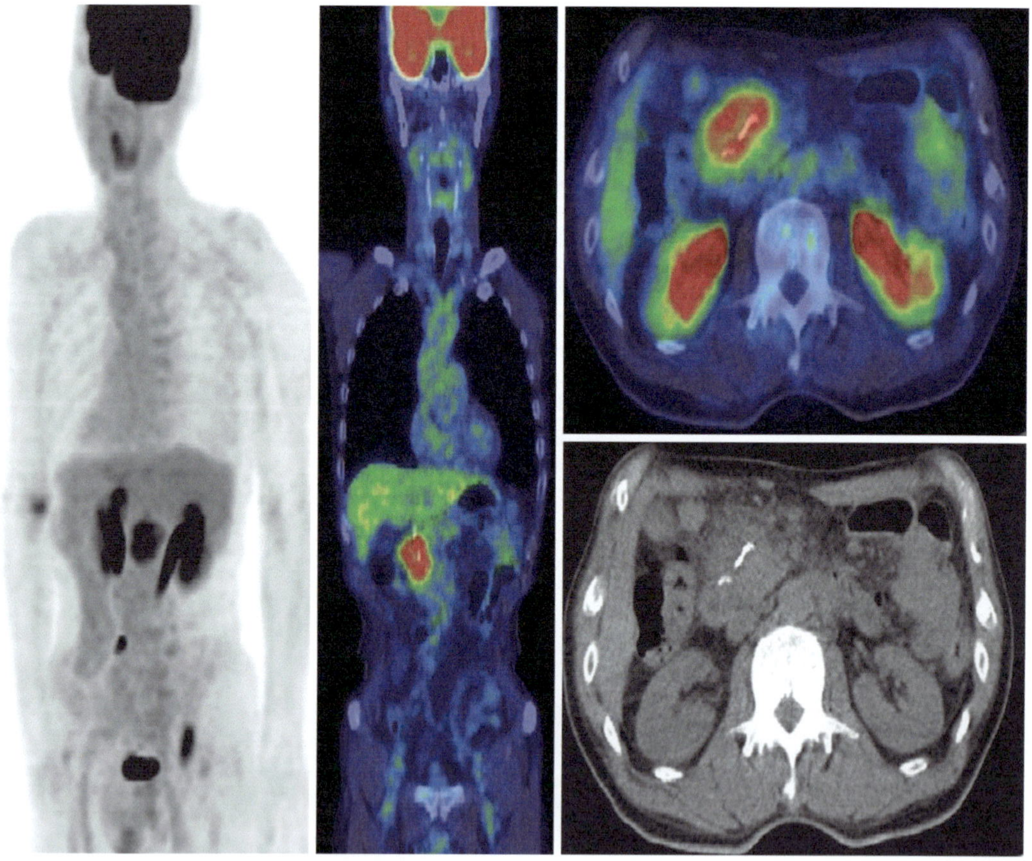

Fig. 7.3 Surgical site infection (duodenum)

7.4   Osteomyelitis

Osteomyelitis is defined as an infection of the bone, can involve any bone, and is caused by *Staphylococcus aureus*. Inflammatory markers, plain radiograph, and blood culture are commonly used for the diagnosis of osteomyelitis, although they are not specific for this condition. The presence of inflammatory cells in osteomyelitis results in increased 2-[¹⁸F]FDG uptake [17, 18] and contrasts well with low 2-[¹⁸F]FDG uptake in normal cortical bone. For acute limb osteomyelitis, clinical evaluation, serum markers of inflammation, and conventional imaging (plain radiographs, magnetic resonance imaging (MRI), or three-phase [⁹⁹ᵐTc]Tc-hydroxymethylene diphosphonate scintigraphy) have been sufficient to reach a diagnosis. However, 2-[¹⁸F]FDG PET has much higher sensitivity and specificity (more than 90%) for the diagnosis of chronic limb osteomyelitis compared to traditional radionuclide and morphological imaging [19–21]. Nonetheless, increased osseous 2-[¹⁸F]FDG activity has also been observed in inflammatory arthritis, in acute fractures, with significant metal artifacts, and when assessing the postoperative status (persisting 4–6 weeks after the procedure) [22] (Fig. 7.4).

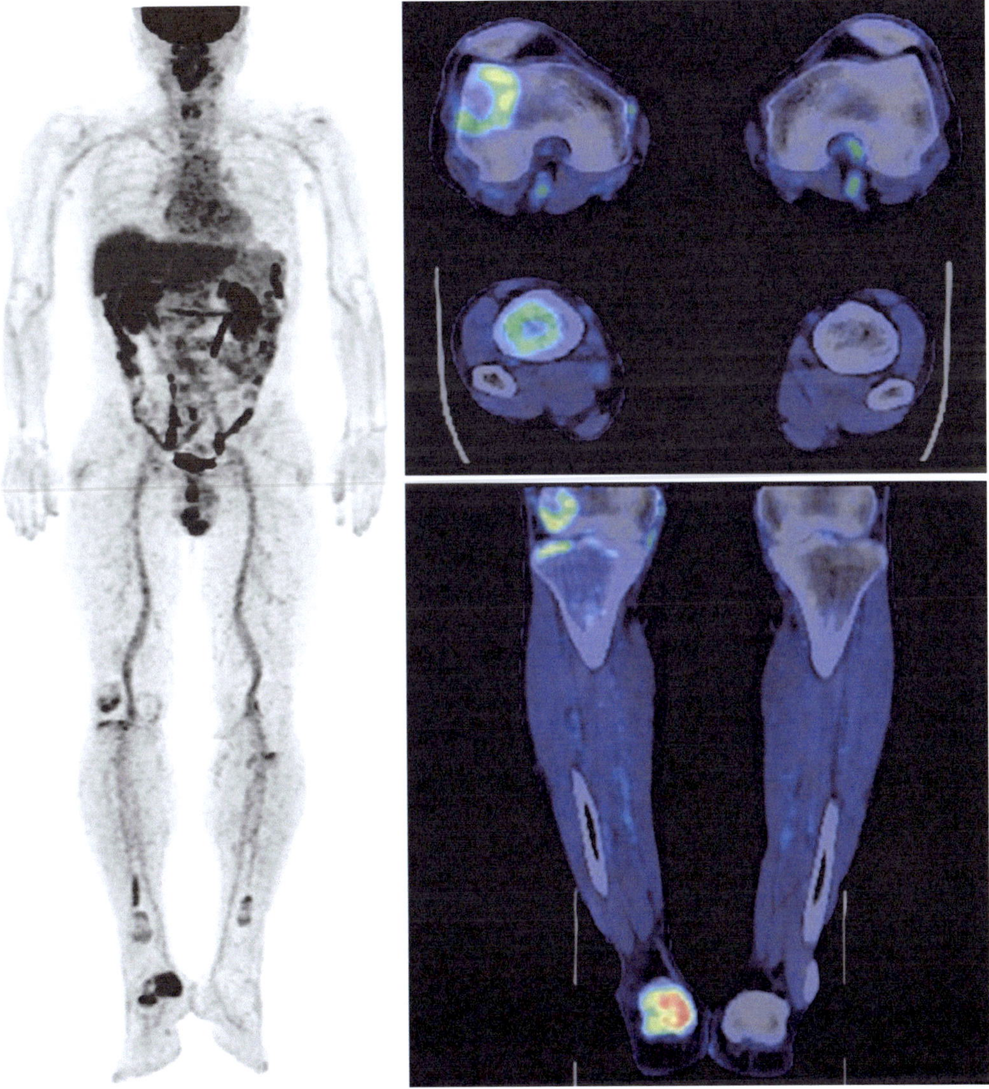

Fig. 7.4 Osteomyelitis. Focal 2-[¹⁸F]FDG uptake in the right femur, bilateral tibia, and right talus demonstrates osteomyelitis

Spinal osteomyelitis and discitis are usually caused by direct extension into the spine from adjacent foci or by hematogenous spread. MRI is considered the imaging technique of choice in spinal osteomyelitis with an accuracy of 90%, especially for delineating the extent of soft-tissue, epidural, and spinal cord involvement [23]. 2-[18F]FDG PET is useful in these patients as marrow uptake of 2-[18F]FDG is low, leading to a high target-to-background contrast ratio. 2-[18F]FDG PET shows a higher sensitivity (96%) and specificity (91%) for diagnosing and excluding chronic osteomyelitis compared to combined bone and leukocyte scintigraphy (78% and 84%, respectively) and MRI (84% and 60%, respectively) [24] (Figs. 7.5 and 7.6).

Spinal infection often involves the intervertebral disk, vertebral body, or both due to hemato-genic spread or a postsurgical origin. The high spatial resolution of 2-[18F]FDG PET/CT can usually discern bone and soft tissue involvement [25] and is thus used for the diagnosis of osteomyelitis [26]. In a meta-analysis, 2-[18F]FDG PET/CT showed a sensitivity of 97% and specificity of 88% for the diagnosis of spondylodiscitis [27].

For the evaluation of the therapeutic response in patients with osteomyelitis, 2-[18F]FDG PET/CT has a huge potential for making clinical decisions regarding initiation or prolongation of antibiotic therapy or recourse to surgical intervention in 52% of patients with infection [28]. Inflammatory changes in MRI scans can be seen long after the disappearance of the infection, and therefore, 2-[18F]FDG PET appears to be superior to MRI [29].

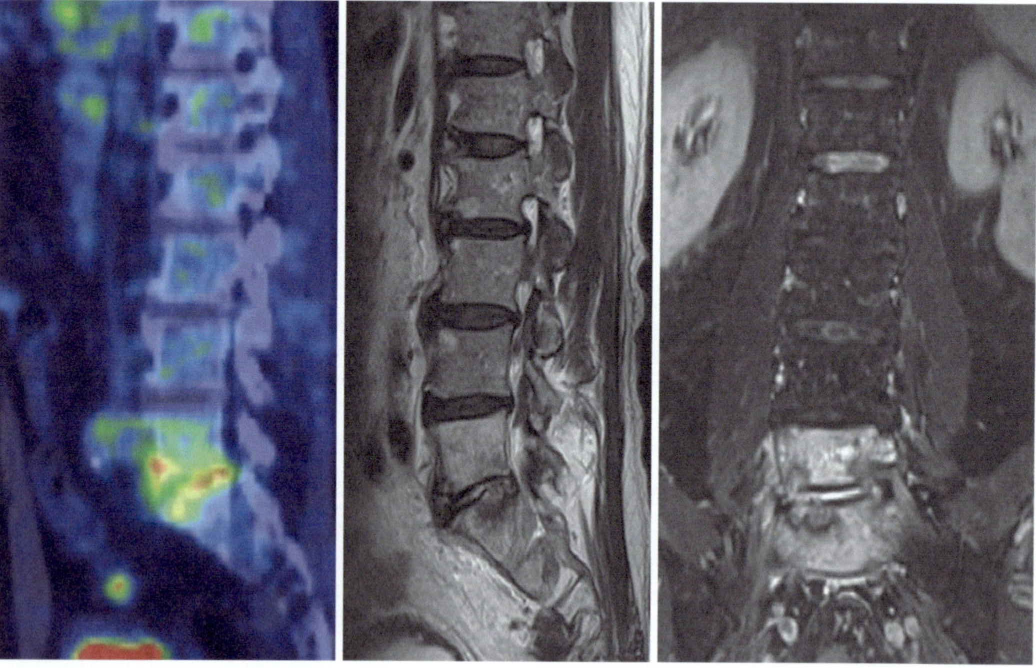

Fig. 7.5 Discitis. 2-[18F]FDG uptake is evident at the site of discitis. 2-[18F]FDG PET/CT and MRI images reveal that the inflammation is spread to the upper and lower vertebra

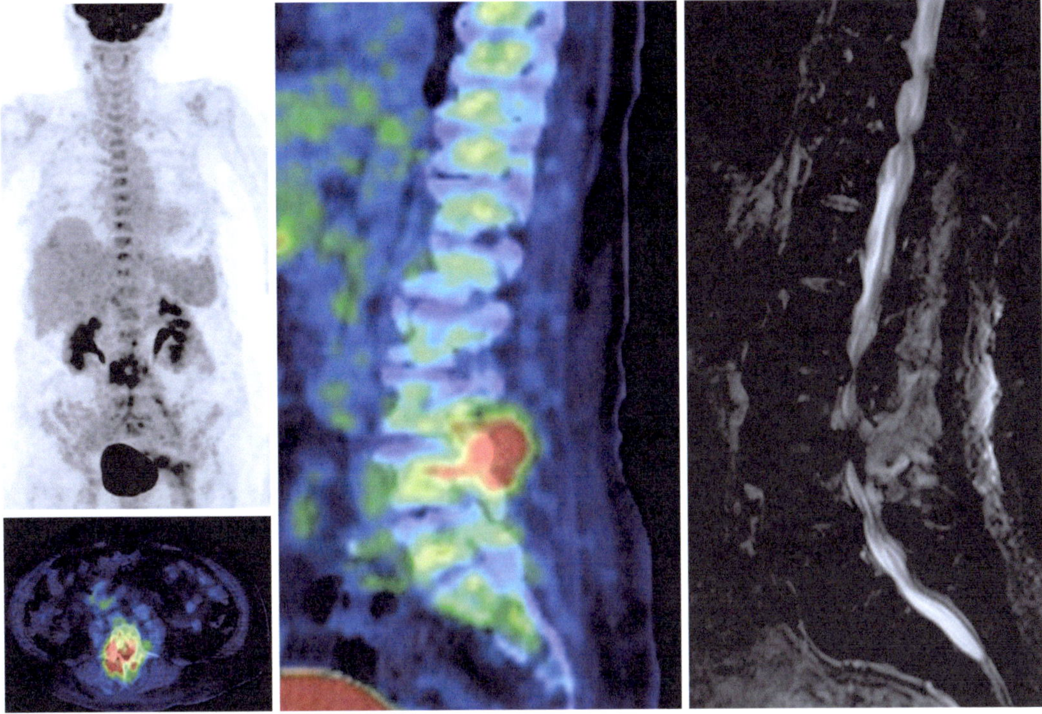

Fig. 7.6 Pyogenic spondylitis. 2-[¹⁸F]FDG uptake in the lumber pyogenic spondylitis

7.5   Cardiac Device Infection and Inflammatory Diseases of the Heart

2-[¹⁸F]FDG PET has a huge potential for the diagnosis of cardiovascular implantable electronic device (CIED) infection. 2-[¹⁸F]FDG PET/CT demonstrated a sensitivity of 96% and specificity of 97% for the diagnosis of pocket infections [30] compared to a lower pooled sensitivity of 76% and specificity of 83% for lead infections [31] (Fig. 7.7).

2-[¹⁸F]FDG PET/CT has a sensitivity of 73–100%, specificity of 71–100%, positive predictive value of 67–100%, and negative predictive value of 50–100% for prosthetic valve endocarditis [32]. The application of 2-[¹⁸F] FDG PET/CT and the Duke criteria increases the sensitivity from 52–70% to 91–97% without compromising specificity [33, 34]. Infective endocarditis is an infection of the endocardial surface of the heart, mainly due to *Staphylococcus* spp. Transthoracic echocardiography and transesophageal echocardiography have been used for detecting endocardial vegetations with a sensitivity of 40–63% and specificity of 90–100%. Unlike prosthetic valve endocarditis, the role of 2-[¹⁸F]FDG PET/CT for the diagnosis of native valve infective endocarditis is limited, with a sensitivity of 14% [35]. In a meta-analysis, 2-[¹⁸F]FDG PET/CT showed a sensitivity of 61% for the diagnosis of infective endocarditis [36], which is lower than with the modified Duke criteria (80%) advo-

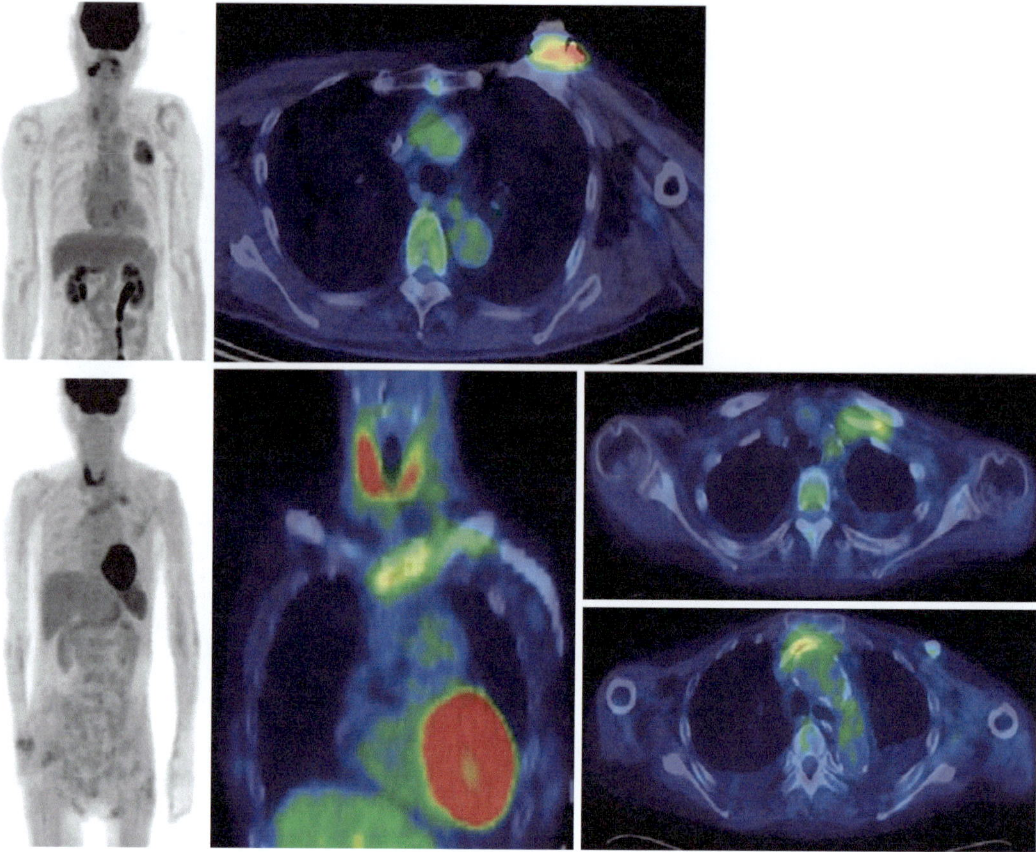

Fig. 7.7 Cardiovascular implantable electronic device (CIED) infection. Upper row, pocket infections; lower row, lead infection

cated in the European Society of Cardiology (ESC) guidelines [37]. 2-[^{18}F]FDG PET/CT is a valid diagnostic procedure for visualization of infective cardiac valve vegetation and can contribute to the identification of the primary extracardiac infection source or infective emboli in patients with native valve endocarditis, which leads to appropriate intervention and a reduction in the incidence of relapsed infective endocarditis [38].

Pericarditis is caused by viruses in most cases. Other etiologies include tuberculosis (TB), autoimmune diseases, and malignancy [39]. 2-[^{18}F]FDG PET/CT can indicate the existence of active pericarditis. 2-[^{18}F]FDG uptake in TB as an acute infectious disease is higher than in idiopathic pericarditis [40] (Fig. 7.8).

Myocarditis is an inflammatory disease of the heart muscle and an important cause of acute heart failure, sudden death, and cardiomyopathy. Echocardiogram is the first-line investigation, and cardiac MRI can provide functional and structural information, useful for further investigation of myocarditis. The role of 2-[^{18}F]FDG PET/CT is not specified and is thus not recommended as a diagnostic strategy for myocarditis.

A 2-[^{18}F]FDG PET study should be performed after a dietary preparation with a meal of high fat and low carbohydrates to suppress the physiologic cardiac 2-[^{18}F]FDG uptake. Moreover, 2-[^{18}F]FDG PET should generally be performed at least 3 months after the surgical placement of a device [37].

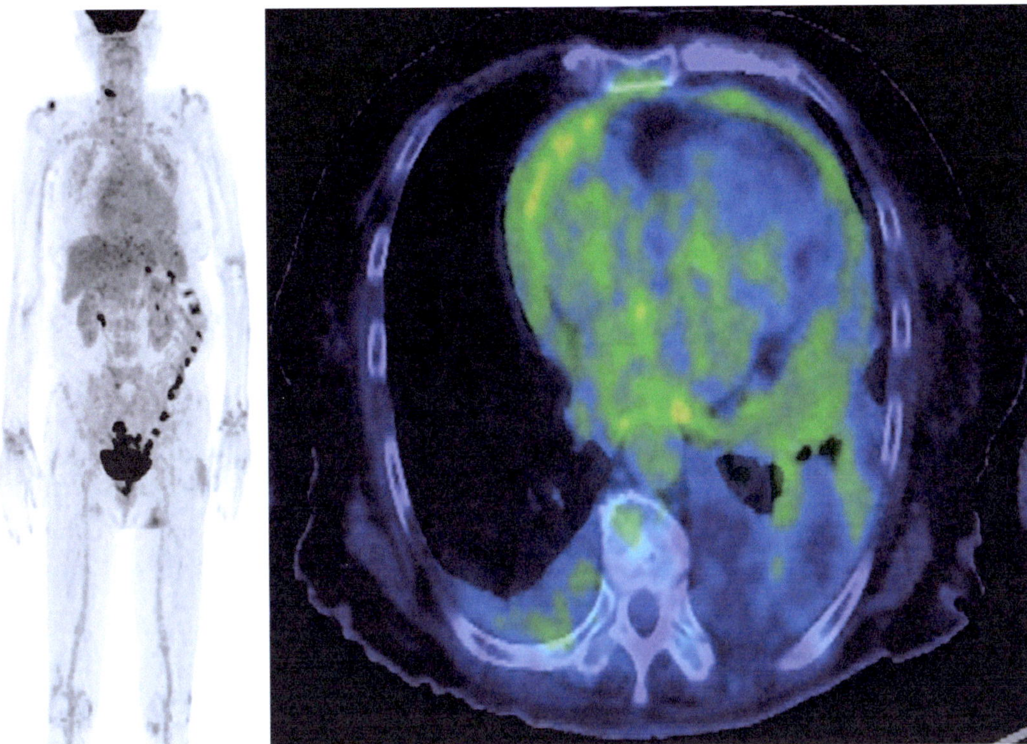

Fig. 7.8 Pericarditis. Diffuse 2-[¹⁸F]FDG uptake in the epicardium indicates pericarditis

7.6 Vascular Graft Infection (Vascular Prosthesis Infection)

Although vascular prosthesis infection (VPI) is quite a rare occurrence, it is associated with a significant increase in morbidity and mortality risk [41, 42]. Complications regarding early-onset infection include fever, bacteremia, graft dysfunction, thrombosis, and bleeding [43]. Graft infection as a late complication occurs months to years after the procedure and causes graft erosion and pseudoaneurysm. Therefore, long and close observation and early and accurate diagnosis are crucial for the management of patients with suspected VPI (Fig. 7.9).

Focal, heterogeneous 2-[¹⁸F]FDG uptake around the prosthesis is highly suggestive of VPI. Irregular graft boundaries, soft tissue thick-

ening, or peri-graft fluid collections on concomitant CT also suggest VPI [44]. 2-[¹⁸F]FDG PET shows high sensitivity and specificity for the diagnosis (93% sensitivity, 70–91% specificity) of VPI [45]. Several reports showed that image quality assessment using a three-point scale combined with the semiquantitative assessment [46] and a maximum standardized uptake value (SUVmax) cutoff can improve the diagnostic accuracy [47]. Mild to moderate diffuse physiological 2-[¹⁸F] FDG uptake has been confirmed in 92% of noninfected vascular prostheses, and this tends to remain in a region of anastomosis [44]. VPI consists of an infected hematoma or a lymphocele around the site of the graft, which leads to decreased specificity of 2-[¹⁸F]FDG PET/CT for identifying graft infection. Focal or segmental 2-[¹⁸F]FDG uptake is more likely to occur with infection than diffuse uptake [45]. 2-[¹⁸F]FDG often accumulates in scar

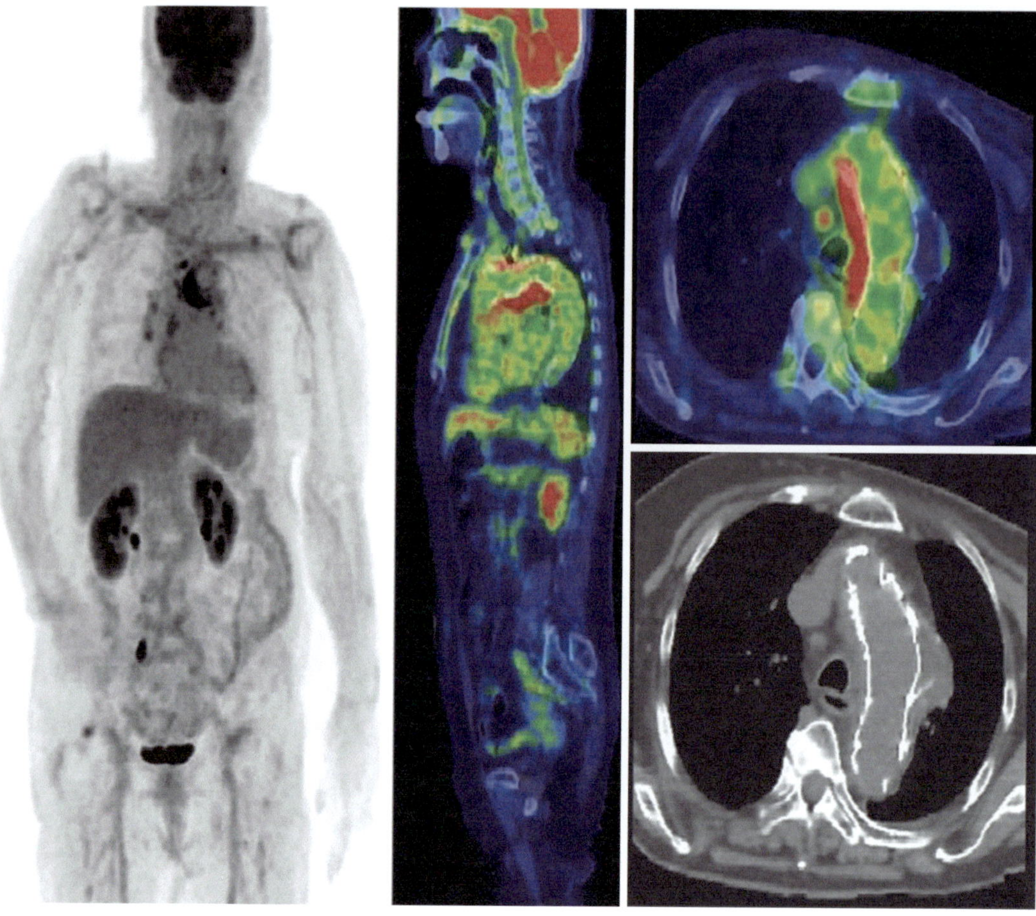

Fig. 7.9 Vascular prosthesis infection (VPI). 2-[¹⁸F]FDG uptake seen along the vascular graft indicates VPI; slight 2-[¹⁸F]FDG uptake is also seen in the aortic arch aneurysm

tissue and postoperative site, which can result in false-positive interpretation [48].

7.7 Joint Prosthesis Infection

More than a quarter of patients who have undergone a primary hip or knee arthroplasty will eventually develop symptoms of mechanical loosening after a decade of use. Although prosthetic infection is an uncommon complication that occurs in less than 1% of patients after primary hip or knee arthroplasty, distinguishing between prosthetic infection and mechanical loosening is crucial since the prosthetic infection is a major complication for the patient in terms of prognosis and multistep revision surgery. 2-[¹⁸F]

FDG PET shows significant heterogeneity in the cumulative test performance for infected prostheses, with sensitivity that ranges from 28% to 91% and specificity that ranges from 9% to 97% [36, 49]. The typical 2-[¹⁸F]FDG uptake pattern of prosthetic infection for hip implants is the presence of 2-[¹⁸F]FDG uptake between the bone and the prosthesis in the mid-shaft portion of the prosthesis; an accuracy of over 90% has been reported with this pattern [50] (Fig. 7.10). On the other hand, nonspecific 2-[¹⁸F]FDG uptake around the head and neck of prostheses frequently occurs and can remain for many years [51]. The site of 2-[¹⁸F]FDG uptake is essential for establishing an accurate diagnosis and minimizing false-positive results in patients suspected of having prosthetic infection. However, semi-

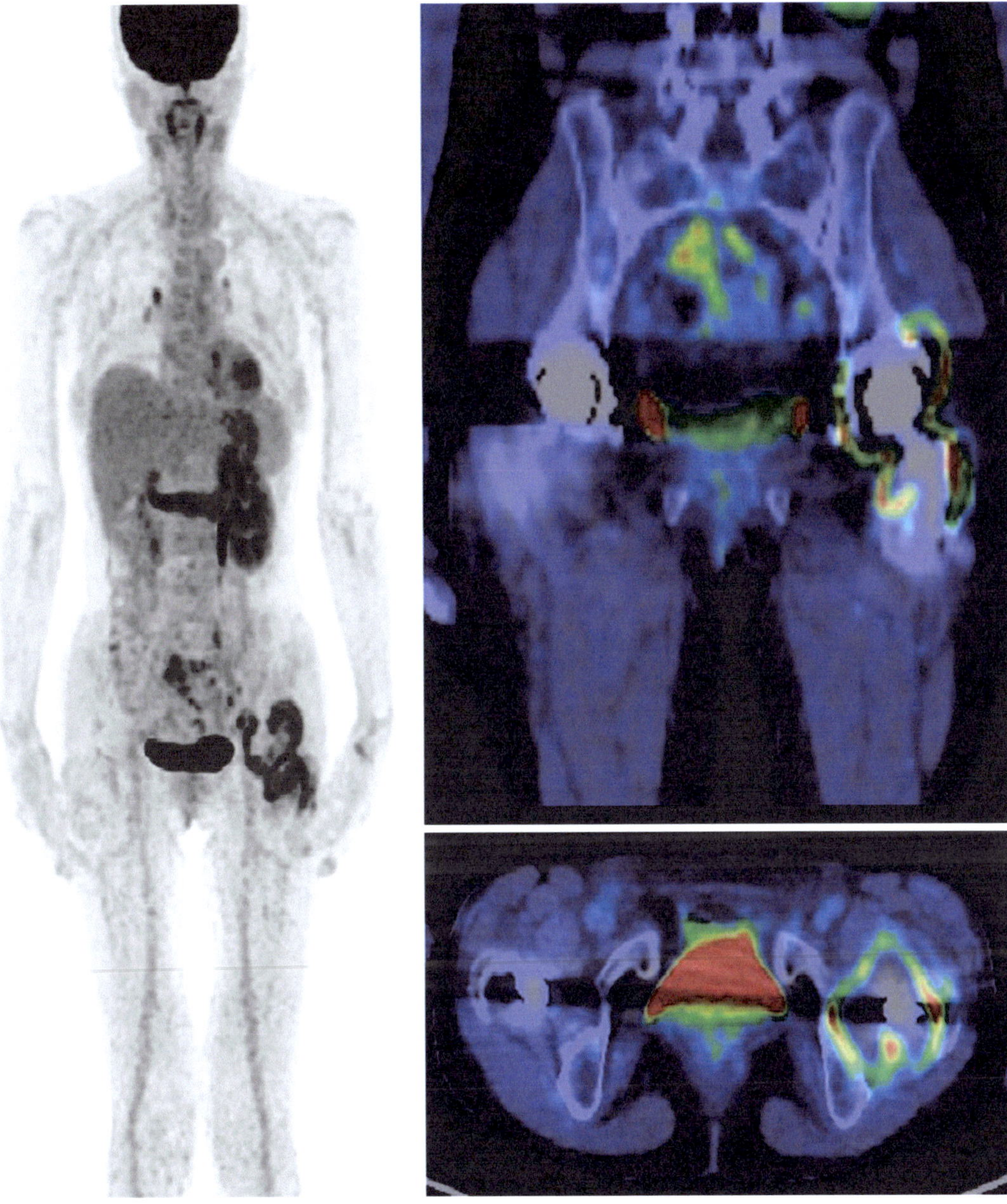

Fig. 7.10 Suspected left hip prosthesis infection. 2-[¹⁸F] FDG PET/CT shows 2-[¹⁸F]FDG uptake around the neck but negative findings at bone-prosthesis interface. The uptake pattern suggests nonspecific 2-[¹⁸F]FDG uptake around the head and neck of prostheses

quantitative assessment of 2-[¹⁸F]FDG uptake in prostheses is not reliable for differentiating septic and aseptic loosening.

The test of choice for diagnosing infected prostheses has remained combined labeled leukocyte/ marrow imaging over three decades, with an estimated sensitivity of 92–100%, specificity of 91–100%, and accuracy of 91–95% [52–54]. 2-[¹⁸F]FDG PET shows almost identical sensitivity as labeled leukocyte/marrow imaging, but the specificity is thought to be insufficient using this modality. Thus, at present, although 2-[¹⁸F]FDG PET is a worthwhile preoperative modality, the development of better diagnostic criteria is still required.

7.8   Tuberculosis (TB)

TB can involve any organ by hematogenous and/or lymphatic spread. The most commonly involved site of active TB lesions is the lung parenchyma [55, 56], particularly tuberculoma, which typically manifests as a rather discrete nodule or mass with central caseous necrosis surrounded by a mantle of epithelial cells and collagen with peripheral inflammatory cell infiltration [57]. Due to the large number of activated inflammatory cells with high glycolytic rates, active TB lesions are usually represented as areas of intense 2-[^{18}F]FDG uptake. Therefore, the sensitivity of 2-[^{18}F]FDG PET is very high for identifying active granulomatous foci (Fig. 7.11).

TB lesions do not have any characteristic 2-[^{18}F]FDG PET features but show variable 2-[^{18}F]FDG uptake according to the grade of inflammatory activity [55]. Due to the lack of specificity of 2-[^{18}F]FDG PET for distinguishing granulomatous disease from malignancy, TB should be considered in the differential diagnosis of 2-[^{18}F]FDG-avid thoracic lesions, and biopsy and histopathological examination are still essential for the final diagnosis.

Nontuberculous mycobacterial (NTM) infection is caused by a group of opportunistic bacterial pathogens such as *Mycobacterium avium intracellular* complex that is hard to isolate and is characterized by nonspecific clinical signs. In the same manner as TB, NTM might represent a broad range of radiological patterns, comprising parenchymal consolidation, nodular or pseudonodular lesions, cavitary lesions, pleural effusions, pleural thickenings, or a mixed pattern

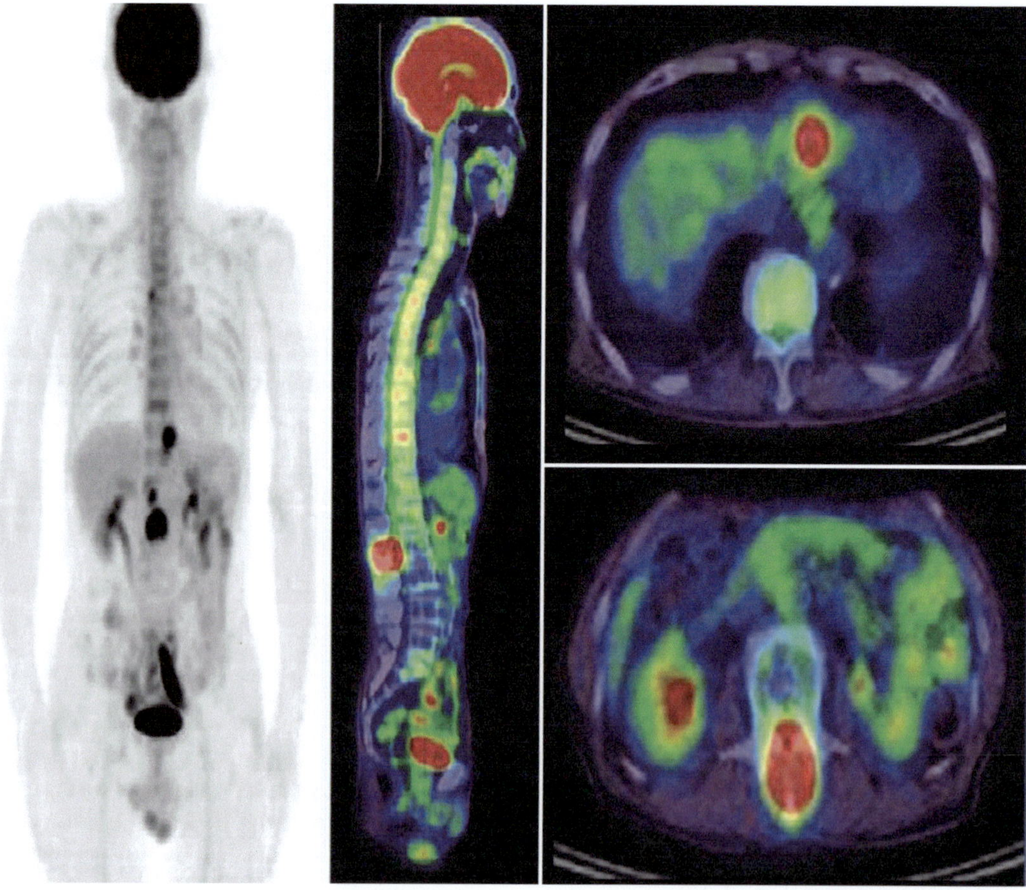

Fig. 7.11 Tuberculosis. 2-[^{18}F]FDG PET/CT shows tuberculous abscess around the vertebral body and liver

[58–60]. 2-[¹⁸F]FDG PET/CT could reflect the activity and extent of disease by monitoring metabolic activity not only in nodular lesions but also in a broad range of radiologically visible lung lesions in NTM. Despite these uncertainties, an important aspect of PET/CT imaging is its potential role in assessing the extent of disease, its evolution, and follow-up of NTM patients [61].

7.9   Sarcoidosis

Sarcoidosis is regarded as a systemic noncaseating granulomatous disease of unknown etiology. Typical clinical features are bilateral active lymph nodes in the mediastinal and hilar regions. Sarcoidosis also appears as pulmonary lymphoreticular opacities and lesions in the skin, muscle, joints, eyes, and other organs including the myocardium, liver, and spleen [62].

Serum angiotensin converting enzyme is produced by epithelial cells derived from activated macrophages and is a known marker for sarcoidosis that reflects the amount of whole-body granuloma. However, the use of angiotensin converting enzyme (ACE) in sarcoidosis is limited due to its poor sensitivity and specificity [63].

Malignant lymphoma and TB are major differential diagnoses of sarcoidosis; therefore, typical clinicoradiological findings with the histopathological hallmark of noncaseating granulomas are required for the diagnosis of sarcoidosis. 2-[¹⁸F]FDG PET/CT is a less-invasive test that can be used to determine targets for tissue sampling and evaluation of the extent of the disease (Fig. 7.12). Compared to gallium-67 scanning, 2-[¹⁸F]FDG PET is more sensitive and accurate for detecting pulmonary sarcoidosis, is better for identification of extrapulmonary sarcoidosis, and has higher interobserver agreement [64, 65]. 2-[¹⁸F]FDG uptake is correlated with disease activity and the clinical course [66]. 2-[¹⁸F]FDG PET is useful for monitoring the treatment response in the early phase, which can be an indication of the success of the management of patients with sarcoidosis [67].

Myocardial involvement of sarcoidosis is reported in approximately 5% of patients and

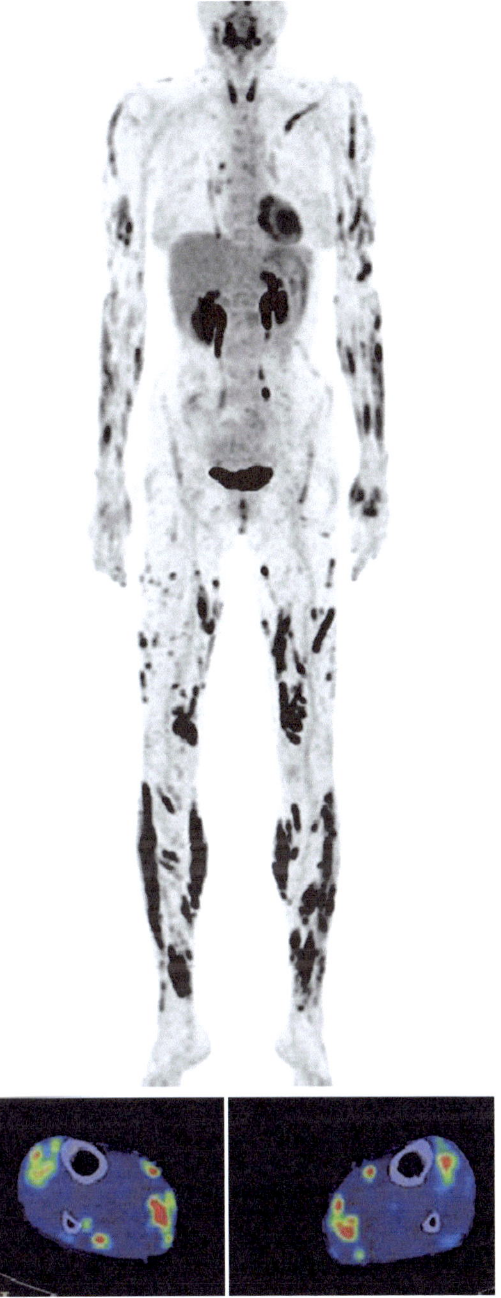

Fig. 7.12 Sarcoidosis. Muscular invasion of sarcoidosis

may lead to a life-threatening condition. Although an endomyocardial biopsy has been conducted for the definitive diagnosis, a sampling error may end in a false-negative result. Therefore, a sensitive imaging technique is required for the diagnosis and monitoring of cardiac sarcoidosis.

Delayed gadolinium enhancement in cardiac MRI is a hallmark finding of existing lesions and a poor prognostic factor [68, 69]. 2-[18F]FDG PET and cardiac MRI in patients with suspected cardiac sarcoidosis show a sensitivity comparable to 2-[18F]FDG PET (87.5% versus 75%, respectively) but with lower specificity (38.5% versus 76.9%, respectively) [70]. 2-[18F]FDG PET/CT can be implemented in cardiac sarcoidosis patients with a cardiac device unable to undergo MRI.

Focal heterogeneous 2-[18F]FDG uptake in the myocardium indicates active myocardial sarcoidosis (Fig. 7.13). However, myocardial physiological 2-[18F]FDG uptake shows a variable pattern; therefore, special preparation to suppress glucose consumption in the myocardium is required to reduce background physiological myocardial 2-[18F]FDG uptake. During fasting states in aerobic conditions, the human myocardium preferentially utilizes energy derived from free fatty acids. Therefore, focal patchy myocardial uptake reflecting active myocardial sarcoidosis will emerge [71]. A prolonged interval of fasting for more than 12 h (recommended 18 h or more) leads to a decrease in blood glucose and insulin levels and an increase in blood free fatty acid levels, minimizing physiological 2-[18F]FDG uptake in the normal myocardium [8]. As dietary modification prior to 2-[18F]FDG PET, a low-carbohydrate diet of less than 5 g the night before 2-[18F]FDG PET is recommended to reduce blood glucose and insulin levels [72, 73]. An Atkins-style low-carbohydrate diet (less than 3 g) on the day before PET together with overnight fasting effectively suppresses myocardial 2-[18F]FDG uptake compared to overnight fasting alone [74]. False-positive nonhomogeneous 2-[18F]FDG uptake in the myocardium due to poor patient preparation results in a characteristic pattern of 2-[18F]FDG uptake in the basal and lateral walls [75].

7.10 Autoimmune Diseases

7.10.1 Vasculitis

Systemic vasculitis is characterized by inflammation with infiltration of leukocytes into the blood vessels and reactive damage to mural structures. Classification of vasculitis was first advocated in the Chapel Hill Consensus Conference (CHCC1994) with consensus on names for the most common forms of vasculitides and to construct a specific definition for each type [76]. Due to the emergence of new knowledge about vasculitis, the International Chapel Hill Consensus Conference (CHCC2012) was advocated to improve the CHCC1994. In CHCC2012, names and definitions of vasculitides were changed, and important categories of vasculitides were newly added [77].

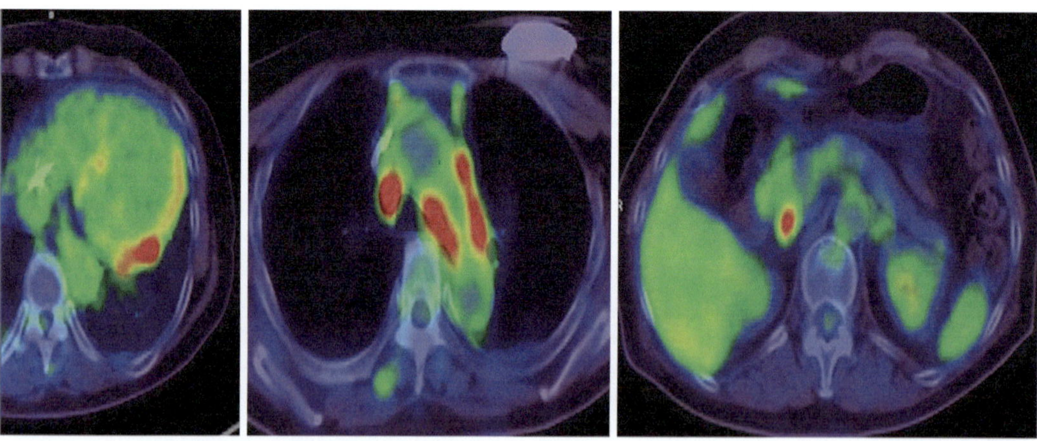

Fig. 7.13 Sarcoidosis. 2-[18F]FDG PET/CT demonstrates mediastinal and abdominal lymphadenopathies accompanied by cardiac sarcoidosis

Vasculitis is difficult to diagnose due to the absence of specific symptoms. For the diagnosis of large vessel vasculitis (LVV), CT is useful for detecting wall thickening, calcification, and mural thrombi. CT angiography demonstrates luminal changes (stenosis, occlusion, dilatation, and aneurysm). MRI can provide detailed information about structural vascular abnormalities (aneurysms, stenosis) but does not identify inflammation in structurally normal blood vessels.

Because of the limited spatial resolution of the PET/CT scanner, 2-[18F]FDG PET/CT can only visualize LVV, which is defined as a disease mainly affecting the large arteries, with two major variants, Takayasu arteritis (TA) and giant cell arteritis (GCA) (Fig. 7.14). However, the advantage of 2-[18F]FDG PET/CT is that it can detect areas affected by vasculitis in the early phase prior to structural changes. TA and GCA are different diseases with different ages of onset, ethnic distributions, immunogenic backgrounds [78], and response to therapies [79, 80]. TA mainly affects the aorta and its main branches, namely, the carotid arteries, brachiocephalic trunk, and subclavian arteries. GCA can involve

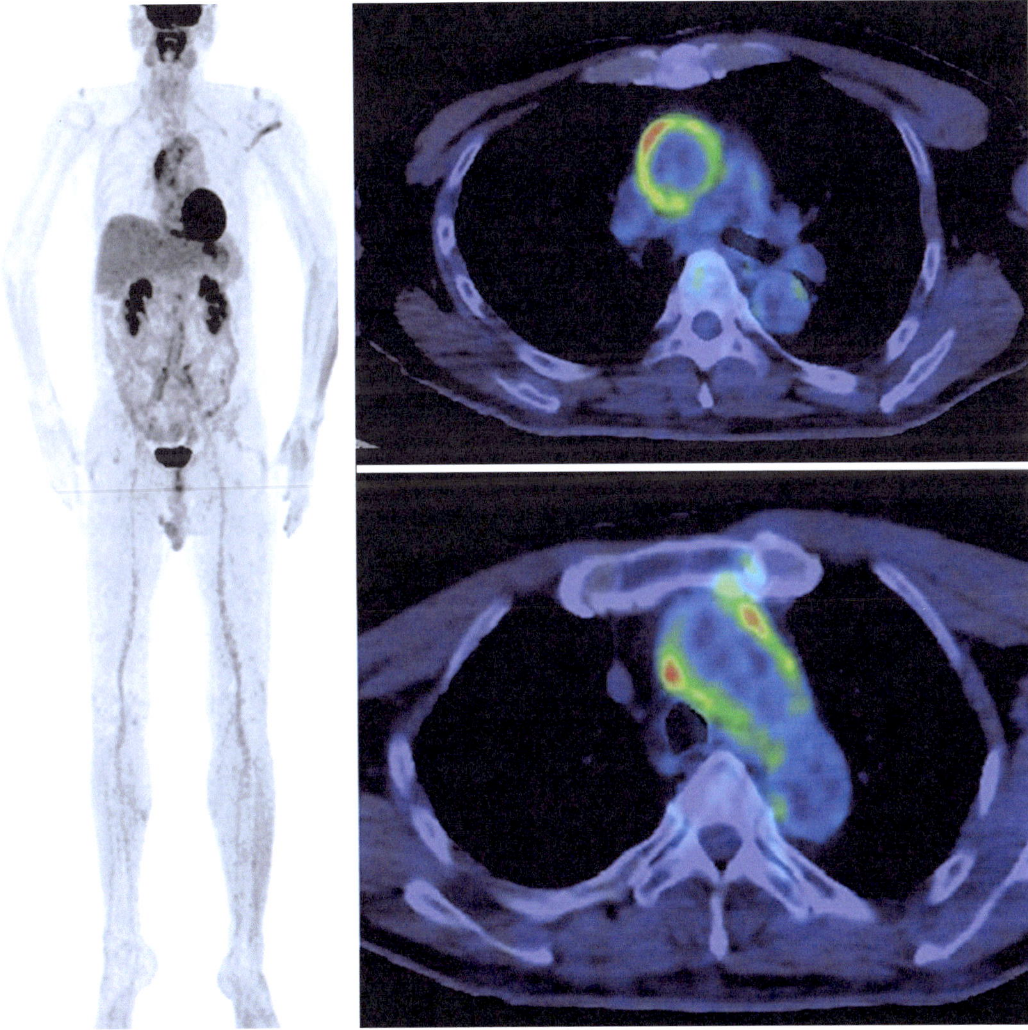

Fig. 7.14 Vasculitis (Takayasu arteritis). Smooth liner 2-[18F]FDG uptake in the aortic arch and abdominal aorta, which is a typical 2-[18F]FDG uptake pattern in large vessel arteritis

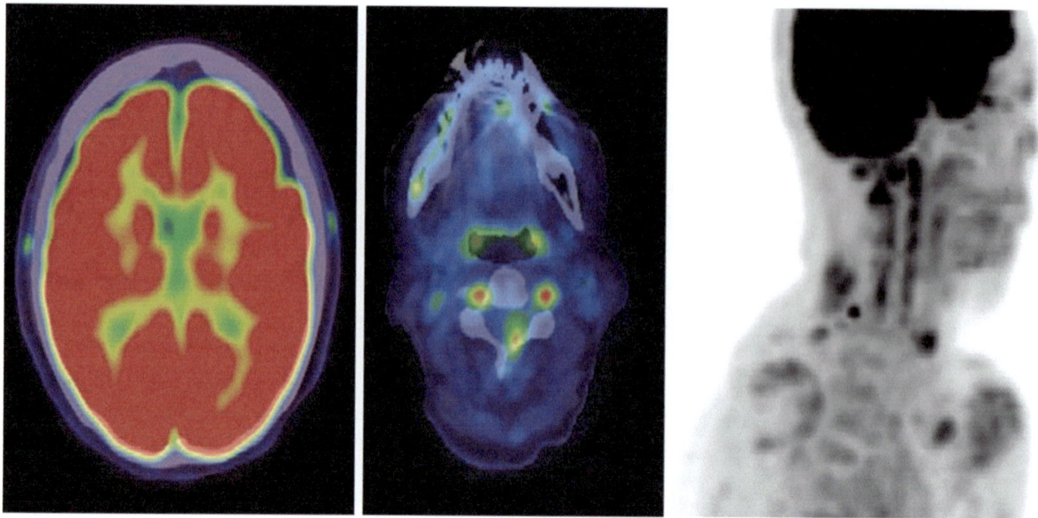

Fig. 7.15 Vasculitis (giant cell arteritis). 2-[^{18}F]FDG uptake in the temporal arteries and cervical arteries. 2-[^{18}F]FDG uptake in the temporal arteries is frequently seen in giant cell arthritis

the temporal artery as well as the aorta and its main branches (Fig. 7.15). However, GCA and TA also show some overlap regarding the histopathology of arterial lesions, reflecting shared pathways in tissue inflammation [79, 81].

The sensitivity and specificity of 2-[^{18}F]FDG PET for the diagnosis of TA are 92% and 100%, respectively. The sensitivity and specificity of 2-[^{18}F]FDG PET for the diagnosis of GCA are 77–92% and 89–100%, respectively [80, 82].

GCA is associated with polymyalgia rheumatica (PMR), an inflammatory disease around the joints that causes pain and stiffness. Typical 2-[^{18}F]FDG image patterns of PMR include uptake in glenohumeral synovia, subacromial-subdeltoid bursa, supraspinatus tendinitis, and biceps synovitis (shoulder); trochanteric/ischial bursa; hip synovia; interspinous regions of the cervical and lumbar vertebrae; or the synovial tissue of the knees [83] (Fig. 7.16). Nearly half of the patients with GCA can present with PMR as a complication, whereas approximately 20% of patients with PMR might develop GCA [84, 85].

Interpretation criteria proposed to assess the vasculitides have a visual 0 to 3 grading scale (0 = no uptake (≤mediastinum); 1 = low-grade uptake (<liver); 2 = intermediate-grade uptake (= liver), 3 = high-grade uptake (>liver)), with grade 2 possibly indicative of and grade 3 considered

positive for active LVV [86]. A total vascular score that includes the visual grading scale is another reasonable method that can be used to evaluate not only the activity of vasculitis but also the extent of the disease by summing up the 2-[^{18}F]FDG uptake scores at seven different vascular regions (thoracic aorta, abdominal aorta, subclavian arteries, axillary arteries, carotid arteries, iliac arteries, and femoral arteries) [83, 87]. The target-to-background ratio, using the blood pool as a reference, is a possible semiquantitative method for the evaluation of vasculitis [88, 89], whereas SUV itself is not recommended due to the large overlap between patients with vasculitis and normal cases and the low specificity [88, 90].

Although 2-[^{18}F]FDG PET has the potential for monitoring the response to therapy, no definitive result has led to such recommendation. Several reports showed a difference in 2-[^{18}F]FDG uptake between baseline and post-corticosteroid therapy. 2-[^{18}F]FDG uptake is reduced several months after the initiation of therapy, but it has no evidence of utility in further 2-[^{18}F]FDG scans or for prediction of disease relapse [91, 92].

Atherosclerotic vascular uptake is observed with aging and can result in false-positive findings in the evaluation of LVV. Typical 2-[^{18}F]

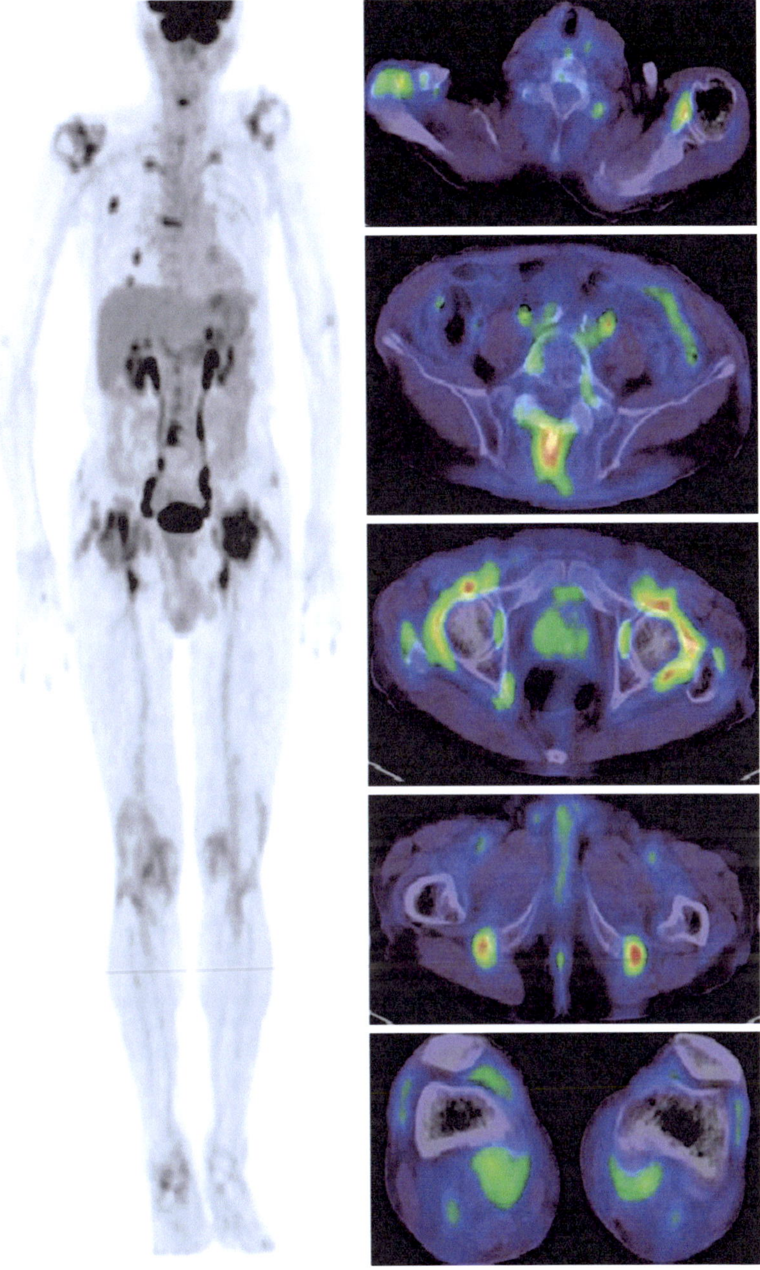

Fig. 7.16 Polymyalgia rheumatica (PMR). PMR often coexists with giant cell arteritis

FDG PET finding is uptake in iliofemoral arteries, a feature of atherosclerosis. This should be taken into consideration in the assessment of LVV [93, 94].

Polyarteritis *nodosa* is a systemic necrotizing vasculitis, which occurs in the medium- and small-sized arteries and causes multiple aneurysms. A recent report shows the utility of 2-[¹⁸F]FDG PET/CT for the early diagnosis of polyarteritis *nodosa* [95].

Vasculitis is often accompanied by other autoimmune diseases, and therefore, careful observation of whole-body PET imaging should be done to monitor other disease etiologies [96–99].

7.10.2 Inflammatory Bowel Diseases (IBD)

IBD is a chronic immune-mediated inflammatory disease that occurs in the gastrointestinal tract. Crohn's disease and ulcerative colitis are the representative diseases of IBD. 2-[18F]FDG PET/CT is a highly sensitive method to detect areas of active IBD. A meta-analysis revealed overall pooled sensitivity and specificity of 85% and 87% for 2-[18F]FDG PET, respectively [100] (Fig. 7.17). Another indication for 2-[18F]FDG PET may be for children, adolescents, and high-risk patients with IBD who appear to have difficulty undergoing an invasive endoscopy. Visual analysis of PET images is most accurate for diagnosis, whereas SUVs of 2-[18F]FDG are not correlated with any indicators of Crohn's disease activity (C-reactive protein or inflamed segments confirmed with endoscopy) [101].

However, variable physiological 2-[18F]FDG uptake in the bowel, such as uptake at the ileocecal junction, uptake in areas of small bowel peristalsis, and diffuse uptake in the ascending colon [102], might be observed. Therefore, detection of IBD with 2-[18F]FDG PET/CT still has major limitations. The specificity of 2-[18F]FDG PET can be increased by combining 2-[18F]FDG uptake with the anatomical accuracy of CT [100, 103]. The presence of certain features, such as bowel wall thickening, loop separation, mesenteric injection, and fat stranding, on concomitant CT, helps discern physiological from pathological uptake. The addition of intravenous iodinated contrast enhancement can provide more precise information about mural enhancement or increased thickness of the bowel wall [104]. 2-[18F]FDG PET/CT shows the potential for treatment monitoring of IBD with steroids or infliximab [105].

7.10.3 IgG4-Related Disease

The IgG4-related disease is characterized by the formation of mass-forming lesions in various organs that consist of lymphoplasmacytic infiltrates and fibrosclerosis [106, 107]. This disease was traditionally thought to consist of disparate clinical entities, such as autoimmune pancreatitis, Mikulicz disease, and primary sclerosing cholangitis. The IgG4-related disease is highly

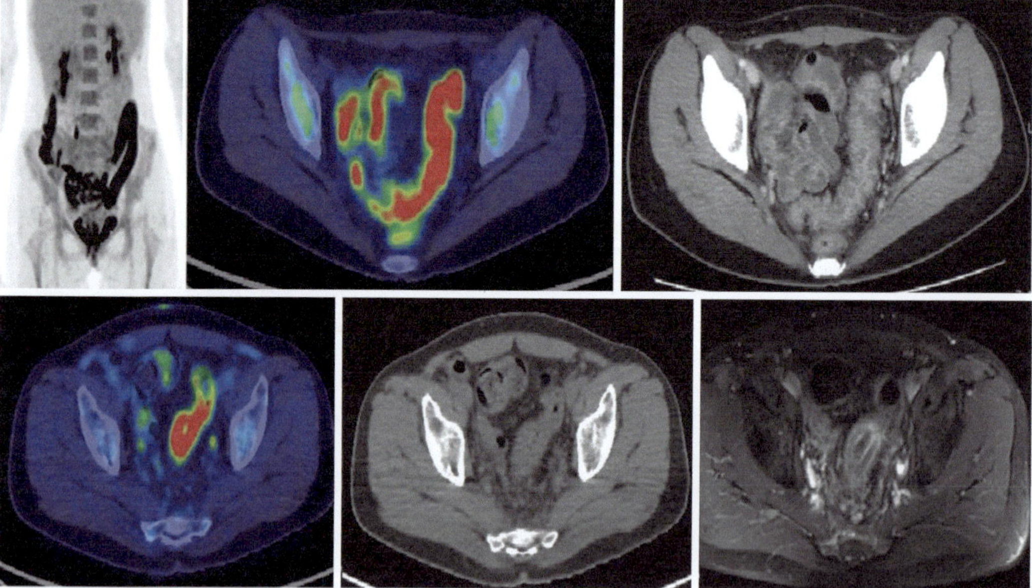

Fig. 7.17 Inflammatory bowel disease (IBD). Upper row, Crohn's disease (small intestine); lower row, ulcerative colitis (sigmoid colon)

sensitive to corticosteroids. However, it mimics malignancy that may require surgery or chemoradiotherapy, and therefore, accurate diagnosis is crucial for the management of patients. Increased serum immunoglobulin (Ig)G4 was initially thought to be the major diagnostic criterion for IgG4-related disease. Now, clinicians know that elevated IgG4 is not present in all patients with histologically proven IgG4-related disease and that the IgG4 is not specific for this disease. 2-[¹⁸F]FDG PET/CT can identify the disease distribution and activity in IgG4-related disease and is also useful for determining biopsy sites for pathological diagnosis. PET/CT indicates a larger extent of organ involvement than assumed before imaging in 70% of patients with IgG4-related disease [108] (Fig. 7.18).

Autoimmune pancreatitis (AIP) is one of the major IgG4-related diseases and should be distinguished from pancreatic cancer. Compared to pancreatic cancer, AIP tends to show extra-

pancreatic lesions and multiple foci of 2-[¹⁸F]FDG uptake in the pancreas [51]. Mikulicz disease and primary sclerosing cholangitis are also major IgG4-related diseases. The other reported sites of IgG4-related involvement include the meninges, lacrimal gland, salivary gland, thyroid gland, lung, breast, liver, kidney, prostate, and skin [107].

IgG4-related vasculitis is thought to be categorized as a primary type of vasculitis and a secondary form of vascular involvement characterized by periaortic or periarterial involvement [109]. Macrovascular manifestations of IgG4-related disease have been reported as inflammatory aortic aneurysm [110], coronary periarteritis [111], and periaortitis/arteritis in the setting of retroperitoneal fibrosis [112, 113]. IgG4-related vasculitis can lead to morbidity and mortality in the form of aortic dissection and sudden cardiac death [114]. 2-[¹⁸F]FDG uptake is confirmed in the area of IgG4-related soft tissue thickening

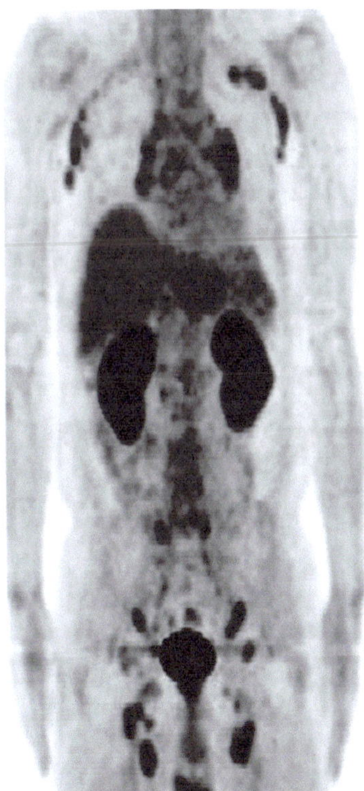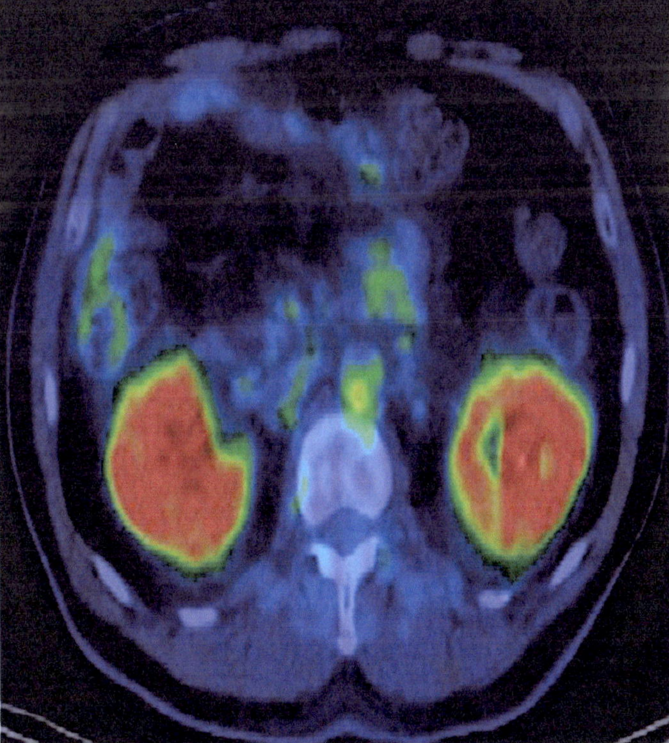

Fig. 7.18 IgG4-related disease (interstitial nephritis). 2-[¹⁸F]FDG uptake in bilateral kidneys without a clear border between the cortex and medulla of the kidneys

with active inflammation around arteries such as coronary arteries [115–117].

The differential diagnosis of IgG4-related disease is malignant lymphoma, which requires different treatment than IgG4-related disease. IgG4-related lymphadenopathy with atypical lymphoplasmacytic and immunoblastic proliferation shows histological characteristics that are often confused with malignant lymphoma, especially angioimmunoblastic T-cell lymphoma, which typically presents with polyclonal hypergammaglobulinemia [107, 118]. IgG4-related mucosa-associated lymphoid tissue lymphoma and IgG4-producing lymphoma in ocular adnexal regions have also been reported [119].

Glucocorticoids have been considered first-line therapy for active, untreated IgG4-related disease [120]. PET/CT is a promising tool not only for the diagnosis of IgG4-related disease but also for monitoring of disease activity. However, hyperglycemia due to diabetes mellitus induced by steroid therapy may influence 2-[^{18}F]FDG uptake, and steroid therapy itself could lead to overestimation of the response (Fig. 7.19).

7.10.4 Rheumatoid Arthritis (RA)

RA is an autoimmune chronic inflammatory disorder that mainly affects the joints with synovitis, pannus formation, and cartilage erosion and sometimes affects the skin, eyes, lungs, heart, and blood vessels. 2-[^{18}F]FDG uptake has been confirmed at the sites affected by RA with higher sensitivity early after the onset of clinical symptoms (Fig. 7.20). The degree of 2-[^{18}F]FDG uptake in affected joints reflects disease activity, which correlates with serum blood markers of inflammation (erythrocyte sedimentation rate [ESR], C-reactive protein), disease activity score, symptoms such as swelling and tenderness of joints, ultrasonography findings of synovitis and synovial thickening, and power Doppler studies for neovascularization [121–123].

Although little evidence exists for the utility of 2-[^{18}F]FDG PET/CT for the evaluation of therapeutic response, several reports show promising results in predicting the outcome of traditional treatment [124] and treatment with biologicals such as anti-tumor necrosis factor-α [123, 125,

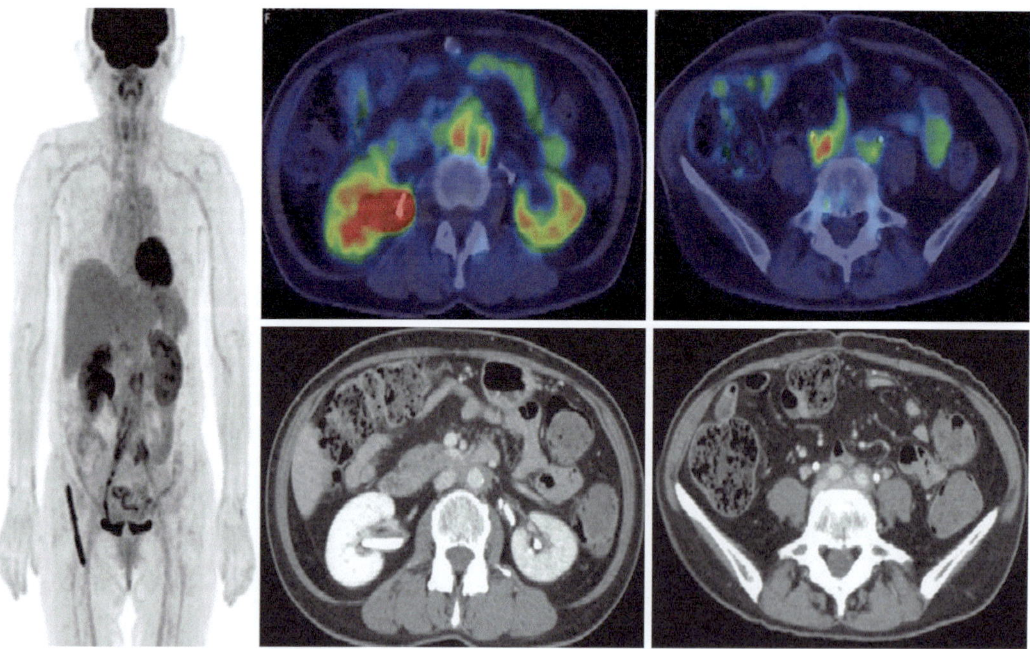

Fig. 7.19 IgG4-related vasculitis. 2-[^{18}F]FDG uptake is seen in the outer part of large vessels

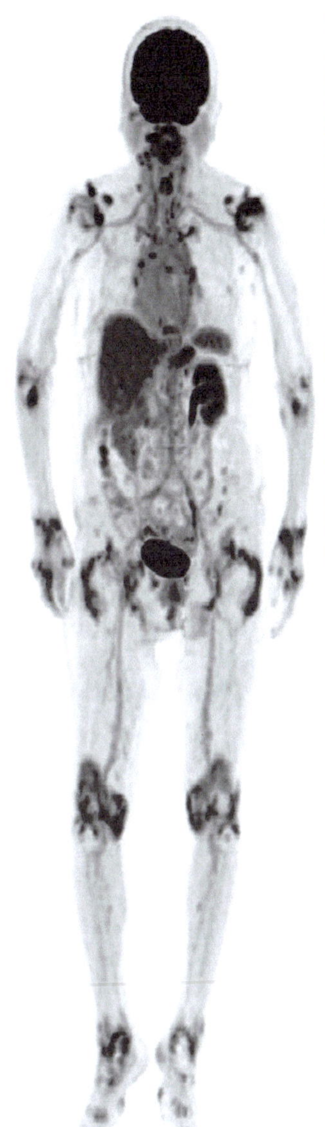

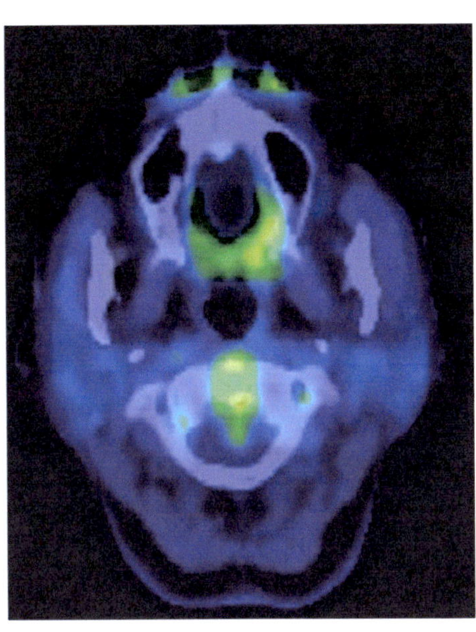

Fig. 7.20 Rheumatoid arthritis. Symmetrical 2-[¹⁸F]FDG uptake in large joints is a typical feature of rheumatoid arthritis. 2-[¹⁸F]FDG uptake at atlantoaxial joint may suggest the future occurrence of atlantoaxial subluxation which is an important and potentially life-threatening complication of rheumatoid arthritis

126]. Moreover, 2-[¹⁸F]FDG PET/CT can predict the outcome earlier than other types of morphological imaging [123, 126]. Due to insufficient evidence and according to the European League Against Rheumatism (EULAR) recommendation, 2-[¹⁸F]FDG PET is not recommended as an imaging tool for the diagnosis or therapy evaluation in RA [127].

7.10.5 Other Autoimmune Diseases

Limbic encephalitis is mainly caused by a viral infection (typically herpes simplex virus) and an autoimmune response against the limbic system. Autoimmune limbic encephalitis has two types: the paraneoplastic and non-paraneoplastic. The specific feature seen on 2-[¹⁸F]FDG

PET imaging is hypermetabolism in the temporal and orbitofrontal cortices and hypometabolism in the occipital lobe and bilateral basal ganglia [128, 129].

Multiple sclerosis is thought to be an autoimmune disease that leads to demyelination in the central nervous system. 2-[¹⁸F]FDG PET shows hypometabolism at demyelinated sites in the white matter, in addition to changes in glucose metabolism in the cortex [130].

7.11 Immune Deficiency (HIV-Related Disease)

Approximately 36.9 million people worldwide were living with HIV/AIDS in 2017. An estimated 1.8 million individuals worldwide became newly infected with HIV in 2017 [131]. AIDS-related morbidity and mortality have decreased due to advanced treatment options, advances in treatment access, and the establishment of effective prevention strategies, in addition to the low rate of new infections even in high-burden countries. The clinical manifestations of patients with HIV are variable and include a wide range of infections, malignancies, neurological disorders, and lifestyle diseases [132].

2-[¹⁸F]FDG uptake in lymph nodes of HIV patients is positively correlated with viral replication and inversely correlated with CD4 counts [133, 134]. This specific 2-[¹⁸F]FDG uptake is often misleading in the assessment of HIV-associated malignancies in patients with HIV infection (Fig. 7.21). 2-[¹⁸F]FDG PET is useful for distinguishing primary central nervous system lymphoma from opportunistic infections such as toxoplasmosis [135, 136].

In immunosuppressed patients, pulmonary TB occurs in an atypical pattern and increases the risk of extrapulmonary lesions. 2-[¹⁸F]FDG PET can be used to evaluate the distribution of TB lesions in the whole body [137, 138]. 2-[¹⁸F]FDG PET/CT has proven useful for ascertaining the source of infection in HIV-related FUO [139].

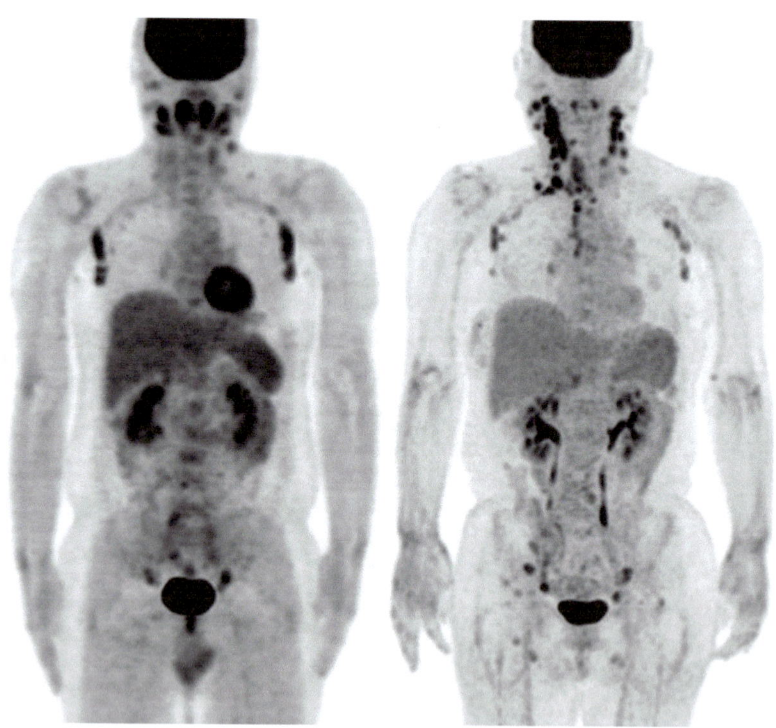

Fig. 7.21 HIV infection. The image on the left side shows nonspecific lymphadenopathies frequently seen in a patient with HIV infection. The image on the right side shows angioimmunoblastic T-cell lymphoma in a patient with HIV infection

7.12   Conclusion

This chapter introduces the impact of 2-[18F]FDG PET for the diagnosis and assessment of treatment in infections, inflammatory, and autoimmune diseases. 2-[18F]FDG PET can provide higher resolution images than conventional nuclear medicine examinations. Moreover, 2-[18F]FDG PET has the advantage of completing a whole-body scan in a short time. However, the utility of 2-[18F]FDG PET varies greatly, and the underlying mechanism of each disease still remains to be elucidated. Compared to malignancy, evidence for the usefulness of 2-[18F]FDG PET is still weak for assessing infections, inflammatory, and autoimmune diseases. Therefore, further evaluation will be required to determine the role of 2-[18F]FDG PET in these contexts.

References

1. Bell GI, Burant CF, Takeda J, Gould GW. Structure and function of mammalian facilitative sugar transporters. J Biol Chem. 1993;268(26):19161–4.
2. Pauwels EK, Ribeiro MJ, Stoot JH, McCready VR, Bourguignon M, Maziere B. FDG accumulation and tumor biology. Nucl Med Biol. 1998;25(4):317–22.
3. Zhuang H, Alavi A. 18-Fluorodeoxyglucose positron emission tomographic imaging in the detection and monitoring of infection and inflammation. Semin Nucl Med. 2002;32(1):47–59. https://doi.org/10.1053/snuc.2002.29278.
4. Mochizuki T, Tsukamoto E, Kuge Y, Kanegae K, Zhao S, Hikosaka K, et al. FDG uptake and glucose transporter subtype expressions in experimental tumor and inflammation models. J Nucl Med. 2001;42(10):1551–5.
5. O'Neill LA, Hardie DG. Metabolism of inflammation limited by AMPK and pseudo-starvation. Nature. 2013;493(7432):346–55. https://doi.org/10.1038/nature11862.
6. Basu S, Kwee TC, Surti S, Akin EA, Yoo D, Alavi A. Fundamentals of PET and PET/CT imaging. Ann N Y Acad Sci. 2011;1228:1–18. https://doi.org/10.1111/j.1749-6632.2011.06077.x.
7. Ohba K, Sasaki S, Oki Y, Nishizawa S, Matsushita A, Yoshino A, et al. Factors associated with fluorine-18-fluorodeoxyglucose uptake in benign thyroid nodules. Endocr J. 2013;60(8):985–90.
8. Vaidyanathan S, Patel CN, Scarsbrook AF, Chowdhury FU. FDG PET/CT in infection and inflammation—current and emerging clinical applications. Clin Radiol. 2015;70(7):787–800. https://doi.org/10.1016/j.crad.2015.03.010.
9. Bental M, Deutsch C. Metabolic changes in activated T cells: an NMR study of human peripheral blood lymphocytes. Magn Reson Med. 1993;29(3):317–26.
10. Marjanovic S, Skog S, Heiden T, Tribukait B, Nelson BD. Expression of glycolytic isoenzymes in activated human peripheral lymphocytes: cell cycle analysis using flow cytometry. Exp Cell Res. 1991;193(2):425–31. https://doi.org/10.1016/0014-4827(91)90116-c.
11. Kubota R, Yamada S, Kubota K, Ishiwata K, Tamahashi N, Ido T. Intratumoral distribution of fluorine-18-fluorodeoxyglucose in vivo: high accumulation in macrophages and granulation tissues studied by microautoradiography. J Nucl Med. 1992;33(11):1972–80.
12. Irmler IM, Opfermann T, Gebhardt P, Gajda M, Brauer R, Saluz HP, et al. In vivo molecular imaging of experimental joint inflammation by combined (18)F-FDG positron emission tomography and computed tomography. Arthritis Res Ther. 2010;12(6):R203. https://doi.org/10.1186/ar3176.
13. Rakesh Kumar MRN, Balakrishnan V, Bal C, Malhotra A. FDG-PET imaging in infection and inflammation. Indian J Nucl Med. 2006;21(4):10.
14. Tseng JR, Chen KY, Lee MH, Huang CT, Wen YH, Yen TC. Potential usefulness of FDG PET/CT in patients with sepsis of unknown origin. PLoS One. 2013;8(6):e66132. https://doi.org/10.1371/journal.pone.0066132.
15. Bleeker-Rovers CP, Vos FJ, de Kleijn EM, Mudde AH, Dofferhoff TS, Richter C, et al. A prospective multicenter study on fever of unknown origin: the yield of a structured diagnostic protocol. Medicine (Baltimore). 2007;86(1):26–38. https://doi.org/10.1097/MD.0b013e31802fe858.
16. Besson FL, Chaumet-Riffaud P, Playe M, Noel N, Lambotte O, Goujard C, et al. Contribution of (18)F-FDG PET in the diagnostic assessment of fever of unknown origin (FUO): a stratification-based meta-analysis. Eur J Nucl Med Mol Imaging. 2016;43(10):1887–95. https://doi.org/10.1007/s00259-016-3377-6.
17. Guhlmann A, Brecht-Krauss D, Suger G, Glatting G, Kotzerke J, Kinzl L, et al. Chronic osteomyelitis: detection with FDG PET and correlation with histopathologic findings. Radiology. 1998;206(3):749–54. https://doi.org/10.1148/radiology.206.3.9494496.
18. Sugawara Y, Braun DK, Kison PV, Russo JE, Zasadny KR, Wahl RL. Rapid detection of human infections with fluorine-18 fluorodeoxyglucose and positron emission tomography: preliminary results. Eur J Nucl Med. 1998;25(9):1238–43.
19. Bleeker-Rovers CP, Vos FJ, Corstens FH, Oyen WJ. Imaging of infectious diseases using [18F] fluorodeoxyglucose PET. Q J Nucl Med Mol Imaging. 2008;52(1):17–29.
20. de Winter F, van de Wiele C, Vogelaers D, de Smet K, Verdonk R, Dierckx RA. Fluorine-18

fluorodeoxyglucose-position emission tomography: a highly accurate imaging modality for the diagnosis of chronic musculoskeletal infections. J Bone Joint Surg Am. 2001;83(5):651–60. https://doi.org/10.2106/00004623-200105000-00002.

21. Hartmann A, Eid K, Dora C, Trentz O, von Schulthess GK, Stumpe KDM. Diagnostic value of 18F-FDG PET/CT in trauma patients with suspected chronic osteomyelitis. Eur J Nucl Med Mol Imaging. 2007;34(5):704–14. https://doi.org/10.1007/s00259-006-0290-4.

22. El-Haddad G, Zhuang H, Gupta N, Alavi A. Evolving role of positron emission tomography in the management of patients with inflammatory and other benign disorders. Semin Nucl Med. 2004;34(4): 313–29.

23. Palestro CJ. FDG-PET in musculoskeletal infections. Semin Nucl Med. 2013;43(5):367–76. https://doi.org/10.1053/j.semnuclmed.2013.04.006.

24. Termaat MF, Raijmakers PG, Scholten HJ, Bakker FC, Patka P, Haarman HJ. The accuracy of diagnostic imaging for the assessment of chronic osteomyelitis: a systematic review and meta-analysis. J Bone Joint Surg Am. 2005;87(11):2464–71. https://doi.org/10.2106/JBJS.D.02691.

25. Stumpe KD, Zanetti M, Weishaupt D, Hodler J, Boos N, Von Schulthess GK. FDG positron emission tomography for differentiation of degenerative and infectious endplate abnormalities in the lumbar spine detected on MR imaging. AJR Am J Roentgenol. 2002;179(5):1151–7. https://doi.org/10.2214/ajr.179.5.1791151.

26. Jamar F, Buscombe J, Chiti A, Christian PE, Delbeke D, Donohoe KJ, et al. EANM/SNMMI guideline for 18F-FDG use in inflammation and infection. J Nucl Med. 2013;54(4):647–58. https://doi.org/10.2967/jnumed.112.112524.

27. Prodromou ML, Ziakas PD, Poulou LS, Karsaliakos P, Thanos L, Mylonakis E. FDG PET is a robust tool for the diagnosis of spondylodiscitis: a meta-analysis of diagnostic data. Clin Nucl Med. 2014;39(4):330–5. https://doi.org/10.1097/RLU.0000000000000336.

28. Ito K, Kubota K, Morooka M, Hasuo K, Kuroki H, Mimori A. Clinical impact of (18)F-FDG PET/CT on the management and diagnosis of infectious spondylitis. Nucl Med Commun. 2010;31(8):691–8. https://doi.org/10.1097/MNM.0b013e32833bb25d.

29. Gemmel F, Rijk PC, Collins JM, Parlevliet T, Stumpe KD, Palestro CJ. Expanding role of 18F-fluoro-D-deoxyglucose PET and PET/CT in spinal infections. Eur Spine J. 2010;19(4):540–51. https://doi.org/10.1007/s00586-009-1251-y.

30. Sollini M, Raffaella B, Bandera F, Lazzeri E, Erba PA. Detection of device infection using nuclear cardiology imaging. Ann Nucl Cardiol. 2018;4(1):52–9. https://doi.org/10.17996/anc.18-00078.

31. Mahmood M, Kendi AT, Farid S, Ajmal S, Johnson GB, Baddour LM, et al. Role of (18)F-FDG PET/CT in the diagnosis of cardiovascular implantable electronic device infections: a meta-analysis. J Nucl Cardiol. 2019;26(3):958–70. https://doi.org/10.1007/s12350-017-1063-0.

32. Gomes A, Glaudemans A, Touw DJ, van Melle JP, Willems TP, Maass AH, et al. Diagnostic value of imaging in infective endocarditis: a systematic review. Lancet Infect Dis. 2017;17(1):e1–e14. https://doi.org/10.1016/S1473-3099(16)30141-4.

33. Saby L, Laas O, Habib G, Cammilleri S, Mancini J, Tessonnier L, et al. Positron emission tomography/computed tomography for diagnosis of prosthetic valve endocarditis: increased valvular 18F-fluorodeoxyglucose uptake as a novel major criterion. J Am Coll Cardiol. 2013;61(23):2374–82. https://doi.org/10.1016/j.jacc.2013.01.092.

34. Pizzi MN, Roque A, Fernandez-Hidalgo N, Cuellar-Calabria H, Ferreira-Gonzalez I, Gonzalez-Alujas MT, et al. Improving the diagnosis of infective endocarditis in prosthetic valves and intracardiac devices with 18F-fluordeoxyglucose positron emission tomography/computed tomography angiography: initial results at an infective endocarditis referral center. Circulation. 2015;132(12):1113–26. https://doi.org/10.1161/CIRCULATIONAHA.115.015316.

35. Salomaki SP, Saraste A, Kemppainen J, Bax JJ, Knuuti J, Nuutila P, et al. (18)F-FDG positron emission tomography/computed tomography in infective endocarditis. J Nucl Cardiol. 2017;24(1):195–206. https://doi.org/10.1007/s12350-015-0325-y.

36. Yan J, Zhang C, Niu Y, Yuan R, Zeng X, Ge X, et al. The role of 18F-FDG PET/CT in infectious endocarditis: a systematic review and meta-analysis. Int J Clin Pharmacol Ther. 2016;54(5):337–42. https://doi.org/10.5414/CP202569.

37. Habib G, Lancellotti P, Iung B. 2015 ESC guidelines on the management of infective endocarditis: a big step forward for an old disease. Heart. 2016;102(13):992–4. https://doi.org/10.1136/heartjnl-2015-308791.

38. Kestler M, Munoz P, Rodriguez-Creixems M, Rotger A, Jimenez-Requena F, Mari A, et al. Role of (18)F-FDG PET in patients with infectious endocarditis. J Nucl Med. 2014;55(7):1093–8. https://doi.org/10.2967/jnumed.113.134981.

39. Adler Y, Charron P, Imazio M, Badano L, Baron-Esquivias G, Bogaert J, et al. 2015 ESC guidelines for the diagnosis and management of pericardial diseases: the task force for the Diagnosis and Management of Pericardial Diseases of the European Society of Cardiology (ESC) endorsed by: The European Association for Cardio-Thoracic Surgery (EACTS). Eur Heart J. 2015;36(42):2921–64. https://doi.org/10.1093/eurheartj/ehv318.

40. Dong A, Dong H, Wang Y, Cheng C, Zuo C, Lu J. (18)F-FDG PET/CT in differentiating acute tuberculous from idiopathic pericarditis: preliminary study. Clin Nucl Med. 2013;38(4):e160–5. https://doi.org/10.1097/RLU.0b013e31827a2537.

41. Kilic A, Arnaoutakis DJ, Reifsnyder T, Black JH III, Abularrage CJ, Perler BA, et al. Management of infected vascular grafts. Vasc Med. 2016;21(1):53–60. https://doi.org/10.1177/1358863X15612574.

42. Darouiche RO. Treatment of infections associated with surgical implants. N Engl J Med. 2004;350(14):1422–9. https://doi.org/10.1056/NEJMra035415.

43. Perera GB, Fujitani RM, Kubaska SM. Aortic graft infection: update on management and treatment options. Vasc Endovasc Surg. 2006;40(1):1–10. https://doi.org/10.1177/153857440604000101.

44. Keidar Z, Pirmisashvili N, Leiderman M, Nitecki S, Israel O. 18F-FDG uptake in noninfected prosthetic vascular grafts: incidence, patterns, and changes over time. J Nucl Med. 2014;55(3):392–5. https://doi.org/10.2967/jnumed.113.128173.

45. Fukuchi K, Ishida Y, Higashi M, Tsunekawa T, Ogino H, Minatoya K, et al. Detection of aortic graft infection by fluorodeoxyglucose positron emission tomography: comparison with computed tomographic findings. J Vasc Surg. 2005;42(5):919–25. https://doi.org/10.1016/j.jvs.2005.07.038.

46. Spacek M, Belohlavek O, Votrubova J, Sebesta P, Stadler P. Diagnostics of "non-acute" vascular prosthesis infection using 18F-FDG PET/CT: our experience with 96 prostheses. Eur J Nucl Med Mol Imaging. 2009;36(5):850–8. https://doi.org/10.1007/s00259-008-1002-z.

47. Tokuda Y, Oshima H, Araki Y, Narita Y, Mutsuga M, Kato K, et al. Detection of thoracic aortic prosthetic graft infection with 18F-fluorodeoxyglucose positron emission tomography/computed tomography. Eur J Cardiothorac Surg. 2013;43(6):1183–7. https://doi.org/10.1093/ejcts/ezs693.

48. Cook GJ, Fogelman I, Maisey MN. Normal physiological and benign pathological variants of 18-fluoro-2-deoxyglucose positron-emission tomography scanning: potential for error in interpretation. Semin Nucl Med. 1996;26(4):308–14.

49. van der Bruggen W, Bleeker-Rovers CP, Boerman OC, Gotthardt M, Oyen WJ. PET and SPECT in osteomyelitis and prosthetic bone and joint infections: a systematic review. Semin Nucl Med. 2010;40(1):3–15. https://doi.org/10.1053/j.semnuclmed.2009.08.005.

50. Manthey N, Reinhard P, Moog F, Knesewitsch P, Hahn K, Tatsch K. The use of [18 F]fluorodeoxyglucose positron emission tomography to differentiate between synovitis, loosening and infection of hip and knee prostheses. Nucl Med Commun. 2002;23(7):645–53.

51. Zhuang H, Chacko TK, Hickeson M, Stevenson K, Feng Q, Ponzo F, et al. Persistent non-specific FDG uptake on PET imaging following hip arthroplasty. Eur J Nucl Med Mol Imaging. 2002;29(10):1328–33. https://doi.org/10.1007/s00259-002-0886-2.

52. Love C, Marwin SE, Palestro CJ. Nuclear medicine and the infected joint replacement. Semin Nucl Med. 2009;39(1):66–78. https://doi.org/10.1053/j.semnuclmed.2008.08.007.

53. Palestro CJ, Kim CK, Swyer AJ, Capozzi JD, Solomon RW, Goldsmith SJ. Total-hip arthroplasty: periprosthetic indium-111-labeled leukocyte activity and complementary technetium-99m-sulfur colloid imaging in suspected infection. J Nucl Med. 1990;31(12):1950–5.

54. Mulamba L, Ferrant A, Leners N, de Nayer P, Rombouts JJ, Vincent A. Indium-111 leucocyte scanning in the evaluation of painful hip arthroplasty. Acta Orthop Scand. 1983;54(5):695–7.

55. Soussan M, Brillet PY, Mekinian A, Khafagy A, Nicolas P, Vessieres A, et al. Patterns of pulmonary tuberculosis on FDG-PET/CT. Eur J Radiol. 2012;81(10):2872–6. https://doi.org/10.1016/j.ejrad.2011.09.002.

56. Yang CM, Hsu CH, Lee CM, Wang FC. Intense uptake of [F-18]-fluoro-2 deoxy-D-glucose in active pulmonary tuberculosis. Ann Nucl Med. 2003;17(5):407–10.

57. Goo JM, Im JG, Do KH, Yeo JS, Seo JB, Kim HY, et al. Pulmonary tuberculoma evaluated by means of FDG PET: findings in 10 cases. Radiology. 2000;216(1):117–21. https://doi.org/10.1148/radiology.216.1.r00jl19117.

58. Spiliopoulou I, Foka A, Bounas A, Marangos MN. Mycobacterium kansasii cutaneous infection in a patient with sarcoidosis treated with anti-TNF agents. Acta Clin Belg. 2014;69(3):229–31. https://doi.org/10.1179/0001551214Z.00000000052.

59. Hollings NP, Wells AU, Wilson R, Hansell DM. Comparative appearances of non-tuberculous mycobacteria species: a CT study. Eur Radiol. 2002;12(9):2211–7. https://doi.org/10.1007/s00330-001-1282-1.

60. Kim JS, Tanaka N, Newell JD, Degroote MA, Fulton K, Huitt G, et al. Nontuberculous mycobacterial infection: CT scan findings, genotype, and treatment responsiveness. Chest. 2005;128(6):3863–9. https://doi.org/10.1378/chest.128.6.3863.

61. Martinez V, Castilla-Lievre MA, Guillet-Caruba C, Grenier G, Fior R, Desarnaud S, et al. (18)F-FDG PET/CT in tuberculosis: an early non-invasive marker of therapeutic response. Int J Tuberc Lung Dis. 2012;16(9):1180–5. https://doi.org/10.5588/ijtld.12.0010.

62. Iannuzzi MC, Rybicki BA, Teirstein AS. Sarcoidosis. N Engl J Med. 2007;357(21):2153–65. https://doi.org/10.1056/NEJMra071714.

63. Studdy PR, Bird R. Serum angiotensin converting enzyme in sarcoidosis—its value in present clinical practice. Ann Clin Biochem. 1989;26(Pt 1):13–8. https://doi.org/10.1177/000456328902600102.

64. Prager E, Wehrschuetz M, Bisail B, Woltsche M, Schwarz T, Lanz H, et al. Comparison of 18F-FDG and 67Ga-citrate in sarcoidosis imaging. Nuklearmedizin. 2008;47(1):18–23.

65. Keijsers RG, Grutters JC, Thomeer M, Du Bois RM, Van Buul MM, Lavalaye J, et al. Imaging the inflammatory activity of sarcoidosis: sensitivity and inter observer agreement of (67)Ga imaging and (18)F-FDG PET. Q J Nucl Med Mol Imaging. 2011;55(1):66–71.

66. Keijsers RG, Verzijlbergen EJ, van den Bosch JM, Zanen P, van de Garde EM, Oyen WJ, et al. 18F-FDG PET as a predictor of pulmonary function

in sarcoidosis. Sarcoidosis Vasc Diffuse Lung Dis. 2011;28(2):123–9.

67. Mortensen J, Loft A, Baslund B. 18F-fluoro-deoxyglucose PET for monitoring treatment in sarcoidosis. Clin Respir J. 2007;1(2):124–6. https://doi.org/10.1111/j.1752-699X.2007.00035.x.

68. Shafee MA, Fukuda K, Wakayama Y, Nakano M, Kondo M, Hasebe Y, et al. Delayed enhancement on cardiac magnetic resonance imaging is a poor prognostic factor in patients with cardiac sarcoidosis. J Cardiol. 2012;60(6):448–53. https://doi.org/10.1016/j.jjcc.2012.08.002.

69. Schatka I, Bengel FM. Advanced imaging of cardiac sarcoidosis. J Nucl Med. 2014;55(1):99–106. https://doi.org/10.2967/jnumed.112.115121.

70. Teirstein AS, Machac J, Almeida O, Lu P, Padilla ML, Iannuzzi MC. Results of 188 whole-body fluorodeoxyglucose positron emission tomography scans in 137 patients with sarcoidosis. Chest. 2007;132(6):1949–53. https://doi.org/10.1378/chest.07-1178.

71. Ohira H, Tsujino I, Ishimaru S, Oyama N, Takei T, Tsukamoto E, et al. Myocardial imaging with 18F-fluoro-2-deoxyglucose positron emission tomography and magnetic resonance imaging in sarcoidosis. Eur J Nucl Med Mol Imaging. 2008;35(5):933–41. https://doi.org/10.1007/s00259-007-0650-8.

72. Ishida Y, Yoshinaga K, Miyagawa M, Moroi M, Kondoh C, Kiso K, et al. Recommendations for (18) F-fluorodeoxyglucose positron emission tomography imaging for cardiac sarcoidosis: Japanese Society of Nuclear Cardiology recommendations. Ann Nucl Med. 2014;28(4):393–403. https://doi.org/10.1007/s12149-014-0806-0.

73. Lum DP, Wandell S, Ko J, Coel MN. Reduction of myocardial 2-deoxy-2-[18F]fluoro-D-glucose uptake artifacts in positron emission tomography using dietary carbohydrate restriction. Mol Imaging Biol. 2002;4(3):232–7.

74. Coulden R, Chung P, Sonnex E, Ibrahim Q, Maguire C, Abele J. Suppression of myocardial 18F-FDG uptake with a preparatory "Atkins-style" low-carbohydrate diet. Eur Radiol. 2012;22(10):2221–8. https://doi.org/10.1007/s00330-012-2478-2.

75. Maurer AH, Burshteyn M, Adler LP, Gaughan JP, Steiner RM. Variable cardiac 18FDG patterns seen in oncologic positron emission tomography computed tomography: importance for differentiating normal physiology from cardiac and paracardiac disease. J Thorac Imaging. 2012;27(4):263–8. https://doi.org/10.1097/RTI.0b013e3182176675.

76. Jennette JC, Falk RJ, Andrassy K, Bacon PA, Churg J, Gross WL, et al. Nomenclature of systemic vasculitides. Proposal of an international consensus conference. Arthritis Rheum. 1994;37(2):187–92. https://doi.org/10.1002/art.1780370206.

77. Jennette JC, Falk RJ, Bacon PA, Basu N, Cid MC, Ferrario F, et al. 2012 revised International Chapel Hill Consensus Conference Nomenclature of Vasculitides. Arthritis Rheum. 2013;65(1):1–11. https://doi.org/10.1002/art.37715.

78. Carmona FD, Coit P, Saruhan-Direskeneli G, Hernandez-Rodriguez J, Cid MC, Solans R, et al. Analysis of the common genetic component of large-vessel vasculitides through a meta-Immunochip strategy. Sci Rep. 2017;7:43953. https://doi.org/10.1038/srep43953.

79. Maksimowicz-McKinnon K, Clark TM, Hoffman GS. Takayasu arteritis and giant cell arteritis: a spectrum within the same disease? Medicine (Baltimore). 2009;88(4):221–6. https://doi.org/10.1097/MD.0b013e3181af70c1.

80. Cheng Y, Lv N, Wang Z, Chen B, Dang A. 18-FDG-PET in assessing disease activity in Takayasu arteritis: a meta-analysis. Clin Exp Rheumatol. 2013;31(1 Suppl 75):S22–7.

81. Gravanis MB. Giant cell arteritis and Takayasu aortitis: morphologic, pathogenetic and etiologic factors. Int J Cardiol. 2000;75(Suppl 1):S21–33; discussion S5–6.

82. Besson FL, Parienti JJ, Bienvenu B, Prior JO, Costo S, Bouvard G, et al. Diagnostic performance of (1) (8)F-fluorodeoxyglucose positron emission tomography in giant cell arteritis: a systematic review and meta-analysis. Eur J Nucl Med Mol Imaging. 2011;38(9):1764–72. https://doi.org/10.1007/s00259-011-1830-0.

83. Slart R, Writing group; Reviewer group; Members of EANM Cardiovascular; Members of EANM Infection & Inflammation; Members of Committees, SNMMI Cardiovascular; Members of Council, PET Interest Group; Members of ASNC; EANM Committee Coordinator. FDG-PET/CT(A) imaging in large vessel vasculitis and polymyalgia rheumatica: joint procedural recommendation of the EANM, SNMMI, and the PET Interest Group (PIG), and endorsed by the ASNC. Eur J Nucl Med Mol Imaging. 2018;45(7):1250–69. https://doi.org/10.1007/s00259-018-3973-8.

84. Blockmans D, Stroobants S, Maes A, Mortelmans L. Positron emission tomography in giant cell arteritis and polymyalgia rheumatica: evidence for inflammation of the aortic arch. Am J Med. 2000;108(3):246–9. https://doi.org/10.1016/s0002-9343(99)00424-6.

85. Ernst D, Baerlecken NT, Schmidt RE, Witte T. Large vessel vasculitis and spondyloarthritis: coincidence or associated diseases? Scand J Rheumatol. 2014;43(3):246–8. https://doi.org/10.3109/03009742.2013.850737.

86. Lensen KD, Comans EF, Voskuyl AE, van der Laken CJ, Brouwer E, Zwijnenburg AT, et al. Large-vessel vasculitis: interobserver agreement and diagnostic accuracy of 18F-FDG-PET/CT. Biomed Res Int. 2015;2015:914692. https://doi.org/10.1155/2015/914692.

87. Blockmans D, de Ceuninck L, Vanderschueren S, Knockaert D, Mortelmans L, Bobbaers H. Repetitive 18F-fluorodeoxyglucose positron emission tomography in giant cell arteritis: a prospective study of 35 patients. Arthritis Rheum. 2006;55(1):131–7. https://doi.org/10.1002/art.21699.

88. Besson FL, de Boysson H, Parienti JJ, Bouvard G, Bienvenu B, Agostini D. Towards an optimal semi-quantitative approach in giant cell arteritis: an (18) F-FDG PET/CT case-control study. Eur J Nucl Med Mol Imaging. 2014;41(1):155–66. https://doi.org/10.1007/s00259-013-2545-1.

89. Tezuka D, Haraguchi G, Ishihara T, Ohigashi H, Inagaki H, Suzuki J, et al. Role of FDG PET-CT in Takayasu arteritis: sensitive detection of recurrences. JACC Cardiovasc Imaging. 2012;5(4):422–9. https://doi.org/10.1016/j.jcmg.2012.01.013.

90. Lehmann P, Buchtala S, Achajew N, Haerle P, Ehrenstein B, Lighvani H, et al. 18F-FDG PET as a diagnostic procedure in large vessel vasculitis-a controlled, blinded re-examination of routine PET scans. Clin Rheumatol. 2011;30(1):37–42. https://doi.org/10.1007/s10067-010-1598-9.

91. Cimmino MA, Zampogna G, Parodi M. Is FDG-PET useful in the evaluation of steroid-resistant PMR patients? Rheumatology (Oxford). 2008;47(6):926–7. https://doi.org/10.1093/rheumatology/ken098.

92. Pipitone N, Versari A, Salvarani C. Role of imaging studies in the diagnosis and follow-up of large-vessel vasculitis: an update. Rheumatology (Oxford). 2008;47(4):403–8. https://doi.org/10.1093/rheumatology/kem379.

93. Ben-Haim S, Kupzov E, Tamir A, Israel O. Evaluation of 18F-FDG uptake and arterial wall calcifications using 18F-FDG PET/CT. J Nucl Med. 2004;45(11):1816–21.

94. Dunphy MP, Freiman A, Larson SM, Strauss HW. Association of vascular 18F-FDG uptake with vascular calcification. J Nucl Med. 2005;46(8):1278–84.

95. Schollhammer R, Schwartz P, Jullie ML, Pham-Ledard A, Mercie P, Fernandez P, et al. 18F-FDG PET/CT imaging of popliteal vasculitis associated with polyarteritis nodosa. Clin Nucl Med. 2017;42(8):e385–e7. https://doi.org/10.1097/RLU.0000000000001711.

96. Demir S, Sag E, Dedeoglu F, Ozen S. Vasculitis in systemic autoinflammatory diseases. Front Pediatr. 2018;6:377. https://doi.org/10.3389/fped.2018.00377.

97. Geraldino-Pardilla L, Zartoshti A, Ozbek AB, Giles JT, Weinberg R, Kinkhabwala M, et al. Arterial inflammation detected with (18) F-fluorodeoxyglucose-positron emission tomography in rheumatoid arthritis. Arthritis Rheumatol. 2018;70(1):30–9. https://doi.org/10.1002/art.40345.

98. Kemna MJ, Bucerius J, Drent M, Voo S, Veenman M, van Paassen P, et al. Aortic (1)(8)F-FDG uptake in patients suffering from granulomatosis with polyangiitis. Eur J Nucl Med Mol Imaging. 2015;42(9):1423–9. https://doi.org/10.1007/s00259-015-3081-y.

99. Mooij CF, Hermsen R, Hoppenreijs EP, Bleeker-Rovers CP, IJland MM, de Geus-Oei LF. Fludeoxyglucose positron emission tomography-computed tomography scan showing polyarthritis in a patient with an atypical presentation of Henoch-Schonlein vasculitis without clinical signs of arthritis: a case report. J Med Case Rep. 2016;10(1):159. https://doi.org/10.1186/s13256-016-0913-8.

100. Treglia G, Quartuccio N, Sadeghi R, Farchione A, Caldarella C, Bertagna F, et al. Diagnostic performance of Fluorine-18-Fluorodeoxyglucose positron emission tomography in patients with chronic inflammatory bowel disease: a systematic review and a meta-analysis. J Crohns Colitis. 2013;7(5):345–54. https://doi.org/10.1016/j.crohns.2012.08.005.

101. Neurath MF, Vehling D, Schunk K, Holtmann M, Brockmann H, Helisch A, et al. Noninvasive assessment of Crohn's disease activity: a comparison of 18F-fluorodeoxyglucose positron emission tomography, hydromagnetic resonance imaging, and granulocyte scintigraphy with labeled antibodies. Am J Gastroenterol. 2002;97(8):1978–85. https://doi.org/10.1111/j.1572-0241.2002.05836.x.

102. Shreve PD, Anzai Y, Wahl RL. Pitfalls in oncologic diagnosis with FDG PET imaging: physiologic and benign variants. Radiographics. 1999;19(1):61–77; quiz 150-1. https://doi.org/10.1148/radiographics.19.1.g99ja0761.

103. Bicik I, Bauerfeind P, Breitbach T, von Schulthess GK, Fried M. Inflammatory bowel disease activity measured by positron-emission tomography. Lancet. 1997;350(9073):262. https://doi.org/10.1016/S0140-6736(05)62225-8.

104. Groshar D, Bernstine H, Stern D, Sosna J, Eligalashvili M, Gurbuz EG, et al. PET/CT enterography in Crohn disease: correlation of disease activity on CT enterography with 18F-FDG uptake. J Nucl Med. 2010;51(7):1009–14. https://doi.org/10.2967/jnumed.109.073130.

105. Meisner RS, Spier BJ, Einarsson S, Roberson EN, Perlman SB, Bianco JA, et al. Pilot study using PET/CT as a novel, noninvasive assessment of disease activity in inflammatory bowel disease. Inflamm Bowel Dis. 2007;13(8):993–1000. https://doi.org/10.1002/ibd.20134.

106. Deshpande V, Zen Y, Chan JK, Yi EE, Sato Y, Yoshino T, et al. Consensus statement on the pathology of IgG4-related disease. Mod Pathol. 2012;25(9):1181–92. https://doi.org/10.1038/modpathol.2012.72.

107. Nakatani K, Nakamoto Y, Togashi K. Utility of FDG PET/CT in IgG4-related systemic disease. Clin Radiol. 2012;67(4):297–305. https://doi.org/10.1016/j.crad.2011.10.011.

108. Ozaki Y, Oguchi K, Hamano H, Arakura N, Muraki T, Kiyosawa K, et al. Differentiation of autoimmune pancreatitis from suspected pancreatic cancer by fluorine-18 fluorodeoxyglucose positron emission tomography. J Gastroenterol. 2008;43(2):144–51. https://doi.org/10.1007/s00535-007-2132-y.

109. Perugino CA, Wallace ZS, Meyersohn N, Oliveira G, Stone JR, Stone JH. Large vessel involvement by IgG4-related disease. Medicine (Balti-

more). 2016;95(28):e3344. https://doi.org/10.1097/MD.0000000000003344.

110. Kasashima S, Zen Y, Kawashima A, Konishi K, Sasaki H, Endo M, et al. Inflammatory abdominal aortic aneurysm: close relationship to IgG4-related periaortitis. Am J Surg Pathol. 2008;32(2):197–204. https://doi.org/10.1097/PAS.0b013e3181342f0d.

111. Matsumoto Y, Kasashima S, Kawashima A, Sasaki H, Endo M, Kawakami K, et al. A case of multiple immunoglobulin G4-related periarteritis: a tumorous lesion of the coronary artery and abdominal aortic aneurysm. Hum Pathol. 2008;39(6):975–80. https://doi.org/10.1016/j.humpath.2007.10.023.

112. Zen Y, Kasashima S, Inoue D. Retroperitoneal and aortic manifestations of immunoglobulin G4-related disease. Semin Diagn Pathol. 2012;29(4):212–8. https://doi.org/10.1053/j.semdp.2012.07.003.

113. Inoue D, Zen Y, Abo H, Gabata T, Demachi H, Yoshikawa J, et al. Immunoglobulin G4-related periaortitis and periarteritis: CT findings in 17 patients. Radiology. 2011;261(2):625–33. https://doi.org/10.1148/radiol.11102250.

114. Patel NR, Anzalone ML, Buja LM, Elghetany MT. Sudden cardiac death due to coronary artery involvement by IgG4-related disease: a rare, serious complication of a rare disease. Arch Pathol Lab Med. 2014;138(6):833–6. https://doi.org/10.5858/arpa.2012-0614-CR.

115. Yabusaki S, Oyama-Manabe N, Manabe O, Hirata K, Kato F, Miyamoto N, et al. Characteristics of immunoglobulin G4-related aortitis/periaortitis and periarteritis on fluorodeoxyglucose positron emission tomography/computed tomography co-registered with contrast-enhanced computed tomography. EJNMMI Res. 2017;7(1):20. https://doi.org/10.1186/s13550-017-0268-1.

116. Settepani F, Monti L, Antunovic L, Torracca L. IgG4-related aortitis: multimodality imaging approach. Ann Thorac Surg. 2017;103(3):e289. https://doi.org/10.1016/j.athoracsur.2016.09.040.

117. Mavrogeni S, Markousis-Mavrogenis G, Kolovou G. IgG4-related cardiovascular disease. The emerging role of cardiovascular imaging. Eur J Radiol. 2017;86:169–75. https://doi.org/10.1016/j.ejrad.2016.11.012.

118. Sato Y, Kojima M, Takata K, Morito T, Asaoku H, Takeuchi T, et al. Systemic IgG4-related lymphadenopathy: a clinical and pathologic comparison to multicentric Castleman's disease. Mod Pathol. 2009;22(4):589–99. https://doi.org/10.1038/modpathol.2009.17.

119. Sato Y, Notohara K, Kojima M, Takata K, Masaki Y, Yoshino T. IgG4-related disease: historical overview and pathology of hematological disorders. Pathol Int. 2010;60(4):247–58. https://doi.org/10.1111/j.1440-1827.2010.02524.x.

120. Khosroshahi A, Wallace ZS, Crowe JL, Akamizu T, Azumi A, Carruthers MN, et al. International Consensus Guidance Statement on the Management and Treatment of IgG4-Related Disease. Arthritis Rheumatol. 2015;67(7):1688–99. https://doi.org/10.1002/art.39132.

121. Carey K, Saboury B, Basu S, Brothers A, Ogdie A, Werner T, et al. Evolving role of FDG PET imaging in assessing joint disorders: a systematic review. Eur J Nucl Med Mol Imaging. 2011;38(10):1939–55. https://doi.org/10.1007/s00259-011-1863-4.

122. Kubota K, Ito K, Morooka M, Minamimoto R, Miyata Y, Yamashita H, et al. FDG PET for rheumatoid arthritis: basic considerations and whole-body PET/CT. Ann N Y Acad Sci. 2011;1228:29–38. https://doi.org/10.1111/j.1749-6632.2011.06031.x.

123. Beckers C, Ribbens C, Andre B, Marcelis S, Kaye O, Mathy L, et al. Assessment of disease activity in rheumatoid arthritis with (18)F-FDG PET. J Nucl Med. 2004;45(6):956–64.

124. Roivainen A, Hautaniemi S, Mottonen T, Nuutila P, Oikonen V, Parkkola R, et al. Correlation of 18F-FDG PET/CT assessments with disease activity and markers of inflammation in patients with early rheumatoid arthritis following the initiation of combination therapy with triple oral antirheumatic drugs. Eur J Nucl Med Mol Imaging. 2013;40(3):403–10. https://doi.org/10.1007/s00259-012-2282-x.

125. Okamura K, Yonemoto Y, Arisaka Y, Takeuchi K, Kobayashi T, Oriuchi N, et al. The assessment of biologic treatment in patients with rheumatoid arthritis using FDG-PET/CT. Rheumatology (Oxford). 2012;51(8):1484–91. https://doi.org/10.1093/rheumatology/kes064.

126. Elzinga EH, van der Laken CJ, Comans EF, Boellaard R, Hoekstra OS, Dijkmans BA, et al. 18F-FDG PET as a tool to predict the clinical outcome of infliximab treatment of rheumatoid arthritis: an explorative study. J Nucl Med. 2011;52(1):77–80. https://doi.org/10.2967/jnumed.110.076711.

127. Colebatch AN, Edwards CJ, Ostergaard M, van der Heijde D, Balint PV, D'Agostino MA, et al. EULAR recommendations for the use of imaging of the joints in the clinical management of rheumatoid arthritis. Ann Rheum Dis. 2013;72(6):804–14. https://doi.org/10.1136/annrheumdis-2012-203158.

128. Fisher RE, Patel NR, Lai EC, Schulz PE. Two different 18F-FDG brain PET metabolic patterns in autoimmune limbic encephalitis. Clin Nucl Med. 2012;37(9):e213–8. https://doi.org/10.1097/RLU.0b013e31824852c7.

129. Rey C, Koric L, Guedj E, Felician O, Kaphan E, Boucraut J, et al. Striatal hypermetabolism in limbic encephalitis. J Neurol. 2012;259(6):1106–10. https://doi.org/10.1007/s00415-011-6308-2.

130. Faria Dde P, Copray S, Buchpiguel C, Dierckx R, de Vries E. PET imaging in multiple sclerosis. J Neuroimmune Pharmacol. 2014;9(4):468–82. https://doi.org/10.1007/s11481-014-9544-2.

131. gov. H. 2019. https://www.hiv.gov/hiv-basics/overview/data-and-trends/global-statistics.

132. Wagner TBS. PET/CT in infection and inflammation. Switzerland: Springer; 2018.

133. Iyengar S, Chin B, Margolick JB, Sabundayo BP, Schwartz DH. Anatomical loci of HIV-associated immune activation and association with viraemia. Lancet. 2003;362(9388):945–50. https://doi.org/10.1016/S0140-6736(03)14363-2.

134. Sathekge M, Maes A, Kgomo M, Van de Wiele C. Fluorodeoxyglucose uptake by lymph nodes of HIV patients is inversely related to CD4 cell count. Nucl Med Commun. 2010;31(2):137–40. https://doi.org/10.1097/MNM.0b013e3283331114.

135. Villringer K, Jager H, Dichgans M, Ziegler S, Poppinger J, Herz M, et al. Differential diagnosis of CNS lesions in AIDS patients by FDG-PET. J Comput Assist Tomogr. 1995;19(4):532–6.

136. Hoffman JM, Waskin HA, Schifter T, Hanson MW, Gray L, Rosenfeld S, et al. FDG-PET in differentiating lymphoma from nonmalignant central nervous system lesions in patients with AIDS. J Nucl Med. 1993;34(4):567–75.

137. Vorster M, Sathekge MM, Bomanji J. Advances in imaging of tuberculosis: the role of (1)(8)F-FDG PET and PET/CT. Curr Opin Pulm Med. 2014;20(3):287–93. https://doi.org/10.1097/MCP.0000000000000043.

138. Ankrah AO, van der Werf TS, de Vries EF, Dierckx RA, Sathekge MM, Glaudemans AW. PET/CT imaging of Mycobacterium tuberculosis infection. Clin Transl Imaging. 2016;4:131–44. https://doi.org/10.1007/s40336-016-0164-0.

139. Martin C, Castaigne C, Tondeur M, Flamen P, De Wit S. Role and interpretation of fluorodeoxyglucose-positron emission tomography/computed tomography in HIV-infected patients with fever of unknown origin: a prospective study. HIV Med. 2013;14(8):455–62. https://doi.org/10.1111/hiv.12030.

2-[^{18}F]FDG PET/CT in Fever of Unknown Origin

Ilse J. E. Kouijzer, Chantal P. Bleeker-Rovers, and Lioe-Fee de Geus-Oei

Contents

8.1   Introduction

Fever of unknown origin (FUO) refers to a prolonged febrile illness without an established etiology despite broad evaluation and diagnostic testing. In 1961, FUO was defined by Petersdorf and Beeson as an illness of more than 3 weeks duration with fever higher than 38.3 °C (101 °F) on several occasions and uncertain diagnosis after 1 week of hospitalization [1]. In 1992, this definition has been changed by removing the requirement that the evaluation must take place during hospitalization and also by excluding immunocompromised patients [2] because these patients need a different approach in diagnosis and therapy [3]. Later, the quantitative criterion of *diagnosis uncertain after a certain time period* was changed to a qualitative criterion that requires a certain set of diagnostic investigations to be performed [4–6].

FUO is characterized as conditions with (1) temperature ≥38.3 °C (101 °F) on a minimum of two occasions, (2) duration of illness ≥3 weeks or multiple febrile episodes during ≥3 weeks, (3) not immunocompromised (characterized as neutropenia for at least 1 week in the 3 months

I. J. E. Kouijzer (✉) · C. P. Bleeker-Rovers
Department of Internal Medicine and Radboud
Center for Infectious Diseases, Radboud University
Medical Center, Nijmegen, the Netherlands
e-mail: Ilse.Kouijzer@radboudumc.nl;
Chantal.Bleeker-Rovers@radboudumc.nl

L.-F. de Geus-Oei
Department of Radiology, Leiden University Medical
Center, Leiden, the Netherlands
e-mail: L.F.de_Geus-Oei@lumc.nl

© Springer Nature Switzerland AG 2022
S. Harsini et al. (eds.), *Nuclear Medicine and Immunology*,
https://doi.org/10.1007/978-3-030-81261-4_8

before the initiation of the fever, known hypogammaglobulinemia, known HIV-infection, or administration of 10 mg prednisone or equivalent for at least 2 weeks in the 3 months prior to the start of fever), and (4) indeterminate diagnosis despite comprehensive history taking, physical examination, and the following investigations: erythrocyte sedimentation rate or C-reactive protein, platelet count, leukocyte count and differentiation, hemoglobin, electrolytes, total serum protein, protein electrophoresis, creatinine, aspartate aminotransferase, alanine aminotransferase, alkaline phosphatase, creatine kinase, lactate dehydrogenase, antinuclear antibodies, rheumatoid factor, ferritin, three blood cultures, microscopic urinalysis, urine culture, abdominal ultrasonography, chest X-ray, and tuberculin skin test or interferon gamma release assay.

Having similar causes and workup, FUO is closely related to inflammation of unknown origin (IUO) [7]. The differential diagnosis of FUO can be categorized as infections, noninfectious inflammatory diseases (NIID), malignancies, and miscellaneous causes [6, 8]. In most cases of FUO, there is an uncommon manifestation of a common disease.

In diagnosing FUO, it is very important to search for potential diagnostic clues (PDCs). PDCs can be found by taking complete and repeated medical history, physical examination, and essential investigations. PDCs encompass all localizing signs, symptoms, and abnormalities possibly specifying a certain diagnosis. A limited list of probable diagnoses based on these PDCs should then be made. Further diagnostic measures should be limited to specific studies to corroborate or rule out these potential diseases since the majority of investigations are helpful only when performed in patients presenting with PDCs for the diagnosis searched for. When PDCs are absent, 2-[^{18}F]FDG PET/CT should be performed to guide additional diagnostic tests. In this chapter, the role of 2-[^{18}F]FDG PET/CT in patients with FUO is reviewed.

8.2 Morphological and Molecular Imaging

2-[^{18}F]FDG accumulates in cells with an increased rate of glycolysis. All activated leukocytes show increased 2-[^{18}F]FDG uptake leading to the delineation of acute and chronic inflammatory and infectious processes. The mechanism of 2-[^{18}F]FDG uptake in these activated leukocytes is related to the usage of glucose as the primary energy source only upon activation during the metabolic burst of these cells. 2-[^{18}F]FDG PET can be used to evaluate abnormalities throughout the body but has limitations for assessment of the urinary tract due to 2-[^{18}F]FDG excretion into the urine, of the brain due to high physiological accumulation of 2-[^{18}F]FDG, and potentially of the gastrointestinal tract due to diffuse or focal uptake as a result of peristalsis. Accumulation of 2-[^{18}F]FDG may be observed in the myocardium, which can be decreased by using a prior low-carbohydrate fat-allowed diet [9, 10] and additional heparin pre-administration [11].

In patients with fever, bone marrow uptake is frequently increased because of nonspecific activation of proliferating bone marrow cells due to the interleukin-dependent upregulation of glucose transporters [12]. Also, 2-[^{18}F]FDG uptake in the spleen may be diffusely increased in patients with fever, probably due to a shift in oxidative metabolism to glycolysis in the metabolism of proliferating effector T cells in the spleen which require high metabolic flux through growth-promoting pathways [13].

For 2-[^{18}F]FDG PET/CT, improved anatomical resolution by direct integration with CT has further boosted the accuracy of 2-[^{18}F]FDG PET. Focal infectious and inflammatory processes can also be detected by radiological techniques, such as CT, magnetic resonance imaging (MRI), and ultrasound. 2-[^{18}F]FDG PET/CT has some advantages compared to CT and MRI: (1) 2-[^{18}F]FDG PET/CT is more suitable as a screening method when clues for specific sites of infection are absent because it provides whole-body imaging in a single session without increasing radiation exposure; (2) it detects early metabolic activity rather than the relatively late anatomical changes as visualized by CT or MRI and does not rely on nonspecific signs such as edema or increased perfusion; (3) there are fewer artifacts due to metallic hardware; and (4) there are no contrast-related reactions. In contrast to conventional nuclear imaging techniques, 2-[18F]FDG PET/CT has the advantages of higher resolution, higher sensitivity in chronic low-grade infections, and high accuracy in the central skeleton, as well as the short time period between injection of the radiopharmaceutical and the moment of imaging [14]. Important disadvantages of conventional nuclear imaging, such as [67Ga]Ga-citrate scintigraphy and 111In-labeled or 99mTc-labeled leukocyte scintigraphy, are handling of potentially infected blood products (labeled leukocyte scintigraphy), high-radiation burden (111In-labeled leukocyte and [67Ga]Ga-citrate scintigraphy), instability of the labeling (99mTc-labeled leukocyte scintigraphy), and the relatively long time span between injection of the radiopharmaceutical and diagnosis ([67Ga]Ga-citrate scintigraphy).

8.3   2-[18F]FDG PET/CT in FUO

Because 2-[18F]FDG PET/CT provides whole-body imaging in a single session with relatively low radiation exposure, it plays an important role in the diagnostic investigation of FUO in clinical practice. Many studies on the value of 2-[18F]FDG PET and 2-[18F]FDG PET/CT in the diagnosis of FUO have been published. In these studies, authors have often referred to the effectiveness of imaging techniques in terms of sensitivity, specificity, and clinical helpfulness. However, calculating sensitivity and specificity in patients with FUO is difficult or even misleading due to the lack of a true gold standard. In addition, a final diagnosis cannot be established in a relatively high number of patients, and nonspecific 2-[18F]FDG uptake could result in false-positive findings and in limitations in the follow-up of these results. Therefore, in FUO, it is more useful to investigate the clinical helpfulness of 2-[18F]FDG PET/CT rather than sensitivities and specificities [12]. 2-[18F]FDG PET/CT is helpful when the 2-[18F]FDG PET/CT contributes to the final causal diagnosis of FUO. In case of negative 2-[18F]FDG PET/CT and persisting

FUO, it is probably more rewarding to wait for new PDCs to appear than immediately performing more screening investigations [15].

The value of 2-[18F]FDG PET/CT has been investigated in several studies (Table 8.1). Keidar et al. performed a prospective study on the value of 2-[18F]FDG PET/CT in 48 patients with FUO [16]. In this study, 2-[18F]FDG PET/CT identified the underlying etiology of FUO in 22 patients (46%). In 90% of patients, 2-[18F]FDG PET/CT contributed clinically important information to the diagnosis by exclusion of a focal etiology. Another prospective study in 240 patients with either FUO or IUO was performed by Schonau et al. [17]. 2-[18F]FDG PET/CT was helpful in 56.7% of all patients and 71.6% of patients with a final diagnosis. The likelihood of a helpful 2-[18F]FDG PET/CT was increased in case of the absence of intermittent fever, higher age, and elevated CRP level. Hung et al. [18] included 58 patients with FUO who both underwent gallium-67 single photon emission tomography computed tomography (SPECT)/CT and 2-[18F]FDG PET/CT within 7 days from each other. 2-[18F]FDG PET/CT was helpful in 57% of patients versus 33% for gallium-67 SPECT/CT. Pereira et al. [19] retrospectively investigated the value of 2-[18F]FDG PET/CT in 76 patients with FUO, which turned out to be helpful in 60% of patients. Another retrospective study on the value of 2-[18F]FDG PET/CT in FUO was performed by Gafter-Gvili et al. [20]. In this study in 112 patients with FUO, 2-[18F]FDG PET/CT was helpful in 46% of patients. Singh et al. [21] included 47 patients with FUO and found that 2-[18F]FDG PET/CT was helpful in 38% of patients. In this study, a final diagnosis could be established in 53% of patients. Tokmak et al. [22] concluded 2-[18F]FDG PET/CT to be helpful in 60% of 21 patients with FUO. In the study of Buch-Olsen et al. [23], 2-[18F]FDG PET/CT was helpful in 53% of 57 patients with FUO. Another study on 103 FUO patients by Manohar et al. [24] found that 2-[18F]FDG PET/CT was helpful in 60% of patients and all 63 patients with a final diagnosis, and 2-[18F]FDG PET/CT contributed to this diagnosis in 98%. Pedersen et al. [25] included 22 patients with FUO, and 2-[18F]FDG PET/CT successfully identified the cause of FUO in

Table 8.1 Review of the literature of 2-[^{18}F]FDG PET/CT in patients with FUO

Reference	Study design (number of patients)	FUO definition	Helpfulness of 2-[^{18}F]FDG PET/CT (%)
Keidar et al. 2008 [16]	Prospective (48)	Fever >38.3 °C > 3 weeks; no diagnosis after 1 week of inpatient investigations	46
Balink et al. 2009 [33]	Retrospective (68)	Not specified	56
Federici et al. 2010 [30]	Retrospective (10)	Fever >38.3 °C > 3 weeks; no diagnosis after 1 week of inpatient investigations	50
Ferda et al. 2010 [31]	Retrospective (48)	Not specified	54
Kei et al. 2010 [32]	Retrospective (12)	Fever >38.3 °C > 3 weeks; no diagnosis after >3 days inpatient investigations or 2 weeks outpatient investigations	42
Sheng et al. 2011 [28]	Retrospective (48)	Not specified	67
Pelosi et al. 2011 [29]	Retrospective (24)	Not specified	46
Pedersen et al. 2012 [25]	Retrospective (22)	Fever >38.3 °C > 3 weeks; no diagnosis after 3 days of inpatient investigations	45
Crouzet et al. 2012 [26]	Retrospective (79)	Not specified	75
Kim et al. 2012 [27]	Retrospective (48)	Not specified	52
Manohar et al. 2013 [24]	Retrospective (103)	Fever >38.3 °C > 3 weeks; no diagnosis after >1 week of inpatient or outpatient investigations	60
Tokmak et al. 2014 [22]	Retrospective (21)	Fever >38.3 °C > 3 weeks; no diagnosis after >1 week of inpatient investigations	60
Buch-Olsen et al. 2014 [23]	Retrospective (57)	Not specified	53
Singh et al. 2015 [21]	Retrospective (47)	Fever >38.3 °C > 3 weeks; no diagnosis after >1 week of inpatient investigations	38
Gafter-Gvili et al. 2015 [20]	Retrospective (112)	Fever >38.3 °C > 3 weeks; no diagnosis after >1 week of inpatient or outpatient investigations	46
Pereira et al. 2016 [19]	Retrospective (76)	Fever >38.3 °C > 3 weeks	60
Hung et al. 2017 [18]	Retrospective (58)	Fever >38.3 °C > 3 weeks; no diagnosis after >1 week of inpatient investigations	57
Schonau et al. 2018 [17]	Prospective (240)	Fever >38.3 °C > 3 weeks; no diagnosis after specific inpatient or outpatient investigations	57

45%. Crouzet et al. [26] investigated the diagnostic value of 2-[^{18}F]FDG PET/CT in 79 patients with FUO. 2-[^{18}F]FDG PET/CT was helpful in 57% of all FUO patients. In patients with a final diagnosis, 2-[^{18}F]FDG PET/CT contributed to this diagnosis in 74%. The study of Kim et al. [27] on 48 patients with FUO showed 2-[^{18}F] FDG PET/CT to be helpful in 52%. Sheng et al. [28] included 48 patients with FUO, and 2-[^{18}F] FDG PET/CT was helpful in 67% of cases. In 36 patients (75%), a final diagnosis was established,

and in 89%, 2-[^{18}F]FDG PET/CT contributed to this final diagnosis. The study of Pelosi et al. [29] on 24 patients with FUO showed 2-[^{18}F] PET/CT to be helpful in 46%. Federici et al. [30] investigated the value of 2-[^{18}F]FDG PET/CT in 10 FUO patients and 4 IUO patients. In this study, 2-[^{18}F]FDG PET/CT was helpful in 50% of both groups of patients. Ferda et al. [31] performed a retrospective study on 48 patients with FUO, and 2-[^{18}F]FDG PET/CT was concluded to be helpful in 54% of cases. The study of Kei et al. [32] in 12 patients with FUO showed 2-[¹⁸F]FDG PET/CT to be helpful in 42% of patients. Balink et al. [33] retrospectively included 68 patients with FUO who underwent 2-[¹⁸F]FDG PET/CT which was helpful in 56%. In this study, in 93% of positive studies, 2-[¹⁸F]FDG PET/CT led to the causal source of FUO, either by identifying the etiology of the FUO or by guiding further management.

Comparing these studies, however, is difficult as the definition of FUO was not further specified in all studies. The precise definition of FUO generally varied in all studies. In the study of Pereira et al. [19], immunocompromised patients were included, although these patients need a different approach and are difficult to compare with non-immunocompromised patients with FUO. In most of the studies, duration of follow-up was not mentioned. Furthermore, because the majority of these studies were retrospective in design, there may be inclusion bias as patients with negative findings on conventional imaging techniques are more likely to undergo 2-[¹⁸F]FDG PET/CT than patients with positive findings. The difference in timing of 2-[¹⁸F]FDG PET/CT and the selection of patients could also have affected the calculation of clinical helpfulness.

8.4   Timing of 2-[¹⁸F]FDG PET/CT in FUO

Several studies have been performed on timing of 2-[¹⁸F]FDG PET/CT in patients with FUO and/or IUO. One study showed that 2-[¹⁸F]FDG PET (without combined CT) did not contribute to the final diagnosis of FUO in case of normal C-reactive protein (CRP) and/or erythrocyte sedimentation rate (ESR) [15]. In a large study on 498 patients with FUO and IUO, a final diagnosis was established with 2-[¹⁸F]FDG PET/CT in 331 patients [34]. 2-[¹⁸F]FDG PET/CT had a diagnostic accuracy of 89%. Elevated CRP reflected the presence and degree of inflammation more reliably compared to ESR. 2-[¹⁸F]FDG PET/CT was 100% true negative only in patients with CRP less than 5 mg/l. Another retrospective investigation of 76 patients with FUO reported that 2-[¹⁸F]

FDG PET/CT was helpful and contributed toward the final diagnosis of FUO in patients with higher levels of CRP and ESR [35]. One prospective study on 240 patients with either FUO or IUO showed that elevated CRP level increased the likelihood for a diagnostic 2-[¹⁸F]FDG PET/CT [17]. A recent retrospective study on 104 patients with FUO or IUO showed that 2-[¹⁸F]FDG PET/CT was never contributive to the diagnosis when both inflammatory parameters and body temperature were normal [36].

8.5   Cost-Effectiveness

The cost-effectiveness of 2-[¹⁸F]FDG PET/CT has been investigated in two studies. In a Spanish study on the cost-effectiveness of 2-[¹⁸F]FDG PET/CT in 20 patients with FUO, the mean costs per patient of the diagnostic procedures preceding 2-[¹⁸F]FDG PET/CT were €11,167, which included the costs of 11 days of hospitalization on average and which also included outpatient checks [37]. When 2-[¹⁸F]FDG PET/CT had been performed earlier in the diagnostic process of FUO, €5471 per patient would have been saved on costs concerning hospitalization days as well as on costs concerning diagnostic tests. The second study on the cost-effectiveness of 2-[¹⁸F]FDG PET/CT was performed in 46 patients with IUO [38]. In this retrospective study, all patients underwent 2-[¹⁸F]FDG PET/CT and were compared with 46 patients with IUO using a diagnostic algorithm without 2-[¹⁸F]FDG PET/CT. Of all patients who underwent 2-[¹⁸F]FDG PET/CT, a final diagnosis was established in 32 patients (70%). The estimated mean costs per patient of all diagnostic procedures with 2-[¹⁸F]FDG PET/CT were €1821. When costs of mean number of hospitalization days per patient (6.9 days, range 0–32 days) were added, the mean costs increased to €5298 per patient. In patients in whom no 2-[¹⁸F]FDG PET/CT was performed, a diagnosis on IUO was reached in 14 patients (30%). Estimated mean costs per patient of all diagnostic procedures without 2-[¹⁸F]FDG PET/CT were €2051. Following adding costs of mean number of hospitalization days per patient (21 days, unknown range), the mean costs increased to €12,614 per patient. Therefore, 2-[¹⁸F]FDG PET/CT appears to be a cost-effective routine imaging technique for diagnostic decision-making by avoiding further unnecessary, invasive, and expensive investigations and also by reducing total hospitalization duration (Fig. 8.1).

8.6 Conclusion

In patients with FUO, 2-[¹⁸F]FDG PET/CT is a very helpful imaging technique with favorable characteristics that appears to be a cost-effective routine imaging modality by avoiding unnecessary investigations and reducing the duration of hospitalization. 2-[¹⁸F]FDG PET/CT should be a routine procedure in the FUO workup when diagnostic clues are absent.

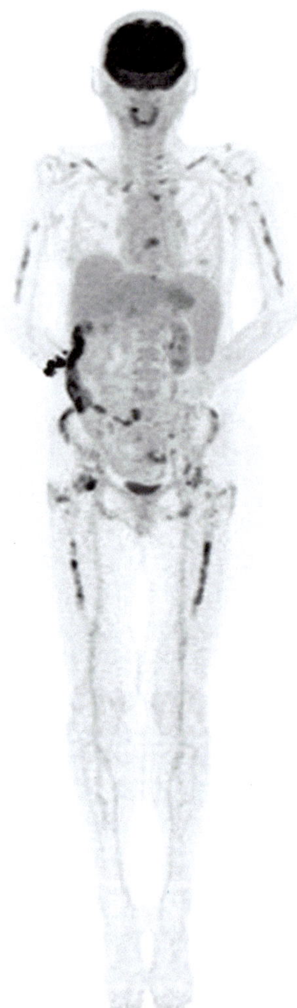

Fig. 8.1 A 63-year-old woman presented with fever, malaise, weight loss, and night sweats. Physical examination was unremarkable. Laboratory results showed increased ESR (88 mm/h) and anemia (Hb 6.1 mmol/l) with low reticulocyte count (14%). Blood cultures were negative. Random bone marrow biopsy showed reactive changes without other abnormalities. 2-[¹⁸F]FDG PET/CT showed a patchy 2-[¹⁸F] FDG uptake pattern in the musculoskeletal system, suspicious for lymphoma. Bone biopsy of the femur where increased 2-[¹⁸F]FDG uptake was present showed an extended localization of large B-cell lymphoma

References

1. Petersdorf RG, Beeson PB. Fever of unexplained origin: report on 100 cases. Medicine (Baltimore). 1961;40:1–30.
2. Petersdorf RG. Fever of unknown origin. An old friend revisited. Arch Intern Med. 1992;152(1):21–2.
3. Durack DT, Street AC. Fever of unknown origin—reexamined and redefined. Curr Clin Top Infect Dis. 1991;11:35–51.
4. de Kleijn EM, Vandenbroucke JP, van der Meer JW. Fever of unknown origin (FUO). I. A prospective multicenter study of 167 patients with FUO, using fixed epidemiologic entry criteria. The Netherlands FUO Study Group. Medicine. 1997;76(6):392–400.
5. de Kleijn EM, van Lier HJ, van der Meer JW. Fever of unknown origin (FUO). II. Diagnostic procedures in a prospective multicenter study of 167 patients. The Netherlands FUO Study Group. Medicine. 1997;76(6):401–14.
6. Bleeker-Rovers CP, Vos FJ, de Kleijn EM, Mudde AH, Dofferhoff TS, Richter C, et al. A prospective multicenter study on fever of unknown origin: the yield of a structured diagnostic protocol. Medicine (Baltimore). 2007;86(1):26–38.
7. Vanderschueren S, Del Biondo E, Ruttens D, Van Boxelaer I, Wauters E, Knockaert DD. Inflammation of unknown origin versus fever of unknown origin: two of a kind. Eur J Intern Med. 2009;20(4):415–8.
8. Vanderschueren S, Knockaert D, Adriaenssens T, Demey W, Durnez A, Blockmans D, et al. From prolonged febrile illness to fever of unknown origin: the challenge continues. Arch Intern Med. 2003;163(9):1033–41.
9. de Groot M, Meeuwis AP, Kok PJ, Corstens FH, Oyen WJ. Influence of blood glucose level, age and fasting period on non-pathological FDG uptake in heart and gut. Eur J Nucl Med Mol Imaging. 2005;32(1):98–101.
10. Balink H, Hut E, Pol T, Flokstra FJ, Roef M. Suppression of 18F-FDG myocardial uptake using a fat-allowed, carbohydrate-restricted diet. J Nucl Med Technol. 2011;39(3):185–9.
11. Scholtens AM, Verberne HJ, Budde RP, Lam MG. Additional heparin preadministration improves

cardiac glucose metabolism suppression over low-carbohydrate diet alone in (1)(8)F-FDG PET imaging. J Nucl Med. 2016;57(4):568–73.

12. Meller J, Sahlmann CO, Scheel AK. 18F-FDG PET and PET/CT in fever of unknown origin. J Nucl Med. 2007;48(1):35–45.

13. Ahn SS, Hwang SH, Jung SM, Lee SW, Park YB, Yun M, et al. Evaluation of spleen glucose metabolism using (18)F-FDG PET/CT in patients with febrile autoimmune disease. J Nucl Med. 2017;58(3): 507–13.

14. Bleeker-Rovers CP, Boerman OC, Rennen HJ, Corstens FH, Oyen WJ. Radiolabeled compounds in diagnosis of infectious and inflammatory disease. Curr Pharm Des. 2004;10(24):2935–50.

15. Bleeker-Rovers CP, Vos FJ, Mudde AH, Dofferhoff ASM, de Geus-Oei LF, Rijnders AJ, et al. A prospective multi-centre study of the value of FDG-PET as part of a structured diagnostic protocol in patients with fever of unknown origin. Eur J Nucl Med Mol Imaging. 2007;34(5):694–703.

16. Keidar Z, Gurman-Balbir A, Gaitini D, Israel O. Fever of unknown origin: the role of 18F-FDG PET/CT. J Nucl Med. 2008;49(12):1980–5.

17. Schonau V, Vogel K, Englbrecht M, Wacker J, Schmidt D, Manger B, et al. The value of (18)F-FDG-PET/CT in identifying the cause of fever of unknown origin (FUO) and inflammation of unknown origin (IUO): data from a prospective study. Ann Rheum Dis. 2018;77(1):70–7.

18. Hung BT, Wang PW, Su YJ, Huang WC, Chang YH, Huang SH, et al. The efficacy of (18)F-FDG PET/CT and (67)Ga SPECT/CT in diagnosing fever of unknown origin. Int J Infect Dis. 2017;62:10–7.

19. Pereira AM, Husmann L, Sah BR, Battegay E, Franzen D. Determinants of diagnostic performance of 18F-FDG PET/CT in patients with fever of unknown origin. Nucl Med Commun. 2016;37(1): 57–65.

20. Gafter-Gvili A, Raibman S, Grossman A, Avni T, Paul M, Leibovici L, et al. [18F]FDG-PET/CT for the diagnosis of patients with fever of unknown origin. QJM. 2015;108(4):289–98.

21. Singh N, Kumar R, Malhotra A, Bhalla AS, Kumar U, Sood R. Diagnostic utility of fluorodeoxyglucose positron emission tomography/computed tomography in pyrexia of unknown origin. Indian J Nucl Med. 2015;30(3):204–12.

22. Tokmak H, Ergonul O, Demirkol O, Cetiner M, Ferhanoglu B. Diagnostic contribution of (18)F-FDG-PET/CT in fever of unknown origin. Int J Infect Dis. 2014;19:53–8.

23. Buch-Olsen KM, Andersen RV, Hess S, Braad PE, Schifter S. 18F-FDG-PET/CT in fever of unknown origin: clinical value. Nucl Med Commun. 2014;35(9):955–60.

24. Manohar K, Mittal BR, Jain S, Sharma A, Kalra N, Bhattacharya A, et al. F-18 FDG-PET/CT in evalu-ation of patients with fever of unknown origin. Jpn J Radiol. 2013;31(5):320–7.

25. Pedersen TI, Roed C, Knudsen LS, Loft A, Skinhoj P, Nielsen SD. Fever of unknown origin: a retrospective study of 52 cases with evaluation of the diagnostic utility of FDG-PET/CT. Scand J Infect Dis. 2012;44(1):18–23.

26. Crouzet J, Boudousq V, Lechiche C, Pouget JP, Kotzki PO, Collombier L, et al. Place of (18)F-FDG-PET with computed tomography in the diagnostic algorithm of patients with fever of unknown origin. Eur J Clin Microbiol Infect Dis. 2012;31(8):1727–33.

27. Kim YJ, Kim SI, Hong KW, Kang MW. Diagnostic value of 18F-FDG PET/CT in patients with fever of unknown origin. Intern Med J. 2012;42(7):834–7.

28. Sheng JF, Sheng ZK, Shen XM, Bi S, Li JJ, Sheng GP, et al. Diagnostic value of fluorine-18 fluorodeoxyglucose positron emission tomography/computed tomography in patients with fever of unknown origin. Eur J Intern Med. 2011;22(1):112–6.

29. Pelosi E, Skanjeti A, Penna D, Arena V. Role of integrated PET/CT with [(1)(8)F]-FDG in the management of patients with fever of unknown origin: a single-centre experience. Radiol Med. 2011;116(5):809–20.

30. Federici L, Blondet C, Imperiale A, Sibilia J, Pasquali JL, Pflumio F, et al. Value of (18)F-FDG-PET/CT in patients with fever of unknown origin and unexplained prolonged inflammatory syndrome: a single centre analysis experience. Int J Clin Pract. 2010;64(1): 55–60.

31. Ferda J, Ferdova E, Zahlava J, Matejovic M, Kreuzberg B. Fever of unknown origin: a value of (18) F-FDG-PET/CT with integrated full diagnostic isotropic CT imaging. Eur J Radiol. 2010;73(3):518–25.

32. Kei PL, Kok TY, Padhy AK, Ng DC, Goh AS. [18F] FDG PET/CT in patients with fever of unknown origin: a local experience. Nucl Med Commun. 2010;31(9):788–92.

33. Balink H, Collins J, Bruyn GA, Gemmel F. F-18 FDG PET/CT in the diagnosis of fever of unknown origin. Clin Nucl Med. 2009;34(12):862–8.

34. Balink H, Veeger NJ, Bennink RJ, Slart RH, Holleman F, van Eck-Smit BL, et al. The predictive value of C-reactive protein and erythrocyte sedimentation rate for 18F-FDG PET/CT outcome in patients with fever and inflammation of unknown origin. Nucl Med Commun. 2015;36(6):604–9.

35. Okuyucu K, Alagoz E, Demirbas S, Ince S, Karakas A, Karacalioglu O, et al. Evaluation of predictor variables of diagnostic [18F] FDG-PET/CT in fever of unknown origin. Q J Nucl Med Mol Imaging. 2018;62(3):313–20.

36. Mulders-Manders CM, Kouijzer IJE, Janssen MJR, Oyen WJG, Simon A, Bleeker-Rovers CP. Optimal use of [18F]FDG-PET/CT in patients with fever or inflammation of unknown origin. Q J Nucl Med Mol Imaging. 2021;65(1):51–8.

37. Nakayo EMB, Vicente AMG, Castrejon AMS, Narvaez JAM, Rubio MPT, Garcia VMP, et al. Analysis of cost-effectiveness in the diagnosis of fever of unknown origin and the role of F-18-FDG PET-CT: a proposal of diagnostic algorithm. Rev Esp Med Nucl Imagen Mol. 2012;31(4):178–86.

38. Balink H, Tan SS, Veeger NJGM, Holleman F, van Eck-Smit BLF, Bennink RJ, et al. F-18-FDG PET/CT in inflammation of unknown origin: a cost-effectiveness pilot-study. Eur J Nucl Med Mol Imaging. 2015;42(9):1408–13.

Tumor-Targeting Agents

9

Dhritiman Chakraborty, Abhijit Das, and C. S. Bal

Contents

D. Chakraborty
Department of Nuclear and Experimental Medicine,
Institute of PGMER, Kolkota, India

A. Das
Department of Pathology, Janakpuri Superspeciality
Hospital Society, New Delhi, India

C. S. Bal (✉)
Department of Nuclear Medicine, All India Institute
of Medical Sciences, New Delhi, India

© Springer Nature Switzerland AG 2022
S. Harsini et al. (eds.), *Nuclear Medicine and Immunology*,
https://doi.org/10.1007/978-3-030-81261-4_9

9.1 Introduction

Targeted therapy with monoclonal antibody involves a greater understanding of the underlying pathology of cancer development and metastases, interaction of tumor cells with its microenvironment, and advancements in molecular techniques determining the underlying metabolic and enzymatic processes. The unique targets could be a membrane receptor, an enzyme, and a part of the signaling pathway present specifically or over-expressed in a tumor cell or the tumor micro-environment [1, 2]. Targeting involves either specific monoclonal antibodies or other novel constructs, including small molecule inhibitors. Hence, understanding the pathogenesis of tumor development, metastases, and interaction of cells with its microenvironment is important for dis-covering targeted therapeutics [3, 4]. The tumor comprises parenchymal components (formed by the malignant cells in different stages of devel-opment) and stromal components. Stromal com-ponent is composed of supporting connective tissue extracellular matrix (ECM) formed by the mesh of polysaccharides and fibrous proteins, cells including inflammatory/immune cells (lym-phocytes, natural killer cells, tumor-associated macrophages), fibroblast, mesenchymal stromal cells, pericytes, blood and lymphatic network channels, and occasionally adipocytes [5].

The metastases from the primary tumor mass after initial growth of malignant cells involve a series of steps, including extensive vasculariza-tion (by angiogenesis factors), local invasion in the stroma, invasion into the blood vessels, detachment and embolization of cells, aggrega-tion in the capillary bed of distant organs, extrav-asation from the vessels, and proliferation within distant organs. All the steps are tightly regulated by tumor cells' interaction with the tumor micro-environment (TME) [6].

With the development of newer technologies, like DNA sequencing technologies, discovering the unique genetic and molecular alterations in the tumor cells and a greater understanding of the role of different signaling pathways affected in the tumor cells, the use of the targeted therapies seems possible. Characteristic targets within the tumor cell and the TME, like vascular and the immune component, have been identified and utilized for targeted therapy (Table 9.1). Most of the currently used targeting agents include either the monoclonal antibodies or the small molecule inhibitors. Further advancements in this field have occurred, and many new novel constructs for targeting have been discovered.

Table 9.1 Different targets in tumor cell or tumor micro-environment utilized for developing targeted therapies [7]

Tyrosine kinase
• BCR-ABL tyrosine kinase
• ALK fusion protein
• EGFR
• PDGFR
• HER2
• VEGF
• Rapidly Accelerated Fibrosarcoma (RAF)/ mitogen extracellular kinase (MEK)/extracellular signal-related kinase (ERK) signal transduction pathway
The mammalian target of rapamycin (mTOR) pathway serine/threonine kinase
Proteasome
Histone deacetylase
PARP1/2
CTLA-4
PD1/PD-L1
Antigens overexpressed on cells such as CD20, CD30, CD52, etc.

ALK anaplastic lymphoma kinase, *EGFR* epidermal growth factor receptor, *PDGFR* platelet-derived growth factor receptor, *HER2* human epidermal growth factor receptor 2, *VEGF* vascular endothelial growth factor, *PARP* poly ADP ribose polymerase, *CTLA-4* cytotoxic T-lymphocyte-associated protein 4, *PD1* programmed cell death protein 1, *PD-L1* programmed death-ligand 1, *CD* cluster of differentiation

9.2 Ligand Targeted Therapy

The use of targeted drugs (e.g., monoclonal anti-body, small molecule inhibitor) directed toward particular physiologic processes (Fig. 9.1) in tumor cell (which are required for tumor growth, e.g., targeting signaling pathways, angiogenesis) or tagging any toxic drug with other ligand targeting component (e.g., monoclonal antibody or polymer) or ligand targeted nano-drug reservoirs containing active drug (e.g., liposome) ultimately results in increased exposure of drugs to tumor cells rather than the normal cell in the body (Table 9.2) [8, 9]. Few points should be considered before selecting a target in the tumor cell (Table 9.3).

Particle size has significant effects on clear-ance time and tumor penetrability (Fig. 9.2). Monoclonal antibodies (mAbs) and antibody fragments are given intravenously. Considering renal threshold of ~70 kDa, intact mAbs with

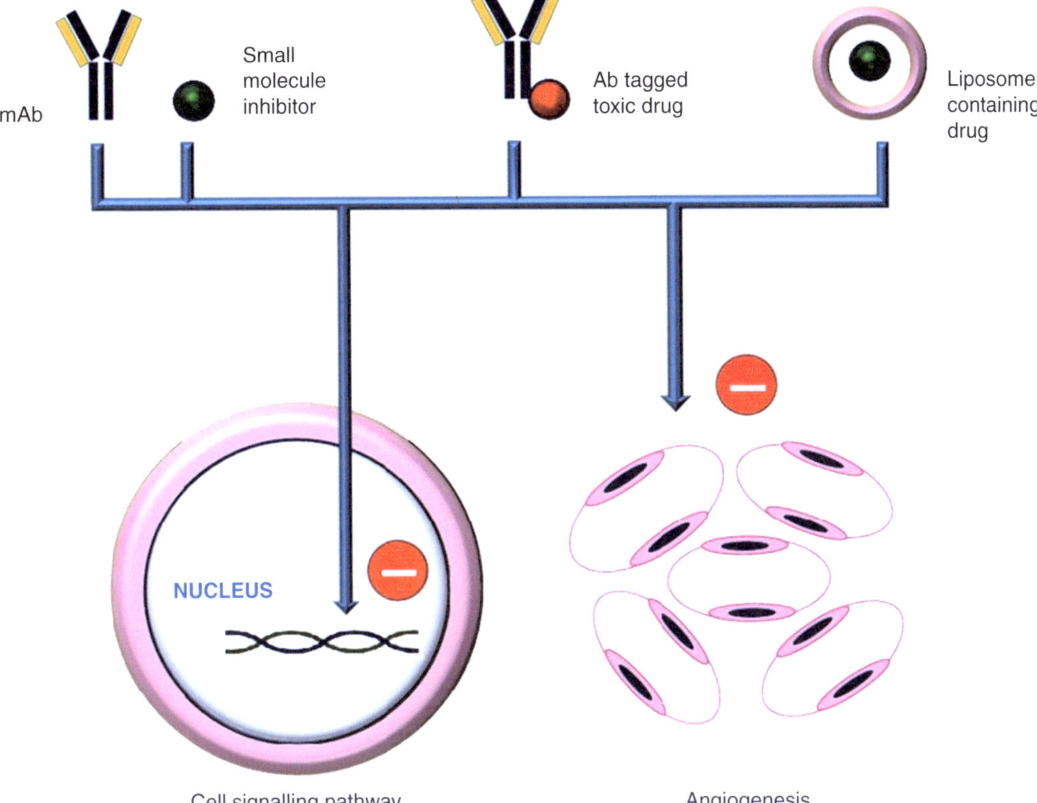

Fig. 9.1 Basic overview of ligand targeted therapy

Table 9.2 Ligand (antibody/non-antibody)-based therapy spectrum

As targeted drug
- Monoclonal antibody/small molecule inhibitors

As vehicle
- Immunotoxin/immunoconjugate/fusion protein conjugate

As part of nano-drug reservoir containing active drug (e.g., liposome)

Table 9.3 Issues to be considered prior to selection of targets

Targeted antigen/receptor should have high density [10] and less heterogeneous expression, and the cell should not shed or downregulate the targeted antigen.

Internalization of target-ligand complex
- Might increase or decrease the efficacy of the therapeutic molecule
- Immunoliposome complex, immunotoxins, radiometal-labeled antibody (e.g., [^{177}Lu] Lu-rituximab) will be benefited from the internalization
- Deiodinase, an ubiquitous enzyme that is present in most of the tissues, shall break the carbon-iodine bond to release free radioiodine from the labeled antibody (e.g., [^{131}I]I-tositumomab)
- Internalization will hamper the effect of antibody-directed enzyme/prodrug therapy because enzyme must be present at the surface of the cell for the conversion of prodrug to an active drug [11]

molecular weight of ~150 kDa stay in circulation for a longer time, whereas different antibody fragments which have a molecular weight less than the glomerular threshold limit (scFv, 25 kDa; Fab, 50 kDa; F(ab)$_2$, 100 kDa) stay in circulation for less time [12, 13].

Small molecule inhibitor drugs are usually much smaller in size (≤500 Da), translocate easily through plasma membranes, and are amenable

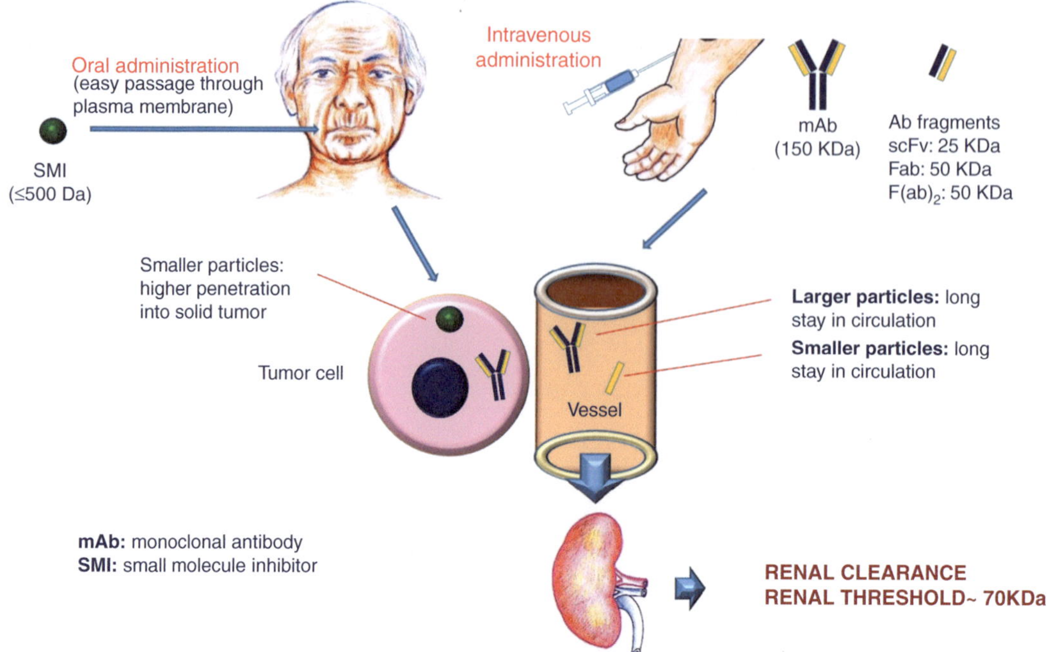

Fig. 9.2 The impact of particle size on tumor penetrability and renal clearance

to oral administration. In general, smaller particles have higher penetration into solid tumor tissue, considering their size criteria, which changes the kidney filtration. Larger particles, such as immunoliposomes (approximately 100–150 nm in diameter), can take 48 h or longer to reach peak levels in the tumor. For these nanocarriers, it is important not only that the particles circulate for sufficient time in circulation to allow for maximum tumor localization, but also stability of construct to retain their drug contents during this process is important [14].

9.3 Antibody

Antibodies are the immunoglobulins (Igs) secreted by differentiated B cells called plasma cells, which form the adaptive immune system. There are two physical forms of antibodies present in the body, soluble form (present free in the blood plasma) and the membrane-bound form (attached to the surface of a B cell) and is also referred to as the B-cell receptor.

There are five types of antibodies named IgA, IgD, IgE, IgG, and IgM present. These are classed according to the heavy chain (alpha, delta, epsilon, gamma, or mu, respectively) present in the structure. These antibodies differ in the sequence, constant domains, hinge structure, and valencies.

IgG is the most common type. It is composed of a pair of heavy and light polypeptide chains assembled to form a "Y"-shaped structure. The light and heavy polypeptide chains fold into repeated immunoglobulin folds and create either constant or variable domains (Fig. 9.3). Functionally, it can be divided into two parts:

- Fab fragment (antigen-binding fragment) recognizes the antigen and consists of two variable and two constant domains. Two variable domains form the variable fragment (Fv). Each variable domain contains three hypervariable loops, known as complementarity determining regions (CDRs), which provide a specific antigen recognition site called paratope, binding to the antigen's epitope [15].

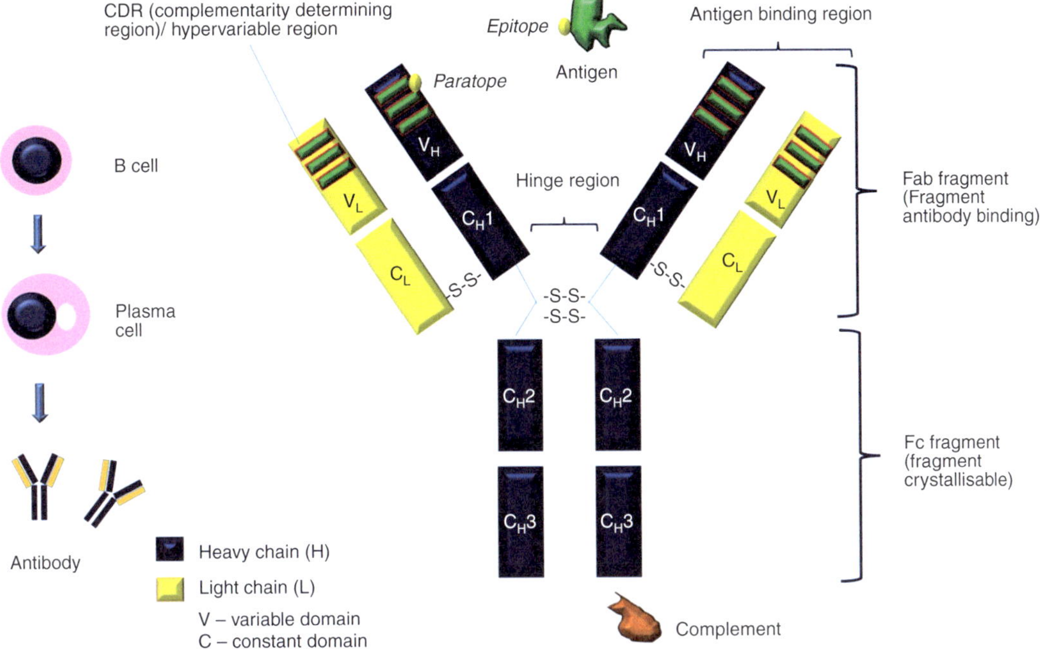

Fig. 9.3 Antibody structure

- Fc fragment (crystallizable fragment). It is the tail region of an antibody that consists of four constant domains. Constant domain interacts with other elements of the immune system, such as phagocytes or components of the complement pathway [16].

9.3.1 Monoclonal Antibody

Monoclonal antibodies (mAbs) are antibodies with specificity for one particular epitope on an antigen. Large quantities of monoclonal antibodies can be produced by the hybridoma technique (Fig. 9.4). The fusion of an isolated mouse lymphocyte with a malignant mouse plasma (myeloma) cell was done. This hybridoma could produce large amounts of the specific immunoglobulin against the antigen for which the lymphocyte had been encoded by earlier immunization [17].

9.3.1.1 Immune Response to Monoclonal Antibodies

The patients' immune systems recognize mouse antibodies as foreign proteins, result-ing in a neutralizing immune response called the human anti-mouse antibody (HAMA) response. This phenomenon can alter the pharmacokinetics of subsequent therapeutic antibody infusion by increasing the clearance from circulation. The lack of efficacy of subsequent therapeutic antibody can occur due to the generation of neutralizing antibodies, which will block the antigen-binding site of the therapeutic antibody [18].

To minimize HAMA (i.e., to overcome immunogenicity risk), new techniques were developed based on the thought that a reduction in the mAb molecule size will decrease the immunogenicity. The size reduction could be accomplished through methods such as enzymatic cleavage or genetic engineering techniques, including digestion of an antibody with enzyme pepsin, which produces F(ab)$_2$ fragment (100 kDa), that retain two antigen-binding sites and digestion with papain enzyme resulting in Fab (50 kDa) with one antigen-binding site. However, further advancement in the biotechnology field resulted in other different techniques to decrease immunogenicity [19].

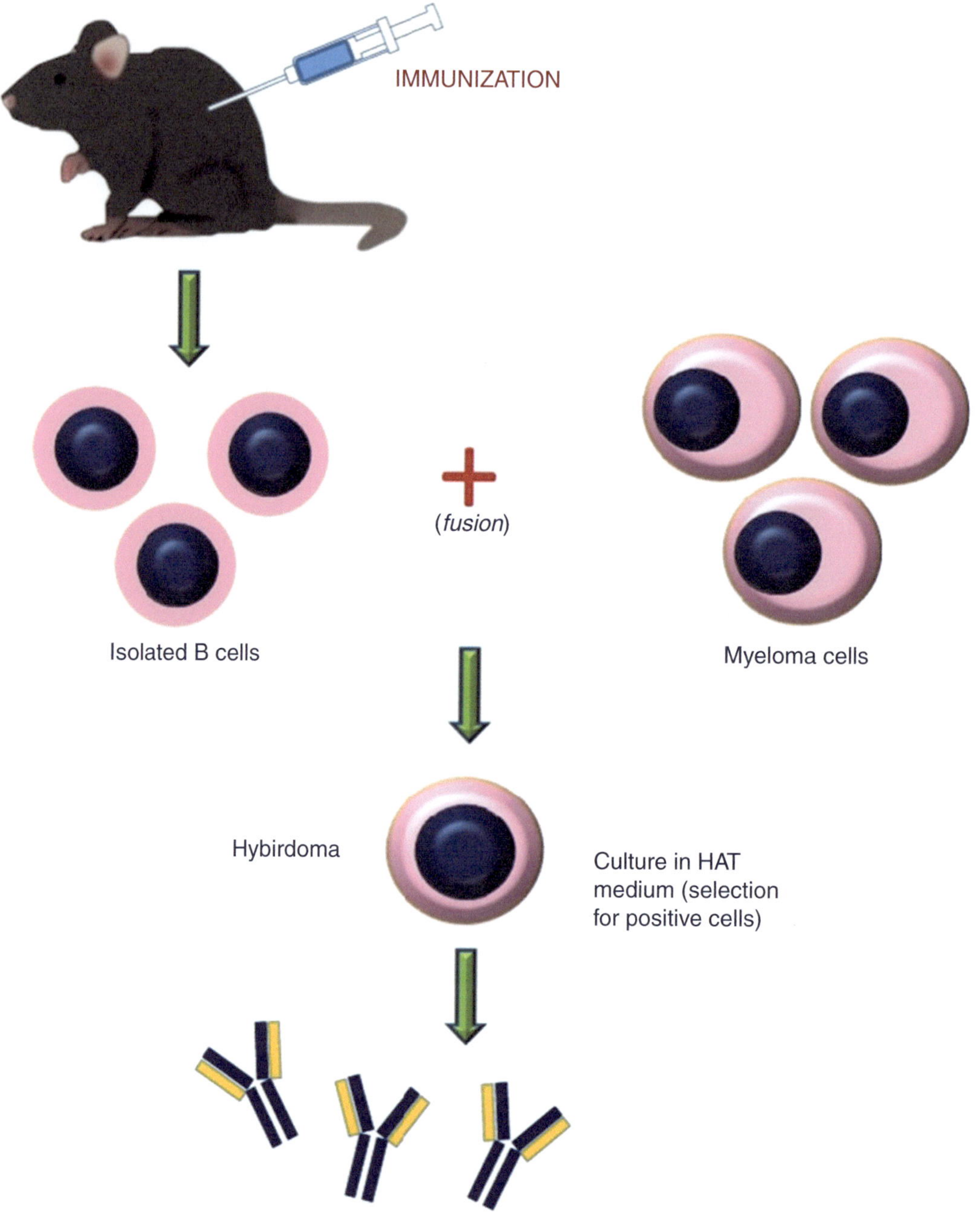

Fig. 9.4 Antibody engineering—hybridoma technique (*HAT* hypoxanthine-aminopterin-thymidine)

9.3.1.2 Antibody Engineering

Antibody engineering encompasses new techniques in which by retaining only the immune-specific portion of murine antibody and replacing a large portion of the remainder of the murine IgG molecule with a human IgG sequence, mixed sequence antibodies, called chimeric antibody (70–90% replacement) [20], and humanized antibody (by CDR grafting, approximately 98% replacement) could be achieved (Fig. 9.5) [21].

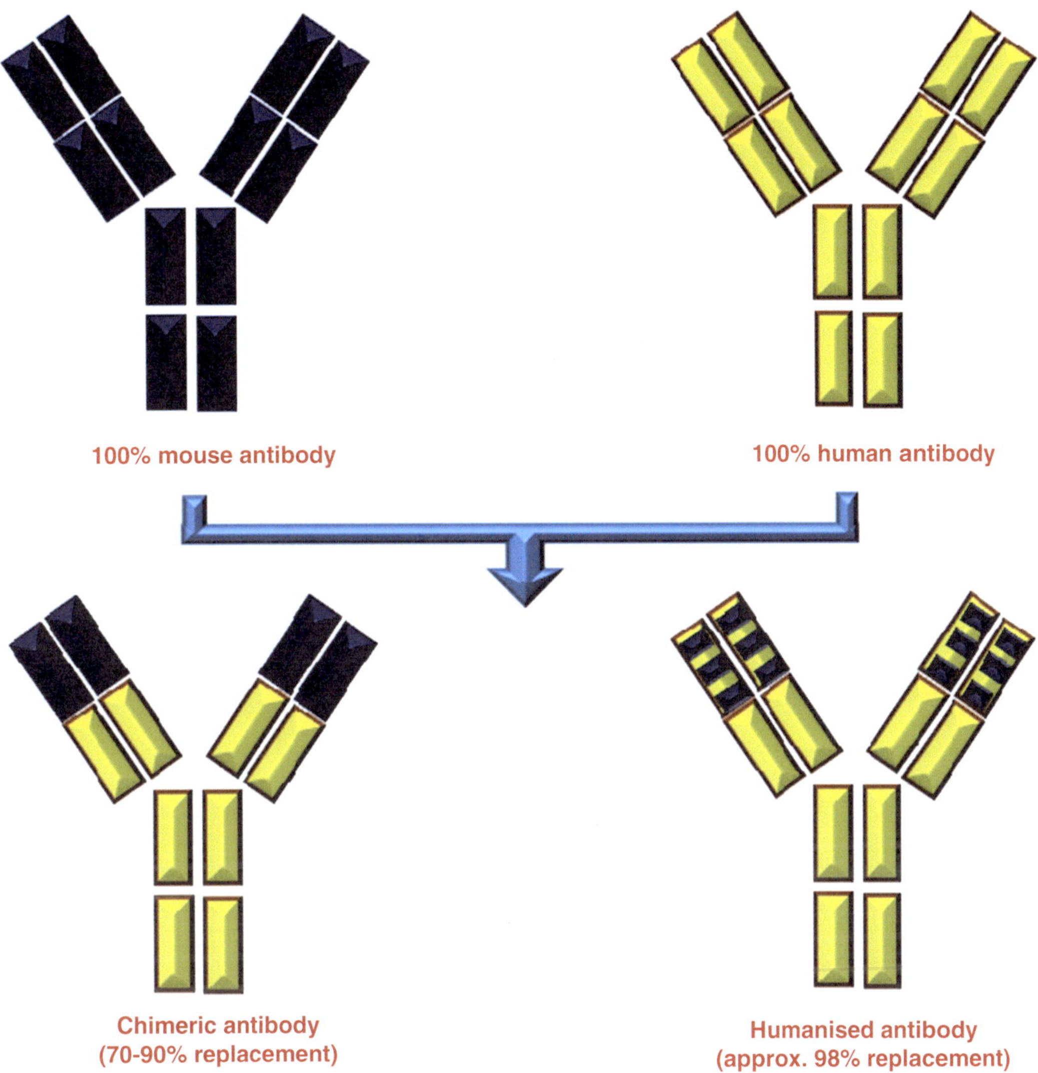

Fig. 9.5 Chimeric and humanized antibody

Chimeric antibodies still have a significant amount of murine sequence (in Fv region) that is immunogenic and can even evoke immune response called human anti-chimeric antibody response (HACA). A humanized antibody, though only the murine CDRs are grafted onto a wholly human immunoglobulin framework, still rarely can evoke human anti-humanized antibody response (HAHA) [22]. Further development in this field resulted in fully human antibodies using recombinant DNA technology [23, 24].

Intact mAb (full IgG, 150 kDa) with molecular weight more than the glomerular filtration threshold (~70 kDa) has a long serum half-life and remains in circulation for 3–4 weeks. The intact antibody is dissected into smaller antigen-binding fragments by different techniques, including proteolysis and genetic engineering. The smallest fragment, the single-chain variable fragment (scFv, 25 kDa), has a blood clearance time of fewer than 10 h, primarily by renal excretion in 2–4 h [25, 26].

9.3.2 Antibody Fragments Variations

Different variations of small fragments of antibodies include (Fig. 9.6):

- **Nanobody** is the smallest antigen-binding region or fragment of naturally occurring heavy-chain antibodies [27, 28].
- **scFv (single-chain variable fragment)** (25 kDa) consists of the VL and VH domains of the antibody molecule joined by a peptide linker [29].
- **dsFv (disulfide variable fragment)**. In this type of fragment, the stability to VL and VH domain is provided by a disulfide bridge rather than a peptide linker [30].
- **scdsFv (single-chain disulfide variable fragment)**. Here, the combination of peptide linker and disulfide bridge provides structural stability [31].
- **Diabodies** are multimeric forms of scfv, i.e., noncovalent dimers of scFv fragments formed using short peptide linkers (3–12 amino acids) that promote cross-pairing of the VH and VL domains of two polypeptides. Molecular weight is around 60 kDa [32].
- **Triabody** is a multimeric form of scFv with a noncovalent trimer of scFv.
- **Tetrabody** is a multimeric form of scFv with a noncovalent tetramer of scFv.
- **Mini body** is another multimeric form constructed by ligating the gene encoding the scFv to the human IgG1 CH3 domain, leading to the dimerization of two polypeptide chains as a result of interactions between the two CH3 domains [33].

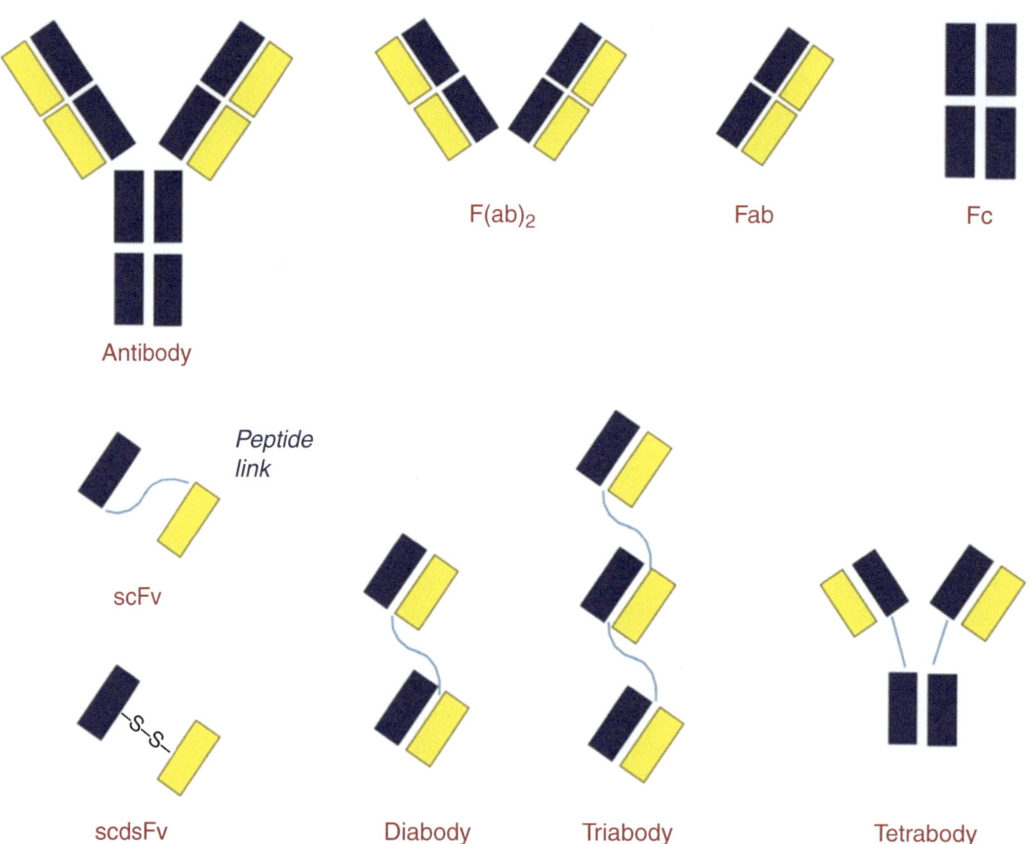

Fig. 9.6 Various antibody fragments

9.3.2.1 Characteristics of Antibody Fragments

These smaller antigen-binding fragments retain tumor-targeting properties, are less immunogenic, clear rapidly from the circulation, enable deeper penetration in the tumor, and permit imaging at earlier times. But limitations are used as a therapeutic option (reduced half-life, typically in hours to days instead of weeks for a typical IgG, may result in lesser tumor uptake time), and renal excretion greatly increases the risk for renal toxicity. The production method must be optimized for each mAb. Monoclonal antibodies or antibody fragments can be used in cancer management in the following forms [34]:

- **Unconjugated antibody**—as targeted therapy by itself.
- **Conjugated antibody**—immunotoxin, immuno-drug conjugate, immune-directed prodrug therapy, and radiolabeled antibodies.
- **Targeting nano-drug reservoir.**

The unconjugated antibody can function by the different mechanisms which include blocking ligand-receptor interaction, complement-dependent cytotoxicity (CDC), antibody-dependent cellular cytotoxicity (ADCC) by the interaction of Fc receptors on effector cells (natural killer cells, macrophages, monocytes, and eosinophils), and opsonization (Table 9.4) [35].

Conjugated Antibody

Immunotoxins are composed of targeting mAbs (or other targeting ligands) linked to potent toxins or active toxin subunits. There are three types of peptide cytotoxins, namely, type 1, which are intracellular enzymes that act by altering the intracellular environment; type 2 that bind to the cell surface and act by altering signaling pathways; and type 3 that are pore-forming peptides which mediate cell membrane leakage and cause cell death. These toxins can be derived from plants, fungi, or bacteria, e.g., ricin toxin, diphtheria toxin, or *Pseudomonas* exotoxin [36]. As an example, HD37-dgA is an anti-CD22/dgA (deglycosylated ricin A), which is being evaluated in refractory B-cell lymphoma (Phase I) [37].

Table 9.4 Examples of individual antibodies

EGFR targeting antibodies
- Cetuximab
- Panitumumab

HER2-targeting antibodies
- Trastuzumab
- Pertuzumab

VEGF-targeting antibody
- Bevacizumab

CD52-targeting antibody
- Alemtuzumab

CD20-targeting antibodies
- Obinutuzumab
- Ofatumumab
- Rituximab

CTLA-4 (CD152)-targeting antibodies
- Ipilimumab
- Tremelimumab

PD1-targeting antibodies
- Pembrolizumab
- Nivolumab

PD-L1-targeting antibody
- Avelumab

EGFR epidermal growth factor receptor, *HER2* human epidermal growth factor receptor 2, *VEGF* vascular endothelial growth factor, *CD* cluster of differentiation, *CTLA-4* cytotoxic T-lymphocyte-associated protein 4, *PD1* programmed cell death protein 1, *PD-L1* programmed death-ligand 1

mAb drug conjugate is composed of targeting mAbs linked to a chemotherapy drug, which mediates cell killing. Different chemotherapy drugs have been linked to antibodies, including methotrexate, the vinca alkaloids, and the anthracyclines (Table 9.5).

Antibody-directed prodrug therapy is a stepwise approach. It can be utilized for the enzyme-labeled antibody, which can be given first to localize the enzyme at the target. The prodrug can then be administered, which will become activated close to the tumor. Few examples include enzyme β-lactamase (which activates paclitaxel and doxorubicin by releasing cleavage of β-lactam rings) and cytosine deaminase (which converts prodrug 5-fluorocytosine to the active drug 5-fluorouracil) [11].

The antibody fusion protein as decoy receptors method uses the Fc portion of the antibody, not to provide the specificity of Fv fragment. Rather, it allows modulation of size

Table 9.5 Monoclonal antibody drug conjugates

Gemtuzumab ozogamicin
• It consists of a humanized anti-CD33 that is linked to calicheamicin (approved for use in AML) [38]
Ado-trastuzumab emtansine
• mAb directed at HER2 conjugated with microtubule inhibitor DM1 (approved for HER2-positive breast cancer)
Brentuximab vedotin
• mAb directed at CD30 with microtubule inhibitor drug monomethyl auristatin (MMAE) (approved for Hodgkin's lymphoma and anaplastic large cell lymphoma after failure to prior therapies)

CD cluster of differentiation, *AML* acute myelogenous leukemia, *mAb* monoclonal antibody, *HER2* human epidermal growth factor receptor 2

Table 9.6 Examples of radiolabeled antibodies for diagnostic use

Satamomab pentedide
• [^{111}In]In-anti TAG72 (OncoScint) in colorectal and ovarian malignancies
Arcitumomab
• [^{99m}Tc]Tc-anti CEA fab in colorectal carcinoma
Capromab pentedide
• [^{111}In]In-anti-PSMA (7E11) in prostate cancer
[^{64}Cu]Cu-trastuzumab
• Against HER2
[^{89}Zr]Zr-J591
• Against PSMA
[^{89}Zr]Zr-pembrolizumab
• Against PD1
[^{89}Zr]Zr-atezolizumab
• Against PD-L1
[^{89}Zr]Zr-bevacizumab
• Against VEGF

CEA carcinoembryonic antigen, *PSMA* prostate-specific membrane antigen, *PD1* programmed cell death protein 1, *PD-L1* programmed death-ligand 1, *VEGF* vascular endothelial growth factor

and pharmacokinetic of the fusion protein molecule. Since the Fc part can bind to the Fc receptor (FcR), which is responsible for the recycling of antibody, favorable pharmacokinetics is provided to fusion protein as well as, e.g., aflibercept formed by genetic fusion of domain 2 of vascular endothelial growth factor receptor-1 (VEGFR1) to domain 3 of VEGFR2 with the Fc portion of human IgG1. It works like a composite soluble decoy receptor for VEGF and hence prevents VEGFR binding/activation (approved for use in macular degeneration and colorectal carcinoma) [39].

Radioimmunoconjugates—Monoclonal antibody (mAb) is labeled with radionuclides for diagnostic or therapeutic purposes (theranostic use).

Diagnostic—Single-photon emission computed tomography (SPECT) radionuclides, technetium-99m (^{99m}Tc), indium-111 (^{111}In), iodine-123 (^{123}I), iodine-131 (^{131}I) and positron emission tomography (PET) radionuclides, gallium-68 (^{68}Ga), fluorine-18 (^{18}F), yttrium-86 (^{86}Y), zirconium-89 (^{89}Zr), and iodine-124 (^{124}I) can be used to radiolabel antibodies (Table 9.6).

Therapeutic—In radioimmunotherapy (RIT), mAb labeled with auger electron, β, or α particle emitting radionuclides can be used for therapy. RIT of hematological malignancies have resulted in good responses compared to solid tumor RIT.

Many different antibodies have been tried for therapeutic use in hematological and solid tumors. Two radiolabeled antibodies against CD20$^+$ low-grade follicular lymphoma that have been approved by the US Food and Drug Administration (FDA) include:

• [^{131}I]I-tositumomab (Bexxar)
• [^{90}Y]Y-ibritumomab tiuxetan (Zevalin)

Both of these radiolabeled antibodies have shown higher objective response rates compared to the unlabeled anti-CD20 antibody used alone [40, 41]. In a randomized controlled trial, Witzig et al. reported an overall response rate (ORR) of 80% for 73 patients treated with single-cycle [^{90}Y]Y-ibritumomab tiuxetan versus 56% in 70 patients who received rituximab weekly for 4 weeks. The complete response (CR) rates were 30% and 16%, respectively. The duration of response for [^{90}Y]Y-ibritumomab tiuxetan was 14.2 months compared with 12.1 months for rituximab immunotherapy [40].

Apart from the FDA-approved anti-CD20 antibodies ([^{131}I]I-tositumomab, [^{90}Y]Y-ibritumomab tiuxetan), other radiolabeled anti-CD20 antibodies have been evaluated in clinical studies, including [^{131}I]I-rituximab, [^{177}Lu]Lu-DOTA rituximab, and [^{90}Y]Y-rituximab, though they still are not FDA approved [42, 43].

Other B-cell antigens have also been targeted for RIT, including CD22, CD33, and human leukocyte antigen (HLA)-DR10. Many solid tumor RITs have also been tried though they have resulted in less success than hematological malignancies.

Different new approaches have been tried to improve the results, including the use of small fragments which have shown better tumor permeability and different approaches labeled as affinity enhancement system, which utilizes other methods of pretargeting, including the use of bi-specific antibodies or avidin-biotin-based pretargeting [44].

9.3.3 Pretargeting

Pretargeting depends on three steps. The first step involves designing and injecting the target vector capable of binding with the target antigen and small radiolabeled molecule; in the second step, after accumulating in the target site, the majority is cleared from the blood. The third step involves the injection of a small radiolabeled molecule. When it encounters the target vector, binding takes place and forms in vivo radioimmunoconjugate. In some cases, clearing agents are injected to remove the unbound targeting vector from the circulation before injecting the small radiolabeled molecule. Four commonly used pretargeting approaches are as follows (Fig. 9.7):

1. Streptavidin biotin approach
2. Bi-specific antibody approach
3. Oligonucleotide hybridization approach
4. Click chemistry approach

Pretargeting is a challenging multistep process. Each of the strategies stands at a different stage in its scientific development, having its advantages and disadvantages.

9.4 Small Molecule Inhibitors Targeting Kinases

Posttranslational modifications, including phosphorylation, are responsible for various aspects of normal physiology and pathological conditions [45]. Phosphorylation is carried out by kinases, which cause the transfer of gamma phosphate of adenosine triphosphate (ATP) onto hydroxyl groups of various substrates, including lipids, sugars, or amino acids.

Protein kinases in eukaryotes include either tyrosine kinases (TKs), serine/threonine kinases (STKs), or both tyrosine and threonine (dual-specificity) protein kinases [46].

TKs are subdivided into two main classes, receptor tyrosine kinase (RTK) and nonreceptor TKs. Physiologically, RTK transmits the signal from extracellular ligands to the cell nucleus and hence alters the DNA synthesis. They have an extracellular domain that binds to the ligand, lipophilic transmembrane, and an intracellular domain that contains the catalytic site. In the absence of ligand, RTK is present in an unphosphorylated, monomeric inactive state. Ligand binding results in inactivation; it induces dimerization, which results in autophosphorylation of the intracellular domain, which causes recruitment of multiple signaling proteins to membrane and activation of signaling cascade transmitting information to nucleus, e.g., epidermal growth factor receptor (EGFR) (ErbB/HER) family, vascular endothelial growth factor receptors (VEGFR), and platelet-derived growth factor receptors (PDGFR).

Nonreceptor tyrosine kinases are located in intracellular regions and play a role in the intracellular signals transduction, e.g., BCR-ABL, c-kit (also referred to as stem cell factor receptor or CD117), and c-Src. Another important kinase is phosphatidyl-inositol kinase (PI3K). It phosphorylates phosphatidyl inositol (PI) together with the atypical serine-threonine PK (mTOR) [47].

These kinases are part of signal transduction pathways organized in cascades. Signals initiated by various receptors, including receptor

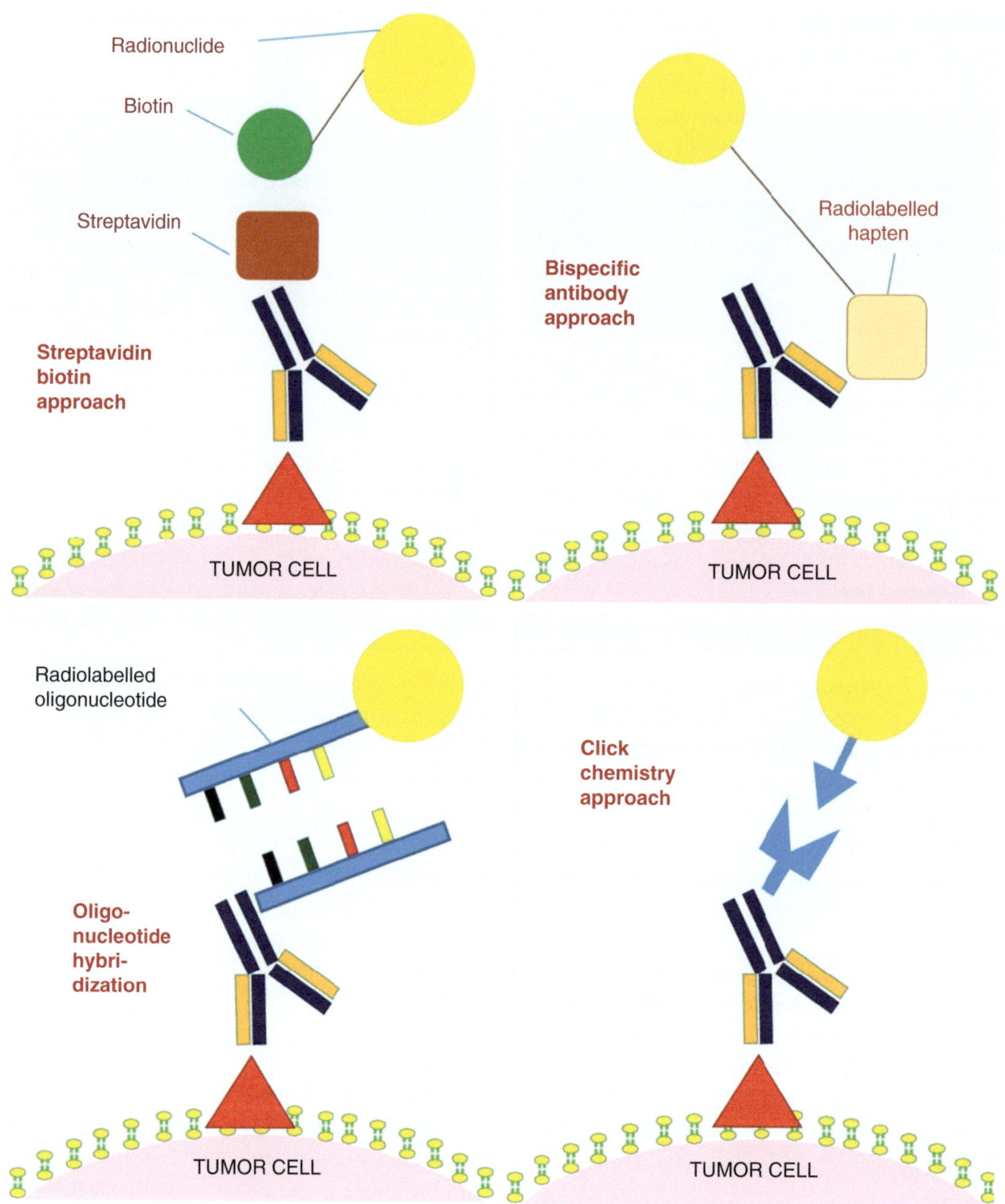

Fig. 9.7 Various tumor pretargeting approaches

and nonreceptor TKs or STKs, pass downstream through effectors such as the PI3K/mTOR, the RAS-RAF-MAPK, SMAD, and STAT ultimately to the nucleus (the cell cycle kinases and kinases regulating transcription) [48].

Many human malignancies are associated with aberrant regulation of protein or lipid kinases, which could be because of activating mutations, chromosomal rearrangements, and/or gene amplification [47, 49, 50]. Hence, these become an important target for using targeted therapies.

Small molecule inhibitors are used to target the extracellular (cell surface receptors) or intracellular proteins which are critical cancer targets such as serine/threonine/tyrosine kinases, matrix metalloproteinases (MMPs), heat-shock proteins (HSPs), proteosomes, and other proteins playing a role in signal transduction pathways. These molecules are small in size ($\leq$500 Da), can cross the plasma membrane, are amenable to oral administration, and are comparatively cost-effective compared to mAbs, which are large molecular weight proteins (~150 kDa) given intravenously [51].

9.4.1 Structure and Mode of Action of Small Molecule Inhibitors

These agents share the similarity in their three-dimensional (3D) structures, especially in their catalytically active kinase domain, where the ATP-binding pocket is located. They consist of a small, mostly N-lobe connected by a short hinge region to a larger C-lobe. The N-lobe mainly has a β-stranded structure, and C-lobe has mainly an α-helical structure [52]. ATP binds in the cleft between the N- and C-terminal lobes. A flexible activation loop starting with a conserved amino acid sequence Aspartate-Glycine-Phenylalanine (Asp-Phe-Gly) (DFG) controls access to the active site. The ATP binding site's conservation might cause different inhibitors to cross-react with other different kinases and hence called multikinase inhibitors, e.g., sunitinib [53]. Based on the inhibition mechanism, different classes of inhibitors are present (Table 9.7) [7, 54].

After the FDA approval of the first kinase inhibitor, imatinib, in 2001, many other kinase inhibitors have been evaluated. There are approximately 175 different orally effective protein kinase inhibitors in clinical trials worldwide [56]. The US FDA has approved many small molecule protein kinase inhibitors; some of the commonly used examples in oncology practice are mentioned in Table 9.8.

Table 9.7 Small molecule inhibitors' classification

Noncovalent inhibitors (reversible)
- *Type I inhibitors*: Bind to the active protein kinase conformation (DFG or Asp-Phe-Gly are the most frequent sites of these type of inhibitor binding)
- *Type I1/2 inhibitors:* Bind to a DFG (Asp-Phe-Gly) motif in inactive kinase conformation (e.g., vemurafenib) [55]
- *Type II inhibitors*: Bind to an inactive enzyme and hydrophobic site formed by conserved amino acid sequence, DFG motif (Asp-Phe-Gly) (e.g., sorafenib)
- *Type III inhibitors*: Bind to an allosteric site (non-ATP site) that does not overlap the ATP binding site (e.g., MEK inhibitors)
- *Type IV inhibitors*: Form irreversible bond to a cysteine residue within active site (e.g., Bruton's tyrosine kinase (BTK) inhibitor, ibrutinib)
- *Type V inhibitors*: Bivalent compounds that bind to two distinct regions of the protein kinase

Covalent inhibitors (irreversible): Form covalent bonds with their target enzyme (e.g., afatinib)

Table 9.8 Examples of small molecule protein kinase inhibitors approved by the US FDA

Reversible nonreceptor TK inhibitor
- BCR-ABL tyrosine kinase inhibitors—imatinib, bosutinib, dasatinib, nilotinib, and ponatinib

Reversible receptor TK inhibitor
- EGFR/ErbB tyrosine kinase inhibitors—gefitinib, erlotinib, lapatinib (dual EGFR and ErbB2), and vandetanib (multiple kinase inhibitor against EGFR, VEGFR, RET)
- VEGFR inhibitor—sorafenib, sunitinib, pazopanib, axitinib, regorafenib, nintedanib, and lenvatinib
- ALK inhibitor—crizotinib and ceritinib
- MET inhibitor (HGFR)—crizotinib and cabozantinib (dual MET and VEGFR2)

Irreversible (covalent) inhibitor
- Receptor TK (EGFR/ErbB TK) inhibitor—afatinib
- Nonreceptor TK inhibitor—Bruton's tyrosine kinase (BTK) and ibrutinib

(continued)

Table 9.8 (continued)

Serine-threonine TK inhibitor
• RAF tyrosine kinase inhibitor—vemurafenib and dabrafenib
• MEK inhibitor—trametinib
• mTOR inhibitor (serine/threonine kinase)—sirolimus, everolimus, and temsirolimus
• CDK4-CDK6 inhibitors—palbociclib and abemaciclib
Lipid kinase inhibitor (PI3K inhibitors)—idelalisib and copanlisib
HER2 inhibitor—Lapatinib
Proteasome inhibitor—bortezomib and carfilzomib
Histone deacetylase inhibitor—romidepsin and vorinostat

TK tyrosine kinase, *EGFR* epidermal growth factor receptor, *VEGFR* vascular endothelial growth factor receptor, *RET* rearranged during transfection, *ALK* anaplastic lymphoma kinase, *MET* mesenchymal-epithelial transition, *HGFR* hepatocyte growth factor receptor, *CDK* cyclin-dependent kinase, *HER2* human epidermal growth factor receptor 2

9.4.2 Limitations of Small Molecule Inhibitors as Targeted Cancer Therapy

Many of these drugs are multikinase inhibitors, which have both implications. The multiple targets are advantageous when the therapeutic effect is related to inhibition of different kinase targets (e.g., sunitinib and cabozantinib, which have potent AXL off-target activity). Limitation when inhibiting nontarget kinases results in side effects, e.g., mTOR inhibitor everolimus [57]. Hence, the word magic shotgun is used in analogy to the magic bullet used for monoclonal antibodies [58].

As we already discussed, the small molecule inhibitor drugs act on one particular target in the tumor carcinogenesis pathway. Still, most tumors do not seem to respond to a highly selective inhibitor of a single critical kinase, which can be explained by the fact that tumorigenesis is the result of multiple concomitant alterations. Firstly, decreased efficacy can be because the drug does not reach the desired target; secondly, the development of resistance to these drugs eventually can be because of acquired mutations and signal transduction plasticity. The question arises as how to deal with such problems. Investigators are working on anticancer resistance issue by blocking the MAP kinase pathways at different levels, namely, for vemurafenib, a selective BRAF inhibitor. Resistance of this drug can be dealt with combining dabrafenib or trametinib (potent MEK 1 inhibitors) in the treatment regime [59].

9.5 Development of Newer Drugs

New drug discovery utilizes screening of historical inhibitors and more unique computer-aided drug-designing techniques. Techniques like protein crystallography and nuclear magnetic resonance spectroscopy determine the three-dimensional structure of the proteins (more than 6000 X-ray crystal structures of protein kinase in the public domain), and structure-based drug-designing methods are used for newer drug discovery.

9.5.1 Selective High-Affinity Ligand (SHAL)

As further advancement to unique target binding by individual ligand concept, these selective high-affinity ligands (SHALs) have been developed. These are small molecule proteins targeting agents that consist of two or three small molecule recognition elements (which bind to their unique target protein surface) linked together in a common molecule to increase the affinity of the molecule.

By attaching different tags to these molecules, they can be utilized as diagnostic or therapeutic agents similar to antibodies. They have characteristics similar to antibodies, such as selectivity for a protein target, high-affinity binding (nanomolar to picomolar range), being tagged with radionuclides or other reporters, inherent cytotoxicity, and ability to bind mono- or bivalently to their target; however, they provide added advantages of small molecules like rapid clearance and lack of immunogenicity. Their properties can be altered by varying the individual recognition elements and linker lengths [60, 61].

They are created using a structure-based designing technique involving computational and experimental technologies. Several SHALs have been developed against HLA-DR10 and shown tumor-selective cytotoxicity and promise as imaging agents for non-Hodgkin's lymphoma and other B-cell-derived malignancies preclinical studies [61].

9.5.2 Phage Display Technique for New Targeting Ligands

Phage display is a selection technique in which a peptide or protein is expressed as a fusion with a bacteriophage coat protein. The fusion allows discovering different specific antigens, studying protein-protein interactions, and selecting peptides which are bound to receptors or target proteins, and can be used for targeted therapy [62, 63].

9.6 Selective Small Molecule Targeted Radionuclide Imaging/Therapy

Similar to radiolabeled monoclonal antibodies, different small molecule agents have been radiolabeled and used for imaging and therapy of the tumor (theranostics as "therapy plus diagnostic").

9.6.1 Tumor Receptor Targeting with Radiolabeled Peptides

Many different radiolabeled peptides that bind with high affinity and specificity to the receptors overexpressed in tumor cells have been developed. These receptors (molecular targets) are located on the plasma membrane. Upon binding to the radiolabeled ligand, the receptor-ligand complex is internalized, resulting in longer retention of radioactivity in tumor cells for the efficient killing of cancer cells [64]. Examples of these molecular targets are somatostatin, bombesin, vasoactive intestinal peptide, gastrin, neurotensin, exendin, and RGD (Arginine-Glycine-Aspartate), which can be radiolabeled for diagnostic as well therapeutic uses.

Compared to monoclonal antibodies (large protein molecules), peptides have several advantages, including small size, rapid pharmacokinetics (faster clearance), better targeting characteristics (tumor permeability), easy synthesis, less immunogenicity, and the capability to tolerate harsher conditions compared to antibodies [65].

Structure-based design is used for synthesis. The peptides are synthesized using solid-phase peptide synthesis (SPPS) methods. The design is generally based on the endogenous ligand (natural peptide ligand), modified to produce a stable analog, which is radiolabeled with bifunctional chelators' help.

Among the available radiolabeled peptides, radiolabeled octreotide has been extensively evaluated. The first approved radiolabeled peptide imaging agent was somatostatin analog, $[^{111}\text{In}]$ In-DTPA-octreotide ($[^{111}\text{In}]$In-OctreoScan), for imaging somatostatin receptor (SSTR)-positive tumors such as neuroendocrine tumors (NETs) and small cell lung cancer [66]. SSTR imaging can be performed by SPECT tracer $[^{111}\text{In}]$In-DTPA-octreotide or PET tracers $[^{68}\text{Ga}]$Ga-DOTA-octreotide and $[^{64}\text{Cu}]$Cu-TETA-octreotide.

The basis of SSTR therapy (targeted radionuclide therapy in NET) is the same. The peptide ligand is radiolabeled with a therapeutic radionuclide, which delivers high radiation doses to receptor-specific disease sites (tumor lesions). For therapeutic use, auger electron or β or α particle emitting radionuclides can be used. Auger electron-emitting $[^{111}\text{In}]$In-DTPA-octreotide, β particle emitting $[^{90}\text{Y}]$Y-DOTATOC and $[^{177}\text{Lu}]$ Lu-DOTATATE (FDA approved), and α particle emitting $[^{213}\text{Bi}]$Bi-DOTATOC [67] and $[^{225}\text{Ac}]$ Ac-DOTATOC [68] are the commonly used radiopharmaceuticals.

9.6.2 Radioligand Targeted Diagnosis and Therapeutics in Prostate Cancer

Prostate-specific membrane antigen (PSMA) is a membrane protein expressed on prostate epithelial cells. PSMA acts as a glutamate carboxypeptidase (GCPII) on small molecule substrates, including folate and neuropeptide *N*-acetyl-L-aspartyl-L-glutamate (NAAG). Studies have shown that PSMA expression is upregulated in prostate carcinoma. The degree of upregulation increases progressively in higher-grade cancers, metastatic disease, and hormone-refractory prostate cancer, making it a useful therapeutic target for use in targeted therapy [69, 70]. It has extracellular, transmembrane, and intracellular components.

The targeting of PSMA has been tried with both monoclonal antibodies and small molecule inhibitors.

9.6.2.1 Monoclonal Antibodies

- [^{111}In]In-anti Capreomabpentetide (Prostascint) (7E11) which targets intracellular portion of PSMA [71]
- [^{111}In]In-DOTA-J591, [^{90}Y]Y-, or [^{177}Lu]Lu-DOTA-J591 act against the external domain of PSMA [72]

9.6.2.2 Small Molecule Inhibitors

Structure-based designing of compounds targeting the binding cavity of the PSMA has resulted in different peptide-mimetic ligands. Three types of compounds, phosphorus-based, thiol-based, and urea-based, have been developed. Urea-based inhibitors have a high affinity and specificity for PSMA and show fast and efficient internalization. The urea-based PSMA ligands consist of three components, the binding motif (glutamate-urea-lysine [Glu-urea-Lys]), a linker, and a radiolabel-bearing moiety. Many of these ligands have entered into clinical study phases (Table 9.9) [73].

9.7 The Use of Nano-Drug Carrier

Targeting particle (mAb or small molecules) can be used in cancer therapy. The nano-drug carriers are the vehicles carrying the cytotoxic drugs to the target site without producing systemic toxicity.

Table 9.9 PSMA targeting small molecule inhibitors

Diagnostic agents
• SPECT: [^{123}I]I-MIP-1072, [^{123}I]I-MIP-1095, [^{99m}Tc]Tc-MIP-1404, [^{99m}Tc]Tc-MIP-1405 [74]
• PET: [^{68}Ga]Ga-PSMA-11/HBED-CC [75], [^{18}F]F-DCFBC [76]
Therapeutic agents
• [^{131}I]I-MIP-1095 [77]
• [^{177}Lu]Lu-PSMA-I&T, [^{177}Lu]Lu-PSMA-617 [78]
• [^{225}Ac]Ac-PSMA-617 [79], [^{213}Bi]Bi-PSMA-617 [80]

SPECT single-photon emission computed tomography, *PET* positron emission tomography, *PSMA* prostate-specific membrane antigen

Nanocarriers allow a higher concentration of the anticancer agents at the tumor site, less concentrations in nontargeted areas, reduced toxicity, protection of the drug from degradation, reduced renal clearance, and increased circulation time of the drug [81, 82].

Nanocarriers are of two broad types, polymer conjugates or particulate type. Polymer conjugates are linear polymeric macromolecular structures conjugated to antitumor proteins/drugs via cleavable linkers. They are water-soluble. In particulate nanocarriers, the drug is physically entrapped within the structure. Few types of particulate-type nanocarrier include polymeric micelles, dendrimers, polymeric nanoparticles, lipid-based liposomes, and organometallic compounds like carbon nanotubes [83].

For active targeting, these nanocarriers can be labeled with targeting moieties, which include monoclonal antibodies, antibody fragments, and small molecules like peptides, growth factors, carbohydrates, biotin, transferrin, folate, glycoproteins, or receptor ligands which are overexpressed or selectively expressed on cancer cells or its microenvironment [84–87].

9.8 Aptamers

Aptamers are short nucleic acid-based ligands that fold into unique three-dimensional conformations and bind to their respective targets (proteins, nucleic acids, or small molecules) by noncovalent interactions. Since each aptamer with its unique structure will bind specifically to its target, it can also target the tumor cells [88].

As targeting agents, these agents provide specificities like monoclonal antibodies or peptides and provide added advantages in conditions where they can be screened for a range of targets, even poorly immunogenic (where generating mAb is difficult or where peptide screening by phage display is difficult). Advancements in nucleic acid chemistry; automated DNA/RNA synthesizer; efficient, cost-effective aptamer screening methods; easy large-scale production; chemical modification of aptamer; and stable structure with typical long shelf life make them an efficient targeting tool [89]. Many different aptamers against target molecules such as EGFR, HER2, VEGF, and PSMA have been developed. Other ways in which they can be used in anticancer therapy include acting as a therapeutic agent by themselves such as AS1411, developed and tested for treatment of AML, as drug conjugate, radiolabeled conjugate, photoconjugate, immunotherapy (against cytotoxic T-lymphocyte-associated protein 4 (CTLA-4), programmed cell death protein 1 (PD1), and programmed death-ligand 1 (PD-L1)) [90], and for labeling nano-drug carriers similar to monoclonal antibodies, such as nanoparticle conjugated with A10 aptamer (against PSMA) which has been tried to deliver chemotherapy drug cisplatin in prostate cancer (capable of delivering 80 times more drug to prostate cancer cells) [91].

9.9 Conclusion

Antibodies and tumor targeting is a complex and promising procedure. Several issues are taken into consideration regarding antibodies and targets. If the target expresses an adequate amount of surface molecules, the target tissue can be differentiated from the background by imaging. Pretargeted strategies have not yet been implemented in the clinical practice on a large scale despite its immense promise. It's an exciting time for clinical translation of antibody fragments and alternative affinity scaffolds for tumor targeting

with improved properties such as rapid blood clearance. Newer strategies will stimulate the pretargeting approach in a novel way. Small molecule inhibitors, either alone or in combination, may play an immense role in managing cancers. Aptamers have high molecular weights and complex synthesis procedures. With newer development, further cost reduction and improved pharmacokinetics may provide exciting therapeutic approaches.

References

1. DeVita VT Jr, Hellman S, Rosenberg SA, editors. Biologic therapy of cancer. 2nd ed. Philadelphia, PA: J.B. Lippincott; 1995. p. 295–327.
2. Oldham RK. Biologicals and biological response modifiers: the fourth modality of cancer treatment. Cancer Treat Rep. 1984;68:221–32.
3. Eberhard A, Kahlert S, Goede V, et al. Heterogeneity of angiogenesis and blood vessel maturation in human tumors: implications for antiangiogenic tumor therapies. Cancer Res. 2000;60:1388–93.
4. Ferrara N, Gerber HP, LeCouter J. The biology of VEGF and its receptors. Nat Med. 2003;9:669–76.
5. Yeo TK, Dvorak HF. Tumor stroma. In: Colvin R, Bhan A, McCluskey R, editors. Diagnostic immunopathology. New York: Raven Press; 1995. p. 485–697.
6. Fidler IJ, Kim SJ, Langley RR. The role of the organ microenvironment in the biology and therapy of cancer metastasis. J Cell Biochem. 2007;101:927–36.
7. Hojjat-Farsangi M. Small molecule inhibitors: suitable drugs for targeted-based cancer therapy. Am J Leuk Res. 2017;1:1005.
8. Carter P. Improving the efficacy of antibody-based cancer therapies. Nat Rev Cancer. 2001;1:118–29.
9. Huston JS, George AJ. Engineered antibodies take center stage. Hum Antibodies. 2001;10:127–42.
10. Park JW, et al. Anti-HER2 immunoliposomes: enhanced efficacy attributable to targeted delivery. Clin Cancer Res. 2002;8:1172–81.
11. Senter PD, Springer CJ. Selective activation of anticancer prodrugs by monoclonal antibody-enzyme conjugates. Adv Drug Deliv Rev. 2001;53:247–64.
12. Nelson AL, Reichert JM. Development trends for therapeutic antibody fragments. Nat Biotechnol. 2009;27:331–7.
13. Holliger P, Hudson PJ. Engineered antibody fragments and the rise of single domains. Nat Biotechnol. 2005;23:1126–36.
14. Allen TM, Hansen CB, Stuart DD. In: Lasic DD, Papahadjopoulos D, editors. Medical applications of liposomes. 1st ed. Amsterdam: Elsevier Science; 1998. p. 297–323.

15. Leder P. The genetics of antibody diversity. Sci Am. 1980;243:102–15.
16. Gessner JE, Heiken H, Tamm A, et al. The IgG Fc receptor family. Ann Hematol. 1998;76:231–48.
17. Köhler G, Milstein C. Continuous cultures of fused cells secreting antibody of predefined specificity. Nature. 1975;256:495–7.
18. Khazaeli MB, Conry RM, LoBuglio AF. Human immune response to monoclonal antibodies. J Immunother. 1994;15:42–52.
19. Waller M, Curry N, Mallory J. Immunochemical and serological studies of enzymatically fractionated human IgG globulins. I. Hydrolysis with pepsin, papain, ficin and bromelin. Immunochemistry. 1968;5:577–83.
20. Morrison SL, Johnson MJ, Herzenberg LA, et al. Chimeric human antibody molecules: mouse antigen-binding domains with human constant region domains. Proc Natl Acad Sci U S A. 1984;81:6851–5.
21. Jones PT, Dear PH, Foote J, et al. Replacing the complementarity-determining regions in a human antibody with those from a mouse. Nature. 1986;321(6069):522–5.
22. Foon KA, Yang XD, Weiner LM, et al. Preclinical and clinical evaluations of ABX-EGF, a fully human anti-epidermal growth factor receptor antibody. Int J Radiat Oncol Biol Phys. 2004;58(3):984–90.
23. Moroney SPA. Modern antibody technology: the impact on drug development. 1st ed. Weinheim: Wiley-VCH Verlag GmbH & Co KGaA; 2005. p. 49–70.
24. Green LL, Hardy MC, Maynard-Currie CE, et al. Antigen-specific human monoclonal antibodies from mice engineered with human Ig heavy and light chain YACs. Nat Genet. 1994;7:13–21.
25. Lane DM, Eagle KF, Begent RH, et al. Radioimmunotherapy of metastatic colorectal tumors with iodine-131-labeled antibody to carcinoembryonic antigen: phase I/II study with comparative biodistribution of intact and F(ab)2 antibodies. Br J Cancer. 1994;70:521–5.
26. Colcher D, Bird R, Roselli M, et al. In vivo tumor targeting of a recombinant single-chain antigen-binding protein. J Natl Cancer Inst. 1990;82:1191–7.
27. Revets H, De Baetselier P, Muyldermans S. Nanobodies as novel agents for cancer therapy. Expert Opin Biol Ther. 2005;5:111–24.
28. Gainkam LO, Huang L, Caveliers V, et al. Comparison of the biodistribution and tumor targeting of two 99mTc-labeled anti-EGFR nanobodies in mice, using pinhole SPECT/micro-CT. J Nucl Med. 2008;49:788–95.
29. Bird RE, Hardman KD, Jacobson JW, et al. Single-chain antigen-binding proteins. Science. 1988;242:423–6.
30. Almog O, Benhar I, Vasmatzis G, et al. Crystal structure of the disulfide-stabilized Fv fragment of anticancer antibody B1: conformational influence of an engineered disulfide bond. Proteins. 1998;31:128–38.
31. Rajagopal V, Pastan I, Kreitman RJ. A form of anti-Tac(Fv), which is both single-chain and disulfide stabilized: comparison with its single-chain and disulfide-stabilized homologs. Protein Eng. 1997;10:1453–9.
32. Holliger P, Prospero T, Winter G. "Diabodies": small bivalent and bispecific antibody fragments. Proc Natl Acad Sci U S A. 1993;90:6444–8.
33. Hu S, Shively L, Raubitschek A, et al. Mini body: a novel engineered anti-carcinoembryonic antigen antibody fragment (single-chain Fv-CH3) which exhibits rapid, high-level targeting of xenografts. Cancer Res. 1996;56:3055–61.
34. Oldham RK. Monoclonal antibodies in cancer therapy. J Clin Oncol. 1983;1:582–90.
35. Dillman RO. Monoclonal antibodies in the treatment of cancer. Crit Rev Oncol Hematol. 1984;1:357–86.
36. Sears CL, Kaper JB. Enteric bacterial toxins: mechanisms of action and linkage to intestinal secretion. Microbial Rev. 1996;60:167–215.
37. Schindler J, Sausville EA, Messmann R, et al. The toxicity of deglycosylated ricin A chain containing immunotoxins in patients with non-Hodgkin's lymphoma is exacerbated by prior radiotherapy: a retrospective analysis of patients in five clinical trials. Clin Cancer Res. 2001;7:255–8.
38. Jurcic JG. Antibody therapy for residual disease in acute myelogenous leukemia. Crit Rev Oncol Hematol. 2001;38:37–45.
39. Scartozzi M, et al. Aflibercept, a new way to Target angiogenesis in the second-line treatment of metastatic colorectal cancer (mCRC). Target Oncol. 2016;11:489–500.
40. Witzig TE, Gordon LI, Cabanillas F, et al. Randomized controlled trial of yttrium-90-labeled ibritumomab tiuxetan radioimmunotherapy versus rituximab immunotherapy for patients with relapsed or refractory low-grade, follicular, or transformed B-cell non-Hodgkin's lymphoma. J Clin Oncol. 2002a;20:2453–246.
41. Davis TA, Kaminski MS, Leonard JP, et al. The radioisotope contributes significantly to the activity of radioimmunotherapy. Clin Cancer Res. 2004;10:7792–8.
42. Yadav MP, Singla S, Thakral P, et al. Dosimetric analysis of 177Lu-DOTA-rituximab in patients with relapsed/refractory non-Hodgkin's lymphoma. Nucl Med Commun. 2016;37(7):735–42.
43. Thakral P, Singla S, Vashist A, et al. Preliminary experience with yttrium-90-labelled rituximab (chimeric anti CD-20 antibody) patients with relapsed and refractory B cell non-Hodgkin's lymphoma. Curr Radiopharm. 2016;9(2):160–8.
44. Barbet J, et al. Pretargeting with the affinity enhancement system for radioimmunotherapy. Cancer Biother Radiopharm. 1999;14:153–66.
45. Walsh CT, Garneau-Tsodikova S, Gatto GJ Jr. Protein post-translational modifications: the chemistry of proteome diversifications. Angew Chem Int Ed Engl. 2005;44:7342–72.

46. Cohen P. The role of protein phosphorylation in human health and disease. The Sir Hans Krebs Medal Lecture. Eur J Biochem. 2001;268:5001–10.

47. Kannan N, Taylor SS, Zhai Y, Venter JC, Manning G. Structural and functional diversity of the microbial kinome. PLoS Biol. 2007;5:e17.

48. Lahiry P, Torkamani A, Schork NJ, Hegele RA. Kinase mutations in human disease: interpreting genotype-phenotype relationships. Nat Rev Genet. 2010;11: 60–74.

49. Engelman JA. Targeting PI3K signaling in cancer: opportunities, challenges, and limitations. Nat Rev Cancer. 2009;9:550–62.

50. Courtney KD, Corcoran RB, Engelman JA. The PI3K pathway as a drug target in human cancer. J Clin Oncol. 2010;28:1075–83.

51. Carter PJ. Potent antibody therapeutics by design. Nat Rev Immunol. 2006;6:343–57.

52. Nolen B, Taylor S, Ghosh G. Regulation of protein kinases; controlling activity through activation segment conformation. Mol Cell. 2004;15:661–75.

53. Motzer RJ, Hoosen S, Bello CL, et al. Sunitinib malate for the treatment of solid tumors: a review of current clinical data. Expert Opin Investig Drugs. 2006;15:553–61.

54. Kokhaei P, Jadidi-Niaragh F, SotoodehJahromi A, et al. Ibrutinib-A double-edged sword in cancer autoimmune disorders. J Drug Target. 2016;24(5): 373–85.

55. Roskoski R Jr. Classification of small molecule protein kinase inhibitors based upon the structures of their drug-enzyme complexes. Pharmacol Res. 2016;103:26–48.

56. Carles F, Bourg S, Meyer C, et al. PKIDB: a curated, annotated, and updated database of protein kinase inhibitors in clinical trials. Molecules. 2018;23(4): E908. https://doi.org/10.3390/molecules23040908.

57. Myers SH, Brunton VG, Unciti-Broceta A. AXL inhibitors in cancer: a medicinal chemistry perspective. J Med Chem. 2016;59:3593–608.

58. Roth BL, Sheffler DJ, Kroeze WK. Magic shotguns versus magic bullets: selectively nonselective drugs for mood disorders and schizophrenia. Nat Rev Drug Discov. 2004;3:353–9.

59. King AJ, Arnone MR, Bleam MR, et al. Dabrafenib; preclinical characterization, increased efficacy when combined with trametinib, while BRAF/MEK tool combination reduced skin lesions. PLoS One. 2013;8:e67583.

60. Balhorn R, Hok S, Burke PA, et al. Selective high-affinity ligand antibody mimics for cancer diagnosis and therapy: initial application to lymphoma/leukemia. Clin Cancer Res. 2007;13:5621s–8s.

61. DeNardo GL, Hok S, Van Natarajan A, et al. Characteristics of dimeric (bis) bidentate selective high-affinity ligands as HLA-DR10 beta antibody mimics targeting non-Hodgkin's lymphoma. Int J Oncol. 2007a;31:729–40.

62. D'Mello F, Partidos CD, Steward MW, et al. Definition of the primary structure of hepatitis B virus (HBV) pre-S hepatocyte binding domain using random peptide libraries. Virology. 1997;237:319–26.

63. Wrighton NC, Farrell FX, Chang R, et al. Small peptides as potent mimetics of the protein hormone erythropoietin. Science. 1996;273:458–64.

64. Mariani G, Erba PA, Signore A. Receptor-mediated tumor targeting radiolabeled peptides: there is more to it than somatostatin analogs. J Nucl Med. 2006;47:1904–7.

65. Fani M, Maecke HR. Radiopharmaceutical development of radiolabelled peptides. Eur J Nucl Med Mol Imaging. 2012b;39:S11–30.

66. Kaltsas GA, Papadogias D, Makras P, et al. Treatment of advanced neuroendocrine tumors with radiolabelled somatostatin analogs. Endocr Relat Cancer. 2005;12:683–99.

67. Norenberg JP, Krenning BJ, Konings IR, et al. 213Bi-[DOTA0, Tyr3]octreotide peptide receptor radionuclide therapy of pancreatic tumors in a preclinical animal model. Clin Cancer Res. 2006;12:897–903.

68. Miederer M, Henriksen G, Alke A, et al. Preclinical evaluation of the alpha-particle generator nuclide 225Ac for somatostatin receptor radiotherapy neuroendocrine tumors. Clin Cancer Res. 2008;14: 3555–61.

69. Sokoloff RL, Norton KC, Gasior CL, et al. A dual-monoclonal sandwich assay for prostate-specific membrane antigen: levels in tissues, seminal fluid, and urine. Prostate. 2000;43:150–7.

70. Bostwick DG, Pacelli A, Blute M, et al. Prostate-specific membrane antigen expression in prostatic intraepithelial neoplasia and adenocarcinoma: a study of 184 cases. Cancer. 1998;82:2256–61.

71. Kahn D, Williams RD, Manyak MJ, et al. 111Indium-capromab pendetide in evaluating patients with residual or recurrent prostate cancer after radical prostatectomy. The ProstaScint study group. J Urol. 1998a;159:2041–6.

72. Smith-Jones PM, Vallabhajosula S, Navarro V, et al. Radiolabeled monoclonal antibodies specific to the extracellular domain of prostate-specific membrane antigen: preclinical studies in nude mice bearing LNCaP human prostate tumor. J Nucl Med. 2003;44:610–7.

73. Mease RC, Foss CA, Pomper MG. PET imaging in prostate cancer: focus on prostate-specific membrane antigen. Curr Top Med Chem. 2013;13:951–62.

74. Barrett JA, Coleman RE, Goldsmith SJ, et al. First-in-man evaluation of 2 high-affinity PSMA-avid small molecules for imaging prostate cancer. J Nucl Med. 2013;54:380–7.

75. Eder M, Neels O, Müller M, et al. Novel preclinical and radiopharmaceutical aspects of [68Ga] Ga-PSMA-HBED-CC: a new PET tracer for imaging of prostate cancer. Pharmaceuticals (Basel). 2014;7: 779–96.

76. Cho SY, Gage KL, Mease RC, et al. Biodistribution, tumor detection, and radiation dosimetry of 18F-DCFBC, a low-molecular-weight inhibitor prostate-specific membrane antigen, in patients with

metastatic prostate cancer. J Nucl Med. 2012;53: 1883–91.

77. Zechmann CM, Afshar-Oromieh A, Armor T, et al. Radiation dosimetry and first therapy results with a 124I/131I-labeled small molecule (MIP-1095) targeting PSMA for prostate cancer therapy. Eur J Nucl Med Mol Imaging. 2014;41:1280–92.

78. Rahbar K, Ahmadzadehfar H, Kratochwil C, et al. German multicenter study investigating 177Lu-PSMA-617 radioligand therapy in advanced prostate cancer patients. J Nucl Med. 2017;58:85–90.

79. Kratochwil C, Bruchertseifer F, Giesel FL, et al. 225Ac-PSMA-617 for PSMA-targeted alpha radiation therapy of metastatic castration-resistant prostate cancer. J Nucl Med. 2016;57:1941–4.

80. Sathekge M, Knoesen O, Meckel M, et al. 213Bi-PSMA-617 targeted alpha-radionuclide therapy in metastatic castration-resistant prostate cancer. Eur J Nucl Med Mol Imaging. 2017;44:1099–100.

81. Danhier F, Feron O, Preat V. To exploit the tumor microenvironment: passive and active tumor targeting of nanocarriers for anticancer drug delivery. J Control Release. 2010;148:135–46.

82. Davis ME, Chen Z, Shin DM. Nanoparticle therapeutics: an emerging treatment modality for cancer. Nat Rev Drug Discov. 2008;7:771–82.

83. Farokhzad OC, Langer R. Impact of nanotechnology on drug delivery. ACS Nano. 2009;3:16–20.

84. Sapra P, Allen TM. Improved outcome when B-cell lymphoma is treated with combinations of immunoliposomal anticancer drugs targeted to both the CD19 and CD20 epitopes. Clin Cancer Res. 2004;10: 2530–7.

85. Choi KY, Saravanakumar G, Park JH, et al. Hyaluronic acid-based nanocarriers for intracellular targeting: interfacial interactions with proteins in cancer. Colloids Surf B Biointerfaces. 2012;99:82–94.

86. Na K, Bum Lee T, Park KH, et al. Self-assembled nanoparticles of hydrophobically-modified polysaccharide bearing vitamin H as a targeted anticancer drug delivery system. Eur J Pharm Sci. 2003;18: 165–73.

87. Ponka P, Lok CN. The transferrin receptor: role in health and disease. Int J Biochem Cell Biol. 1999;31:1111–37.

88. Gu FX, Karnik R, Wang AZ, et al. Targeted nanoparticles for cancer therapy. Nano Today. 2007;2:14–21.

89. Keefe AD, Pai S, Ellington A. Aptamers as therapeutics. Nat Rev Drug Discov. 2010;9:537–50.

90. Huang BT, Lai WY, Chang YC, et al. A CTLA-4 antagonizing DNA aptamer with antitumor effect. Mol Ther. 2017;8:520–8.

91. Dhar S, Gu FX, Langer R, et al. Targeted delivery of 3441 cisplatin to prostate cancer cells by aptamer functionalized Pt(IV) prodrug-3442 PLGA-PEG nanoparticles. Proc Natl Acad Sci U S A. 2008;105:17356–61.

Tumor Architecture and Targeted Delivery

10

Dhritiman Chakraborty, Abhijit Das,
Meghana Prabhu, Konudula Sreenivasa Reddy,
Saurabh Arora, and C. S. Bal

Contents

D. Chakraborty
Department of Nuclear and Experimental Medicine,
Institute of PGMER, Kolkota, India

A. Das
Department of Pathology, Janakpuri Superspeciality
Hospital Society, New Delhi, India

M. Prabhu · K. S. Reddy · S. Arora · C. S. Bal (✉)
Department of Nuclear Medicine, All India Institute
of Medical Sciences, New Delhi, India

© Springer Nature Switzerland AG 2022
S. Harsini et al. (eds.), *Nuclear Medicine and Immunology*,
https://doi.org/10.1007/978-3-030-81261-4_10

10.1 Introduction

Advances in molecular imaging developed targeted imaging agents that are specific in binding to intracellular or extracellular targets. They can predict the responses to therapeutic interventions and are used in the diagnosis and treatment planning of the disease. Targeted imaging agents need access to the tumor tissue space and then will be retained by individual cells through binding and uptake. After absorption, drugs circulate throughout the body. The drug molecules distribute in various types of tissues. The extent of the particle penetration into the tissue depends on both the biophysical characteristics of the tissues and the biochemical features of the particles. Investigators who are developing new drugs, antibodies, or improved radionuclides should have some knowledge of the tumor architecture so that they may appreciate the barriers that may limit the delivery of antibodies or other circulating macromolecules to target tumor cells.

10.2 Organization of the Solid Tumor

Tumors are comprised of two distinct but interdependent compartments (Fig. 10.1), the malignant cells (parenchyma) and the supporting connective tissue (stroma) that they induce and in which they are dispersed [1]. Cell compartments are differentiated from the stromal compartment by a basement membrane, which is often incomplete, especially in aggressive and poorly differentiated varieties. Even if cancer originates from stromal cells, these two compartments can be distinguished.

10.2.1 Parenchymal Component

Initially, tumor cell units are formed by sheets and nests of tumor cells, which form the tumor mass along with stromal cells. Tumor cell units are separated from each other by abundant or scant stromal tissue. It provides the vascular supply necessary for tumor cell nutrition and waste disposal.

Tumor cells encompass different cell populations in different stages of differentiation arising from cancer stem cells, which are the least differentiated cells in cancer and lack specific marker [2]. The stem cells are capable of self-renewal and population renewal. It should be noted that the differentiation might be arrested at any step along the line in tumors and that full maturity may never be achieved.

Cells in a tumor can generate a new tumor by the property of population renewal, and these should be eliminated to reach successful treat-

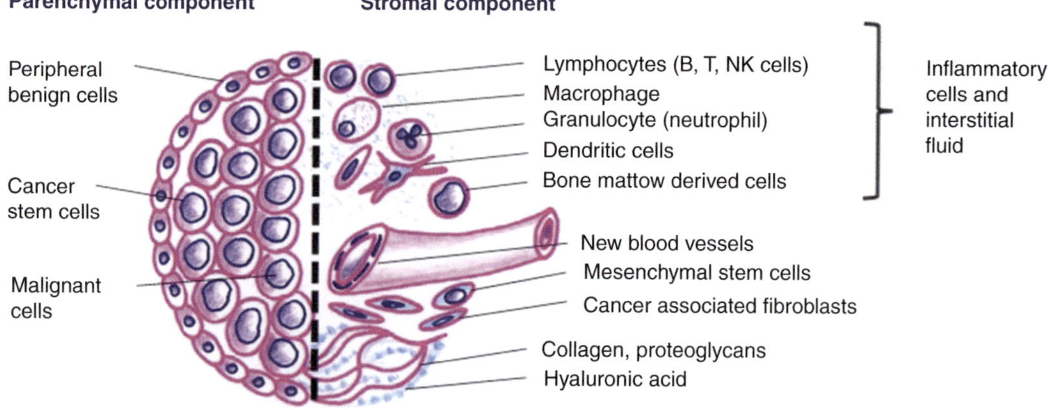

Fig. 10.1 Basic tumor architecture and tumor microenvironment (TME)

ment. Many monoclonal antibodies prepared against an antigenic markers of the differentiated cells, which are not present over stem cells, may not result in cure. The crossfire of beta particle radioimmunoconjugates does provide for bystander killing.

10.2.2 Stromal Component

Connective tissue components essential for tumor growth and generated from the host elements mainly consist of inflammatory cells and interstitial fluids, fibroblast and new blood vessels, as well as collagens, hyaluronic acid, and proteoglycan. Stroma as a whole may be regarded as a three-dimensional sieve formed by an interlocking meshwork of polysaccharides and fibrous proteins, which shapes a gel, provides support to the cellular mass, and regulates the passage of small molecules (including drugs), macromolecules, and inflammatory, mesenchymal, and tumor cell [3]. Tumor stroma is poorly organized and functionally deficient; it resembles more closely the connective tissue of a healing wound [4].

Fibronectin, an Arg-Gly-Asp (RGD)-containing adhesive protein, is much more abundant in tumor stroma, facilitating cell adherence and migration [5]. The glycosaminoglycans (GAGs) are highly viscous, negatively charged polymers. Most of the GAGs are covalently linked to core proteins, forming proteoglycans (PGs), also known as mucopolysaccharides. The necessary GAGs for the generation of tumor stroma include hyaluronic acid, chondroitin sulfate, heparin, heparan sulfate, and keratan sulfate. Another RGD-containing structural protein synthesized locally in tumor stroma by fibroblasts is tenascin, which is prominent in fetal connective tissue and facilitates cell migration. Osteopontin and thrombospondin are the other RGD-containing proteins synthesized by tumor stroma.

Extracellular matrix (ECM) remodeling is required for tumor growth. The tumor cells frequently recruit fibroblasts, endothelial cells, smooth muscle cells, and immune cells into the ECM matrix [6].

Fibroblasts in the stroma, also known as cancer-associated fibroblasts (CAFs), found as heterogeneous and highly abundant cell populations (Fig. 10.2), are master regulators orchestrating the structural organization of the TME. Various factors activate CAFs via tumor-derived signals or mechanical stress. Numerous studies have demonstrated that CAFs have prominent roles in cancer pathogenesis, having significant clinical implications [7]. CAFs are regarded as the sources of extracellular matrix, cytokines, chemokines, nutrients, and other signaling factors.

Fibroblasts are generally quiescent in normal tissues. However, during wound healing or tissue fibrosis, they can become activated and form smooth muscle reactive fibroblasts, which signals in tissue repair and scar formation [8]. Numerous preclinical studies have targeted CAFs in various mouse models; however, there are a few clinical trials performed with CAFs as direct targets. It is of utmost importance for oncologists and drug developers to fully recognize the functional importance and molecular mechanisms used by CAFs.

Small tumors, less than 2 mm in diameter, are perfused by the vasculature of the surrounding host tissues [9]. New blood vessels are necessary for tumors to obtain nutrients, exchange gas, and dispose waste materials. Successful tumors grow by protrusion and outgrowth of preexisting blood vessels, known as angiogenesis, resulting in the establishment of vascular networks. Vascular density varies widely from tumor to tumor and also within different portions of the same tumor [10].

Among the critical contents of the tumor stroma are the protein-rich interstitial fluid and plasma filtrates, especially fibrinogen. Fibrinogen clots to form fibrin, which serves as a significant component of the provisional tumor stroma. It can be replaced eventually by durable, mature connective tissue stroma. Other RGD-containing proteins may also be synthesized locally in the tumor stroma.

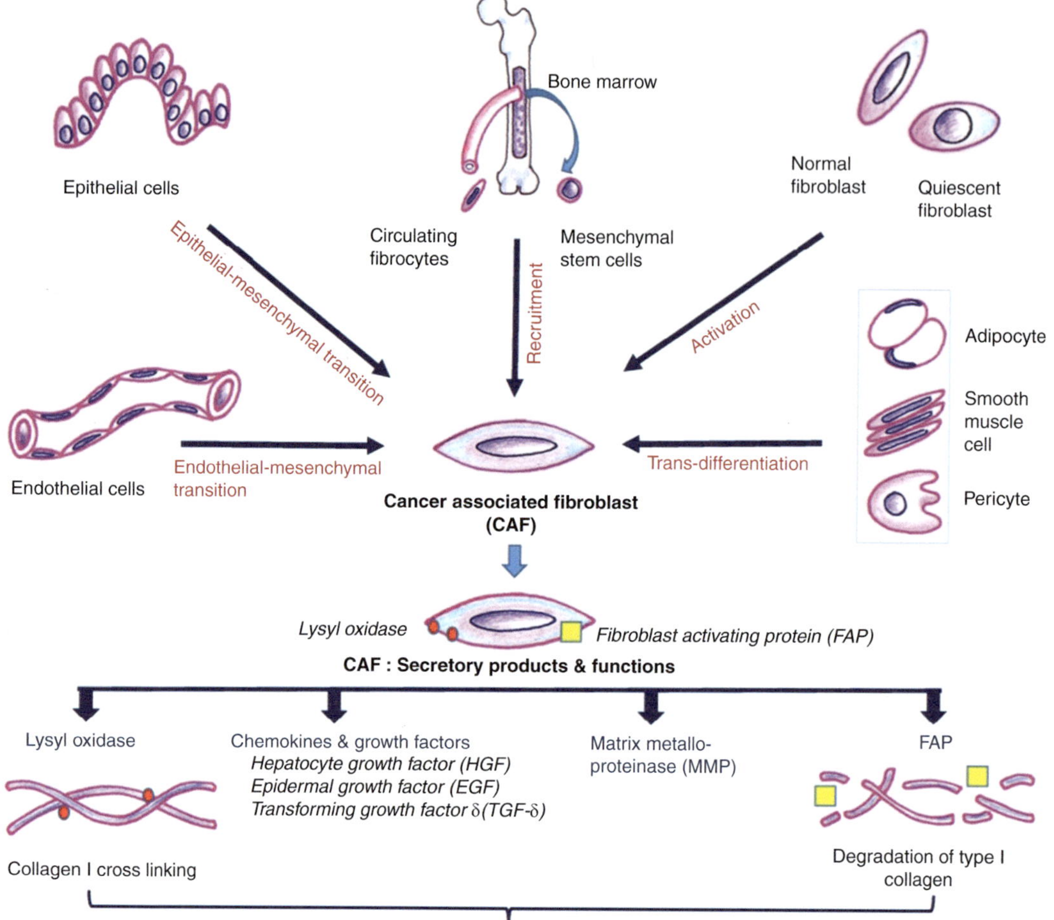

Fig. 10.2 Sources and basic functions of cancer-associated fibroblasts (CAFs)

10.2.3 Cancer-Associated Fibroblasts (CAF)

CAFs constitute the most abundant cell population in the stroma of many solid tumors. Activated CAFs exhibit enhanced proliferative and migratory properties (Fig. 10.2). They are responsible for the desmoplastic reaction, leading to ECM synthesis and remodeling. Highly dense tumors such as pancreatic, prostate, and breast cancer have more CAFs, whereas brain and renal tumors have less content. CAFs are a complex and heterogeneous cell population derived from various cell types, including resident tumor fibroblasts, epithelial cells via epithelial-to-mesenchymal transition (EMT), endothelial cells via endothelial-to-mesenchymal transition (EndMT), bone marrow-derived cells (BMDCs), adipocytes, and stellate cells, and are subsequently reprogrammed by malignant and nonmalignant cells [11, 12]. CAFs contain biological markers with particular expression patterns in the context of specific TMEs. The alpha-smooth muscle actin (α SMA), fibroblast activation protein alpha (FAP-α), podoplanin, fibroblast-specific protein-1 (FSP-1) (also known as S100A4), and platelet-derived growth factor beta receptor (PDGFβR) have also been proposed as biomarkers of a CAF phenotype [13]. None of these markers are exclusively specific for CAFs.

Though they are not exclusive, in combination, they might be useful to identify CAFs.

CAFs are responsible for cancer initiation, tumorigenesis, angiogenesis, and metastasis. They secrete proteins of extracellular matrix such as hyaluronic acid, collagens, and tenascin C; specific enzyme lysyl oxidase causing cross-linking of collagen I; and metalloproteinases (MMP) that degrade the matrix [11, 12]. Dense ECM laid by CAFs increases the interstitial fluid pressure and acts as a barrier to drug delivery. This is known as one of the causes of the reduced accumulation and failure of chemotherapy [11, 12].

CAFs release chemokines and growth factors which act as tumorigenic stimuli, namely, hepatocyte growth factor (HGF), epidermal growth factor (EGF), transforming growth factor beta (TGF-β), and stromal-derived factor-1 alpha (SDF-1α) [14]. Cancer cells may take part in epithelial-to-mesenchymal transition (EMT) highly invasive phenotype, which originated as a result of the transdifferentiation program. CAFs travel with cancer cells in the bloodstream, facilitating survival and extravasation at metastatic sites [15].

The inhibition of signaling pathways by TGF-β, hedgehog, or the angiotensin II receptor promotes a reduction in CAF and ECM content and thereby improves drug delivery and inhibits tumor growth and metastasis [16, 17]. A marker protein of CAFs is the fibroblast-activating protein (FAP), a type II transmembrane cell surface proteinase that belongs to the dipeptidyl peptidase (DPP) family, which consists of the enzymes DPP4, FAP, DPP8, and DPP9 [18]. All members have a DPP activity, cleaving two amino acids after a proline residue of the N terminus of a protein.

FAP has an additional endopeptidase activity that allows cleavage after a glycine-proline motif, making it different from other DPP family members. FAP causes denaturation and degradation of type I collagen, α2-antiplasmin, and several neuropeptides and is related to many pathologic processes. Over 90% of epithelial cancers express FAP, and its overexpression is associated with worse prognosis in solid tumors [19]. Targeting of this enzyme for imaging and endoradiotherapy can be considered a promising strategy for detecting and treating malignant tumors. Clinical trials using talabostat, a selective DPP inhibitor, showed insufficient clinical activity in various cancers. Sibrotuzumab, an anti-FAP antibody, labeled with iodine-131 for therapeutic use suffered from low clearance and lack of clinical activity [20, 21]. Haberkorn's group [22, 23] developed a series of quinoline-based radiopharmaceuticals for diagnostic and therapeutic use. The generated inhibitors bind human and murine FAPs with rapid and almost complete internalization and, importantly, without cross-reactivity to the DPP family members. A high tumor uptake rate in tumor-engrafted mice and, eventually, in patients with metastatic epithelial cancers were described using [^{68}Ga] Ga-FAPI-04.

Further, theranostic use was approached in two patients with metastasized breast cancer using [^{90}Y]Y-FAPI-04, which led to a reduction in pain symptoms at a considerably low dose. Quantification of the tumor uptake on [^{68}Ga]Ga-FAPI positron emission tomography (PET)/computed tomography (CT) of various primary and metastatic tumors was carried out by Kratochwil et al. (Haberkorn's group) in a group of 80 patients with 28 different tumor entities (54 primary tumors and 229 metastases). They noted the highest average maximum standardized uptake value (SUVmax) (average SUVmax >12) in cholangiocarcinoma, sarcoma, esophageal, breast, and lung cancers. The lowest [^{68}Ga]Ga-FAPI uptake (average SUVmax <6) was observed in pheochromocytoma, renal cell carcinoma, differentiated thyroid cancer, adenoid cystic carcinoma, and gastric cancer. The average SUVmax of hepatocellular, colorectal, head and neck, ovarian, pancreatic, and prostate cancers was intermediate (SUVmax of 6–12) [24].

Targeting the stroma with FAP-binding molecules may lead to highly promising new applications for noninvasive tumor characterization, staging examinations, and theranostic approaches with enormous potential and sets the stage to target the interaction between cancer cells, host cells, and ECM.

10.3 Cancer Metastasis

The neoplastic cells residing within the primary tumor primarily exhibit epithelial characteristics. Tumor cells must acquire, at least transiently, mesenchymal properties in order to invade and disseminate to distant sites and subsequently form metastatic deposits. This complex biological cellular program of attaining mesenchymal properties from epithelial phenotype is known as "epithelial-mesenchymal transition" (EMT). Cancer metastasis involves multiple steps starting from EMT signals through stromal invasion, tumor dissemination, and finally culminating in the mesenchymal-epithelial transition to form macrometastasis at distal sites (Fig. 10.3).

10.4 Angiogenesis

Angiogenesis causes the vascularization of the tumor, which is essential for tumor progression. The process is mediated by vascular endothe-lial growth factor (VEGF) and basic fibroblast growth factor (bFGF) [25, 26]. It occurs by the interplay of pro- and antiangiogenic molecules that are released by cancer cells and some other cells, such as the endothelial cells, stromal cells, and cellular components of the ECM. The angiogenic process involves degradation of the blood vessel basement membrane and associated ECM, endothelial cell proliferation, early tube formation, and differentiation of newly formed blood vessels into arterioles and venules with the remodeling of the ECM.

10.5 Tumor Vascular Architecture

Tumor vasculature is generally characterized by a lack of smooth muscle cells and pericytes in the vessel walls, compared to normal tissue vasculature (Fig. 10.4). These vessels, having irregular basement membrane and discontinuous endothelial lining, do not have sinusoidal vessel plexuses, adrenergic innervation, and lymphatic

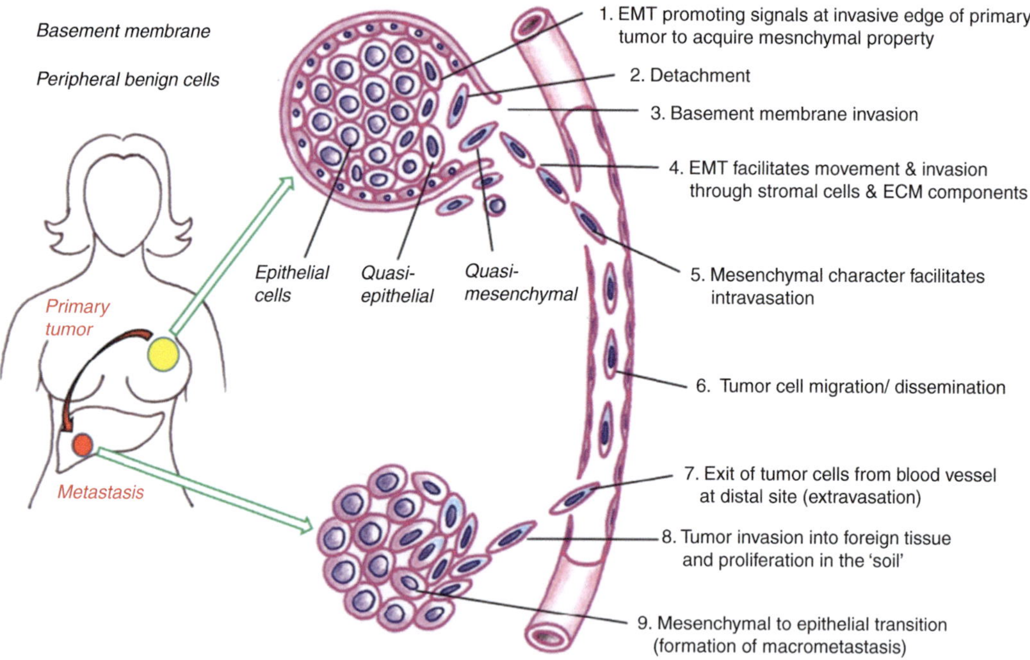

Fig. 10.3 Cancer metastasis-invasion-metastasis cascade in cancer

drainage [27–30]. Tumor vasculature shows intricate branching patterns and lacks the hierarchy of blood vessels found in the normal tissues [30]. Growth of tumor vasculature is poorly regulated; hence, the vascular growth is vigorous but disordered in all possible directions, termed as invasion percolation [31]. Penetration of blood vessels into the solid tumor causes intra-tumoral differences in the vascularization; consequently, the border of tumor-normal tissue is usually highly vascularized, while the interior most parts of the tumor may remain avascular [32]. Tumor vascular network appears irregular with significantly high tortuosity, leading to resistance to blood flow, high vascular density in specific regions, and complete lack of vasculature in others. Arteries and veins have never been observed in the center of a tumor. All tumor vessels have shown a capillary wall construction with variations in the height and densities of the endothelial cells.

10.6 Transport Across the Microvascular Wall

Tumor microvessels are hyperpermeable to circulating macromolecules due to intermittent widened intercellular spaces with overlapping endothelial cells and multiple cellular processes.

Leakiness of the tumor vasculature could also be related to vasodilation and elevated levels of growth factors. Tumor blood vessels have greater diameter and volume compared to the normal vasculature due to overexpression of VEGF, bFGF, bradykinin, and nitric oxide. The net result of leaky vasculature and lack of lymphatic drainage is enhanced accumulation of particulate and macromolecules at the tumor site. This phenomenon is called the enhanced permeation and retention (EPR) effect (Fig. 10.4).

10.7 Transport Across the Stroma

After extravasation from leaky blood vessels, molecules make their way through the tumor stroma before interacting with the cancer cells. Extensive stroma is found in many common human cancers, and molecules pass through convection and/or diffusion.

In convection, molecules move down a pressure gradient and are thought to contribute significantly to the passage of circulating macromolecules across normal microvessels and in extravascular connective tissue [33]. Active extravasation of circulating therapeutic molecules is prevented based on convection due to sufficiently high interstitial pressures within the tumors, which may be present to balance the intravascular pressures. Indeed,

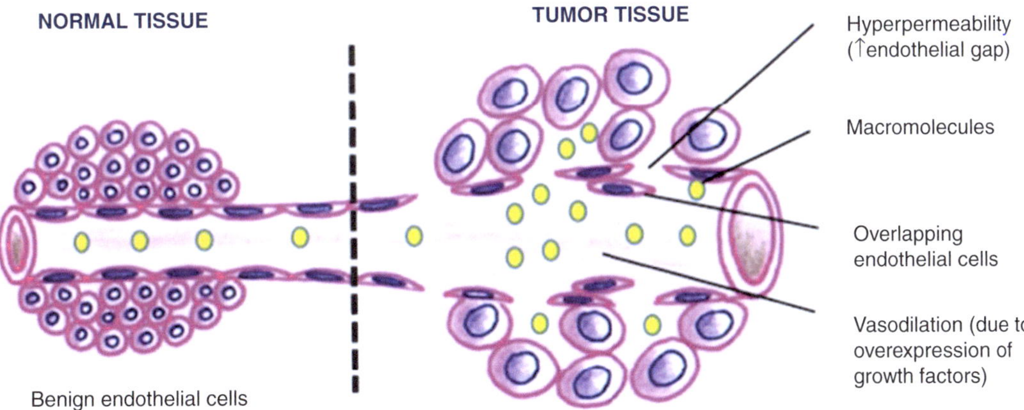

Fig. 10.4 Tumor microvascular architecture and "enhanced permeation and retention" (EPR) effect

since molecules flow down a pressure gradient, the high interstitial pressure of tumors directs convective flow away from the tumor center toward the periphery [34].

Diffusion is driven by solute concentration gradients, and these may be expected to favor the passage of the blood-delivered molecules across the stroma. However, the movement of large molecules across significant distances by diffusion is extremely slow. Jain has estimated that a macromolecule such as immunoglobulin (Ig)G can diffuse a distance of ~100 µm in 1 h but would require some days to cover a distance of ~1 mm [35]. Even though the diffusion is regarded as a useful mechanism for the delivery of small molecules that diffuse rapidly, these mechanisms would not permit therapeutic macromolecules to reach tumor cells in a timely fashion.

10.8 Transport Across the Parenchyma

Apart from the convection and diffusion through the parenchyma, an additional barrier is provided by the intercellular junctions between tumor cells. Depending on the particular cell type and the degree of tumor differentiation, carcinoma cells form various secure attachments with each other, whereas lymphoma and melanoma cells do not. Unlike endothelial cells junctions, interepithelial cell junctions, when present, might restrict the passage of even small molecules such as salts or water and limit the passage of macromolecules. Different regions of the same tumor show extensively different level of differentiation and the complexity of tumor cell junctions. This heterogeneity indicates that the passage of large and small molecules will vary considerably from one region to another within the same tumor, in the same manner as the blood flow.

10.9 Strategies to Reduce the Barriers for the Macromolecules to Reach Their Target

Reduction of the size of the particles, with the development of engineered small antibody fragments, leads to diffusion across tumor vessels, stroma, and parenchyma. Smaller fragments can still be designed, capable of retaining specificity and avidity for tumor antigen targets. Disadvantages of small size are shorter circulation time, more extensive extravasation across normal microvessels, and hence higher concentrations of potentially toxic molecules in normal tissues. Hyperpermeability of macromolecules is exploited in the therapy of solid tumors with monoclonal antibodies. Approaches that reduce the interstitial pressure will help in the entry of macromolecules in the tumor stroma.

Difficulties of delivery would be significantly reduced through targeting the tumor vasculature and the endothelial cells lining tumor vessels by selective targeting and/or destruction instead. Targeting vascular endothelium, specifically VEGF and its receptors VEGFR-1 and VEGFR-2, αvβ3 integrin, vascular cell adhesion molecule-1 (VCAM-1), and matrix metalloproteinases (MMPs), obviates the need for the extravasation of drug delivery carriers and is generally applicable to all tumor types. Besides, the risk of developing drug resistance is lower since endothelial cells are genetically more stable compared to tumor cells [36].

10.10 Drug Delivery in Cancer

Most of the anticancer agents are chemotherapeutic agents that are small molecules. Higher molecular weight antitumor agents include monoclonal antibodies, cytokines, and oligonucleotides. The transport process depends on drug properties such as size, diffusivity, electrostatic charge, nonspecific binding, plasma half-life as well as tumor characteristics including interstitial fluid pressure, ECM components, cellular density, and the vascular architecture.

During the early phase studies, molecules are tested in cell culture models, followed by animal toxicology studies. During preclinical and early clinical development, a candidate drug is characterized for its solubility in common solvents and under different pH conditions in aqueous buffers. With successful passage, larger quantities of the compound become available and are used for the development of clinical formulations.

For rapid initiation of action, the alleviation of drug action, bioavailability, and accurate dosing intravenous (IV) route of administration are preferred for anticancer drugs. IV dosage forms are preferred as simple solutions with minimal use of excipients and preservatives. Other formulations are oral tablets or capsules and the less commonly used delivery systems such as gels, implants, and aerosols.

10.10.1 Drug Delivery Targeting Tumor Vasculature

10.10.1.1 Passive Targeting

Here, the distribution of the drug is based on its physical characteristics, not due to other specific features, and this way, it extravasates into the interstitial tumor fluid due to increased vascular permeability of the tumor vasculature. EPR effect contributes to the targeting of the tumor and the prolonged retention of drug in the tumor. Passive targeting involves a process to achieve high tumor drug levels and/or overall exposure and avoids body sites or tissues that may be particularly sensitive to the drug and contribute to its toxic effects [37].

10.10.1.2 Active Targeting

This class of drugs acts as antiangiogenic molecules that can cause tumor growth arrest or as vasoactive agents that may induce hyperabnormalization of the tumor vasculature and accumulation of drug and cause vessel congestion resulting in tumor necrosis. VEGF and its receptors VEGFR-1 and VEGFR-2, $\alpha v \beta 3$ integrin, VCAM-1, and MMPs are the different antigens and receptors on vascular endothelial cells. In addition to antibodies, ligands such as peptides, aptamers, and small organic molecules can be exploited for tumor vasculature targeting.

10.10.2 Increase in Blood Circulation Time and Reduced Immunogenicity

An increase in blood circulation time modifies the overall tumor accumulation, achieved by covalent conjugation of synthetic polymers, such as polyethylene glycol (PEG), on the surface of the drug delivery system, termed as PEGylated drug delivery systems. PEGylation of proteins also reduces their immunogenicity and improves patient response in cases with allergy to the non-PEGylated native protein.

10.10.3 Drug Release Based on the Tumor Microenvironment

Extracellular pH in the tumor microenvironment (5.7–7.8) differs significantly from the normal tissue pH (7.4), leading to the different behavior of ionizable anticancer drugs, resulting in significant differences in the activity of organic molecules in the tumor microenvironment and the feasibility of making pH-responsive micelles for tumor drug delivery [38, 39].

10.10.4 Prodrug Mechanism

Prodrug strategies target specific features of the tumor, like differences in the interstitial pH of the tumor tissue, and can lead to the release of the drug in the tumor interstitium from the nanoparticulate drug carriers or high enzymatic activity in the tumor environment that can result in the tumor-specific cleavage of the prodrug and the release of the active moiety.

10.10.5 Drug Delivery by Modulation of Tumor Vasculature

Tumor necrosis factor-α (TNF-α) can cause increased tumor drug penetration by endothelial cell damage and reduce interstitial tumor pressure [40]. Coadministration of tiny doses of TNF-α can increase the therapeutic index of cytotoxic agents by increasing drug efficacy at low doses.

10.11 Conclusion

Properly targeted drug delivery, be it cytotoxic agents or molecularly targeted agents, from the systemic circulation to the cancer cells, increases the efficacy of the drug and reduces toxicities. Understanding of tumor pathophysiology, which depends upon dynamic tumor microenvironment with changes in its angiogenesis potential, cell mass, and the extracellular environment, will help to overcome the barriers to the drug entry process in the tumor cells and help targeted drug delivery.

References

1. Yeo TK, Dvorak HF. Tumor stroma. In: Colvin R, Bhan A, McCluskey R, editors. Diagnostic immunopathology. New York: Raven Press; 1995. p. 485–697.
2. Knudson AG. Stem cell regulation, tissue ontogeny, and oncogenic events. Semin Cancer Biol. 1992;3(3):99–106.
3. Campbell NE, Kellenberger L, Greenaway J, Moorehead RA, Linnerth-Petrik NM, Petrik J. Extracellular matrix proteins and tumor angiogenesis. J Oncol. 2010;2010:586905. Epub 2010 Jun 29. https://doi.org/10.1155/2010/586905.
4. Dvorak HF. Tumors: wounds that do not heal. Similarities between tumor stroma generation and wound healing. N Engl J Med. 1986;315(26):1650–9.
5. Yamada K. Fibronectin and other cell interactive glycoproteins. In: Hay E, editor. Cell biology of extracellular matrix. 2nd ed. New York: Plenum Press; 1991. p. 111–46.
6. Radisky D, Hagios C, Bissell MJ. Tumors are unique organs defined by abnormal signaling and context. Semin Cancer Biol. 2001;11:87–95.
7. Su S, et al. CD10(+)GPR77(+) cancer-associated fibroblasts promote cancer formation and chemoresistance by sustaining cancer stemness. Cell. 2018;172:841–56.
8. Mueller MM, Fusenig NE. Friends or foes - bipolar effects of the tumour stroma in cancer. Nat Rev Cancer. 2004;4(11):839–49.
9. Gimbrone MA Jr, Leapman SB, Cotran RS, Folkman J. Tumor dormancy in vivo by prevention of neovascularization. J Exp Med. 1972;136(2):261–76.
10. Weidner N, Folkman J. Tumoral vascularity as a prognostic factor in cancer. In: De Vita VT, Hellman S, Rosenberg SA, editors. Important advances in oncology. Philadelphia: Lippincott-Raven; 1996. p. 167–90.
11. Ohlund D, et al. Fibroblast heterogeneity in the cancer wound. J Exp Med. 2014;211:1503–23.
12. Cirri P, Chiarugi P. Cancer associated fibroblasts: the dark side of the coin. Am J Cancer Res. 2011;1:482–97.
13. Kalluri R. The biology and function of fibroblasts in cancer. Nat Rev Cancer. 2016;16:582–98.
14. Scherz-Shouval R, et al. The reprogramming of tumor stroma by HSF1 is a potent enabler of malignancy. Cell. 2014;158:564–78.
15. Duda DG, et al. Malignant cells facilitate lung metastasis by bringing their own soil. Proc Natl Acad Sci U S A. 2010;107:21677–82.
16. Liu J, et al. TGF-b blockade improves the distribution and efficacy of therapeutics in breast carcinoma by normalizing the tumor stroma. Proc Natl Acad Sci U S A. 2012;109:16618–23.
17. Olive KP, et al. Inhibition of hedgehog signalling enhances delivery of chemotherapy in a mouse model of pancreatic cancer. Science. 2009;324:1457–61.
18. Hamson EJ, Keane FM, Tholen S, Schilling O, Gorrell MD. Understanding fibroblast activation protein (FAP): substrates, activities, expression and targeting for cancer therapy. Proteomics Clin Appl. 2014;8:454–63.
19. Liu F, Qi L, Liu B, et al. Fibroblast activation protein overexpression and clinical implications in solid tumors: a meta-analysis. PLoS One. 2015;10:e0116683.
20. Scott AM, Wiseman G, Welt S, et al. A phase I dose-escalation study of sibrotuzumab in patients with advanced or metastatic fibroblast activation protein-positive cancer. Clin Cancer Res. 2003;9:1639–47.
21. Kloft C, Graefe EU, Tanswell P, et al. Population pharmacokinetics of sibrotuzumab, a novel therapeutic monoclonal antibody, in cancer patients. Investig New Drugs. 2004;22:39–52.
22. Lindner T, Loktev A, Altmann A, et al. Development of quinoline-based theranostic ligands for the targeting of fibroblast activation protein. J Nucl Med. 2018;59:1415–22.

23. Loktev A, Lindner T, Mier W, et al. A tumor-imaging method targeting cancer-associated fibroblasts. J Nucl Med. 2018;59:1423–9.

24. Kratochwil C, Flechsig P, Lindner T, Abderrahim L, Altmann A, Mier W, Adeberg S, Rathke H, Röhrich M, Winter H, Plinkert PK, Marme F, Lang M, Kauczor HU, Jäger D, Debus J, Haberkorn U, Giesel FL. 68Ga-FAPI PET/CT: tracer uptake in 28 different kinds of cancer. J Nucl Med. 2019;60: 801–5.

25. Ferrara N, Houck K, Jakeman L, Leung DW. Molecular and biological properties of the vascular endothelial growth factor family of proteins. Endocr Rev. 1992;13:18–32.

26. Compagni A, Wilgenbus P, Impagnatiello MA, Cotten M, Christofori G. Fibroblast growth factors are required for efficient tumor angiogenesis. Cancer Res. 2000;60:7163–9.

27. Dvorak HF, Nagy JA, Dvorak JT, Dvorak AM. Identification and characterization of the blood vessels of solid tumors that are leaky to circulating macromolecules. Am J Pathol. 1988;133:95–109.

28. Eberhard A, Kahlert S, Goede V, Hemmerlein B, Plate KH, Augustin HG. Heterogeneity of angiogenesis and blood vessel maturation in human tumors: implications for antiangiogenic tumor therapies. Cancer Res. 2000;60:1388–93.

29. Paku S, Paweletz N. First steps of tumor-related angiogenesis. Lab Investig. 1991;65:334–46.

30. Konerding MA, Malkusch W, Klapthor B, van Ackern C, Fait E, Hill SA, Parkins C, Chaplin DJ, Presta M, Denekamp J. Evidence for characteristic vascular patterns in solid tumours: quantitative studies using corrosion casts. Br J Cancer. 1999;80:724–32.

31. Baish JW, Gazit Y, Berk DA, Nozue M, Baxter LT, Jain RK. Role of tumor vascular architecture in nutrient and drug delivery: an invasion percolation-based network model. Microvasc Res. 1996;51:327–46.

32. Ahlstrom H, Christofferson R, Lorelius LE. Vascularization of the continuous human colonic cancer cell line LS 174 T deposited subcutaneously in nude rats. APMIS. 1988;96:701–10.

33. Eppe B, Haraldsson B. Transport of macromolecules across microvascular walls: the two-pore theory. Physiol Rev. 1994;74:163–219.

34. Butler TP, Grantham FH, Gullinr PM. Bulk transfer of fluid in the interstitial compartment of mammary tumors. Cancer Res. 1975;35:3084–8.

35. Jain RK. Delivery of novel therapeutic agents in tumors: physiological barriers and strategies. J Natl Cancer Inst. 1989;81:570–6.

36. Gosk S, Moos T, Gottstein C, Bendas G. VCAM-1 directed immunoliposomes selectively target tumor vasculature in vivo. Biochim Biophys Acta. 2008;1778:854–63. https://doi.org/10.1016/j.bbamem.2007.12.021.

37. Lammers T, Hennink WE, Storm G. Tumour-targeted nanomedicines: principles and practice. Br J Cancer. 2008;99:392–7.

38. van Sluis R, Bhujwalla ZM, Raghunand N, Ballesteros P, Alvarez J, Cerdan S, Galons JP, Gillies RJ. In vivo imaging of extracellular pH using 1H MRSI. Magn Reson Med. 1999;41:743–50.

39. Simon SM. Role of organelle pH in tumor cell biology and drug resistance. Drug Discov Today. 1999;4:32–8.

40. Kristensen CA, Nozue M, Boucher Y, Jain RK. Reduction of interstitial fluid pressure after TNF-alpha treatment of three human melanoma xenografts. Br J Cancer. 1996;74:533–6.

Radionuclide Therapy and Immunomodulation

11

Rachel Anderson and Katherine Vallis

Contents

11.1 Introduction

Since its discovery in the late nineteenth century, external beam radiation therapy (EBRT) has become a cornerstone in oncology and is used around the world. Today, as many as 60% of cancer patients receive EBRT for both curative and palliative treatment. This localized treatment delivers high doses of radiation to the defined tumor or at-risk volumes but is limited by exposure of surrounding normal tissues. Historically, the prevailing explanation for the antitumor effects of EBRT has been the induction of complex DNA damage leading to cell death and abrogated clonogenic survival, ultimately providing local disease control. Alongside this, the general view of EBRT for some time suggested it was in fact immunosuppressive. This arose predominantly from observations of lymphopenia following radiation therapy (RT) and the widespread use of total body irradiation as an immunosuppressant to prevent immunologic rejection during bone marrow transplantation. However, in

R. Anderson · K. Vallis (✉)
Oxford Institute for Radiation Oncology, Department of Oncology, University of Oxford, Oxford, UK
e-mail: rachel.anderson@oncology.ox.ac.uk;
katherine.vallis@oncology.ox.ac.uk

© Springer Nature Switzerland AG 2022
S. Harsini et al. (eds.), *Nuclear Medicine and Immunology*,
https://doi.org/10.1007/978-3-030-81261-4_11

recent years, it has become increasingly clear that the immune system is key to EBRT efficacy, with a plethora of mechanisms inducing a functional antitumor immune response as well as direct tumor cell killing.

Despite its widespread use, the potency of EBRT as a stimulus of the immune response may be limited by a number of factors, such as the inability to target all sites of disseminated disease. This may be addressed using an alternative form of radiotherapy known as targeted radionuclide therapy (TRT). This increasingly common form of therapy employs therapeutic radioisotopes conjugated to targeting moieties. These small molecules, antibodies, or other ligands specifically recognize and bind to tumor antigens and thus enable specific accumulation within the tumor site following systemic administration. As the isotope decays, it delivers protracted, low-dose rate radiation to the tumor site, which is analogous to EBRT and may stimulate an antitumor immune response. Importantly, the use of systemic radiotherapy enables the treatment of all sites of metastatic disease which should promote induction of a functional immune response. Other differences such as dose, dose rate, and radiation quality are also likely to impact the landscape of the immune response in various ways as discussed in this chapter.

11.2 The Role of the Immune System in Radiotherapy

11.2.1 External Beam Radiation Therapy and Abscopal Responses

In the early years of radiotherapy, very few investigators considered its interaction with the immune response. In 1917, a few years after the establishment of radiotherapy as a treatment for cancer, Ewing noted the exudation of lymphocytes and polymorphonuclear leukocytes within days of administration of radium. However, more direct assessment of the effects of irradiation on immunity was lacking until much later

[1]. Almost 40 years after this initial observation, Cohen and Cohen conducted a number of studies demonstrating that administration of ex vivo irradiated tumor samples improved the efficacy of irradiation of preestablished murine xenografts [2, 3]. They went on to suggest such a response *could be explained only on the basis of a systemic resistance mechanism, possibly in the nature of a circulating iso-antibody arising in the host.* Again, there was a long wait before further studies provided conclusive evidence for this hypothesis, but in the 1970s, both Suit et al. and Slone et al. observed that the radiosensitivity of murine xenografts was significantly affected by the immune status of the mouse host, with additional effects on the likelihood of developing metastases [4, 5]. Unfortunately, this aspect of radiotherapy then received little attention for some time, perhaps because of reports that appeared to rule out a radiation-induced immune response. For example, Hewitt et al. assessed the immunization capacity of lethally irradiated murine tumor cells of spontaneous origin and observed no induction of resistance in isogenic recipient mice. Based on this, Hewitt suggested that the literature showing otherwise was an artifact of immunity associated with the viral or chemical induction of the tumors that were used in these studies [6]. In hindsight, while this appreciation of the importance of tumor immunogenicity was undoubtedly insightful, the erroneous rejection of the evidence that irradiation can directly cause immune effects likely impeded advancement in the field for years.

Slowly, the recognition that EBRT may induce an antitumor immune response arose from observations, across a range of malignancies, of therapeutic responses outside the irradiated field [7–9]. Such a response was first described in 1953 [10], although occurrences remained scarce with two cases in papillary adenocarcinoma and melanoma described in 1973 and 1975, respectively [8, 9]. Due to the local nature of the treatment, these systemic responses were unexpected and could not be explained by the accepted principle that direct induction of cytotoxic DNA and cellular damage is necessary for cell killing by radiation. This phenomenon, coined the abscopal effect [10], has since been shown to be a function of the immune response induced by EBRT [11–13]. While such cases are rare and anecdotal, it is becoming increasingly clear that radiation commonly induces an immune response. However, concurrent immunosuppressive effects—particularly in tumors outside the radiation field—may have thus far limited the effectiveness of this response [14]. Indeed, despite the millions of patients treated with EBRT between 1969 and 2014, only 46 cases of abscopal effects have been reported [15]. While observation of abscopal effects is rare, more widespread clinical evidence for the importance of immune activation by EBRT includes the observed effect of immunosuppressants, genetic mutations, and low lymphocyte count on the efficacy of EBRT [16].

Importantly, the induction of an immune response provides the possibility of systemic, long-lasting protection, highlighting the potential for synergistic responses to combined radiotherapy-immunotherapy combinations. Consistently, since the introduction of immune checkpoint inhibitors into the clinic, reports of abscopal responses have been increasing. One key case report from Memorial Sloan Kettering Cancer Center in 2012 described a metastatic melanoma patient with progressive disease on ipilimumab, who was subsequently treated with palliative EBRT to alleviate back pain caused by a paraspinal mass [17]. Following RT, there was significant regression of both the treated lesion and nontargeted lesions, with stable disease 10 months later. Another patient with metastatic melanoma who had been treated with ipilimumab and stereotactic body radiotherapy to two of seven liver metastases was recently reported to be in complete remission, with no evidence of disease or recurrence 6.5 years after treatment [18]. As a result, a number of clinical trials have been undertaken to test combinations of EBRT with immunotherapeutics to explore whether the frequency of abscopal effects could be increased. With many trials ongoing, a number of success stories have already been described. In 2015, a proof-of-principle study was published showing that the immunoadjuvant granulocyte-macrophage colony-stimulating factor (GM-CSF) could stimulate otherwise rare abscopal responses to occur in approximately 30% of patients with multiple metastatic solid tumors [19]. Preclinical evidence is also emerging, for example, showing that fractionated EBRT combined with anti-cytotoxic T-lymphocyte-associated protein 4 (CTLA-4) antibody caused an abscopal effect in both a murine TS/A breast carcinoma model and the murine MCA38 colon carcinoma model [20].

11.2.2 Immunomodulation by EBRT Can Contribute to Therapeutic Efficacy

Given this new understanding that in rare cases EBRT can induce a functional systemic immune response, it is of growing interest to investigate how widespread this immune induction is and whether it more generally contributes to the therapeutic efficacy of EBRT. As well as the evidence of abscopal effects, a growing pool of both preclinical and clinical observations supports the importance of a functional immune response. A standout study by Lee et al. strikingly demonstrated the loss of B16 tumor radiosensitivity in immunocompromised (nude) mice, compared to wild-type (WT) mice, suggesting that at least in some cases, immune activation is not only a contributing factor but is essential to therapeutic efficacy [21]. These investigators went on to show that this loss of response is due to the need for an intact immune system, and not a result of the differing strains, using antibody mediated CD8$^+$ T-cell depletion to dramatically reduce tumor response in WT mice (Fig. 11.1) [21]. A similar trend was demonstrated in both EG7 and LLC-OVA tumor-bearing mice [22], as well as in EL4 tumor-bearing mice where the loss of response in immunosuppressed mice was accompanied by loss of cytokine and antibody production [23]. These studies highlight the potential importance of the EBRT-induced immune response to both locoregional tumor control and its role in mediating abscopal effects.

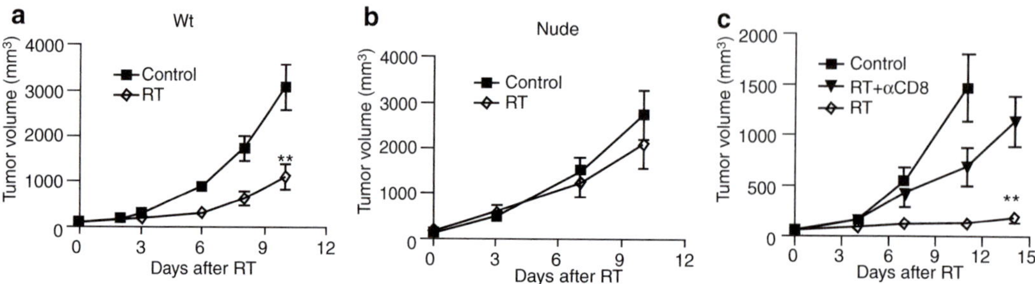

Fig. 11.1 Lee et al., 2009, demonstrate radiosensitivity of B16 tumors observed in wild-type (WT) mice (**a**) is lost in mice lacking a thymus and thus immunodeficient (**b**). To show this is not due to the different mice strains, this is then repeated in WT mice using anti-CD8 antibodies to deplete cluster of differentiation (CD)8+ T cells, demonstrating a significant reduction in therapeutic efficacy (**c**). (Adapted from Lee et al., 2009 [21])

Antitumor Immunity

An antitumor immune response is generated by the immune system that fights against pathogens (bacteria, viruses, etc.). This system is comprised of a large number of highly specialized cells and molecules that act together to eliminate foreign matter from the body. Central to this are T cells—in particular cytotoxic CD8+ T cells—which exert their cytotoxic effects upon recognition of a specific antigen. This recognition occurs via specific T-cell receptors (TCRs).

During development, a large population of T cells is generated, each possessing a different receptor capable of recognizing a small number of cognate antigens. T cells recognizing self-antigens are destroyed, leaving a T-cell repertoire capable only of recognizing and eliminating foreign matter. The bulk T-cell population remains in a naïve state within lymph nodes, incapable of exerting cytotoxic effects until a cell becomes activated by recognition of its cognate antigen in a special complex with a major histocompatibility complex (MHC)-II molecule, along with an additional activation signal, on the surface of an antigen-presenting cell (APC).

During tumorigenesis, aberrant protein expression leads to the generation of tumor antigens that can be recognized by cognate TCRs leading to targeted elimination of cancer cells. This destruction requires an APC, typically a dendritic cell (DC), to first engulf tumor cells or tumor cell debris and process the antigens for exposure on their surface with the MHC-II complex. These activated DCs travel to the lymph nodes where they interact with and activate cognate T cells. The activated T cells return to the circulation and infiltrate the tumor through a process promoted by chemokines and adhesion molecules produced by local inflammation. Here, they are able to locate and kill target cells expressing their cognate tumor antigen in a process that can be further promoted by the presence of other cytokines and stimulatory signals. Unfortunately, during the process of tumorigenesis, the tumor evolves to overcome the barrier of the immune system. A number of mechanisms act to create an immunosuppressive tumor microenvironment (TME) that enables the tumor to develop. Such mechanisms include exclusion of lymphocytes from the TME and polarization of immune cells to immunosuppressive subtypes, such as Treg cells and M2 macrophages, along with the expression of checkpoint inhibitors such as CTLA-4 that inhibit T-cell action (Fig. 11.2).

11.2.3 Molecular Understanding of Immunomodulation by EBRT

Given the clinical and preclinical evidence for the importance of the immune response to RT efficacy, there is now accumulating literature that reports the mechanisms underlying these effects. Such work has revealed a plethora of changes induced by EBRT that act at various stages of the cancer immunity cycle: promoting changes to the tumor cells to increase their susceptibility to T-cell killing, promoting DC activation and subsequent T-cell priming, further stimulation of T-cell activation, and recruitment of lymphocytes to the tumor site, to name but a few (Fig. 11.2).

11.2.3.1 Increasing Sensitivity of Tumor Cells to Cytotoxic Immune Cells

There have been a number of observations suggesting that treatment with EBRT can increase sensitivity of tumor cells to immune-mediated killing. This increased sensitivity is a result of a number of factors including upregulation of various cell surface proteins involved in cytotoxic T lymphocyte (CTL) interactions with target cells. One such protein, Fas, is increased in a dose-dependent fashion in response to EBRT [24]. This protein binds Fas-ligand expressed on CTLs inducing death of the tumor cell.

RT can also increase the expression of MHC class I complexes [25]. It is these complexes that expose antigens from within the cell, including tumor antigens (TAs), to the surveying immune cells in the tumor microenvironment (TME). Only when expressed in this way are T cells able to recognize their cognate antigens and exert their cytolytic activity on the cancer cell. Perhaps unsurprisingly then, tumor cells often downregulate these molecules during the process of tumorigenesis, masking themselves from immune surveillance. Consequently, radiation-induced upregulation enables recog-

nition and destruction of TA-expressing cells. Upregulation of DNA damage response and cell cycle regulation genes by radiotherapy may also promote this process. These newly transcribed proteins are more likely to be processed for MHC loading, and as these proteins are often mutated in cancer, their increased presentation on the cell surface provides neoantigens for recognition by T cells [25, 26]. As well as enabling recognition of existing TAs, it is also possible that radiation induces neoantigen generation via its DNA-damaging effects, increasing the number of tumor-specific antigens available for recognition.

11.2.3.2 Lymphocyte Activation

Together with increasing tumor cell susceptibility, RT can also promote the activation of lymphocytes within the TME. Perhaps the best understood mechanism of immune cell activation by EBRT is immunogenic cell death (ICD). This highly immunogenic form of programmed cell death results in the release of a number of immunostimulatory compounds that go on to activate and prime an antitumor immune response. Three key molecular determinants of immunogenic cell death (ICD) have been defined: exposure of calreticulin (CRT) on the cell surface, release of high mobility group box 1 (HMGB1), and release of adenosine triphosphate (ATP).

Relocation of CRT, an endoplasmic reticulum protein, to the cell surface allows it to interact with the TME. In this context, it acts as a potent "eat-me" signal, promoting uptake of the tumor cell by macrophages and DCs, with subsequent processing and presentation of TAs. HMGB1 released from the cell further stimulates this process via action on several APC receptors, including toll-like receptor 4 (TLR-4). This results in a number of downstream effects, for example, inhibition of lysosome-dependent degradation of phagosomes, thus enabling antigen processing and degradation rather than breakdown and ultimately driving

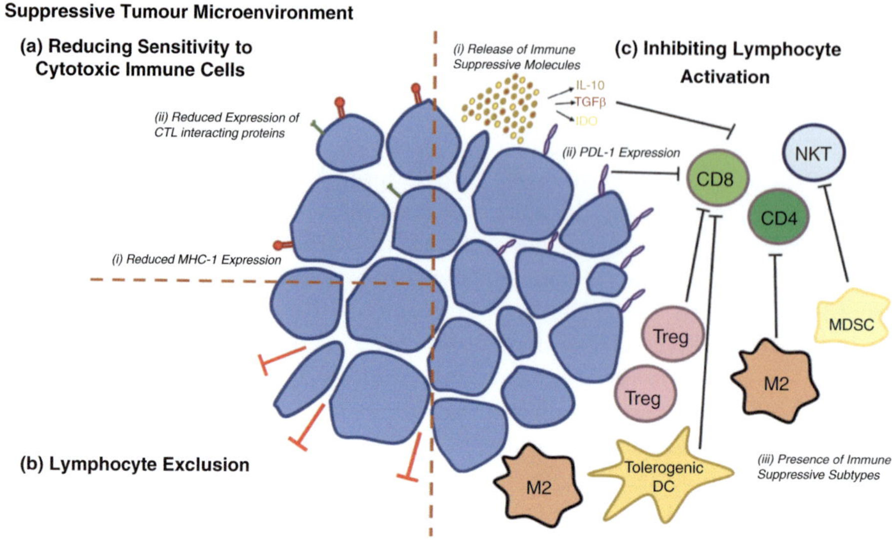

Fig. 11.2 Tumoral immunosuppression and the immune response to EBRT. (1) Suppressive tumor microenvironment: Tumorigenesis requires the formation of an immunosuppressive microenvironment to enable tumor growth unhindered by the immune system. The major mechanisms employed by the tumor to generate this environment produce three key changes: (a) Reduction in sensitivity to cytotoxic immune cells including CD8+ T cells and NKT cells. This is achieved via a number of mechanisms, including (i) reduced expression of MHC class I complexes, which are required to present peptides derived from intracellular proteins on the cell surface in a format recognizable by cognate T-cell receptor of cytotoxic T cells activating them to kill the target cell. (ii) Tumor cells also downregulate other cell surface proteins involved in these cytotoxic interactions, including Fas-L. (b) Tumors also create either "immune desert" or "immune excluded" microenvironments, characterized by poor infiltration of T cells with high myeloid-derived suppressor cell (MDSC) counts, or high tumor-infiltrating lymphocytes in the surrounding stroma but no infiltration into the tumor parenchyma. (c) For those cells that do enter the tumor, there are a plethora of mechanisms waiting to inhibit lymphocyte activation. They include (i) the production of immunosuppressive molecules by both tumor cells and immune cells, (ii) high expression of immune checkpoint molecules such as PD-L1, which inhibits programmed cell death protein 1 (PD-1) positive T cells, and (iii) the presence of various immunosuppressive subtypes, including regulatory T cells, M2 macrophages, and MDSCs, which can facilitate angiogenesis, immunosuppression, and inflammation. (2) Immune activation by EBRT is achieved via abrogation of these immunosuppressive effects in various ways. (a) Increasing sensitivity to cytotoxic immune cells by restoring/increasing (i) MHC-1 and (ii) other immune cell-interacting molecules. (iii) Alongside this, the release of tumor-associated antigens leads to increased T-cell priming and recruitment of cognate T cells. (b) Lymphocyte recruitment converts "immune desert" or "immune excluded" tumors into "immune inflamed" tumors with high numbers of tumor infiltrating T cells. This is achieved by (i) secretion of chemokines that are recognized by chemokine receptors on immune cells recruiting them to the tumor site and (ii) normalization of aberrant vasculature, enabling access to previously excluded tumor sites. (c) (i) Lymphocytes are then activated by (i) immunostimulatory cytokines released by the tumor and immune cells. (ii) Reduced immune checkpoint expression may also help to "release the breaks" on the antitumor immune response. (iii) Changes in the ratios of immune subtypes, for example, Treg: CD8+ T cells, M2: M1 macrophages, and tolerogenic: mature DCs, shift to the immune-activating cells, alongside activation and various immune-promoting mechanisms such as (iv) immunogenic cell death and (v) the cGAS STING pathway to produce further immune-stimulating molecules. (3) Immunosuppression by EBRT unfortunately occurs alongside the immune-activating mechanisms and may limit response. These inhibitory changes predominantly act to inhibit lymphocyte activation and may compete with immune-activating mechanisms in a dose-dependent manner. Major changes that have been observed under certain settings include (i) increases in MDSCs and M2 macrophages and (ii) immunosuppressive effects of cGas/STING activation

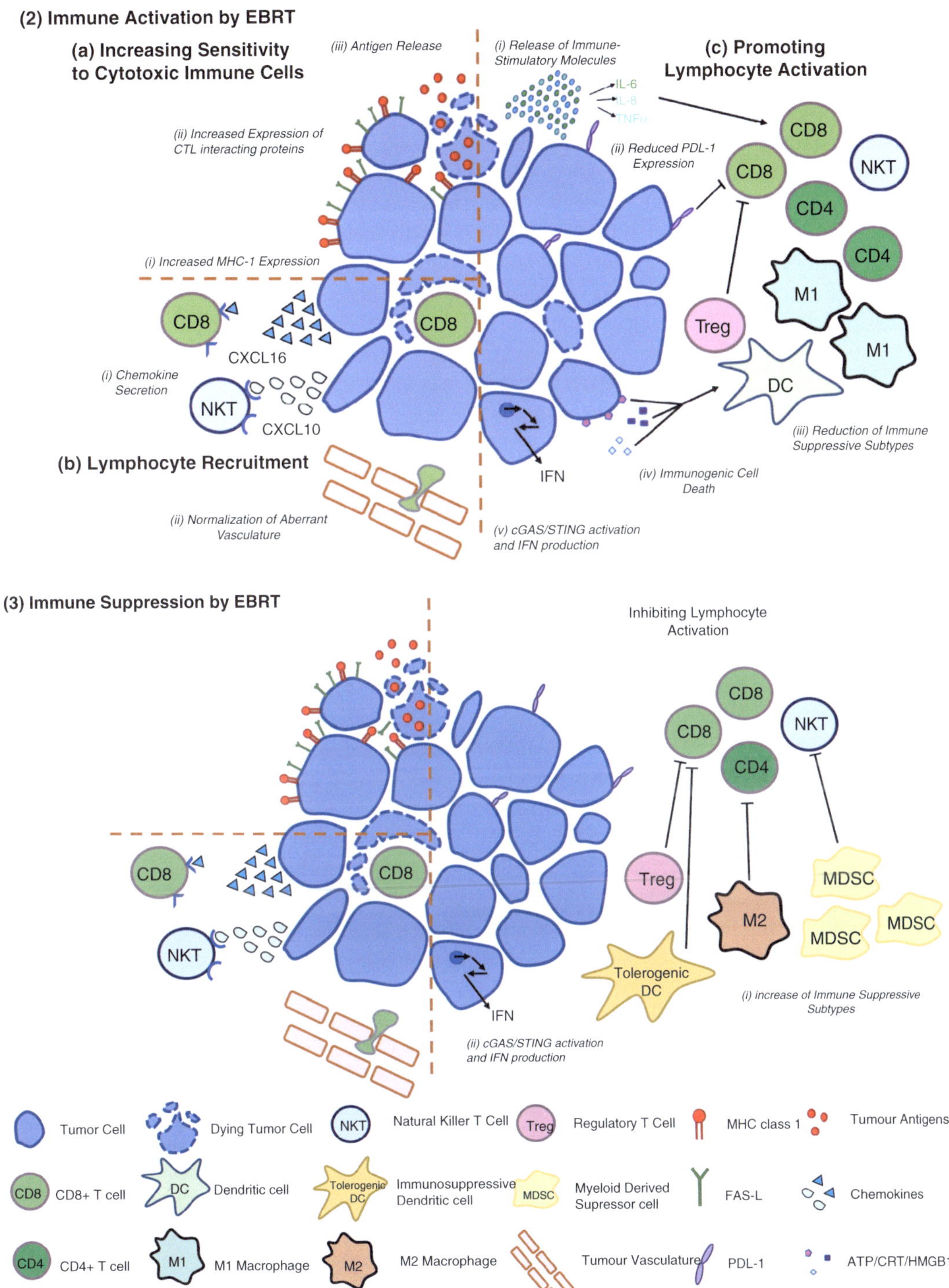

Fig. 11.2 (continued)

DC activation [27]. Meanwhile, released ATP acts as a key cell-cell signaling factor via activation of P2X7 purinergic receptors on DCs, triggering inflammasome activation and thus interleukin (IL)-1β production. This cytokine subsequently primes CD8$^+$ T cells, key mediators of the antitumor immune response. The importance of these processes has been highlighted by work demonstrating that for various ICD inducers, loss of these key mediators prevents induction of an immune response and thus limits efficacy. For instance, Apetoh et al. demonstrated that loss of the HMGB1/TLR4 axis in Tlr4$^{-/-}$ mice could significantly diminish the efficacy of RT [28].

Alongside the key mediators of ICD, a number of other immunostimulatory factors capable of stimulating immune cells in the TME are released by the stressed and dying tumor cells following irradiation. These include a range of cytokines such as granulocyte-macrophage colony-stimulating factor (GM-CSF), IL-6, IL-8, and tumor necrosis factor-α (TNF-α) which can all contribute to activation of immune cells [29–31]. Natural killer group 2 member D (NKG2D) ligands are also induced in tumor cells exposed to radiation, enabling interaction with NKG2D on various lymphocytes including NKT cells, macrophages, and some CD4$^+$ and CD8$^+$ T cells [32]. This interaction can again promote lymphocyte activation prompting an immune response against the tumor cells.

Another key family of cytokines stimulated by RT are interferons (IFNs), which can be induced via the cGAS/STING pathway. This mechanism has been receiving much attention recently following a number of studies highlighting how important this activation may be and leading to the development of STING agonists [33, 34]. DNA damage induced by radiation causes the generation of micronuclei and/or accumulation of DNA in the cytoplasm [35–37]. This activates the cytoplasmic DNA-binding protein cyclic GMP-AMP synthase (cGAS).

Activated cGAS produces the secondary messenger cyclic GMP-AMP (cGAMP) from ATP and GTP, which in turn activates stimulator of interferon genes (STING) [38–40]. Downstream pathways then result in the expression and secretion of interferons I, II, and III, which may be key to RT efficacy [35, 41–43]. For example, in B16 melanoma, the antitumor effects of RT were abolished in type I IFN nonresponsive murine hosts [35, 42]. Despite this apparent benefit, there is also accumulating evidence that cGAS/STING activation and interferon responses may also be immunosuppressive in certain circumstances [44–46]. Indeed, activation of interferon-stimulated genes (ISGs) may be associated with resistance to RT through both programmed death-ligand 1 (PD-L1)-dependent and PD-L1-independent mechanisms [44]. There is also evidence that STING activation by RT can cause infiltration of myeloid-derived suppressor cells (MDSCs) which contribute to the generation of an immunosuppressive environment [45].

Alongside its effects on T-cell activation, radiation can also reduce the presence of immunosuppressing cells, such as Treg cells and M2 macrophages which commonly populate the TME to generate an immunosuppressive environment [47, 48]. Reducing the number of these cells thus alleviates their immunosuppressive effects, enabling a functional immune environment to develop within the tumor.

11.2.3.3 Lymphocyte Recruitment

In conjunction with increased lymphocyte activation, RT additionally promotes recruitment of lymphocytes to the tumor site, enabling access to otherwise poorly infiltrated tumors. For example, *in vitro* irradiation of human and mouse breast tissue resulted in elevated C-X-C motif chemokine ligand (CXCL)16 secretion [49]. As a ligand for C-X-C motif chemokine receptor (CXCR)6 on T-helper and CD8$^+$ effector T cells, this chemokine participates in the recruitment of these immune cells to sites of inflammation. Similarly, CXCL10, a ligand for the CXCR3 receptor on monocytes, natural killer (NK) cells and T cells, was significantly elevated following RT treatment in mice. Furthermore, prevention of CXCL10 upregulation correlated with loss of RT-induced T-cell infiltration in a B16 melanoma model [50]. Concurrent radiation-induced normalization of the aberrant tumor vasculature can further trigger efficient recruitment of otherwise excluded immune cells [47].

11.2.3.4 Innate Immune Activation

Aside from the adaptive immune response, innate immunity has also been seen to play a role in antitumor effects of EBRT. In particular, activation of complement with local production of proinflammatory anaphylatoxins C3a and C5a is critical for tumor responses in both human and murine tumor models [51].

Ultimately, these combined pro-immunogenic mechanisms go on to elicit changes to the immune landscape of the tumor microenvironment (TME), promoting recruitment and activation of cytotoxic CD8+ T cells, dendritic cells (DC), and other immune effector cells that ultimately promote antitumor immunity [52].

11.2.3.5 Concurrent Immunosuppressive Effects

While the mechanisms described above have the potential to produce a curative systemic immune response, this is rarely the case with RT alone. Activation of immunosuppressive mechanisms that limit the immune response may contribute to this. Alongside pro-immunogenic changes, EBRT is also known to induce a wound repair response at the site of irradiation. This response, primarily mediated by macrophages, is predominantly immunosuppressive. Macrophages of the suppressive M2 phenotype accumulate in the tumor following RT

[53], though it is worth noting that this accumulation is dose-dependent, with low dose RT causing M1 polarization as mentioned above [47]. The immunostimulatory M1 phenotype produces high levels of proinflammatory cytokines and nitric oxide and present antigens to kill unhealthy cells. Meanwhile, M2 cells are characterized by low production of proinflammatory cytokines and do not produce nitric oxide, instead expressing arginase I and IL-10, which promote the building of extracellular matrix that enhances rather than prevents tumor growth.

RT may also drive development of various other immunosuppressive cells, including Tregs, MDSCs, tolerogenic DCs, and tumor-associated neutrophils [54–61]. Again, the treatment regimen appears key, with ablative hypofractionated RT reducing rather than increasing MDSCs [62].

Another major immunosuppressive mechanism employed by tumors is the expression of immune checkpoint molecules that bind receptors on T cells to inhibit T-cell function. There is evidence that RT may promote expression of such checkpoints. For example, in a murine carcinoma model, fractionated EBRT caused an increase in tumor cell PD-L1 expression [63]. Similar observations were made in a number of cell lines following chemoradiation [64].

Ultimately, the balance must be tipped to create an immune-promoting environment within the tumor to overcome the limiting factors. There is therefore a strong rationale for combining other therapeutics with EBRT to provide a multipronged approach that can overcome the abundant immunosuppressive mechanisms present in a tumor. Another possibility is modulation of RT to promote the immune-activating mechanisms and simultaneously avoid immunosuppression. Tipping the scales may be possible with alteration of dose and fractionation or through the use of other forms of RT such as TRT.

11.3 Targeted Radionuclide Therapy and the Immune System

TRT represents a distinct form of radiotherapy, which unlike EBRT provides systemic treatment enabling targeting of multiple tumor sites. Imaging and/or therapeutic radioisotopes can be conjugated to targeting moieties such as small molecules, antibodies, or other ligands to promote specific accumulation within the tumor site following systemic administration. These isotopes then provide protracted, low-dose rate irradiation to the tumor as the isotope decays. Importantly, this form of therapy is becoming increasingly widespread with the Food and Drug Administration (FDA) approval of lutetium-177 dotatate (LUTATHERA®) for the treatment of gastroenteropancreatic neuroendocrine tumors in 2018. Despite growing understanding of the role of immune engagement by EBRT, little is known about how these mechanisms may contribute to TRT. Given its similarity to EBRT, it follows that TRT is likely to also be capable of promoting an antitumor immune response, with the potential for this activation to contribute to the observed efficacy. Indeed, there is accumulating evidence that the closely related modality, brachytherapy, where a sealed radiation source is placed in or beside the treatment site, also acts via modulation of the immune response [65–68]. However, differences in various factors such as dose rate and treatment duration are likely to shape this immune response (Fig. 11.3).

One potential benefit comes from the systemic nature of the treatment. There is mounting evidence that treatment of multiple tumor sites is an important factor for generating a systemic immune response with EBRT [14]. The reasons for this are multifold including lack of expression of the same tumor antigens (TAs) in all lesions, lack of infiltration at non-irradiated sites, and persistent local immunosuppression at non-irradiated sites.

Firstly, the immunosuppressive effects of the TME may only be alleviated by RT locally, and thus while activated antitumor T cells may be in circulation, their action at non-irradiated lesions may be limited, for example, because of the continued presence of M2 macrophages and Treg, along with expression of immune checkpoints. Secondly, the TME may continue to exclude immune cells from non-irradiated sites. While irradiation can cause changes in the tumor vasculature and expression of immune cell-recruiting chemokines locally, non-targeted tumors may remain poorly infiltrated by antitumor immune cells. A third consideration is that heterogeneity of the tumor cells themselves may also pose an issue for single-site irradiation. The activated immune response will be directed against the subset of TAs released form the irradiated lesion. Should the TAs of other sites differ, they will not be targeted by the activated cytotoxic T cells.

It has also been shown that the microenvironment of disseminated tumors can continue to modulate the immune response in the primary tumor affecting response to immunotherapies [69], again pointing to reduced efficacy when only a single site is treated. All of these problems associated with single-site irradiation may be overcome when systemically administered TRT is used, enabling simultaneous irradiation of all lesions.

The protracted irradiation associated with TRT may also have an effect, though this is somewhat difficult to predict and may well be impacted by the half-life and tumor retention of any given radiopharmaceutical. For example, lymphocytes are highly radiosensitive, and thus immunosuppressive TILs present in the tumor may be killed by any form of RT (EBRT or TRT). This may be beneficial, enabling repopulation with activated

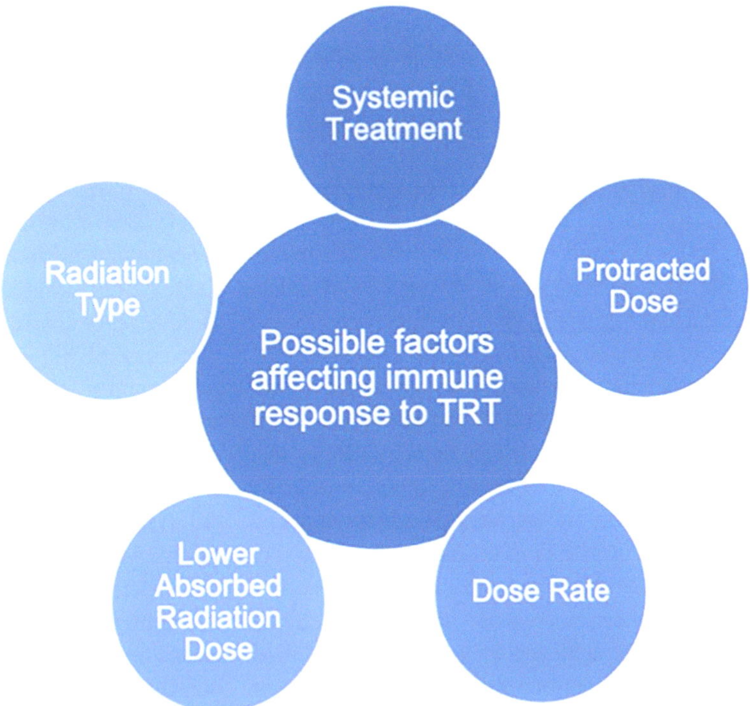

Fig. 11.3 Possible factors affecting the immune response to TRT

lymphocytes; however, the prolonged irradiation by TRT may limit this repopulation due to retention of radioactivity in the tumor. In general, TRT results in lower total radiation absorbed dose compared with EBRT, which is another interesting factor to consider, with conflicting evidence as to the benefits of high versus low dose irradiation for immune activation [70]. Other factors such as treatment delivery and radiation quality may also impact the interaction between radiation and the immune response. Questions arise over the extent to which TRT, like EBRT, will be capable of inducing pro-immunogenic changes such as ICD, cGAS/STING, and vascular changes. Equally important will be consideration of how TRT may impact on immunosuppressive mechanisms such as macrophage polarization and myeloid-derived suppressor cell (MDSC) recruitment, with the ultimate balance between these pro- and anti-immunogenic processes defining the resulting immune response. Understanding the immune landscape of the tumor following TRT may ultimately inform decisions on TRT-immunotherapy combinations.

A range of emerging preclinical and clinical research addresses the question of the immune response to TRT and is beginning to illuminate the details of this response. This work is complicated by the plethora of targeting agents and radioisotopes available that will likely result in variations in the immune responses they evoke. Existing work in this area—discussed in the following sections—is thus far relatively limited compared with studies of EBRT but already suggests that TRT can indeed induce a functional antitumor immune response.

11.3.1 Understanding the Mechanisms of Immune Activation by TRT (Preclinical Evidence)

Accumulating preclinical data has begun to establish a role for the immune system in the response to TRT. As predicted, various radiopharmaceuticals have been shown to be capable of inducing pro-immunogenic changes both *in vitro* and *in vivo*. In keeping with studies evaluating EBRT, it is becoming clear that T cells are central to this response. There is already evidence that a range of radiopharmaceuticals can induce changes that ultimately promote T-cell killing of tumor cells, by either promoting DC activation, T-cell recruitment, and T-cell activation or increasing the susceptibility of the cancer cell to cytotoxic T cells [71–84].

As has been seen with EBRT, one way in which this is achieved is via the upregulation of various cell surface molecules on the tumor cells that can promote T-cell activity in various ways. For example, a key surface molecule shown to be upregulated by β- and γ-emitting samarium-153 chelated to bone-seeking ethylene diamine tetramethylene phosphonate (EDTMP) and α-emitting radium-223 dichloride (^{223}Ra) is MHC class I [71, 72].

[^{153}Sm]Sm-EDTMP has also been shown to cause upregulation of intercellular adhesion molecule 1 (ICAM-1), an adhesion molecule thought to increase T-cell binding and thus enhancing cytolytic activity, along with Fas which binds Fas ligand on CTLs mediating direct tumor cell killing [71]. Along with these changes in expression of surface receptors, [^{153}Sm]Sm-EDTMP can also increase the expression of TAs and thus increase tumor immunogenicity. Ultimately, these changes were shown to produce an increase in susceptibility to killing by TA-specific CTLs, demonstrating a functional response. Similar effects on promoting TA-specific T-cell-mediated lysis have also been observed for α-emitting, bone-seeking radium-223 dichloride (^{223}Ra) in human prostate, breast, and lung carcinoma cells [72].

As well as direct effects on the susceptibility of the tumor cells to CTLs, radiopharmaceuticals have also been shown to promote mechanisms that can stimulate T-cell priming. As described above, one key mechanism for immune stimulation by EBRT is via activation of ICD. While comprehensive analysis of ICD activation by TRT is thus far lacking, various studies have hinted at activation of this process by a number of radiopharmaceuticals. Both Iodine-131 and Radium-223 have been shown to promote calreticulin upregulation and exposure on the cell surface [72, 85], while Gorin et al. demonstrated that another alpha emitter, bismuth-213, is capable of inducing HMGB1 release in a murine model of adenocarcinoma [86]. Moreover, this work, along with work by Hernandez et al., using a tumor-targeting alkylphosphocholine (NM600) radiolabeled with yttrium-90 in murine lymphoblastic lymphoma (EL4) tumors [74], demonstrated induction of ICD *in vivo* via the gold standard rechallenge experiment. Here, cells are treated *in vitro* to induce 95% cell killing before injection into one flank of a syngeneic murine host. Subsequently, healthy non-irradiated cells are injected into the contralateral flank. The treated cells, undergoing ICD, are predicted to produce a vaccination effect, preventing growth of contralateral, untreated cells to form a tumor. Gorin et al. also tested the animals at later time points to assess the longevity of the immune response, demonstrating a long-lived immune response. Using a similar experimental setup, the authors went on to show that, again analogous to EBRT, this immune response is T-cell-dependent, being absent in athymic nude mice. Hernandez et al., similarly verified that T cells are required for the response to [^{90}Y]Y-NM600 using immunocompromised Rag2 KO mice of the same syngeneic C57BL/6 genetic background but lacking mature T and B lymphocytes. The authors went one step further, transplanting the mice with T cells from either naïve WT mice or WT mice previously cured of EL4 tumors by [^{90}Y]Y-NM600 TRT. Both showed significant initial tumor regression following a single 9.25 MBq [^{90}Y]Y-NM600 dose. However, 80% of the naïve T-cell-transplanted mice experienced tumor recurrence, compared with only 20% of those mice that had received adoptive T-cell transfer from complete responders. These percentages were similar to durable response rates in immunocompetent mice confirming the crucial role of T cells in producing a systemic antitumor immune response.

Alongside these effects on T-cell activation, there is some evidence that TRT can promote TIL recruitment. Wu et al. addressed this question in a study investigating [^{177}Lu]Lu-DOTATATE in a mouse model of a human neuroendocrine tumor [75]. However, as the tumors were human, nude mice that are athymic and thus lack T cells and mature B cells of the adaptive immune response were used, restricting this study to assessment of the innate compartment including dendritic cells (DCs). While this prevents assessment of the complete immune response, the authors were able to show an increase in CD86 expression and increased infiltration of CD86$^+$ APCs into the tumor. Given that expression of this co-stimulatory molecule has been shown to be both necessary for and correlated to the efficacy of APC-mediated CD8$^+$ T-cell activation [76, 77], this suggests that [^{177}Lu]Lu-DOTATATE has the potential to induce a CD8$^+$-mediated antitumor immune response as has been observed for EBRT. This impact was assessed more directly by Rouanet et al., who demonstrated that [^{131}I]ICF01012 induces adaptive and innate immune cell recruitment in the tumor microenvironment, and this translated into increased survival in immune-competent animals compared with immune-deficient [85].

An increase in CD8$^+$ T cells following TRT has also been directly observed using a syngeneic model of T-cell non-Hodgkin's lymphoma treated with [^{90}Y]Y-NM600 [74]. Alongside the increased CD8$^+$ T-cell presence, a reduction of tumor-associated immunosuppressive Treg cells was observed, suggesting TRT may be able to further promote an antitumor immune response by removing this suppressive barrier.

Following this early work demonstrating the ability of various radiopharmaceuticals to induce an immune response, there is now increasing interest in developing combination protocols with immunotherapeutic agents, as for EBRT. As with EBRT, immune checkpoint blockades have been tested as possible combination therapeutics. Combination of an anti-CTLA4 antibody plus a novel radioisotope-based therapy has been tested *in vivo*. Here, ^{131}I-labelled catalase enzyme was injected intratumorally with sodium alginate which then produces a homogeneously distributed hydrogel at the physiological concentration of Ca^{2+} within the tumor. The addition of anti-CTLA4 demonstrated that this combination could effectively induce abscopal effects accompanied by a significant increase in tumor-infiltrating CD8$^+$ T cells and a reduction in Tregs [78]. This radioisotope treatment was also tested in combination with the immune adjuvant CpG, an oligodeoxynucleotide that can activate the TLR9 receptor of innate immune cells, demonstrating that local treatment with this [^{131}I]I-Cat/CpG/ALG mixture could generate a strong systemic antitumor immune response with robust resistance to tumor rechallenge. This combination was similarly effective with diffusing α-emitters radiation therapy (DaRT) [79].

DaRT has also demonstrated initial success preclinically in combination with various other TLR agonists (TLR3, TLR1,2) in the CT26 colon cancer mouse model [87]. This combination is further enhanced by concurrent treatment with the MDSC inhibitor, sildenafil. Moreover, this treatment regimen provided long-term immunologic memory, protecting from tumor rechallenge. Although this treatment is a form of brachytherapy rather than TRT—utilizing implantable seeds embedded with low activity radium-224—it still indicates the ability of radioisotopes to induce an antitumor immune response.

Traditional TRTs have also been employed in combination studies. Choi et al. first combined immune checkpoint inhibitors with lutetium-177 TRT in 2018, making use of very late antigen 4 (VLA-4) targeting with [^{177}Lu]Lu-LLP2 (LLP2 is a peptidomimetic with very high affinity for VLA-4) [88]. This demonstrated a significant enhancement of overall survival compared with TRT or ICIs alone in B16F10 murine melanoma models. However, it is worth noting that this study was impacted by significant immune cell targeting by the radiopharmaceutical. Using a different targeting moiety to target cell surface receptor integrin αvβ3 of murine MC38 colon carcinoma, Chen et al. showed a similar synergistic response with ^{177}Lu-radiopharmaceuticals ([^{177}Lu]Lu-EB-RGD) combined with anti-PD-L1 treatment, going on to show the importance of scheduling with an improved response achieved using concurrent rather than sequential treatment [89]. Indeed, this treatment schedule resulted in immunologic memory that protected mice from tumor rechallenge.

Alpha-emitting TRT has also demonstrated successful combination with immunotherapy in the form of adoptive T-cell therapy in preclinical assessment [80]. Here, a multiple myeloma murine model expressing the tumor antigen CD138 and ovalbumin (OVA) was treated with α-emitting ^{213}Bi-conjugated anti-CD138 antibody, followed by adoptive transfer of OVA-specific CD8$^+$ T cells producing significant tumor growth control and improved survival. Czernin et al., have also demonstrated efficacy when combining alpha-emitting [225Ac]PSMA-617 with anti-PDL1 [90].

While these preclinical studies have begun to reveal the potential of combined TRT-immunotherapy (TRT-IT) combinations, it will be important to expand our understanding of the immune landscape following TRT to inform rational selection of combinations to achieve the best possible responses. This is of course further complicated by differences in the physico-chemical properties of radioisotopes and their pharmacokinetics that will likely impact the characteristics of the induced immune response. However, comprehensive analysis of the effect of different isotopes or carriers is thus far lacking.

11.3.2 Clinical Evidence for an Immune Response

Along with the preclinical studies described above, a small number of reports suggest immune activation by TRT occurs in the clinical setting. In particular, observations of abscopal effects—while generally not possible because of the systemic nature of most TRTs—have been described for a small number of related therapies. For example, ^{90}Y-radio-embolization (RE), a treatment that is delivered directly to tumors in the liver via injection into the hepatic artery, was noted to cause complete regression of a nontargeted, left hepatic lobe lesion in a patient following targeted [^{90}Y]Y-RE of a right lobar lesion [81].

There is also evidence of possible abscopal effects with the α-emitter radium-223. The highly bone-seeking nature of radium-223 combined with the short range of the emitted α-particles means it is not expected to act on carcinomas in soft tissue. However, there have been multiple observations of regression of tumors at distant sites indicative of an abscopal effect [82, 83].

Recent work has also directly probed the immune effects of various TRTs, also supporting the hypothesis of immune activation. Again in the case of [^{90}Y] Y-RE, Chew et al. employed a noteworthy combination of time-of-flight mass cytometry and next-generation sequencing to demonstrate local immune activation in [^{90}Y] Y-RE treated tumors [84]. Using this combination, they were not only able to observe an enrichment of CD8$^+$ and CD4$^+$ T cells and NKT cells alongside a reduction in immunosuppressive Treg cells but were also able to probe the immune activation pathways stimulated by [^{90}Y]Y-RE. This analysis demonstrated a number of mechanisms including MHC upregulation, CD28-dependent T-cell activation pathways, and upregulation of the adhesion molecule ICAM-1 which is important for lymphocyte recruitment. The authors went on to show that upregulation of chemokines CXCL16 and C-C motif chemokine ligand 5 (CCL5) correlated with the increased CD8$^+$ T-cell infiltration. Furthermore, the response to [^{90}Y]Y-RE could be effectively predicted based on peripheral blood immune status highlighting the potential importance of immune activation for TRT response.

While there is still work to be done to bring our understanding of the immune response to TRT to the same level as that of EBRT, the evidence so far has been sufficient to stimulate the initiation of clinical trials combining TRT with immunotherapeutics. Following on from the promising data for [^{90}Y]Y-RE, multiple studies are investigating combination of [^{90}Y]Y-RE with immunotherapeutic (NCT03802747 and NCT03033446). Beyond this, studies are also underway to investigate other systemically delivered radiopharmaceuticals; one phase I study is looking into combining [^{177}Lu] Lu-PSMA, a small molecule targeting the prostate-specific membrane antigen (PSMA), with the anti-PD1 immunotherapeutic pembrolizumab (NCT03805594). In another phase I/II study, the combination of another anti-PD1 immunotherapeutic nivolumab, with [^{177}Lu]Lu-DOTA-TATE, is being tested in patients with relapsed or refractory extensive-stage small cell lung cancer or grade I–II lung neuroendocrine tumors (NCT03325816).

11.4 Conclusion

For decades, the immunomodulating properties of RT were largely ignored, but now the essential nature of immune activation by RT is widely acknowledged. Changes in the immune landscape following EBRT are increasingly well understood, leading to combination regimens with immunotherapeutic agents. However, the role of immune activation by TRT remains largely unexplored. Here, we have summarized the early work in this area which has already demonstrated the potential for TRT to instigate immune-activating mechanisms, including increasing sensitivity to cytotoxic immune cells, promoting lymphocyte recruitment, and promoting lymphocyte activation, analogous to EBRT (Fig. 11.2(2)). What is yet to be identified is how this radiation modality may differ to EBRT in terms of immune activation, and whether these differences could be exploited in certain settings.

Continuing this work to better comprehend immune activation by TRT will enable the development of rational RT-IT combinations, by identifying the key factors still limiting immune activation following RT and using a targeted immunotherapeutic to abolish this limitation. Moreover, the plethora of immune-activating mechanisms observed following RT suggests it may be an optimal agent for combination with targeted immunotherapy, which, despite showing unprecedented responses in a number of cancer types, has failed to demonstrate these striking response rates in a majority of cancers. This is perhaps due to the abundance of immunosuppressive mechanisms employed by the tumor microenvironment (Fig. 11.2(1)) limiting the potential for efficacy by a single targeted agent, alongside the significant capacity for the development of resistance against a targeted agent. The wide-reaching effects of RT may help to overcome these limitations, enabling the unprecedented response rates of immunotherapy to reach more patients across a wide range of cancer types.

References

1. Ewing J. Radium therapy in cancer. J Am Med Assoc. 1917;LXVIII:1238–47.
2. Cohen A, Cohen L. Radiobiology of the C3H mouse mammary carcinoma: the effect of body dose on the radiocurability of the tumor treated in situ. Br J Cancer. 1953;7:452–5.
3. Cohen A, Cohen L. Radiobiology of the c3h mouse mammary carcinoma: increased radiosensitivity of the tumor induced by inoculation of the host with radiation attenuated isografts. Br J Cancer. 1956;10: 312–7.
4. Slone HB, Peters LJ, Milas L. Effect of host immune capability on radiocurability and subsequent transplantability of a murine fibrosarcoma. J Natl Cancer Inst. 1979;63:1229–35.
5. Suit HD, Kastelan A. Immunologic status of host and response of a methylcholanthrene-induced sarcoma to local x-irradiation. Cancer. 1970;26:232–8.
6. Hewitt HB, Blake ER, Walder AS. A critique of the evidence for active host defence against cancer, based on personal studies of 27 murine tumors of spontaneous origin. Br J Cancer. 1976;33:241–59.
7. Nobler MP. The abscopal effect in malignant lymphoma and its relationship to lymphocyte circulation. Radiology. 1969;93:410–2.
8. Ehlers G, Fridman M. Abscopal effect of radiation in papillary adenocarcinoma. Br J Radiol. 1973;46: 220–2.
9. Kingsley DPE. An interesting case of possible abscopal effect in malignant melanoma. Br J Radiol. 1975;48:863–6.
10. Mole RH. Whole body irradiation; radiobiology or medicine? Br J Radiol. 1953;26:234–41.
11. Demaria S, Ng B, Devitt ML, Babb JS, Kawashima N, Liebes L, Formenti SC. Ionizing radiation inhibition of distant untreated tumors (abscopal effect) is immune mediated. Int J Radiat Oncol Biol Phys. 2004;58:862–70.
12. Stamell EF, Wolchok JD, Gnjatic S, Lee NY, Brownell I. The abscopal effect associated with a systemic anti-melanoma immune response. Int J Radiat Oncol Biol Phys. 2013;85:293–5.
13. Chakravarty PK, Alfieri A, Thomas EK, Beri V, Tanaka KE, Vikram B, Guha C. Flt3-ligand administration after radiation therapy prolongs survival in a murine model of metastatic lung cancer. Cancer Res. 1999;59:6028–32.
14. Brooks ED, Chang JY. Time to abandon single-site irradiation for inducing abscopal effects. Nat Rev Clin Oncol. 2019;16:123–35.
15. Abuodeh Y, Venkat P, Kim S. Systematic review of case reports on the abscopal effect. Curr Probl Cancer. 2016;40:25–37.

16. Tseng YD, Nguyen MH, Baker K, et al. Effect of patient immune status on the efficacy of radiation therapy and recurrence-free survival among 805 patients with merkel cell carcinoma. Int J Radiat Oncol Biol Phys. 2018;102:330–9.

17. Postow MA, Callahan MK, Barker CA, et al. Immunologic correlates of the abscopal effect in a patient with melanoma. N Engl J Med. 2012;366:925–31.

18. Gutkin PM, Hiniker SM, Swetter SM, Reddy SA, Knox SJ. Complete response of metastatic melanoma to local radiation and immunotherapy: 6.5 year follow-up. Cureus. 2018;10:e3723.

19. Golden EB, Chhabra A, Chachoua A, et al. Local radiotherapy and granulocyte-macrophage colony-stimulating factor to generate abscopal responses in patients with metastatic solid tumors: a proof-of-principle trial. Lancet Oncol. 2015;16:795–803.

20. Dewan MZ, Galloway AE, Kawashima N, Dewyngaert JK, Babb JS, Formenti SC, Demaria S. Fractionated but not single-dose radiotherapy induces an immune-mediated abscopal effect when combined with anti-CTLA-4 antibody. Clin Cancer Res. 2009;15:5379–88.

21. Lee Y, Auh SL, Wang YY, et al. Therapeutic effects of ablative radiation on local tumor require CD8+ T cells: Changing strategies for cancer treatment. Blood. 2009;114:589–95.

22. Takeshima T, Chamoto K, Wakita D, Ohkuri T, Togashi Y, Shirato H, Kitamura H, Nishimura T. Local radiation therapy inhibits tumor growth through the generation of tumor-specific CTL: its potentiation by combination with Th1 cell therapy. Cancer Res. 2010;70:2697–706.

23. Yoshimoto Y, Suzuki Y, Mimura K, et al. Radiotherapy-induced anti-tumor immunity contributes to the therapeutic efficacy of irradiation and can be augmented by CTLA-4 blockade in a mouse model. PLoS One. 2014;9:92572.

24. Morisada M, Moore EC, Hodge R, Friedman J, Cash HA, Hodge JW, Mitchell JB, Allen CT. Dose-dependent enhancement of T-lymphocyte priming and CTL lysis following ionizing radiation in an engineered model of oral cancer. Oral Oncol. 2017;71:87–94.

25. Reits EA, Hodge JW, Herberts CA, et al. Radiation modulates the peptide repertoire, enhances MHC class I expression, and induces successful antitumor immunotherapy. J Exp Med. 2006;203:1259–71.

26. Lhuillier C, Rudqvist N-P, Elemento O, Formenti SC, Demaria S. Radiation therapy and anti-tumor immunity: exposing immunogenic mutations to the immune system. Genome Med. 2019;11:40.

27. Delamarre L, Couture R, Mellman I, Trombetta ES. Enhancing immunogenicity by limiting susceptibility to lysosomal proteolysis. J Exp Med. 2006;203:2049–55.

28. Apetoh L, Ghiringhelli F, Tesniere A, et al. Toll-like receptor 4-dependent contribution of the immune system to anticancer chemotherapy and radiotherapy. Nat Med. 2007;13:1050–9.

29. Akashi M, Hachiya M, Koeffler HP, Suzuki G. Irradiation increases levels of GM-CSF through RNA stabilization which requires an AU-rich region in cancer cells. Biochem Biophys Res Commun. 1992;189:986–93.

30. Ao X, Zhao L, Davis MA, Lubman DM, Lawrence TS, Kong F-M. Radiation produces differential changes in cytokine profiles in radiation lung fibrosis sensitive and resistant mice. J Hematol Oncol. 2009;2:6.

31. Van der Meeren A, Monti P, Vandamme M, Squiban C, Wysocki J, Griffiths N. Abdominal radiation exposure elicits inflammatory responses and abscopal effects in the lungs of mice. Radiat Res. 2005;163:144–52.

32. Kim J-Y, Son Y-O, Park S-W, Bae J-H, Chung JS, Kim HH, Chung B-S, Kim S-H, Kang C-D. Increase of NKG2D ligands and sensitivity to NK cell-mediated cytotoxicity of tumor cells by heat shock and ionizing radiation. Exp Mol Med. 2006;38:474–84.

33. Li A, Yi M, Qin S, Song Y, Chu Q, Wu K. Activating cGAS-STING pathway for the optimal effect of cancer immunotherapy. J Hematol Oncol. 2019;12:35.

34. Ramanjulu JM, Pesiridis GS, Yang J, et al. Design of amidobenzimidazole STING receptor agonists with systemic activity. Nature. 2018;564:439–43.

35. Deng L, Liang H, Xu M, et al. STING-dependent cytosolic DNA sensing promotes radiation-induced type I interferon-dependent antitumor immunity in immunogenic tumors. Immunity. 2014;41:543–852.

36. Gekara NO. DNA damage-induced immune response: micronuclei provide key platform. J Cell Biol. 2017;216:2999–3001.

37. Härtlova A, Erttmann SF, Raffi FA, et al. DNA damage primes the Type I Interferon system via the cytosolic DNA sensor STING to promote anti-microbial innate immunity. Immunity. 2015;42:332–43.

38. Mackenzie KJ, Carroll P, Martin C-A, et al. cGAS surveillance of micronuclei links genome instability to innate immunity. Nature. 2017;548:461–5.

39. Harding SM, Benci JL, Irianto J, Discher DE, Minn AJ, Greenberg RA. Mitotic progression following DNA damage enables pattern recognition within micronuclei. Nature. 2017;548:466–70.

40. Bartsch K, Knittler K, Borowski C, et al. Absence of RNase H2 triggers generation of immunogenic micronuclei removed by autophagy. Hum Mol Genet. 2017;26:3960–72.

41. Lugade AA, Moran JP, Gerber SA, Rose RC, Frelinger JG, Lord EM. Local radiation therapy of B16 melanoma tumors increases the generation of tumor antigen-specific effector cells that traffic to the tumor. J Immunol. 2005;174:7516–23.

42. Burnette BC, Liang H, Lee Y, Chlewicki L, Khodarev NN, Weichselbaum RR, Fu YX, Auh SL. The efficacy of radiotherapy relies upon induction of type I interferon-dependent innate and adaptive immunity. Cancer Res. 2011;71:2488–96.

43. Vanpouille-Box C, Formenti SC, Demaria S. TREX1 dictates the immune fate of irradiated cancer cells. Oncoimmunology. 2017;6(9):e1339857.

44. Benci JL, Xu B, Qiu Y, et al. Tumor interferon signaling regulates a multigenic resistance program to immune checkpoint blockade. Cell. 2016;167:1540–1554.e12.

45. Liang H, Deng L, Hou Y, et al. Host STING-dependent MDSC mobilization drives extrinsic radiation resistance. Nat Commun. 2017;8:1736.

46. Post AEM, Smid M, Nagelkerke A, Martens JWM, Bussink J, Sweep FCGJ, Span PN. Interferon-stimulated genes are involved in cross-resistance to radiotherapy in tamoxifen-resistant breast cancer. Clin Cancer Res. 2018;24:3397–408.

47. Klug F, Prakash H, Huber PE, et al. Low-dose irradiation programs macrophage differentiation to an iNOS+/M1 phenotype that orchestrates effective T Cell immunotherapy. Cancer Cell. 2013;24:589–602.

48. Zhang T, Yu H, Ni C, et al. Hypofractionated stereotactic radiation therapy activates the peripheral immune response in operable stage I non-small-cell lung cancer. Sci Rep. 2017;7:4866.

49. Matsumura S, Wang B, Kawashima N, et al. Radiation-induced CXCL16 release by breast cancer cells attracts effector T cells. J Immunol. 2008;181:3099–107.

50. Lim JYH, Gerber SA, Murphy SP, Lord EM. Type I interferons induced by radiation therapy mediate recruitment and effector function of CD8(+) T cells. Cancer Immunol Immunother. 2014;63:259–71.

51. Surace L, Lysenko V, Fontana AO, et al. Complement is a central mediator of radiotherapy-induced tumor-specific immunity and clinical response. Immunity. 2015;42:767–77.

52. Walle T, Martinez Monge R, Cerwenka A, Ajona D, Melero I, Lecanda F. Radiation effects on antitumor immune responses: current perspectives and challenges. Ther Adv Med Oncol. 2018;10:1758834017742575.

53. Tsai CS, Chen FH, Wang CC, Huang HL, Jung SM, Wu CJ, Lee CC, McBride WH, Chiang CS, Hong JH. Macrophages from irradiated tumors express higher levels of iNOS, Arginase-I and COX-2, and promote tumor growth. Int J Radiat Oncol Biol Phys. 2007;68:499–507.

54. Xu J, Escamilla J, Mok S, David J, Priceman S, West B, Bollag G, McBride W, Wu L. CSFR1 signaling blockade stanches tumor-infiltrating myeloid cells and improves the efficacy of radiotherapy in prostate cancer. Cancer Res. 2013;73:2782–94.

55. Kalbasi A, Komar C, Tooker GM, Liu M, Lee JW, Gladney WL, Ben-Josef E, Beatty GL. Tumor-derived CCL2 mediates resistance to radiotherapy in pancreatic ductal adenocarcinoma. Clin Cancer Res. 2017;23:137–48.

56. Melsens E, Verberckmoes B, Rosseel N, Vanhove C, Descamps B, Pattyn P, Ceelen W. The VEGFR inhibitor cediranib improves the efficacy of fractionated radiotherapy in a colorectal cancer xenograft model. Eur Surg Res. 2017;58:95–108.

57. Golden EB, Frances D, Pellicciotta I, Demaria S, Helen Barcellos-Hoff M, Formenti SC. Radiation fosters dose-dependent and chemotherapy-induced immunogenic cell death. Onco Targets Ther. 2014;3:28518.

58. Jobling MF, Mott JD, Finnegan MT, et al. Isoform-specific activation of latent transforming growth factor β (LTGF-β) by reactive oxygen species. Radiat Res. 2006;166:839–48.

59. Fridlender ZG, Sun J, Kim S, Kapoor V, Cheng G, Ling L, Worthen GS, Albelda SM. Polarization of tumor-associated neutrophil phenotype by TGF-β: "N1" versus "N2" TAN. Cancer Cell. 2009;16:183–94.

60. Tanaka H, Shinto O, Yashiro M, Yamazoe S, Iwauchi T, Muguruma K, Kubo N, Ohira M, Hirakawa K. Transforming growth factor β signaling inhibitor, SB-431542, induces maturation of dendritic cells and enhances anti-tumor activity. Oncol Rep. 2010;24:1637–43.

61. Kachikwu EL, Iwamoto KS, Liao YP, Demarco JJ, Agazaryan N, Economou JS, McBride WH, Schaue D. Radiation enhances regulatory T cell representation. Int J Radiat Oncol Biol Phys. 2011;81:1128–35.

62. Lan J, Li R, Yin L-M, et al. Targeting myeloid-derived suppressor cells and programmed death ligand 1 confers therapeutic advantage of ablative hypofractionated radiation therapy compared with conventional fractionated radiation therapy. Int J Radiat Oncol. 2018;101:74–87.

63. Dovedi SJ, Cheadle EJ, Popple AL, et al. Fractionated radiation therapy stimulates antitumor immunity mediated by both resident and infiltrating polyclonal T-cell populations when combined with PD-1 blockade. Clin Cancer Res. 2017;23:5514–26.

64. Derer A, Spiljar M, Bäumler M, Hecht M, Fietkau R, Frey B, Gaipl US. Chemoradiation increases PD-L1 expression in certain melanoma and glioblastoma cells. Front Immunol. 2016;7:610.

65. Kubo M, Satoh T, Ishiyama H, et al. Enhanced activated T cell subsets in prostate cancer patients receiving iodine-125 low-dose-rate prostate brachytherapy. Oncol Rep. 2018;39:417–24.

66. Keam SP, Caramia F, Gamell C, Paul PJ, Arnau GM, Neeson PJ, Williams SG, Haupt Y. The transcriptional landscape of radiation-treated human prostate cancer: analysis of a prospective tissue cohort. Int J Radiat Oncol Biol Phys. 2018;100:188–98.

67. Hodge JW, Sharp HJ, Gameiro SR. Abscopal regression of antigen disparate tumors by antigen cascade after systemic tumor vaccination in combination with local tumor radiation. Cancer Biother Radiopharm. 2012;27:12–22.

68. Eric A, Juranic Z, Tisma N, Plesinac V, Borojevic N, Jovanovic D, Milovanovic Z, Gavrilovic D, Ilic B. Radiotherapy-induced changes of peripheral blood lymphocyte subpopulations in cervical cancer patients: relationship to clinical response. J BUON. 2009;14(1):79–83.

69. Morris ZS, Guy EI, Werner LR, et al. Tumor-specific inhibition of in situ vaccination by distant

untreated tumor sites. Cancer Immunol Res. 2018;6: 825–34.

70. Garnett CT, Palena C, Chakarborty M, Tsang K-YY, Schlom J, Hodge JW, Hodge JW. Sublethal irradiation of human tumor cells modulates phenotype resulting in enhanced killing by cytotoxic T lymphocytes. Cancer Res. 2004;64:7985–94.

71. Chakraborty M, Wansley EK, Carrasquillo JA, Yu S, Paik CH, Camphausen K, Becker MD, Goeckeler WF, Schlom J, Hodge JW. The use of chelated radionuclide (samarium-153-ethylenediaminetetramethylenephosphonate) to modulate phenotype of tumor cells and enhance T cell-mediated killing. Clin Cancer Res. 2008;14:4241–9.

72. Malamas AS, Gameiro SR, Knudson KM, Hodge JW. Sublethal exposure to alpha radiation (223Ra dichloride) enhances various carcinomas sensitivity to lysis by antigen-specific cytotoxic T lymphocytes through calreticulin-mediated immunogenic modulation. Oncotarget. 2016;7:86937–47.

73. Gorin J-B, Ménager J, Gouard S, et al. Antitumor immunity induced after α irradiation. Neoplasia. 2014;16:319–28.

74. Hernandez R, Walker KL, Grudzinski JJ, et al. 90Y-NM600 targeted radionuclide therapy induces immunologic memory in syngeneic models of T-cell non-Hodgkin's lymphoma. Commun Biol. 2019;2:79.

75. Wu Y, Pfeifer A, Myschetzky R, Garbyal R, Rasmussen P, Knigge U, Bzorek M, Kristensen M, Kjaer A. Induction of anti-tumor immune responses by peptide receptor radionuclide therapy with 177Lu-dotatate in a murine model of a human neuroendocrine tumor. Diagnostics. 2013;3:344–55.

76. Mukai T, Maeda Y, Tamura T, Matsuoka M, Tsukamoto Y, Makino M. Induction of cross-priming of naive CD8+ T lymphocytes by recombinant Bacillus Calmette-Guérin that secretes heat shock protein 70-major membrane protein-II fusion protein. J Immunol. 2009;183:6561–8.

77. Oizumi S, Strbo N, Pahwa S, Deyev V, Podack ER. Molecular and cellular requirements for enhanced antigen cross-presentation to CD8 cytotoxic T lymphocytes. J Immunol. 2007;179:2310–7.

78. Chao Y, Xu L, Liang C, Feng L, Xu J, Dong Z, Tian L, Yi X, Yang K, Liu Z. Combined local immunostimulatory radioisotope therapy and systemic immune checkpoint blockade imparts potent antitumor responses. Nat Biomed Eng. 2018;2:611–21.

79. Confino H, Schmidt M, Efrati M, Hochman I, Umansky V, Kelson I, Keisari Y. Inhibition of mouse breast adenocarcinoma growth by ablation with intratumoral alpha-irradiation combined with inhibitors of immunosuppression and CpG. Cancer Immunol Immunother. 2016;65:1149–58.

80. Ménager J, Gorin JB, Maurel C, et al. Combining α-radioimmunotherapy and adoptive T cell therapy to potentiate tumor destruction. PLoS One. 2015;10:e0130249.

81. Ghodadra A, Bhatt S, Camacho JC, Kim HS. Abscopal effects and Yttrium-90 radioembolization. Cardiovasc Intervent Radiol. 2016;39:1076–80.

82. Kwee SA, Lim J, Coel MN. Soft tissue response on 18F-fluorocholine PET/CT in metastatic castrate-resistant prostate cancer treated with 223Ra-dichloride: a possible abscopal effect? Clin Nucl Med. 2017;42:868–71.

83. Poon DMC, Wong KCW. Lymph node response in a patient with metastatic castration-resistant prostate cancer treated with Radium-223. Clin Genitourin Cancer. 2018;16:e397–401.

84. Chew V, Lee YH, Pan L, et al. Immune activation underlies a sustained clinical response to Yttrium-90 radioembolisation in hepatocellular carcinoma. Gut. 2018;68(2):335–46.

85. Rouanet J, Benboubker V, Akil H, Hennino A, Auzeloux P, Besse S, Pereira B, Delorme S, Mansard S, D'Incan M, Degoul F, Rouzaire PO. Immune checkpoint inhibitors reverse tolerogenic mechanisms induced by melanoma targeted radionuclide therapy. Cancer Immunol Immunother. 2020;69:2075–88.

86. Gorin JB, Ménager J, Gouard S, et al. Antitumor immunity induced after α irradiation. Neoplasia (United States). 2014;16:319–28.

87. Domankevich V, Cohen A, Efrati M, Schmidt M, Rammensee HG, Nair SS, Tewari A, Kelson I, Keisari Y. Combining alpha radiation-based brachytherapy with immunomodulators promotes complete tumor regression in mice via tumor-specific long-term immune response. Cancer Immunol Immunother. 2019;68:1949–58.

88. Choi J, Beaino W, Fecek RJ, Fabian KPL, Laymon CM, Kurland BF, Storkus WJ, Anderson CJ. Combined VLA-4–targeted radionuclide therapy and immunotherapy in a mouse model of melanoma. J Nucl Med. 2018;59:1843–9.

89. Chen H, Zhao L, Fu K, et al. Integrin αvβ3-targeted radionuclide therapy combined with immune checkpoint blockade immunotherapy synergistically enhances anti-tumor efficacy. Theranostics. 2019;9:7948–60.

90. Czernin J, Current K, Mona CE, Nyiranshuti L, Hikmat F, Radu CG, Lückerath K. Immune-checkpoint blockade enhances 225Ac-PSMA617 efficacy in a mouse model of prostate cancer. J Nucl Med. 2021;62:228–31.

Translational Development and Testing of Theranostics in Combination with Immunotherapies

12

Peter M. Carlson and Zachary S. Morris

Contents

P. M. Carlson · Z. S. Morris (✉)
Department of Human Oncology, School of Medicine and Public Health, University of Wisconsin-Madison, Madison, WI, USA
e-mail: pcarlson2@wisc.edu;
zmorris@humonc.wisc.edu

12.1 Introduction

One of the most profound breakthroughs in our understanding of cancer biology in the last three decades has been the illumination of the complex interplay between cancer and the immune system. It is clear that the immune system plays a critical role in surveilling normal tissues and is

© Springer Nature Switzerland AG 2022
S. Harsini et al. (eds.), *Nuclear Medicine and Immunology*,
https://doi.org/10.1007/978-3-030-81261-4_12

capable of eliminating neoplastic cells [1]. Yet tumor cells may engage regulatory and immunosuppressive capabilities of the immune system to evade immune-mediated eradication and may even leverage immune response to promote tumor growth, angiogenesis, and metastatic spread [2, 3]. This role of the immune system in tumorigenesis is described in the cancer immunoediting hypothesis, which is summarized by the "three Es": Elimination, Equilibrium, and Escape [4]. In certain settings, the immune system can identify and *E*liminate cancer cells. In other settings, accumulated tumor mutations and phenotypes result in *E*quilibrium between neoplastic cell division and immune-mediated elimination. This may last for years, creating a microcosm of natural selection for those cancer clones "fit" to resist elimination by the immune system. Eventually, persisting tumor cells may *E*scape immune detection, resulting in clinically detectable emergence or progression of cancer [4]. With treatments and adaptive immune response, cancer immunoediting becomes a dynamic continuum that may exist in different states in different regions of a tumor, in different locations in the body, and at different times throughout the disease course.

Cancer immunotherapies have been developed as treatment strategies to tip the balance of immunoediting toward equilibrium or elimination. Cancer patients present with tumors having varying degrees of immune recognition of tumor antigens, tumor infiltration by immune cells, and activation of tumor-infiltrating immune cells. Those tumors with a high degree of lymphocytic infiltration are termed immunologically "hot," whereas those devoid of tumor-infiltrating lymphocytes are referred to as immunologically "cold" tumors [5]. In addition to patient-to-patient variation, immune recognition and infiltration can vary based on the type or location of the tumor. Though both hot and cold tumors clearly represent a failure of the immune system to adequately control the tumor, the mechanism of tumor escape may be different in these two situations. In a "hot" tumor, there may be a predominance of immunosuppressive mechanisms in the tumor microenvironment that prevents tumor-specific effector T cells from eradicating the tumor. In contrast, "cold" tumors may not have been effectively recognized by effector T cells, possibly due to poor processing and presentation of tumor antigens by antigen-presenting cells and/or due to low tumor mutation burden resulting in few mutation-created tumor neoantigens [5, 6]. A critical challenge now is the development of therapeutic strategies that augment response against immunologically hot tumors and those that initiate immune recognition of immunologically cold tumors.

12.2 Rationale for Combining Radiation and Immunotherapy

The interaction between radiation therapy and immune response has been described for nearly 100 years. In 1921, Murphy and colleagues demonstrated that radiated mouse skin had an increased degree of lymphoid infiltration and that attempting to engraft a tumor into radiated skin was much less successful compared to unirradiated skin [7]. In the 1970s, Helen Stone and colleagues showed in murine models that the dose of radiation required to eradicate an implanted flank tumor was twice as high in immune-deficient mice compared to immune-competent mice [8]. This demonstrates that an intact immune system contributes to the local killing of tumor cells following radiation.

The abscopal effect is a rare but well-documented phenomenon in radiation oncology whereby patients with metastatic disease may experience partial or complete responses at distant, unirradiated tumor sites following radiation of a separate tumor location. This phenomenon is mediated by systemic activation of an antitumor immune response [9]. Thus, the immune system has always been a critical component of radiation therapy, and radiation has the potential to drive antitumor immunity.

Radiation elicits both immune stimulatory and immunosuppressive effects, which can be heterogeneous and dynamic within both the tumor and the body. These can be categorized as (1) direct effects on tumor cells and (2) effects on the tumor microenvironment including fibroblasts, endothelial cells, and tumor-infiltrating immune cells. As a cumulative result of these influences on tumor immune tolerance and functional immunogenicity, focal external beam radiation can elicit in situ tumor vaccination effect—converting a patient's own tumor into a nidus for the presentation of tumor-specific antigens in a way that stimulates and diversifies the patient's antitumor T-cell response [10, 11].

12.2.1 Immunomodulatory Effects of Radiation on Tumor Cells

The tumor-killing effect of radiation is traditionally thought to result from the accumulation of DNA damage in malignant cells leading to tumor cell death by mitotic catastrophe [12]. Recent studies demonstrate that the tumor cell death triggered by radiation is immunogenic. Several unique features characterize immunogenic tumor cell death. While apoptosis, autophagy, and even necrosis exert limited inflammation in surrounding normal tissues, immunogenic cell death results in a strong inflammatory mechanisms [13–15]. In cells undergoing immunogenic cell death following radiation therapy, calreticulin is translocated to the cell surface. Calreticulin is a well-known endoplasmic reticulum chaperone protein that is upregulated during times of stress and is a potent activator of dendritic cell (DC) phagocytosis [16]. High mobility box group 1 (HMGB1) protein is also released from the nuclear compartment of cells dying following radiation and is released to the extracellular tumor microenvironment [17]. HMGB1 is classified as a damage associated molecular pattern (DAMP) and can activate innate immune cell inflammatory response by binding toll-like receptor (TLR) family members, including TLR2 and TLR4 [18, 19]. Immunogenic cell death following radiation is also associated with the extracellular release of adenosine triphosphate (ATP), and this has been shown to activate the P2RX7 purinergic receptor pathway and the DC inflammasome [20]. This leads to increased secretion of inflammatory cytokines including interleukin (IL)-1B,

tumor necrosis factor (TNF)-α, and IL-12 [21], culminating in DC activation, enhanced antigen processing, and cluster of differentiation (CD)8+ T-cell recruitment and activation [14].

Radiation is also known to have a broad effect on tumor cells receiving a sublethal dose. For instance, doses of external beam radiation as low as 2–4 Gy have been shown to increase expression of the major histocompatibility complex class I (MHC-I) on the surface of cancer cells both in vitro and in vivo. Formenti and colleagues demonstrated that 4 Gy of radiation caused an increase in MHC-I expression through increased synthesis of the beta-2 microglobulin subunit in GL621 glioma cells [22]. This increase in expression correlated with the observed increase in CD4+ and CD8+ T-cell infiltration, though did not by itself extend survival in mice. This effect has been observed in numerous cancer cell lines including human lung adenocarcinoma, hepatocellular carcinoma, prostate adenocarcinoma, melanoma, and many others [23]. Interestingly, the dose of radiation required to optimally induce MHC-I upregulation is different for different tumor cell lines, which emphasizes the heterogeneity in tumor radiobiology and radiosensitivity. This radiation-induced effect on MHC-I is also observed following treatment with of alpha-emitting radium-223 (^{223}Ra) [24]. This has important implications for radionuclide-based, theranostic platforms. Increased tumor cell MHC-I expression renders these tumor cells more recognizable by tumor-specific CD8+ T cells recruited and activated as sequelae of immunogenic cell death.

Tumor cells surviving radiation are also modified in their susceptibility to the immune response by increased expression of cell death pathway proteins including FAS [25], which is a target of T-cell killing. Radiation also activates a type I interferon (IFN) response in surviving cells. cGAS is a cytosolic sensor of DNA that, upon detection of cytosolic DNA (as during viral infection), activates STING leading to phosphorylation of IFN regulatory factor (IRF)3/7, production of type I IFN, and upregulated expression of IFN-stimulated genes (e.g., *MX1*, *OAS2*, *OAS3*). Ionizing radiation elicits double-strand

DNA breaks that may result in chromosome fragments lacking a centromere, leading to formation of micronuclei when such cells progress through mitosis [26, 27]. The compromised nuclear envelope of these micronuclei enables detection by cGAS and activation of a type I IFN response that increases with a radiation dose up to ~8–12 Gy (single fraction). At higher doses, this effect of radiation is negatively regulated by expression of the exonuclease TREX1 (three prime repair exonuclease 1), which may degrade the cytoplasmic and micronuclear DNA that activates cGAS [27].

12.2.2 Immunomodulatory Effects of Radiation on the Tumor Microenvironment

Radiation also directly affects components of the tumor microenvironment, and this has both positive and negative influences on antitumor immunity. For instance, radiation increases the expression of vascular and matrix adhesion proteins including vascular cell adhesion molecule 1 (VCAM1), intercellular adhesion molecule 1 (ICAM1), and CD31, which facilitate immune cell infiltration into the tumor [25]. Radiation further stimulates tumor infiltration by an activation of immune cells through an immediate local release of inflammatory cytokines. This includes reported effects on the production of IL-10, IL-12, IL-15, IL-17, IL-18, IFN-α, IFN-γ, IFN-β, and transforming growth factor (TGF)-β [28]. Importantly, this effect is observed at low doses (between 2 and 5 Gy) and at low dose rates [29, 30]. Radiation also modifies the tumor microenvironment at low doses (1–4 Gy) through a rapid and direct cytotoxic effect on radiation-sensitive tumor-infiltrating lymphocytic lineages. This may create a window of opportunity by locally and temporarily depleting exhausted, anergic, and suppressive lymphocytes enabling subsequent reconstitution of the tumor microenvironment with a more favorable infiltrate [14]. T lymphocytes are among the most sensitive mammalian cells to radiation. Doses of 0.5, 2, and 3 Gy trigger apoptosis in 10%, 50%, and 90% of naïve T lymphocytes within 2–8 h of radiation therapy

exposure, respectively [31]. Activated T effector cells (Teffs) and immunosuppressive regulatory T cells (Tregs) may be slightly less sensitive to radiation therapy compared to naïve T cells [32, 33]. Nevertheless, both Teff and Tregs are highly radiosensitive relative to most tumor cells [31, 33]. Notably, compared to most other cell types, which commonly exhibit reduced response to low-dose rate radiation, lymphocytes show little change in radiation therapy sensitivity with reduced dose rate [29]. This implies that low-dose rate radiation delivered by targeted radionuclide therapy (TRT) can modify the lymphocytic infiltrate in the tumor microenvironment.

Conversely, radiation also triggers immunosuppressive effects in the tumor microenvironment including delayed recruitment of suppressive immune lineages including Tregs, M2-polarized macrophages, and myeloid-derived suppressor cells (MDSCs) [34, 35]. Moreover, negative feedback pathways may also be activated after radiation therapy with increased expression of immunosuppressive ligands including programmed death-ligand 1 (PD-L1) on tumor cells and T-cell exhaustion markers including programmed cell death protein 1 (PD1), T-cell immunoglobulin- and mucin domain-containing protein 3 (TIM3), and lymphocyte activating 3 (LAG-3) on tumor infiltrating lymphocytes (TILs) [36]. Finally, large-volume external beam radiation may irradiate a significant portion of the blood pool and bone marrow, leading to radiation-induced systemic lymphopenia, which is associated with reduced survival in cancer patients [37, 38].

12.3 Rationale for Combining Targeted Radionuclide Therapies and Immunotherapy

While focal external beam radiation consistently induces a local inflammatory response, this alone rarely leads to a sustained and systemic antitumor immune response. Without other immune stimuli, focal external beam radiation therapy has a poor capacity for stimulating an abscopal antitumor immune response at non-radiated tumor sites [39]. This may reflect a negative impact of distant tumor sites on the priming and propagation of systemic antitumor immunity from a focal in situ vaccine site. For example, in murine tumor models, we previously demonstrated a combination of focal external beam radiation synergized with local injections of a tumor-targeted hu14.18-IL2 immunocytokine to generate a greater in situ vaccine [40]. However, this same in situ vaccine was substantially less effective when delivered to a single tumor site in mice-bearing multiple tumors [41]. The presence of a distant, *untreated* tumor in this model prevented the generation of an immune response at *any* tumor including the site targeted by in situ vaccination. This phenomenon, coined "concomitant immune tolerance," is only observed when the two tumors are of the same type. This suggests that the tolerizing effect of CIT from a distant, untreated tumor is specific to the antigens of that tumor. Though the mechanisms of CIT are not fully elucidated, Tregs are necessary for the effect [41]. While focal external beam radiotherapy can dramatically alter the immune landscape in a targeted tumor, it does not alter the landscape within *all* tumors. Immunosuppressive cells and pathways in these unaltered non-radiated tumors may quench the activation of effector immune cells emerging from the in situ vaccination site or may circulate between tumor sites and reconstitute a suppressive tumor microenvironment at the radiated site. Consequently, to engage radiation in effectively priming and propagating antitumor immunity, it may be necessary to deliver immunomodulatory radiation to the *collective* tumor microenvironment at *all* tumor sites. In fact, CIT is overcome by delivering radiation to all tumor sites, and even low doses of radiation at these distant tumor sites may restore the systemic antitumor efficacy of in situ vaccination [41, 42].

In metastatic settings, radiation therapy has historically been reserved for palliative indications targeting symptomatic lesions. In patients with limited or oligometastatic disease, recent studies demonstrate the feasibility and even a survival benefit from delivering radiation to all tumor sites [43]. This supports the notion that metastatic disease may be managed by delivering some form of radiation in combination with other therapies to all sites of disease. Radiating all tumor sites using external beam radiation is often not possible in settings of widely metastatic disease due to (1) normal tissue toxicity, and (2) radiating radiographically occult tumor sites in this context would require whole-body radiation resulting in systemic bone marrow suppression. On the other hand, TRTs enable effective delivery of radiation to all tumor sites in settings of metastatic disease. TRT is a systemic form of radiation therapy that combines a tumor-selective vector or mechanism with a therapeutic radioisotope. These vectors can include antibodies, antibody fragments, peptides, lipids, and small molecules [44]. TRT has been used for nearly a century [45], and a growing number of TRT agents are approved for the treatment of cancers [46, 47]. As a monotherapy, TRTs generally have limited efficacy in most solid tumors [46]. In part, this reflects the difficulty in delivering high-dose radiation to an entire tumor using TRT while sparing other tissues in the body. Heterogeneity in targeting moiety expression, tumor vascular supply, and cell radiosensitivity also contribute to a lack of effective response to TRT monotherapy in clinical settings for many common solid tumors [48]. Combining TRT with immunotherapies may overcome these limitations, and in turn, the delivery of radiation to all tumor microenvironments may prime and propagate a more effective response to immunotherapies.

12.4 Translational Development and Testing of TRT in Combination with Immunotherapies

12.4.1 TRT in Combination with Immune Checkpoint Inhibitors

Immune checkpoint inhibitors are a class of therapeutic antibodies that modulate tumor tolerance by recognizing and blocking specific inhibitory receptors on the surface of immune cells and thereby enhancing T-cell activation. These checkpoint receptors normally function in co-regulatory pathways that inhibit T-cell activation following antigen recognition by the T-cell receptor (TCR). Such mechanisms, normally involved in the maintenance of self-tolerance, can be co-opted by tumor cells to avoid immune detection. Antibodies targeting checkpoint receptors have shown therapeutic benefits for a variety of tumor types. These include antibodies targeting cyto-toxic T-lymphocyte antigen-4 (CTLA-4) as well as programmed cell death-1 (PD-1) and its ligand PD-L1. CTLA-4 is constitutively expressed at low levels on the surface of naïve effector and regulatory T cells among other immune lineages. The ligands of CTLA-4, B7-1/2 (CD80/CD86), also bind the co-stimulatory CD28 receptor on the surface of immune cells resulting in enhanced T-cell activation. In the context of strong or pro-longed TCR signaling, CTLA-4 expression is upregulated, and CTLA-4 competes with CD28 for binding of B7-1/2 resulting in inhibition of further T-cell activation. By blocking the interaction of CTLA-4 and B7-1/2, anti-CTLA-4 antibodies promote T-cell activation. PD-1 is expressed on activated T cells as well as B cells and monocytes. Its ligands, PD-L1 and PD-L2, are expressed on antigen-presenting cells, tumor cells, placenta, and cells in an inflammatory microenvironment. Binding of PD-1 by its ligands results in inhibi-tion of T-cell activation. Importantly, tumor cell expression of PD-L1 is correlated with dimin-ished tumor-infiltrating lymphocytes and poor clinical outcome for multiple cancer types [49]. Antibodies targeting PD-1 or PD-L1 have been approved in the treatment of many different types of cancer. A consistent theme from clinical stud-ies of immune checkpoint inhibitors is that a subgroup of patients who respond to treatment experience durable regression of disease. This raises hope that further augmenting the immune response in the context of these treatments may yield higher clinical response rates with a dra-matic impact on survival.

Preclinical studies demonstrated the potential for TRT to augment response to immune check-point inhibitors. The alkylphosphocholine analog NM600, which can chelate radiometals and pref-erentially accumulates in malignant cells [50], has been used to deliver yttrium-90 (^{90}Y) to the tumor microenvironment in a variety of synge-neic murine tumor models and consistently aug-ments response to anti-PD-1 and anti-CTLA-4 [51]. These studies delivered only low-dose radia-tion to the tumor microenvironment (2–5 Gy) and demonstrated that the combination of TRT and checkpoint blockade enhanced CD8$^+$ T-cell infil-tration of tumor, increased expression of numer-ous pro-inflammatory cytokines, and increased clonal expansion of tumor-infiltrating T cells [52]. In other preclinical studies, a peptide-based TRT, [^{177}Lu]Lu-Arg-Gly-Asp ([^{177}Lu]Lu-RGD), which targets $\alpha_v\beta_3$ integrin on activated angio-genic endothelial cells, was found to be coopera-tive with anti-PD-L1 in controlling the growth of extending survival of mice-bearing syngeneic MC38 tumors [53]. These investigators observed that [^{177}Lu]Lu-RGD increased PD-L1 expres-sion on surviving tumor cells, and the combina-tion of [^{177}Lu]Lu-RGD plus anti-PD-L1 resulted in increased tumor infiltration by CD8$^+$ T cells [53]. A separate preclinical study demonstrated that a small molecule TRT ([^{177}Lu]Lu-LLP2A) targeting $\alpha_4\beta_1$ integrin (also called Very Late Antigen-4, VLA-4) enhanced tumor response in B16F10 melanoma tumors when combined with anti-PD-1, anti-PD-L1, and anti-CTLA-4 anti-bodies [54]. Collectively, these studies demon-strate the potential for TRT to enhance response to immune checkpoint inhibition and begin to shed light on mechanisms of cooperative thera-peutic interaction.

Clinical trials are now testing the safety and efficacy of combining TRT and immune checkpoint inhibition. Among these is a prom-ising ongoing study conducted jointly between research teams in the United Kingdom, Germany, and the United States evaluating the combina-tion of [^{131}I]metaiodobenzylguanidine (MIBG), nivolumab (anti-PD-1 antibody), and dinutux-imab (anti-GD-2 antibody) in pediatric patients with neuroblastoma [55]. Colloquially referred to as the MiNivAN study (NCT02914405), the objective of this study is to evaluate efficacy. MIBG is actively transported into neuroblas-toma cells, and [^{131}I]MIBG is already in use for the treatment of neuroblastoma, heightening the translational potential of this combined modality approach. For men with metastatic castrate-resistant prostate cancer (mCRPC), radium-223 (^{223}Ra, Xofigo) is approved for treatment. Radium is a calcium mimetic that naturally accumulates in the bony metastatic tumor sites that typify mCRPC. At least two studies are now evaluating the addition of an anti-PD-1 antibody to radium-223 in mCRPC [56, 57]. These studies will test the hypothesis that immunogenic tumor cell death triggered by radium-223 will improve response to PD-1 blockade. Also in mCRPC, a small molecule TRT targeting prostate-specific membrane antigen (^{177}Lu-PSMA) is being tested in combination with an anti-PD-1 antibody in a phase Ib/II study evaluating safety and efficacy [58]. It will be intriguing to compare the relative efficacy of TRT in stimulating response to anti-PD-1 in these mCRPC studies because the high linear energy transfer (LET), very short range alpha particles emitted by radium-223, may have quite distinct effects on tumor cells and the tumor microenvironment compared to the lower LET, longer-range beta particles, and gamma rays emitted by lutetium-177.

12.4.2 TRT in Combination with In Situ Vaccine

In immunologically cold tumors that are poorly recognized by the immune system, simply "taking the brakes off" of the immune response with immune checkpoint inhibitors is generally ineffective. In these settings, it may be critical to implement treatment strategies such as in situ vaccination to increase tumor antigen recognition. External beam radiation can elicit an in situ vaccine and may prime immune recognition of tumor antigens not recognized prior to radiation [59, 60]. In immunologically cold tumors, it may be advantageous to combine external beam radiation and TRT to prime and propagate antitumor immunity, respectively, in combination with immune checkpoint inhibitors. Combination Internal and External RadioTherapy (CIERT) has long been hypothesized as a strategy for enhanc-

ing dose to tumors and improving the treatment of patients with metastatic disease [61]. The combination of TRT and external beam radiation therapy delivers radiation dose to a target volume while affecting two different sets of off-target organs. External beam radiation therapy tends to demonstrate toxicity in tissues neighboring the target volume, while TRT typically affects distant organs showing off-target TRT uptake. There is also a theorized synergy between the two different dose rates of external beam radiation and TRT, namely, that low-dose rate TRT may further sensitize cells to the effects of high-dose rate external beam radiation therapy [62, 63]. These radiation modalities have been studied in the context of maximizing dose to a target tumor but have not been thoroughly explored as a combinatorial approach to enhancing response to immunotherapy [64]. Early preclinical studies of this approach suggest promise and indicate that delivering low-dose radiation to all tumor sites with TRT can enhance the systemic antitumor response to an external beam radiation therapy-based in situ vaccine regimen [42] and to a combination of an external beam radiation therapy in situ vaccine and immune checkpoint inhibition [52, 65].

Oncolytic viruses are a class of immunotherapy with the capacity to deliver genetic payloads to targeted tumor cells while also triggering apoptosis and lytic release of additional virus particles [66]. By priming immune recognition of tumor antigens from lysed tumor cells, oncolytic viruses may elicit an in situ vaccine effect. Preclinical studies have begun to evaluate combinations of TRT and oncolytic virus. Sorensen and colleagues have engineered an oncolytic herpes virus to deliver the noradrenaline transporter (NAT), which selectively transports MIBG into infected cells [67]. This oncolytic virus renders infected tumors susceptible to MIBG while also stimulating an antitumor immune response. This combination is effective in controlling the growth of UWV and SK-MEL-3 xenograft tumor models [67]. Similarly, Peerlinck and colleagues have engineered an adenoviral vector that delivers the Na/I importer gene to colorectal carcinoma cells [68]. This importer promotes iodine-131 uptake into infected cancer cells, and a combination of the Na/I adenovirus and a single dose of iodine-131 is capable of shrinking HCT116 tumor xenografts [68].

12.4.3 TRT in Combination with Other Immunotherapies

DNA vaccines for cancer are designed to be taken up by antigen-presenting cells, affect the synthesis of a tumor antigen encoded in the DNA, and present those protein fragments through MHC-I-mediated pathways to T cells in the immune system [69]. In preclinical studies of prostate cancer, Olsen and colleagues demonstrate that a DNA vaccine encoding the androgen receptor ligand binding domain increases tumor infiltration by tumor-specific $CD8^+$ T cells and controls growth of syngeneic prostate cancer in mice [70, 71]. In a MyC-CaP murine prostate tumor model, these investigators observed that TRT increased T-cell infiltrate and that TRT combined with DNA vaccination controlled tumor growth to a greater degree than either agent alone [72].

Sipuleucel-T is an autologous cellular therapy for the treatment of mCRPC. This therapy uses leukopheresis to isolate antigen-presenting cells, which are incubated with granulocyte-macrophage colony-stimulating factor (GM-CSF) and a prostate cancer-specific antigen prostatic acid phosphatase (PAP). These cells are then reinfused back into the patient with the goal of stimulating the patient's T cells to destroy prostate cancer cells [73]. In 2010, the US Food and Drug Administration (FDA) approved sipuleucel-T, after a phase III randomized trial demonstrated a 4-month survival increase in patients with mCRPC [74]. A phase II study is now testing the combination of radium-223 with sipuleucel-T. That study recently completed accrual of 36 patients, half of whom received six courses of radium-223 during treatment with sipuleucel-T [75]. The primary endpoint for this study is the degree of antitumor T-cell proliferation and results are pending.

12.5 Challenges in Translational Testing of TRT in Combination with Immunotherapy

12.5.1 Determining Macro-dosimetry

A number of unique challenges arise in the preclinical and clinical testing of combinations of TRT and immunotherapies [76–78]. In the past, TRT agents have generally been delivered at maximum tolerated doses in order to maximize tumor cell death. However, in combination with immunotherapy, the goal of using TRT is not necessarily to cause maximal tumor cell death. Rather, in this context, the goal of TRT may be to modulate the collective tumor microenvironment and stimulate phenotypic changes within tumor cells to better enable the response to immunotherapy. With this approach, it becomes critical to understand patient-specific dosimetry with spatial and temporal resolution. Traditional approaches to studying pharmacokinetics and pharmacodynamics can be limited in this application because of the impact of spatial and temporal heterogeneity on TRT dose deposition. Such heterogeneity of TRT uptake may be influenced by the type of tumor, tumor heterogeneity, and dynamics of tumor perfusion [78]. Time resolution is important in discerning the cumulative dose deposited by the exponential decay of radionuclides. While ex vivo biodistribution studies can be used in preclinical models to estimate dose distribution as a function of time, this is not feasible in clinical settings. Rather, imaging-based dosimetry approaches are essential in this context, and single photon emission tomography computed tomography/computed tomography (SPECT)/CT or positron emission tomography (PET)/CT of theranostic agents can be paired with advanced dosimetry calculation platforms to determine patient-specific dosimetry for tumors and organs at risk [79]. These approaches can be applied in preclinical and clinical settings [80]. Given the potential for radiation to enhance tumor susceptibility to immune response but also to deplete lymphocytic effector cells, it is important to engage dosimetry studies in all translational studies optimizing the sequencing, timing, and dosing of TRT and immunotherapy combinations.

Even with appropriate dosimetry, our understanding of how to optimally prescribe TRT in combination with immunotherapies is limited. It is unknown whether a minimum threshold dose, mean dose, or maximum dose will be most important for immune activation. It is further unknown whether such dose must be delivered to all, a majority, or some other proportion of tumor sites and tumor volumes. Larger tumors tend to have hypoxic, necrotic, avascular cores that often do not significantly take up TRT. These are often sites of radioresistance that are rich with innate immune infiltrate (e.g., neutrophils and macrophages). Delivering TRT dose to these necrotic sites may be important in driving an antitumor immune response, or it may simply be critical to delivering dose to viable cells at the tumor periphery. Additional studies are needed to determine how such dose heterogeneity from TRT may affect cooperative interaction with immunotherapies. The dose-limiting organs at risk for combinations of TRT and immunotherapy are also yet to be defined. In these combinations, draining lymph node, spleen, blood pool, and bone marrow dose may be critical and could exhibit lower functional limits than those recognized under maximum tolerated dosing paradigms. Further complicating this challenge is the fact that preclinical murine tumor models, which are commonly used for translational cancer research, do not recapitulate the spatial separation of human tumors and normal tissues. While these geometries scale approximately to the size of the host animal, the range or path length of radiation emitted from radionuclides is fixed. Veterinary trials of TRT and immunotherapy combinations may overcome this challenge and could be offered to pet owners of companion canines with spontaneously arising cancers. The heterogeneity of this veterinary patient population strengthens the translatability of any findings emerging from such studies by mirroring the heterogeneity observed clinically among patients with the same tumor type.

12.5.2 Determining Micro-dosimetry

It is unclear how the microscale dosimetry of TRT may influence its ability to modulate the efficacy of cancer immunotherapies. Radionuclides emitting short-range radiation (e.g., alpha particles, Auger electrons) will deliver dose to the cell taking up TRT and to cells directly in contact with that cell. Such radionuclides, which may be optimal for triggering immunogenic cell death and DNA damage-dependent phenotypic changes in tumor cells, may be less effective in modulating cytokine production and infiltrating immune cells in the tumor microenvironment compared with radionuclides that emit longer-range radiation (e.g., beta particles, gamma rays). Conversely, radionuclides emitting longer-range radiation may not be effective in delivering dose to the individual cell of TRT uptake, relying instead on "crossfire" radiation from TRT uptake in neighboring cells. This may limit the effect of such agents against isolated or circulating tumor cells without such neighbors. It is unclear whether it is necessary to deliver immunomodulatory radiation to such tumor cells in order to optimize the effect of TRT in enhancing response to immunotherapies.

Time resolution of micro-dosimetry is also important to optimize the sequencing of TRT with immunotherapy. In these settings, an initial dose from TRT may be needed to trigger immunogenic tumor cell death, depletion of radiosensitive-suppressive lymphocyte populations in the tumor microenvironment, and activation of a type I IFN response [31]. Following this, the goal of immunotherapy would be to repopulate the tumor microenvironment with activated, antitumor effector lymphocytes capable of facilitating tumor destruction. If, at the time of immunotherapy administration, residual TRT decay emits enough radiation to deplete effector T cells, this could hinder the development of an effective antitumor response. This makes optimized sequencing of TRT and immunotherapy critical and highlights the need for understanding the microscopic scale of the dose delivered to tumor cells and the surrounding microenvironment from TRT. Similarly, micro-dosimetry is needed in order to optimize the activation of molecular pathways that increase the immune susceptibility of tumor cells. For instance, activation of a type I IFN response following external beam radiation is optimal at single fraction doses of 8–12 Gy [27]. It is unclear what the dose response relationship between TRT and activation of a type I IFN response will be, and understanding TRT micro-dosimetry in tumor cells is needed to clarify this.

12.5.3 Performing Advanced Immunophenotyping on Radioactive Tissues

Standard approaches for evaluating immune cell infiltration of tumors include the use of flow cytometry on disaggregated tumor specimens. These studies are generally performed on fresh tissue, and this can pose a challenge to studies involving TRT in which fresh tumor specimens are radioactive. Performing flow cytometry on radioactive tissues requires a dedicated facility and may generate considerable volumes of radioactive waste. To overcome this challenge, we have developed flow cytometry methods that enable the labeling of disaggregated tumor specimens and subsequent freezing of these until specimen radioactivity has decayed to background levels—at which point specimens can be analyzed using standard flow cytometry methods [81]. Similar innovations may be required with other techniques to allow safe use of state-of-the-art methods for tumor immunophenotyping.

12.5.4 Developing Fundamental Understanding of the Immunogenic Effects of TRT

Performing comparative studies evaluating the effects of different radionuclides on tumor immunogenicity is challenging because for each radionuclide, there is a simultaneous change in the half-life, LET, type of radioactive decay, and daughter radionuclides. This inherent challenge cannot be avoided, and it limits the design of well-controlled studies evaluating the independent impact of these distinct physical parameters of radionuclides on tumor immunogenicity. Rather, such mechanistic studies will need to compare the relative capacities of individual radionuclides to one another. With increasing experience using diverse radionuclides, it may then be possible to infer conclusions about the potential effects of a given physical property of radionuclides on tumor immune susceptibility.

A similar challenge arises in attempting to perform comparative studies evaluating the effects of TRT in different tumor types. The vectors used to deliver TRT are typically specific for a single or a select few tumor types. Because the dosimetry and off-target uptake of TRT changes with each vector, the specificity of TRT vectors for tumor types limits the ability to perform controlled studies testing the generalizability across tumor types of findings on the effects of a TRT on tumor immunogenicity. This challenge may be overcome with TRT vectors that are more broadly specific for malignant cells rather than a single tumor type. Alkylphosphocholine analogs such as NM600 are one example of such a vector, and these will be critical to translational studies that seek to advance a fundamental understanding of the immunogenic effects of TRT.

12.6 Conclusion

By engaging a patient's immune system to attack cancer cells, immunotherapies have the potential to cure even advanced or metastatic cancers. However, the response rate to immunotherapies remains low in most solid tumors. Radiation not only triggers an immunogenic form of tumor cell death, but tumor cells surviving radiation commonly exhibit phenotypic changes that increase susceptibility to immune detection and elimination. Radiation also modifies components of the tumor microenvironment in a manner that can promote immune cell infiltration and activation. By delivering radiation to all tumor sites while limiting dose to immune organs including lymph nodes, blood, spleen, and bone marrow, TRTs have the potential to increase the response rates to immunotherapies and in this way may have a tremendous impact on the survival of cancer patients. To achieve this will require well-designed preclinical and clinical studies that provide a mechanistic understanding of the therapeutic interaction between TRTs and antitumor immunity. This will be critical to translational studies that seek to develop and optimize combinations of TRTs and immunotherapies in the treatment of patients with metastatic cancers.

References

1. Emens LA, Ascierto PA, Darcy PK, et al. Cancer immunotherapy: opportunities and challenges in the rapidly evolving clinical landscape. Eur J Cancer. 2017;81:116–29. https://doi.org/10.1016/j.ejca.2017.01.035.
2. Seelige R, Searles S, Jack BD. Mechanisms regulating immune surveillance of cellular stress in cancer. Cell Mol Life Sci. 2018;75:225–40. https://doi.org/10.1007/s00018-017-2597-7.
3. Bates JP, Derakhshandeh R, Jones L, Webb TJ. Mechanisms of immune evasion in breast cancer. BMC Cancer. https://doi.org/10.1186/s12885-018-4441-3.
4. Dunn GP, Old LJ, Schreiber RD. The three Es of cancer immunoediting. Annu Rev Immunol. 2004;22(1):329–60. https://doi.org/10.1146/annurev.immunol.22.012703.104803.
5. Galon J, Bruni D. Approaches to treat immune hot, altered and cold tumours with combination immunotherapies. Nat Rev Drug Discov. 2019;18(3):197–218. https://doi.org/10.1038/s41573-018-0007-y.
6. Vareki SM. High and low mutational burden tumors versus immunologically hot and cold tumors and response to immune checkpoint inhibitors. J Immunother Cancer. https://doi.org/10.1186/s40425-018-0479-7.
7. Murphy JB, Hussey RG, Nakahara W, Sturm E. Studies on x-ray effects: VI. Effect of the cellular reaction induced by x-rays on cancer grains. J Exp Med. 1921;33(3):299–313. https://doi.org/10.1084/jem.33.3.299.
8. Slone HB, Peters LJ, Milas L. Effect of host immune capability on radiocurability and subsequent transplantability of a murine fibrosarcoma. J Natl Cancer Inst. 1979;63(5):1229–35. https://doi.org/10.1093/jnci/63.5.1229.
9. Law AW, Mole RH. Direct and abscopal effects of X-radiation on the thymus of the weanling rat. Int J Radiat Biol Relat Stud Phys Chem Med. 1961;3(3):233–48. https://doi.org/10.1080/09553006114551161.
10. Brody JD, Ai WZ, Czerwinski DK, et al. In situ vaccination with a TLR9 agonist induces systemic lymphoma regression: a phase I/II study. J Clin Oncol. 2010; https://doi.org/10.1200/JCO.2010.28.9793.
11. Marabelle A, Tselikas L, de Baere T, Houot R. Intratumoral immunotherapy: using the tumor as the remedy. Ann Oncol. 2017; https://doi.org/10.1093/annonc/mdx683.
12. Kinner A, Wu W, Staudt C, Iliakis G. Gamma-H2AX in recognition and signaling of DNA double-strand breaks in the context of chromatin. Nucleic Acids Res. 2008; https://doi.org/10.1093/nar/gkn550.
13. Krysko DV, Garg AD, Kaczmarek A, Krysko O, Agostinis P, Vandenabeele P. Immunogenic cell death and DAMPs in cancer therapy. Nat Rev Cancer. 2012; https://doi.org/10.1038/nrc3380.
14. Golden EB, Apetoh L. Radiotherapy and immunogenic cell death. Semin Radiat Oncol. 2015; https://doi.org/10.1016/j.semradonc.2014.07.005.
15. Green DR, Ferguson T, Zitvogel L, Kroemer G. Immunogenic and tolerogenic cell death. Nat Rev Immunol. 2009; https://doi.org/10.1038/nri2545.
16. Panaretakis T, Kepp O, Brockmeier U, et al. Mechanisms of pre-apoptotic calreticulin exposure in immunogenic cell death. EMBO J. 2009;28:578–90. https://doi.org/10.1038/emboj.2009.1.
17. Golden EB, Frances D, Pellicciotta I, Demaria S, Helen Barcellos-Hoff M, Formenti SC. Radiation fosters dose-dependent and chemotherapy-induced immunogenic cell death. Onco Targets Ther. 2014;3(4):e28518. https://doi.org/10.4161/onci.28518.
18. Apetoh L, Ghiringhelli F, Tesniere A, et al. Toll-like receptor 4-dependent contribution of the immune system to anticancer chemotherapy and radiotherapy. Nat Med. 2007;13(9):1050–9. https://doi.org/10.1038/nm1622.
19. Lotze MT, Tracey KJ. High-mobility group box 1 protein (HMGB1): nuclear weapon in the immune arsenal. Nat Rev Immunol. 2005;5(4):331–42. https://doi.org/10.1038/nri1594.
20. Ohshima Y, Tsukimoto M, Takenouchi T, et al. γ-Irradiation induces P2X7 receptor-dependent ATP release from B16 melanoma cells. Biochim Biophys Acta Gen Subj. 2010;1800(1):40–6. https://doi.org/10.1016/j.bbagen.2009.10.008.
21. Ghiringhelli F, Apetoh L, Tesniere A, et al. Activation of the NLRP3 inflammasome in dendritic cells induces IL-1B-dependent adaptive immunity against tumors. Nat Med. 2009;15(10):1170–8. https://doi.org/10.1038/nm.2028.
22. Newcomb EW, Demaria S, Lukyanov Y, et al. The combination of ionizing radiation and peripheral vaccination produces long-term survival of mice bearing established invasive GL261 gliomas. Clin Cancer Res.

2006;12(15):4730–7. https://doi.org/10.1158/1078-0432.CCR-06-0593.

23. Son CH, Lee HR, Koh EK, et al. Combination treatment with decitabine and ionizing radiation enhances tumor cells susceptibility of T cells. Sci Rep. 2016; https://doi.org/10.1038/srep32470.

24. Malamas AS, Gameiro SR, Knudson KM, Hodge JW. Sublethal exposure to alpha radiation (223Ra dichloride) enhances various carcinomas' sensitivity to lysis by antigen specific cytotoxic T lymphocytes through calreticulin-mediated immunogenic modulation. Oncotarget. 2016;7(52):86937–47. https://doi.org/10.18632/oncotarget.13520.

25. Chakraborty M, Abrams SI, Camphausen K, et al. Irradiation of tumor cells up-regulates Fas and enhances CTL lytic activity and CTL adoptive immunotherapy. J Immunol. 2003; https://doi.org/10.4049/jimmunol.170.12.6338.

26. Benci JL, Xu B, Qiu Y, et al. Tumor interferon signaling regulates a multigenic resistance program to immune checkpoint blockade HHS public access. Cell. 2016;167(6):1540–54. https://doi.org/10.1016/j.cell.2016.11.022.

27. Vanpouille-Box C, Alard A, Aryankalayil MJ, et al. DNA exonuclease Trex1 regulates radiotherapy-induced tumour immunogenicity. Nat Commun. 2017;8:15618. https://doi.org/10.1038/ncomms15618.

28. Di Maggio FM, Minafra L, Forte GI, et al. Portrait of inflammatory response to ionizing radiation treatment. J Inflamm (United Kingdom). 2015; https://doi.org/10.1186/s12950-015-0058-3.

29. Liu S-Z. Nonlinear dose-response relationship in the immune system following exposure to ionizing radiation: mechanisms and implications. Nonlinearity Biol Toxicol Med. 2003; https://doi.org/10.1080/15401420390844483.

30. Rodriguez-Ruiz ME, Garasa S, Rodriguez I, et al. Intercellular adhesion molecule-1 and vascular cell adhesion molecule are induced by ionizing radiation on lymphatic endothelium. Int J Radiat Oncol Biol Phys. 2017;97(2):389–400. https://doi.org/10.1016/j.ijrobp.2016.10.043.

31. Nakamura N, Kusunoki Y, Akiyama M. Radiosensitivity of CD4 or CD8 positive human T-lymphocytes by an in vitro colony formation assay. Radiat Res. 1990; https://doi.org/10.2307/3577549.

32. Balogh A, Persa E, Bogdándi EN, et al. The effect of ionizing radiation on the homeostasis and functional integrity of murine splenic regulatory T cells. Inflamm Res. 2013; https://doi.org/10.1007/s00011-012-0567-y.

33. Liu R, Xiong S, Zhang L, Chu Y. Enhancement of antitumor immunity by low-dose total body irradiation is associated with selectively decreasing the proportion and number of T regulatory cells. Cell Mol Immunol. 2010; https://doi.org/10.1038/cmi.2009.117.

34. Xu J, Escamilla J, Mok S, et al. CSF1R signaling blockade stanches tumor-infiltrating myeloid cells and improves the efficacy of radiotherapy in prostate cancer. Cancer Res. 2013; https://doi.org/10.1158/0008-5472.CAN-12-3981.

35. Chiang CS, Fu SY, Wang SC, et al. Irradiation promotes an M2 macrophage phenotype in tumor hypoxia. Front Oncol. 2012; https://doi.org/10.3389/fonc.2012.00089.

36. Schaue D, Ratikan JA, Iwamoto KS, McBride WH. Maximizing tumor immunity with fractionated radiation. Int J Radiat Oncol Biol Phys. 2012; https://doi.org/10.1016/j.ijrobp.2011.09.049.

37. Lin AJ, Gang M, Rao YJ, et al. Association of posttreatment lymphopenia and elevated neutrophil-to-lymphocyte ratio with poor clinical outcomes in patients with human papillomavirus-negative oropharyngeal cancers. JAMA Otolaryngol Head Neck Surg. 2019;145(5):413–21. https://doi.org/10.1001/jamaoto.2019.0034.

38. Kim DY, Kim IS, Park SG, Kim H, Choi YJ, Seol YM. Prognostic value of posttreatment neutrophil-lymphocyte ratio in head and neck squamous cell carcinoma treated by chemoradiotherapy. Auris Nasus Larynx. https://doi.org/10.1016/j.anl.2016.05.013.

39. Abuodeh Y, Venkat P, Kim S. Systematic review of case reports on the abscopal effect. Curr Probl Cancer. 2016; https://doi.org/10.1016/j.currproblcancer.2015.10.001.

40. Morris ZS, Guy EI, Francis DM, et al. In situ tumor vaccination by combining local radiation and tumor-specific antibody or immunocytokine treatments. Cancer Res. 2016;76(13):3929–41. https://doi.org/10.1158/0008-5472.CAN-15-2644.

41. Morris ZS, Guy EI, Werner LR, et al. Tumor-specific inhibition of *in situ* vaccination by distant untreated tumor sites. Cancer Immunol Res. 2018;6(7):825–34. https://doi.org/10.1158/2326-6066.CIR-17-0353.

42. Carlson PM, Heinze C, Grudzinski J, Hernandez R, Gillies SD, Loibner H, Rakhmilevich AL, Otto M, Bednarz B, Weichert J, Sondel PM, Morris ZS. Molecular targeted radiotherapy facilitates in situ vaccination in a syngeneic murine melanoma model. J Immunother Cancer. 2017;5. https://jitc.biomedcentral.com/articles/10.1186/s40425-017-0288-4.

43. Gomez DR, Blumenschein GR, Lee JJ, et al. Local consolidative therapy versus maintenance therapy or observation for patients with oligometastatic non-small-cell lung cancer without progression after first-line systemic therapy: a multicentre, randomised, controlled, phase 2 study. Lancet Oncol. 2016;17(12):1672–82. https://doi.org/10.1016/S1470-2045(16)30532-0.

44. Gill MR, Falzone N, Du Y, Vallis KA. Review Targeted radionuclide therapy in combined-modality regimens. Lancet Oncol. 2019;18(7):e414–23. https://doi.org/10.1016/S1470-2045(17)30379-0.

45. Divgi C. The current state of radiopharmaceutical therapy. J Nucl Med. 2018;59(11):2018–20. https://doi.org/10.2967/jnumed.118.214122.

46. Dolgin E. Radioactive drugs emerge from the shadows to storm the market. Nat Biotechnol. 2018; https://doi.org/10.1038/nbt1218-1125.

47. Czernin J. Molecular imaging and therapy with a purpose: a renaissance of nuclear medicine. J Nucl Med. 2017;58(1):21A–2A.

48. Zukotynski K, Jadvar H, Capala J, Fahey F. Targeted radionuclide therapy: practical applications and future prospects supplementary issue: biomarkers and their essential role in the development of personalised therapies (A). Biomark Cancer. 2016;8 https://doi.org/10.4137/BiC.s31804.

49. Hino R, Kabashima K, Kato Y, et al. Tumor cell expression of programmed cell death-1 ligand 1 is a prognostic factor for malignant melanoma. Cancer. 2010;116(7):1757–66. https://doi.org/10.1002/cncr.24899.

50. Weichert JP, Clark PA, Kandela IK, et al. Alkylphosphocholine analogs for broad-spectrum cancer imaging and therapy. Sci Transl Med. 2014;6:240ra75. https://doi.org/10.1126/scitranslmed.3007646.

51. Patel RB, Hernandez R, Carlson P, Grudzinski J, Bates AM, Jagodinsky JC, Erbe A, Marsh IR, Arthur I, Aluicio-Sarduy E, Sriramaneni RN, Jin WJ, Massey C, Rakhmilevich AL, Vail D, Engle JW, Le T, Kim K, Bednarz B, Sondel PM, Weichert J, Morris ZS. Low-dose targeted radionuclide therapy renders immunologically cold tumors responsive to immune checkpoint blockade. Sci Transl Med. 2021;13(602). PMID: 34261797.

52. Patel R, Hernandez R, Carlson P, Brown R, Zangl L, Bates A, Arthur I, Jagodinsky J, Grudinski J, Erbe A, Weichert J, Sondel PM, Morris ZS. Mechanistic insights into combination low dose targeted radionuclide and checkpoint blockade treatment to turn a "cold" tumor "hot". J Immunother Cancer. 2019;7. https://jitc.biomedcentral.com/articles/10.1186/s40425-019-0764-0.

53. Chen H, Zhao L, Fu K, et al. Integrin αvβ3-targeted radionuclide therapy combined with immune checkpoint blockade immunotherapy synergistically enhances anti-tumor efficacy. Theranostics. 2019;9(25): 7948–60. https://doi.org/10.7150/thno.39203.

54. Choi J, Beaino W, Fecek RJ, et al. Combined VLA-4–targeted radionuclide therapy and immunotherapy in a mouse model of melanoma. J Nucl Med. 2018;59(12):1843–9. https://doi.org/10.2967/jnumed.118.209510.

55. ClinicalTrials.gov. Phase I study of investigational medicinal products in children with relapsed/refractory neuroblastoma. https://clinicaltrials.gov/ct2/show/NCT02914405.

56. ClinicalTrials.gov. Study evaluating the addition of pembrolizumab to Radium-223 in mCRPC. https://clinicaltrials.gov/ct2/show/NCT03093428.

57. ClinicaTrials.gov. Safety and tolerability of Atezolizumab in combination with Radium-223 Dichloride in metastatic castrate resistant prostate cancer progressed following treatment with an androgen pathway inhibitor. https://clinicaltrials.gov/ct2/show/NCT02814669.

58. ClinicalTrials.gov. PRINCE (PSMA-lutetium Radionuclide Therapy and ImmuNotherapy in Prostate CancEr). https://clinicaltrials.gov/ct2/show/NCT03658447.

59. Victor CT-S, Rech AJ, Maity A, et al. Radiation and dual checkpoint blockade activate nonredundant immune mechanisms in cancer. Nature. 2015;520(7547):373–7. https://doi.org/10.1038/nature14292.

60. Formenti SC, Rudqvist N, Golden E, et al. Radiotherapy induces responses of lung cancer to CTLA-4 blockade. Nat Med. 2018;24(12):1845–51. https://doi.org/10.1038/s41591-018-0232-2.

61. Dietrich A, Koi L, Zöphel K, et al. Improving external beam radiotherapy by combination with internal irradiation. Br J Radiol. 2015;88(1051):20150042. https://doi.org/10.1259/bjr.20150042.

62. Nevedomskaya E, Baumgart SJ, Haendler B. Recent advances in prostate cancer treatment and drug discovery. Int J Mol Sci. 2018;19(5):1359. https://doi.org/10.3390/ijms19051359.

63. Hall EJ, Brenner DJ. The dose-rate effect revisited: radiobiological considerations of importance in radiotherapy. Int J Radiat Oncol Biol Phys. 1991; https://doi.org/10.1016/0360-3016(91)90314-T.

64. Dietrich A, Koi L, Sihver W, Kotzerke J, Baumann M, Krause M. Improving external beam radiotherapy by combination with internal irradiation. J Radiol. 2015;88:20150042. https://doi.org/10.1259/bjr.20150042.

65. Jagodinsky JC, Bates AM, Hernandez R, Grudzinski JJ, Marsh IR, Chakravarty I, Arthur IA, Zangl LM, Brown RJ, Nystuen EJ, Emma SE, Kerr C, Jin WJ, Carlson PM, Engle JW, Aluicio-Sarduy E, Barnhart TE, Le T, Kim KM, Bednarz BP, Weichert JP, Patel RB, Morris ZS. Temporal analysis of type 1 interferon activation in tumor cells following external beam radiotherapy or targeted radionuclide therapy. Theranostics. 2021;11(13):6120–37. PMID: 33995649; PMCID: PMC8120207.

66. Kaufman HL, Kohlhapp FJ, Zloza A. Oncolytic viruses: a new class of immunotherapy drugs. Nat Rev Drug Discov. 2015; https://doi.org/10.1038/nrd4663.

67. Sorensen A, Mairs RJ, Braidwood L, et al. In vivo evaluation of a cancer therapy strategy combining HSV1716-mediated oncolysis with gene transfer and targeted radiotherapy. J Nucl Med. 2012;53(4):647–54. https://doi.org/10.2967/jnumed.111.090886.

68. Peerlinck I, Merron A, Baril P, et al. Targeted radionuclide therapy using a wnt-targeted replicating adenovirus encoding the Na/I symporter. Clin Cancer Res. 2009;15(21):6595–601. https://doi.org/10.1158/1078-0432.CCR-09-0262.

69. Rekoske BT, Smith HA, Olson BM, Maricque BB, McNeel DG. PD-1 or PD-L1 blockade restores antitumor efficacy following SSX2 epitope-modified DNA

vaccine immunization. Cancer Immunol Res. 2015; https://doi.org/10.1158/2326-6066.CIR-14-0206.

70. Olson BM, Johnson LE, McNeel DG. The androgen receptor: a biologically relevant vaccine target for the treatment of prostate cancer. Cancer Immunol Immunother. 2013; https://doi.org/10.1007/s00262-012-1363-9.

71. Olson BM, McNeel DG. CD8+ T cells specific for the androgen receptor are common in patients with prostate cancer and are able to lyse prostate tumor cells. Cancer Immunol Immunother. 2011; https://doi.org/10.1007/s00262-011-0987-5.

72. Potluri H, Hernandez R, Zahm C, Grudzinski J, Massey C, Jamey Weichert DM. Molecularly targeted radionuclide therapy modulates the composition of the murine prostate cancer microenvironment. J Immunother Cancer. 2019;7. https://jitc.biomedcentral.com/articles/10.1186/s40425-019-0764-0.

73. Kantoff PW, Higano CS, Shore ND, et al. Sipuleucel-T immunotherapy for castration-resistant prostate cancer. N Engl J Med. 2010; https://doi.org/10.1056/NEJMoa1001294.

74. Small EJ, Schellhammer PF, Higano CS, et al. Placebo-controlled phase III trial of immunologic therapy with Sipuleucel-T (APC8015) in patients with metastatic, asymptomatic hormone refractory prostate cancer. J Clin Oncol. 2006; https://doi.org/10.1200/JCO.2005.04.5252.

75. ClinicalTrials.gov. Study of Sipuleucel-T with or without Radium-223 in men with asymptomatic or minimally symptomatic MCRPC. https://clinicaltrials.gov/ct2/show/NCT02463799.

76. Pouget JP, Lozza C, Deshayes E, Boudousq V, Navarro-Teulon I. Introduction to radiobiology of targeted radionuclide therapy. Front Med. 2015;2(MAR):12. https://doi.org/10.3389/fmed.2015.00012.

77. Jadvar H. Targeted radionuclide therapy: an evolution toward precision cancer treatment. Am J Roentgenol. 2017;209(2):277–88. https://doi.org/10.2214/AJR.17.18264.

78. Lassmann M, Chiesa C, Flux G, Bardiès M. EANM Dosimetry Committee guidance document: good practice of clinical dosimetry reporting. Eur J Nucl Med Mol Imaging. 2011; https://doi.org/10.1007/s00259-010-1549-3.

79. Besemer AE, Yang YM, Grudzinski JJ, Hall LT, Bednarz BP. Development and validation of RAPID: a patient-specific Monte Carlo three-dimensional internal dosimetry platform. Cancer Biother Radiopharm. 2018;33(4):155–65. https://doi.org/10.1089/cbr.2018.2451.

80. Bednarz B, Grudzinski J, Marsh I, et al. Murine-specific internal dosimetry for preclinical investigations of imaging and therapeutic agents. Health Phys. 2018;114(4):450–9. https://doi.org/10.1097/HP.0000000000000789.

81. Carlson P, Mohan M, Patel R, Nettenstrom L, Sheerar D, Fox K, Rodriguez M, Hoefges A, Hernandez R, Zahm C, McNeel D, Weichert J, Morris Z, Sondel P. Labeling method for flow cytometric analysis of radioactive tumors following immunotherapy and molecular targeted radionuclide therapy (mTRT): demonstration of augmented immune infiltrate. In: 34th Annual Meeting of the Society for Immunotherapy of Cancer; 2019. https://jitc.biomedcentral.com/track/pdf/10.1186/s40425-019-0764-0.

Radioimmunotherapy 13

Majid Assadi and Ali Gholamrezanezhad

Contents

M. Assadi (✉)
Nuclear Medicine and Molecular Imaging Research Center, School of Medicine, Bushehr University of Medical Sciences, Bushehr, Iran
e-mail: asadi@bpums.ac.ir

A. Gholamrezanezhad
Division of Emergency Radiology, Department of Radiology, Keck School of Medicine, University of Southern California (USC), Los Angeles, CA, USA
e-mail: gholamre@usc.edu

© Springer Nature Switzerland AG 2022
S. Harsini et al. (eds.), *Nuclear Medicine and Immunology*,
https://doi.org/10.1007/978-3-030-81261-4_13

13.1   Introduction

Every year, many people die from various types of cancer. However, the specialist efforts that have been made in this field and in the study of the molecular biology of cancer have resulted in advancements in the successful treatment of the disease and the augmentation of the quality and longevity of patients' lives. For decades, external beam radiation therapy (EBRT) and chemotherapy after surgery have been implemented as the most practical methods in the treatment of cancer.

However, external beam radiation therapy (EBRT) and chemotherapy are not targeted enough and therefore cause damage to healthy tissue in addition to cancerous tissue [1]. To address this issue, research has focused on understanding the molecular differences between normal and cancerous tissue in order to improve the therapeutic index as a critical aim of treatment. A therapeutic index is a tool related to measuring whether maximum damage is done to tumorous tissue while minimum damage is done to normal tissue. Several efforts have been applied to augment the desired result, and positive results in cancer therapy have been achieved through some strategies that seek to provide more targeted treatments.

One of these challenging new methods is radioimmunotherapy (RIT), which involves the conjugation of a therapeutic radionuclide with anticancer antibodies [2]. RIT applies antibodies as a therapeutic tracer or target. Clinically, RIT is primarily utilized to treat radiosensitive tumors, including lymphoma and leukemia. Solid tumors are relatively rather resistant to radiation and, for a complete response, require almost five to ten times the deposited radiation required by hematological malignancies. After the injection of the radioimmunoconjugate drug in RIT, radioantibodies are spread out by blood flow and conveyed to the specific target, such as antigen-associated tumor cells. In this technique, the adverse effects on surrounding normal tissue are diminished when compared with chemotherapy and EBRT. These radioantibodies, which are created specifically as drugs, are injected intravenously directly into the target tissue or body cavities, such as the intrathecal space, peritoneum, or pleura. Based on different factors, such as the kind of tumor and staging, the time interval between injection sessions varies. In RIT, radiation damage in tumor cells occurs through the huge energy release that arises during radioactive nucleus decay (such as alpha [α] and beta [β] particles), resulting in DNA damage that causes the death of tumor cells. Further, RIT is one of the most energy-efficient processes. The comparative radioresistance and radiosensitivity are intrinsic features of cancer cells that correlate with the cell of origin of a tumor. Hypoxia and the ability to repair radiation-induced destruction are two factors that can increase cells' radiation resistance [3].

The second component of the drug used in RIT is a monoclonal antibody (mAb). Before their application in RIT, these therapeutic antibodies were used in immunotherapy. Immunotherapy is a type of biological therapy that helps the immune system to fight cancer and applies substances made from living organisms to treat malignant tissues; it includes such therapies as checkpoint inhibitors, adoptive cell transfer, treatment vaccines, and monoclonal or therapeutic antibodies.

Pressman and Keighley were the first researchers to use radiolabeled antibody (Ab) in vivo in RIT. At this time, radiolabeled Ab was evaluated in radioimmunodiagnosis applications and was then implemented to aid in the delivery of curative doses of radiation to malignant tissues [4]. In 1975, Köhler and Milstein invented hybridoma technology and were the pioneer researchers in the production of rodent antibodies with single specificity; it was at this point that the name "mAb" was introduced. Next, mAbs were employed as a delivery transporter for radioactive nuclides to tumor-associated antigen [5]. Many factors affect the biological response of a tumor in RIT, some of which include the properties of the radionuclide, cell cycle kinetics, dose rate, target tissue radiosensitivity, radiation repair capacity, kind of antibody, and condition of dose absorption within the tumor [6]. Recent advances in antibody technology, radiochemistry, radiobiology, and genetic engineering have provided important tools for the RIT procedure. In this chapter, we define key terms and expressions related to RIT and review important developments that have been made in the technique.

13.2 Antibodies

Antibodies, also known as an immunoglobulin (Ig), are Y-shaped glycoproteins that release from plasma B cells and are implemented through the immune system to recognize and eliminate microbial toxins and foreign pathogens such as viruses and bacteria [7]. A full-throughout antigen-antibody category does not exist, but cluster of differentiation 22 (CD22), CD20, and human leukocyte antigen-DR isotope (HLA-DR) have been successfully targeted on B-cell lymphomas, CD33 and CD45 have shown acceptable results in clinical trials for treating acute myeloid leukemia (AML), and preliminary studies have proposed that CD38 is advantageous for targeting multiple myeloma (MM) [8]. After that the certain region of antigens attaches to antibody, the antibody can interact with it and operate its biological function. Antigens are molecular components or structures that bind specifically to an antibody or cell antigen receptor, and also it is described as a molecule that binds to the product of immune response whereas immunogen molecule that is capable of inducing an immune response by an organism's immune system. So an immunogen is undoubtedly an antigen, but an antigen may not inevitably be an immunogen inducing. The molecular types of antigens include proteins, polysaccharides, lipids, and nucleic acids. Choosing the most favorable cell surface antigen and targeting antibody is crucial to the successful result of a therapeutic program. An ideal antigen for RIT must be expressed infinite and high density on the surface of all tumors cells [9]. The identification of tumor antigens is carried out via screening expression collection—specifically, through the in vitro sensitization of peripheral blood mononuclear cells (PBMCs) or through an in vitro culture with tumor-infiltrating lymphocytes (TILs) of the autologous malignant cells or autologous healthy cells (which were either transfected with genetic settings encoding candidate antigens or pulsed with candidate T-cell epitopes). When antigen expression appears all over a tumor, it is possible that it is a heterogeneous type that causes the trivial distribution of the absorbed dose of radionuclide throughout the tumor, decreasing the therapeutic improvements [10].

Antigenic targets in malignant tissues include hematopoietic clusters of differentiation (CD) antigens; enzymes such as carbonic anhydrase IX (CAIX) and prostate-specific membrane antigen (PSMA); cell surface glycoproteins such as mucins; glycolipids such as GD2; stromal components; blood vessel constituents, such as the vascular endothelial growth factor receptor (VEGFR), integrin, or the amino domain of fibronectin; carbohydrates such as Lewis; and cell membrane receptors associated with the direction of several signaling pathways such as growth factor receptors, epidermal growth factor receptor (EGFR), and the human epidermal growth factor receptor-2 (HER2) [9, 11].

Monoclonal antibodies (mAb) are the individual antibodies specific to a single antigen. The basic method of making mAb is the combination of B cells from an immunized mouse with a myeloma cell line (as the tumor cell line); then the cells are grown in conditions in which unfused healthy and non-healthy cells cannot survive but in which cells that are fused can grow; the cells that can grow in such an environment are called "hybridoma." The important properties of antibodies that have been changed to optimize efficacy include affinity and avidity, size, and immunogenicity. "Affinity" is defined as the strength and an amount of binding of the antibody to the single antigen, while "avidity" is the collected strength of multiple affinities that summed up from multiple binding reciprocal actions and is commonly mentioned to as a functional affinity.

13.2.1 Structure of Antibodies

Although antibodies have different structures and figures, all Ig antibodies have identical Y structures (Fig. 13.1). Below are explained the different parts of the antibody.

- *Light and heavy chain*: A standard antibody consists of four polypeptide chains, including two light and two heavy chains. Each light and the heavy chain have variable and constant regions.
- *Variable and constant regions*: The amino variable (V) parts at the end of even heavy and light chains are important in antigen identification. Effector operators are conducted by

carboxy-terminal constant (C) parts of the heavy chains. Two heavy and light chains are made up of Ig domain, forming a protein domain. The Ig domain consists of folded and regularity units, including 110 amino acids situated lengthwise among two layers of β-pleated foils. These β-pleated foils stick together via a disulfide bridge, and there are some short loops that link the adjacent strings of every β sheet. Amino acids in some of these loops are highly necessary for antigen recognition. Light and heavy chain arrangements are nearly identical. However, in a light chain, there is one variable region (VL) and one constant region (CL) Ig domain, while in a heavy chain, there are one V region (VH) of one Ig domain and three or four C region (CH) domains. The antigen-binding site includes a V region of a light chain and the adjacent V region of a heavy chain [13]. The types of Ig are IgM, IgG, IgE, IgA, and IgD.

- Heavy and light chains slightly connect through the non-covalent connections between the VH and VL domains and between the CH1 and CL domains. The two heavy chains in every antibody are completely conjoined covalently through disulfide bonds. In addition, in IgG antibodies, disulfide bonds are constructed in the middle of cysteine residues in the CH2 region. Hinge regions are flexible links between the fragment antigen binding (Fab) arms and the fragment crystallizable (Fc) part. Flexibility and the length of the hinge region can differ among the various IgG classifications [14].
- The Fc region, a distal region of an antibody, is composed of two similar disulfide-linked peptides, including the CH2 and CH3 domains of the heavy chain (Fig. 13.1). Fc regions interact with certain cell surface receptors, as well as called "Fc receptors," and this property of Fc regions helps antibodies to incite the immune system. The biological properties of antibodies are carried out through Fc regions. Moreover, Fab (Fragment, antigen-binding) division of antibody that makes the possibility

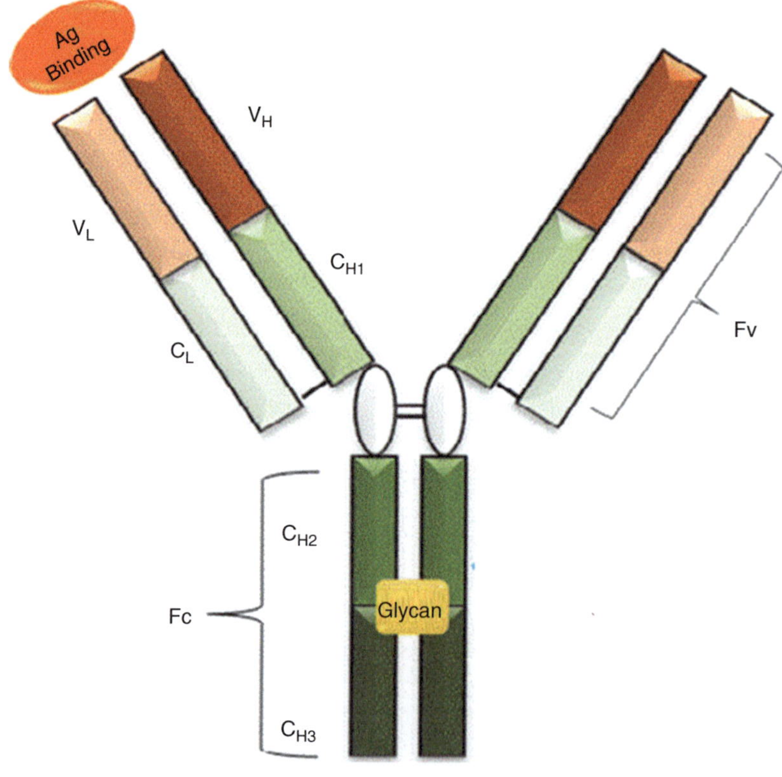

Fig. 13.1 Structure of mAb antibodies. (Adapted from Kizhedath et al., 2017, Archives of toxicology) [12]

for attaching to an antigen is composed of one CL and one VL domain for each heavy and light chain.

- *Hinge region*: The hinge region is a very flexible area of the antibody, located between CH1 and CH2, and is responsible for the Y formation of the antibody.
- *Haptens*: Haptens are small antigenic molecules that, alone, cannot induce immunoreactivity.
- *Epitope*: This determinant is the part of an antigen that is recognized by the immune system (such as antibodies, T cells, and B cells). This specific part of the antigen binds to an antibody.
- *Affinity and avidity*: The interaction between antigens and antibodies is a reversible connection process that requires multiple non-covalent interactions, including electrostatic forces, hydrogen bonds, and hydrophobic interactions. There are two important properties that play a significant role in the interaction between antigens and antibodies, one of which is affinity or the strength of the binding between antigens and antibodies. Affinity is determined by the power of the reciprocation between a specific epitope and its synthesis with the antibody. Wittrup et al. developed a practical pattern for selecting targeting functions for optimal uptake with the use of chemical engineering principles. They concluded that the role of high binding affinity in tumor uptake is crucial for small peptides, less important for antibodies, and insignificant for nanoparticles [15]. The next term, "avidity," relates to the general potential and possibility of a connection between an antigen with several epitopes and a multifunctional antibody. Avidity is qualified by three major factors: the valence of both the antigen and the antibody, antibody-epitope affinity, and the structural regulation of the interacting segments.
- *Specificity*: This term refers to the ability of a single antibody-combining site to react with just one epitope or antigenic determinant. With this property (especially in mAbs), antibodies can identify differences between the primary structure, isomeric forms, and secondary and tertiary structures of an antigen.

13.3 Consideration of RIT Approach

The choice of the optimum cell surface antigen and attacking antibody are very important for the successful implementation of a therapeutic plan. As such, the following aspects must be considered:

- The tumor specificity of antigen expression must be considered as this indicates whether the antigen expresses extraordinary and uniform density on tumor cells versus normal tissues (i.e., more than 100,000 sites per cancer cell).
- The antigen does not shed into the bloodstream.
- Antigens are easily accessible from the blood and from the extracellular liquid.
- The type of metabolism of the radionuclide of the target cell is a crucial matter. Retaining or disposing of the lysosome organelle from the cell increases and decreases, respectively, the radiation effects of radionuclide and anticancer properties.
- The uptake and in vivo biodistribution in critical organs, such as the kidney, liver, and spleen, must also be considered. A radiolabeled antibody must show low uptake and a high therapeutic index ratio between the tumor and radiosensitive tissues, such as the kidney and bone marrow (>10 and >50, respectively).
- The immune response of radioimmunoconjugates should be stimulated as much as possible (>90%).

13.4 Selection of Radionuclides

The use of only antibodies is not sufficient for complete treatment response in tumor malignancies; therefore, for a more durable remission, radionuclide materials must conjugate to Abs. Radioactive cargo decays and emits therapeutic radiation in tumor cells. The utilization of Abs conjugated with proper radioisotopes emerged in the early 1950s [16]. Then, after substantial clinical research, the first radioimmunolabels were approved for therapeutic application in non-Hodgkin lymphoma (NHL) in the early twenty-first century. In the early years of this application, most efforts were devoted to the discovery and production of the proper antibodies and also radiolabeling techniques. These developments are being continued by different organizations to expand the engineered monoclonal antibodies that have specific properties such as a low level of toxicity [17].

Therapeutic radionuclide particles emit radiation and make a single- or double-strand break in DNA beyond the DNA's capacity to repair itself; this destroys the target cell using a special antigen. Different existing radionuclides emit particle radiation, including α, β, and Auger emission, and deposit a significant quantity of their radiation energy within the malignancy mass for the purpose of treatment. The selection of the most favorable radionuclide for use in RIT is dictated by its effectiveness and by practical considerations related to its specific treatment applications [9].

The number of ionizations per track stated as linear energy transfer (LET) is an important property expressing the power of ionization particles. The benefits of high LET radiation include (1) causes more molecular damage per path-length unit, (2) the high capability to make hypoxic cells, (3) have a high therapeutic index (i.e., the maximum damage is caused to target tissue versus the minimum adverse effects in surrounding or healthy tissues), (4) more quickly attenuation as well as making shielding more impressive and preventing deep penetration, and (5) being fewer differences between radiation sensitivity when compared to the normal cell cycle [18].

Three radioactive emissions have been applied in RIT: β or electron particles, with a wide range of tumor applications and lower toxicity; α particles (i.e., with helium nuclei), with a low range but high toxicity; and Auger electrons, with a low range and high toxicity (but only when produced in the cell, ideally adjacent to the nucleus). Until now, β emitters have been applied most extensively in RIT. They have significant practical

benefits, such as good accessibility and cost-effectiveness. Attachment to the proteins of β particles under good physiological conditions is ideal due to the good chemistry between them. Their physical half-lives make their distribution from a production center convenient. Conventionally, the β particles used in RIT therapies (e.g., iodine-131 (^{131}I), yttrium-90 (^{90}Y), rhenium-188 (^{188}Re), rhenium-186 (^{186}Re), lutetium-177 (^{177}Lu), and copper-67 (^{67}Cu)) produce low LET radiation, with almost identical features (Table 13.1). β particles have different radiation levels between 30 keV and 2.3 MeV energies, with length paths of between 0.5 and 12 mm in the tissue, in the form of β^- particles, internal conversion electrons, and X or Gamma rays. These sparse ionization radiations are scattered throughout an extensive region of the body and release energies in nontargeted and surrounding cells (known as the "crossfire effect") [11]. So β particles cannot be used to treat leukemias, single-cell metastatic diseases, or dispersive diseases [19]. These particles are instead the most popular radionuclides for use in the treatment of bulky diseases and in the case of hematopoietic stem cell transplantation [20].

The α-particle emitters, as high LET radionuclides, are an appropriate option in the treatment of small-volume malignancies or minimal residual leukemia [20]. These emitters (e.g., asta-

Table 13.1 Therapeutic features of radionuclides used in RIT

Radionuclide	E_{max} (MeV)	$T_{1/2}$	Mean range (mm)
Alpha emitter			
^{211}At	8.87	7.21 h	0.04–0.1
^{225}Ac	5.83	9.92 day	0.04–0.1
^{213}Bi	5.87	45.59 min	0.04–0.1
Auger electron emitter			
^{125}I	0.35	60.1 day	0.001–0.02
^{123}I	0.16	13.2 h	0.001–0.02
^{195m}Pt	0.13	4.0 day	0.001–0.02
Beta emitter			
^{131}I	0.8	80.02 day	0.4
^{67}Cu	0.57	2.6 day	0.6
^{90}Y	2.3	2.67 day	2.76
^{177}Lu	0.5	6.65 day	0.28
^{186}Re	1.1	3.72 day	0.92
^{188}Re	2.1	17.01 h	2.43

tine-211 (^{211}At), actinium-225 (^{225}Ac), and bismuth-213 (^{213}Bi)) move in a short path (40–100 µm) with a restricted crossfire effect, and they deposit high-energy particles (4–9 MeV). Moreover, these nuclei can selectively kill single cancer cells with one round of nuclear decay and little damage to neighboring tissues [19, 21].

Auger electron emitters include iodine-123 (^{123}I), gallium-67 (^{67}Ga), iodine-125 (^{125}I), and platinum-195 (^{195m}Pt), and these recently emerged in RIT. Due to the generally accepted supposition of their extreme cytotoxicity, the efficacy of these emitters is limited, based on the prerequisite emissions particles that occur within the cell nucleus. Despite the evident limitation, researchers have demonstrated that Auger emitters have a potentially crucial role as therapeutics, even if only in situations in which microscopic residual disease must be irradiated [22, 23].

Finally, Auger electron-emitting radionuclides and α-particles are preferred in RIT because of their high potency and lower toxicity to nontarget healthy tissues, such as bone marrow. The short length path in this emitter makes it a treatment option for individual cells, such as in the treatment of leukemia and small-volume malignancies; β emitters, with their longer range, are more often applied in the treatment of tumor masses of a greater volume [24]. Moreover, Auger electrons are utilized in the treatment of B-cell lymphomas and AML. Examples of molecular targets of Auger electrons include EGFR and HER2. Many preclinical and clinical evaluations have been done with different antibodies labeled with emission nuclides.

Further development in RIT requires the use of quantitative procedures to determine the absorbed dose of radiation in tumorous and healthy tissue. To achieve this, the theranostics approach has emerged in RIT. In this approach, one radionuclide is used both for diagnostic goals (at low quantities) and therapeutic goals (at high quantities). Nuclear imaging approaches implement a theranostics technique, especially in recently developed high-resolution devices such as positron emission tomography (PET) and PET/computerized tomography (CT) imaging for precise dosimetry and the definition of staging information for improving treatment planning.

13.5 Molecular Pharmacology in RIT

The molecular pharmacology of antigens and antibodies is dependent on their biodistribution in physiological spaces after drug injection. "Pharmacodynamics" and "pharmacokinetics" are two important terms in this area. "Pharmacokinetics" is defined as the study of the period of drug absorption, spreading, metabolism, and excretion. The primary goals of clinical pharmacokinetics include enhancing treatment results and minimizing the toxicity of drug therapies for individual patients. In this subject, a mathematical model characterizes the immunokinetics of complex radioactive antibody targeting, allowing for a determination and explanation of the therapeutic index or the absorbed radiation dose for malignant tissue. This modeling scheme leads to the optimization of the therapeutic index of RIT for each condition. For example, in one study done using [^{131}I]I-3F8 mAb injected intrathecally into the cerebrospinal fluid (CSF) for leptomeningeal and parenchymal metastases in neuroblastoma patients, researchers examined every parameter that could affect the RIT, using two-compartment models and comparing them to one-compartment models. This pharmacokinetic modeling showed that the therapeutic ratio is significantly influenced by immunoreactivity affinity and the optimal programming of antibody injections, while the effects of specific activities and half-life are much lower [25].

"Pharmacodynamics" is defined as the relationship between drug concentration at the site of action and the subsequent effects that occur. The effect of a drug at the site of action is determined by that drug's binding with a receptor. In RIT, in contrast with immunotherapy, the therapeutic goal is realized with regard to the radiation effects of the radioactive substance and not just the antigen-antibody targeting. As such, the antibody plays a tracer role in radioactive material.

13.6 Estimation of Deposited Radiation in Tumors and Normal Tissue with RIT

"Dosimetry" is defined as a calculation and measurement of the ionization radiation dose. Biological effects on tissues are caused by the release of energy through radioactive nuclide decay. In RIT, the two types of radiation, high and low LET, have a different relative biological effectiveness (RBE). Dosimetry is a vital function in RIT for the correlation of absorbed dose to clinical results, for treatment planning for individual patients, and for the prediction of dose distribution and treatment for moderate toxicity. The doses calculated for use in RIT are less accurate than those calculated for use in EBRT because of the relative uncertainty related to dose computation, inhomogeneous dose distributions, limited dose input data, and the calculation procedures used to estimate RIT doses [26, 27]. Internal radiation doses are calculated using mathematical equations that convert the deposited energy in tissue to radiation-absorbed units, including radiation-absorbed dose (RAD) and centigray (cGy). Generally, radiation treatment is accompanied by unwanted radiation to critical organs; the dose is limited to the level that can be withstood by these organs. The optimization of RIT is dependent on anticipation of the radiation dose distributions in both the target tissues and critical organs. Through the utilization of quantities, radionuclide imaging in patients provides the necessary data.

Over time, with continued advancements in human RIT, quantitative procedures have been developed to estimate the absorbed dose, caused by released radiation, for normal and tumor tissues; this estimate has been used in designing individualized treatment plans for patients to avoid the toxicity, especially in high radiation exposure situations. In the situation of specific molecular targeting, probes (such as antibodies) are applied and labeled with diagnostic or killer isotopes (i.e., low and high doses, respectively) in nuclear medicine; these probes suggest the most beneficial devices to use in theranostic medicine.

Due to its quantitative nature, PET imaging has been recommended as an optimal device for theranostics imaging to compute the RAD of normal and tumorous tissues [28]. These procedures facilitate greater precision in medical treatment. Precision medicine is an emerging approach in which patients are treated based on individual variabilities. Using this modality, physicians can more accurately predict the proper treatment strategies to use [29, 30]. The most fundamental information needed for the purpose of dose estimation calculation in RIT is the volume of the region of interest (e.g., tumors and normal organs), the cumulative radioactivity absorbed by special organs, and the pharmacokinetics of the administered radionuclides. The necessary data is collected by PET, gamma camera imaging or SPECT scans, and renal excretion.

Furthermore, because radioimmunoconjugate animal studies provide almost identical dose biodistribution to human biodistribution, animal models have commonly been used in this research. Normal absorbed doses have been considered to range between 0.2 and 2.2 mGy/MBq, with notable interpatient variation in most clinical studies [31]. All dose biodistribution calculations in nuclear medicine have been done according to the specifications of the Committee on Medical Internal Radiation Dosimetry (MIRD). In their technique, a phantom-validated method has been developed that is appropriate and enforceable for normal organs. This procedure has been accepted by the Food and Drug Administration (FDA) as a foundation for estimating and assessing radiation doses for all normal organs [9]. Organs are comprised of multiple types of cells and tissues, so currently, microdosimetry is being applied to develop more accurate dose estimation calculations. Radiobiologists emphasize that the tumor response is dependent on the total absorbed doses and the sensitivity of the tumor tissue [3].

13.7 Clinical Application

13.7.1 Hematological Cancers

RIT is an acceptable and eminent treatment method for hematological malignancies (including lymphoma, leukemia, and multiple myeloma). High-level cell-surface-associated antigens of these tumors are not available for other cells; furthermore, there are many accessible antibodies to these types of malignancies. The most favorable outcomes are observed when treating lymphomas with RIT, as treating solid tumors with RIT is associated with high radiosensitivity, a susceptibility to antibody-induced apoptosis and low-dose rate radiation, and, in some situations, the potential for unwanted immune mechanisms [31]. Total body external radiation therapy for hematological malignancies (especially the spread of NHL) causes critical toxicity and bone marrow suppression; as such, in acute situations, stem cell transplant must be conducted. The development of RIT for these tumors can allow for tumor cells to be specifically targeted while normal tissues, such as bone marrow, are spared. In this method, dose fractionation can be used to increase dose administration after the recovery of bone marrow, according to the intervals between the treatment sessions.

Many preclinical and clinical research has been done about antibodies in different types of lymphomas. So far, as a result of these clinical trials, just two RIT products have been approved by the FDA, both of which are murine anti-CD20 mAbs that are conjugated with yttrium-90 and/or iodine-131, as [^{90}Y]Y-ibritumomab tiuxetan (Zevalin) and [^{131}I]I-tositumomab (Bexxar), respectively [32]. [^{131}I]I-tositumomab is a theranostics radioimmunoconjugate because of the role of iodine-131 in imaging and therapy applications. Some RIT methods have confirmed promising findings in specific clinical settings, especially for small-volume tumors dispersed to bone marrow or at an early minimal residual disease phase [33]. Because of the common characteristics in lymphoma and leukemia, similar treatment choices tend to be implemented in the two diseases. Rituximab and epratuzumab, human-specific versions of anti-CD22 and lumiliximab, are under development in chronic lymphocytic leukemia (CLL). Other treatments for leukemia include therapy with α and β emitters as an option to treat residual diseases, along with other standard therapies, including chemotherapy and whole-body irradiation in EBRT.

The occurrence of myelodysplasia and late second malignancies related to RIT in patients with hematological malignancy treated by [^{90}Y]Y-ibritumomab tiuxetan or [^{131}I]I-tositumomab has been reported as 2.5% and 3.5%, respectively [34, 35]. In spite of the benefits of the RIT method, the medical community faces a number of limitations in adopting this therapeutic approach, including concerns regarding the possibility of myelodysplasia and unexpected side effects, the availability of multiple novel competing targeted agents (e.g., brentuximab vedotin, idelalisib, and ibrutinib), the complexity and difficulty of referring patients to other clinical departments, and problems associated with coordination between hematologists and oncologists to administer the necessary elements in their respective offices. So notwithstanding the many studies touting the efficacy and safety of RIT for lymphomas and the existence of two FDA-approved radiopharmaceuticals, this treatment approach seems to be used less frequently than do other nonradioactive treatments, such as chemotherapy [36]. The question of whether future technology and developments (such as α emitters, pretargeting, and antibody-drug conjugates) will adequately overcome these practical restrictions remains uncertain. In this regard, preclinical and clinical studies have recommended that some chemotherapy drugs be combined with RIT; the results of these studies showed great advantages from combining the two techniques. For example, one substitute method is using veltuzumab (anti-CD20) combined with [^{90}Y]Y-epratuzumab tetraxetan (anti-CD22) [37]. Examples such as this show that the incorporation of RIT into the preferred therapy for treating NHL (i.e., chemotherapy) produces stable and positive results, with median remission duration of more than 6 years in many cases (Fig. 13.2).

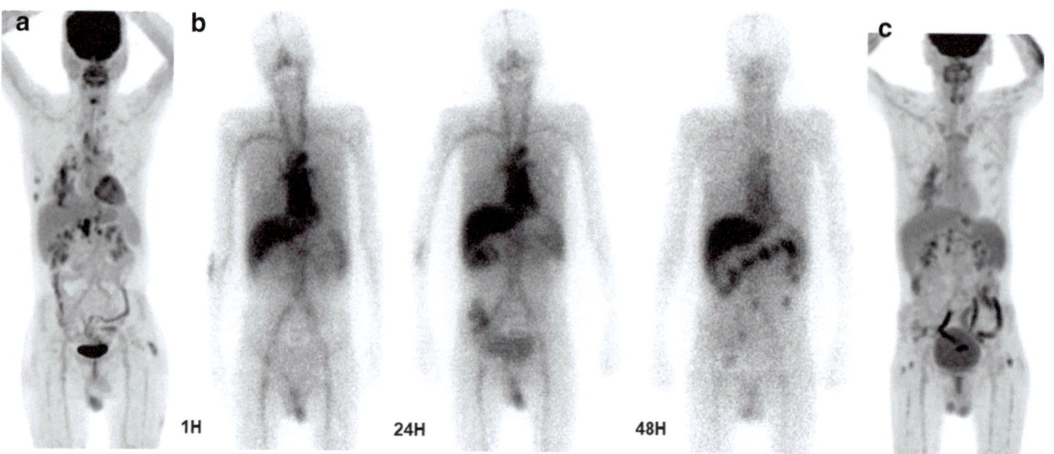

Fig. 13.2 Follicular lymphoma in a 63-year-old patient with relapsing disease after four previous regimens. He was treated with [177Lu]Lu-DOTA-rituximab. (**a**) 2-[18F] FDG PET shows multiple hypermetabolic tumoral residues especially in the lung. (**b**) Lutetium-177 scintigram up to 2 days after [177Lu]Lu-DOTA-rituximab depicts distribution of lutetium-177 throughout the body. (**c**) Repeated 2-[18F]FDG PET about 1 month after radioimmunotherapy shows partial response

13.7.2 Non-hematological (Solid) Cancers

Solid tumors are mostly radioresistant and need more irradiation and deposited radiation energy for complete tumor response when compared with leukemias and lymphomas. The success rate in using RIT in the treatment of solid tumors is lower than it is in treating hematological cancers. Clinical RIT trials in patients with solid tumors have involved a wide variety of cancers, including prostate, colorectal, renal, brain, head and neck, and breast. Improvements in disease-associated markers of prostate cancer have been reported in clinical trials of castration-resistant prostate cancers. For example, the use of RIT with [177Lu]Lu-J591 leads to a decrease and stabilization in the prostate-specific antigen (PSA) level. Moreover, pain relief and reduction in tumor size have been seen in phase II metastatic prostate cancer with [131I]I-CC49 [38–40].

In 2001, Meredith et al. examined the possibility of combining the radiolabeled mAb, [177Lu] Lu-CC49, with chemotherapy and observed that this new modality was well tolerated in this patient groups when using bone marrow suppression as the dose-limiting toxicity [41]. Some studies have reported the application of RIT in breast cancer with various antibodies; in these studies, the role of HER2 has been remarkable [42, 43]. Although primary colorectal cancers are usually removed surgically, in metastatic stages, surgical interventions can lead to a poor prognosis. Recently, RIT has been used with other adjuvant therapies, but promising and practical results have not yet been observed. As such, more research in the area of colorectal cancer is required [44, 45]. Also, RIT with [90Y]Y-biotin and [131I]I-α-tenascin antibodies have shown improvements in the treatment of brain tumors, especially when used in combination with chemotherapy drugs [46–48]. However, certain kinds of radiation-resistant tissues, such as the bronchial epithelium or brain tissues, cause intense resistance to radiation. In solid malignancies, tumor contraction, with a positive effect on survival rates, has been observed when the conjugated radionuclide is injected directly into the part of the body in which tumors are restricted.

In particular, there are three techniques currently being studied for increasing the therapeutic index in solid tumors that show positive results in preclinical studies: the combination of chemotherapy and RIT modalities, pretargeted radioimmunotherapy (PRIT), and the utilization of appropriate radionuclides with suitable emissions, particularly α emitters [9].

13.8 PRIT

Conventional RIT has been tested at preclinical and clinical levels with the intravenous injection of radiolabeled antibodies. The main complicating issue is that radionuclide-antibody conjugates are highly stable in blood circulation, and consequently, everywhere the antibody is diffused, the radionuclide follows. In addition, a radionuclide that is separated from the antibody has insufferable and undesirable properties.

The efficiency of RIT is limited in cases of large solid tumors (except in the case of NHL, due to its radiosensitivity and according to need for a low absorbed dose for a complete response). One of the important challenges in treating large tumors with RIT is that the mAb molecule must pass a long path for the destruction of cancer cells and, after more, the physiological obstacles such as pharmacokinetics and solubility of radiotracers which prohibit the quick biodistribution of an antibody within the tumor. After reaching the tumor, the antibody molecule requires a high binding affinity for attaching the tumor strongly; on the other hand, it also requires a low binding affinity to keep it from penetrating the tumor too deeply [32]. Finally, in general, a trivial fraction of the injected radioactive material will localize to the tumor, showing a modest response amount.

The most favorable tumor targeting requires a high tumor uptake and a low upkeep time of radioactivity in healthy tissues. A new method that can help to solve this issue is the pretargeting technique. Briefly, the theory of PRIT includes the separating of the transference of tumor-individual antibody from the delivery of the radioactive nuclide. In other words, tumors in the PRIT method are targeted through a large amount of bispecific non-radiolabeled mAb. After the distribution of antibody throughout the whole body, the mAb binds to the specific antigen on the tumor cells and is cleared from other tissues through blood flow. In the next step, exactly at the time of highest absorbance of the antibody into tumor cell and the minimum amount of absorbance in other tissues, a small radioactive molecule is injected, which is identified by the bispecific antibody; finally, the unbound radiolabeled compound quickly binds to pre-localized antibody and cumulates in the tumor or excretes rapidly through the blood flow [49].

PRIT has been developed as a technique that decreases toxicity while augmenting the therapeutic index when compared to the direct injection of radiolabeled antibody, especially in situations in which there are several macroscopic tumor targets that are larger than 3–4 cm in diameter without hematological toxicities. PRIT was developed over the past 20 years and includes four distinct approaches that feature (1) avidin or streptavidin (StAv) used for targeting radiolabeled biotin (avidin-biotin and StAv-biotin), (2) bispecific monoclonal antibodies (bsMAb) with radiolabeled haptens, (3) antibody-oligonucleotide conjugates for aiming at radiolabeled supplementary oligonucleotides, and (4) antibody-directed enzyme prodrug therapy [46, 50]. Recently, in addition to solid tumors, pilot PRIT clinical trials have been conducted in patients with lymphoma [51, 52]. In human PRIT studies, normal tissues are almost always affected, resulting in a suboptimal therapeutic index (i.e., tumor-to-healthy ratio), so the method must be used carefully. To evaluate the technique, the imaging and dosimetry of healthy tissues are done at the same time as treatment (e.g., the use of the theranostics approach).

Table 13.2 summarizes some examples of outlined radioimmunoconjugates evaluated in clinical trials up to 2019.

13.9 Concluding Remarks and Future Prospects

RIT individuality targets and delivers radionuclides—emitting α particles, β particles, or Auger electrons—to malignant tissues, using labeled monoclonal antibodies that identify disease- or tumor-associated receptors (i.e., antigens). The efficacy of RIT depends on a number of factors, including the properties of the tumor (such as

Table 13.2 Examples of the outlined radioimmunoconjugates in clinical trials (up to 2019)

Antigen target	Radioimmunoconjugates	Disease	Clinical trials status
CD20	[^{90}Y]Y-ibritumomab tiuxetan (Zevalin) [53, 54]	NHL	FDA approved
	[^{131}I]I-tositumomab (Bexxar) [55–57]		FDA approved
	[^{90}Y]Y-DOTA [52]		Phase II
DNA	[^{131}I]I-chTNT-1/B (Cotara)	Glioblastoma multiform and anaplastic astrocytoma	Phase II
PSMA	[^{177}Lu]Lu-J591 [58]	mCRPC	Phase II
TROP-2	[^{177}Lu]Lu-IMP288		Phase II
CEA	[^{111}In]In-Labetuzumab (CEA-Cide)	Colorectal, breast, lung, pancreatic, and stomach carcinoma	
CD22	[^{90}Y]Y-epratuzumab (Lymphocide) [59]	NHL	Phase II
HER2	[^{89}Zr]Zr-trastuzumab [60]	Breast	Phase I/II
G250	[^{131}I]I-cG250 [61]	Renal cell carcinoma	Phase I/II
HLA-DR10 (Oncolym)	[^{131}I]I-Lym-1	NHL and CLL	Phase I
PEM	[^{90}Y]Y-Pemtumomab (Theragyn)	Ovarian and primary peritoneal cavity cancer	Phase III

CD cluster of differentiation, *NHL* non-Hodgkin lymphoma, *FDA* Food and Drug Administration, *PSMA* prostate-specific membrane antigen, *TROP-2* tumor-associated calcium signal transducer 2, *mCRPC* metastatic castration-resistant prostate cancer, *CEA* carcinoembryonic antigen, *HER2* human epidermal growth factor receptor 2, *HLA* human leukocyte antigen, *CLL* chronic lymphocytic leukemia, *PEM* Pemetrexed

blood circulation, vascularity, and permeability), the features of the targeted antigen (such as rate of accumulation, accessibility, shedding, and heterogeneity of appearance), and the mAb (such as affinity, avidity, specificity of the binding site, immunoreactivity, and being stable in vivo). One advantage of RIT is its potential ability to target small metastatic damage that has not been detected usual scanning and therefore remains untreated. Currently, nearly all the preclinical models and some new clinical studies of NHL that compare traditional drugs with RIT verify that RIT has more efficiency than chemotherapy. Further, it has been verified that a combination of RIT and chemotherapy is even more beneficial than either procedure performed alone. For solid tumors, a combination of RIT and chemotherapy also shows a better outcome.

In RIT, radiolabeled antibodies are directed against different antigens overexpressed in blood vessels that form during the angiogenesis of tumor cells. Modern RIT procedures and the evolution of novel radioimmunoconjugates have resulted in the development of personalized medicine, mostly in terms of the multimodality strategies for the treatment of poor-prognosis malignancies that are resistant to typical treatments. The application of RIT enhances the opportunity to destroy the primary tumor cells and other subsequent lesions that are caused by systemically metastasizing them. Toxicity in hematological RIT depends on previous treatment and bone marrow involvement. These agents are a dose-limiting index, but in non-hematological malignancies, toxicity is trivial. New reported studies have evaluated RIT procedures and revealed new implications for resistant and aggressive tumors through molecular imaging and medicine, especially PET molecular imaging (immune-PET) with a theranostics approach.

To summarize the previous section, more effort has been given to increase the remaining radionuclides at the target cells and augment their cytotoxicity. Some of this clinical research into RIT relates to dose fractionation (i.e., dose administration in multiple treatment sessions), multivalences (i.e., retaining the radionuclide for longer periods in the radiosensitive external parts of the tumor), PRIT (i.e., the multistep strategy in

RIT for decreasing nontargeted cells' exposure by separating the tumor-targeting segment from the radioactive ligand), pre-scouting (i.e., the use of the nuclide with special emissions for imaging or the injection of a small amount of radionuclide into patient to confirm the exact site of the tumor and to supply dosimetry data for patient-specific treatment), and reducing kidney uptake. Future studies should investigate the potential combined effect of PRIT with small molecule inhibitors, radiosensitizing an agent's polymerase inhibitors, and the important role of bispecific PRIT in stem cell transplantation. In conclusion, improving the efficacy of PRIT will help make it more available and accessible in comprehensive clinical trials, which can then further evaluate the implementation of bispecific antibody seen in preclinical projects and which will be crucial in the future development and studies conducted in this field.

References

1. Vaidyanathan G, Zalutsky MR. Targeted therapy using alpha emitters. Phys Med Biol. 1996;41(10):1915.
2. Milenic DE, Brady ED, Brechbiel MW. Antibody-targeted radiation cancer therapy. Nat Rev Drug Discov. 2004;3(6):488.
3. Hall EJ, Giaccia AJ. Radiobiology for the radiologist. Philadelphia: Lippincott Williams & Wilkins; 2006.
4. Milenic DE. Radioimmunotherapy: designer molecules to potentiate effective therapy. Semin Radiat Oncol. 2000;10:139–55.
5. Köhler G, Milstein C. Continuous cultures of fused cells secreting antibody of predefined specificity. Nature. 1975;256(5517):495.
6. Buras RR, Wong JY, Kuhn JA, Beatty BG, Williams LE, Wanek PM, et al. Comparison of radioimmunotherapy and external beam radiotherapy in colon cancer xenografts. Int J Radiat Oncol Biol Phys. 1993;25(3):473–9.
7. Kawashima H. Radioimmunotherapy: a specific treatment protocol for cancer by cytotoxic radioisotopes conjugated to antibodies. ScientificWorldJournal. 2014;2014:492061.
8. Green DJ, Press OW. Whither radioimmunotherapy: To be or not to be? Cancer Res. 2017;77:2191–6.
9. Larson SM, Carrasquillo JA, Cheung N-KV, Press OW. Radioimmunotherapy of human tumours. Nat Rev Cancer. 2015;15(6):347.
10. Dearling J, Pedley R. Technological advances in radioimmunotherapy. Clin Oncol. 2007;19(6):457–69.
11. Martins CD, Kramer-Marek G, Oyen WJ. Radioimmunotherapy for delivery of cytotoxic radioisotopes: current status and challenges. Expert Opin Drug Deliv. 2018;15(2):185–96.
12. Kizhedath A, Wilkinson S, Glassey J. Applicability of predictive toxicology methods for monoclonal antibody therapeutics: status Quo and scope. Arch Toxicol. 2017;91(4):1595–612.
13. Kumar S. Cellular and molecular immunology. Philadelphia: Elsevier; 2014.
14. Irani V, Guy AJ, Andrew D, Beeson JG, Ramsland PA, Richards JS. Molecular properties of human IgG subclasses and their implications for designing therapeutic monoclonal antibodies against infectious diseases. Mol Immunol. 2015;67(2):171–82.
15. Wittrup KD, Thurber GM, Schmidt MM, Rhoden JJ. Practical theoretic guidance for the design of tumor-targeting agents. Methods Enzymol. 2012;503:255–68.
16. Wissler R, Barker P, Flax M, La Via M, Talmage D. A study of the preparation, localization, and effects of antitumor antibodies labeled with I131. Cancer Res. 1956;16(8):761–73.
17. Goldenberg D, Sharkey R. Advances in cancer therapy with radiolabeled monoclonal antibodies. Q J Nucl Med Mol Imaging. 2006;50(4):248.
18. Richter MP, Laramore GE, Griffin TW, Goodman RL. Current status of high linear energy transfer irradiation. Cancer. 1984;54(S2):2814–22.
19. Humm JL. Dosimetric aspects of radiolabeled antibodies for tumor therapy. J Nucl Med. 1986;27(9):1490–7.
20. Amadori S, Stasi R. Monoclonal antibodies and immunoconjugates in acute myeloid leukemia. Best Pract Res Clin Haematol. 2006;19(4):715–36.
21. Jurcic JG, Larson SM, Sgouros G, McDevitt MR, Finn RD, Divgi CR, et al. Targeted α particle immunotherapy for myeloid leukemia. Blood. 2002;100(4):1233–9.
22. Kassis AI, Harapanhalli RS, Adelstein SJ. Comparison of strand breaks in plasmid DNA after positional changes of Auger electron-emitting iodine-125. Radiat Res. 1999;151(2):167–76.
23. Michel RB, Brechbiel MW, Mattes MJ. A comparison of 4 radionuclides conjugated to antibodies for single-cell kill. J Nucl Med. 2003;44(4):632.
24. Larson SM. Choosing the right radionuclide and antibody for intraperitoneal radioimmunotherapy. J Natl Cancer Inst. 1991;83:1602–4.
25. He P, Kramer K, Smith-Jones P, Zanzonico P, Humm J, Larson SM, et al. Two-compartment model of radioimmunotherapy delivered through cerebrospinal fluid. Eur J Nucl Med Mol Imaging. 2011;38(2):334–42.
26. Buchsbaum DJ, Wessels BW. Introduction: radiolabeled antibody tumor dosimetry. Med Phys. 1993;20(2):499–501.
27. Knox SJ, Meredith RF. Clinical radioimmunotherapy. Semin Radiat Oncol. 2000;10:73–93.
28. Yordanova A, Eppard E, Kürpig S, Bundschuh RA, Schönberger S, Gonzalez-Carmona M, et al.

Theranostics in nuclear medicine practice. Onco Targets Ther. 2017;10:4821.

29. Ghasemi M, Nabipour I, Omrani A, Alipour Z, Assadi M. Precision medicine and molecular imaging: new targeted approaches toward cancer therapeutic and diagnosis. Am J Nucl Med Mol Imaging. 2016;6(6):310.

30. Assadi M, Nabipour I. The future of molecular imaging in paradigm shift from reactive to proactive (P4) medicine: predictive, preventive, personalized and participatory. Nucl Med Commun. 2014;35:1193–6.

31. Siegel J, Goldenberg D, Badger C. Radioimmunotherapy dose estimation in patients with B-cell lymphoma. Med Phys. 1993;20(2):579–82.

32. Sharkey RM, Goldenberg DM. Perspectives on cancer therapy with radiolabeled monoclonal antibodies. J Nucl Med. 2005;46(1):115S.

33. Kraeber-Bodéré F, Barbet J, Chatal J-F. Radioimmunotherapy: from current clinical success to future industrial breakthrough? J Nucl Med. 2016;57(3):329–31.

34. Bennett JM, Kaminski MS, Leonard JP, Vose JM, Zelenetz AD, Knox SJ, et al. Assessment of treatment-related myelodysplastic syndromes and acute myeloid leukemia in patients with non-Hodgkin lymphoma treated with tositumomab and iodine I131 tositumomab. Blood. 2005;105(12):4576–82.

35. Czuczman MS, Emmanouilides C, Darif M, Witzig TE, Gordon LI, Revell S, et al. Treatment-related myelodysplastic syndrome and acute myelogenous leukemia in patients treated with ibritumomab tiuxetan radioimmunotherapy. J Clin Oncol. 2007;25(27):4285–92.

36. Schaefer NG, Ma J, Huang P, Buchanan J, Wahl RL. Radioimmunotherapy in non-Hodgkin lymphoma: opinions of US medical oncologists and hematologists. J Nucl Med. 2010;51(6):987.

37. Witzig TE, Tomblyn MB, Misleh JG, Kio EA, Sharkey RM, Wegener WA, et al. Anti-CD22 90Y-epratuzumab tetraxetan combined with anti-CD20 veltuzumab: a phase I study in patients with relapsed/refractory, aggressive non-Hodgkin lymphoma. Haematologica. 2014;99(11):1738–45.

38. Milowsky MI, Nanus DM, Kostakoglu L, Vallabhajosula S, Goldsmith SJ, Bander NH. Phase I trial of yttrium-90—labeled anti—prostate-specific membrane antigen monoclonal antibody J591 for androgen-independent prostate cancer. J Clin Oncol. 2004;22(13):2522–31.

39. Meredith RF, Khazaeli M, Macey DJ, Grizzle WE, Mayo M, Schlom J, et al. Phase II study of interferon-enhanced 131I-labeled high affinity CC49 monoclonal antibody therapy in patients with metastatic prostate cancer. Clin Cancer Res. 1999;5(10):3254s–8s.

40. Khan A, Shergill I, Arya M, Barua JM, Kaisary AV. Radioimmunotherapy and prostate cancer: a promising new therapy in the management of metastatic disease. BJU Int. 2006;98(1):8–9.

41. Meredith RF, Alvarez RD, Partridge EE, Khazaeli M, Lin C-Y, Macey DJ, et al. Intraperitoneal radioimmunochemotherapy of ovarian cancer: a phase I study. Cancer Biother Radiopharm. 2001;16(4):305–15.

42. Wong J, Somlo G, Odom-Maryon T, Williams L, Liu A, Yamauchi D, et al. Initial results of a phase I trial evaluating 90yttrium (90Y)-chimeric T84. 66 (cT84. 66) anti-CEA antibody and autologous stem cell support in CEA-producing metastatic breast cancer. Cancer Biother Radiopharm. 1998;13:314.

43. Brechbiel MW, Waldmann TA. Anti-HER2 radioimmunotherapy. Breast Dis. 1999;11(1):125–32.

44. Wong JY, Shibata S, Williams LE, Kwok CS, Liu A, Chu DZ, et al. A phase I trial of 90Y-anti-carcinoembryonic antigen chimeric T84. 66 radioimmunotherapy with 5-fluorouracil in patients with metastatic colorectal cancer. Clin Cancer Res. 2003;9(16):5842–52.

45. Buchegger F, Gillet M, Doenz F, Vogel C, Achtari C, Mach J, et al. Biodistribution of anti-CEA F (ab′) 2 fragments after intra-arterial and intravenous injection in patients with liver metastases due to colorectal carcinoma. Nucl Med Commun. 1996;17(6):500–3.

46. Paganelli G, Bartolomei M, Ferrari M, Cremonesi M, Broggi G, Maira G, et al. Pre-targeted locoregional radioimmunotherapy with 90Y-biotin in glioma patients: phase I study and preliminary therapeutic results. Cancer Biother Radiopharm. 2001;16(3):227–35.

47. Riva P, Arista A, Franceschi G, Frattarelli M, Sturiale C, Riva N, et al. Local treatment of malignant gliomas by direct infusion of specific monoclonal antibodies labeled with 131I: comparison of the results obtained in recurrent and newly diagnosed tumors. Cancer Res. 1995;55(23 Suppl):5952s–6s.

48. Kalofonos H, Pawlikowska T, Hemingway A, Courtenay-Luck N, Dhokia B, Snook D, et al. Antibody guided diagnosis and therapy of brain gliomas using radiolabeled monoclonal antibodies against epidermal growth factor receptor and placental alkaline phosphatase. J Nucl Med. 1989;30(10):1636.

49. Frampas E, Rousseau C, Bodet-Milin C, Barbet J, Chatal J-F, Kraeber-Bodéré F. Improvement of radioimmunotherapy using pretargeting. Front Oncol. 2013;3:159.

50. Reilly RM. Monoclonal antibody and peptide-targeted radiotherapy of cancer. Hoboken, NJ: John Wiley & Sons; 2010.

51. Walter RB, Press OW, Pagel JM. Pretargeted radioimmunotherapy for hematologic and other malignancies. Cancer Biother Radiopharm. 2010;25(2):125–42.

52. Forero A, Weiden PL, Vose JM, Knox SJ, LoBuglio AF, Hankins J, et al. Phase 1 trial of a novel anti-CD20 fusion protein in pretargeted radioimmunotherapy for B-cell non-Hodgkin lymphoma. Blood. 2004;104(1):227–36.

53. Witzig TE, Flinn IW, Gordon LI, Emmanouilides C, Czuczman MS, Saleh MN, et al. Treatment with ibritumomab tiuxetan radioimmunotherapy in patients with rituximab-refractory follicular non-Hodgkin's lymphoma. J Clin Oncol. 2002;20(15):3262–9.

54. Witzig TE, Gordon LI, Cabanillas F, Czuczman MS, Emmanouilides C, Joyce R, et al. Randomized controlled trial of yttrium-90–labeled ibritumomab tiuxetan radioimmunotherapy versus rituximab immunotherapy for patients with relapsed or refractory low-grade, follicular, or transformed B-cell non-Hodgkin's lymphoma. J Clin Oncol. 2002;20(10):2453–63.
55. Kaminski MS, Zelenetz AD, Press OW, Saleh M, Leonard J, Fehrenbacher L, et al. Pivotal study of iodine I 131 tositumomab for chemotherapy-refractory low-grade or transformed low-grade B-cell non-Hodgkin's lymphomas. J Clin Oncol. 2001;19(19):3918–28.
56. Kaminski MS, Zasadny KR, Francis IR, Milik AW, Ross CW, Moon SD, et al. Radioimmunotherapy of B-cell lymphoma with [131I] anti-B1 (anti-CD20) antibody. N Engl J Med. 1993;329(7):459–65.
57. Horning SJ, Younes A, Jain V, Kroll S, Lucas J, Podoloff D, et al. Efficacy and safety of tositumomab and iodine-131 tositumomab (Bexxar) in B-cell lymphoma, progressive after rituximab. J Clin Oncol. 2005;23(4):712–9.
58. Simone CB, Hahn SM. What's in a label? Radioimmunotherapy for metastatic prostate cancer. Clin Cancer Res. 2013;19(18):4908–10.
59. Morschhauser F, Kraeber-Bodéré F, Wegener WA, Harousseau J-L, Petillon M-O, Huglo D, et al. High rates of durable responses with anti-CD22 fractionated radioimmunotherapy: results of a multicenter, phase I/II study in non-Hodgkin's lymphoma. J Clin Oncol. 2010;28(23):3709–16.
60. Chatal J-F. Theranostic radioimmunotherapy (RIT) combined with immunotherapy: the best way to go? Med Res Innov. 2017;1:4.
61. Brouwers AH, Buijs WC, Mulders PF, de Mulder PH, van den Broek WJ, Mala C, et al. Radioimmunotherapy with [131I] cG250 in patients with metastasized renal cell cancer: dosimetric analysis and immunologic response. Clin Cancer Res. 2005;11(19):7178s–86s.

Radiolabeled Antibodies for Cancer Radioimmunotherapy

14

Julie Rousseau, Joseph Lau, and François Bénard

Contents

J. Rousseau · J. Lau
Department of Molecular Oncology, BC Cancer
Research Institute, Vancouver, BC, Canada
e-mail: jrousseau@bccrc.ca; jlau@bccrc.ca

F. Bénard (✉)
Department of Molecular Oncology, BC Cancer
Research Institute, Vancouver, BC, Canada

Department of Radiology, University of British
Columbia, Vancouver, BC, Canada
e-mail: fbenard@bccrc.ca

14.1   Introduction

Monoclonal antibodies (mAb) are molecules that have been widely investigated for cancer diagnosis and treatment because they can target antigens with high affinity and specificity. This targeting property results in less toxicity than with conventional chemotherapy. The advent of hybridoma technology by Köhler and Milstein in 1975 was a major impetus for antibody-based therapeutics [1], by allowing the production of an unlimited range of mAb targeting different antigens including known and new cancer targets. mAbs and their derivatives are a rapidly expanding group of

© Springer Nature Switzerland AG 2022
S. Harsini et al. (eds.), *Nuclear Medicine and Immunology*,
https://doi.org/10.1007/978-3-030-81261-4_14

anticancer drugs and are considered as one of the most successful strategies for improving patient outcomes [2]. The therapeutic strategies using mAb include naked functional antibodies, bispecific antibodies, engineered antibody constructs, antibody-drug conjugates, and radiolabeled antibodies [3].

Radiolabeled antibodies have been used for cancer imaging and therapy for decades. In 1978, Goldenberg et al. radiolabeled polyclonal antibodies targeting carcinoembryonic antigen (CEA) with iodine-131 (^{131}I) for immunoscintigraphy [4]. In 1981, the use of a radiolabeled monoclonal antibody (mAb) was reported by Mach et al. [5]. This marked the beginning of cancer imaging and radioimmunotherapy (RIT). Antibodies were radiolabeled with iodine-131, a radionuclide already used in clinical practice for imaging and treatment of differentiated thyroid carcinomas [6]. This led to the development of radioimmunoconjugates such as [^{131}I]I-Tositumomab, a ^{131}I-labeled mouse mAb targeting CD20. [^{131}I]I-Tositumomab was approved for RIT of patients with non-Hodgkin's lymphoma (NHL) [7]. However, these labeled mAb were met with challenges. First, images showed poor contrast due to the physical gamma emission of iodine-131. Some did not show any significant signal due to the rapid release of the radionuclide, which escapes from cancer cells after the internalization of the target-antibody complex [8, 9]. Human anti-mouse antibody responses [10] and rare allergic reactions with murine mAb [11] were observed with some products. ProstaScint for imaging of prostate-specific membrane antigen (PSMA) had moderate success despite the poor choice of intracellular epitope [12–14]. Finally, the emergence of positron emission tomography (PET) and 2-[^{18}F]fluoro-2-deoxy-D-glucose ([^{18}F]FDG) imaging replaced interest in conventional nuclear medicine approaches.

Many approaches have been used to overcome these issues. Metallic radionuclides which are trapped inside cells after internalization and with more suitable physical properties for imaging were proposed as an alternative to iodine isotopes [15]. As an example, indium-111 (^{111}In) showed superiority over iodine-131 for cancer detection [16]. For RIT, additional radionuclides were also identified. The anti-CD20 Ibritumomab tiuxetan labeled with yttrium-90 (^{90}Y) became the standard for RIT in NHL [17]. The concern of immunogenicity was addressed by the introduction of chimeric, humanized, and human antibodies [18]. Finally, mAb are now labeled with metallic PET isotopes [19] such as zirconium-89 (^{89}Zr) that yield high-resolution images [20].

In addition to the adoption of alternative radionuclides, other developments have also revived the interest in using antibodies or antibody derivatives for cancer diagnosis and RIT. Highly potent antibodies were developed and validated for immunotherapy and antibody-drug conjugates (ADC), offering new opportunities to develop imaging and/or RIT agents [21]. The number of identified targets has increased over the past decade in large part of next-generation sequencing and bioinformatics [2, 22]. New strategies also emerged to increase the safety and efficacy of radioimmunoconjugates [23]. Finally, the use of PET imaging enables patient management prior to and during treatment for RIT and other mAb-based therapeutic strategies [20].

This chapter provides an overview of target selection, mAb structure, and properties in addition to conjugation/radiolabeling strategies for the development of radioimmunoconjugates. The principle of RIT, main achievements, and new investigations in hematological malignancies and solid tumors are presented. Finally, we offer our perspectives for the further improvement of RIT.

14.2 Development of Efficient Radioimmunoconjugates

The efficacy of radioimmunoconjugates for RIT lies in the ability to maximize the delivery of a radionuclide to tumor lesions while sparing normal tissues. The selection of a mAb with high specificity and affinity is not the sole determinant of accumulation in lesions [24]. The identification of a valid target and the selection of a radionuclide and labeling strategy dictate the safety and effectiveness of the radioimmunoconjugate (Fig. 14.1). Each of these different parameters will be described in the following sections.

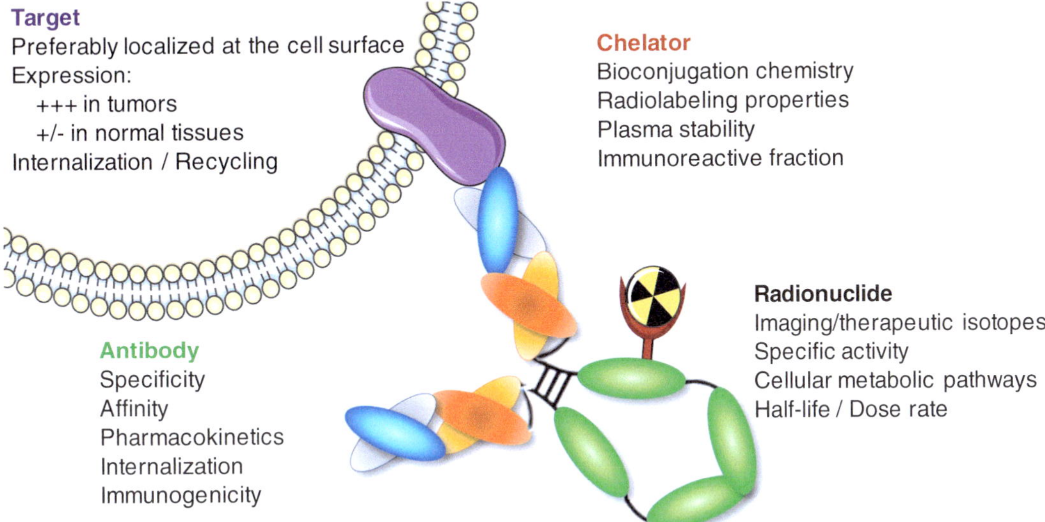

Fig. 14.1 Components that influence the safety and efficacy of radiolabeled mAb. Identification of a target expressed by cancer cells, selection of a mAb, and the use of an adequate radiolabeling strategy are the key parameters for the development and optimization of radioimmunoconjugates (some graphical elements were adapted from Servier Medical Art (www.servier.com))

14.2.1 Target Selection

The first step in the development of radiolabeled mAb is to identify a biological target. The target should be exclusively expressed or overexpressed by tumor cells with minimal expression in healthy tissues. The antigen is preferably localized at the cell surface with an extracellular domain that is accessible for mAb binding. Although an extracellular epitope for binding is preferred, successful targeting of intracellular antigens with mAb has been reported [25]. In a preclinical study, the addition of a cell-penetrating peptide to a radiolabeled mAb allowed targeting of the phosphorylated H2A histone family member X (γH2AX) for PET imaging [26]. Regardless of the target localization, the existence of a secreted form of the target is disadvantageous as this can compete for binding.

The minimum number of targets per cell that is needed to allow efficient therapeutic response is unclear. For ADC, 10^4–10^6 copies/cells were reported as the minimum threshold for different targets [27]. For radiolabeled mAb, Wu proposed that 0.5–1×10^5 copies/cells is a more realistic

range [28]. Higher target expression is favored; however, discordances between target protein expression and mAb accumulation in tumors have been observed [29]. Due to the long biological half-life ($t_{1/2}$) of mAbs (1–3 weeks), the endosomal recycling of the target back to the plasma membrane after internalization of the target-mAb complex offers the possibility for increased binding events enhancing tumor irradiation dose.

The most studied targets are cell membrane receptors involved in signal transduction like the human epidermal growth factor receptor 2 (HER2) in breast cancers; the epidermal growth factor receptor (EGFR) in colorectal, lung, and head and neck cancers; the PSMA in prostate cancers; and the cluster of differentiation (CD) antigens, e.g., CD20 in NHL and chronic lymphocytic leukemia or CD33 in acute myeloid leukemia (AML). Other strategies target proteins involved in the tumor microenvironment such as blood vessel components like the vascular endothelial growth factor A (VEGF-A) in breast, lung, renal, cervical, ovarian, and colorectal cancers, gliomas, and neuroendocrine tumors or immune checkpoint inhibitors, especially the programmed cell death protein 1 (PD-1) in non-small cell lung cancers and melanomas and its ligand programmed death-ligand 1 (PD-L1) in non-small cell lung cancers, bladder cancers, and triple-negative breast cancers [30, 31]. In 2020, numerous mAbs, approved by the United States Food and Drug Administration (FDA) and/or the European Medicines Agency (EMA), are available for cancer immunotherapy or imaging. Representative examples of these mAbs and their corresponding targets are listed in Table 14.1. This includes radiolabeled mAbs [^{131}I] I-Tositumomab and [^{90}Y]Y-Ibritumomab tiuxetan (both anti-CD20) for the treatment of NHL [35].

The most commonly used method to identify targets is through genomic and proteomic data mining using literature search like PubMed or free online databases such as The Human Protein Atlas. Additional web resources are available and were provided by Nimmagadda et al. [36]. In addition to these tools, mass spectrometry-based quantitative proteomics and phage display-based functional proteomics can also be used [37]. Although, personalized mAb against tumor-specific antigens exclusively expressed by tumor cells can be developed, e.g., by targeting mutations, proteins fusions, or altered glycosylation [38–42], only a small subset of patients would be able to benefit from this strategy [43]. The main targets and emerging targets for RIT are therefore more likely selected based on their overexpression by cancer cells.

14.2.2 Antibody Structure and Pharmacokinetic

The mAb is the backbone for RIT, as it is the delivery vector. The in vivo behavior, safety, and efficacy of mAb are determined by the type of mAb, antigen specificity, binding affinity, immunogenicity, internalization capacity, dose, and route of administration in addition to the tumor physiology [15, 28].

14.2.2.1 Antibody Structure

Among the different antibody isotypes, the immunoglobulins G (IgG) are most commonly used for imaging and RIT. IgG are selected over IgA and IgM for immunotherapy and ADC because of their longer serum $t_{1/2}$ that ensures the maximum accumulation at tumor sites. IgG are large "Y"-shaped proteins (~150 kDa), composed of two pairs of identical heavy chains and light chains bound by disulfide and noncovalent bonds (Fig. 14.2). The IgG structure can be divided into two parts: the fragment antigen-binding (Fab) and the fragment crystallizable (Fc). The Fab consists in the pairing of one constant and one variable domain of each of the heavy and light chain, which is responsible for antigen binding. The Fc corresponds to the two constant domains of the heavy chains [44] and is involved in effector functions by interacting with Fc gamma receptors (FcγR) and proteins of the complement system. It is also responsible for binding to the Fc neonatal receptor (FcRn) [33], which regulates IgG pharmacokinetics. IgG are composed of 4 subclasses: IgG1, IgG2, IgG3, and IgG4. Despite being 90% identical on the amino acid level, they differ by the location and number of the interchain-disulfide bonds, the structure of the constant domains (especially the N-terminal CH2 domain), and the hinge regions which impact their effector functions (i.e., the different subclasses have different affinities for the FcγR, FcRn, and proteins involved in the complement cascade) [45]. Within the four subclasses of IgG, IgG1 is the most abundant in human serum and has a superior ability to engage the immune system; its backbone was therefore preferred to develop therapeutic antibodies [46, 47].

Undesired immune responses were observed with the first generation of therapeutic mouse-derived mAb, resulting in pharmacokinetic, safety, and efficacy issues. Engineered mAb constructs with mouse sequence-derived amino acids replaced by human ones were therefore developed [48]. First, constant regions were replaced to generate constructs called chimeric mAb such as Rituximab (anti-CD20). Additional replacements lead to recombinant humanized mAb where only the complementary determining regions of the variable chains remain mouse sequences, e.g., Trastuzumab (anti-HER2).

Table 14.1 Representative targets and approved mAb currently available for cancer therapy or imaging

Target	Name	Type	Indication	FDA	EMA
Hematologic malignancies					
CD20	Rituximab (Rituxan®, MabThera®)	Chimeric IgG1	NHL and CLL	1997	1998
	^{90}Y-Ibritumomab tiuxetan (Zevalin®)	Murine IgG1 as RIT	NHL	2002	2004
	Tositumomab and ^{131}I-Tositumomab (Bexxar®)	Murine IgG2a as RIT	NHL	2003	N/A
	Ofatumumab (Arzerra®)	Human IgG1	CLL	2009	2010
	Obinutuzumab (Gazyva®)	Humanized IgG1	CLL	2013	2014
CD22	Inotuzumab ozogamicin (Besponsa)	Humanized IgG4/κ as ADC	B-cell ALL	2017	2017
CD30	Brentuximab (Adcetris®)	Chimeric IgG1 as ADC	HL, ALCL	2011	2012
CD33	Gemtuzumab ozogamicin (Mylotarg)	Humanized IgG4 as ADC	AML	2017	2018
CD38	Daratumumab (Darzalex®)	Human IgG1/κ	Multiple myeloma	2015	2016
	Isatuximab-irfc (Sarclisa®)	Chimeric IgG1	Multiple myeloma	2020	2020
CD52	Alemtuzumab (Campath®, MabCampath®, Lemtrada®)	Humanized IgG1	B-cell CLL	2014	2013
CD19/CD3	Blinatumomab (Blincyto®)	BiTEs	Precursor cell lymphoblastic leukemia-lymphoma	2014	2015
CD79b	Polatuzumab vedotin (Polivy®)	Humanized IgG1 as ADC	B-cell lymphoma	2019	2020
CCR4	Mogamulizumab (Poteligo®)	Humanized IgG1	Cutaneous T-cell lymphoma	2018	2018
SLAMF7	Elotuzumab (Empliciti®)	Humanized IgG1	Multiple myeloma	2015	2016
Solid tumors					
HER2	Trastuzumab (Herceptin®)	Humanized IgG1	Breast cancer Metastatic gastric or gastroesophageal junction adenocarcinoma	1998	2000
	Ado-Trastuzumab emtansine (Kadcyla®)	Humanized IgG1 as ADC	Metastatic breast cancer	2013	2013
	Pertuzumab (Perjeta®)	Humanized IgG1	Metastatic breast cancer Locally advanced, inflammatory, or early-stage breast cancer	2012	2013
	[fam]-Trastuzumab deruxtecan (Enhertu®)	Humanized IgG1 as ADC	Breast cancer	2019	N/A
PD-1	Pembrolizumab (Keytruda®)	Human IgG4	Unresectable or metastatic melanoma; metastatic NSCLC, recurrent or metastatic HNSCC	2014	2015
	Nivolumab (Opdivo®)	Human IgG4	Metastatic squamous NSCLC, metastatic NSCLC; advanced renal cell carcinoma; recurrent and metastatic HNSCC; melanoma (unresectable, metastatic)	2014	2015
	Cemiplimab (Libtayo®)	Human mAb	Cutaneous squamous cell carcinoma	2018	2019
	Durvalumab (IMFINZI®)	Human IgG1	Bladder cancer	2017	2018

(continued)

Table 14.1 (continued)

Target	Name	Type	Indication	FDA	EMA
PD-L1	Atezolizumab (Tecentriq®)	Human IgG1	Metastatic NSCLC, locally advanced or metastatic urothelial carcinoma	2016	2017
	Avelumab (Bavencio®)	Human IgG1/κ	Metastatic Merkel cellcarcinoma	2017	2017
	Durvalumab (Imfinzi®)	Human IgG1/κ	Metastatic urothelial carcinoma	2017	N/A
EGFR	Cetuximab (Erbitux®)	Chimeric IgG1	HNSCC; metastatic colorectal cancer	2004	2004
	Panitumumab (Vectibix®)	Human IgG2	Metastatic colorectal carcinoma	2006	2007
	Necitumumab (Portrazza®)	Human IgG1	Metastatic squamous NSCLC	2015	2015
VEGF-A	Bevacizumab (Avastin®)	Humanized IgG1	Metastatic colorectal cancer; NSCLC; metastic renal cell carcinoma; metastatic cervical cancer; glioblastoma multiforme; recurrent ovarian, fallopian, or peritoneal cancer	2004	2005
VEGFR	Ramucirumab (Cyramza®)	Human IgG1	Advanced or metastatic gastric or gastroesophageal junction adenocarcinoma; metastatic NSCLC and CRC	2014	2014
PSMA	Capromab (ProstaScint®)	Murine mAb	Prostate adenocarcinoma*	1996	N/A
CTLA-4	Ipilimumab (Yervoy®)	Human IgG1	Melanoma (unresectable, metastatic, cutaneous)	2011	2011
PDGFR-α	Olaratumab (Lartruvo)	Human IgG1	Soft tissue sarcoma	2016	2016
RANKL	Denosumab (Xgeva®)	Human IgG2	Bone metastases	2011	2011
GD2	Dinutuximab (Unituxin®)	Human IgG1/κ	Pediatric high risk neuroblastoma	2015	2015
	Catumaxomab (Proxinium®)	Humanized mAb	HNSCC	2005	2005
EpCAM and CD3	Catumaxomab (Removab®)	Trifunctional chimeric mAb IgG2a/IgG2b	Malignant ascites in patients with EpCAM-positive carcinomas	N/A	2009
TAG-72	Satumomab (OncoScint®)	Murine mAb	Colorectal and ovarian cancers*	1992	N/A
EGP-1	Sacituzumab govitecan (Trodelvy®)	Humanized IgG1 as ADC	Triple-negative breast cancer	2020	N/A
Nectin-4	Enfortumab vedotin (Padcev®)	Human IgG1 as ADC	Urothelial cancer	2019	N/A

This list was generated according to the FDA, the EMA, the animal cell technology industrial platform and literature [32–34]

IgG immunoglobulin G, *HL* Hodgkin's lymphoma, *NSCLC* non-small cell lung cancer, *ALCL* systemic anaplastic large cell lymphoma, *CLL* chronic lymphocytic leukemia, *HNSCC* head and neck squamous cell carcinoma, *NSCLC* non-small cell lung cancer, *ALL* acute lymphoblastic leukemia, *BiTEs* bispecific T-cell engagers; *CCR4* C-C motif chemokine receptor 4; *SLAMF7* signaling lymphocytic activation molecule family member 7; VEGFR, vascular endothelial growth factor receptor; *CTLA-4* cytotoxic T-lymphocyte-associated protein 4, *PDGFR-α*, platelet-derived growth factor receptor-α, *RANKL*, receptor activator of NFκB ligand, *GD2 disialoganglioside 2; EpCAM* epithelial cellular adhesion molecule, *TAG-72* tumor-associated glycoprotein 72; *EGP-1* epithelial glycoprotein 1. *For diagnostic purpose only

Finally, fully humanized mAb can be produced by phage display or transgenic mice, e.g., Panitumumab (anti-EGFR) [49]. Chimeric, humanized, and fully humanized constructs have a lower risk of immune response [50], allowing for multiple injections over time in the same patient. They constitute the vast majority of the currently commercialized mAbs.

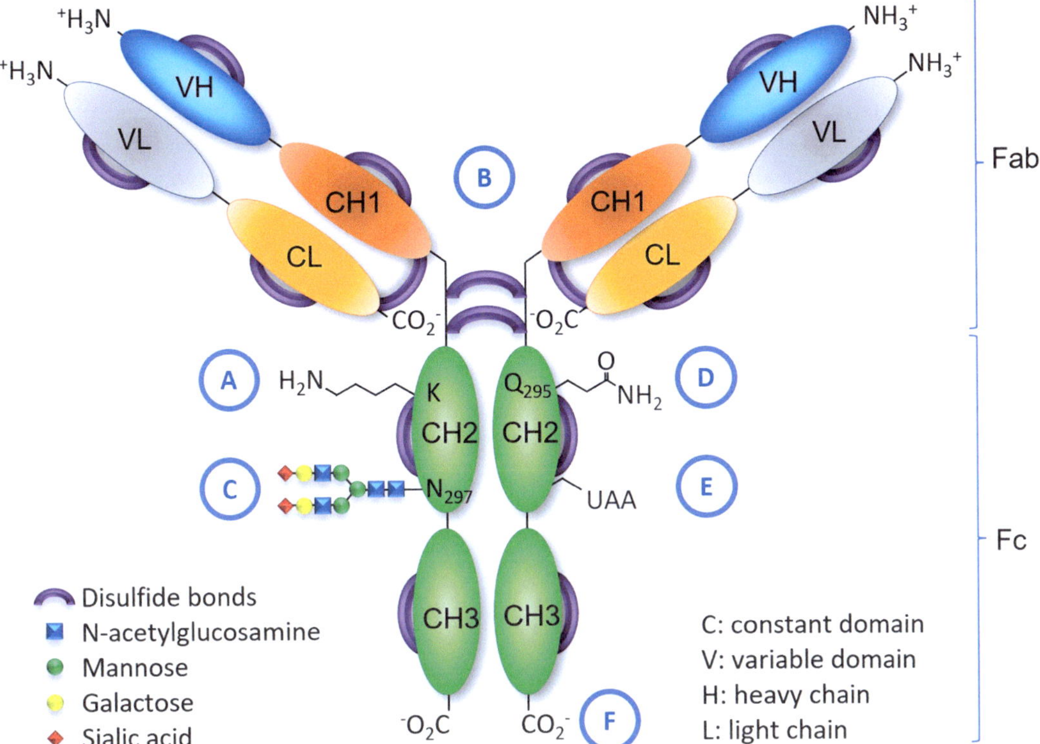

Fig. 14.2 mAb structure and conjugation strategies to add a chelating agent. The Y shape structure of human IgG_1 consisting in the two pairs of light and heavy chains is shown. Constant and variable domains in addition to the fragment antigen-binding (Fab) and the fragment crystallizable (Fc) regions are highlighted. The main reaction sites for conjugation that will be later described are also shown. They include random coupling via primary amines from lysine side chains (**A**), reduced thiol coupling (**B**), the targeting of modified glycans (**C**), enzymatic conjugation such as transglutaminase coupling (**D**), the introduction of unnatural amino acid (UAA) by genetic engineering (**E**), or a His_6 tag at the C-terminus (**F**)

14.2.2.2 mAb Immunological Function

The biological mechanisms of the mAb are mediated by the Fc portion of the IgG and can engage effector cells that can lead to complement-mediated cytotoxicity (CMC), antibody-dependent cellular toxicity (ADCC), and/or antibody-dependent cellular phagocytosis (ADCP) [51]. Briefly, CMC results in the lysis of the target cells due to IgG bound to surface antigens that will activate the formation of the membrane attack complex. ADCC is engaged by effector cells, mainly the natural killer (NK) cells that will recognize and kill IgG-coated target cells. ADCP is similar to ADCC but involves macrophages that express different Fc receptors which lead to phagocytosis [52]. In addition to these mechanisms, the binding of the mAb to its target could result in the removal of a critical protein from the cell surface and/or alter signal transduction for molecular pathways involved in tumor survival, proliferation, and dissemination [53]. In the case of a radiolabeled mAb, these immunological functions will be combined to the radiobiological processes that will be later described.

14.2.2.3 Pharmacokinetic of Radiolabeled mAb

mAbs are preferably administered intravenously. After absorption, their pharmacokinetic is characterized by a relatively fast distribution followed by a slower clearance. The intravenous injection makes them directly available for cell uptake. mAb can be rescued from cellular catabolism by binding to FcRn expressed by endothelial cells in blood vessels, hepatocytes, and some white blood cells [54]. By protecting and releasing the mAb back to the blood circulation, the mAb-FcRn interaction increases the biological $t_{1/2}$ of the mAb [55]. For RIT, the long biological blood $t_{1/2}$ of IgG could expose tumor lesions and normal tissue to higher doses of radiation. Antibody fragments, which do not contain any Fc fragments, will therefore have shorter biological $t_{1/2}$.

After extravasation, mAbs distribute into tissues, including tumor lesions, by diffusion and convection. Their volume of distribution is low and reflects the volume of blood vessels and interstitial spaces [56]. mAb may also accumulate in the spleen since this organ is relatively permissive to large plasma proteins [57]. mAbs are eliminated by either excretion or catabolism. Lysosomal degradation of the mAb-target complex occurs after internalization. In addition to this target-mediated clearance, nonspecific clearance of mAb also occurs via proteolysis in the liver and the reticuloendothelial system [33, 56]. Antibody fragments are smaller and will predominantly be excreted through the kidneys [58].

14.2.2.4   Factors Influencing mAb Pharmacokinetics

In addition to antigen-dependent parameters such as the antigen expression profile (density, turnover rate, and endogenous expression in nontarget organs), the pharmacokinetics of the mAb depends also on the mAb specificity, binding affinity to the target, internalization rate, dose levels, and immunogenicity.

A specific mAb avoids cross-reactivity with other molecules that can result in slower clearance and higher toxicity [59, 60]. In terms of affinity, previous studies have shown that binding affinity in the nanomolar range ensures tumor accumulation [27]. However, if a mAb binds too tightly to its target, the binding-site barrier phenomenon may occur. Following extravasation, the mAb binds immediately to its antigen result-

ing in perivascular accumulation and/or peripheral uptake in solid tumors [61, 62]. This limited penetration into the central part of the tumor reduces treatment efficiency and possibly increases the risk of acquired resistance [63]. Lower binding affinity mAb can penetrate deeper into tumors leading to a more homogeneous distribution. Interactions at the site of initial contact are reduced because they can dissociate from the antigen after binding and subsequently diffuse farther into the tissue [63–65]. Other mAb parameters such as immunogenicity, isoelectric pH, blood concentration, overall charge, or hydrophobicity/hydrophilicity can also influence the magnitude of penetration in the tissue and/or the mAb clearance [56].

Over the years, several methods have been developed to adjust the biological $t_{1/2}$ of mAb in order to improve the mAb distribution in tumors and overall contrast. As an example, injection of a higher quantity of mAb [66] or preinjection of non-radiolabeled mAb prior to the radiolabeled one tend to improve tumor accumulation [67, 68] up to a certain extent. Other strategies consist of modifying the mAb itself. Vivier et al. reported mutant constructs that have been generated to either increase or decrease the binding affinity to FcRn. Faster clearance can be obtained by using Fc-dependent low pH-independent binding mAb or IgG that cannot bind to FcRn. The biological $t_{1/2}$ can also decrease if it is glycosylated or if its isoelectric point decreases [15].

For preclinical development of new radioimmunoconjugates, it is important to consider the immunodeficiency status of the mouse strain and the biological origin of the mAb of interest, as they can both impact the mAb pharmacokinetics. In high immunodeficient mice (e.g., NSG), mAb with a human Fc fragment shows a faster blood clearance and can be hijacked to nontargeted organs (liver, spleen, and bone), leading to a decreased tumor uptake, as compared to lower immunodeficient mice (e.g., Nu/Nu) or murine mAb. It has been attributed to the lack of endogenous mAb production and an avid-Fc mediated binding in nontargeted organs [69].

14.2.3 Radionuclides

The choice of radionuclide depends on the intended application. Radionuclides that emit gamma rays (γ from single-photon emitters) such as iodine-125 (^{125}I), technetium-99 m (^{99m}Tc), or indium-111 can be used for single-photon emission computed tomography (SPECT), while those that emit positrons (followed by β$^+$ annihilation) like iodine-124 (^{124}I) or zirconium-89 are suitable for PET imaging. For RIT, radionuclides associated with more damaging radiations are needed (e.g., α, β, or auger electron) [70]. The physical half-life ($t_{1/2}$) of the radioisotope should match the biological $t_{1/2}$ of the pharmacophore. This maximizes the contrast ratio for imaging or irradiation dose to lesions for therapy.

In general, radionuclides with $t_{1/2}$ of a few days are preferable for labeling intact mAb, while radionuclides with shorter $t_{1/2}$ in a range of hours are more suitable for antibody fragments and smaller constructs. For therapy, the type of particle that is emitted by the radionuclide will dictate the therapeutic dose rate and the total dose received by the patient [71]. Factors like production method, cost, and availability of the radionuclide and/or the starting material also influence radioisotope selection. The most commonly used radionuclides for RIT are listed in Table 14.2. For detailed information on the physical properties, production, and purification methods of the different radionuclides, we invite the reader to refer to more detailed reviews [72, 75, 76].

14.2.3.1 β$^-$-Emitters

β$^-$-Emitters have a low linear energy transfer (LET), which refers to the amount of deposited energy per unit of track length (0.2 keV/μm).

Table 14.2 Examples of therapeutic radionuclides for mAb and antibody derivatives labeling

Isotope	Daughter isotopes[a]	$T_{1/2}$ (h)	β/α (Emax keV)	Maximum range	γ/X (Emax keV)	SPECT
β$^-$-particle emitters (LET 0.2 keV/μm)						
^{188}Re	–	17.0	β$^-$ (2120)	10.4 mm	γ (155)	Yes
^{67}Cu	–	61.8	β$^-$ (561)	2.1 mm	γ (184)	Yes
^{90}Y	–	64.0	β$^-$ (2280)	11.3 mm	–	No
^{47}Sc	–	80.4	β$^-$ (441 600)	NA	γ (159)	Yes
^{177}Lu	–	159.5	β$^-$ (498)	2.0 mm	γ (208)	Yes
^{131}I	–	192.6	β$^-$ (606)	2.9 mm	γ (364)	Yes
Auger electrons emitters (LET 4–26 keV/μm)						
^{99m}Tc	–	6.0	–	NA	γ (140)	Yes
^{123}I	–	13.2	–	20 μm	γ (159)	Yes
^{111}In	–	67.3	–	17 μm	γ (171, 245)	Yes
^{67}Ga	–	78.3	–	3 μm	γ (93, 185, 300)	Yes
^{195m}Pt	–	96.5	–	76 μm	γ (98.9)	Yes
^{125}I	–	1442.4	–	20 μm	γ (35)	Yes
α-Particle emitters (LET 50-260 keV/μm)						
^{213}Bi	^{213}Po (YNS 4.2 μs)	0.76	α (5,875) β$^-$ (1423)	0.1 mm	γ (440)	Yes[b]
^{212}Pb/^{212}Bi[c]	^{212}Po (YNS 0.3 μs)	10.6/1.0	α (6,207) β$^-$ (2252)	51 μm	γ (727)	Yes[b]
^{211}At	^{211}Po (YNS 516 ms)	7.2	α (5,870)	55 μm	γ (79)	Yes[b]
^{225}Ac	^{221}Fr (α 4.9 min) ^{217}At (α 32 ms) ^{213}Bi (α + γ 45.6 min) ^{213}Po (YNS 4.2 μs)	240.0	α (5,830)	48 μm	–	Yes[b] (daughters)

Half-life ($t_{1/2}$), type of emission (both from https://www.nndc.bnl.gov/nudat2/), and maximum range within tissues are provided. Some isotopes can be used for therapy and imaging [6, 72–74]. *YNS* yield not significant, *NA* not available.
[a]Generated after the decay of parental radionuclide
[b]Can be detected by SPECT but will require the injection of high amount of activity
[c]^{212}Pb is used as an in vivo generator of ^{212}Bi which is the α-emitter particle.

Low LET leads to single-strand DNA breaks but delivers energy over longer distances (0.05–12 mm) which makes them more suited for the treatment of solid tumors. The main β^--emitters developed for RIT using full IgG are iodine-131, yttrium-90, and more recently lutetium-177 (^{177}Lu) and rhenium-188 (^{188}Re).

Iodine-131, produced by neutron irradiation of a natural tellurium target (^{130}Te(n,γ)^{131}Te → ^{131}I), was first used to synthesize ^{131}I-labeled anti-CD20 mAb Tositumomab for the treatment and imaging of NHL [7]. mAb could be easily labeled with iodine-131 by direct labeling of tyrosines [77], but iodine-131 is excreted from the cells after internalization. Even though mAb internalization is not mandatory for therapeutic efficiency, iodine-131 is preferable for mAb/antigen systems that have a prolonged retention on the cellular membrane. In general, the release of free isotopes could reduce the dose to tumor and induce toxicity due to their circulation in the blood and/or accumulation in normal tissues (i.e., thyroid tissue for iodine radionuclides).

Residualizing isotopes like yttrium-90, rhenium-188, and lutetium-177 are better-suited for internalizing targets such as PSMA, CD5, or CD22 [78]. Yttrium-90 is easily obtained in pure form via chemical separation from the long-lived strontium-90 (^{90}Sr, 28.8 years) in ^{90}Sr/^{90}Y generators, allowing nearly unlimited access to this isotope [79]. This isotope is the one used to label Ibritumomab tiuxetan (Zevalin) for NHL [17]. Yttrium-90 is widely used in β^- RIT and is readily chelated using 1, 4, 7, 10-tetraazacyclododecane-1, 4, 7, 10-tetraacetic acid (DOTA) [80, 81]. Due to its $t_{1/2}$ of 2.67 days and its long-range β emission (11.3 mm), this pure β^- emitter (100% β^- decay) provides a longer penetration range than many other β^- emitters. This property makes it efficient for the treatment of bulky and poorly vascularized tumors [73, 82]. In addition, due to its high β^- emission energy, yttrium-90 can deliver high-dose deposition. Rhenium-188 has a similar track range, and its γ emission can be imaged by SPECT which is an advantage over yttrium-90 [83]. mAb can be labeled with rhenium-188 either directly by targeting reduced disulfide bridges or using chelating agents.

Long-range emissions may deposit dose in normal tissue beyond the boundaries of smaller tumors or micrometastases. The shorter emission range of copper-67 (^{67}Cu), scandium-47 (^{47}Sc), or lutetium-177 (~2 mm) is more adequate in these cases [84–87]. The emission of β^- particles with lower LET and low-energy γ photons results in relatively low relative biological effectiveness; i.e., higher injected activities might be needed [88]. Among these 3 radioisotopes, the physical $t_{1/2}$ of ^{177}Lu (6.6 days) best matches the pharmacokinetics of mAb. Its γ emission can be efficiently image by SPECT making lutetium-177 an interesting isotope for theranostic applications. Lutetium-177 can be produced by direct and indirect reactor production routes both via single thermal neutron capture using highly enriched lutetium-176 or ytterbium-176 (^{176}Yb) targets, respectively (^{176}Lu(n,γ)^{177}Lu and ^{176}Yb(n,γ)^{177}Yb → ^{177}Lu). Macrocyclic DOTA-based chelators are the gold standard for lutetium-177 mAb radiolabeling [89]. Some preclinical studies have shown the superiority of yttrium-90 over lutetium-177 for RIT in hematological malignancies models [90, 91]. Nevertheless, radionuclide efficiency comparison is not straightforward as parameters including the absorbed dose and the dose rate need to be considered. None of these radionuclides is superior to others, but in the case of yttrium-90 and lutetium-177, the former has been postulated to be more adapted to bulky and poor vascularized tumor lesions, and the latter allows treatment of smaller tumors or metastases [92].

14.2.3.2 α-Emitters

α-Emitters, on the other hand, have a shorter range in tissue (40–100 μm) but are more potent because of higher LET (50–260 keV/μm). These properties make them more suitable for disseminated disease and micrometastases [93]. In addition to the generation of DNA double-strand breaks that are more difficult to repair than single-strand breaks, the effect of α particles does not depend either on the dose rate or the oxygenation of the irradiated tissue [74]. As the relative biological effectiveness of α-emitters is much higher than β$^-$-emitters, α-RIT can potentially kill more cells than β-RIT at the same administered dose [94, 95]. Marcu et al. recently reviewed preclinical and clinical studies comparing the efficacy of α-RIT and β-RIT and found that α-RIT was superior within the tolerated dose [96]. However, it should be noted that the number of α-RIT studies is small and large randomized clinical trials are still needed.

Bismuth-213 (^{213}Bi) is easily obtained from ^{225}Ac[actinium]/^{213}Bi generators and has been used widely. However, its very short $t_{1/2}$ (45.6 min) makes it challenging to work with and is not amenable to the biological $t_{1/2}$ of mAb. Astatine-211 (^{211}At) has a significantly longer $t_{1/2}$ than bismuth-213 (7.2 h), but is still not well matched to the biological half-life of mAb. Nonetheless, tumor therapeutic efficacy in RIT protocols using either bismuth-213 or astatine-211 has been reported in preclinical studies [97–100]. Thus far, bismuth-213 has been more studied for RIT because the use of astatine-211 is constrained by its limited availability [101].

With a $t_{1/2}$ of 10 days, actinium-225 is a very attractive radioisotope for α-RIT. It is available from only a few institutions, and the current main source is thorium-229 generators (^{229}Th, 7.3 years). The global production of actinium-225 is approximately 63 GBq/year [72]. Efforts to increase the production and purification of actinium-225 are actively being investigated [102, 103]. The irradiation of a thorium target with high-energy protons (>70 MeV) or the use of ^{225}Ra[radium]/^{225}Ac generators are promising short-term approaches. Actinium-225 decays to a cascade of 6 daughters, including bismuth-213 described above, for a total of 4 α and 3 β$^-$ emissions. While this enhances cytotoxicity, it concomitantly increases toxicity to normal tissues if those daughters are released from the chelating agent during circulation. Jurcic et al. investigated the use of Lintuzumab (anti-CD33) labeled either with ^{213}Bi or ^{225}Ac for AML treatment and observed better therapeutic response with actinium-225 [104–106].

14.2.3.3 Auger Electron Emitters

Auger electrons are emitted by radionuclides decaying by electron capture and/or internal conversion. Auger electron emitters can be imaged by SPECT and include technetium-99 m, indium-111, iodine-123 (^{123}I), iodine-125, gallium-67 (^{67}Ga), and platinum-195 m (^{195m}Pt). While short $t_{1/2}$ of technetium-99 m and iodine-123 will provide higher dose rate, longer $t_{1/2}$ will be more adapted to label IgG such as indium-111 ($t_{1/2}$: 67.3 h), gallium-67 ($t_{1/2}$: 78.3 h), platinum-195 m ($t_{1/2}$: 96.5 h), and iodine-125 ($t_{1/2}$: 59.5 days). Indium-111 is the classical radioisotope used for immuno-SPECT imaging [107, 108].

Auger electrons are associated with intermediate LET (4–26 keV/μm) as compared to β$^-$- and α-emitters, with a significantly shorter particle range in tissues (< 1 μm). Auger electrons can be highly cytotoxic by inducing DNA double-strand breaks but need to be located near the DNA or even be incorporated into the DNA itself [74]. In this context, most radiopharmaceuticals that have been developed need to be internalized and target the DNA such as [^{125}I]I-IudR (iododeoxyuridine) [109]. For RIT using mAb, strategies focus on targeting receptors containing a nuclear localization sequence (NLS) such as EGFR to promote the delivery of the Auger electrons close to the nucleus. Using this strategy, the internalizing anti-EGFR ^{125}I-mAb 425 significantly increased the overall survival of patients with brain tumors [110–112]. For other receptors, the incorporation of a NLS in the mAb itself can promote nuclear uptake, as reported with the anti-HER2 [^{111}In] In-NLS-Trastuzumab [113]. Auger electrons can also damage cell membranes. Even if the best cytotoxic effects are obtained with nuclear targeting, Pouget et al. reported that cell surface antigen targeting can still be efficient to kill tumor cells [114].

14.2.4 Antibody Bioconjugation with Chelating Agents for Labeling with Metallic Radionuclides

The two main strategies to label mAb are direct and indirect labeling. In the case of direct labeling, radioiodine is used to label tyrosine residues [77]. For indirect labeling, prosthetic groups such as a metal chelator is used [115]. While direct labeling is associated with minimal alteration of the protein backbone, the addition of prosthetic groups can negatively impact binding properties [116]. The addition of chelators on a mAb should therefore preserve the quaternary structure of the mAb, be stable over time, and maintain the binding affinity and specificity of the mAb to its target. Ideally, the immunoreactive fraction after conjugation needs to be as high as possible, ideally at least 50–80% [117]. For conjugation conditions, pH and temperature are the most important considerations to ensure stability. Neutral or slightly neutral pH conditions (pH 5–9), temperatures around 37 °C (should not exceed the melting temperature), and nonreducing conditions are preferable. These recommendations also hold true for the radiolabeling process. Price and Orvig provided a guide detailing the ideal combinations of radiometals and chelators [115].

Currently, the most common conjugation methods target native residues in a nonspecific manner [118]. Among them, lysine-based bioconjugation reactions are the most prevalent. With over 80 lysines in the IgG scaffold including 20 considered highly accessible for conjugation [119], targeting primary amines of lysine side chains has been used widely with *N*-hydroxysuccinimide ester, isothiocyanate derivatives, or anhydrides. As these strategies are nonselective, they yield a heterogeneous mixture of mAb in terms of conjugation ratios and site of conjugation [120]. This strategy can also be associated with a decrease of the immunoreactive fraction [121, 122], especially if the conjugation site is close to the binding region of the mAb. Using [^{89}Zr] Zr-DFO-Trastuzumab (DFO:desferoxamine), Sharma et al. recently demonstrated that increasing DFO:trastuzumab molecular ratios from 5:1 to 200:1, which results in 1.4–10.9 chelator per mAb on average, increases the radiolabeling efficacy but decreases the binding affinity (3.5–4.6 lower) and the immunoreactive fraction from 90% to 50%, which lead to nonoptimal in vivo biodistribution, i.e., decrease of tumor uptake and increase of accumulation in the liver [123]. Quality controls for each generated batch of immunoconjugate are therefore highly mandatory, and chelator:mAb molecular ratios of 5–10 have been recommended to maintain the mAb binding [122, 124], although it could be dependent on the chelator and the mAb. Conjugations that are more site-specific have been developed [121]. These include reaction thiol chemistry with free cysteines, enzyme-mediated conjugation, enzyme-mediated glycan modification, unnatural amino acid addition, and click chemistry.

The targeting of cysteines is commonly used for ADC such as Brentuximab vedotin (FDA-approved anti-CD30 mAb). Thiol groups present on cysteine side chains can react with maleimides, with a chelator attached, via Michael addition [118]. However, the in vivo stability is limited due to the possibility of retro-Michael reaction that either releases the payload or exchanges it with other molecules containing free thiols [125, 126]. Alternatives to maleimides have been developed to optimize the C–S bond stability. For example, Adumeau et al. reported a higher in vivo stability of radiolabeled ^{89}Zr- and ^{177}Lu-labeled Trastuzumab (anti-HER2) and HuA33 (anti-A33) for imaging and/or therapy using a phenyloxadiazole-based reagent for thiol conjugations (methylsulfonyl phenyloxadiazole) in xenograft models [127]. Even if this targeting approach is less random than lysine-based conjugation methods, it does not allow control over which disulfide bonds are involved in the conjugation.

The glycosylation sites present naturally in IgG on a specific asparagine residue (N297 within the CH$_2$ domain) can be modified to enable site-selective addition of chelators with minimal risk of affecting binding properties as these sites are not close to the Fab region [118]. The most common strategy relies on the oxidation of the sugar to create an aldehyde that will be able to form covalent linkages with nucleophiles including amines, hydrazide, and aminooxy groups. This strategy was reported to enhance tumor accumulation and tumor-to-background ratios [128]. A chelator can also be added via an enzymatic reaction by reacting with a modified galactose terminal unit containing a reactive functional group. The incorporation of azide-modified N-acetylgalactosamine monosaccharides in the glycans of an anti-PSMA mAb (J591) showed good labeling efficiency to yield [^{89}Zr] Zr-DFO-J591, with high immunoreactivity, in vivo stability, and selective tumor uptake in mice bearing human prostate tumors [129]. Another example is the use of bacterial transglutaminase that allows a reaction between the side chain of glutamine (Q295) within a deglycosylated mAb and chelators with a free primary amine [130]. Using this strategy, higher target to nontarget ratios were reported for [$^{64/67}$Cu] Cu-CPTA-Rituximab (anti-CD20) and ^{67}Ga/^{89}Zr-DFO-chCE7 (anti-L1-CAM) in subcutaneous xenograft models of lymphoma and ovarian tumors, respectively [131].

The incorporations of unnatural amino acids or peptide tags are other strategies for developing highly selective radioimmunoconjugates. Wu et al. reported efficient labeling of Rituximab by first appending an azido group-bearing amino acid followed by the addition of the chelator by click chemistry [132]. Peptide tags can also be incorporated such as a hexahistidine sequence (His$_6$ tag), a peptide tag composed of several glycines, and a terminal cysteine ((Gly)$_x$Cys Tag) or fusion proteins bearing metallothioneins [133]. These methods are used mostly for mAb derivatives instead of full IgG [121].

In general, site-specific conjugations are attractive but require more complicated modifications and antibody engineering. Therefore, they are not as well adapted as nonspecific conjugation methods that target native residues such as lysine side chains for antibody screening in preclinical development. Indeed, the targeting of lysines remains the most prevalent method used for antibody conjugation even for clinical studies [134]. However, site-specific conjugations can ensure antibody bioactivity and better uniformity and reproducibility of immunoconjugate batches, which can be beneficial for clinical development. Future techniques for site-specific conjugation methods might be inspired by new developments in the ADC field and could be applied to radioimmunoconjugates [134–137]. The different strategies described above are summarized in Fig. 14.2.

14.3 Radioimmunotherapy (RIT)

14.3.1 Principle

The use of a mAb labeled with a particle-emitting radioisotope to deliver low-dose damaging radiation directly to tumor cells is an alternative to external beam radiotherapy (EBRT) for local tumors and especially for diffuse disease [138–140]. RIT's mechanisms of action combine the immunological function of the mAb (CMC, ADCC, and/or ADCP, previously described) and the radiobiological processes. Ionizing radiation can affect cells within the targeted tissue by (A) direct irradiation, the radiolabeled mAb irradiates the cell it is bound to; (B) crossfire effect, irradiation from the radionuclide bound to adjacent cells; or (C) bystander effect, a similar effect on nonirradiated cells mediated by signals received from nearby irradiated cells [74]. Cellular response to irradiation includes activation of growth factor receptors, death receptors, and some membrane-bound tyrosine kinases, but the main consequence is DNA damage. The type of DNA damage (single- or double-strain breaks) is based on the LET, as described previously. In addition, it has been demonstrated that ionizing radiation can stimulate host immunity to kill distant untargeted cancer cells [141–143].

In RIT, the bone marrow (BM) is often considered as the dose-limiting organ when using intact mAb [144–149]. This well-vascularized tissue contains hematopoietic progenitors, and stem cells that are highly radiosensitive. Due to the slow blood clearance of radiolabeled IgG, the BM gets irradiated as the mAb circulates in the blood. This affects the hematopoietic function of this tissue leading to a decline in blood cell counts. For a patient, this leads to a higher risk of developing treatment-associated myelodysplastic syndrome and/or acute myelogenous leukemia [150, 151]. Nevertheless, myelotoxicity is not always an issue for continuing RIT treatments. Indeed, blood transfusions, BM, or hematopoietic stem cell supports can be performed to help the patients to recover. In addition, high-dose myeloablative regimens could be beneficial in the treatment of hematological malignancies.

Hematological malignancies are sensitive to radiation and present a broad variety of antigens on their cellular surface which makes them the ideal target for RIT. Besides [^{90}Y]Y-Ibritumomab tiuxetan and [^{131}I]I-Tositumomab which both target CD20 for patients with NHL, RIT has been tested in other malignancies. First-line therapy or fractionated RIT, to increase the dose to the tumor while sparing the normal tissues, has been used in multiple myelomas and AML. Solid tumors are more resistant to radiation and are less accessible to large molecules such as mAb. Nevertheless, promising results have been obtained, and numerous preclinical studies and clinical trials are currently ongoing to assess and develop RIT. Even though the treatment of solid tumors remains a challenge, RIT has the advantage over EBRT to be able to treat systemic malignancies, including circulating tumor cells [78, 117]. Many targets have now been explored for RIT as shown in Fig. 14.3.

14.3.2 Tumor-Associated Antigens for RIT of Hematological Malignancies

Hematological malignancies are particularly attractive targets for RIT approaches for multiple reasons. In addition to being extremely radiation-sensitive, many lineage-specific cell surface antigens have been identified on malignant cells. Hematopoietic CD are expressed during the maturation of distinct cell lineages. CD3, CD7, or CD5 are associated with T lymphocytes lineage; CD19, CD20, CD22, or CD10 are expressed by B lymphocytes lineage; and CD13, CD14, and CD33 are present on the surface of cells from myeloid lineage [158]. Additional targets that are not restricted to a lineage are also under investigations such as CD45 or HLA-DR. High-affinity mAbs that bind to some of these antigens were developed and are available, which makes them even more attractive for the development of RIT applications. The inherent immunosuppressive nature of hematopoietic malignancies prevents immune reactions against the radioimmunoconjugate, especially for nonhuman or nonhuman-

ized mAb. Finally, the potent BM toxicity induced by RIT could actually be beneficial for patients in the context of myeloablative RIT, as previously mentioned. Autologous and allogeneic stem cell transplants have become part of routine hematological oncology practice [117]. Hematological malignancies have therefore been actively studied for the development of RIT and for NHL.

14.3.2.1 Non-Hodgkin's Lymphoma

The first evidence of the superiority of RIT versus naked mAb was obtained in NHL, a heterogeneous group of lymphoid neoplasm of B cell, T cell, or NK cell origin, by targeting CD20 [159]. CD20 is a 35 kDa non-glycosylated phosphoprotein expressed only by mature B cells and most malignant B cells (>90%) and plays a role in B-cell activation and proliferation [160–162]. This antigen is absent from other hematopoietic lineages and is not excreted in any soluble forms. By using [^{131}I]I-Tositumomab (Bexxar), higher overall response (60–80%) and complete response (CR) rates (15–40%) than non-radiolabeled anti-CD20 mAb were observed for patients with relapsed or refractory NHL [117, 163]. Nevertheless, the production and use of this radiolabeled anti-CD20 mAb were discontinued in 2013, most likely due to economic reasons [155].

[^{90}Y]Y-Ibritumomab tiuxetan (Zevalin) is an approved RIT for NHL. The current protocol (Fig. 14.4a) consists of an initial intravenous injection of 250 mg/m^2 of Rituximab (naked anti-CD20) to deplete B cells from the peripheral circulation. A SPECT scan after injection of ^{111}In-labeled Zevalin can be performed 48–72 h after Rituximab preinjection to detect altered biodistribution of the radiolabeled mAb [168, 169]. Seven to nine days later, patients receive a second injection of Rituximab followed by the administration of Zevalin within 4 h with the injected activity depending on the patient's platelet counts prior to treatment [170]. In general, the maximum injected activity of [^{90}Y]Y-Ibritumomab tiuxetan is 1.2 GBq [6, 171]. Treatment-induced myelodysplastic syndrome or AML was reported in 2.5% of the treated patients [172]. [^{90}Y]Y-Ibritumomab tiuxetan is

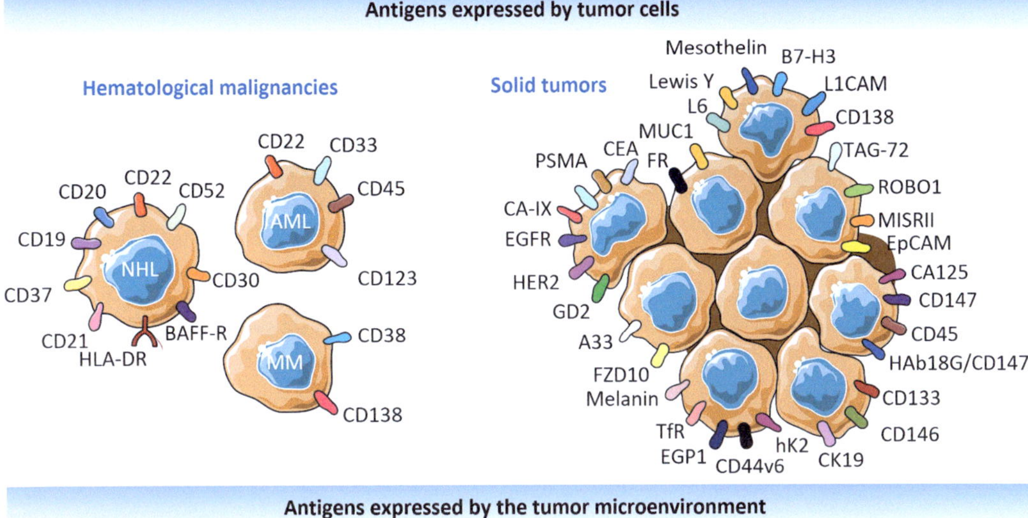

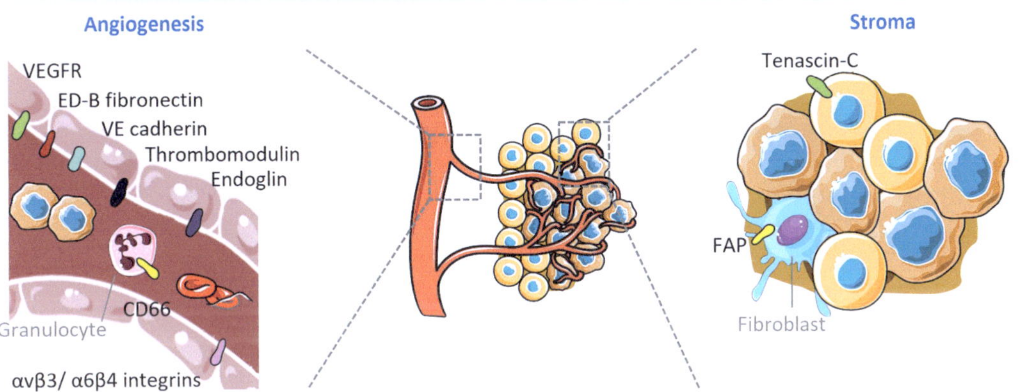

Fig. 14.3 Examples of targets investigated for RIT studies in hematological malignancies and solid tumors. Antigens can be either expressed by the tumor cells themselves and/or by cells within the tumor microenvironment. In hematological malignancies, most of the targets correspond to CD overexpressed by the tumor cells such as CD20 for NHL, CD33 for AML, or CD138 for multiple myeloma (MM). For solid tumors, the most common targets include the carcinoembryonic antigen (CEA), TAG-72, PSMA, GD2, and the carbonic anhydrase IX (CA-IX). Other targets are also investigated such as proteins involved in tumor angiogenesis, VEGFR or the extra domain B-containing fibronectin (ED-B fibronectin), and antigens expressed by cells within the tumor microenvironment, CD66 expressed by granulocytes for AML RIT and the fibroblast activation protein (FAP) for solid tumors. (Some graphical elements were adapted from Servier Medical Art (www.servier.com), and the cited targets were summarized from recent reviews [73, 78, 117, 152–157]). BAFF-R, a receptor for B-cell activating factor; HLA-DR, MHC class II cell surface receptor; MUC1, mucin 1; FZD10, frizzled-10; TfR, transferrin receptor; CD44v6, CD44 variant isoform 6; hK2, human kallikrein 2; CK19, cytokeratin 19; ROBO1, roundabout guidance receptor 1; L1CAM, L1 cell adhesion molecule; B7-H3, CD276; L6, tumor-associated antigen L6; FR, folate receptor; VE-cadherin, vascular endothelial cadherin; CD138, syndecan-1; CD133, prominin-1; MISRII, Müllerian-inhibiting substance receptor type I; CD147, extracellular matrix metalloproteinase inducer; CD146, melanoma cell adhesion molecule (MCAM)

well-tolerated and associated with a higher overall response rate as compared to the naked Rituximab (Fig. 14.4b) and an increase in survival [165, 173]. An example of a patient with CR is shown in Fig. 14.4c.

In clinical practice, Zevalin is used in combination with other therapies. Consolidation therapy, i.e., short-course treatment of Zevalin given after completion of the standard therapeutic protocol, was shown to be beneficial. In phase III

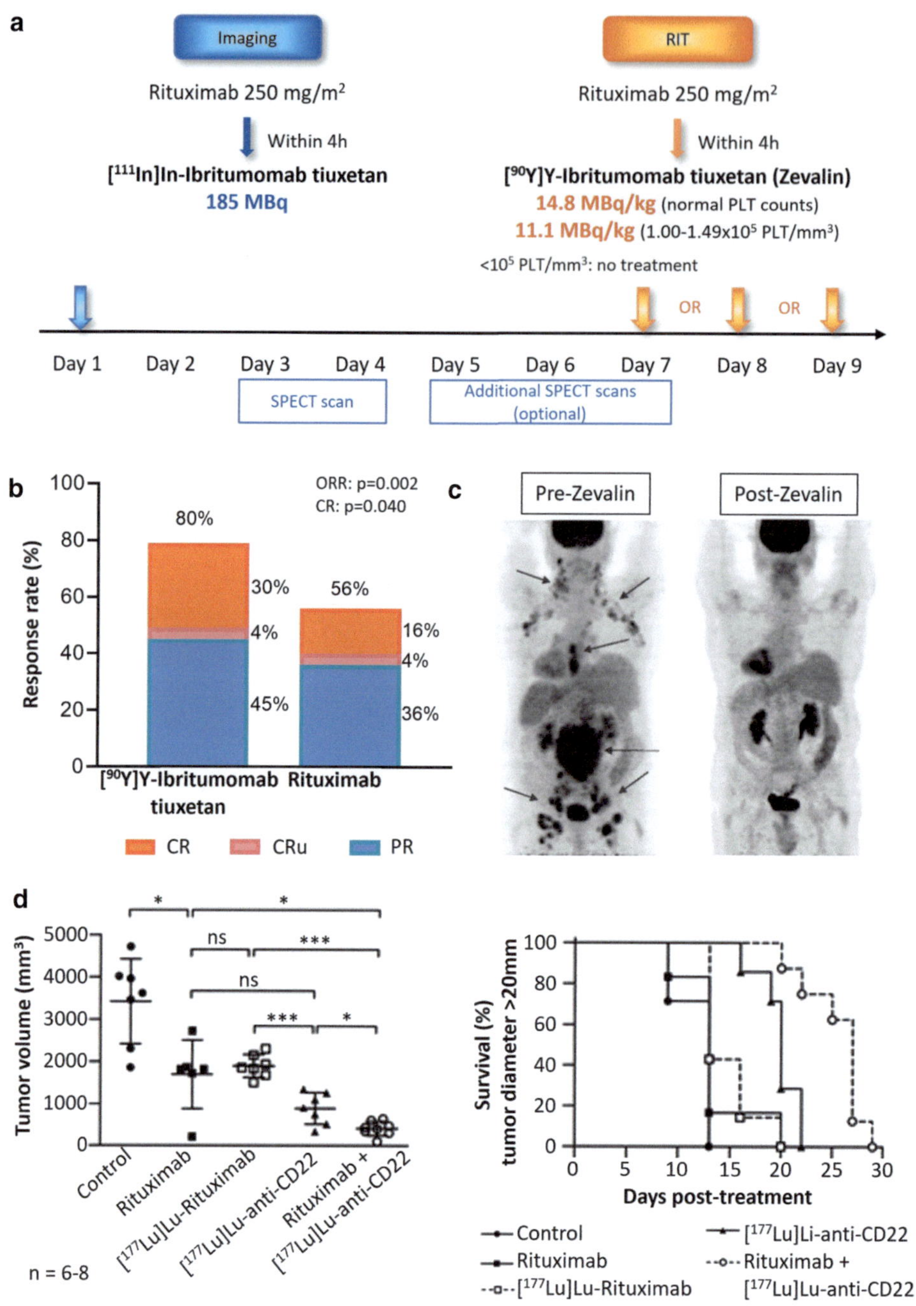

Fig. 14.4 RIT in NHL. (**a**) The [⁹⁰Y]Y-Ibtritumomab tiuxetan (Zevalin) treatment protocol with imaging prior to treatment is shown (adapted with permission from Kawashima [164]). PLT, platelets. (**b**) Response rates observed after treatment of relapsed or refractory low-grade, follicular, or transformed NHL with Zevalin as compared to naked Rituximab from a pivotal phase III study (ORR, overall response rate). (Adapted with permission from Marcus [165]). (**c**) [¹⁸F]FDG PET scan showed abnormal positive nodes (arrows) pre-Zevalin. Three months posttreatment, CR was observed. (Adapted with permission from Jacobs et al. [166]). (**d**) Demonstration of the higher efficiency of a ¹⁷⁷Lu-labeled anti-CD22 mAb as compared to the anti-CD20 [¹⁷⁷Lu] Lu-Rituximab in a preclinical model of Burkitt's lymphoma (another NHL subtype) (adapted with permission from Weber et al. [167])

first-line indolent trial of Zevalin with 409 patients with advanced-stage follicular lymphoma in the first remission, an 8-year overall progression-free survival (PFS) of 41% was estimated with Zevalin consolidation versus 22% with no treatment. For patients with unconfirmed CR (Cru), 8-year PFS was 48% versus 32%, and 33% versus 10% for patients with partial response (PR) [174]. However, other consolidation protocols are used more often than RIT as they are considered safer for patients with BM involvement and more favorable in terms of cost and logistics [17]. Combination of RIT and high-dose chemotherapy for preparative conditioning protocol before allogeneic or autologous hematopoietic stem cell transplantation have also been investigated and showed promising results for patients with lymphomas as well as other hematological malignancies. The aim of this combination is to prevent the relapse of the primary disease while decreasing the morbidity and non-relapse mortality associated with stem cell transplantation strategies [175, 176]. More recently, β-RIT targeting CD20 has successfully been evaluated as first-line treatment [177–180]. The feasibility for α-RIT for NHL has been evaluated but only in few preclinical studies using ^{213}Bi- or ^{211}At-labeled mAb [100, 181, 182].

Efforts to improve NHL RIT mostly aim at identifying and testing alternative targets to CD20 such as other clusters of differentiation: CD19, CD21, CD22, CD37, CD45, CD2, CD80, and CD52; members of the tumor necrosis factor (TNF) family: CD30, CD40, receptors of the TNF-related apoptosis-inducing ligand (TRAIL); receptors of the B-cell activating factor (BAFF) and of a proliferation-inducing ligand (APRIL); and HLA-DR and surface immunoglobulin (sIg) [117, 183]; some have been already tested for RIT developments [156, 184]. The most popular one is CD22, a B-cell-specific transmembrane glycoprotein that modulates B-cell function, survival, and apoptosis. It is expressed in 60–70% of B-cell malignancies [185, 186]. The anti-CD22 [^{90}Y]Y-Epratuzumab tetraxetan demonstrated durable remission rates for patients with relapsed or refractory B-NHL with or without anti-CD20 mAb combination [187–189]. ^{177}Lu-labeled anti-CD22 huRFB4 mAb showed a

higher therapeutic response and increase in survival than [^{177}Lu]Lu-Rituximab in a preclinical study (Fig. 14.4d) [167].

In addition to CD22, CD37, and tenascin-C have also been proposed as new targets for NHL. The results obtained by targeting these two proteins were reviewed in 2019 by Bailly et al. and showed promise for further pursuit [190]. CD37 is a highly glycosylated transmembrane antigen selectively expressed by normal B cells and overexpressed in most B-cell malignancies [191]. The ^{177}Lu-labeled anti-CD37 mAb, [^{177}Lu]Lu-Lilotomab satetraxetan, is currently in clinical trials for relapsed/refractory lymphomas [192]. Kolstad et al. reported an overall response rate of 61% with 26% CR in a phase I/II study [192]. Tenascin-C is an extracellular hexameric matrix glycoprotein expressed by embryonic and adult extracellular matrices [193]. It was also shown to be present in the lymph nodes of patients with B cell and T cell NHL in addition to Hodgkin's lymphoma. [^{131}I]I-81C6 anti-tenascin-C mAb-induced transient or manageable hematological toxicity with stem cell infusion [194]. In a phase I trial, 1 patient out of 9 showed a CR, and 1 showed a PR [195]. Other targets have been evaluated in preclinical studies such as CD19, a transmembrane glycoprotein expressed by normal and malignant B cells [196]. ^{90}Y-labeled anti-CD19 mAb showed antitumor activity after a single injection and was comparable to ^{90}Y-labeled anti-CD20 mAb [184, 197].

14.3.2.2 Acute Leukemia

Acute leukemia is an aggressive malignant disease of the hematopoietic system characterized by the accumulation of immature cells in the BM and a reduction of blood cell production. The main types of acute leukemia are acute myeloid leukemia (AML), the most common type, and acute lymphoid leukemia (ALL) that differs from AML by the lineage of origin that was malignantly transformed. The main RIT strategies for acute leukemia target proteins such as CD33 and CD45, expressed directly by the blasts [157, 198].

To date, most efforts have been focused on targeting CD33 for the treatment of AML with radiolabeled mAb. CD33 is a myeloid differentiation antigen. Its expression is restricted to early multilineage hematopoietic progenitors, myelomonocytic precursors, and more mature myeloid cells and is absent on normal pluripotent hematopoietic stem cells. CD33 is also present on the surface of myeloid leukemias and clonogenic leukemia progenitors and was shown to be expressed by 85–90% of AML [199–201]. Its expression is associated with poor prognosis, poor therapeutic response to chemotherapy, and higher recurrence rate [202]. M195, an anti-CD33 mAb, and its humanized version HuM195 (Lintuzumab) have been labeled with therapeutic isotopes and studied in clinical trials [203]. It was first labeled with iodine-131 with benefits observed for patients with a relapse or chemotherapy-refractory AML when [^{131}I]I-Lintuzumab was given as a single agent or as part of the preparative regimen for allogenic BM transplantation [203–205]. Nevertheless, [^{131}I]I-Lintuzumab had limitations as multiple injections were needed to deliver enough irradiation dose to the tumor cells, treatment required hospitalization and isolation of the injected patients, the long physical $t_{1/2}$ of iodine-131 delayed the time for stem cell infusion, the labeling strategy affected binding of the mAb, and iodine-131 was not trapped into the tumor cells after internalization. Anti-CD33 mAb was therefore labeled with yttrium-90 as an alternative to iodine-131 and showed a significant reduction in the number of BM blasts [206]. More recently, α-emitters have been evaluated for AML treatment. The results obtained with bismuth-213 and actinium-225 have been reviewed by Jurcic in 2018 [104]. [^{213}Bi]Bi-Lintuzumab can accumulate effectively in leukemic lesions and is safe and associated with remissions in AML patients in combination with chemotherapy. [^{225}Ac]Ac-Lintuzumab was also found to be safe with significant antileukemic effect even when used in a fractionated protocol in combination with low-dose chemotherapy [104, 105, 207, 208].

However, targeting CD33 for the treatment of AML can be challenging as it is also expressed by normal myeloid progenitors, and the level of expression on AML cells is relatively low compared to other targets such as CD20 for NHL. The number of copies of CD33 per AML cells was estimated at 10–20,000 copies depending on the subtype [209, 210]. Other targets with higher levels of expression are being investigated. With 100–300,000 copies of CD45 per leukemic stem cells, this pan-leukocyte protein was suggested as a promising target. It is associated with tyrosine phosphatase activity that regulates signal transduction in hematopoiesis. With the exception of mature erythrocytes and platelets, all hematopoietic cells express CD45 [211]. More than 90% of primary patient samples of ALL express this antigen [212]. After binding, CD45 does not get internalized but remains stable on the cell surface. Anti-CD45 mAbs were first labeled with iodine-131, and the main radioimmunoconjugate was [^{131}I]I-BC8. A study showed the safety and efficiency of the radiolabeled mAb in patients with AML and ALL. [^{131}I]I-BC8 was also used in combination with therapy and in myeloablative conditioning regimens [212–214].

Similar to anti-CD33, yttrium-90 and lutetium-177 were suggested as alternatives to iodine-131 for anti-CD45 mAb. In a syngeneic disseminated leukemia model, yttrium-90 was shown to be more effective than lutetium-177. Despite similar targeting efficiencies, the lower efficacy of lutetium-177 was explained by differences in the radiation properties leading to lower dose and dose rate to the tumor cells [91]. More recently, preclinical investigations of myelosuppression obtained with an anti-CD45 mAb labeled with α-emitters such as bismuth-213 and astatine-211 were reported [215, 216]. A phase I/II clinical trial to assess the side effects and optimal dose of the ^{211}At-labeled BC8-BC10 anti-CD45 mAb followed by donor stem cell transplant is currently ongoing for patients with a relapse or refractory AML, ALL, and myelodysplastic syndrome at the National Cancer Institute, NIH.

Targets studied for mAb-based therapies in AML were recently reviewed [217, 218]. In addition to the ones cited above, current efforts include using mAb to target the alpha chain of the interleukin 2 receptor (CD25), the tumor necrosis factor receptor (CD27), the cyclic ADP-ribose hydrolase (CD38), the cell surface gly-coprotein CD44, the receptor tyrosine kinase (FLT3 or CD135), the BM stromal antigen 1 (CD157), and the type II membrane glycoprotein CLEC12A. Some aim to target leukemic stem cells that seem to be involved in AML relapse [219, 220]. An ^{111}In-labeled mAb targeting the interleukin 3 receptor (CD123, overexpressed by leukemic stem cells) allowed visualization of engrafted primary human AML specimens and showed efficacy in eradicating leukemia in BM of mice (Fig. 14.5) [221–223].

14.3.3 RIT of Solid Tumors

Compared to hematological malignancies, the development of RIT in solid tumors remains a challenge. Numerous studies have been reported over the past three decades but most result in insufficient therapeutic indices [155, 224]. This could be explained by differences in the biology and radiobiology between hematological and solid malignancies. Solid tumors are more radio-resistant, i.e., a higher delivered dose of radia-tion is needed to obtain a therapeutic response equivalent to that of hematological malignan-cies, but injected activity is limited by toxicity. Nonhomogeneous dose distribution has been reported within the tumor tissue because of the binding-site barrier but also because some tumors are poorly vascularized. For tumors that are vascularized, tumor neoangiogenesis is often abnormal, and vessels are more permissive to the accumulation of macromolecules. Nevertheless, the disorganized vessel structure or blood flow and the increased hydrostatic pressure within the tumor tissue can also limit the penetration capac-ity of large molecules such as mAb [225–227]. Hypoxia can also explain the limited efficacy of low LET beta emitters that have been mainly used in RIT. Numerous clinical trials were carried out, but only a few went beyond phase II testing. The cost of RIT clinical trials, its limited access, and

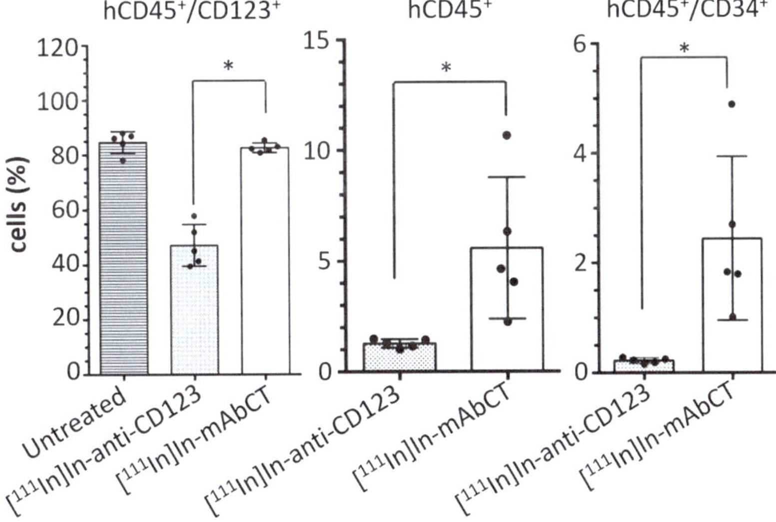

Fig. 14.5 RIT by targeting leukemic stem cells in preclinical models of AML. Injection of [111In] In-anti-CD123 mAb decreased the number of leukemic cells (B). [111In]In-anti-CD123 decreased the percentage of leukemic hCD45+/CD123+ cells in the BM of treated mice as compared to untreated mice or mice that received a control mAb: [111In]In-mAbCT (left panel). Viable cells from the treated mice were inoculated into additional recipient mice, and the repopulation capacity of the BM in the recipient mice was assessed by determining the percentage of leukemic hCD45+ and progenitors cells hCD45+/CD34+ (middle and right panel respectively) (adapted with permission from Leyton et al. [221])

restrictive eligibility criteria might have limited the number of mAb that can progress to phase III [153]. New targets and optimized protocols are therefore needed to treat solid tumors.

14.3.3.1 Targeting of Tumor Cells in Solid Tumors

Some of the most common tumor-associated antigens in solid tumors are the transmembrane glycoprotein A33 for colorectal cancers; EGFR in various tumor types; GD2 expressed by neuroblastomas and melanomas; MUC1 expressed by epithelial cells and that shows aberrant glycosylation in colorectal, pancreatic, breast, and ovarian cancers; TAG-72 in ovarian, pancreatic and colorectal cancer; HER2 in breast cancers; and CA-IX in renal cell carcinoma [154]. In addition to these targets, the two well-studied ones for RIT of solid malignancies are CEA, which is highly expressed in epithelial tumors from the digestive tract, including colorectal, gastric, and pancreatic cancers, and PSMA, which is strongly expressed in prostate cancers. Examples of RIT responses for patients with solid tumors by targeting these targets among others are presented in Table 14.3.

CEA (also known as CD66e) was discovered in the early 1960s [232]. This antigen is expressed in 90% of colorectal cancers and is the recommended prognostic marker for tumor diagnosis and monitoring response to therapy. In colorectal cancers, CEA is involved in cell survival, metastatic behavior, and angiogenesis [233]. Colorectal cancers are sensitive to radiation, and anti-CEA mAbs were available by the late 1990s. The efficacy of RIT was therefore evaluated with mAb labeled first with iodine-131 and subsequently with rhenium-188 or yttrium-90 [234, 235]. After resection of colorectal metastases, single and repeated administrations of [^{131}I]

Table 14.3 Examples of radioimmunoconjugates used for patient treatment with solid tumors

Target	mAb	Radionuclides	Application	Main findings
A33	A33	^{131}I, ^{125}I	Colorectal cancer	Modest antitumor activity, no toxicity
CA-IX	cG250	^{90}Y, ^{177}Lu, ^{131}I	Renal cell carcinoma	Transient toxicity, lack of therapeutic efficacy with ^{131}I, other radionuclides can stabilize disease progression
CEA	hMN-14	^{131}I	Colorectal cancer	Overall response rate of 58% and mean duration response of 9 months in patients with small metastasis refractory to treatment and patients with surgical resection of liver metastases
CEA	T84.66	^{90}Y	Colorectal cancer	No-low response, toxicity
EGFR	425	^{125}I	Brain and CNS tumors	Therapeutic response
EpCAM	NR-LU-10	^{186}Re	Ovarian cancer	Acceptable hematological toxicity, objective response with a single injection
GD2	3F8	^{131}I	Brain and CNS tumors	Significant response of soft tissue lesions and BM disease without improvement of overall survival in neuroblastoma, promising results for patients with brain metastases, durable survival benefit for patients with medulloblastoma
Melanin	PTI-6D2	^{188}Re	Melanoma	Well tolerated and antitumor activity, median overall survival of 13 months
MUC-1	HMFG1	^{90}Y	Ovarian cancer	Prolongation of PFS (80% at 5 years) for tumor nodules less than 2 cm
PSMA	HuJ591	^{177}Lu	Prostate cancer	Well tolerated with reversible myelosuppression, longer overall survival (43.9 months), dose-response relationship
Tenascin-C	81C6	^{90}Y, ^{131}I	Brain and CNS tumors	Prolong median survival after surgery for glioblastomas, ^{90}Y > ^{131}I for bulky disease
TAG72	CC-49	^{177}Lu	Ovarian cancer	Well tolerated, antitumor activity for chemotherapeutic resistant tumors >5 mm or micrometastases

The main findings from clinical studies in different cancer types were summarized from literature [228–231]
CNS central nervous system

I-Labetuzumab (anti-CEA) improved the survival of patients [236, 237]. In advanced medullary thyroid cancer, [^{90}Y]Y-Labetuzumab in combination with chemotherapy and peripheral blood stem cell support showed encouraging therapeutic benefits [238]. More recently, a preclinical study demonstrated that fractionation of a ^{90}Y-labeled anti-CEA mAb could enhance the therapeutic effects observed in CEA-positive cancers [239]. ^{90}Y-labeled mAbs targeting CEA have been also studied in combination strategies with systemic or regional therapies to further improve the therapeutic response [240].

Prostate cancers are a very appealing indication for RIT as these tumors are known to be radiosensitive, and the fact that they can spread to lymph nodes or within the BM makes them accessible to radiolabeled mAb [152]. PSMA is considered as the most established antigen in prostate cancer. PSMA is expressed in 90% of prostate cancers with up to 1000-fold overexpression in tumor cells and metastases as compared to normal prostate. PSMA is expressed at the cell membrane and is not secreted, with increased expression in higher-grade cancers, metastases, and hormone-refractory prostate cancer [241]. Multiple anti-PSMA agents have been described in the literature for targeted radionuclide therapy using a plethora of peptidomimetics [242]. Anti-PSMA mAb were also developed and radiolabeled for RIT applications in prostate cancer, the most commonly studied one is the humanized J591 mAb which binds to the extracellular domain of PSMA and was shown to be nonimmunogenic [84, 138, 243]. For RIT clinical trials, this mAb was labeled with yttrium-90 and later with lutetium-177 [138, 244]. A single dose of [^{177}Lu]Lu-J591 is associated with PSA stabilization in serum and stable disease [84]. However, β-RIT seems to be limited by myelosuppression, especially thrombocytopenia. Nevertheless, in 2013, Tagawa et al. reported complete neutrophil and platelet count recovery from long-term follow-up of 150 patients treated with either ^{177}Lu- or ^{90}Y-J591 [245]. To decrease the BM dose, fractionation has been proposed. A recent phase I/II study reported a higher cumulative dose of [^{177}Lu]Lu-J591 delivered to the tumors, dose-response relationship, increase overall survival, and manageable neutropenia and thrombocytopenia by fractionation [246]. The use of α-emitters as an alternative to β-emitters was also proposed to further reduce the myelotoxicity and therefore allow delivering higher radiations doses to the tumor cells. In this context, [^{225}Ac]Ac-J591 induced tumor regression, decreased PSA level in the serum, and improved survival in preclinical models [247]. A phase I dose-escalation study of the [^{225}Ac]Ac-J591 is currently recruiting to determine the maximum tolerated injected activity in a single-dose protocol for patients with progressive metastatic prostate cancer [248].

A plethora of other potent targets have been evaluated in preclinical models, and some of them led to clinical trials for RIT for different solid tumors using radiolabeled mAb (Table 14.3). In parallel, new targets were proposed and tested in preclinical RIT studies (examples since 2015 are presented in Table 14.4). Some of these targets are already established ones such as EGFR or HER2. Other studies aim to investigate recently identified marker as potent target for RIT of solid tumors. One example is CD133 for the treatment of hepatocellular carcinoma. The biological function of CD133 is unclear, but it has drawn significant attention as a surface marker of primary and metastatic liver cancer stem cells in recent years [276]. CD146, a tumor-associated cell surface glycoprotein has also been suggested for the treatment of melanoma and osteosarcoma using RIT [267, 277].

14.3.3.2 Indirect RIT by Targeting Antigens Within the Tumor Microenvironment

Most targeted strategies in oncology focus on targeting cancer cells. Tumor tissues are not only composed of malignant cells but should be considered as an ecosystem where the stroma also plays crucial roles in tumor initiation, progression, and dissemination [278]. For these reasons, some RIT strategies were developed to target other components of the tumor tissue, including stroma and vasculature. Some cells within the microenvironment have been targeted in the past such as activated fibroblasts that express the

Table 14.4 Examples of tumor cell expressed antigens targeted by radiolabeled mAb in preclinical RIT studies since 2015

Target	mAb	Radionuclides	Tumor models	References
EGFR	Panitumumab, cetuximab	^{212}Pb, ^{131}I, ^{177}Lu, ^{213}Bi, ^{188}Re	Colon adenocarcinoma, squamous cell carcinoma, oral squamous cell carcinoma, bladder carcinoma, lung cancer	[249–255]
HER2	Trastuzumab	^{177}Lu, ^{188}Re, ^{211}At	Breast carcinoma, colon adenocarcinoma, gastric cancer	[85, 256, 257]
hK2	11B6, hu11B6	^{177}Lu, ^{225}Ac	Prostate cancer, breast cancer	[258–261]
Melanin	Benzamide, h8C3	^{131}I, ^{177}Lu, ^{213}Bi	Melanoma	[250, 262]
B7-H3	376.96	^{212}Pb	Ovarian cancer, pancreatic ductal adenocarcinoma	[263, 264]
L1-CAM	chCE7	^{177}Lu, ^{67}Cu, ^{161}Tb	Ovarian carcinoma	[265]
CA-IX	Girentuximab	^{177}Lu	Metastatic renal cell carcinoma	[266]
CD146	OI-3	^{125}I, ^{177}Lu	Osteosarcoma	[267]
ROBO1	Anti-ROBO1 IgG	^{90}Y	Small cell lung cancer	[268]
TfR	TSP-A01	^{90}Y	Pancreatic cancer	[269]
CD138	B-B4	^{213}Bi	Epithelial ovarian carcinoma	[270]
CD133	AC133, AC133.1	^{131}I	Colorectal cancer	[271, 272]
MISRII	16F12	^{177}Lu, ^{213}Bi	Ovarian cancer	[273]
CD147	059-053	^{90}Y	Refractory pancreatic cancer	[274]
FZD10	OTSA101	^{211}At	Synovial sarcoma	[275]

fibroblast activation protein (FAP). FAP is a serine protease that is highly expressed in primary and metastatic colorectal carcinomas [279]. It was proposed as a potent target for RIT using an anti-FAP mAb: [^{131}I]I-F19. Unfortunately, the treatment was not associated with clinical benefit. Some promising results were obtained in a preclinical study where the injection of ^{177}Lu-labeled anti-FAP mAb delayed tumor growth and/or extended survival of the treated groups [280]. New strategies are now focusing on targeting FAP by small molecule inhibitors for targeted radionuclide therapy [281].

Other markers within the microenvironment have also been identified as potent targets, especially proteins involved in neoangiogenesis [282]. The most common one is the vascular endothelial growth factor (VEGF) and its receptor VEGFR. The biodistribution of an anti-VEGFR mAb labeled with lutetium-177 showed high specific tumor uptake and high tumor-to-blood ratios in a model of non-small cell lung cancer [283]. Many other cell surface receptors and extracellular adhesion molecules that regulate angiogenic processes have been identified for targeted therapies [282]. The extra domain B of fibronectin (ED-B fibronectin) is a promising target present in the perivascular space of many aggressive solid tumors, especially in the modified extracellular matrix surrounding newly formed blood vessels [284]. Radiolabeled mAbs targeting ED-B fibronectin have demonstrated efficacy in tumor xenografts of head and neck cancers, gliomas, and colorectal cancers [285–287]. Endoglin (CD150) is an accessory protein of the transforming growth factor β receptor family expressed by proliferating cells in the activated endothelium [288]. ^{177}Lu-labeled TRC105, an anti-endoglin mAb, inhibited tumor growth and increased survival in breast tumor-bearing mice [289].

It should be noted that some of these targets are also expressed on the tumor cells themselves. This can actually help to further increase the dose of radiation delivered to the tumor. For instance, FAP and VEGFR are known to be expressed by some cancer cells in addition to the cells within the microenvironment [290, 291]. Another example is the integrins, a family of transmembrane glycoproteins composed of many α and β subunit heterodimers; they were first identified on active angiogenic endothelium but were later shown to be expressed by tumor cells as well. ^{90}Y-labeled anti-$\alpha_6\beta_4$ or anti-$\alpha_v\beta_3$ mAbs showed promising therapeutic benefits in murine pancreatic cancer and glioblastoma multiforme xenografts, respectively [292, 293].

14.3.4 Prospects to Improve Radioimmunotherapy Efficacy and Reduce Toxicity

Despite the safety and efficacy of the radiolabeled anti-CD20 mAb approved by the FDA and the EMA for the treatment of NHL, RIT is not commonly applied in routine clinical practice. Multiple factors can explain the limited use of these radiopharmaceuticals including availability, concerns about radiation toxicity, and the development of competing therapeutic strategies. We will focus on recent developments that address RIT limitations for both hematological malignancies and solid tumors [23, 117, 153, 155, 224]. Some aim to further increase the efficacy of RIT on the tumor cells, while others aim to decrease toxicity to normal tissues.

14.3.4.1 Locoregional Approaches

Locoregional approaches have been proposed for tumors that tend to grow in a defined compartment such as astrocytoma, liver, ovarian, bladder, and head and neck cancers [224]. Locoregional administration of radiolabeled mAb is particularly appealing for brain tumors [294]. When tight junctions are disrupted leading to an opening of the blood-brain barrier, systemic administration of mAb can be performed. However, the recurrence of brain tumors such as primary malignant gliomas is indicative of eradication failure. To improve the local control and patient outcome, local administration of radiolabeled mAb has been tested, especially by targeting tenascin-C [295]. These methods consist of bolus injections into the tumor or tumor resection cavity after surgery [296]. In general, local administration of radiolabeled mAb showed improved targeting as compared to intravenous administration [297]. It also resulted in less toxicity than systemic delivery and was therefore proposed for other tumor types. In a murine model of gastric cancer, intraperitoneal injections of a ^{213}Bi-labeled mAb targeting the mutant d9-E-cadherin significantly increased the survival of treated mice [298]. Nevertheless, this approach cannot be applied to every tumor type and is not suitable for disseminated cancers.

14.3.4.2 RIT in Combination Regimens

RIT can be combined with other therapeutic strategies to improve the therapeutic index. Chemotherapeutic drugs or EBRT, in addition to fractionation of the injected activity, have been proposed and were demonstrated to be efficient, as described previously. In addition, physical methods such as hyperthermia or pulsed high-intensity focused ultrasound seem to be able to increase the efficacy of RIT [153]. Chemical methods to further enhance the internalization of the radiolabeled mAb have been investigated by using cell-penetrating peptides or vasoactive agents such as angiotensin II [299]. Inhibitors of poly(ADP-ribose) polymerases (PARP) compromise the cell ability to repair DNA damage [300]; thus, they can increase the response to radiopharmaceuticals [301] including radiolabeled mAb. The triple combination of a ^{177}Lu-anti-EGFR mAb, conventional chemotherapy (docetaxel + doxorubicin), and a PARP inhibitor (rucaparib) eradicated tumors and metastasis in orthotopic and metastatic xenograft models of triple-negative breast cancer [302].

In addition, RIT can be combined with traditional immunotherapy for better efficacy such as naked mAb. Repetto-Llamazares et al. recently showed that [^{177}Lu]Lu-Lilotomab (anti-CD37) interact synergistically with Rituximab to improve tumor suppression and increase survival in a murine model of NHL [303]. To overcome nonuniform dose distribution in solid tumors, the use of a radiolabeled mAb cocktail has also been proposed. Therapeutic benefits were observed when combining ^{131}I-labeled anti-CEA and ^{131}I-labeled anti-CSAp (color-specific antigen-p) in colorectal cancer xenografts or by using a mixture of an anti-HER-2 with an anti-TAG-72 both labeled with bismuth-213 in mice bearing intraperitoneal human colon carcinoma xenografts [304, 305]. In contrast, radiolabeled anti-CD20, anti-HLA-DR, or anti-CD22 alone delivered higher absolute uptake than the combination of the three in lymphoma xenograft models [306].

Other strategies combining radiotherapy and stimulation of the immune system could in theory also be associated with RIT. They involve combination with checkpoint inhibitors targeting PD-1, its ligand PDL-1 or CTLA-4, oncolytic viruses, or chimeric antigen receptor T cells (CAR T cells). These strategies enable new options to improve overall patient outcomes, especially for previously untreatable tumors [307, 308], to be considered for future studies. For example, therapeutic vaccines designed to induce the activation of T cells against tumor antigens have also been combined with radioactive molecules and showed a significant increase in progression-free survival [142, 309].

14.3.4.3 mAb Fragments

Reducing hematological toxicity implies reducing BM exposure. One way to achieve this is by increasing the blood clearance of the radioimmunoconjugate. Enzymatically cleaved mAb fragments (F(ab')$_2$, F(ab'), Fab), genetically engineered protein scaffolds such as minibodies, diabodies or single-chain variable fragments (scFv), and smaller molecules like nanobodies or affibodies have been investigated for this purpose in preclinical models (Fig. 14.6). The smaller the antibody derivative, the faster its blood clearance will be. Faster clearance is also attributed in part by the inability of the mAb fragments to bind to the FcRn receptors. At 150 kDa, IgG exhibit the longest circulation times with serum $t_{1/2}$ of 1–3 weeks, fragments at 50–110 kDa have $t_{1/2}$ of 3–10 h, and smaller protein scaffolds (7–28 kDa) have even shorter $t_{1/2}$ of 0.5–4 h [310]. The size of the fragment will also affect its excretion route. Proteins with molecular weight above 60 kDa will be eliminated by the liver whereas smaller ones will be excreted through the kidneys. Consequently, the radionuclide used should be adapted to these shorter $t_{1/2}$.

The other advantage of using smaller fragments is their ability to cross the vascular wall of the tumor blood vessels and diffuse through the extracellular matrix [311]. However, a faster clearance limits the time frame for target interaction. Moreover, the ability to cross the vascular wall more efficiently also means that the radiopharmaceutical may diffuse back into the circulation and compromise tumor retention. Consequently, this can result in a decrease in cumulative radioactivity in tumor tissues as compared to full mAb. In general, higher injected activities are required to compensate for the loss of activity retention, which increases potent renal toxicity [78].

Therapeutic efficacy has been reported in the literature using mAb fragments. In a metastatic mouse model of ovarian cancer, intraperitoneal

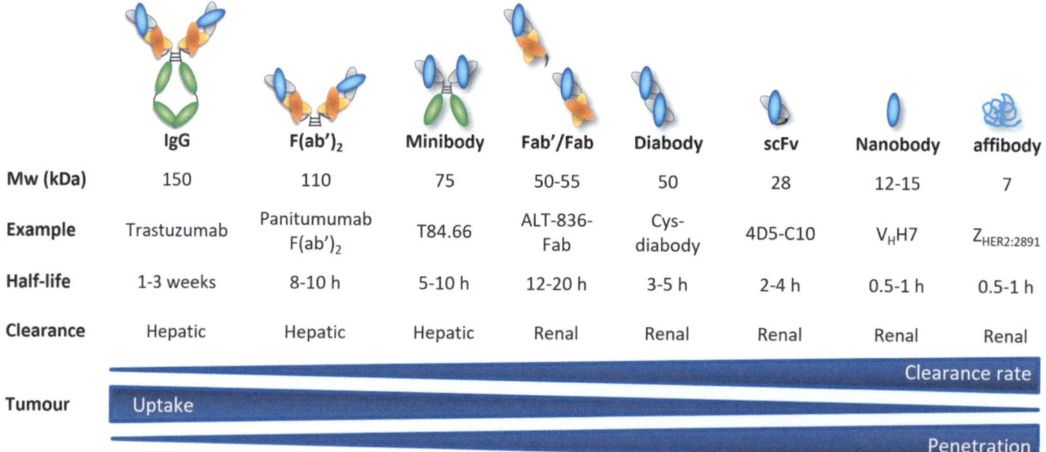

	IgG	F(ab')$_2$	Minibody	Fab'/Fab	Diabody	scFv	Nanobody	affibody
Mw (kDa)	150	110	75	50-55	50	28	12-15	7
Example	Trastuzumab	Panitumumab F(ab')$_2$	T84.66	ALT-836-Fab	Cys-diabody	4D5-C10	V$_H$H7	Z$_{HER2:2891}$
Half-life	1-3 weeks	8-10 h	5-10 h	12-20 h	3-5 h	2-4 h	0.5-1 h	0.5-1 h
Clearance	Hepatic	Hepatic	Hepatic	Renal	Renal	Renal	Renal	Renal

Fig. 14.6 Antibody derivatives. For the different constructs, the molecular weight (Mw), an example of a validated compound, the serum half-life, and the clearance route and rate, in addition to the tumor uptake and penetration, are given (adapted with permission from Fu et al. [310] in accordance with the Creative Commons Attribution License (CC BY 4.0))

injections of [²¹¹At]At-MX35-F(ab′)₂, which recognizes the sodium-dependent phosphate transport protein 2b (NaPi2b), were able to decrease the number of macroscopic and microscopic tumors and ascites [312]. A dose-dependent response was observed using a fractionation approach with this mAb fragment, but complete remission was achieved only with high injected activity [313]. Affibodies present high target specificity and a rapid blood clearance with favorable tumor uptake. A radiolabeled anti-HER2 affibody ($Z_{HER2:342}$) showed fast extravasation and efficient tumor penetration by imaging [314]. The fusion of this affibody labeled with lutetium-177 with the albumin-binding domain, to prolong its circulation, prevented tumor formation in animals bearing human ovarian cancer xenografts [315]. The results obtained with mAb fragments in general have not been as successful as full mAb, and more studies are needed to determine if these molecules could improve RIT outcomes. Because they clear predominantly through the kidneys, there are concerns about increased irradiation dose to this organ. Nevertheless, mAb fragments and derivatives are also studied as highly potent tracers for imaging purposes [28, 310, 316–319].

14.3.4.4 Pre-Targeting

In conventional RIT, the radiolabeled mAb (or mAb fragment) is injected in one step (Fig. 14.7a). In pre-targeting strategies (PRIT) the injection of the mAb and the therapeutic radionuclide is separated into two steps (Fig. 14.7b). The nonradioactive mAb is first injected allowing for tumor accumulation and slow clearance of the unbound mAb from the blood over a few days. In the second step, a radioactive small molecule that binds with the tumor-bound mAb is injected. This molecule will be cleared rapidly from the blood [320] increasing the tumor-to-normal tissue ratio but decreasing the overall tumor uptake as compared to conventional RIT. Between the two steps, an optional clearing agent can be injected to optimize the elimination of the unbound circulating mAb. The main goal of PRIT is to achieve the same targeting performance as that of peptidomimetics and small molecules used in targeted radionuclide therapy, which have a fast blood clearance and reduced side effects. But compared to targeted radionuclide therapy using peptides and small molecules, mAb can target a wider range of antigens and have higher specificity and affinity, meaning that PRIT could in theory be more powerful [321].

PRIT was first developed in the 1980s and was further optimized over the years [321–327]. At least four pre-targeting mechanisms have been developed and tested: (A) (strep)avidin-biotin interaction, (B) bispecific mAb, (C) oligonucleotides hybridization, and (D) click chemistry (Fig. 14.7c) [323]. For all these strategies, the optimal dosage of the mAb, the optional clearing agent, and the radioligand, in addition to the time frame for the different injections, are key parameters that need to be determined.

The first mechanism is based on the biological interaction between biotin and avidin or streptavidin which has a strong noncovalent interaction ($Kd = 10^{-15}$ M). A conjugated mAb with avidin or streptavidin, which possesses four binding sites for biotin is first injected, followed by the injection of a clearing agent and then the radiolabeled biotin molecule. Streptavidin was shown to be more adapted for pre-targeting strategies than avidin because of its higher in vivo stability. Another streptavidin-biotin configuration uses biotinylated mAb instead of (strep)avidin ones in a three-step protocol. Glycosylated avidin is injected as a scavenger, then non-glycosylated streptavidin that will bind to the biotin-mAb, and finally the radiolabeled biotin is given resulting in a "sandwich approach" [328, 329]. The avidin-biotin strategy has been extensively studied and has shown significant benefits over traditional RIT [330]. In patients with NHL, PRIT against CD20 led to better therapeutic responses than RIT as higher injected activities of the radioligand were tolerated [331]. Similar observations were reported in preclinical studies with solid tumors [332]. Using an α-emitter, PRIT with an avidin-conjugated MX35 mAb (anti-NaPi2b) and a ²¹¹At-labeled biotinylated succinylated poly-L-lysine was shown to be more efficient than RIT in a preclinical model of intraperitoneal ovarian tumors [333]. Nevertheless, the use of this PRIT strategy for clinical applica-

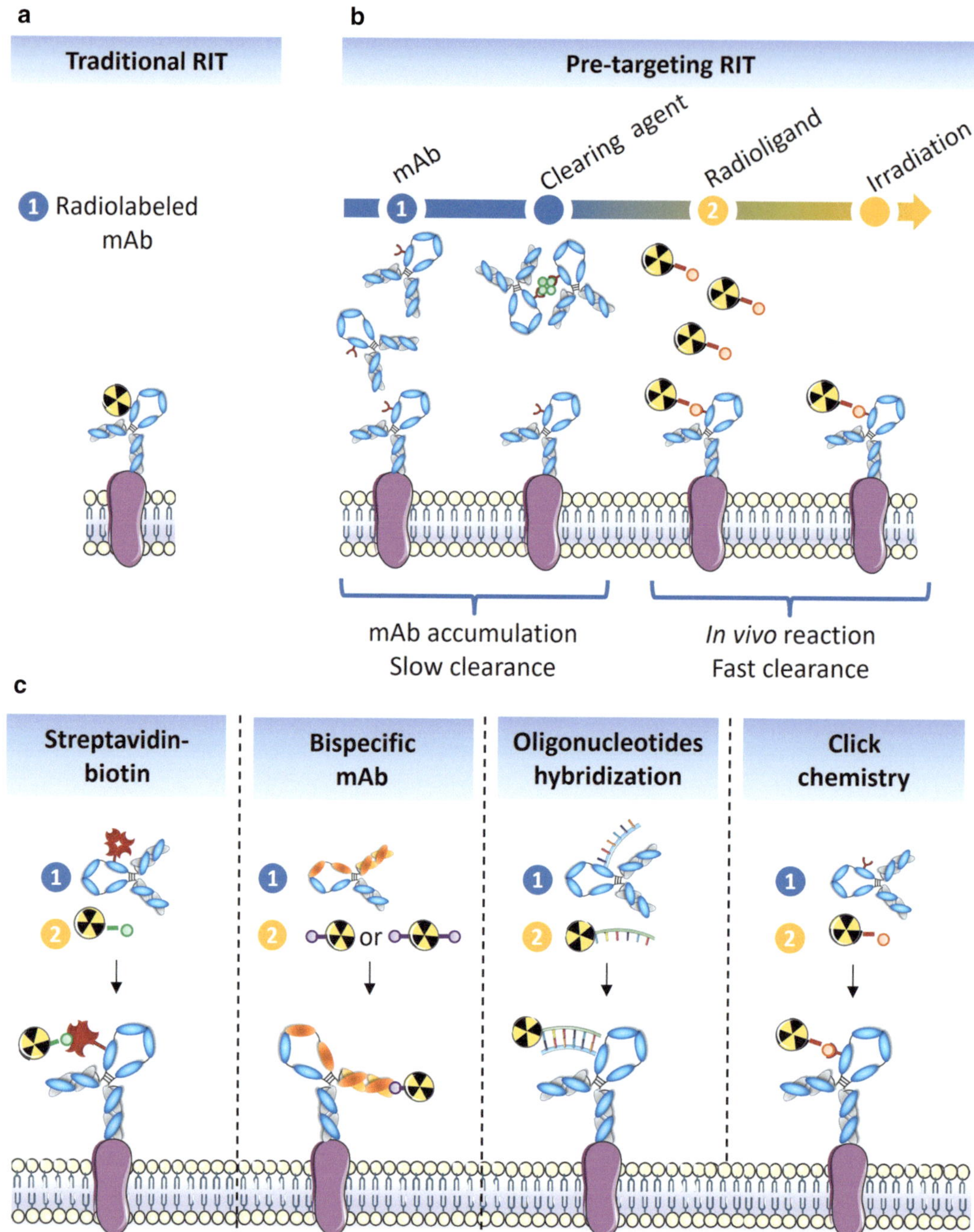

Fig. 14.7 PRIT strategies versus traditional RIT. (**a**) Traditional RIT consists of injecting a radioimmunoconjugate that will accumulate in tumor tissue. The unbound radiolabeled mAb fraction will be cleared slowly from the blood, which could be associated to potent myelotoxicity. (**b**) In pre-targeting strategies, first the nonradioactive mAb is administered with optimal accumulation into the tumors accomplished within 24–48 h. A clearing agent could also be injected to accelerate the clearance of the unbound circulating mAb (optional). In a second step, the radioligand is injected and will bind to the tumor-bound mAb and will be cleared rapidly from the blood by the kidneys or the liver. (**c**) Using the previously described two-step protocol, different PRIT strategies have been developed and are presented in the bottom panel: the (strept)avidin-biotin approach, bispecific mAb with one arm that will recognize the cancer target and the second one a radiolabeled monovalent or bivalent hapten, the oligonucleotide hybridization, and the click chemistry technology (some graphical elements were adapted from Servier Medical Art (www.servier.com))

tion has declined. The development of immunogenic responses, difficulties in producing streptavidin conjugates, and interference of endogenous biotin complicate translation [326].

Another strategy developed in the 1980s involves bispecific mAb and radiolabeled haptens. One arm of the bispecific mAb will bind to the target antigen expressed by the tumor cells, and the other arm will recognize a radiolabeled hapten [334]. Hapten is a nonimmunogenic small molecule such as a peptide that is characterized by a high affinity and specificity for the second binding site of the bispecific mAb. Given its low molecular weight, haptens allow for fast distribution and rapid clearance [335]. Since high-affinity hapten may preferably bind to the circulating mAb fraction than the cell-bound fraction, mAb-clearing agents are recommended to optimize the tumor uptake [335]. Using this strategy, the injection of an anti-GPA33 (glycoprotein A33) bispecific mAb followed by the injection of a clearing agent and then a [^{177}Lu]Lu-DOTA-Bn eradicated tumor growth (100% CR) and increased survival in a colorectal cancer xenograft model [336]. The use of bivalent haptens that can cross-link two cell-bound bispecific mAb results in an "enhanced affinity system" which increases tumor uptake and retention and avoid to inject mAb-clearing agents [337, 338]. This strategy has been extensively studied in animal models and in patients, with ongoing clinical trials [339–342]. Anti-CD38/[^{90}Y]Y-DOTA bispecific construct showed 100% complete remission and superiority to the strepatividin-biotin-based CD38 PRIT in multiple myeloma and NHL xenograft models [340]. TF2, a trivalent mAb with two binding sites for CEA and one for a radiolabeled peptide (IMP288) accumulates efficiently in different cancer types in patients (Fig. 14.8a, b), is safe and shows significant inhibition of tumor growth using either ^{177}Lu- or ^{213}Bi-IMP288 in preclinical and clinical studies [95, 343]. DOTA-PRIT can also be performed to target internalizing membrane antigens such as HER2 as shown in Fig. 14.8c. In a preclinical breast cancer xenografts model, a fractionated PRIT protocol was well tolerated and showed efficient accumulation of [^{177}Lu]Lu-DOTA-Bn after each treatment cycle and led to CR [345].

The PRIT method based on the hybridization of an oligonucleotide conjugated to a mAb and a radiolabeled complementary oligonucleotide was introduced in the 1990s [348]. This strategy uses synthetic DNA analogs, phosphorodiamidate morpholino oligomers (MORFs) to enhance in vivo stability [349]. In a preclinical PRIT study, a MORF-conjugated mAb was first injected in mice bearing TAG-72 expressing tumors, followed by the injection of a ^{188}Re-labeled complementary MORF. No evidence of toxicity was observed and effective tumor growth inhibition was reported [350].

The most recent strategy employed for PRIT is based on in vivo bioorthogonal click chemistry. These chemical reactions can occur in vivo without interfering with native biochemical processes. The most popular click chemistry technique is the inverse-demand Diels-Alder cycloaddition reaction between trans-cyclooctene (TCO) and tetrazine (Tz). By targeting A33 in colorectal carcinoma mouse models, the administration of huA33-TCO mAb followed by the injection of either [^{64}Cu]Cu-Tz-SarAr or [^{177}Lu]Lu-DOTA-PEG$_7$-Tz led to clear tumor visualization by PET imaging and CR in PRIT studies, respectively (Fig. 14.8d, e) [346, 347]. Dose-dependent therapeutic response was obtained with TCO-conjugated anti-CA19.9 mAb and [^{177}Lu]Lu-DOTA-PEG$_7$-Tz [351]. The same mAb in ^{225}Ac-PRIT showed a significant therapeutic response and prolonged median survival of mice with pancreatic ductal adenocarcinoma [352]. A-PRIT showed higher dose delivered to the tumor and lower absorbed doses in the blood, liver, spleen, or bone. In a preclinical colorectal cancer model, the same strategy using a TCO-anti-TAG-72 mAb with [^{212}Pb]Pb-Tz-labeled radioligands reduced tumor growth rate and improved median survival with minimal toxicity [353]. In 2018, Stéen et al. concluded that among all PRIT strategies, the TCO-Tz strategy is the most attractive system for PRIT because of fast reaction kinetics, high specificity, advantages of small molecule, synthetic accessibility, irreversibility of the reaction, bioorthogonality of the ligation, and no immunogenicity issues reported so far [326].

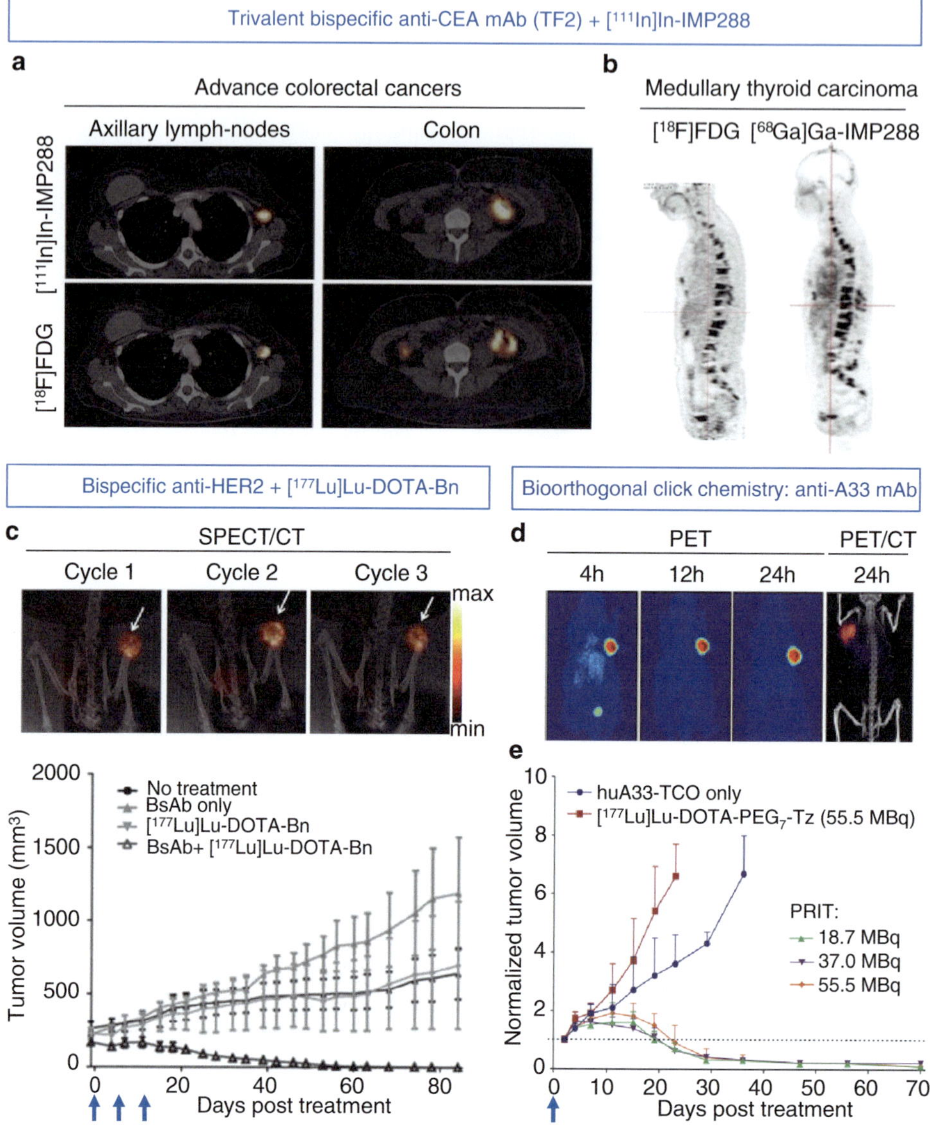

Fig. 14.8 Examples of PRIT results obtained in solid tumors. (**a**) Similar to [18F]FDG PET scans, pre-targeted SPECT images with the trivalent bispecific anti-CEA TF2 mAb and [111In]In-IMP288 show accumulation in axillary lymph-node metastasis (left panels) and primary colon tumor (right panels) with low background in normal tissues in a patient with advance colorectal cancer. Adapted with permission from Schoffelen et al. [343]. (**b**) Using the same strategy, a higher number of spine bone lesions can be seen using the TF2/[68Ga]Ga-IMP288 strategy as compared to [18F]FDG PET (533 versus 425, respectively) (adapted from Bodet-Milin et al. [344], copyright in accordance with the CC BY 4.0.) (**c**) Using a bispecific mAb, fractionated anti-HER2 PRIT of three injection cycles showed efficient accumulation of [177Lu] Lu-DOTA-Bn (top panel: SPECT/CT images obtained 24 h after each cycle of injection) and led to CR (bottom graph, injection cycles are highlighted with arrows) in all mice bearing breast tumors (reproduced with permission from Cheal et al. [345] in accordance with CC BY 4.0.). By targeting A33, bioorthogonal in vivo click chemistry is also efficient for imaging (**d**) and therapy (**e**). (**d**) The injection of a huA33-TCO mAb followed by [64Cu] Cu-Tz-SarAr shows high tumor-to-background imaging contrast in a preclinical model of colorectal carcinoma (adapted with permission from Zeglis et al. [346]). (**e**) In a colorectal carcinoma model as well, a similar PRIT strategy using a huA33-TCO/[177Lu]Lu-DOTA-PEG7-Tz led to complete tumor responses (adapted with permission from Membreno et al. [347])

14.3.4.5 Imaging and Dosimetry Prior to RIT

In EBRT, treatment planning is aimed at delivering predefined doses to tumors while sparing healthy organs [354]. In contrast, radionuclide therapy including RIT has most commonly been based on a "one-dose-fits-all" approach in which the same amount of radioactivity is injected into all patients, sometimes adjusted to patient weight or body surface area [355]. This amount of radioactivity has been empirically determined based on results from phase I/II studies designed to assess the maximum tolerated dose. Even if this is not optimal, the use of similar injected activity for all patients has yielded therapeutic responses for hematological malignancies. In contrast, the higher repair capability of solid tumors may require a personalized approach and a better understanding of the dose-response relationships. Many clinical trials using the "one-dose-fits-all" approach for solid tumors have failed to achieve a therapeutic response. By considering a dosimetric approach prior to treatment, better results might have been obtained [78, 153].

Dosimetry aims at estimating the radiation dose delivered to healthy organs and tumors to obtain the optimal biological effect, i.e., the maximum eradication of tumor cells with tolerable and/or manageable toxicity. This has the potential of limiting unnecessary toxicity in patients that would require a lower injected activity or improving the outcome for those for which a higher injected activity would be required to achieve the same biological effect [23]. The procedure requires the knowledge of the physical properties of the radioisotope and the pharmacokinetic behavior of the radiopharmaceutical. For the latter, sequential imaging studies prior to treatment can be performed by imaging the therapeutic radiolabeled mAb or using an imaging companion.

Multiple studies tried to correlate the tumor response to the radiation absorbed dose, as it was already established for EBRT, but with less success [356]. The biological mechanisms involved in RIT (CMC, ADCC, and/or ADCP, described earlier in this chapter) can actually modify the expected response. Furthermore, RIT delivers heterogeneous dose irradiation with a constantly changing dose rate. Dose-response relationships are also difficult to achieve for hematological toxicity [149].

The presence of target cells within the BM and/or the effects of prior therapies that might have already compromised the hematopoietic cell reserve making it difficult to predict hematological toxicity. Thus, the accurate calculation of the absorbed dose in nuclear medicine can be challenging [357] but imaging can be an asset. Nevertheless, the accuracy of the absorbed dose calculation is also impacted by the uncertainty of each step in the process such as the uncertainty of the injected activity, registration, reconstruction, segmentation of volume of interest, or the integration to determine the cumulated activity [358–360].

Imaging and dosimetry calculations prior to treatments have already been shown to improve the prediction of the safety and effectiveness of radiopharmaceuticals including mAb [361–364]. Improved dose-response correlations were indeed observed when accurate dosimetry assessments were performed for RIT with the anti CD20 [^{131}I] I-Tositumomab, for example [365]. Individualized iodine-124 PET image-based dosimetry could also be an asset for the optimization of RIT in patients with renal cancer (CA-IX targeting) or colorectal cancer (anti-A33 RIT) [366]. Using ^{177}Lu-labeled mAb that can be imaged by SPECT, dosimetry can also be performed [354]. In a PRIT clinical study using an anti-CEA bispecific mAb that also recognizes a ^{177}Lu-labeled peptide, the use of a Monte Carlo-based dosimetric method prior to PRIT allowed identifying patients at risk of developing toxicity [367]. In general, the accuracy of quantitative images will be impacted by factors such as spatial resolution, accurate attenuation and scatter correction, and sensitivity of the system, in addition to the use of an adequate collimator (based on the energy of the emissions for SPECT).

In addition to providing support information for dosimetry for treatment and dose planning for RIT, imaging can be used for patient selection for other targeted therapies including mAb-based strategies prior to treatment. With an improved spatial resolution allowing better delineation of tumors and organs in general and a higher sensitivity, PET is superior over SPECT and more popular [23]. In 2017, Moek et al. reported 24 antibodies or antibody-related therapeutics labeled with PET radionuclides for theranostic purposes that are used in patients [31]. Among all

PET isotopes, zirconium-89 is the most popular radionuclide for immunoPET imaging [368]. Its $t_{1/2}$ of 78.4 h is adequate for IgG labeling, and its very short range in tissues before annihilation (less than 0.5 mm in water) leads to good image quality and high spatial resolution. In the past 5 years, multiple clinical studies reported the feasibility of using ^{89}Zr-immunoPET and are summarized in Table 14.5. Many targets are being investigated. For most of the studies, the radiopharmaceutical is based on a validated mAb already used in the clinic. The most frequently investigated therapeutic mAb is the anti-HER2 Trastuzumab. [^{89}Zr]Zr-Trastuzumab can detect unsuspected HER2 expressing metastases in some patients with HER2-negative primary breast cancer and can also be used to monitor alteration of HER2 expression over time [387, 388]. Also, the anti-PSMA mAb, [^{89}Zr]Zr-J591, was able to detect bone lesions that were not highlighted by [^{18}F]FDG or other imaging techniques in patients with prostate cancer (Fig. 14.9) [374].

Table 14.5 Summary of ^{89}Zr-immunoPET clinical studies using mAb in cancer patients over the past 5 years

Target	mAb	Cancer type	References
CD20	Rituximab	Diffuse large B-cell lymphoma	[369, 370]
HER2	Trastuzumab	Esophagogastric cancer	[371]
	Pertuzumab	Breast cancer	[372]
HER3	GSK2849330	Breast, head and neck, cervical, ovarian, prostate colorectal cancers	[373]
PSMA	J591	Prostate cancer	[374]
VEGF-A	Bevacizumab	Glioma, renal cell carcinoma	[375–377]
CA-IX	Girentuximab	Renal cell carcinoma	[378]
TGFβ	Fresolimumab	Glioma	[379]
EGFR	Cetuximab	Head and neck, colorectal cancer	[380–382]
MSLN	MMOT0530A	Pancreatic, ovarian cancer	[383]
PD-L1	Atezolizumab	Solid tumors	[384]
PD-1	Nivolumab	Non-small-cell lung cancer	[385]
STEAP1	MSTP2109A	Prostate cancer	[386]

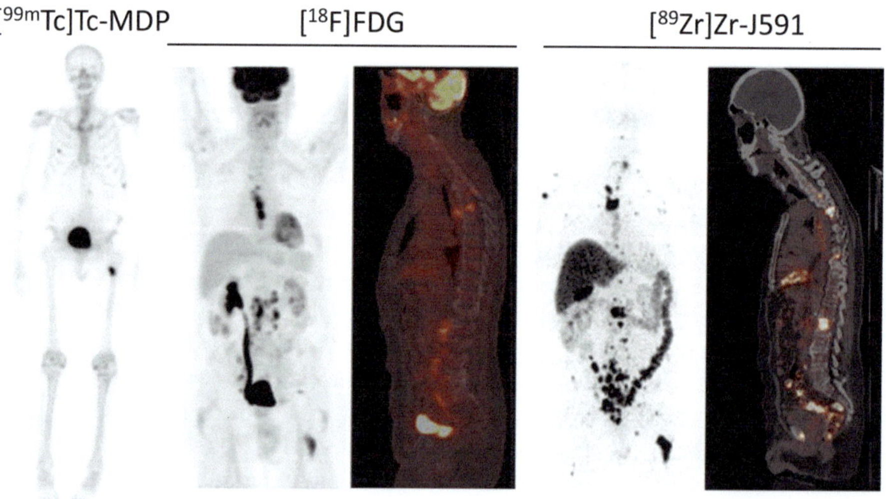

Fig. 14.9 Example of [^{89}Zr]Zr-J591 (anti-PSMA) immunoPET images in a patient with advanced metastatic prostate cancer. By targeting PSMA with the [^{89}Zr] Zr-J591, additional osseous metastases were observed as compared to the gold standard [^{18}F]FDG using PET and as compared to SPECT images with the bone-seeking agent: [^{99m}Tc]Tc-methyldiphosphonate (MDP) (Adapted with permission from Pandit-Taskar et al. [389])

^{89}Zr-ImmunoPET images can also be used for dosimetry prior RIT, and methods have been proposed to improve the accuracy of absorbed dose calculation using zirconium-89 images [390].

14.4 Conclusions

Radiolabeled mAbs have been used for more than 30 years for cancer imaging and therapy. The success of radioimmunoconjugates relies on the identification of a valid target expressed by the tumor cells, the selection of a suitable mAb, and its effective radiolabeling with an adapted radionuclide, leading to a radiolabeled mAb with good antigen binding, no/low immunogenicity, good tumor penetration and retention, and suitable rate of clearance to spare normal tissues. The optimal in vivo behavior of the radioimmunoconjugate depends on the biochemical processes related to the protein target, the properties of the mAb, and the tumor microenvironment. Preclinical studies and their design have a critical role in in vivo mAb selection, development, and optimization. The selection of the most relevant animal species and tumor models, the screening of various radioimmunoconjugate candidates, the design of the studies including multiple adequate time points biodistribution, specificity assessment (i.e., by comparing to an irrelevant mAb and/or using knockout/knock-in models), optimal dosage to ensure high tumor-to-background ratios, sufficient number of mice for statistical analysis, and whole-body imaging, in addition to quality controls of the radioimmunoconjugate (e.g., aggregation, radiolysis, and immunoreactive fraction) are important parameters to consider for efficient in vivo validation. Furthermore, the use of multiple tumor cell lines and/or cancer types with different expression levels of the target but still showing the efficacy in RIT studies further increases the robustness and justification of the radiolabeled mAb development.

The first successes of radiolabeled mAb were obtained in hematological malignancies with the anti-CD20 mAb Bexxar and Zevalin, in combination strategies, but also in first-line treatment. Despite their successes, these strategies are not widely used since other therapeutic strategies were judged to have a higher impact on patient survival and could be easier to implement on-site than radiopharmaceuticals. Nevertheless, mAbs have emerged as a leading class of biological drugs with evidence of clinical benefits. A diversity of new targets was investigated and the development of radiolabeled mAb was extended to other hematological malignancies and solid tumors. Despite the first challenges faced in solid tumors, the success of newly validated immunoconjugates and development of new labeling methods with new radionuclides in addition to new strategies to improved RIT are all in favor of large-scale use of radiopharmaceuticals in clinical practice for cancer RIT. Further improvements in the use of radiolabeled mAb might be achieved by better target selection based on improved understanding of cancer biology in addition to the development of new ADC strategies and recombinant protein engineering to improve uptake and pharmacokinetics.

Conflicts of Interest The authors report no conflict of interest with the material presented in this study. Dr. François Bénard is co-founder, director, and shareholder of Alpha-9 Theranostics, a radiopharmaceutical company. No other potential conflicts of interest relevant to this article exist.

References

1. Köhler G, Milstein C. Continuous cultures of fused cells secreting antibody of predefined specificity. Nature. 1975;256(5517):495–7. https://doi.org/10.1038/256495a0.
2. Scott AM, Allison JP, Wolchok JD. Monoclonal antibodies in cancer therapy. Cancer Immun. 2012;12:14.
3. Dobrenkov K, Cheung N-KV. 30 – Therapeutic antibodies and immunologic conjugates. In: Niederhuber JE, Armitage JO, Kastan MB, Doroshow JH, Tepper JE, editors. Abeloff's clinical oncology. 6th ed. Philadelphia: Sanders; 2020. p. 486–99. e8.
4. Goldenberg DM, DeLand F, Kim E, Bennett S, Primus FJ, van Nagell JR Jr, et al. Use of radiolabeled antibodies to carcinoembryonic antigen for the detection and localization of diverse cancers by external photoscanning. N Engl J Med. 1978;298(25):1384–6. https://doi.org/10.1056/NEJM197806222982503.

5. Mach JP, Buchegger F, Forni M, Ritschard J, Berche C, Lumbroso JD, et al. Use of radiolabelled monoclonal anti-CEA antibodies for the detection of human carcinomas by external photoscanning and tomoscintigraphy. Immunol Today. 1981;2(12):239–49. https://doi.org/10.1016/0167-5699(81)90011-6.

6. Barbet J, Bardies M, Bourgeois M, Chatal JF, Cherel M, Davodeau F, et al. Radiolabeled antibodies for cancer imaging and therapy. Methods Mol Biol. 2012;907:681–97. https://doi.org/10.1007/978-1-61779-974-7_38.

7. Shimoni A, Zwas ST. Radioimmunotherapy and autologous stem-cell transplantation in the treatment of B-cell non-Hodgkin lymphoma. Semin Nucl Med. 2016;46(2):119–25. https://doi.org/10.1053/j.semnuclmed.2015.10.009.

8. Sharkey RM, Behr TM, Mattes MJ, Stein R, Griffiths GL, Shih LB, et al. Advantage of residualizing radiolabels for an internalizing antibody against the B-cell lymphoma antigen, CD22. Cancer Immunol Immunother. 1997;44(3):179–88.

9. DeNardo GL, DeNardo SJ, O'Donnell RT, Kroger LA, Kukis DL, Meares CF, et al. Are radiometal-labeled antibodies better than iodine-131-labeled antibodies: comparative pharmacokinetics and dosimetry of copper-67-, iodine-131-, and yttrium-90-labeled Lym-1 antibody in patients with non-Hodgkin's lymphoma. Clin Lymphoma. 2000;1(2):118–26.

10. Schroff RW, Foon KA, Beatty SM, Oldham RK, Morgan AC Jr. Human anti-murine immunoglobulin responses in patients receiving monoclonal antibody therapy. Cancer Res. 1985;45(2):879–85.

11. van der Linden EF, van Kroonenburgh MJ, Pauwels EK. Side-effects of monoclonal antibody infusions for the diagnosis and treatment of cancer. Int J Biol Markers. 1988;3(3):147–53.

12. Liu H, Moy P, Kim S, Xia Y, Rajasekaran A, Navarro V, et al. Monoclonal antibodies to the extracellular domain of prostate-specific membrane antigen also react with tumor vascular endothelium. Cancer Res. 1997;57(17):3629–34.

13. Sodee DB, Malguria N, Faulhaber P, Resnick MI, Albert J, Bakale G. Multicenter ProstaScint imaging findings in 2154 patients with prostate cancer. ProstaScint Imaging Centers Urol. 2000;56(6):988–93.

14. Han M, Partin AW. Current clinical applications of the in-capromab Pendetide scan (ProstaScint(R) scan, Cyt-356). Rev Urol. 2001;3(4):165–71.

15. Vivier D, Sharma SK, Zeglis BM. Understanding the in vivo fate of radioimmunoconjugates for nuclear imaging. J Labelled Comp Radiopharm. 2018;61(9):672–92. https://doi.org/10.1002/jlcr.3628.

16. Carrasquillo JA, Mulshine JL, Bunn PA Jr, Reynolds JC, Foon KA, Schroff RW, et al. Indium-111 T101 monoclonal antibody is superior to iodine-131 T101 in imaging of cutaneous T-cell lymphoma. J Nucl Med. 1987;28(3):281–7.

17. Rizzieri D. Zevalin((R)) (ibritumomab tiuxetan): after more than a decade of treatment experience, what have we learned? Crit Rev Oncol Hematol. 2016;105:5–17. https://doi.org/10.1016/j.critrevonc.2016.07.008.

18. Teillaud JL. Engineering of monoclonal antibodies and antibody-based fusion proteins: successes and challenges. Expert Opin Biol Ther. 2005;5(Suppl 1):S15–27. https://doi.org/10.1517/14712598.5.1.S15.

19. Wei W, Rosenkrans ZT, Liu J, Huang G, Luo Q-Y, Cai W. ImmunoPET: concept, design, and applications. Chem Rev. 2020;120(8):3787–851. https://doi.org/10.1021/acs.chemrev.9b00738.

20. McKnight BN, Viola-Villegas NT. (89)Zr-ImmunoPET companion diagnostics and their impact in clinical drug development. J Labelled Comp Radiopharm. 2018;61(9):727–38. https://doi.org/10.1002/jlcr.3605.

21. Beck A, Dumontet C, Joubert N. Antibody-drug conjugates in oncology. Recent success of an ancient concept. Med Sci (Paris). 2019;35(12):1034–42. https://doi.org/10.1051/medsci/2019227.

22. Scott AM, Wolchok JD, Old LJ. Antibody therapy of cancer. Nat Rev Cancer. 2012;12(4):278–87. https://doi.org/10.1038/nrc3236.

23. Bailly C, Bodet-Milin C, Guérard F, Rousseau C, Chérel M, Kraeber-Bodéré F, et al. Prospects for enhancing efficacy of Radioimmunotherapy. In: Hosono M, Chatal J-F, editors. Resistance to Ibritumomab in lymphoma. Cham: Springer International Publishing; 2018. p. 139–53.

24. Ricart AD. Immunoconjugates against solid tumors: mind the gap. Clin Pharmacol Ther. 2011;89(4):513–23. https://doi.org/10.1038/clpt.2011.8.

25. Slastnikova TA, Ulasov AV, Rosenkranz AA, Sobolev AS. Targeted intracellular delivery of antibodies: the state of the art. Front Pharmacol. 2018;9:1208. https://doi.org/10.3389/fphar.2018.01208.

26. Poty S, Mandleywala K, O'Neill E, Knight JC, Cornelissen B, Lewis JS. (89)Zr-PET imaging of DNA double-strand breaks for the early monitoring of response following alpha- and beta-particle radioimmunotherapy in a mouse model of pancreatic ductal adenocarcinoma. Theranostics. 2020;10(13):5802–14. https://doi.org/10.7150/thno.44772.

27. Carmon KS, Azhdarinia A. Application of immunoPET in antibody-drug conjugate development. Mol Imaging. 2018;17:1536012118801223. https://doi.org/10.1177/1536012118801223.

28. Wu AM. Engineered antibodies for molecular imaging of cancer. Methods. 2014;65(1):139–47. https://doi.org/10.1016/j.ymeth.2013.09.015.

29. Aerts HJ, Dubois L, Perk L, Vermaelen P, van Dongen GA, Wouters BG, et al. Disparity between in vivo EGFR expression and 89Zr-labeled cetuximab uptake assessed with PET. J Nucl Med. 2009;50(1):123–31. https://doi.org/10.2967/jnumed.108.054312.

30. Colombo I, Overchuk M, Chen J, Reilly RM, Zheng G, Lheureux S. Molecular imaging in drug development: update and challenges for radiolabeled antibodies and nanotechnology. Methods. 2017;130:23–35. https://doi.org/10.1016/j.ymeth.2017.07.018.

31. Moek KL, Giesen D, Kok IC, de Groot DJA, Jalving M, Fehrmann RSN, et al. Theranostics using antibodies and antibody-related therapeutics. J Nucl Med. 2017;58(Suppl 2):83S–90S. https://doi.org/10.2967/jnumed.116.186940.

32. Chiavenna SM, Jaworski JP, Vendrell A. State of the art in anti-cancer mAbs. J Biomed Sci. 2017;24(1):15. https://doi.org/10.1186/s12929-016-0311-y.

33. Ryman JT, Meibohm B. Pharmacokinetics of monoclonal antibodies. CPT Pharmacometrics Syst Pharmacol. 2017;6(9):576–88. https://doi.org/10.1002/psp4.12224.

34. Cui Y, Cui P, Chen B, Li S, Guan H. Monoclonal antibodies: formulations of marketed products and recent advances in novel delivery system. Drug Dev Ind Pharm. 2017;43(4):519–30. https://doi.org/10.1080/03639045.2017.1278768.

35. Boyiadzis M, Foon KA. Approved monoclonal antibodies for cancer therapy. Expert Opin Biol Ther. 2008;8(8):1151–8. https://doi.org/10.1517/14712598.8.8.1151.

36. Nimmagadda S, Shelake S, Pomper MG. Preclinical experimentation in oncology. In: Lewis JS, Windhorst AD, Zeglis BM, editors. Radiopharmaceutical chemistry. Cham: Springer International Publishing; 2019. p. 569–82.

37. Dimastromatteo J, Kelly KA. Target identification, lead discovery, and optimization. In: Lewis JS, Windhorst AD, Zeglis BM, editors. Radiopharmaceutical chemistry. Cham: Springer International Publishing; 2019. p. 555–67.

38. Beraud E, Collignon A, Franceschi C, Olive D, Lombardo D, Mas E. Investigation of a new tumor-associated glycosylated antigen as target for dendritic cell vaccination in pancreatic cancer. Onco Targets Ther. 2012;1(1):56–61. https://doi.org/10.4161/onci.1.1.18459.

39. Vankemmelbeke M, Chua JX, Durrant LG. Cancer cell associated glycans as targets for immunotherapy. Onco Targets Ther. 2016;5(1):e1061177. https://doi.org/10.1080/2162402X.2015.1061177.

40. Lu Z, Kamat K, Johnson BP, Yin CC, Scholler N, Abbott KL. Generation of a fully human scFv that binds tumor-specific Glycoforms. Sci Rep. 2019;9(1):5101. https://doi.org/10.1038/s41598-019-41567-6.

41. Hakomori S. Glycosylation defining cancer malignancy: new wine in an old bottle. Proc Natl Acad Sci U S A. 2002;99(16):10231–3. https://doi.org/10.1073/pnas.172380699.

42. Hauselmann I, Borsig L. Altered tumor-cell glycosylation promotes metastasis. Front Oncol. 2014;4:28. https://doi.org/10.3389/fonc.2014.00028.

43. Schietinger A, Philip M, Schreiber H. Specificity in cancer immunotherapy. Semin Immunol. 2008;20(5):276–85. https://doi.org/10.1016/j.smim.2008.07.001.

44. Chiu ML, Goulet DR, Teplyakov A, Gilliland GL. Antibody structure and function: the basis for engineering therapeutics. Antibodies (Basel). 2019;8(4). https://doi.org/10.3390/antib8040055.

45. Vidarsson G, Dekkers G, Rispens T. IgG subclasses and allotypes: from structure to effector functions. Front Immunol. 2014;5:520. https://doi.org/10.3389/fimmu.2014.00520.

46. Hoffmann RM, Coumbe BGT, Josephs DH, Mele S, Ilieva KM, Cheung A, et al. Antibody structure and engineering considerations for the design and function of antibody drug conjugates (ADCs). Onco Targets Ther. 2018;7(3):e1395127. https://doi.org/10.1080/2162402X.2017.1395127.

47. Irani V, Guy AJ, Andrew D, Beeson JG, Ramsland PA, Richards JS. Molecular properties of human IgG subclasses and their implications for designing therapeutic monoclonal antibodies against infectious diseases. Mol Immunol. 2015;67(2, Part A):171–82. https://doi.org/10.1016/j.molimm.2015.03.255.

48. Stern M, Herrmann R. Overview of monoclonal antibodies in cancer therapy: present and promise. Crit Rev Oncol Hematol. 2005;54(1):11–29. https://doi.org/10.1016/j.critrevonc.2004.10.011.

49. Weiner LM. Fully human therapeutic monoclonal antibodies. J Immunother. 2006;29(1):1–9. https://doi.org/10.1097/01.cji.0000192105.24583.83.

50. Harding FA, Stickler MM, Razo J, DuBridge RB. The immunogenicity of humanized and fully human antibodies: residual immunogenicity resides in the CDR regions. MAbs. 2010;2(3):256–65. https://doi.org/10.4161/mabs.2.3.11641.

51. Gómez Román VR, Murray JC, Weiner LM. Chapter 1 - antibody-dependent cellular cytotoxicity (ADCC). In: Ackerman ME, Nimmerjahn F, editors. Antibody Fc. Boston: Academic Press; 2014. p. 1–27.

52. Weiskopf K, Weissman IL. Macrophages are critical effectors of antibody therapies for cancer. MAbs. 2015;7(2):303–10. https://doi.org/10.1080/19420862.2015.1011450.

53. Adams GP, Weiner LM. Monoclonal antibody therapy of cancer. Nat Biotechnol. 2005;23(9):1147–57. https://doi.org/10.1038/nbt1137.

54. Keizer RJ, Huitema AD, Schellens JH, Beijnen JH. Clinical pharmacokinetics of therapeutic monoclonal antibodies. Clin Pharmacokinet. 2010;49(8):493–507. https://doi.org/10.2165/11531280-000000000-00000.

55. Liu L. Antibody glycosylation and its impact on the pharmacokinetics and pharmacodynamics of monoclonal antibodies and fc-fusion proteins. J Pharm Sci. 2015;104(6):1866–84. https://doi.org/10.1002/jps.24444.

56. Ovacik M, Lin K. Tutorial on monoclonal antibody pharmacokinetics and its considerations in early development. Clin Transl Sci. 2018;11(6):540–52. https://doi.org/10.1111/cts.12567.

57. Cataldi M, Vigliotti C, Mosca T, Cammarota M, Capone D. Emerging role of the spleen in the pharmacokinetics of monoclonal antibodies, nanoparticles and exosomes. Int J Mol Sci. 2017;18(6) https://doi.org/10.3390/ijms18061249.

58. Batra SK, Jain M, Wittel UA, Chauhan SC, Colcher D. Pharmacokinetics and biodistribution of genetically engineered antibodies. Curr Opin Biotechnol. 2002;13(6):603–8.

59. Senter PD. Potent antibody drug conjugates for cancer therapy. Curr Opin Chem Biol. 2009;13(3):235–44. https://doi.org/10.1016/j.cbpa.2009.03.023.

60. Tolcher AW, Sugarman S, Gelmon KA, Cohen R, Saleh M, Isaacs C, et al. Randomized phase II study of BR96-doxorubicin conjugate in patients with metastatic breast cancer. J Clin Oncol. 1999;17(2):478–84. https://doi.org/10.1200/JCO.1999.17.2.478.

61. Juweid M, Neumann R, Paik C, Perez-Bacete MJ, Sato J, van Osdol W, et al. Micropharmacology of monoclonal antibodies in solid tumors: direct experimental evidence for a binding site barrier. Cancer Res. 1992;52(19):5144–53.

62. Weinstein JN, van Osdol W. Early intervention in cancer using monoclonal antibodies and other biological ligands: micropharmacology and the "binding site barrier". Cancer Res. 1992;52(9 Suppl):2747s–51s.

63. Rudnick SI, Adams GP. Affinity and avidity in antibody-based tumor targeting. Cancer Biother Radiopharm. 2009;24(2):155–61. https://doi.org/10.1089/cbr.2009.0627.

64. Thurber GM, Schmidt MM, Wittrup KD. Antibody tumor penetration: transport opposed by systemic and antigen-mediated clearance. Adv Drug Deliv Rev. 2008;60(12):1421–34. https://doi.org/10.1016/j.addr.2008.04.012.

65. Thurber GM, Schmidt MM, Wittrup KD. Factors determining antibody distribution in tumors. Trends Pharmacol Sci. 2008;29(2):57–61. https://doi.org/10.1016/j.tips.2007.11.004.

66. Wittrup KD, Thurber GM, Schmidt MM, Rhoden JJ. Practical theoretic guidance for the design of tumor-targeting agents. Methods Enzymol. 2012;503:255–68. https://doi.org/10.1016/B978-0-12-396962-0.00010-0.

67. Sharkey RM, Press OW, Goldenberg DM. A reexamination of radioimmunotherapy in the treatment of non-Hodgkin lymphoma: prospects for dual-targeted antibody/radioantibody therapy. Blood. 2009;113(17):3891–5. https://doi.org/10.1182/blood-2008-11-188896.

68. Mattes MJ, Sharkey RM, Karacay H, Czuczman MS, Goldenberg DM. Therapy of advanced B-lymphoma xenografts with a combination of 90Y-anti-CD22 IgG (epratuzumab) and unlabeled anti-CD20 IgG (veltuzumab). Clin Cancer Res. 2008;14(19):6154–60. https://doi.org/10.1158/1078-0432.CCR-08-0404.

69. Sharma SK, Chow A, Monette S, Vivier D, Pourat J, Edwards KJ, et al. Fc-mediated anomalous biodistribution of therapeutic antibodies in Immunodeficient mouse models. Cancer Res. 2018;78(7):1820–32. https://doi.org/10.1158/0008-5472.CAN-17-1958.

70. Bhattacharyya S, Dixit M. Metallic radionuclides in the development of diagnostic and therapeutic radiopharmaceuticals. Dalton Trans. 2011;40(23):6112–28. https://doi.org/10.1039/c1dt10379b.

71. Wolf W, Shani J. Criteria for the selection of the most desirable radionuclide for radiolabeling monoclonal antibodies. Int J Radiation Appl Instrum Part B, Nucl Med Biol. 1986;13(4):319–24.

72. Boros E, Holland JP. Chemical aspects of metal ion chelation in the synthesis and application antibody-based radiotracers. J Labelled Comp Radiopharm. 2018;61(9):652–71. https://doi.org/10.1002/jlcr.3590.

73. Kraeber-Bodere F, Rousseau C, Bodet-Milin C, Mathieu C, Guerard F, Frampas E, et al. Tumor immunotargeting using innovative radionuclides. Int J Mol Sci. 2015;16(2):3932–54. https://doi.org/10.3390/ijms16023932.

74. Pouget JP, Navarro-Teulon I, Bardies M, Chouin N, Cartron G, Pelegrin A, et al. Clinical radioimmunotherapy—the role of radiobiology. Nat Rev Clin Oncol. 2011;8(12):720–34. https://doi.org/10.1038/nrclinonc.2011.160.

75. Mikolajczak R, van der Meulen NP, Lapi SE. Radiometals for imaging and theranostics, current production and future perspectives. J Labelled Comp Radiopharm. 2019; https://doi.org/10.1002/jlcr.3770.

76. Wilbur DS. The radiopharmaceutical chemistry of alpha-emitting radionuclides. In: Lewis JS, Windhorst AD, Zeglis BM, editors. Radiopharmaceutical chemistry. Cham: Springer International Publishing; 2019. p. 409–24.

77. Tolmachev V, Orlova A, Andersson K. Methods for radiolabelling of monoclonal antibodies. Methods Mol Biol. 2014;1060:309–30. https://doi.org/10.1007/978-1-62703-586-6_16.

78. Martins CD, Kramer-Marek G, Oyen WJG. Radioimmunotherapy for delivery of cytotoxic radioisotopes: current status and challenges. Expert Opin Drug Deliv. 2018;15(2):185–96. https://doi.org/10.1080/17425247.2018.1378180.

79. Wester DW, Steele RT, Rinehart DE, DesChane JR, Carson KJ, Rapko BM, et al. Large-scale purification of 90Sr from nuclear waste materials for production of 90Y, a therapeutic medical radioisotope. Appl Radiation Isotopes. 2003;59(1):35–41.

80. Chakravarty R, Chakraborty S, Sarma HD, Nair KV, Rajeswari A, Dash A. (90) Y/(177) Lu-labelled Cetuximab immunoconjugates: radiochemistry optimization to clinical dose formulation. J Labelled Comp Radiopharm. 2016;59(9):354–63. https://doi.org/10.1002/jlcr.3413.

81. Papi S, Martano L, Garaboldi L, Rossi A, Cremonesi M, Grana CM, et al. Radiolabeling optimization and reduced staff radiation exposure for high-dose 90Y-ibritumomab tiuxetan (HD-Zevalin). Nucl Med Biol. 2010;37(1):85–93. https://doi.org/10.1016/j.nucmedbio.2009.08.012.

82. Kassis AI. Therapeutic radionuclides: biophysical and radiobiologic principles. Semin Nucl Med. 2008;38(5):358–66. https://doi.org/10.1053/j.semnuclmed.2008.05.002.

83. Kuo WI, Cheng KH, Chang YJ, Wu TT, Hsu WC, Chen LC, et al. Radiolabeling, characteristics and NanoSPECT/CT Imaging of 188Re-cetuximab in NCI-H292 human lung cancer xenografts. Anticancer Res. 2019;39, 183(1):–190. https://doi.org/10.21873/anticanres.13096.

84. Vallabhajosula S, Nikolopoulou A, Jhanwar YS, Kaur G, Tagawa ST, Nanus DM, et al. Radioimmunotherapy of metastatic prostate cancer with (1)(7)(7)Lu-DOTAhuJ591 anti prostate specific membrane antigen specific monoclonal antibody. Curr Radiopharm. 2016;9(1):44–53.

85. Yong KJ, Milenic DE, Baidoo KE, Brechbiel MW. Mechanisms of cell killing response from Low Linear Energy Transfer (LET) radiation originating from (177)Lu radioimmunotherapy targeting disseminated intraperitoneal tumor xenografts. Int J Mol Sci. 2016;17(5) https://doi.org/10.3390/ijms17050736.

86. Muller C, Bunka M, Haller S, Koster U, Groehn V, Bernhardt P, et al. Promising prospects for 44Sc-/47Sc-based theragnostics: application of 47Sc for radionuclide tumor therapy in mice. J Nucl Med. 2014;55(10): 1658–64. https://doi.org/10.2967/jnumed.114.141614.

87. Novak-Hofer I, Schubiger PA. Copper-67 as a therapeutic nuclide for radioimmunotherapy. Eur J Nucl Med Mol Imaging. 2002;29(6):821–30. https://doi.org/10.1007/s00259-001-0724-y.

88. Dash A, Pillai MR, Knapp FF Jr. Production of (177)Lu for targeted radionuclide therapy: available options. Nucl Med Mol Imaging. 2015;49(2):85–107. https://doi.org/10.1007/s13139-014-0315-z.

89. Guleria M, Das T, Kumar C, Amirdhanayagam J, Sarma HD, Banerjee S. Preparation of clinical-scale (177) Lu-rituximab: optimization of protocols for conjugation, radiolabeling, and freeze-dried kit formulation. J Labelled Comp Radiopharm. 2017;60(5):234–41. https://doi.org/10.1002/jlcr.3493.

90. Frost SH, Frayo SL, Miller BW, Orozco JJ, Booth GC, Hylarides MD, et al. Comparative efficacy of 177Lu and 90Y for anti-CD20 pretargeted radioimmunotherapy in murine lymphoma xenograft models. PLoS One. 2015;10(3):e0120561. https://doi.org/10.1371/journal.pone.0120561.

91. Orozco JJ, Balkin ER, Gooley TA, Kenoyer A, Hamlin DK, Wilbur DS, et al. Anti-CD45 radioimmunotherapy with 90Y but not 177Lu is effective treatment in a syngeneic murine leukemia model. PLoS One. 2014;9(12):e113601. https://doi.org/10.1371/journal.pone.0113601.

92. de Jong M, Breeman WA, Valkema R, Bernard BF, Krenning EP. Combination radionuclide therapy using 177Lu- and 90Y-labeled somatostatin analogs. J Nucl Med. 2005;46(Suppl 1):13s–7s.

93. Guerard F, Barbet J, Chatal JF, Kraeber-Bodere F, Cherel M, Haddad F. Which radionuclide, carrier molecule and clinical indication for alpha-immunotherapy? Q J Nucl Med Mol Imaging. 2015;59(2):161–7.

94. Wild D, Frischknecht M, Zhang H, Morgenstern A, Bruchertseifer F, Boisclair J, et al. Alpha- versus beta-particle radiopeptide therapy in a human prostate cancer model (213Bi-DOTA-PESIN and 213Bi-AMBA versus 177Lu-DOTA-PESIN). Cancer Res. 2011;71(3):1009–18. https://doi.org/10.1158/0008-5472.CAN-10-1186.

95. Heskamp S, Hernandez R, Molkenboer-Kuenen JDM, Essler M, Bruchertseifer F, Morgenstern A, et al. Alpha- versus beta-emitting radionuclides for pretargeted radioimmunotherapy of carcinoembryonic antigen-expressing human colon cancer xenografts. J Nucl Med. 2017;58(6):926–33. https://doi.org/10.2967/jnumed.116.187021.

96. Marcu L, Bezak E, Allen BJ. Global comparison of targeted alpha vs targeted beta therapy for cancer: in vitro, in vivo and clinical trials. Crit Rev Oncol Hematol. 2018;123:7–20. https://doi.org/10.1016/j.critrevonc.2018.01.001.

97. McDevitt MR, Barendswaard E, Ma D, Lai L, Curcio MJ, Sgouros G, et al. An alpha-particle emitting antibody ([213Bi]J591) for radioimmunotherapy of prostate cancer. Cancer Res. 2000;60(21):6095–100.

98. McDevitt MR, Sgouros G, Sofou S. Targeted and nontargeted alpha-particle therapies. Annu Rev Biomed Eng. 2018;20:73–93. https://doi.org/10.1146/annurev-bioeng-062117-120931.

99. Qiu H, Santos EB, Storb RF, Hamlin DK, Wilbur DS, Sandmaier BM. Addition of astatine-211-labeled anti-CD45 antibody to Total Body Irradiation (TBI) As conditioning for DLA-identical marrow transplantation: a novel strategy to overcome graft rejection in a canine presensitization model. Blood. 2016;128(22):2152.

100. Green DJ, Shadman M, Jones JC, Frayo SL, Kenoyer AL, Hylarides MD, et al. Astatine-211 conjugated to an anti-CD20 monoclonal antibody eradicates disseminated B-cell lymphoma in a mouse model. Blood. 2015;125(13):2111–9. https://doi.org/10.1182/blood-2014-11-612770.

101. Zalutsky MR, Pruszynski M. Astatine-211: production and availability. Curr Radiopharm. 2011;4(3):177–85.

102. Griswold JR, Medvedev DG, Engle JW, Copping R, Fitzsimmons JM, Radchenko V, et al. Large scale accelerator production of (225)Ac: effective cross sections for 78-192MeV protons incident on (232) Th targets. Appl Radiat Isot. 2016;118:366–74. https://doi.org/10.1016/j.apradiso.2016.09.026.

103. Robertson AKH, Ramogida CF, Schaffer P, Radchenko V. Development of (225)ac radiopharmaceuticals: TRIUMF perspectives and experiences. Curr Radiopharm. 2018;11(3):156–72. https://doi.org/10.2174/1874471011666180416161908.

104. Jurcic JG. Clinical studies with Bismuth-213 and Actinium-225 for hematologic malignancies. Curr Radiopharm. 2018;11(3):192–9. https://doi.org/10.2174/1874471011666180525102814.

105. Jurcic JG, Rosenblat TL. Targeted alpha-particle immunotherapy for acute myeloid leukemia. Am

Soc Clin Oncol Educ Book. 2014:e126–31. https://doi.org/10.14694/EdBook_AM.2014.34.e126.

106. Jurcic JG. Radioimmunotherapy for hematopoietic cell transplantation. Immunotherapy. 2013;5(4):383–94. https://doi.org/10.2217/imt.13.11.

107. Hnatowich DJ. Recent developments in the radiolabeling of antibodies with iodine, indium, and technetium. Semin Nucl Med. 1990;20(1):80–91.

108. Halpern SE. The advantages and limits of indium-111 labeling of antibodies. Experimental studies and clinical applications. Int J Rad Appl Instrum B. 1986;13(2):195–201.

109. Speth PAJ, Kinsella TJ, Chang AE, Klecker RW Jr, Belanger K, Collins JM. Selective incorporation of iododeoxyuridine into DNA of hepatic metastases versus normal human liver. Clin Pharmacol Ther. 1988;44(4):369–75. https://doi.org/10.1038/clpt.1988.166.

110. Cornelissen BA, Vallis K. Targeting the nucleus: an overview of auger-electron radionuclide therapy. Curr Drug Discov Technol. 2010;7(4):263–79. https://doi.org/10.2174/157016310793360657.

111. Emrich JG, Brady LW, Quang TS, Class R, Miyamoto C, Black P, et al. Radioiodinated (I-125) monoclonal antibody 425 in the treatment of high grade glioma patients: ten-year synopsis of a novel treatment. Am J Clin Oncol. 2002;25(6):541–6.

112. Kim JH, Li L, Quang TS, Emrich JG, Yaeger TE, Jenrette JM, et al. Phase II trial of anti-epidermal growth factor receptor radioimmunotherapy in the treatment of anaplastic astrocytoma. J Radiat Oncol. 2013;2(1):7–13. https://doi.org/10.1007/s13566-012-0071-6.

113. Costantini DL, Chan C, Cai Z, Vallis KA, Reilly RM. (111)in-labeled trastuzumab (Herceptin) modified with nuclear localization sequences (NLS): an auger electron-emitting radiotherapeutic agent for HER2/neu-amplified breast cancer. J Nucl Med. 2007;48(8):1357–68. https://doi.org/10.2967/jnumed.106.037937.

114. Pouget JP, Santoro L, Raymond L, Chouin N, Bardiès M, Bascoul-Mollevi C, et al. Cell membrane is a more sensitive target than cytoplasm to dense ionization produced by auger electrons. Radiat Res. 2008;170(2):192–200. https://doi.org/10.1667/rr1359.1.

115. Price EW, Orvig C. Matching chelators to radiometals for radiopharmaceuticals. Chem Soc Rev. 2014;43(1):260–90. https://doi.org/10.1039/c3cs60304k.

116. Lindmo T, Boven E, Cuttitta F, Fedorko J, Bunn PA Jr. Determination of the immunoreactive fraction of radiolabeled monoclonal antibodies by linear extrapolation to binding at infinite antigen excess. J Immunol Methods. 1984;72(1):77–89.

117. Larson SM, Carrasquillo JA, Cheung NK, Press OW. Radioimmunotherapy of human tumours. Nat Rev Cancer. 2015;15(6):347–60. https://doi.org/10.1038/nrc3925.

118. Adumeau P, Sharma SK, Brent C, Zeglis BM. Site-specifically labeled immunoconjugates for molecular imaging--part 1: cysteine residues and Glycans. Mol Imaging Biol. 2016;18(1):1–17. https://doi.org/10.1007/s11307-015-0919-4.

119. Chari RV. Targeted cancer therapy: conferring specificity to cytotoxic drugs. Acc Chem Res. 2008;41(1):98–107. https://doi.org/10.1021/ar700108g.

120. McCombs JR, Owen SC. Antibody drug conjugates: design and selection of linker, payload and conjugation chemistry. AAPS J. 2015;17(2):339–51. https://doi.org/10.1208/s12248-014-9710-8.

121. Morais M, Ma MT. Site-specific chelator-antibody conjugation for PET and SPECT imaging with radiometals. Drug Discov Today Technol. 2018;30:91–104. https://doi.org/10.1016/j.ddtec.2018.10.002.

122. Kukis DL, DeNardo GL, DeNardo SJ, Mirick GR, Miers LA, Greiner DP, et al. Effect of the extent of chelate substitution on the immunoreactivity and biodistribution of 2IT-BAT-Lym-1 immunoconjugates. Cancer Res. 1995;55(4):878–84.

123. Sharma SK, Glaser JM, Edwards KJ, Khozeimeh Sarbisheh E, Salih AK, Lewis JS, et al. A systematic evaluation of antibody modification and (89) Zr-radiolabeling for optimized Immuno-PET. Bioconjug Chem. 2020; https://doi.org/10.1021/acs.bioconjchem.0c00087.

124. Vosjan MJ, Perk LR, Visser GW, Budde M, Jurek P, Kiefer GE, et al. Conjugation and radiolabeling of monoclonal antibodies with zirconium-89 for PET imaging using the bifunctional chelate p-isothiocyanatobenzyl-desferrioxamine. Nat Protoc. 2010;5(4):739–43. https://doi.org/10.1038/nprot.2010.13.

125. Christie RJ, Tiberghien AC, Du Q, Bezabeh B, Fleming R, Shannon A, et al. Pyrrolobenzodiazepine antibody-drug conjugates designed for stable thiol conjugation. Antibodies (Basel). 2017;6(4) https://doi.org/10.3390/antib6040020.

126. Sussman D, Westendorf L, Meyer DW, Leiske CI, Anderson M, Okeley NM, et al. Engineered cysteine antibodies: an improved antibody-drug conjugate platform with a novel mechanism of drug-linker stability. Protein Eng Des Sel. 2018;31(2):47–54. https://doi.org/10.1093/protein/gzx067.

127. Adumeau P, Davydova M, Zeglis BM. Thiol-reactive bifunctional chelators for the creation of site-selectively modified radioimmunoconjugates with improved stability. Bioconjug Chem. 2018;29(4):1364–72. https://doi.org/10.1021/acs.bioconjchem.8b00081.

128. Maguire RT, Pascucci VL, Maroli AN, Gulfo JV. Immunoscintigraphy in patients with colorectal, ovarian, and prostate cancer. Results with site-specific immunoconjugates. Cancer. 1993;72(11 Suppl):3453–62.

129. Zeglis BM, Davis CB, Aggeler R, Kang HC, Chen A, Agnew BJ, et al. Enzyme-mediated methodology

for the site-specific radiolabeling of antibodies based on catalyst-free click chemistry. Bioconjug Chem. 2013;24(6):1057–67. https://doi.org/10.1021/bc 400122c.

130. Anami Y, Tsuchikama K. Transglutaminase-mediated conjugations. Methods Mol Biol. 2020;2078:71–82. https://doi.org/10.1007/978-1-4939-9929-3_5.

131. Jeger S, Zimmermann K, Blanc A, Grunberg J, Honer M, Hunziker P, et al. Site-specific and stoichiometric modification of antibodies by bacterial transglutaminase. Angew Chem. 2010;49(51):9995–7. https://doi.org/10.1002/anie.201004243.

132. Wu Y, Zhu H, Zhang B, Liu F, Chen J, Wang Y, et al. Synthesis of site-specific radiolabeled antibodies for radioimmunotherapy via genetic code expansion. Bioconjug Chem. 2016;27(10):2460–8. https://doi.org/10.1021/acs.bioconjchem.6b00412.

133. Adumeau P, Sharma SK, Brent C, Zeglis BM. Site-specifically labeled immunoconjugates for molecular imaging—part 2: peptide tags and unnatural amino acids. Mol Imaging Biol. 2016;18(2):153–65. https://doi.org/10.1007/s11307-015-0920-y.

134. Fay R, Holland JP. The impact of emerging bioconjugation chemistries on radiopharmaceuticals. J Nucl Med. 2019;60(5):587–91. https://doi.org/10.2967/jnumed.118.220806.

135. Beck A, Goetsch L, Dumontet C, Corvaia N. Strategies and challenges for the next generation of antibody-drug conjugates. Nat Rev Drug Discov. 2017;16(5):315–37. https://doi.org/10.1038/nrd.2016.268.

136. Falck G, Müller KM. Enzyme-based labeling strategies for antibody–drug conjugates and antibody mimetics. Antibodies. 2018;7(1):4.

137. Tsuchikama K, An Z. Antibody-drug conjugates: recent advances in conjugation and linker chemistries. Protein Cell. 2018;9(1):33–46. https://doi.org/10.1007/s13238-016-0323-0.

138. Bander NH, Milowsky MI, Nanus DM, Kostakoglu L, Vallabhajosula S, Goldsmith SJ. Phase I trial of 177lutetium-labeled J591, a monoclonal antibody to prostate-specific membrane antigen, in patients with androgen-independent prostate cancer. J Clin Oncol. 2005;23(21):4591–601. https://doi.org/10.1200/JCO.2005.05.160.

139. Kim SH. Is radioimmunotherapy a 'magic bullet'? Korean J Hematol. 2012;47(2):85–6. https://doi.org/10.5045/kjh.2012.47.2.85.

140. Chamarthy MR, Williams SC, Moadel RM. Radioimmunotherapy of non-Hodgkin's lymphoma: from the 'magic bullets' to 'radioactive magic bullets'. Yale J Biol Med. 2011;84(4):391–407.

141. Janiak MK, Wincenciak M, Cheda A, Nowosielska EM, Calabrese EJ. Cancer immunotherapy: how low-level ionizing radiation can play a key role. Cancer Immunol Immunother. 2017;66(7):819–32. https://doi.org/10.1007/s00262-017-1993-z.

142. Gorin JB, Menager J, Gouard S, Maurel C, Guilloux Y, Faivre-Chauvet A, et al. Antitumor immunity induced after alpha irradiation. Neoplasia. 2014;16(4):319–28. https://doi.org/10.1016/j.neo.2014.04.002.

143. Gorin JB, Guilloux Y, Morgenstern A, Cherel M, Davodeau F, Gaschet J. Using alpha radiation to boost cancer immunity? Onco Targets Ther. 2014;3(9):e954925. https://doi.org/10.4161/216240 11.2014.954925.

144. Wilderman SJ, Roberson PL, Bolch WE, Dewaraja YK. Investigation of effect of variations in bone fraction and red marrow cellularity on bone marrow dosimetry in radio-immunotherapy. Phys Med Biol. 2013;58(14):4717–31. https://doi.org/10.1088/0031-9155/58/14/4717.

145. Sgouros G. Bone marrow dosimetry for radioimmunotherapy: theoretical considerations. J Nucl Med. 1993;34(4):689–94.

146. Vallabhajosula S, Goldsmith SJ, Hamacher KA, Kostakoglu L, Konishi S, Milowski MI, et al. Prediction of myelotoxicity based on bone marrow radiation-absorbed dose: radioimmunotherapy studies using 90Y- and 177Lu-labeled J591 antibodies specific for prostate-specific membrane antigen. J Nucl Med. 2005;46(5):850–8.

147. Dainiak N. Hematologic consequences of exposure to ionizing radiation. Exp Hematol. 2002;30(6):513–28.

148. Baechler S, Hobbs RF, Jacene HA, Bochud FO, Wahl RL, Sgouros G. Predicting hematologic toxicity in patients undergoing radioimmunotherapy with 90Y-ibritumomab tiuxetan or 131I-tositumomab. J Nucl Med. 2010;51(12):1878–84. https://doi.org/10.2967/jnumed.110.079947.

149. Sas N, Rousseau J, Nguyen F, Bellec E, Larrsson E, Becavin S, et al. A compartmental model of mouse thrombopoiesis and erythropoiesis to predict bone marrow toxicity after internal irradiation. J Nucl Med. 2014;55(8):1355–60. https://doi.org/10.2967/jnumed.113.133330.

150. Peyrade F, Triby C, Slama B, Fontana X, Gressin R, Broglia JM, et al. Radioimmunotherapy in relapsed follicular lymphoma previously treated by autologous bone marrow transplant: a report of eight new cases and literature review. Leuk Lymphoma. 2008;49(9):1762–8. https://doi.org/10.1080/10428190802273278.

151. Cheson BD. Radioimmunotherapy of non-Hodgkin's lymphomas. Curr Drug Targets. 2006;7(10):1293–300.

152. Kraeber-Bodere F, Bodet-Milin C, Rousseau C, Eugene T, Pallardy A, Frampas E, et al. Radioimmunoconjugates for the treatment of cancer. Semin Oncol. 2014;41(5):613–22. https://doi.org/10.1053/j.seminoncol.2014.07.004.

153. Navarro-Teulon I, Lozza C, Pelegrin A, Vives E, Pouget JP. General overview of radioimmunotherapy of solid tumors. Immunotherapy. 2013;5(5):467–87. https://doi.org/10.2217/imt.13.34.

154. Song H, Sgouros G. Radioimmunotherapy of solid tumors: searching for the right target. Curr Drug Deliv. 2011;8(1):26–44.

155. Bartholoma MD. Radioimmunotherapy of solid tumors: approaches on the verge of clinical application. J Labelled Comp Radiopharm. 2018; https://doi.org/10.1002/jlcr.3619.

156. Bodet-Milin C, Ferrer L, Pallardy A, Eugene T, Rauscher A, Alain F-C, et al. Radioimmunotherapy of B-cell non-Hodgkin's lymphoma. Front Oncol. 2013;3:177. https://doi.org/10.3389/fonc.2013.00177.

157. Bodet-Milin C, Kraeber-Bodere F, Eugene T, Guerard F, Gaschet J, Bailly C, et al. Radioimmunotherapy for treatment of acute leukemia. Semin Nucl Med. 2016;46(2):135–46. https://doi.org/10.1053/j.semnuclmed.2015.10.007.

158. Rezaei A, Adib M, Mokarian F, Tebianian M, Nassiri R. Leukemia markers expression of peripheral blood vs bone marrow blasts using flow cytometry. Med Sci Monit. 2003;9(8):CR359–62.

159. Goldenberg DM. Some like it hot: lymphoma radioimmunotherapy. Blood. 2009;113(20):4823–4. https://doi.org/10.1182/blood-2009-02-203166.

160. Santos MAO, Lima MM. CD20 role in pathophysiology of Hodgkin's disease. Rev Assoc Med Bras. 2017;63(9):810–3. https://doi.org/10.1590/1806-9282.63.09.810.

161. Shanehbandi D, Majidi J, Kazemi T, Baradaran B, Aghebati-Maleki L. CD20-based immunotherapy of B-cell derived hematologic malignancies. Curr Cancer Drug Targets. 2017;17(5):423–44. https://doi.org/10.2174/1568009617666170109151128.

162. Tedder TF, Engel P. CD20: a regulator of cell-cycle progression of B lymphocytes. Immunol Today. 1994;15(9):450–4. https://doi.org/10.1016/0167-5699(94)90276-3.

163. Read ED, Eu P, Little PJ, Piva TJ. The status of radioimmunotherapy in CD20+ non-Hodgkin's lymphoma. Target Oncol. 2015;10(1):15–26. https://doi.org/10.1007/s11523-014-0324-y.

164. Kawashima H. Characteristics of Ibritumomab as radionuclide therapy agent. In: Hosono M, Chatal J-F, editors. Resistance to Ibritumomab in lymphoma. Cham: Springer International Publishing; 2018. p. 79–97.

165. Marcus R. Use of 90Y-ibritumomab tiuxetan in non-Hodgkin's lymphoma. Semin Oncol. 2005;32(1 Suppl 1):S36–43. https://doi.org/10.1053/j.seminoncol.2005.01.012.

166. Jacobs SA, Harrison AM, Swerdlow SH, Foon KA, Avril N, Vidnovic N, et al. Radioisotopic localization of 90Yttrium–Ibritumomab Tiuxetan in patients with CD20+ non-Hodgkin's lymphoma. Mol Imaging Biol. 2009;11(1):39–45. https://doi.org/10.1007/s11307-008-0170-3.

167. Weber T, Bötticher B, Mier W, Sauter M, Krämer S, Leotta K, et al. High treatment efficacy by dual targeting of Burkitt's lymphoma xenografted mice with a 177Lu-based CD22-specific radioimmunoconjugate and rituximab. Eur J Nucl Med Mol Imaging. 2016;43(3):489–98. https://doi.org/10.1007/s00259-015-3175-6.

168. Conti PS, White C, Pieslor P, Molina A, Aussie J, Foster P. The role of imaging with (111)in-ibritumomab tiuxetan in the ibritumomab tiuxetan (zevalin) regimen: results from a Zevalin imaging registry. J Nucl Med. 2005;46(11):1812–8.

169. MICAD Research Team. (111)In-Ibritumomab tiuxetan. Bethesda, MD: Molecular Imaging and Contrast Agent Database (MICAD); 2004.

170. Jacobs SA, Vidnovic N, Joyce J, McCook B, Torok F, Avril N. Full-dose 90Y ibritumomab tiuxetan therapy is safe in patients with prior myeloablative chemotherapy. Clin Cancer Res. 2005;11(19 Pt 2):7146s–50s. https://doi.org/10.1158/1078-0432.CCR-1004-0003.

171. Theuer CP, Leigh BR, Multani PS, Allen RS, Liang BC. Radioimmunotherapy of non-Hodgkin's lymphoma: clinical development of the Zevalin regimen. Biotechnol Annu Rev. 2004;10:265–95. https://doi.org/10.1016/S1387-2656(04)10011-2.

172. Czuczman MS, Emmanouilides C, Darif M, Witzig TE, Gordon LI, Revell S, et al. Treatment-related myelodysplastic syndrome and acute myelogenous leukemia in patients treated with ibritumomab tiuxetan radioimmunotherapy. J Clin Oncol. 2007;25(27):4285–92. https://doi.org/10.1200/JCO.2006.09.2882.

173. Iagaru A, Gambhir SS, Goris ML. 90Y-ibritumomab therapy in refractory non-Hodgkin's lymphoma: observations from 111In-ibritumomab pretreatment imaging. J Nucl Med. 2008;49(11):1809–12. https://doi.org/10.2967/jnumed.108.052928.

174. Morschhauser F, Radford J, Van Hoof A, Botto B, Rohatiner AZ, Salles G, et al. 90Yttrium-ibritumomab tiuxetan consolidation of first remission in advanced-stage follicular non-Hodgkin lymphoma: updated results after a median follow-up of 7.3 years from the international, randomized, phase III first-LineIndolent trial. J Clin Oncol. 2013;31(16):1977–83. https://doi.org/10.1200/jco.2012.45.6400.

175. Wagner JY, Schwarz K, Schreiber S, Schmidt B, Wester HJ, Schwaiger M, et al. Myeloablative anti-CD20 radioimmunotherapy +/− high-dose chemotherapy followed by autologous stem cell support for relapsed/refractory B-cell lymphoma results in excellent long-term survival. Oncotarget. 2013, 4(6):899–910. https://doi.org/10.18632/oncotarget.1037.

176. Ali AM, Dehdashti F, DiPersio JF, Cashen AF. Radioimmunotherapy-based conditioning for hematopoietic stem cell transplantation: another step forward. Blood Rev. 2016;30(5):389–99. https://doi.org/10.1016/j.blre.2016.04.007.

177. Sutamtewagul G, Link BK. Novel treatment approaches and future perspectives in follicular lymphoma. Ther Adv Hematol. 2019;10:2040620718820510. https://doi.org/10.1177/2040620718820510.

178. Witzig TE, Flinn IW, Gordon LI, Emmanouilides C, Czuczman MS, Saleh MN, et al. Treatment with ibritumomab tiuxetan radioimmunotherapy in patients

with rituximab-refractory follicular non-Hodgkin's lymphoma. J Clin Oncol. 2002;20(15):3262–9. https://doi.org/10.1200/JCO.2002.11.017.

179. Eskian M, Khorasanizadeh M, Zinzani PL, Rezaei N. Radioimmunotherapy as the first line of treatment in non-Hodgkin lymphoma. Immunotherapy. 2018;10(8):699–711. https://doi.org/10.2217/imt-2017-0169.

180. Hohloch K, Windemuth-Kieselbach C, Kolz J, Zinzani PL, Cacchione R, Jurczak W, et al. Radioimmunotherapy (RIT) for follicular lymphoma achieves long term lymphoma control in first line and at relapse: 8-year follow-up data of 281 patients from the international RIT-registry. Br J Haematol. 2019;184(6):949–56. https://doi.org/10.1111/bjh.15712.

181. Michel RB, Rosario AV, Brechbiel MW, Jackson TJ, Goldenberg DM, Mattes MJ. Experimental therapy of disseminated B-cell lymphoma xenografts with 213Bi-labeled anti-CD74. Nucl Med Biol. 2003;30(7):715–23.

182. Park SI, Shenoi J, Pagel JM, Hamlin DK, Wilbur DS, Orgun N, et al. Conventional and pretargeted radioimmunotherapy using bismuth-213 to target and treat non-Hodgkin lymphomas expressing CD20: a preclinical model toward optimal consolidation therapy to eradicate minimal residual disease. Blood. 2010;116(20):4231–9. https://doi.org/10.1182/blood-2010-05-282327.

183. Fanale MA, Younes A. Monoclonal antibodies in the treatment of non-Hodgkin's lymphoma. Drugs. 2007;67(3):333–50. https://doi.org/10.2165/00003495-200767030-00002.

184. Ma D, McDevitt MR, Barendswaard E, Lai L, Curcio MJ, Pellegrini V, et al. Radioimmunotherapy for model B cell malignancies using 90Y-labeled anti-CD19 and anti-CD20 monoclonal antibodies. Leukemia. 2002;16(1):60–6. https://doi.org/10.1038/sj.leu.2402320.

185. Sullivan-Chang L, O'Donnell RT, Tuscano JM. Targeting CD22 in B-cell malignancies: current status and clinical outlook. BioDrugs. 2013;27(4):293–304. https://doi.org/10.1007/s40259-013-0016-7.

186. Sharkey RM, Karacay H, Goldenberg DM. Improving the treatment of non-Hodgkin lymphoma with antibody-targeted radionuclides. Cancer. 2010;116(4 Suppl):1134–45. https://doi.org/10.1002/cncr.24802.

187. Morschhauser F, Kraeber-Bodere F, Wegener WA, Harousseau JL, Petillon MO, Huglo D, et al. High rates of durable responses with anti-CD22 fractionated radioimmunotherapy: results of a multicenter, phase I/II study in non-Hodgkin's lymphoma. J Clin Oncol. 2010;28(23):3709–16. https://doi.org/10.1200/JCO.2009.27.7863.

188. Chevallier P, Eugene T, Robillard N, Isnard F, Nicolini F, Escoffre-Barbe M, et al. (90)Y-labelled anti-CD22 epratuzumab tetraxetan in adults with refractory or relapsed CD22-positive B-cell acute lymphoblastic leukaemia: a phase 1 dose-escalation study. Lancet Haematol. 2015;2(3):e108–17. https://doi.org/10.1016/S2352-3026(15)00020-4.

189. Witzig TE, Tomblyn MB, Misleh JG, Kio EA, Sharkey RM, Wegener WA, et al. Anti-CD22 90Y-epratuzumab tetraxetan combined with anti-CD20 veltuzumab: a phase I study in patients with relapsed/refractory, aggressive non-Hodgkin lymphoma. Haematologica. 2014;99(11):1738–45. https://doi.org/10.3324/haematol.2014.112110.

190. Bailly C, Bodet-Milin C, Guerard F, Chouin N, Gaschet J, Cherel M, et al. Radioimmunotherapy of lymphomas. In: Giovanella L, editor. Nuclear medicine therapy: side effects and complications. Cham: Springer International Publishing; 2019. p. 113–21.

191. Payandeh Z, Noori E, Khalesi B, Mard-Soltani M, Abdolalizadeh J, Khalili S. Anti-CD37 targeted immunotherapy of B-cell malignancies. Biotechnol Lett. 2018;40(11–12):1459–66. https://doi.org/10.1007/s10529-018-2612-6.

192. Kolstad A, Madsbu U, Beasley M, Bayne M, Illidge TM, O'Rourke N, et al. LYMRIT 37-01: a phase I/II study of 177Lu-Lilotomab Satetraxetan (Betalutin®) antibody-Radionuclide-Conjugate (ARC) for the treatment of relapsed non-Hodgkin's Lymphoma (NHL)—analysis with 6-month follow-up. Blood. 2018;132(Suppl. 1):2879. https://doi.org/10.1182/blood-2018-99-110555.

193. Gritti G, Gianatti A, Petronzelli F, De Santis R, Pavoni C, Rossi RL, et al. Evaluation of tenascin-C by tenatumomab in T-cell non-Hodgkin lymphomas identifies a new target for radioimmunotherapy. Oncotarget. 2018;9(11):9766–75. https://doi.org/10.18632/oncotarget.23919.

194. Aloj L, D'Ambrosio L, Aurilio M, Morisco A, Frigeri F, Caraco C, et al. Radioimmunotherapy with Tenarad, a 131I-labelled antibody fragment targeting the extra-domain A1 of tenascin-C, in patients with refractory Hodgkin's lymphoma. Eur J Nucl Med Mol Imaging. 2014;41(5):867–77. https://doi.org/10.1007/s00259-013-2658-6.

195. Rizzieri DA, Akabani G, Zalutsky MR, Coleman RE, Metzler SD, Bowsher JE, et al. Phase 1 trial study of 131I-labeled chimeric 81C6 monoclonal antibody for the treatment of patients with non-Hodgkin lymphoma. Blood. 2004;104(3):642–8. https://doi.org/10.1182/blood-2003-12-4264.

196. Kochenderfer JN, Dudley ME, Kassim SH, Somerville RP, Carpenter RO, Stetler-Stevenson M, et al. Chemotherapy-refractory diffuse large B-cell lymphoma and indolent B-cell malignancies can be effectively treated with autologous T cells expressing an anti-CD19 chimeric antigen receptor. J Clin Oncol. 2015;33(6):540–9. https://doi.org/10.1200/JCO.2014.56.2025.

197. Vallera DA, Elson M, Brechbiel MW, Dusenbery KE, Burns LJ, Jaszcz WB, et al. Radiotherapy of CD19 expressing Daudi tumors in nude mice with Yttrium-90-labeled anti-CD19 antibody. Cancer Biother Radiopharm. 2004;19(1):11–23. https://doi.org/10.1089/108497804773391630.

198. Burke JM, Jurcic JG. Radioimmunotherapy of leukemia. Adv Pharmacol. 2004;51:185–208. https://doi.org/10.1016/S1054-3589(04)51008-6.

199. De Propris MS, Raponi S, Diverio D, Milani ML, Meloni G, Falini B, et al. High CD33 expression levels in acute myeloid leukemia cells carrying the nucleophosmin (NPM1) mutation. Haematologica. 2011;96(10):1548–51. https://doi.org/10.3324/haematol.2011.043786.

200. Walter RB. Investigational CD33-targeted therapeutics for acute myeloid leukemia. Expert Opin Investig Drugs. 2018;27(4):339–48. https://doi.org/10.1080/13543784.2018.1452911.

201. Garfin PM, Feldman EJ. Antibody-based treatment of acute myeloid leukemia. Curr Hematol Malig Rep. 2016;11(6):545–52. https://doi.org/10.1007/s11899-016-0349-7.

202. Jiang Y, Xu P, Yao D, Chen X, Dai H. CD33, CD96 and Death Associated Protein Kinase (DAPK) expression are associated with the survival rate and/or response to the chemotherapy in the patients with Acute Myeloid Leukemia (AML). Med Sci Monit. 2017;23:1725–32. https://doi.org/10.12659/msm.900305.

203. Scheinberg DA, Lovett D, Divgi CR, Graham MC, Berman E, Pentlow K, et al. A phase I trial of monoclonal antibody M195 in acute myelogenous leukemia: specific bone marrow targeting and internalization of radionuclide. J Clin Oncol. 1991;9(3):478–90. https://doi.org/10.1200/JCO.1991.9.3.478.

204. Jurcic JG, Caron PC, Nikula TK, Papadopoulos EB, Finn RD, Gansow OA, et al. Radiolabeled anti-CD33 monoclonal antibody M195 for myeloid leukemias. Cancer Res. 1995;55(23 Suppl): 5908s–10s.

205. Burke JM, Caron PC, Papadopoulos EB, Divgi CR, Sgouros G, Panageas KS, et al. Cytoreduction with iodine-131-anti-CD33 antibodies before bone marrow transplantation for advanced myeloid leukemias. Bone Marrow Transplant. 2003;32(6):549–56. https://doi.org/10.1038/sj.bmt.1704201.

206. Burke JM, Jurcic JG, Scheinberg DA. Radioimmunotherapy for acute leukemia. Cancer Control: J Moffitt Cancer Center. 2002;9(2):106–13. https://doi.org/10.1177/107327480200900203.

207. Kozempel J, Mokhodoeva O, Vlk M. Progress in targeted Alpha-particle therapy. What we learned about recoils release from in vivo generators. Molecules. 2018;23(3) https://doi.org/10.3390/molecules23030581.

208. Atallah E, Berger M, Jurcic J, Roboz G, Tse W, Mawad R, et al. A phase 2 study of Actinium-225 (225Ac)-lintuzumab in older patients with untreated acute myeloid leukemia (AML). J Med Imaging Radiat Sci. 2019;50(1):S37. https://doi.org/10.1016/j.jmir.2019.03.113.

209. Ehninger A, Kramer M, Rollig C, Thiede C, Bornhauser M, von Bonin M, et al. Distribution and levels of cell surface expression of CD33 and CD123 in acute myeloid leukemia. Blood Cancer J. 2014;4:e218. https://doi.org/10.1038/bcj.2014.39.

210. Jilani I, Estey E, Huh Y, Joe Y, Manshouri T, Yared M, et al. Differences in CD33 intensity between various myeloid neoplasms. Am J Clin Pathol. 2002;118(4):560–6. https://doi.org/10.1309/1WMW-CMXX-4WN4-T55U.

211. Saint-Paul L, Nguyen CH, Buffiere A, Pais de Barros JP, Hammann A, Landras-Guetta C, et al. CD45 phosphatase is crucial for human and murine acute myeloid leukemia maintenance through its localization in lipid rafts. Oncotarget. 2016;7(40):64785–97. https://doi.org/10.18632/oncotarget.11622.

212. Matthews DC, Appelbaum FR, Eary JF, Fisher DR, Durack LD, Hui TE, et al. Phase I study of (131)I-anti-CD45 antibody plus cyclophosphamide and total body irradiation for advanced acute leukemia and myelodysplastic syndrome. Blood. 1999;94(4):1237–47.

213. Matthews DC, Appelbaum FR, Eary JF, Fisher DR, Durack LD, Bush SA, et al. Development of a marrow transplant regimen for acute leukemia using targeted hematopoietic irradiation delivered by ^{131}I-labeled anti-CD45 antibody, combined with cyclophosphamide and total body irradiation. Blood. 1995;85(4):1122–31.

214. Pagel JM, Appelbaum FR, Eary JF, Rajendran J, Fisher DR, Gooley T, et al. 131I-anti-CD45 antibody plus busulfan and cyclophosphamide before allogeneic hematopoietic cell transplantation for treatment of acute myeloid leukemia in first remission. Blood. 2006;107(5):2184–91. https://doi.org/10.1182/blood-2005-06-2317.

215. Nakamae H, Wilbur DS, Hamlin DK, Thakar MS, Santos EB, Fisher DR, et al. Biodistributions, myelosuppression, and toxicities in mice treated with an anti-CD45 antibody labeled with the alpha-emitting radionuclides bismuth-213 or astatine-211. Cancer Res. 2009;69(6):2408–15. https://doi.org/10.1158/0008-5472.CAN-08-4363.

216. Chen Y, Kornblit B, Hamlin DK, Sale GE, Santos EB, Wilbur DS, et al. Durable donor engraftment after radioimmunotherapy using alpha-emitter astatine-211-labeled anti-CD45 antibody for conditioning in allogeneic hematopoietic cell transplantation. Blood. 2012;119(5):1130–8. https://doi.org/10.1182/blood-2011-09-380436.

217. Morsink LM, Walter RB. Novel monoclonal antibody-based therapies for acute myeloid leukemia. Best Pract Res Clin Haematol. 2019;32(2):116–26. https://doi.org/10.1016/j.beha.2019.05.002.

218. Williams BA, Law A, Hunyadkurti J, Desilets S, Leyton JV, Keating A. Antibody therapies for acute myeloid leukemia: unconjugated, toxin-conjugated, radio-conjugated and multivalent formats. J Clin Med. 2019;8(8):1261. https://doi.org/10.3390/jcm8081261.

219. Yabushita T, Satake H, Maruoka H, Morita M, Katoh D, Shimomura Y, et al. Expression of multiple leukemic stem cell markers is associated with poor

prognosis in de novo acute myeloid leukemia. Leuk Lymphoma. 2018;59(9):2144–51. https://doi.org/10.1080/10428194.2017.1410888.

220. Jin L, Hope KJ, Zhai Q, Smadja-Joffe F, Dick JE. Targeting of CD44 eradicates human acute myeloid leukemic stem cells. Nat Med. 2006;12(10):1167–74. https://doi.org/10.1038/nm1483.

221. Leyton JV, Gao C, Williams B, Keating A, Minden M, Reilly RM. A radiolabeled antibody targeting CD123(+) leukemia stem cells - initial radioimmunotherapy studies in NOD/SCID mice engrafted with primary human AML. Leukemia Res Rep. 2015;4(2):55–9. https://doi.org/10.1016/j.lrr.2015.07.003.

222. Leyton JV, Williams B, Gao C, Keating A, Minden M, Reilly RM. MicroSPECT/CT imaging of primary human AML engrafted into the bone marrow and spleen of NOD/SCID mice using 111In-DTPA-NLS-CSL360 radioimmunoconjugates recognizing the CD123+/CD131- epitope expressed by leukemia stem cells. Leuk Res. 2014;38(11):1367–73. https://doi.org/10.1016/j.leukres.2014.09.005.

223. Leyton JV, Hu M, Gao C, Turner PV, Dick JE, Minden M, et al. Auger electron radioimmunotherapeutic agent specific for the CD123+/CD131− phenotype of the leukemia stem cell population. J Nucl Med. 2011;52(9):1465–73. https://doi.org/10.2967/jnumed.111.087668.

224. Steiner M, Neri D. Antibody-radionuclide conjugates for cancer therapy: historical considerations and new trends. Clin Cancer Res. 2011;17(20):6406–16. https://doi.org/10.1158/1078-0432.CCR-11-0483.

225. Baxter LT, Jain RK. Transport of fluid and macromolecules in tumors. I. Role of interstitial pressure and convection. Microvasc Res. 1989;37(1):77–104.

226. Boucher Y, Baxter LT, Jain RK. Interstitial pressure gradients in tissue-isolated and subcutaneous tumors: implications for therapy. Cancer Res. 1990;50(15):4478–84.

227. Jain RK. Physiological barriers to delivery of monoclonal antibodies and other macromolecules in tumors. Cancer Res. 1990;50(3 Suppl):814s–9s.

228. Prasad V, Baum RP, Oliva JP. Radioimmunotherapy. In: Ahmadzadehfar H, Biersack H-J, Freeman LM, Zuckier LS, editors. Clinical nuclear medicine. Cham: Springer International Publishing; 2020. p. 917–49.

229. Lau J, Lin KS, Bénard F. Past, present, and future: development of Theranostic agents targeting carbonic anhydrase IX. Theranostics. 2017;7(17):4322–39. https://doi.org/10.7150/thno.21848.

230. Scott AM, Wiseman G, Welt S, Adjei A, Lee FT, Hopkins W, et al. A phase I dose-escalation study of sibrotuzumab in patients with advanced or metastatic fibroblast activation protein-positive cancer. Clin Cancer Res. 2003;9(5):1639–47.

231. Klein M, Lotem M, Peretz T, Zwas ST, Mizrachi S, Liberman Y, et al. Safety and efficacy of 188-rhenium-labeled antibody to melanin in patients with metastatic melanoma. J Skin Cancer. 2013;2013:828329. https://doi.org/10.1155/2013/828329.

232. Diamandis EP, Bast RC Jr, Gold P, Chu TM, Magnani JL. Reflection on the discovery of carcinoembryonic antigen, prostate-specific antigen, and cancer antigens CA125 and CA19-9. Clin Chem. 2013;59(1):22–31. https://doi.org/10.1373/clinchem.2012.187047.

233. Campos-da-Paz M, Dorea JG, Galdino AS, Lacava ZGM. de Fatima Menezes Almeida Santos M. carcinoembryonic antigen (CEA) and hepatic metastasis in colorectal cancer: update on biomarker for clinical and biotechnological approaches. Recent Pat Biotechnol. 2018;12(4):269–79. https://doi.org/10.2174/1872208312666180731104244.

234. Koppe MJ, Bleichrodt RP, Oyen WJ, Boerman OC. Radioimmunotherapy and colorectal cancer. Br J Surg. 2005;92(3):264–76. https://doi.org/10.1002/bjs.4936.

235. Bertagnolli MM. Radioimmunotherapy for colorectal cancer. Clin Cancer Res. 2005;11(13):4637–8. https://doi.org/10.1158/1078-0432.CCR-05-0485.

236. Sahlmann CO, Homayounfar K, Niessner M, Dyczkowski J, Conradi LC, Braulke F, et al. Repeated adjuvant anti-CEA radioimmunotherapy after resection of colorectal liver metastases: safety, feasibility, and long-term efficacy results of a prospective phase 2 study. Cancer. 2017;123(4):638–49. https://doi.org/10.1002/cncr.30390.

237. Liersch T, Meller J, Bittrich M, Kulle B, Becker H, Goldenberg DM. Update of carcinoembryonic antigen radioimmunotherapy with (131)I-labetuzumab after salvage resection of colorectal liver metastases: comparison of outcome to a contemporaneous control group. Ann Surg Oncol. 2007;14(9):2577–90. https://doi.org/10.1245/s10434-006-9328-x.

238. Wong JY, Shibata S, Williams LE, Kwok CS, Liu A, Chu DZ, et al. A phase I trial of 90Y-anti-carcinoembryonic antigen chimeric T84.66 radioimmunotherapy with 5-fluorouracil in patients with metastatic colorectal cancer. Clin Cancer Res. 2003;9(16 Pt 1):5842–52.

239. Hanaoka H, Kuroki M, Yamaguchi A, Achmad A, Iida Y, Higuchi T, et al. Fractionated radioimmunotherapy with 90Y-labeled fully human anti-CEA antibody. Cancer Biother Radiopharm. 2014;29(2):70–6. https://doi.org/10.1089/cbr.2013.1562.

240. Cahan B, Leong L, Wagman L, Yamauchi D, Shibata S, Wilzcynski S, et al. Phase I/II trial of anti-carcinoembryonic antigen radioimmunotherapy, gemcitabine, and hepatic arterial infusion of fluorodeoxyuridine postresection of liver metastasis for colorectal carcinoma. Cancer Biother Radiopharm. 2017;32(7):258–65.

241. Tagawa ST, Beltran H, Vallabhajosula S, Goldsmith SJ, Osborne J, Matulich D, et al. Anti-prostate-specific membrane antigen-based radioimmunotherapy for prostate cancer. Cancer. 2010;116(4 Suppl):1075–83. https://doi.org/10.1002/cncr.24795.

242. Kuo HT, Merkens H, Zhang Z, Uribe CF, Lau J, Zhang C, et al. Enhancing treatment efficacy of (177)Lu-PSMA-617 with the conjugation of an albumin-binding motif: preclinical dosimetry and Endoradiotherapy studies. Mol Pharm. 2018;15(11):5183–91. https://doi.org/10.1021/acs.molpharmaceut.8b00720.

243. Vallabhajosula S, Goldsmith SJ, Kostakoglu L, Milowsky MI, Nanus DM, Bander NH. Radioimmunotherapy of prostate cancer using 90Y- and 177Lu-labeled J591 monoclonal antibodies: effect of multiple treatments on myelotoxicity. Clin Cancer Res. 2005;11(19 Pt 2):7195s–200s. https://doi.org/10.1158/1078-0432.CCR-1004-0023.

244. Milowsky MI, Nanus DM, Kostakoglu L, Vallabhajosula S, Goldsmith SJ, Bander NH. Phase I trial of yttrium-90-labeled anti-prostate-specific membrane antigen monoclonal antibody J591 for androgen-independent prostate cancer. J Clin Oncol. 2004;22(13):2522–31. https://doi.org/10.1200/JCO.2004.09.154.

245. Tagawa ST, Akhtar NH, Nikolopoulou A, Kaur G, Robinson B, Kahn R, et al. Bone marrow recovery and subsequent chemotherapy following radiolabeled anti-prostate-specific membrane antigen monoclonal antibody j591 in men with metastatic castration-resistant prostate cancer. Front Oncol. 2013;3:214. https://doi.org/10.3389/fonc.2013.00214.

246. Tagawa ST, Vallabhajosula S, Christos PJ, Jhanwar YS, Batra JS, Lam L, et al. Phase 1/2 study of fractionated dose lutetium-177-labeled anti-prostate-specific membrane antigen monoclonal antibody J591 ((177) Lu-J591) for metastatic castration-resistant prostate cancer. Cancer. 2019;125(15):2561–9. https://doi.org/10.1002/cncr.32072.

247. Scheinberg DA, McDevitt MR. Actinium-225 in targeted alpha-particle therapeutic applications. Curr Radiopharm. 2011;4(4):306–20.

248. Tagawa ST, Vallabhajosula S, Jhanwar Y, Ballman KV, Hackett A, Emmerich L, et al. Phase I dose-escalation study of 225Ac-J591 for progressive metastatic castration resistant prostate cancer (mCRPC). J Clin Oncol. 2018;36(6 Suppl):TPS399. https://doi.org/10.1200/JCO.2018.36.6_suppl.TPS399.

249. Milenic DE, Baidoo KE, Kim YS, Barkley R, Brechbiel MW. Targeted alpha-particle radiation therapy of HER1-positive disseminated intraperitoneal disease: An investigation of the human anti-EGFR monoclonal antibody. Panitumumab Transl Oncol. 2017;10(4):535–45. https://doi.org/10.1016/j.tranon.2017.04.004.

250. Melzig C, Golestaneh AF, Mier W, Schwager C, Das S, Schlegel J, et al. Combined external beam radiotherapy with carbon ions and tumor targeting endoradiotherapy. Oncotarget. 2018;9(52):29985–30004. https://doi.org/10.18632/oncotarget.25695.

251. Kim EJ, Kim BS, Choi DB, Chi SG, Choi TH. Enhanced tumor retention of radioiodinated anti-epidermal growth factor receptor antibody using novel bifunctional iodination linker for radio-immunotherapy. Oncol Rep. 2016;35(6):3159–68. https://doi.org/10.3892/or.2016.4706.

252. Milenic DE, Baidoo KE, Kim YS, Brechbiel MW. Evaluation of cetuximab as a candidate for targeted alpha-particle radiation therapy of HER1-positive disseminated intraperitoneal disease. mAbs. 2015;7(1):255–64. https://doi.org/10.4161/19420862.2014.985160.

253. Song IH, Lee TS, Park YS, Lee JS, Lee BC, Moon BS, et al. Immuno-PET imaging and Radioimmunotherapy of ^{64}Cu-/^{177}Lu-labeled anti-EGFR antibody in esophageal squamous cell carcinoma model. J Nucl Med. 2016;57(7):1105–11. https://doi.org/10.2967/jnumed.115.167155.

254. Fazel J, Rotzer S, Seidl C, Feuerecker B, Autenrieth M, Weirich G, et al. Fractionated intravesical radio-immunotherapy with (213)bi-anti-EGFR-MAb is effective without toxic side-effects in a nude mouse model of advanced human bladder carcinoma. Cancer Biol Ther. 2015;16(10):1526–34. https://doi.org/10.1080/15384047.2015.1071735.

255. Chang YJ, Ho CL, Cheng KH, Kuo WI, Lee WC, Lan KL, et al. Biodistribution, pharmacokinetics and radioimmunotherapy of (188)re-cetuximab in NCI-H292 human lung tumor-bearing nude mice. Investig New Drugs. 2019; https://doi.org/10.1007/s10637-018-00718-8.

256. Luo TY, Cheng PC, Chiang PF, Chuang TW, Yeh CH, Lin WJ. 188Re-HYNIC-trastuzumab enhances the effect of apoptosis induced by trastuzumab in HER2-overexpressing breast cancer cells. Ann Nucl Med. 2015;29(1):52–62. https://doi.org/10.1007/s12149-014-0908-8.

257. Li HK, Morokoshi Y, Nagatsu K, Kamada T, Hasegawa S. Locoregional therapy with alpha-emitting trastuzumab against peritoneal metastasis of human epidermal growth factor receptor 2-positive gastric cancer in mice. Cancer Sci. 2017;108(8):1648–56. https://doi.org/10.1111/cas.13282.

258. Timmermand OV, Elgqvist J, Beattie KA, Orbom A, Larsson E, Eriksson SE, et al. Preclinical efficacy of hK2 targeted [(177)Lu]hu11B6 for prostate cancer theranostics. Theranostics. 2019;9(8):2129–42. https://doi.org/10.7150/thno.31179.

259. Timmermand OV, Nilsson J, Strand SE, Elgqvist J. High resolution digital autoradiographic and dosimetric analysis of heterogeneous radioactivity distribution in xenografted prostate tumors. Med Phys. 2016;43(12):6632. https://doi.org/10.1118/1.4967877.

260. Vilhelmsson Timmermand O, Larsson E, Ulmert D, Tran TA, Strand S. Radioimmunotherapy of prostate cancer targeting human kallikrein-related peptidase 2. EJNMMI Res. 2016;6(1):27. https://doi.org/10.1186/s13550-016-0181-z.

261. Thorek DLJ, Ku AT, Mitsiades N, Veach D, Watson PA, Metha D, et al. Harnessing androgen receptor pathway activation for targeted alpha particle Radioimmunotherapy of breast cancer. Clin Cancer Res.

2019;25(2):881–91. https://doi.org/10.1158/1078-0432.CCR-18-1521.

262. Allen KJH, Jiao R, Malo ME, Frank C, Fisher DR, Rickles D, et al. Comparative radioimmunotherapy of experimental melanoma with novel humanized antibody to melanin labeled with [213]Bismuth and [177]Lutetium. Pharmaceutics. 2019;11(7) https://doi.org/10.3390/pharmaceutics11070348.

263. Kasten BB, Arend RC, Katre AA, Kim H, Fan J, Ferrone S, et al. B7-H3-targeted (212)Pb radioimmunotherapy of ovarian cancer in preclinical models. Nucl Med Biol. 2017;47:23–30. https://doi.org/10.1016/j.nucmedbio.2017.01.003.

264. Kasten BB, Gangrade A, Kim H, Fan J, Ferrone S, Ferrone CR, et al. (212)Pb-labeled B7-H3-targeting antibody for pancreatic cancer therapy in mouse models. Nucl Med Biol. 2018;58:67–73. https://doi.org/10.1016/j.nucmedbio.2017.12.004.

265. Lindenblatt D, Terraneo N, Pellegrini G, Cohrs S, Spycher PR, Vukovic D, et al. Combination of lutetium-177 labelled anti-L1CAM antibody chCE7 with the clinically relevant protein kinase inhibitor MK1775: a novel combination against human ovarian carcinoma. BMC Cancer. 2018;18(1):922. https://doi.org/10.1186/s12885-018-4836-1.

266. Basaco T, Pektor S, Bermudez JM, Meneses N, Heller M, Galvan JA, et al. Evaluation of radiolabeled girentuximab in vitro and in vivo. Pharmaceuticals (Basel). 2018;11(4) https://doi.org/10.3390/ph11040132.

267. Westrom S, Bonsdorff TB, Abbas N, Bruland OS, Jonasdottir TJ, Maelandsmo GM, et al. Evaluation of CD146 as target for Radioimmunotherapy against osteosarcoma. PLoS One. 2016;11(10):e0165382. https://doi.org/10.1371/journal.pone.0165382.

268. Fujiwara K, Koyama K, Suga K, Ikemura M, Saito Y, Hino A, et al. 90Y-labeled anti-ROBO1 monoclonal antibody exhibits antitumor activity against small cell lung cancer xenografts. PLoS One. 2015;10(5):e0125468. https://doi.org/10.1371/journal.pone.0125468.

269. Sugyo A, Tsuji AB, Sudo H, Okada M, Koizumi M, Satoh H, et al. Evaluation of efficacy of Radioimmunotherapy with 90Y-labeled fully human anti-transferrin receptor monoclonal antibody in pancreatic cancer mouse models. PLoS One. 2015;10(4):e0123761. https://doi.org/10.1371/journal.pone.0123761.

270. Derrien A, Gouard S, Maurel C, Gaugler MH, Bruchertseifer F, Morgenstern A, et al. Therapeutic efficacy of alpha-RIT using a (213)bi-anti-hCD138 antibody in a mouse model of ovarian peritoneal Carcinomatosis. Front Med. 2015;2:88. https://doi.org/10.3389/fmed.2015.00088.

271. Weng D, Jin X, Qin S, Lan X, Chen C, Sun X, et al. Radioimmunotherapy for CD133(+) colonic cancer stem cells inhibits tumor development in nude mice. Oncotarget. 2017;8(27):44004–14. https://doi.org/10.18632/oncotarget.16868.

272. Lang J, Lan X, Liu Y, Jin X, Wu T, Sun X, et al. Targeting cancer stem cells with an ^{131}I-labeled anti-AC133 monoclonal antibody in human colorectal cancer xenografts. Nucl Med Biol. 2015;42(5):505–12. https://doi.org/10.1016/j.nucmedbio.2015.01.003.

273. Deshayes E, Ladjohounlou R, Le Fur P, Pichard A, Lozza C, Boudousq V, et al. Radiolabeled antibodies against Mullerian-inhibiting substance receptor, type II: new tools for a theranostic approach in ovarian cancer. J Nucl Med. 2018;59(8):1234–42. https://doi.org/10.2967/jnumed.118.208611.

274. Sugyo A, Tsuji AB, Sudo H, Koizumi M, Ukai Y, Kurosawa G, et al. Efficacy evaluation of combination treatment using gemcitabine and radioimmunotherapy with (90)Y-labeled fully human anti-CD147 monoclonal antibody 059-053 in a BxPC-3 xenograft mouse model of refractory pancreatic cancer. Int J Mol Sci. 2018;19(10) https://doi.org/10.3390/ijms19102979.

275. Li HK, Sugyo A, Tsuji AB, Morokoshi Y, Minegishi K, Nagatsu K, et al. Alpha-particle therapy for synovial sarcoma in the mouse using an astatine-211-labeled antibody against frizzled homolog 10. Cancer Sci. 2018;109(7):2302–9. https://doi.org/10.1111/cas.13636.

276. Ma S. Biology and clinical implications of CD133(+) liver cancer stem cells. Exp Cell Res. 2013;319(2):126–32. https://doi.org/10.1016/j.yexcr.2012.09.007.

277. Wei W, Jiang D, Ehlerding EB, Barnhart TE, Yang Y, Engle JW, et al. CD146-targeted multimodal image-guided Photoimmunotherapy of melanoma. Adv Sci (Weinh). 2019;6(9):1801237. https://doi.org/10.1002/advs.201801237.

278. Valkenburg KC, de Groot AE, Pienta KJ. Targeting the tumour stroma to improve cancer therapy. Nat Rev Clin Oncol. 2018;15(6):366–81. https://doi.org/10.1038/s41571-018-0007-1.

279. Welt S, Divgi CR, Scott AM, Garin-Chesa P, Finn RD, Graham M, et al. Antibody targeting in metastatic colon cancer: a phase I study of monoclonal antibody F19 against a cell-surface protein of reactive tumor stromal fibroblasts. J Clin Oncol. 1994;12(6):1193–203. https://doi.org/10.1200/JCO.1994.12.6.1193.

280. Fischer E, Chaitanya K, Wuest T, Wadle A, Scott AM, van den Broek M, et al. Radioimmunotherapy of fibroblast activation protein positive tumors by rapidly internalizing antibodies. Clin Cancer Res. 2012;18(22):6208–18. https://doi.org/10.1158/1078-0432.CCR-12-0644.

281. Guillermina F-F, Blanca O-G, Myrna Luna G, Clara Santos C, Nallely J-M, Erika A-V, et al. Radiolabeled protein-inhibitor peptides with rapid clinical translation towards imaging and therapy. Curr Med Chem. 2020;27:1–15. https://doi.org/10.2174/0929867327666191223121211.

282. Schliemann C, Neri D. Antibody-based vascular tumor targeting. Recent results in cancer research. Fortschritte der Krebsforschung Progres dans les

recherches sur le cancer. 2010;180:201–16. https://doi.org/10.1007/978-3-540-78281-0_12.

283. Lee SY, Hong YD, Pyun MS, Felipe PM, Choi SJ. Radiolabeling of monoclonal anti-vascular endothelial growth factor receptor 1 (VEGFR 1) with (177)Lu for potential use in radioimmunotherapy. Appl Radiat Isot. 2009;67(7-8):1185–9. https://doi.org/10.1016/j.apradiso.2009.02.006.

284. Ebbinghaus C, Scheuermann J, Neri D, Elia G. Diagnostic and therapeutic applications of recombinant antibodies: targeting the extra-domain B of fibronectin, a marker of tumor angiogenesis. Curr Pharm Des. 2004;10(13):1537–49. https://doi.org/10.2174/1381612043384808.

285. Tijink BM, Neri D, Leemans CR, Budde M, Dinkelborg LM, Stigter-van Walsum M, et al. Radioimmunotherapy of head and neck cancer xenografts using ^{131}I-labeled antibody L19-SIP for selective targeting of tumor vasculature. J Nucl Med. 2006;47(7): 1127–35.

286. El-Emir E, Dearling JL, Huhalov A, Robson MP, Boxer G, Neri D, et al. Characterisation and radio-immunotherapy of L19-SIP, an anti-angiogenic antibody against the extra domain B of fibronectin, in colorectal tumour models. Br J Cancer. 2007;96(12):1862–70. https://doi.org/10.1038/sj.bjc.6603806.

287. Spaeth N, Wyss MT, Pahnke J, Biollaz G, Trachsel E, Drandarov K, et al. Radioimmunotherapy targeting the extra domain B of fibronectin in C6 rat gliomas: a preliminary study about the therapeutic efficacy of iodine-131-labeled SIP(L19). Nucl Med Biol. 2006;33(5):661–6. https://doi.org/10.1016/j.nucmedbio.2006.05.001.

288. Dallas NA, Samuel S, Xia L, Fan F, Gray MJ, Lim SJ, et al. Endoglin (CD105): a marker of tumor vasculature and potential target for therapy. Clin Cancer Res. 2008;14(7):1931–7. https://doi.org/10.1158/1078-0432.CCR-07-4478.

289. Ehlerding EB, Lacognata S, Jiang D, Ferreira CA, Goel S, Hernandez R, et al. Targeting angiogenesis for radioimmunotherapy with a (177)Lu-labeled antibody. Eur J Nucl Med Mol Imaging. 2018;45(1):123–31. https://doi.org/10.1007/s00259-017-3793-2.

290. Goel HL, Mercurio AM. VEGF targets the tumour cell. Nat Rev Cancer. 2013;13(12):871–82. https://doi.org/10.1038/nrc3627.

291. Liu F, Qi L, Liu B, Liu J, Zhang H, Che D, et al. Fibroblast activation protein overexpression and clinical implications in solid tumors: a meta-analysis. PLoS One. 2015;10(3):e0116683. https://doi.org/10.1371/journal.pone.0116683.

292. Aung W, Tsuji AB, Sudo H, Sugyo A, Ukai Y, Kouda K, et al. Radioimmunotherapy of pancreatic cancer xenografts in nude mice using 90Y-labeled anti-alpha6beta4 integrin antibody. Oncotarget. 2016;7(25):38835–44. https://doi.org/10.18632/oncotarget.9631.

293. Veeravagu A, Liu Z, Niu G, Chen K, Jia B, Cai W, et al. Integrin $\alpha v\beta_3$-targeted Radioimmunotherapy of glioblastoma Multiforme. Clin Cancer Res. 2008;14(22):7330–9. https://doi.org/10.1158/1078-0432.Ccr-08-0797.

294. Riva P, Franceschi G, Riva N, Casi M, Santimaria M, Adamo M. Role of nuclear medicine in the treatment of malignant gliomas: the locoregional radioimmunotherapy approach. Eur J Nucl Med. 2000;27(5):601–9. https://doi.org/10.1007/s002590050549.

295. Reardon DA, Zalutsky MR, Bigner DD. Antitenascin-C monoclonal antibody radioimmunotherapy for malignant glioma patients. Expert Rev Anticancer Ther. 2007;7(5):675–87. https://doi.org/10.1586/14737140.7.5.675.

296. Raghavan R, Howell RW, Zalutsky MR. A model for optimizing delivery of targeted radionuclide therapies into resection cavity margins for the treatment of primary brain cancers. Biomed Phys Eng Express. 2017;3(3) https://doi.org/10.1088/2057-1976/aa6db9.

297. Aarts F, Bleichrodt RP, Oyen WJ, Boerman OC. Intracavitary radioimmunotherapy to treat solid tumors. Cancer Biother Radiopharm. 2008;23(1):92–107. https://doi.org/10.1089/cbr.2007.0412.

298. Huber R, Seidl C, Schmid E, Seidenschwang S, Becker KF, Schuhmacher C, et al. Locoregional alpha-radioimmunotherapy of intraperitoneal tumor cell dissemination using a tumor-specific monoclonal antibody. Clin Cancer Res. 2003;9(10 Pt 2):3922S–8S.

299. Kinuya S, Yokoyama K, Kawashima A, Hiramatsu T, Konishi S, Shuke N, et al. Pharmacologic intervention with angiotensin II and kininase inhibitor enhanced efficacy of radioimmunotherapy in human colon cancer xenografts. J Nucl Med. 2000;41(7):1244–9.

300. Chen A. PARP inhibitors: its role in treatment of cancer. Chin J Cancer. 2011;30(7):463–71. https://doi.org/10.5732/cjc.011.10111.

301. Gill MR, Falzone N, Du Y, Vallis KA. Targeted radionuclide therapy in combined-modality regimens. Lancet Oncol. 2017;18(7):e414–e23. https://doi.org/10.1016/S1470-2045(17)30379-0.

302. Al-Ejeh F, Shi W, Miranda M, Simpson PT, Vargas AC, Song S, et al. Treatment of triple-negative breast cancer using anti-EGFR-directed radioimmunotherapy combined with radiosensitizing chemotherapy and PARP inhibitor. J Nucl Med. 2013;54(6):913–21. https://doi.org/10.2967/jnumed.112.111534.

303. Repetto-Llamazares AHV, Malenge MM, O'Shea A, Eiriksdottir B, Stokke T, Larsen RH, et al. Combination of (177) Lu-lilotomab with rituximab significantly improves the therapeutic outcome in preclinical models of non-Hodgkin's lymphoma. Eur J Haematol. 2018;101(4):522–31. https://doi.org/10.1111/ejh.13139.

304. Blumenthal RD, Kashi R, Stephens R, Sharkey RM, Goldenberg DM. Improved radioimmunother-

apy of colorectal cancer xenografts using antibody mixtures against carcinoembryonic antigen and colon-specific antigen-p. Cancer Immunol Immunother. 1991;32(5):303–10. https://doi.org/10.1007/bf01789048.

305. Milenic DE, Brady ED, Garmestani K, Albert PS, Abdulla A, Brechbiel MW. Improved efficacy of alpha-particle-targeted radiation therapy: dual targeting of human epidermal growth factor receptor-2 and tumor-associated glycoprotein 72. Cancer. 2010;116(4 Suppl):1059–66. https://doi.org/10.1002/cncr.24793.

306. Pagel JM, Pantelias A, Hedin N, Wilbur S, Saganic L, Lin Y, et al. Evaluation of CD20, CD22, and HLA-DR targeting for radioimmunotherapy of B-cell lymphomas. Cancer Res. 2007;67(12):5921–8. https://doi.org/10.1158/0008-5472.CAN-07-0080.

307. Deutsch E, Chargari C, Galluzzi L, Kroemer G. Optimising efficacy and reducing toxicity of anticancer radioimmunotherapy. Lancet Oncol. 2019;20(8):e452–e63. https://doi.org/10.1016/S1470-2045(19)30171-8.

308. Levy A, Nigro G, Sansonetti PJ, Deutsch E. Candidate immune biomarkers for radioimmunotherapy. Biochim Biophys Acta Rev Cancer. 2017;1868(1):58–68. https://doi.org/10.1016/j.bbcan.2017.02.006.

309. Heery CR, Madan RA, Stein MN, Stadler WM, Di Paola RS, Rauckhorst M, et al. Samarium-153-EDTMP (Quadramet(R)) with or without vaccine in metastatic castration-resistant prostate cancer: a randomized Phase 2 trial. Oncotarget. 2016;7(42):69014–23. https://doi.org/10.18632/oncotarget.10883.

310. Fu R, Carroll L, Yahioglu G, Aboagye EO, Miller PW. Antibody fragment and Affibody ImmunoPET imaging agents: Radiolabelling strategies and applications. ChemMedChem. 2018;13(23):2466–78. https://doi.org/10.1002/cmdc.201800624.

311. Xenaki KT, Oliveira S, van Bergen En Henegouwen PMP. Antibody or antibody fragments: implications for molecular imaging and targeted therapy of solid tumors. Front Immunol. 2017;8:1287. https://doi.org/10.3389/fimmu.2017.01287.

312. Elgqvist J, Andersson H, Bernhardt P, Back T, Claesson I, Hultborn R, et al. Administered activity and metastatic cure probability during radioimmunotherapy of ovarian cancer in nude mice with 211At-MX35 F(ab')2. Int J Radiat Oncol Biol Phys. 2006;66(4):1228–37. https://doi.org/10.1016/j.ijrobp.2006.07.003.

313. Back T, Chouin N, Lindegren S, Kahu H, Jensen H, Albertsson P, et al. Cure of human ovarian carcinoma solid xenografts by fractionated alpha-radioimmunotherapy with (211)at-MX35-F(ab')2: influence of absorbed tumor dose and effect on long-term survival. J Nucl Med. 2017;58(4):598–604. https://doi.org/10.2967/jnumed.116.178327.

314. Tolmachev V, Nilsson FY, Widstrom C, Andersson K, Rosik D, Gedda L, et al. 111In-benzyl-DTPA-ZHER2:342, an affibody-based conjugate for in vivo imaging of HER2 expression in malignant tumors. J Nucl Med. 2006;47(5):846–53.

315. Tolmachev V, Orlova A, Pehrson R, Galli J, Baastrup B, Andersson K, et al. Radionuclide therapy of HER2-positive microxenografts using a 177Lu-labeled HER2-specific Affibody molecule. Cancer Res. 2007;67(6):2773–82. https://doi.org/10.1158/0008-5472.CAN-06-1630.

316. Wiehr S, Buhler P, Gierschner D, Wolf P, Rolle AM, Kesenheimer C, et al. Pharmacokinetics and PET imaging properties of two recombinant anti-PSMA antibody fragments in comparison to their parental antibody. Prostate. 2014;74(7):743–55. https://doi.org/10.1002/pros.22794.

317. Tavare R, McCracken MN, Zettlitz KA, Knowles SM, Salazar FB, Olafsen T, et al. Engineered antibody fragments for immuno-PET imaging of endogenous CD8+ T cells in vivo. Proc Natl Acad Sci U S A. 2014;111(3):1108–13. https://doi.org/10.1073/pnas.1316922111.

318. Lutje S, Franssen GM, Sharkey RM, Laverman P, Rossi EA, Goldenberg DM, et al. Anti-CEA antibody fragments labeled with [(18)F]AlF for PET imaging of CEA-expressing tumors. Bioconjug Chem. 2014;25(2):335–41. https://doi.org/10.1021/bc4004926.

319. Frejd FY, Kim KT. Affibody molecules as engineered protein drugs. Exp Mol Med. 2017;49(3):e306. https://doi.org/10.1038/emm.2017.35.

320. Goodwin DA, Meares CF, McTigue M, Chaovapong W, Diamanti CI, Ransone CH, et al. Pretargeted immunoscintigraphy: effect of hapten valency on murine tumor uptake. J Nucl Med. 1992;33(11):2006–13.

321. Bailly C, Bodet-Milin C, Rousseau C, Faivre-Chauvet A, Kraeber-Bodere F, Barbet J. Pretargeting for imaging and therapy in oncological nuclear medicine. EJNMMI Radiopharm Chem. 2017;2(1):6. https://doi.org/10.1186/s41181-017-0026-8.

322. Verhoeven M, Seimbille Y, Dalm SU. Therapeutic applications of pretargeting. Pharmaceutics. 2019;11(9) https://doi.org/10.3390/pharmaceutics11090434.

323. Liu G. A revisit to the Pretargeting concept-a target conversion. Front Pharmacol. 2018;9:1476. https://doi.org/10.3389/fphar.2018.01476.

324. Altai M, Membreno R, Cook B, Tolmachev V, Zeglis BM. Pretargeted imaging and therapy. J Nucl Med. 2017;58(10):1553–9. https://doi.org/10.2967/jnumed.117.189944.

325. Patra M, Zarschler K, Pietzsch HJ, Stephan H, Gasser G. New insights into the pretargeting approach to image and treat tumours. Chem Soc Rev. 2016;45(23):6415–31. https://doi.org/10.1039/c5cs00784d.

326. Steen EJL, Edem PE, Norregaard K, Jorgensen JT, Shalgunov V, Kjaer A, et al. Pretargeting in nuclear imaging and radionuclide therapy: improving efficacy of theranostics and nanomedicines. Biomate-

rials. 2018;179:209–45. https://doi.org/10.1016/j.biomaterials.2018.06.021.

327. Knight JC, Cornelissen B. Bioorthogonal chemistry: implications for pretargeted nuclear (PET/SPECT) imaging and therapy. Am J Nucl Med Mol Imaging. 2014;4(2):96–113.

328. Paganelli G, Chinol M, Maggiolo M, Sidoli A, Corti A, Baroni S, et al. The three-step pretargeting approach reduces the human anti-mouse antibody response in patients submitted to radioimmunoscintigraphy and radioimmunotherapy. Eur J Nucl Med. 1997;24(3):350–1. https://doi.org/10.1007/bf01728778.

329. Paganelli G, Magnani P, Zito F, Villa E, Sudati F, Lopalco L, et al. Three-step monoclonal antibody tumor targeting in carcinoembryonic antigen-positive patients. Cancer Res. 1991;51(21):5960–6.

330. Paganelli G, Malcovati M, Fazio F. Monoclonal antibody pretargetting techniques for tumour localization: the avidin-biotin system. International workshop on techniques for amplification of tumour targetting. Nucl Med Commun. 1991;12(3):211–34. https://doi.org/10.1097/00006231-199103000-00006.

331. Weiden PL, Breitz HB, Press O, Appelbaum JW, Bryan JK, Gaffigan S, et al. Pretargeted radioimmunotherapy (PRIT) for treatment of non-Hodgkin's lymphoma (NHL): initial phase I/II study results. Cancer Biother Radiopharm. 2000;15(1):15–29. https://doi.org/10.1089/cbr.2000.15.15.

332. Domingo RJ, Reilly RM. Pre-targeted radioimmunotherapy of human colon cancer xenografts in athymic mice using streptavidin-CC49 monoclonal antibody and 90Y-DOTA-biotin. Nucl Med Commun. 2000;21(1):89–96. https://doi.org/10.1097/00006231-200001000-00015.

333. Frost SH, Back T, Chouin N, Hultborn R, Jacobsson L, Elgqvist J, et al. Comparison of 211At-PRIT and 211At-RIT of ovarian microtumors in a nude mouse model. Cancer Biother Radiopharm. 2013;28(2):108–14. https://doi.org/10.1089/cbr.2012.1281.

334. Kontermann RE, Brinkmann U. Bispecific antibodies. Drug Discov Today. 2015;20(7):838–47. https://doi.org/10.1016/j.drudis.2015.02.008.

335. Le Doussal JM, Martin M, Gautherot E, Delaage M, Barbet J. In vitro and in vivo targeting of radiolabeled monovalent and divalent haptens with dual specificity monoclonal antibody conjugates: enhanced divalent hapten affinity for cell-bound antibody conjugate. J Nucl Med. 1989;30(8):1358–66.

336. Cheal SM, Fung EK, Patel M, Xu H, Guo HF, Zanzonico PB, et al. Curative multicycle radioimmunotherapy monitored by quantitative SPECT/CT-based theranostics, using bispecific antibody pretargeting strategy in colorectal cancer. J Nucl Med. 2017;58(11):1735–42. https://doi.org/10.2967/jnumed.117.193250.

337. Chang CH, Sharkey RM, Rossi EA, Karacay H, McBride W, Hansen HJ, et al. Molecular advances in pretargeting radioimunotherapy with bispecific antibodies. Mol Cancer Ther. 2002;1(7):553–63.

338. Gruaz-Guyon A, Janevik-Ivanovska E, Raguin O, De Labriolle-Vaylet C, Barbet J. Radiolabeled bivalent haptens for tumor immunodetection and radioimmunotherapy. Q J Nucl Med. 2001;45(2):201–6.

339. Green DJ, Frayo SL, Lin Y, Hamlin DK, Fisher DR, Frost SH, et al. Comparative analysis of bispecific antibody and streptavidin-targeted radioimmunotherapy for B-cell cancers. Cancer Res. 2016;76(22):6669–79. https://doi.org/10.1158/0008-5472.CAN-16-0571.

340. Green DJ, O'Steen S, Lin Y, Comstock ML, Kenoyer AL, Hamlin DK, et al. CD38-bispecific antibody pretargeted radioimmunotherapy for multiple myeloma and other B-cell malignancies. Blood. 2018;131(6):611–20. https://doi.org/10.1182/blood-2017-09-807610.

341. van Rij CM, Frielink C, Goldenberg DM, Sharkey RM, Lutje S, McBride WJ, et al. Pretargeted radioimmunotherapy of prostate cancer with an anti-TROP-2xAnti-HSG bispecific antibody and a (177)Lu-labeled peptide. Cancer Biother Radiopharm. 2014;29(8):323–9. https://doi.org/10.1089/cbr.2014.1660.

342. van Rij CM, Lutje S, Frielink C, Sharkey RM, Goldenberg DM, Franssen GM, et al. Pretargeted immuno-PET and radioimmunotherapy of prostate cancer with an anti-TROP-2 x anti-HSG bispecific antibody. Eur J Nucl Med Mol Imaging. 2013;40(9):1377–83. https://doi.org/10.1007/s00259-013-2434-7.

343. Schoffelen R, Boerman OC, Goldenberg DM, Sharkey RM, van Herpen CM, Franssen GM, et al. Development of an imaging-guided CEA-pretargeted radionuclide treatment of advanced colorectal cancer: first clinical results. Br J Cancer. 2013;109(4):934–42. https://doi.org/10.1038/bjc.2013.376.

344. Bodet-Milin C, Bailly C, Touchefeu Y, Frampas E, Bourgeois M, Rauscher A, et al. Clinical results in medullary thyroid carcinoma suggest high potential of Pretargeted Immuno-PET for tumor imaging and Theranostic approaches. Front Med. 2019;6:124. https://doi.org/10.3389/fmed.2019.00124.

345. Cheal SM, Xu H, Guo H-F, Patel M, Punzalan B, Fung EK, et al. Theranostic pretargeted radioimmunotherapy of internalizing solid tumor antigens in human tumor xenografts in mice: curative treatment of HER2-positive breast carcinoma. Theranostics. 2018;8(18):5106–25. https://doi.org/10.7150/thno.26585.

346. Zeglis BM, Brand C, Abdel-Atti D, Carnazza KE, Cook BE, Carlin S, et al. Optimization of a pretargeted strategy for the PET imaging of colorectal carcinoma via the modulation of radioligand pharmacokinetics. Mol Pharm. 2015;12(10):3575–87. https://doi.org/10.1021/acs.molpharmaceut.5b00294.

347. Membreno R, Cook BE, Fung K, Lewis JS, Zeglis BM. Click-mediated pretargeted radioimmu-

notherapy of colorectal carcinoma. Mol Pharm. 2018;15(4):1729–34. https://doi.org/10.1021/acs.molpharmaceut.8b00093.

348. Kuijpers WH, Bos ES, Kaspersen FM, Veeneman GH, van Boeckel CA. Specific recognition of antibody-oligonucleotide conjugates by radiolabeled antisense nucleotides: a novel approach for two-step radioimmunotherapy of cancer. Bioconjug Chem. 1993;4(1):94–102. https://doi.org/10.1021/bc00019a013.

349. Liu G, Mang'era K, Liu N, Gupta S, Rusckowski M, Hnatowich DJ. Tumor pretargeting in mice using (99m)Tc-labeled morpholino, a DNA analog. J Nucl Med. 2002;43(3):384–91.

350. Liu G, Dou S, Baker S, Akalin A, Cheng D, Chen L, et al. A preclinical 188Re tumor therapeutic investigation using MORF/cMORF pretargeting and an antiTAG-72 antibody CC49. Cancer Biol Ther. 2010;10(8):767–74. https://doi.org/10.4161/cbt.10.8.12879.

351. Houghton JL, Membreno R, Abdel-Atti D, Cunanan KM, Carlin S, Scholz WW, et al. Establishment of the in vivo efficacy of pretargeted radioimmunotherapy utilizing inverse electron demand Diels-Alder click chemistry. Mol Cancer Ther. 2017;16(1):124–33. https://doi.org/10.1158/1535-7163.Mct-16-0503.

352. Poty S, Carter LM, Mandleywala K, Membreno R, Abdel-Atti D, Ragupathi A, et al. Leveraging bioorthogonal click chemistry to improve (225) Ac-radioimmunotherapy of pancreatic ductal adenocarcinoma. Clin Cancer Res. 2019;25(2):868–80. https://doi.org/10.1158/1078-0432.CCR-18-1650.

353. Shah MA, Zhang X, Rossin R, Robillard MS, Fisher DR, Bueltmann T, et al. Metal-free cycloaddition chemistry driven pretargeted radioimmunotherapy using alpha-particle radiation. Bioconjug Chem. 2017;28(12):3007–15. https://doi.org/10.1021/acs.bioconjchem.7b00612.

354. Loke KS, Padhy AK, Ng DC, Goh AS, Divgi C. Dosimetric considerations in radioimmunotherapy and systemic radionuclide therapies: a review. World J Nucl Med. 2011;10(2):122–38. https://doi.org/10.4103/1450-1147.89780.

355. Flux GD, Sjogreen Gleisner K, Chiesa C, Lassmann M, Chouin N, Gear J, et al. From fixed activities to personalized treatments in radionuclide therapy: lost in translation? Eur J Nucl Med Mol Imaging. 2018;45(1):152–4. https://doi.org/10.1007/s00259-017-3859-1.

356. Brans B, Bodei L, Giammarile F, Linden O, Luster M, Oyen WJG, et al. Clinical radionuclide therapy dosimetry: the quest for the "holy Gray". Eur J Nucl Med Mol Imaging. 2007;34(5):772–86. https://doi.org/10.1007/s00259-006-0338-5.

357. Pouget JP, Lozza C, Deshayes E, Boudousq V, Navarro-Teulon I. Introduction to radiobiology of targeted radionuclide therapy. Front Med. 2015;2:12. https://doi.org/10.3389/fmed.2015.00012.

358. Ljungberg M, Sjogreen GK. Personalized dosimetry for radionuclide therapy using molecular imaging tools. Biomedicines. 2016;4(4) https://doi.org/10.3390/biomedicines4040025.

359. Li T, Ao ECI, Lambert B, Brans B, Vandenberghe S, Mok GSP. Quantitative imaging for targeted radionuclide therapy dosimetry - technical review. Theranostics. 2017;7(18):4551–65. https://doi.org/10.7150/thno.19782.

360. Bardiès M, Buvat I. Dosimetry in nuclear medicine therapy: what are the specifics in image quantification for dosimetry? Q J Nucl Med Mol Imaging. 2011;55(1):5–20.

361. Santoro L, Boutaleb S, Garambois V, Bascoul-Mollevi C, Boudousq V, Kotzki PO, et al. Noninternalizing monoclonal antibodies are suitable candidates for 125I radioimmunotherapy of small-volume peritoneal carcinomatosis. J Nucl Med. 2009;50(12):2033–41. https://doi.org/10.2967/jnumed.109.066993.

362. Ferrer L, Malek E, Bodet-Milin C, Legouill S, Prangere T, Robu D, et al. Comparisons of dosimetric approaches for fractionated radioimmunotherapy of non-Hodgkin lymphoma. Q J Nucl Med Mol Imaging. 2012;56(6):529–37.

363. Morschhauser F, Dekyndt B, Baillet C, Barthelemy C, Malek E, Fulcrand J, et al. A new pharmacokinetic model for (90)Y-ibritumomab tiuxetan based on 3-dimensional dosimetry. Sci Rep. 2018;8(1):14860. https://doi.org/10.1038/s41598-018-33160-0.

364. Kratochwil C, Schmidt K, Afshar-Oromieh A, Bruchertseifer F, Rathke H, Morgenstern A, et al. Targeted alpha therapy of mCRPC: dosimetry estimate of (213)bismuth-PSMA-617. Eur J Nucl Med Mol Imaging. 2018;45(1):31–7. https://doi.org/10.1007/s00259-017-3817-y.

365. Dewaraja YK, Schipper MJ, Shen J, Smith LB, Murgic J, Savas H, et al. Tumor-absorbed dose predicts progression-free survival following (131)I-Tositumomab Radioimmunotherapy. J Nucl Med. 2014;55(7):1047–53. https://doi.org/10.2967/jnumed.113.136044.

366. Schwartz J, Humm JL, Divgi CR, Larson SM, O'Donoghue JA. Bone marrow dosimetry using 124I-PET. J Nucl Med. 2012;53(4):615–21. https://doi.org/10.2967/jnumed.111.096453.

367. Woliner-van der Weg W, Schoffelen R, Hobbs RF, Gotthardt M, Goldenberg DM, Sharkey RM, et al. Tumor and red bone marrow dosimetry: comparison of methods for prospective treatment planning in pretargeted radioimmunotherapy. EJNMMI Phys. 2015;2(1):5. https://doi.org/10.1186/s40658-014-0104-x.

368. La MT, Tran VH, Kim HK. Progress of coordination and utilization of Zirconium-89 for positron emission tomography (PET) studies. Nucl Med Mol Imaging. 2019;53(2):115–24. https://doi.org/10.1007/s13139-019-00584-z.

369. Jauw YW, Zijlstra JM, de Jong D, Vugts DJ, Zweegman S, Hoekstra OS, et al. Performance of 89Zr-labeled-rituximab-PET as an imaging biomarker to assess CD20 targeting: a pilot study in patients with relapsed/refractory diffuse large B cell lymphoma. PLoS One. 2017;12(1):e0169828. https://doi.org/10.1371/journal.pone.0169828.

370. Muylle K, Flamen P, Vugts DJ, Guiot T, Ghanem G, Meuleman N, et al. Tumour targeting and radiation dose of radioimmunotherapy with (90)Y-rituximab in CD20+ B-cell lymphoma as predicted by (89)Zr-rituximab immuno-PET: impact of preloading with unlabelled rituximab. Eur J Nucl Med Mol Imaging. 2015;42(8):1304–14. https://doi.org/10.1007/s00259-015-3025-6.

371. O'Donoghue JA, Lewis JS, Pandit-Taskar N, Fleming SE, Schoder H, Larson SM, et al. Pharmacokinetics, biodistribution, and radiation dosimetry for (89)Zr-Trastuzumab in patients with Esophagogastric cancer. J Nucl Med. 2018;59(1):161–6. https://doi.org/10.2967/jnumed.117.194555.

372. Ulaner GA, Lyashchenko SK, Riedl C, Ruan S, Zanzonico PB, Lake D, et al. First-in-human human epidermal growth factor receptor 2-targeted imaging using (89)Zr-Pertuzumab PET/CT: dosimetry and clinical application in patients with breast cancer. J Nucl Med. 2018;59(6):900–6. https://doi.org/10.2967/jnumed.117.202010.

373. Menke-van der Houven van Oordt CW, McGeoch A, Bergstrom M, McSherry I, Smith DA, Cleveland M, et al. Immuno-PET imaging to assess target engagement: experience from (89)Zr-anti-HER3 mAb (GSK2849330) in patients with solid tumors. J Nucl Med. 2019;60(7):902–9. https://doi.org/10.2967/jnumed.118.214726.

374. Pandit-Taskar N, O'Donoghue JA, Durack JC, Lyashchenko SK, Cheal SM, Beylergil V, et al. A phase I/II study for analytic validation of 89Zr-J591 ImmunoPET as a molecular imaging agent for metastatic prostate cancer. Clin Cancer Res. 2015;21(23):5277–85. https://doi.org/10.1158/1078-0432.CCR-15-0552.

375. van Es SC, Brouwers AH, Mahesh SVK, Leliveld-Kors AM, de Jong IJ, Lub-de Hooge MN, et al. (89)Zr-bevacizumab PET: potential early indicator of Everolimus efficacy in patients with metastatic renal cell carcinoma. J Nucl Med. 2017;58(6):905–10. https://doi.org/10.2967/jnumed.116.183475.

376. Jansen MH, van Zanten SEM V, van Vuurden DG, Huisman MC, Vugts DJ, Hoekstra OS, et al. Molecular drug imaging: (89)Zr-Bevacizumab PET in children with diffuse intrinsic pontine glioma. J Nucl Med. 2017;58(5):711–6. https://doi.org/10.2967/jnumed.116.180216.

377. Oosting SF, Brouwers AH, van Es SC, Nagengast WB, Oude Munnink TH, Lub-de Hooge MN, et al. 89Zr-bevacizumab PET visualizes heterogeneous tracer accumulation in tumor lesions of renal cell carcinoma patients and differential effects of antiangiogenic treatment. J Nucl Med. 2015;56(1):63–9. https://doi.org/10.2967/jnumed.114.144840.

378. Hekman MCH, Rijpkema M, Aarntzen EH, Mulder SF, Langenhuijsen JF, Oosterwijk E, et al. Positron emission tomography/computed tomography with (89)Zr-girentuximab can aid in diagnostic dilemmas of clear cell renal cell carcinoma suspicion. Eur Urol. 2018;74(3):257–60. https://doi.org/10.1016/j.eururo.2018.04.026.

379. den Hollander MW, Bensch F, Glaudemans AW, Oude Munnink TH, Enting RH, den Dunnen WF, et al. TGF-beta antibody uptake in recurrent high-grade glioma imaged with 89Zr-Fresolimumab PET. J Nucl Med. 2015;56(9):1310–4. https://doi.org/10.2967/jnumed.115.154401.

380. Even AJ, Hamming-Vrieze O, van Elmpt W, Winnepenninckx VJ, Heukelom J, Tesselaar ME, et al. Quantitative assessment of Zirconium-89 labeled cetuximab using PET/CT imaging in patients with advanced head and neck cancer: a theragnostic approach. Oncotarget. 2017;8(3):3870–80. https://doi.org/10.18632/oncotarget.13910.

381. Menke-van der Houven van Oordt CW, Gootjes EC, Huisman MC, Vugts DJ, Roth C, Luik AM, et al. 89Zr-cetuximab PET imaging in patients with advanced colorectal cancer. Oncotarget. 2015;6(30):30384–93. https://doi.org/10.18632/oncotarget.4672.

382. Makris NE, Boellaard R, van Lingen A, Lammertsma AA, van Dongen GA, Verheul HM, et al. PET/CT-derived whole-body and bone marrow dosimetry of 89Zr-cetuximab. J Nucl Med. 2015;56(2):249–54. https://doi.org/10.2967/jnumed.114.147819.

383. Lamberts LE, Menke-van der Houven van Oordt CW, ter Weele EJ, Bensch F, Smeenk MM, Voortman J, et al. ImmunoPET with anti-Mesothelin antibody in patients with pancreatic and ovarian cancer before anti-Mesothelin antibody-drug conjugate treatment. Clin Cancer Res. 2016;22(7):1642–52. https://doi.org/10.1158/1078-0432.CCR-15-1272.

384. Bensch F, van der Veen EL, Lub-de Hooge MN, Jorritsma-Smit A, Boellaard R, Kok IC, et al. (89)Zr-atezolizumab imaging as a non-invasive approach to assess clinical response to PD-L1 blockade in cancer. Nat Med. 2018;24(12):1852–8. https://doi.org/10.1038/s41591-018-0255-8.

385. Niemeijer AN, Leung D, Huisman MC, Bahce I, Hoekstra OS, van Dongen G, et al. Whole body PD-1 and PD-L1 positron emission tomography in patients with non-small-cell lung cancer. Nat Commun. 2018;9(1):4664. https://doi.org/10.1038/s41467-018-07131-y.

386. Carrasquillo JA, Fine BM, Pandit-Taskar N, Larson SM, Fleming SE, Fox JJ, et al. Imaging patients with metastatic castration-resistant prostate cancer using (89)Zr-DFO-MSTP2109A anti-STEAP1 antibody. J Nucl Med. 2019;60(11):1517–23. https://doi.org/10.2967/jnumed.118.222844.

387. Ulaner GA, Hyman DM, Lyashchenko SK, Lewis JS, Carrasquillo JA. 89Zr-Trastuzumab PET/CT for detection of human epidermal growth factor receptor 2-positive metastases in patients with human epidermal growth factor receptor 2-negative primary breast cancer. Clin Nucl Med. 2017;42(12):912–7. https://doi.org/10.1097/RLU.0000000000001820.

388. Ulaner GA, Hyman DM, Ross DS, Corben A, Chandarlapaty S, Goldfarb S, et al. Detection of HER2-positive metastases in patients with HER2-negative primary breast cancer using 89Zr-Trastuzumab PET/CT. J Nucl Med. 2016;57(10):1523–8. https://doi.org/10.2967/jnumed.115.172031.

389. Pandit-Taskar N, O'Donoghue JA, Beylergil V, Lyashchenko S, Ruan S, Solomon SB, et al. [89]Zr-huJ591 immuno-PET imaging in patients with advanced metastatic prostate cancer. Eur J Nucl Med Mol Imaging. 2014;41(11):2093–105. https://doi.org/10.1007/s00259-014-2830-7.

390. Makris NE, van Velden FH, Huisman MC, Menke CW, Lammertsma AA, Boellaard R. Validation of simplified dosimetry approaches in [89]Zr-PET/CT: the use of manual versus semi-automatic delineation methods to estimate organ absorbed doses. Med Phys. 2014;41(10):102503. https://doi.org/10.1118/1.4895973.

Dosimetric Principles of Targeted Radiotherapy and Radioimmunotherapy

15

Giuseppe De Vincentis, Viviana Frantellizzi, and Massimiliano Pacilio

Contents

G. De Vincentis (✉)
Department of Radiological Sciences, Oncology and Anatomo-Pathology, Sapienza University of Rome, Rome, Italy
e-mail: giuseppe.devincentis@uniroma1.it

V. Frantellizzi
Department of Molecular Medicine, Sapienza University, Rome, Italy
e-mail: viviana.frantellizzi@uniroma1.it

M. Pacilio
Medical Physics Department, "Policlinico Umberto I" University Hospital, Rome, Italy
e-mail: m.pacilio@policlinicoumberto1.it

15.1 Introduction

The use of radioisotopes in therapy, in the so-called radiometabolic therapy, represents a scenario in constant evolution and growth, so much that at present we talk about theragnostic as a new frontier in cancer therapy. Biologically targeted radiation therapy permits the selective irradiation of tumors through radioactive isotopes bound with molecular vectors that present a certain degree of biological specificity for certain tumor targets. Radioimmunotherapy (RIT) involves the use of antibodies and their fragments

© Springer Nature Switzerland AG 2022
S. Harsini et al. (eds.), *Nuclear Medicine and Immunology*,
https://doi.org/10.1007/978-3-030-81261-4_15

for cell and tissue targeting [1–4]. Compared to external beam radiotherapy, one of the most powerful advantages of RIT is the ability to treat not only primary tumors but also metastatic lesions at a distance.

The energy released in a mass is called absorbed dose and is expressed in Gray (Gy; 1 Gy = 1 J/kg). The therapeutic effect of radionuclide administration must be related to the absorbed dose and not to the simple activity, and this concept represents the founding concept of the individualized dosimetry in the therapeutic field. Personalized dosimetry aims to customize the therapeutic activity in such a way that the dose absorbed at the target corresponds to the value of the prescribed dose. Individual patient dosimetry is essential not only to optimize the activity administered by calculating the minimum effective dose but also to determine a dose-response relationship as the basis for predicting clinical outcomes.

The scope of dosimetry is to optimize the treatment, by choosing an administered activity able to maximize therapeutic efficacy, minimizing toxicity. However, pretreatment dosimetry is rarely performed, due to technical and clinical issues, and a commonly accepted method is to limit the administered activity to the value able to release a maximum tolerated dose of 2 Gy to bone marrow. No information about lesion absorbed dose is deducible with this methodology.

15.2 Radioimmunotherapy

Antibodies (Ab) are glycoproteins used by the immune system to identify and remove external pathogens or cells expressing particular antigens. One of the frontiers of radiometabolic therapy is transporting radionuclides to specific cells or tissues through the binding with antibodies or their fragments. In this way, the radioisotopes are brought to the target tissue with the help of an appropriate vehicle. After the radiolabeled Ab binds to the tumor receptors/antigens expressed on the surface of the cancerous tissue, there will be the effect of cell killing.

RIT involves the application of radiolabeled monoclonal Ab (mAb) for a targeted therapeutic approach. Direct labeling methods for Abs have been developed as well as in vivo labeling methods following binding of Ab to the target [5]. The irradiated cells absorb high amounts of energy in the form of photons or charged particles, which promote both direct macromolecular damage (in particular high linear energy transfer (LET) radiation) and the generation of reactive oxygen species, with subsequent damage to the DNA strand [6] and subsequent induction of necrosis and apoptosis [7]. Since the penetrating power of ionizing radiation in the tissues allows us to have pathways much longer than the size of the single cell, adjacent cells that do not express tumor molecular targets can still be killed by the cross-fire effect. This means that continuous low-dose irradiation produced by radiolabeled Ab causes lethal effects even on nearby normal cells. Furthermore, it has been reported that RIT causes normalization of tumor vasculature [8]. It should be noted that the simultaneous emission of γ or X-rays allows performing imaging and permits the measurement of pharmacokinetic parameters and the dosimetry of radioimmunoconjugates.

Currently, the radionuclides that emit negative beta particles are by far the most used and those in which one has the greatest clinical experience. However, more recently, there is a growing interest in adrotherapy applications in nuclear medicine, using alpha radiation, the so-called targeted alpha therapy (TaT). This radiation therapy does not require the presence of oxygen, a particularly advantageous feature in oncology.

15.3 The Conceptual Approach to Dosimetry

Independently of the radionuclide carrier and regardless of the radionuclides and the biological mechanisms involved, several characteristics of therapeutic agents and biological targets need to be taken into account. This is easily understood by considering how there are no specific targets exclusive to neoplastic cells, so there will always be an accumulation of activity in healthy nontarget tissues. For example, almost all antibodies cross-react with normal cells. Depending on whether intact antibodies or fragments are used, there is generally some degree of hepatic or renal nonspecific radionuclide concentration. Moreover, tumor targeting is typically heterogeneous. Even with the most specific antibodies, it can happen that some tumor areas, even if expressing the antibody target, may be inaccessible to antibodies [9]. This may be due to the high pressure of the interstitial fluid within the tumors [10] or to the existence of a "binding site barrier" [11]. The heterogeneity in the distribution of radionuclides gives rise to a corresponding tumor dose heterogeneity [12, 13].

Many factors affect the therapeutic efficacy such as the radionuclide emission characteristics, the size, radiosensitivity of the tumor target, and, as previously stated, the radiation dose distribution.

15.3.1 Linear Energy Transfer

Another fundamental parameter is the ability of radiations to penetrate the tissues, expressed by the linear energy transfer (LET). High LET leads to largely irreparable DNA double-strand break damage such that individual α-particle interactions with DNA yield a high probability of cell lethality. In contrast, in DNA damage induced by low LET, such as β-particles (and photons), cell death requires the accumulation of many (thousands) of DNA ionization events or "hits" to overcome the cell's DNA repair machinery. On the other hand, the ability to penetrate tissues for millimeters means that radionuclides do not necessarily need to be internalized within the cancer cell to act on it.

It is mentioned here, for example, through the crossfire effect, even cells that do not express the specific target of the therapeutic agent can interact with the radiation emitted by nearby cells. The intensity of crossfire radiation depends on the spatial distribution of tumor cells and the radionuclide emission range. The distance covered in the matter of a β-particle depends on its energy in such a way that higher energy particles have longer paths. The range of emissions, therefore, varies from one radionuclide to another, depending on the energy spectrum. This affects the way the energy is deposited in the vicinity of radioactive sources [13, 14].

The categories described above are intimately related. For example, the use of a radionuclide with a longer emission range will improve the homogeneity of the irradiation, perhaps worsening the specificity of the radiation and influencing therapeutic efficacy.

The main theoretical advantage of radiometabolic therapy is represented by the possibility of irradiating cellular clusters of dimensions not detectable with the usual imaging methods. In these cases, the systemic and selective nature of radiometabolic therapy represents an undeniable advantage towards other systemic therapies, which generally lack selectivity.

It is also necessary to consider how, even in the presence of such uptake levels that do not allow the irradiation of lethal doses for neoplastic lesions, we could imagine using this approach together with the other therapeutic methods, with a mutual enhancement of the effects.

15.3.2 Absorbed Dose

The absorbed dose is the energy absorbed in a given volume divided by the mass of the volume. The greater biological response of α-particles per unit absorbed dose is quantified as their relative biological effectiveness (RBE), which is defined relative to a reference radiation value and a biological endpoint. It is the ratio of a reference radiation-absorbed dose to the α-particle radiation-absorbed dose required to achieve a particular endpoint (Fig. 15.1).

The reference radiation has typically been a beam of cobalt-57 photons. Historically, the RBE has been measured for cells in cell culture using clonogen formation assays and a cell survival endpoint. The RBE under these circumstances ranges from three to seven.

Because α-particle-induced cell death does not depend on the accumulation of α-particle-DNA hits, modulators of DNA repair that reduce or

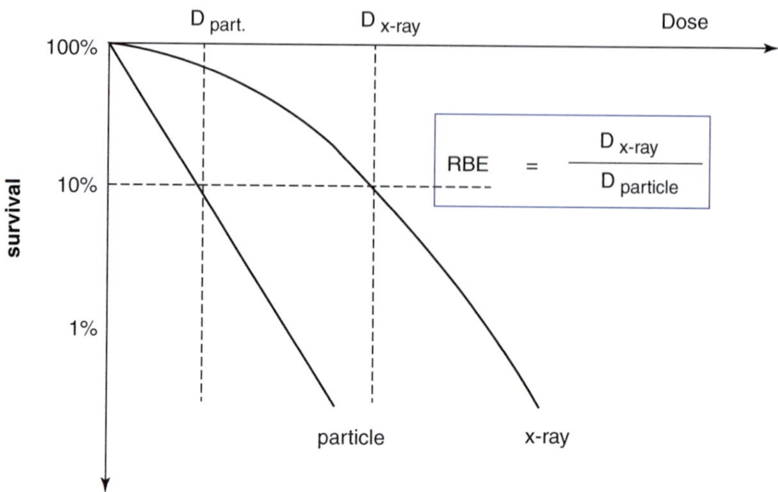

Fig. 15.1 Cell survival curves as a function of absorbed dose for high and low linear energy transfer (LET) emitters. *RBE* relative biological effectiveness

prevent the accumulation of a lethal number of hits do not affect α-particle-induced cell death. Accordingly, hypoxic cells are as radiosensitive to α-particle radiation as well-oxygenated cells. The level of cell death does not depend on the α-particle dose rate; the radiation damage caused by α-particles is considered impervious to conventional cellular resistance mechanisms such as effusion pumps, signaling pathway redundancy, and cell cycle modulation (e.g., cell dormancy, G1/G0 or G2/M block) [15–17].

Another important manifestation of the high LET emission associated with α-particle tracks is that a given absorbed dose of α-particle radiation causes a greater biological response in tissue normal organ toxicity or tumor cell death than the same absorbed dose of β- or γ-particle radiation.

The RBE for α-particles is obtained by calculating the α-particle and β-particle (or photon) absorbed doses required to obtain a particular tissue response. Dosimetry methods for radionuclides that emit β-particles or photons are already established [18].

15.3.2.1 Calculation of the Absorbed Dose Rate: The MIRD Method

The method for calculating the dose rate Medical Internal Radiation Dose (MIRD) has been described by Howell et al. [19], beginning with determining the absorbed dose rate for a very large volume (almost infinite size) tissue equivalent of a material containing in its entirety a uniform distribution of radioactive substances. Because the dose rate is the amount of energy absorbed per unit of time per unit mass of material, it varies directly with the activity per unit of mass absorbing material and the amount of energy released (emitted) by the nuclear transition.

In the example of a huge volume of tissue, all the energy emitted is absorbed, and therefore, if we know the energy issued per unit of time, we also know that energy absorbed per unit of time, expressed as follows:

$$(\text{energy emitted}) / \text{time} = (\text{transitions} / \text{time}) \\ (\text{energy} / \text{transition})$$

Because the activity is the number of transitions per unit of time:

$$(\text{energy emitted}) / \text{time} = (\text{activity}) \\ (\text{energy} / \text{transition})$$

If all the emitted energy is absorbed into the material:

$$\text{dose rate} \propto (\text{activity})(\text{energy} / \text{transition}) / \text{mass}$$

The terms that represent the components of the dose rate can be replaced with the symbols used by the MIRD scheme:

$\check{D}$ = absorbed dose rate
A = quantity of activity

m = mass of the tissue
A/m = activity per unit of mass or concentration
E = energy emitted by nuclear transition

and are indicated as follows:

$$\overset{\lor}{D} \propto \left(\frac{A}{m}\right)(E)$$

In most organs, except in some special cases, such as in small blood vessels or medullary spaces, the beta particles and electrons release their energies within the original organ where the emission takes place.

15.3.2.2 Calculation of the Absorbed Dose

If the amount of activity in a source remains constant during the period of interest, the absorbed dose $\overset{\lor}{D}$ can be calculated as follows:

$$\overset{\lor}{D} = D * t$$

where t = time on which the dose is calculated.

If the amount of activity in a source does not remain constant, the absorbed dose is equal to the integral of the (different) dose rate for the period of interest, expressed as:

$$\overset{\lor}{D} = \int D(t)\,dt$$

The dose rate depends on the activity, which varies with time.

The activity in a source is determined by the biodistribution of the radiopharmaceutical, the metabolism of the person, and the radioactive decay of the radionuclide.

The MIRD scheme uses the cumulative term of the activity $\tilde{A}$ to represent the integral of the activity over time, expressed as follows:

$$\tilde{A} = \int_{0}^{\infty} A(t)\,dt$$

Since the integral of each continuous curve is equal to the area under the curve, the cumulative activity $\tilde{A}$ can be obtained physically by measuring the area under the time-activity curve that tracks the actual disappearance of activity in an organ.

15.3.3 Radiosensitivity

This parameter determines how the response depends on the absorbed dose, while the rate of proliferation determines how it depends on the treatment time. Therefore, generally, higher doses and longer irradiation times correspond to an increase in the intensity of the therapy and consequently a greater response.

In some circumstances, it may be advantageous to use a radionuclide with a shorter half-life to increase the dose rate in earlier periods. This may be appropriate when activity distribution in the tumor is particularly rapid and the number of accessible binding targets is limited. In other cases, a longer half-life element may be better.

Dosimetry methods for therapy and, in particular, therapy with α-particle emitters require consideration of tissue subregions that are defined, in part, by the distribution of the agent at the millimeter scale for β-particle emitters and at the sub-millimeter scale for α-particle emitters [20, 21].

15.4 Clinical Evidence on the Role of Dosimetry

Beta emitters represent the radioisotopes widely used in clinical practice. The radioisotope to be used is selected considering the radiophysical properties (energy and half-life) and the labeling chemistry. For example, yttrium-90 (^{90}Y) has a more energetic β-particle and a shorter half-life than iodine-131 (^{131}I). On the other hand, metal yttrium-90 must be conjugated to antibodies via a chelating agent, while iodine-131 can directly form a carbon-iodine bond. Lutetium-177 (^{177}Lu) has physical properties similar to those of iodine-131 and chemical properties similar to yttrium-90.

However, more recently, RIT methods are being studied using α-particle emitters, since the α-particle (high LET) transfers its energy to the surrounding molecules within a narrow spatial range (<100 µm,), with relative savings of non-target tissues. In addition to the high LET, which leads to the high RBE, recent studies have shown that the cytotoxic efficacy of the particle is independent of the local concentration of oxygen and the state of the cell cycle [22]. Radium-223 (^{223}Ra), bismuth-213 (^{213}Bi), astatine-211 (^{211}At), thorium-227 (^{227}Th), and actinium-225 (^{225}Ac) have been examined [23].

Some examples of the application of dosimetry in the field of nuclear medicine therapy are presented below.

15.4.1 Treatment of Differentiated Thyroid Carcinoma

With iodine-131 activities routinely used (up to 3.7 GBq) on differentiated thyroid carcinoma patient's standard without special conditions (pediatric, dialyzed), there are no hematologic toxicity problems (dosimetry to risk organs is not clinically necessary) and are not reported therapeutic efficacy problems (dosimetry at the target is not clinically necessary). On the other hand, the technical problems for the determination of the target volume are very relevant.

The combination of these conditions makes the verification of dosimetry optional, recommended only in special cases, according to clinical need, typically in patients who are candidates for the administration of radioiodine in pediatric age and patients characterized by particular clinical and genetic conditions and/or comorbidities (dialyzed, immunosuppressed, reduced body weight, etc.).

The particular nature of these patients leads to defining this therapy as nonstandardized. First of all, the determination of the blood dose per unit of activity must be carried out administrable (Gy/GBq) [24]. The dosimetry of the lesions is desirable when it is technically reliable and based on the volume of measurable lesions. A 24-h image is suggested for diagnostic and dosimetric purposes. If the lesions are visible, it is advisable to continue the sequence of scintigraphy for dosimetric purposes according to guidelines and standards of good practice related to dosimetry.

15.4.2 Treatment of Pediatric Tumors Using [^{131}-I]I-mIBG

The dosimetry is feasible in the provisional stage of neural crest-derived childhood malignancies, although difficulties may exist in clinical order with an impact on the methodology. The primary purpose of this dosimetry is to quantitatively support the justification of the treatment. As a method to the state of the art, dosimetry is recommended for both the critical organ and lesions, when technically feasible in pediatric patients. The critical organ dosimetry (hematopoietic marrow) allows the determination of the maximum administrable activity. It can be done either using the whole-body dose as a surrogate of hematopoietic marrow [25], through the calculation of hematopoietic marrow dose by the European Association of Nuclear Medicine (EANM) methodology, based on counts of the whole body and blood samples [24]. In the case of uncooperative pediatric patients, this second strategy might be operationally applicable only in some cases.

The dosimetry of the lesions, which can be performed only if the lesion volume is radiologically measurable, is necessary to ascertain that the expected dose of the lesion is adequate (at least equal to 70 Gy) [26, 27]; otherwise, the opportunity of therapy should be questioned. To calculate the dose to the critical organ and lesions, it is recommended to plan a specific administration of metaiodobenzylguanidine (mIBG) diagnostic activity labeled with iodine-131 followed by single-photon emission computed tomography (SPECT) quantitative serial images of the lesion and counts on the whole body at least up to 4 days after administration. The use of iodine-123, currently administered for diagnostic purposes, is reported in the literature [28], but the accuracy of the dosimetric evaluations is less due to the short half-life compared to the therapeutic isotope. This introduces significant errors in the valuation of long-lasting half-life components with iodine-131 [29].

15.4.3 Treatment of Neuroendocrine Tumors Using Radio-Peptides Labeled with Lutetium-177

There is a registered [^{177}Lu]Lu-DOTATATE (LUTATERA®) radiopharmaceutical that includes a 7.4 GBq dose for four administrations with an 8-week interval approved for gastroenteropancreatic neuroendocrine tumors (GEP-NET). Sundlov et al. demonstrated the safety of a variable number of administrations according to the individual tolerance of the individual patient determined by kidney dosimetry [30]. Garske-Román et al. dealt with a series of patients with the same agent [31]. One group reached the maximum tolerable kidney dose with a maximized number of administrations thanks to dosimetric planning. The other could not reach this limit for clinical reasons. In the first group, the median progression-free interval (PFS) was 33 months compared with 15 months in the second group ($p < 0.0001$). Using peptides labeled with lutetium-177, the cases of renal toxicity are sporadic, unlike the [^{90}Y]Y-DOTATOC. Therefore, the dosimetry of the critical kidney organ results in less clinical impact. The lutetium-177 beta range, much lower than those emitted by yttrium-90, would seem to be the base of the reduced toxicity that characterizes lutetium-177 (microscopic radiation unevenness with glomerulus dose savings). However, in the absence of new dose-toxicity correlation data obtained with lutetium-177, it is advisable to keep the irradiation to the kidneys within these limits. This method allows the number of therapeutic administrations to be individually modulated.

As for the correlation between marrow dose and hematological toxicity, which has a low prevalence among patients treated, the data available in the literature are unclear [32]. The method based on blood samples does not correlate with thrombocytopenia [33]. The method based on tomographic images of vertebral bodies is discussed [34, 35] and has found a correlation only in a restricted class of patients, those in whom there was a spontaneous recovery of the blood crisis. The hematopoietic marrow dosimetry has not yet proved to be useful for clinical purposes,

and therefore additional data are needed. Regarding the dosimetry to lesions, the dose-effectiveness correlations are most strikingly obtained in nuclear medical therapy [36]. As the studies progress, the concrete possibility of optimizing the patient's management based on the dosimetry of the lesions is therefore emerging. An insufficient level of tumor irradiation could in the future constitute a criterion for exclusion from therapy. Therefore, the evaluation of the lesions has today a relevant aspect in the dosimetry in the radio-peptides labeled with lutetium-177. Based on the trends expressed in the literature, the purposes of dosimetry in radio-peptides are, consequently, to modulate the number of administrations based on renal tolerance, with a prognostic evaluation of efficacy. This second aspect could imply a better selection of patients who are candidates for therapy, making economic saving possible.

The method of choice is the use of SPECT/CT (or SPECT corrected for attenuation on a CT basis). A proposed protocol suggests the acquisition of at least one first SPECT/CT the day after the administration (18–24 h), possibly followed by others up to at least 66–72 h (fourth day). The execution of the last scan at 90–96 h (fifth day) would be optimal for the kidney, while even later scans (seventh day) would allow to better define the trend of the time-activity curve for the lesions [37]. Using peptides labeled with lutetium-177, the cases of renal toxicity are sporadic, unlike the [^{90}Y]Y-DOTATOC.

15.4.4 Treatment with Radio-Peptides Labeled with Yttrium-90

The critical kidney organ dosimetry is essential to prevent late and irreversible kidney damage. The correlation between dose to the marrow and hematological toxicity has been reported for ^{177}Lu-labeled radiopharmaceuticals. In the absence of additional data, the marrow dosimetry has not shown a benefit for clinical use. The considerations for ^{177}Lu-labeled radiopharmaceuticals are valid for lesion dosimetry.

In addition to the predictive dosimetry difficulties mentioned for ^{177}Lu-radiolabeled drugs, with yttrium-90 for verification dosimetry, we have the possibility of imaging Bremsstrahlung, which however is of poor quality, and above all not quantitative, unless special methods are applied only in specialized research centers. Yttrium-90 positron emission tomography (PET)/CT imaging is only possible for patients in whom the concentrations in the volumes of interest are greater than 1 MBq/mL [38]. It is therefore recommended to carry out dosimetry following the first therapeutic administration, using the same ^{177}Lu-labeled molecule instead of yttrium-90. This evaluation is provisional of the subsequent administration with yttrium-90 in GEP-NET.

15.4.4.1 Treatment of Non-Hodgkin Lymphoma Using [⁹⁰Y] Y-Ibritumomab Tiuxetan (Zevalin®)

The provisional dosimetry is feasible by the administration of antibody labeled with indium-111, following the same pattern as with the previous administration of rituximab [39–41]. Two cases have been reported in whom this dosimetry has prevented serious overdoses to the liver suspending planned experimental administration with 56 MBq/kg [42]. This is, therefore, the main purpose of this practice: limiting doses to healthy organs. However, the cost of this practice is equal to that of the therapy itself, since it requires the use of the same antibody.

15.4.5 Treatment of Bone Metastasis from Castration-Resistant Prostate Cancer Using [²²³Ra] Ra-Dichloride

The radiopharmaceutical [²²³Ra]Ra-dichloride (Xofigo®) is registered according to a posology of six administrations, 4 weeks apart, with an activity calculated based on the patient's body weight (55 kBq/kg). However, given the very large incidence of the pathology treated, and the type of lesions treated, bone metastases, which are usually the least responsive to radiant treatments, would be of interest to investigate what the additional benefits obtainable with administrations could optimize this therapeutic agent, which has proved successful in increasing the survival from 11 to 14 months with the indicated schedule.

So beyond the current registration (but for now only in clinical trials), in the future, there would be a wide margin of use of the dosimetry to increase the per kilogram activity administered and/or to individualize the number of administrations, in order to optimize the treatment and maximize its effectiveness [43, 44]. Regarding the dosimetry to the organs at risk (bone marrow and intestine) with the posology registered, there is no clinical need. There are aspects of red marrow dosimetry technically more complicated that involves a micro modeling interpretation dosimetric research studies, but that could hardly be addressed in routine clinic through conventional approval of in vivo dosimetry. Dosimetry in routine therapy is therefore only addressable to lesions.

It is by now established that, despite the low abundance of photonic emission (about 1% of abundance) of radium-223 and low administered activity, quantitative in vivo post-administration therapeutic imaging is possible and that the dosimetry to lesions (and sometimes even organs) is technically feasible [43, 45–49]. It is also true that within the standard posology, lesion dosimetry studies have only been conducted and that not all lesions depicted on pretreatment bone scans are visible on the images obtained post-administration of radium-223. According to the current data [49], not all lesions are eligible for dosimetric studies.

From a technical point of view, the dosimetry of bone lesions would be simple and could satisfy treatment verification requirements (as well as "recording" and "reporting" of the dose absorbed by the lesions) and provide data that can be useful in the near future to highlight correlations in terms of local response/control of the lesion or in terms of other clinical endpoints of interest. The search for evidence is underway to personalize the treatment according to dosimetric results.

Due to the low quality of images obtained with radium-223 (low counting statistics and low spatial resolution), the contouring of the lesions cannot be performed directly on the images obtained. Since a good correlation has been demonstrated between the uptake of the [^{223}Ra] Ra-dichloride and the uptake of [^{99m}Tc] Tc-diphosphonates, the lesions must be delineated on the whole-body images with [^{99m}Tc] Tc-diphosphonates performed for diagnostic purposes before therapy. To improve the repositioning of the ROIs on radium-223 images, it is suggested to pre-register a whole-body [^{99m}Tc] Tc-diphosphonate together with static images of [^{223}Ra]Ra-dichloride [44, 46, 47]. Since in the majority of the cases examined, clearance was mono-exponential (and this in any case assumption would introduce a negligible error), the biokinetic sampling can be optimized through three acquisitions with adequate timing (e.g., 24–36 h, 48–60 h, 7–15 days, starting from the moment of administration).

15.5   Conclusion

Market estimates show that the global therapeutic radiopharmaceuticals market will expand at an impressive 9.7% compound annual growth rate over the forecast period 2020–2030. In principle, as is proper practice for therapeutic regimens with ionizing radiation, a dosimetric approach should be performed to optimize and personalize the treatment, allowing a choice based on the dosimetry regimen of administration, paving the way for radionuclide therapy based on dosimetry. Treatment endpoints should be selected based on the relationship between the absorbed dose and the observed biological/clinical effect. In the era of personalized medicine, the dosimetric approach appears to represent the cornerstone of the concept of optimization of the therapeutic approach using radionuclides, a rapidly expanding therapeutic methodology.

References

1. Bruland OS. Cancer therapy with radiolabeled antibodies. An overview. Acta Oncol. 1995;34(8):1085–94.
2. Jurcic JG, Scheinberg DA. Radioimmunotherapy of hematological cancer: problems and progress. Clin Cancer Res. 1995;1(12):1439–46.
3. Kairemo KJ. Radioimmunotherapy of solid cancers: a review. Acta Oncol. 1996;35(3):343–55. https://doi.org/10.3109/02841869609101651.
4. Wilder RB, DeNardo GL, DeNardo SJ. Radioimmunotherapy: recent results and future directions. J Clin Oncol. 1996;14(4):1383–400. https://doi.org/10.1200/jco.1996.14.4.1383.
5. Cremonesi M, Ferrari M, Chinol M, Stabin MG, Grana C, Prisco G, et al. Three-step radioimmunotherapy with yttrium-90 biotin: dosimetry and pharmacokinetics in cancer patients. Eur J Nucl Med. 1999;26(2):110–20.
6. Azzam EI, Jay-Gerin JP, Pain D. Ionizing radiation-induced metabolic oxidative stress and prolonged cell injury. Cancer Lett. 2012;327(1–2):48–60. https://doi.org/10.1016/j.canlet.2011.12.012.
7. Pouget JP, Georgakilas AG, Ravanat JL. Targeted and off-target (Bystander and Abscopal) effects of radiation therapy: redox mechanisms and risk/benefit analysis. Antioxid Redox Signal. 2018;29(15):1447–87. https://doi.org/10.1089/ars.2017.7267.
8. Huang CY, Pourgholami MH, Allen BJ. Optimizing radioimmunoconjugate delivery in the treatment of solid tumor. Cancer Treat Rev. 2012;38(7):854–60. https://doi.org/10.1016/j.ctrv.2011.12.005.
9. Oosterwijk E, Bander NH, Divgi CR, Welt S, Wakka JC, Finn RD, et al. Antibody localization in human renal cell carcinoma: a phase I study of monoclonal antibody G250. J Clin Oncol. 1993;11(4):738–50. https://doi.org/10.1200/jco.1993.11.4.738.
10. Jain RK. Delivery of novel therapeutic agents in tumors: physiological barriers and strategies. J Natl Cancer Inst. 1989;81(8):570–6. https://doi.org/10.1093/jnci/81.8.570.
11. Juweid M, Neumann R, Paik C, Perez-Bacete MJ, Sato J, van Osdol W, et al. Micropharmacology of monoclonal antibodies in solid tumors: direct experimental evidence for a binding site barrier. Cancer Res. 1992;52(19):5144–53.
12. Yorke ED, Williams LE, Demidecki AJ, Heidorn DB, Roberson PL, Wessels BW. Multicellular dosimetry for beta-emitting radionuclides: autoradiography, thermoluminescent dosimetry and three-dimensional dose calculations. Med Phys. 1993;20(2 Pt 2):543–50. https://doi.org/10.1118/1.597050.
13. Humm JL, Macklis RM, Lu XQ, Yang Y, Bump K, Beresford B, et al. The spatial accuracy of cellular dose

estimates obtained from 3D reconstructed serial tissue autoradiographs. Phys Med Biol. 1995;40(1):163–80. https://doi.org/10.1088/0031-9155/40/1/014.

14. Goddu SM, Rao DV, Howell RW. Multicellular dosimetry for micrometastases: dependence of self-dose versus cross-dose to cell nuclei on type and energy of radiation and subcellular distribution of radionuclides. J Nucl Med. 1994;35(3):521–30.

15. Ballangrud AM, Yang WH, Charlton DE, McDevitt MR, Hamacher KA, Panageas KS, et al. Response of LNCaP spheroids after treatment with an alpha-particle emitter (213Bi)-labeled anti-prostate-specific membrane antigen antibody (J591). Cancer Res. 2001;61(5):2008–14.

16. Song H, Hedayati M, Hobbs RF, Shao C, Bruchertseifer F, Morgenstern A, et al. Targeting aberrant DNA double-strand break repair in triple-negative breast cancer with alpha-particle emitter radiolabeled anti-EGFR antibody. Mol Cancer Ther. 2013;12(10):2043–54. https://doi.org/10.1158/1535-7163.Mct-13-0108.

17. Barendsen GW, Beusker TL. Effects of different ionizing radiations on human cells in tissue culture. I. Irradiation techniques and dosimetry. Radiat Res. 1960;13:832–40.

18. Bolch WE, Eckerman KF, Sgouros G, Thomas SR. MIRD pamphlet no. 21: a generalized schema for radiopharmaceutical dosimetry—standardization of nomenclature. J Nucl Med. 2009;50(3):477–84. https://doi.org/10.2967/jnumed.108.056036.

19. Howell RW, Wessels BW, Loevinger R, Watson EE, Bolch WE, Brill AB, et al. The MIRD perspective 1999. Medical Internal Radiation Dose Committee. J Nucl Med. 1999;40(1):3s–10s.

20. Hobbs RF, Song H, Huso DL, Sundel MH, Sgouros G. A nephron-based model of the kidneys for macro-to-micro alpha-particle dosimetry. Phys Med Biol. 2012;57(13):4403–24. https://doi.org/10.1088/0031-9155/57/13/4403.

21. Hobbs RF, Song H, Watchman CJ, Bolch WE, Aksnes AK, Ramdahl T, et al. A bone marrow toxicity model for (2)(2)(3)Ra alpha-emitter radiopharmaceutical therapy. Phys Med Biol. 2012;57(10):3207–22. https://doi.org/10.1088/0031-9155/57/10/3207.

22. McDevitt MR, Barendswaard E, Ma D, Lai L, Curcio MJ, Sgouros G, et al. An alpha-particle emitting antibody ([213Bi]J591) for radioimmunotherapy of prostate cancer. Cancer Res. 2000;60(21):6095–100.

23. Kratochwil C, Bruchertseifer F, Rathke H, Bronzel M, Apostolidis C, Weichert W, et al. Targeted alpha-therapy of metastatic castration-resistant prostate cancer with (225)Ac-PSMA-617: dosimetry estimate and empiric dose finding. J Nucl Med. 2017;58(10):1624–31. https://doi.org/10.2967/jnumed.117.191395.

24. Lassmann M, Hanscheid H, Chiesa C, Hindorf C, Flux G, Luster M. EANM Dosimetry Committee series on standard operational procedures for pre-therapeutic dosimetry I: blood and bone marrow dosimetry in differentiated thyroid cancer therapy. Eur J Nucl Med Mol Imaging. 2008;35(7):1405–12. https://doi.org/10.1007/s00259-008-0761-x.

25. Lashford LS, Lewis IJ, Fielding SL, Flower MA, Meller S, Kemshead JT, et al. Phase I/II study of iodine 131 metaiodobenzylguanidine in chemoresistant neuroblastoma: a United Kingdom Children's Cancer Study Group investigation. J Clin Oncol. 1992;10(12):1889–96. https://doi.org/10.1200/jco.1992.10.12.1889.

26. Matthay KK, DeSantes K, Hasegawa B, Huberty J, Hattner RS, Ablin A, et al. Phase I dose escalation of 131I-metaiodobenzylguanidine with autologous bone marrow support in refractory neuroblastoma. J Clin Oncol. 1998;16(1):229–36. https://doi.org/10.1200/jco.1998.16.1.229.

27. Matthay KK, Panina C, Huberty J, Price D, Glidden DV, Tang HR, et al. Correlation of tumor and whole-body dosimetry with tumor response and toxicity in refractory neuroblastoma treated with (131)I-MIBG. J Nucl Med. 2001;42(11):1713–21.

28. Monsieurs M, Brans B, Bacher K, Dierckx R, Thierens H. Patient dosimetry for 131I-MIBG therapy for neuroendocrine tumours based on 123I-MIBG scans. Eur J Nucl Med Mol Imaging. 2002;29(12):1581–7. https://doi.org/10.1007/s00259-002-0973-4.

29. Flux GD, Guy MJ, Beddows R, Pryor M, Flower MA. Estimation and implications of random errors in whole-body dosimetry for targeted radionuclide therapy. Phys Med Biol. 2002;47(17):3211–23. https://doi.org/10.1088/0031-9155/47/17/311.

30. Sundlov A, Sjogreen-Gleisner K, Svensson J, Ljungberg M, Olsson T, Bernhardt P, et al. Individualised (177)Lu-DOTATATE treatment of neuroendocrine tumours based on kidney dosimetry. Eur J Nucl Med Mol Imaging. 2017;44(9):1480–9. https://doi.org/10.1007/s00259-017-3678-4.

31. Garske-Román U, Sandstrom M, Fross Baron K, Lundin L, Hellman P, Welin S, et al. Prospective observational study of (177)Lu-DOTA-octreotate therapy in 200 patients with advanced metastasized neuroendocrine tumours (NETs): feasibility and impact of a dosimetry-guided study protocol on outcome and toxicity. Eur J Nucl Med Mol Imaging. 2018;45(6):970–88. https://doi.org/10.1007/s00259-018-3945-z.

32. Bergsma H, Konijnenberg MW, Kam BL, Teunissen JJ, Kooij PP, de Herder WW, et al. Subacute haematotoxicity after PRRT with (177)Lu-DOTA-octreotate: prognostic factors, incidence and course. Eur J Nucl Med Mol Imaging. 2016;43(3):453–63. https://doi.org/10.1007/s00259-015-3193-4.

33. Forrer F, Krenning EP, Kooij PP, Bernard BF, Konijnenberg M, Bakker WH, et al. Bone marrow dosimetry in peptide receptor radionuclide therapy with [177Lu-DOTA(0),Tyr(3)]octreotate. Eur J Nucl Med Mol Imaging. 2009;36(7):1138–46. https://doi.org/10.1007/s00259-009-1072-6.

34. Walrand S, Barone R, Pauwels S, Jamar F. Experimental facts supporting a red marrow uptake due to radiometal transchelation in 90Y-DOTATOC therapy and relationship to the decrease of platelet counts. Eur J Nucl Med Mol Imaging. 2011;38(7):1270–80. https://doi.org/10.1007/s00259-011-1744-x.

35. Hartmann H, Oehme L, Kotzerke J. 86Y-DOTATOC uptake in red marrow is not routinely visible. Eur J Nucl Med Mol Imaging. 2011;38(7):1384–5. https://doi.org/10.1007/s00259-011-1825-x.

36. Ilan E, Sandstrom M, Wassberg C, Sundin A, Garske-Roman U, Eriksson B, et al. Dose response of pancreatic neuroendocrine tumors treated with peptide receptor radionuclide therapy using 177Lu-DOTATATE. J Nucl Med. 2015;56(2):177–82. https://doi.org/10.2967/jnumed.114.148437.

37. Gleisner KS, Brolin G, Sundlov A, Mjekiqi E, Ostlund K, Tennvall J, et al. Long-term retention of 177Lu/177mLu-DOTATATE in patients investigated by gamma-spectrometry and gamma-camera imaging. J Nucl Med. 2015;56(7):976–84. https://doi.org/10.2967/jnumed.115.155390.

38. Fabbri C, Bartolomei M, Mattone V, Casi M, De Lauro F, Bartolini N, et al. (90)Y-PET/CT imaging quantification for dosimetry in peptide receptor radionuclide therapy: analysis and corrections of the impairing factors. Cancer Biother Radiopharm. 2015;30(5):200–10. https://doi.org/10.1089/cbr.2015.1819.

39. Cremonesi M, Ferrari M, Grana CM, Vanazzi A, Stabin M, Bartolomei M, et al. High-dose radioimmunotherapy with 90Y-ibritumomab tiuxetan: comparative dosimetric study for tailored treatment. J Nucl Med. 2007;48(11):1871–9. https://doi.org/10.2967/jnumed.107.044016.

40. Chiesa C, Botta F, Coliva A, Maccauro M, Devizzi L, Guidetti A, et al. Absorbed dose and biologically effective dose in patients with high-risk non-Hodgkin's lymphoma treated with high-activity myeloablative 90Y-ibritumomab tiuxetan (Zevalin). Eur J Nucl Med Mol Imaging. 2009;36(11):1745–57. https://doi.org/10.1007/s00259-009-1141-x.

41. Pacilio M, Betti M, Cicone F, Del Mastro C, Montani L, Chiacchiararelli L, et al. A theoretical dose-escalation study based on biological effective dose in radioimmunotherapy with (90)Y-ibritumomab tiuxetan (Zevalin). Eur J Nucl Med Mol Imaging. 2010;37(5):862–73. https://doi.org/10.1007/s00259-009-1333-4.

42. Arico D, Grana CM, Vanazzi A, Ferrari M, Mallia A, Sansovini M, et al. The role of dosimetry in the high activity 90Y-ibritumomab tiuxetan regimens: two cases of abnormal biodistribution. Cancer Biother Radiopharm. 2009;24(2):271–5. https://doi.org/10.1089/cbr.2008.0541.

43. Chittenden SJ, Hindorf C, Parker CC, Lewington VJ, Pratt BE, Johnson B, et al. A phase 1, open-label study of the biodistribution, pharmacokinetics, and dosimetry of 223Ra-dichloride in patients with hormone-refractory prostate cancer and skeletal metastases. J Nucl Med. 2015;56(9):1304–9. https://doi.org/10.2967/jnumed.115.157123.

44. Murray I, Chittenden SJ, Denis-Bacelar AM, Hindorf C, Parker CC, Chua S, et al. The potential of (223)Ra and (18)F-fluoride imaging to predict bone lesion response to treatment with (223)Ra-dichloride in castration-resistant prostate cancer. Eur J Nucl Med Mol Imaging. 2017;44(11):1832–44. https://doi.org/10.1007/s00259-017-3744-y.

45. Hindorf C, Chittenden S, Aksnes AK, Parker C, Flux GD. Quantitative imaging of 223Ra-chloride (Alpharadin) for targeted alpha-emitting radionuclide therapy of bone metastases. Nucl Med Commun. 2012;33(7):726–32. https://doi.org/10.1097/MNM.0b013e328353bb6e.

46. Pacilio M, Ventroni G, De Vincentis G, Cassano B, Pellegrini R, Di Castro E, et al. Dosimetry of bone metastases in targeted radionuclide therapy with alpha-emitting (223)Ra-dichloride. Eur J Nucl Med Mol Imaging. 2016;43(1):21–33. https://doi.org/10.1007/s00259-015-3150-2.

47. Pacilio M, Ventroni G, Cassano B, Ialongo P, Lorenzon L, Di Castro E, et al. A case report of image-based dosimetry of bone metastases with Alpharadin ((223)Ra-dichloride) therapy: inter-fraction variability of absorbed dose and follow-up. Ann Nucl Med. 2016;30(2):163–8. https://doi.org/10.1007/s12149-015-1044-9.

48. Pacilio M, Cassano B, Chiesa C, Giancola S, Ferrari M, Pettinato C, et al. The Italian multicentre dosimetric study for lesion dosimetry in (223)Ra therapy of bone metastases: calibration protocol of gamma cameras and patient eligibility criteria. Phys Med. 2016;32(12):1731–7. https://doi.org/10.1016/j.ejmp.2016.09.013.

49. Pacilio M, Cassano B, Pellegrini R, Di Castro E, Zorz A, De Vincentis G, et al. Gamma camera calibrations for the Italian multicentre study for lesion dosimetry in (223)Ra therapy of bone metastases. Phys Med. 2017;41:117–23. https://doi.org/10.1016/j.ejmp.2017.04.019.

Theranostics of Hematologic Disorders

16

Arif Sheikh, Shazia Fatima, Zain Khurshid, and Zaheer Chiragh

Contents

A. Sheikh (✉)
Division of Nuclear Medicine, Department of
Radiology, Kettering Health, Wright State University,
Kettering, OH, USA
e-mail: arif.sheikh@ketteringhealth.org

S. Fatima · Z. Khurshid
Department of Nuclear Medicine, Nuclear Medicine,
Oncology and Radiotherapy Institute (NORI),
Islamabad, Pakistan

Z. Chiragh
Nuclear Medicine Section, Department of Radiology,
Gurayat General Hospital, Al-Qurayyat Ministry of
Health, Al Qurayyat, Saudi Arabia

© Springer Nature Switzerland AG 2022
S. Harsini et al. (eds.), *Nuclear Medicine and Immunology*,
https://doi.org/10.1007/978-3-030-81261-4_16

16.1 Introduction

Hematologic malignancies rank among the 15 most commonly occurring malignant disorders worldwide with variable demographics and prevalence. Over the last decade, non-Hodgkin lymphomas have increased in incidence by 45%. Conventional treatment options are chemotherapy, radiation therapy, immunotherapy, and autologous stem cell transplant. Aggressive pathologies and recurrent disease are often refractory to conventional treatment and have a high incidence of recurrence. Theranostics is the concept where an imaging-based radiolabeled compound is used to determine the appropriateness of delivering a targeted therapy, which in some cases may be another compound with similar biologic characteristics as the imaging compound or the same compound. The therapeutic compound in some cases is radiolabeled with a cytotoxic radionuclide. In this context, radionuclide-based theranostics have been developed and used to treat hematologic disorders quite effectively and will be the focus of this chapter.

Application of the theranostic concept started over half a century ago with radioactive iodine treatments and has flourished with the addition of new radioisotopes and radiopharmaceuticals. In hematologic malignancies, the concept of theranostics is not new, as radiolabeled compounds have been used as diagnostic and dosimetric tools, as well as for therapeutic purposes. The following is a brief overview of the history and the development of radioimmunotherapy and theranostics in myeloproliferative disorders, lymphomas, chronic leukemias, and multiple myeloma. The historical development, clinical implementation, and efficacy are covered. Additional ongoing and future improvements are discussed to enhance the therapeutic index of these treatments in areas such as molecular and hybrid imaging, newer radionuclides, newer constructs and antibodies, pre-targeting and other strategies, dosimetry, optical imaging, and the emergence of image analysis with radiomics.

There is plenty of research and clinical data showing the effectiveness of radioimmunotherapy, particularly in lymphoma, from frontline, consolidative, and even in salvage scenarios. In fact, these have been cost-effective therapies that are well tolerated by patients. Despite these findings, radioimmunotherapy has not been eagerly incorporated into standard regimens in the care of patients and its limitations are usually overestimated by many referring physicians. Nevertheless, the financial and logistical challenges of these therapies are addressed along with new solutions to these problems that may help to create a renaissance in their use.

16.2 Epidemiology of Lymphomas

Lymphomas are a group of malignant diseases that arise due to the uncontrolled proliferation of lymphoid cells. Lymphoid cells are most abundantly found in lymph nodes, and the disease mostly presents clinically in the form of lymph node enlargement; however, due to the fact that lymphatic tissues are also present elsewhere in the body, extranodal involvement is also noted in the bones, lungs, brain, stomach, etc.

Non-Hodgkin's lymphoma (NHL) is one of the most commonly occurring malignancies of hematologic origin. In 2018, it was the 10th most prevalent cancer in males and the 12th most frequent cancer among females worldwide. The estimated new cases were 509,590 while 248,724 deaths were attributed to it [1, 2]. The United Kingdom data suggest that NHL is mainly a disease of old age with a peak incidence at 75 years [3]. The incidence of NHL varies demographically with a relatively poor survival rate among financially compromised regions [4, 5]. Age, sex, and ethnicity are also noted to be significant variables. Other risk factors include genetic predisposition, Epstein-Barr virus (EBV) infection, occupational exposure, and human immunodeficiency virus (HIV)-induced immunosuppression [6–8].

A comprehensive compilation of the estimated worldwide NHL incidence highlights the various patterns and trends in its occurrence [9]. A higher prevalence was noted among males than females (estimated ratio of 1.1–1.8). In terms of gender, a higher incidence in males was observed in Australia and New Zealand (16.4 per 100,000) followed by North America and Northern Europe (14.8 and 13.5 per 100,000, respectively). In females, North American incidence was the highest (10.4 per 100,000). Data from cancer registries of a few selected countries of the Americas, Europe, and Asia suggested either a stable or decreasing pattern in incidence during 1980–

2012. The observed incidence circa 2008–2012 among various countries depending upon human development index noted the highest incidence in Israeli Jewish males (17.6 per 100,000) followed by Australia and United States (whites) (15.3 and 14.5 per 100,000, respectively). Among females, a similar distribution was seen: Israeli Jews (13), Australia (12.3), and United States (whites, 10.3 per 100,000).

16.3 Biology and Classification of Lymphomas

On the basis of histological differences, lymphomas have been broadly classified into two broad categories, namely, Hodgkin's Lymphoma (HL) and non-Hodgkin's lymphoma (NHL), although the world health organization (WHO) also identifies multiple myeloma (MM) and immunoproliferative diseases in these categories [10–12].

NHL is a group of cancers that primarily evolves from two main types of lymphocytes, i.e., both B cells (B-lymphocytes) and T-cells (T-lymphocytes). The tumor may arise in any of the organs that have an aggregation of lymphoid tissues, such as the bone marrow, lymph nodes, the spleen, Waldeyer's ring, etc. There are a few conditions that resemble the lymphomas and hence are termed as benign/pseudo-lymphomas, but by definition, true lymphomas are always malignant in nature [13]. Lymphomas may have different clinical presentations; for instance, the involvement of Waldeyer's ring is more common in the case of NHL than in HL [14].

Since the 1950s, multiple classifications of lymphomas have been proposed and used in routine clinical practice. These included Rappaport (1956), Lennert/Kiel (1974), BNLI, Working Formulation (1982), and REAL classification (1994). All these classifications fell short of fully integrating the histological, phenotyping, molecular, and cytogenetic characteristics, until the WHO classifications were published in 2001 with further amendments in 2008. This classification has been devised into five major groups, namely, mature B-cell neoplasms, mature T-cell and natural killer (NK) cell neo-plasms, precursor lymphoid neoplasms, HL, and immunodeficiency-associated lymphoproliferative disorders [15, 16].

Aside from clinical, morphologic, and immunophenotypic characteristics, the WHO classification also considers genetic and molecular findings while classifying the lymphoid malignancies. Besides these established classification schemas, lymphoid neoplasms are widely discussed according to the lineage of the cells of origin. A detailed account of the types or classes is beyond the scope of this chapter, which will only focus on common lymphomatous malignancies. Since B-cell lineage malignancies are most commonly encountered, brief details about cell lineage, molecular, and genetic characteristics follow.

16.4 B Cells

B-cell development starts from the fetal liver and passes to the bone marrow. Mature B cells can express both m and L chains on their membranes. Prior to the expression of these chains, it is immature and vulnerable to self-antigens. The mature B cell responds to an antigen and transforms into an antibody-secreting plasma cell or a memory B cell. B-cell development starts when bone marrow stromal cells send signals to lymphoid progenitor cells. The first stage of the development is early pro-B cell, which is formed after D-j joining of cells on H cells. These early pro-B cells express cluster of differentiation (CD)45. Joining of a V segment to the D-JH completes the late pro-B cell stage. Pro-B cells become pre-B cells when they express membrane m chains with surrogate light chains in the pre-B receptor. Pre-B cells have large and small pre B-cell stages. Pre-B cells express CD45, class II, pre-B-R, CD19, and CD40. The next stage in the B-cell development is immature B cell which is formed when the L chain has been synthesized and expressed with M chain on the cell membrane. Immature B cells can bind with antigen at this stage and die. Surviving immature cells express d chain and membrane immunoglobulin (Ig)D with their IgM and leave the marrow. The cells leaving the marrow are mature naive (resting) B cells. The membrane markers for mature B cells are CD45R, class II, IgM, IgD, CD19, CD21, and CD40.

The common CD antigens encountered in hematologic disorders are CD20, CD22, CD37, CD25, and CD45, among others. These antigens play a pivotal role in cell immunity. Based on antigen-antibody reactions, several immuno- and radio-immunotherapies (RIT) have been used to treat lymphoid disorders. Several mechanisms have been proposed for monoclonal antibody (mAb) mediated cell death, irrespective of its conjugation status with radioactivity. These mechanisms include antibody-dependent cell-mediated cytotoxicity (ADCC), complement-enhanced ADCC, complement-mediated cytotoxicity (CDC), induction of apoptosis, immune-effector cells recruitment, and cell proliferation function blocking. All or any of these proposed mechanisms may be involved in cancer cell damage and death. The mechanisms by which a therapeutic mAb damages cell survival is dependent on the target antigen receptors. Apoptosis plays a central role in the hematopoietic cells' response to radiation and is proposed to be responsible for the superiority of RIT in comparison with immunotherapy. Radioligands have additional benefits of damaging cancer cells by virtue of having radiobiological effects and linear energy transfer. The three mechanisms through which cell damage has been reported are either self or direct irradiation, crossfire effect, and bystander effect [17].

16.5 Review of Frequently Used Hematologic CD Antigens

Morphological and physical characteristics, function, and the mechanism of cancer cell destruction of commonly used antigens, which has been targeted for immunotherapy and radio-immunotherapy (RIT) in hematologic malignancies, are described in Table 16.1.

Table 16.1 Comparison of main target surface antigens used in B-cell malignancies

	CD20	CD22	CD37
Size	33–37 kDa	130–150 kDa	40–52 kDa
Target characteristics	Non-glycosylated transmembrane phosphoprotein	Single-spanning membrane glycoprotein	Glycosylated glycoprotein, Tetraspan transmembrane family of proteins
Expression	Mature and naive B cells	Cytoplasmic expression: Pro-B cells and pre-B cells Surface expression: Immature B cells	Mature B cells Low levels on T cells, macrophages/monocytes, granulocytes, and dendritic cells
Expression in malignancies	Majority of B-cell lymphoid malignancies, HCL, B-cell CLL	Lymphoplasmacytic lymphoma, DLCBL, MCL, CLL, prolymphocytic leukemia, HCL, ALL	B-cell NHL, CLL, HCL, lymphoplasmacytic lymphoma
Targeting mAb	Ibritumomab tiuxetan	Epratuzumab tetraxetan (humanized)	Lilotomab satetraxetan (murine mAb HH1)
Commonly labeled radioisotope	Yittrium-90	Yittrium-90	Lutetium-177
Function	B-cell calcium channel activation	Inhibitory receptor for BCR signaling; critical role in establishing a baseline level of B-cell inhibition	Regulates the membrane distribution of α(4)β(1) integrin involved in apoptosis; counteracts death signals by regulating PI3K-dependent survival; promotes IgG1 production and antibody production
Internalization/shedding	No internalization or shedding	Internalization and shedding	Internalizes Modest shedding in transformed B-cells expressing the antigen

CD cluster of differentiation, *kDa* kilodaltons, *DLBCL* diffuse large B-cell lymphoma, *CLL* chronic lymphocytic leukemia, *HCL* hairy cell leukemia, *MCL* mantle cell lymphoma, *ALL* acute lymphoblastic leukemia, *mAb* monoclonal antibody, *Ig* immunoglobulin, *BCR* B-cell receptor

16.5.1 CD20

The CD20 molecule is a non-glycosylated transmembrane phosphoprotein member of the membrane-spanning four-domain family, subfamily A (MS4A) of proteins, which is part of the plasma membrane [18]. Its exact function in cells is not precisely known, but many experimental studies showed it to be a part of ion channels. Lymphoma B cells, whether normal or malignant, have cell surface CD20 antigen expression in 90% of their population [19]. However, CD20 antigen is expressed on mature B-cell lineage and not found on stem or plasma cells. This property makes it an ideal target for unconjugated CD20 mAb. Being part of the membrane, it remains at the cell surface even after cross-linking with mAb and is neither shed from the surface nor internalized or modulated [20–22].

These properties of CD20 mAb allow antibody-dependent cellular cytotoxicity and complement-dependent cytotoxicity (CDC), resulting in the death of cancer cells. Various studies have probed the role of CD20 mAb in controlling growth and triggering cell death in various cancers. Along with CDC, other proposed mechanisms of action are antibody-dependent cellular phagocytosis (ADCP), ADCC, and programmed cell death (PCD) [23, 24]. Since the approval of the first chimeric (murine and human) mAb targeting CD20 (rituximab) by the US Food and Drug Administration (FDA) as a cancer therapeutic mAb, it has become the mainstay of B-cell malignancies' treatment. The landmark clinical trial published in 1998 showed an overall response rate (ORR) of 48% with 6% complete remission (CR) and a 13-month time-to-progression (TTP) in relapsed B-cell NHL, with rituximab. These striking results led to FDA approval of rituximab for B-cell malignancies [25, 26].

16.5.2 CD22

CD22 is a cell surface phosphoglycoprotein of 130–150 kilodaltons (kDa). Cytoplasmic expression of CD22 can be detected in both pro-B- and pre-B-cell stages. However, immature B cells only show the surface expression of CD22. The surface CD22 is seen in normal mature and malignant B-lymphocytes. With the activation of B cells, the levels of CD22 initially increase, and with the transformation of B cells into plasma cells, the CD22 levels are downregulated. B-cell CD22 has two DNA clones, CD22α and CD22β. The CD22 possesses inhibitory function along with its limited expression and is an appealing target for B-cell depletion in cases of B-cell-derived malignancies. The CD22 is expressed in various hematologic neoplasms including B-lymphoblastic leukemia/lymphomas and mature B-cell leukemia/lymphomas, hairy cell leukemia (HCL), and prolymphocytic leukemia [27, 28].

16.5.3 CD37

CD37, as an alternative to CD20, has been becoming popular in recent times. It is a glycosylated glycoprotein which is a member of the Tetraspan internalizing transmembrane protein. CD37 is strongly expressed (>90%) on mature B-lymphocytes of normal and cancerous cells. CD37 is expressed in B-cell NHL, B-cell chronic lymphocytic leukemia (B-CLL), and about 60% of Burkitt's lymphomas [29]. Due to the overexpression in B-lymphocytes, it is considered as an alternative target for RIT especially in relapsed and refractory patients to rituximab therapy.

16.6 Historical Perspective of Lymphoma Treatment: Advent of Radioimmunotherapy

The history of lymphoma treatment can be traced back to the early twentieth century when there were reports of disease regression after X-ray treatment [30, 31]. The chemotherapeutic approach was used in the early 1960s [32]. The history of chemotherapy spans over a century now. The concept put forward by Paul Ehrlich, to introduce "magic bullets" to target tumor cells, has been well refined by researchers [33].

Antibodies are a crucial part of the human immune system for fighting against various pathogens and pathologies. The discovery of multiple mAbs during the last quarter of the previous century has revolutionized the management of various tumors and has been effective in introducing tailored treatment protocols. Widespan efforts put in by the researchers to undergo various investigational and clinical trials for mAb development have resulted in almost 60–70 mAbs gaining FDA approval and have ascended to a multibillion dollar healthcare market [34, 35]. The role of the antigen-antibody reaction was first explored in 1952–1953 [36, 37]. Production of the mAb from hybridomas was documented in a ground-breaking paper in 1975 [38]. The ability of mAbs to bind to antigens expressed on the surface of malignant hematopoietic cells leads to the concept of serotherapy for targeting and destroying hematopoietic cancer cells. The initial enthusiasm about these magic bullets resulted in the treatment of the first ever lymphoma patient in 1979 [39]. However, the treatment results of more than 100 patients were not very encouraging and the initial enthusiasm associated with the mAb treatment quickly dwindled. Despite these initial discouraging results, the interest in ADCC led to the production of various antibodies which were approved for use in various pathologies. Further evolution in antibody structure by conjugating it to cytotoxic drugs, toxins, or radionuclides has resulted in improved efficacy and better patient survival. Nevertheless, it took two more decades for the induction of immunoconjugates into clinical scenarios [40].

16.7 Advantages of RIT in Hematologic Malignancies

Preclinical trials in NHL validated that RIT has a definite therapeutic advantage over conventional chemotherapy and immunotherapy alone. There are several advantages to using RIT for the treatment of hematologic malignancies. Among hematologic malignancies, lymphomas are particularly a favorable target for RIT as they are radiosensitive in a dose-dependent pattern.

Additionally, radioimmunoconjugates kill lymphoma cells by radiation induced cytotoxicity and monoclonal antibody-mediated cell death mechanisms; however, RIT efficacy is attributed predominantly to radioactive emissions and thus can be useful even when the patient has treatment failure with unconjugated monoclonal antibodies. The β-particles used most commonly in clinical settings are currently iodine-131 (I-131), yttrium-90 (Y-90), and lutetium-177 (Lu-177). The cytotoxicity of these β-emitters is effective over a certain range or spherical volume covering a few millimeters. The β-particles can indirectly target tumor volumes of several centimeters or numerous layers of cells through its "crossfire" effect. This crossfire/bystander effect is additionally helpful in targeting tumors where there is no access to an unmodified monoclonal antibody [41–43]. The crossfire or bystander effect is presumed to induce cell injury and death, directly by mAb binding and indirectly by penetrating a reasonable length of surrounding cells. The crossfire effect results in increased efficacy of therapy especially in cases of bulky tumors or poor vascular supply [44]. The bystander effect of cell damage has been explained by many mechanisms, such as the transmission of bystander signals through gap-junctional intercellular communication. Another interesting concept of bystander effect has been explained as the transfer of genetic instability from irradiated cells to neighboring, unirradiated cells. Some investigators have also identified secreted factors, such as transforming growth factor-$\beta 1$ (TGF-$\beta 1$) and interleukin (IL)-8 and tumor necrosis factor α (TNF-α), that mediate bystander effects in vitro but do not require the existence of oxidative metabolites or gap junctions [45].

RIT has physical and biological effects owing to its continuous low-dose rate (LDR) irradiation (0.1–1 Gy/h) over hours and days to the target tissue. LDR has been reported to affect multiple biologic processes that are important determinants of cell survival in both tumors and normal tissues [46]. It has been observed that the toxicity of RIT per unit of absorbed dose in tumor cells is higher than that of a single fraction of radiation delivered at a high-dose rate (HDR), as is the case in external beam radiation therapy (EBRT). Several preclinical studies have addressed the question of the relative efficacy of RIT compared with conventional HDR radiation therapy [46, 47]. LDR total body irradiation preferentially spares non-hematopoietic tissues [48], and toxicity data from RIT trials have demonstrated that normal tissues have a higher tolerance to LDR than HDR irradiation [49, 50].

16.8 Historical Antibody Target Constructs

With rapid advances in genetic engineering, the past two decades have seen a dramatic increase in the production of polyspecific antibodies with more than 120 described formats now in clinical use or undergoing evaluation in clinical trials [51]. While the majority of the early development of polyspecific antibodies was focused on hematologic cancers, there are numerous molecules in clinical development directed towards non-hematologic malignancies. The rationale of using mAbs for RIT in the treatment of lymphomas was its radiosensitivity. Various target constructs were used initially; however, CD20 was the most extensively tested target in the initial days of RIT. About three decades back, many target constructs of CD20, CD22, and CD37 were used for RIT. The first published results of these RIT trials were about Lym-1.

16.9 Historical Target Constructs of Radioimmunotherapy

The concept of treating hematologic malignancies with radioimmunoconjugates took another decade after the introduction of immunoconjugates into clinical trials, which by now was three decades from their initial production, and the first study was published in 1987 by using iodine-131 HLA-DR Lym-1 in NHL patients [52]. Initial phase I and II trials used CD20 in the form of B1 and Y2B8, CD22 as LL2, CD21 as OKB7, and CD37 as MB1 target construct. These phases I and II trials mostly focused on dose escalation

studies, determining the maximum tolerated dose, biodistribution, and efficacy [53–62]. To date, the mainstay of RIT remains anti-CD20 targeting radioimmunoconjugates.

Binding of rituximab with CD20 antigen triggers various cellular pathways that result in apoptosis, antibody-dependent cytotoxicity, and complement-dependent toxicity with an overall improvement in treatment response rates. The use of anti CD20 mAbs was described by Nadler et al., and subsequently the use of iodine-131 and yttrium-90 anti CD20$^+$ mAbs was described. Since then, several modifications and new protocols were reported [39, 63].

16.10 Myeloproliferative Disorders and Phosphorus-32

16.10.1 Phosphorus-32 Phosphate Treatment

The first radionuclide therapy for hematologic disorders was performed using phosphorus-32 (^{32}P), although in elemental form and prior to the development of immunoconjugates. Early on, it was noted that neoplastic tissue had a higher turnover of phosphorus compared to normal tissue, even though the total content was the same between tissues. Thus, [^{32}P]NaH$_2$PO$_4$ (^{32}P) became the first isotope used for treating disease [38, 64, 65]. Phosphorus-32 is a pure β-emitter with a half-life of 14.3 days and mean emission energy of 0.695 MeV. It is generally believed to cause apoptosis of cells like other radioisotopes, which is the result of cellular damage to DNA; however, since it is so abundant in organic chemistry and DNA and decays to sulfur-32 (^{32}S), the chemical conversion after incorporation into organic material—and in particular DNA—may be a contributory mechanism for cell death.

Phosphorus-32 was first used in myelodysplastic syndromes and leukemias as early as 1936 and appeared to be effective in myeloproliferative disorders, which includes polycythemia vera (PCV) and essential thrombocytosis (ET). The approach to the correct diagnosis for PCV and ET, and thereby measuring response to therapy, was formalized with the establishment of the Polycythemia Vera Study Group (PSVG). Untreated PCV has a median survival of only 1.5 years, but the life expectancy for patients with PCV treated initially with phosphorus-32 approaches that of the general population [66, 67]. Although prolonged survival in the PCV groups has been noted with phosphorus-32 treatment when added to phlebotomy, an area of concern was the apparent development of acute leukemia at a mean time of 8.5 years after treatment. Studies showed a rate of 5.5–10% of patients that developed leukemias, lymphomas, or other myelodysplastic syndromes within 10–12 years but possibly up to 30% by 20 years of treatment with phosphorus-32. Second malignancies were observed in 8–15% of patients treated [68–70]. This seemed to compare favorably with other forms of therapy such as phlebotomy added to chlorambucil chemotherapy versus phlebotomy alone. The highest rate of leukemogenesis was with chemotherapy, but the best rate was with phlebotomy alone [71]. Hence, phlebotomy is used as the first-line treatment for PCV, and phosphorus-32 is usually added in the elderly patients or those patients who no longer respond to or tolerate regular phlebotomies.

No specific pre-therapy theranostic imaging is done for phosphorus-32 treatment. A liver-spleen scan might offer some insight on not only the splenic size but also disease burden, and distribution of radiopharmaceutical, but the information is unlikely to change management beyond what is already likely known prior to the patient's referral for therapy. On initial treatment, the recommended amount is 74–111 MBq/m^2 up to a total dosage of 185 MBq and up to a single dosage of less than 259 MBq on subsequent treatments. It is administered intravenously, although an oral route is possible but not recommended given the additional exposure of the gut to radioactivity, and requires an absorptive step not needed in the intravenous route. Blood counts can be checked subsequently every 3–4 weeks to look for a response, with the aim to achieve a more than 25% decrease in counts. Should that not occur and/or there is a rebound in counts, the therapy can be repeated ~12 weeks after the ini-

tial dosage, this time with a 25% dosage escalation. Phlebotomy is often recommended for PCV prior to treatment in order to stimulate precursor marrow cells, which in turn increases their radiopharmaceutical uptake. As with many systemic radionuclide therapies, treatment is withheld for platelets <100,000/mm^3, white blood cell (WBC) counts <3000/mm^3, and absolute neutrophil count <1000/mm^3. If after 1 year of treatment there is still a resistant disease, alternative therapies should be considered.

Phosphorus-32 therapy is generally well tolerated by individuals, with little to no side effects seen. Because of the risk of leukemogenesis, older patients are generally selected to undergo the therapy as that matches the overall mean survival time versus lag time towards leukemic transformation. Patients are generally chosen because they have failed or are intolerant to conventional therapies, particularly hydroxyurea, or may not tolerate the side effects of other therapies such as anagrelide or interferon. They may also be chosen as a bridge to transplantation. Newer agents, such as Janus kinase 2 (JAK2) inhibitors, histone deacetylase inhibitors, and other biotherapeutics may hold some promise, but still do not have well-defined roles in treatment algorithms. Nevertheless, it is important to note that conclusive comparisons between various therapies including phosporus-32 have never been made. Despite multiple large trials having been conducted by the PSVG and European Organization for Research and Treatment of Cancer (EORTC), there was too much patient heterogeneity to be able to form final opinions on optimal treatment approaches. Moreover, there was a suggestion by a French group that phlebotomy only provided temporary relief, and eventually, other therapies would be needed [68].

After phosporus-32 therapy for PCV, approximately 60–85% of patients achieve remission in the range of 3–4 years [72]. About 50% of the patients require only 1 dose, whereas an additional 30% no longer require further phosporus-32 treatments after the second dosage given 3 months later [70]. This is important because phlebotomy requires regular visits, and other medications, which although may be tolerable, may still have side effects. In contrast, phosporus-32 does not have any symptomatic side effects beyond the acute phase following treatment. Furthermore, it is unclear whether hydroxyurea itself might also be leukemogenic [69]. Coupled with relatively mild side effects and symptoms compared to other available therapies, phosporus-32 could arguably be considered as the first-line therapy in all patient populations except women of childbearing age, although the official recommendation has been to use it for patients more than 60 years old.

Unlike PCV, the survival of ET patients is not significantly different from the general population, although they are at a higher risk of complications, such as thrombosis and bleeding, miscarriages, and myeloid transformation of disease. Hence, ET patients must be more carefully selected. For ET, treatment recommendations are to treat when platelet counts are >1,000,000/mm^3 and age >60 years especially those who have had a history of thrombosis. The treatment approach with phosphorus-32 is similar to that for PCV and results in complete response (CR) of 63% and partial response (PR) of 37% a year after therapy [73]. Like PCV, alternative treatments in ET should be considered if disease control is not achieved; however, there is often an additional lifetime limit of 1.295 GBq. Although this therapy is not used anymore, consideration would be to use it not only in patients intolerant of conventional treatment but also in the setting of a bridge towards transplantation in other disorders.

16.11 Lym-1

Lym-1 is a murine IgG2a monoclonal antibody (mAb) which was initially produced by immunizing mice with nuclei of cultured cells from a patient with Burkitt's lymphoma. It is B-cell specific but with a relatively greater affinity for cancerous B cells originally produced. It was established that Lym-1 targets a polymorphic variant of human leukocyte antigen (HLA)-DR, present on the surface of B-lymphoma cells. The Lym-1 mAb is incapable of shedding or undergoing modulation after antibody binding [74], and it

was reported for the first time about the production of two mAbs (Lym-1 and Lym-2) which were produced using tumor cell nuclei preparations as immunogens. These antibodies were reactive with the cell surface of B-lymphocytes and derived tumors. The results of this study showed that these two antibodies were reactive to B-cell lineage lymphoma and leukemia cell lines. This B-cell binding was further confirmed by binding with the lymphoma and leukemia biopsy specimens [74]. Preclinical imaging studies established its localization to sites of lymphomatous disease [75].

A phase I study was carried out to determine the safety and maximum tolerated dose (MTD) of [^{90}Y]Y-2IT-BAD-Lym-1. The study showed partial response in 5 out of 8 patients who had stabilization of disease after the [^{90}Y]Y-2IT-BAD-Lym-1 treatment. The maximum tolerated dose was 0.37 GBq/m^2. The safety and toxicity of [^{90}Y]Y-2IT-BAD-Lym-1 were established in this trial, and it was concluded that this therapy can be used in clinical settings as well [76].

The antibody was also labeled with copper-67, which has ideal properties for being a therapeutic radionuclide given its 62 h half-life, as well as β and γ emissions suitable for RIT and imaging, although it has scarcely been used as a RIT agent. The pharmacokinetic dosimetry and outcome of copper-67 (^{67}Cu) labeled Lym-1 antibody was compared with the iodine-131-labeled Lym-1. TETA was incorporated in the immunoconjugate 2IT-BAT-Lym-1 [77]. There was a selective and rapid binding of copper-67 with complete retention of structural and functional integrity. As compared to [^{131}I]I-Lym-1, [^{67}Cu]Cu-Lym-1 exhibited higher peak concentration in 92% of tumors and a longer biological half-time in every tumors. The mean tumor concentration (%A/g) of [^{67}Cu]Cu-Lym-1 was higher than that of [^{131}I]I-Lym-1. The mean biological half-times of [^{67}Cu]Cu-Lym-1 was 8.8 days, better than [^{131}I]I-Lym-1 which was 2.3 days. Consequently, the mean tumor radiation dose delivered by [^{67}Cu]Cu-Lym-1 was twice that of [^{131}I]I-Lym-1. [^{67}Cu]Cu-Lym-1 delivered a lower marrow radiation dose than [^{131}I]I-Lym-1; hence, the tumor, marrow therapeutic indices were 29 and 9.7, respectively. Except for the liver, which received a higher dose from [^{67}Cu]Cu-Lym-1, radiation doses from [^{67}Cu]Cu-2IT-BAT-Lym-1, and [^{131}I] I-Lym-1 to normal tissues were similar. Images obtained with [^{67}Cu]Cu-2IT-BAT-Lym-1 were superior. This was tested as a therapeutic agent in hematologic malignancies in the form of phase I and II clinical studies in humans. The authors recommended that because of better pharmacokinetics and dosimetry, copper-67 has the potential to be the preferred RIT agent [78, 79].

16.12 [^{90}Y]Y-Ibritumomab Tiuxetan and [^{131}I]I-Tositumomab

16.12.1 Development of Clinical Theranostics in Lymphoma

The development of anti-CD20 antibody therapy initially started in the 1990s with the development of rituximab. Subsequently, therapeutic radiolabeled compounds were developed in the hopes that adding targeted radiation would improve the already excellent clinical response that was seen by adding rituximab to standard chemotherapy. Preclinical studies with tositumomab showed an improvement in response when it was radiolabeled with iodine-131 [80]. Similarly, two early phase trials were carried out using this strategy with yttrium-90 ibritumomab tiuxetan ([^{90}Y]Y-IT), leading to similar conclusions. One used cold ibritumomab before a single dose of [^{90}Y]Y-IT [81] and the subsequent one used rituximab prior to [^{90}Y]Y-IT to reduce HAMA production [82].

Larger studies followed in relapsed or refractory low-grade, follicular, or transformed B-cell NHL patients who were rituximab naive and were randomized to receive either ^{90}Y-labeled ibritumomab or rituximab. The analysis of all 143 patients found that overall response rate (ORR) was, respectively, 80% versus 56%, the CR was 30% versus 16%, and the duration of response was 14.2 months versus 12.1 months. The median duration of response was 14.2 months (0.9–28.9). However, the estimated time to next therapy (TTNT) for patients with

nontransformed histology was significantly longer for [^{90}Y]Y-IT patients as compared to rituximab patients (17.8 months vs. 11.2 months). Reversible myelosuppression was seen [83]. Initial studies looking at those patients already refractory to rituximab still had an excellent response to RIT showing ORR of 65–74%, CR rate of 15–42%, and progression-free survival (PFS) of 7–12 months. The ORR improved to 86% in the case of low-grade follicular lymphomas and disease of smaller than 7 cm [84–86]. When looking at patients who had not responded to rituximab or relapsed within 6 months following treatment, an ORR of 74% and CR of 15% were observed. The time to progression (TTP) was 8.7 months for the responders [87].

Based on these trials, by the early 2000s, there were clinical emergence of two radiolabeled mAbs to CD20, [^{131}I]I-tositumomab (Bexxar, murine IgG2a lambda), and [^{90}Y]Y-IT (Zevalin, murine IgG1 kappa), with the latter getting into the market first. The interest in iodine-131 stemmed from the fact that it was readily available and the most understood radionuclide in its clinical usage, but there was also increasing interest in the emergence of yttrium-90 around that time and its increasing availability for clinical purposes. Both radiopharmaceuticals were approved for indications for relapsed or refractory low-grade B-cell lymphomas. They initially had similar procedural approaches in delivering treatments, but there were important differences in how they evaluated the patient for treatment.

16.12.2 Procedure Development, Dosimetry, and Dosing Strategies

Early clinical trials involving the infusion of radiolabeled antibodies showed increased targeting in the mononuclear phagocytic system (MPS), which meant that a significant amount of the radiolabeled material did not make it to the target tissue, but rather normal tissue. In particular, both normal and lymphomatous circulating B cells had CD20 targets, although not on pluripotent hematopoietic stem cells. Phase I trials were performed with escalating doses of unlabeled anti-CD20 antibodies to try and block the initial uptake by the MPS, although the concern was that this would also block some of the receptor sites on tumors, thereby decreasing targeting of the disease sites. In theory, patients with smaller tumor burdens could have more of their antigen sites blocked by the unlabeled antibodies, thus decreasing the efficacy of the radiolabeled version. Nevertheless, there was an overall greater targeting of the tumor sites of the radiolabeled antibody after the unlabeled antibody was administered [88].

$[^{90}Y]Y$-IT developed its dosing calculation as a weight-based approach, as opposed to the dosimetric-based approach for $[^{131}I]$ I-tositumomab. The latter accounts for the variability of biodistribution between patients, but the approach with $[^{90}Y]Y$-IT leads to some variability in biodistribution between patients, although only modest correlations are demonstrated with hematologic toxicity [89, 90]. Both being mAbs, the clearance for both $[^{131}I]I$-tositumomab and $[^{90}Y]Y$-IT is relatively monoexponential and less variable than that of $[^{131}I]NaI$ clearance in thyroid diseases, and as such modeling dosimetry—specifically for $[^{131}I]I$-tositumomab—is simpler. That may be one of the reasons why toxicities are more predictable than with high-dosage thyroid cancer therapies since the similar dosages can give widely different dose deliveries. For $[^{90}Y]$ Y-IT, the relatively shorter half-life may also contribute to fewer variations of whole-body doses and improved predictability of responses.

More advanced approaches using dosimetry can be used to help model myeloablative high-dose RIT with stem cell support. The theory behind using higher doses is similar to high-dose chemotherapy, where aggressive or refractory disease could be treated, except that increasing radiation doses continue to be increasingly cytotoxic to malignant tissue, whereas higher-dose chemotherapy may only increase side effects without any beneficial tumoricidal effects. For high-dose myeloablative treatments, the toxicity of other nontarget organs has to be considered. In this case, nontarget critical organs have a dose-limiting exposure of 25–27 Gy for $[^{131}I]I$-tositumomab for lung and liver [91, 92], whereas for $[^{90}Y]Y$-IT, a dose of 20 Gy to the liver is considered limiting. This is more easily done with $[^{131}I]I$-tositumomab as the dosimetric evaluation is a part of its routine procedure anyway, but $[^{90}Y]Y$-IT must add the serial imaging and evaluation component with the $[^{111}In]$ In-ibritumomab version prior to therapy to assess whole-body and organ dosimetry. This is because the variations in clearance—even though not extreme at the routine clinically indicated levels—would become a greater issue at the myeloablative doses being applied. Nevertheless, both procedures need to have more accurate estimates, and thus attenuation correction maps have been additionally applied. In fact, additional procedures—such as using $[^{99m}Tc]Tc$-MAA (macroaggregated albumin) images for lungs and $[^{99m}Tc]Tc$-sulfur colloid images for the marrow, liver and spleen—can be registered with the pretherapy $[^{131}I]I$-tositumomab images to help better outline these organs to get the best estimates, as these were the organs considered to have dose-limiting toxicities. Further concerns do arise as a result of myeloablative therapies since they use high specific activity preparations neither ordinarily used in standard-dose treatments nor in the pre-therapy tracer assessment. There is also great variability in the amount of uptake in actual tumors both within and between patients. Whereas the amount of radiation targeting these tumors is only a secondary endpoint when used in the standard clinical approaches, in the case of dosimetry, it is the primary endpoint of the procedure and for which more accurate estimates are needed [93]. As a result, the advantage of such approaches is that for myeloablative treatments, median radiation doses of 38 Gy could be delivered to the tumor, as opposed to just a median of 12 Gy when external total body irradiation is used in the regimen [94]. Clearly, these more advanced techniques for patient-specific modeling are needed over not only simplified methods but also over standardized models, since it has been shown that there are wide variations of estimates of dose delivery to organs between methods of various and increasing complexities. Furthermore, it is clear pre-therapy imaging is needed to perform this and thus allows for more advanced types of therapies [95].

16.12.3 Clinical Procedure

RIT is primarily indicated for the treatment of follicular low-grade B-cell lymphomas, although broader indications are for CD20$^+$ non-Hodgkin's lymphomas that are relapsed, refractory, and transformed or even those that have previously failed rituximab. Clinical pre-therapy assessment of the patient involves confirmation of the presence of CD20$^+$ cells. Consequently, a bone marrow biopsy needs to be performed to confirm that the presence of lymphomatous involvement within the marrow is less than 25%. Of note, marrow biopsies are known to be of limited sensitivity as the site of biopsy could potentially miss the location of the greatest marrow involvement. More recently, 2-[^{18}F]fluoro-2-deoxy-D-glucose (2-[^{18}F]FDG) positron emission tomography (PET) scanning has shown that it may better assess the presence of marrow involvement than biopsy, but it is not known whether that would be sufficient to evaluate the marrow for the purpose of RIT and, when the marrow involvement is more extensive on PET than indicated by biopsy, whether there is increased toxicity seen in those cases. Other standard laboratory studies involve checking a complete blood count (especially for platelet levels) and renal function (creatinine). Women who are pregnant have an absolute contraindication to treatment. Those who are contemplating pregnancy should be counseled to avoid it for more than a year after therapy. Male patients undergoing treatment should also be counseled to avoid impregnating partners for more than a year after therapy. They have a theoretical low risk of infertility, and pre-treatment sperm banking could be considered if there is concern from patients with regard to the long-term effects of radiation exposure [96]. Notably, treatment with systemic radionuclide therapies has never been shown to have caused any adverse outcomes in offspring born to parents who have had systemic radionuclide therapy exposures, so fertility

advice can be tempered based on this information [97, 98]. For patients undergoing evaluation for [^{131}I]I-tositumomab therapy, thyroid function testing should be done in order to follow potential thyrotoxicities after therapy. The indications and contraindications for [^{90}Y]Y-IT therapy are depicted in Table 16.2.

The basic clinical procedure was similar for both. In essence, an unlabeled anti-CD20 antibody is infused, followed by a radiolabeled compound for imaging. Up to three scans are obtained over the next few days. A week after the initial infusion, the patient is again given an unlabeled anti-CD20 antibody but then followed by the radiolabeled compound at therapeutic dosages. Figure 16.1 represents the administration scheme for [^{90}Y]Y-IT therapy.

For [^{90}Y]Y-IT, the procedure starts with an infusion of unlabeled 250 mg/m^2 rituximab and was followed by 185 MBq ^{111}In-labeled ibritumomab tiuxetan for the purposes of imaging. The imaging was clinically done for the purpose of predicting biodistribution for [^{90}Y]Y-IT but not for dosimetry. It should be noted that the require-

Table 16.2 Indications and contraindications for ibritumomab tiuxetan [^{90}Y]Y-IT therapy [108]

Indications (adult patients)
- Rituximab-relapsed or rituximab-refractory CD20$^+$ follicular B-cell NHL
  - Relapsed/refractory (RR) indolent B-cell NHL (iNHL)
  - Diffuse large B-cell lymphoma (DLBCL)
  - Indolent lymphoma in the frontline setting
  - Mantle cell lymphoma (MCL)

Contraindications
- Pregnancy and continuing breastfeeding
- Known hypersensitivity to [^{90}Y]Y-ibritumomab tiuxetan, yttrium chloride, other murine proteins, or any of their components
- Children and adolescents under 18 years of age
- Marked bone marrow suppression (<1.5 × 10^9/L leukocytes; <100 × 10^9/L thrombocytes)
- Greater than 25% bone marrow infiltration by lymphoma cells, as judged by bone marrow biopsy
- Previous external beam radiation involving >25% of the active bone marrow
- Prior bone marrow or stem cell transplantation
- Detectable HAMA, depending on titer

NHL non-Hodgkin's lymphoma, *HAMA* human anti-murine antibody

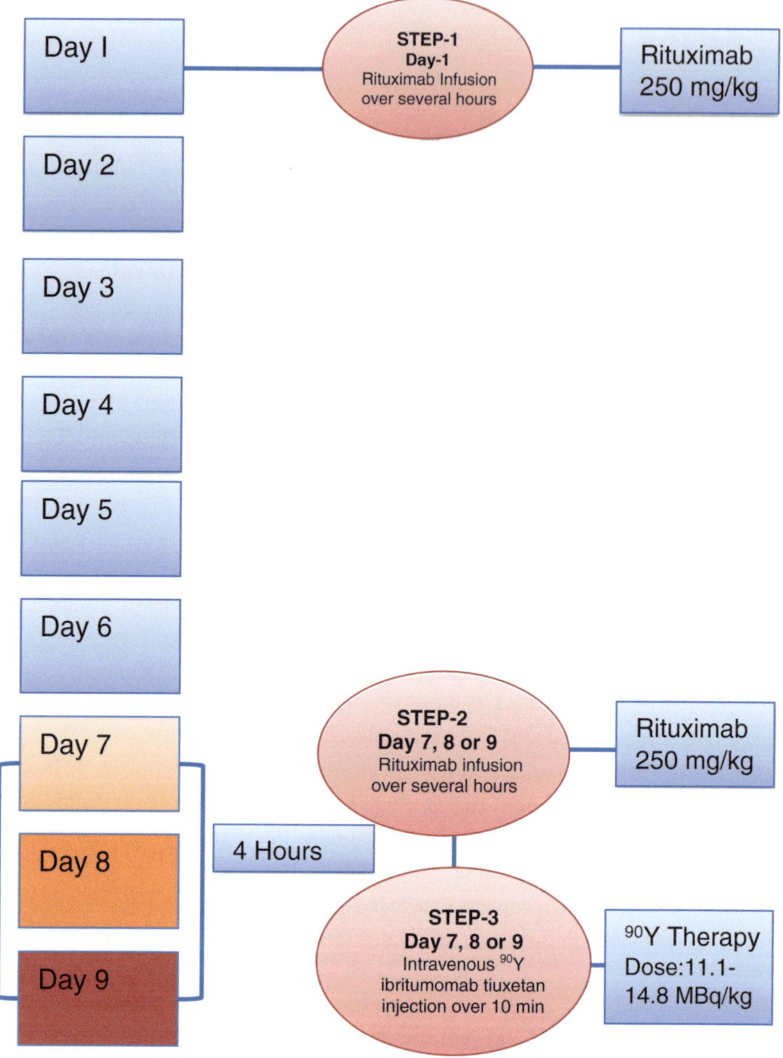

Fig. 16.1 Administration scheme for ibritumomab tiuxetan (Zevalin) therapy

ment for the biodistribution scan was only in a handful of countries including the United States, but not for most other countries. In the case the biodistribution appeared altered, the therapeutic version was not given since this would mean that the patient had inherent antibodies to the material, which would prevent targeting to the sites of interest. This was only seen in 0.6% of the patients [90]. A meta-analysis also found there was no difference in the incidence of serious adverse events or bone marrow failure in the United States and Japan if the biodistribution scan was not performed [99]. Consequently, the requirement for a biodistribution scan was removed, although the initial infusion with rituximab a week prior to the therapy remained.

Analogous to [^{90}Y]Y-IT, [^{131}I]I-tositumomab treatment evaluation also started with an infusion of unlabeled tositumomab, followed by a diagnostic dosage of the radiolabeled radiopharmaceutical [^{131}I]I-tositumomab. Subsequently, three scans were required over the following week to evaluate not only the biodistribution, but also to calculate patient-specific dosimetry.

The two radiopharmaceuticals have used different approaches to calculate the administered dosages. For [^{90}Y]Y-IT administration, the therapeutic dosage is calculated based on platelet count and patient weight, being given at 14.8 MBq/kg if platelets were $\geq$150,000/mm^3 but at 11.1 MBq/kg if platelets were 100,000–149,000/mm^3. The [^{131}I]I-tositumomab calculated a dosage to deliver 75 cGy of whole-body dose if the platelets were $\geq$150,000/mm^3 but at 65 Gy if the platelets were 100,000–149,000/mm^3.

One week following the initial infusion, the patient is again infused with the respective anti-CD20 antibody, but this time followed by the therapeutic radiopharmaceutical. Since [^{131}I]I-tositumomab can be imaged, a post-therapy scan could optionally be done also around a week after the therapy if there were potential questions it could address; however, this was rarely done as there did not seem to be any utility of getting the post-therapy scan as is routine in thyroid cancer. [^{90}Y]Y-IT could not be similarly imaged, and hence none was clinically attempted. Currently, only [^{90}Y]Y-IT is commercially available, and [^{131}I]I-tositumomab has been discontinued.

Following treatment, the most common side effect noted is a drop in the hematologic counts, which can occur as early as 1 week, and could nadir more than 6–8 weeks out. In most cases, the counts do recover, usually around a month to 12 weeks after dropping. Grade III–IV toxicities have been noted in ~60–70% but with ~15–32% requiring hematologic support in the earlier clinical trials. Usually, this is experienced with a drop in platelet counts but can also be seen with leukopenia. Neutropenia-related infections are rare. Drops in hematocrit are less common, and bleeding complications are also rare. Unlike chemotherapy, hematologic drops and recovery tend to occur more gradually, and thus these drops are less likely to lead to major clinical complications requiring intervention. Management strategy posttreatment includes periodical blood counts to timely counteract cytopenias.

Acute or subacute side effects generally may not be as severe as experienced with chemotherapy. There is minimal fatigue, asthenia, nausea and vomiting, abdominal pain, cough, diarrhea, and pyrexia, but in fact, patients may not frequently elicit any noticeable side effects on follow-up. Other side effects often associated with external radiation or chemotherapy, such as alopecia, are not present. Also noted was the presence of human anti-murine antibody (HAMA) response in ~4–11% of patients previously treated with RIT, possibly due to the already relative immunocompromised state and prior therapies, but without any side effects. This appears to occur more frequently in patients treated with [^{131}I]I-tositumomab [85, 88, 100, 101].

There are, however, long-term complications that have been noted. RIT has been associated with myelodysplastic syndromes and acute leukemias in ~2–4% of patients and has thus led to more cautious use of this therapy [102, 103]. What is not clear is whether these complications are solely as a result of the exposure to radiation from RIT, are as a result of the disease itself, or are due to other prior hematotoxic therapies. In many of the earlier trials, the patient had already received multiple rounds of other cytotoxic therapies prior to undergoing RIT. The expected annualized incidences after initial diagnosis of lymphoma are 0.3% per year and 0.7% per year after treatment. The median time to development of hematologic malignancy with [^{90}Y]Y-IT in heavily pre-treated patients is 5.6 years and thus somewhat similar to other patients treated with other approaches [102]; however, all these patients were being carefully monitored as part of a clinical trial, and none in the non-RIT arm had developed malignancy, which raised some concern that the RIT arm could be causing an increase in secondary malignancies [104]. Still, the rate of malignancy is similar to that of alkylating chemotherapy agents, which most of these patients have had previously. Another study evaluated patients who had been treated with [^{131}I]I-tositumomab as frontline therapy and found no incidences of progression to hematologic malignancies with a median follow-up of 5.1 years [105].

There were several practical advantages to [^{90}Y]Y-IT over [^{131}I]I-tositumomab. The weight-based dosage calculation of the former did not need the more extensive dosimetric procedure of the latter. The elimination of the pre-therapy management scan with [^{90}Y]Y-IT also reduced the steps and complexity of the procedure, leading to decreased costs of the procedure, and reduced dependence on a nuclear medicine facility on site, since no imaging component was needed. This then allowed the therapy to be given at outpatient facilities with minimal requirements for equipment. The former also did not need the more restrictive radiation safety precautions of the latter after treatment that patients had to follow of being around their family or the general public. Moreover, the therapy itself could be delivered in a room without the need for shielding, which considerably opened up possibilities of where the therapy could be conducted.

Additionally, $[^{90}Y]Y$-IT is not associated with the thyrotoxicity associated with $[^{131}I]$I-tositumomab, for which the latter needs to have super saturated potassium iodide (SSKI), Lugol's solution, potassium iodide tablets, or any source of concentrated iodide prior to each infusion to decrease the uptake of free radioiodine into the thyroid, which could cause unwanted increased radiation exposure to it and resultant hypothyroidism in up to ~7% of patients [106]. This also raises the theoretic risk of thyroid malignancy due to low-grade, non-ablative level radiation exposure to the thyroid. The presence of low levels of free iodide with $[^{131}I]$I-tositumomab can also be taken up by exocrine glands, such as lacrimal and salivary glands, and leads to toxicities, which can be seen with high-dosage $[^{131}I]$ NaI administration in thyroid cancers; however, the combination of low levels of free iodide and low uptake (compared to normal thyroid tissue) of these glands has not been reported as one of the more concerning adverse effects from the therapy.

The theoretic advantages for $[^{131}I]$I-tositumomab are that its dosage is based on patient-specific whole-body radiation doses and might make it slightly less toxic to the marrow than $[^{90}Y]Y$-IT. Since yttrium-90 is a metal, any free radioisotope could therefore be absorbed into the bone, potentially increasing marrow toxicity as well. Additionally, its longer β-particle path length could lead to greater damage to nontarget tissue. Such an observation has been reported in different groups of patients treated with these therapies, but not in a randomized trial [107]. Another logistical advantage of $[^{131}I]$I-tositumomab is that given the long half-life of iodine-131, it can

be constituted and shipped over longer distances and times, whereas the shorter-lived yttrium-90 often has to be constituted at a short distance from the site of therapy delivery, possibly in the facility itself. Thus, for the latter, there may be additional costs the facility may have to absorb to do this, which may not necessarily be reimbursed.

The overall outcomes in terms of therapeutic efficacy and survival have not been noted to be significantly different between them, as has been noted in this chapter. There is no head-to-head trials comparing between these therapies to show which one might have an edge, but a large reason for this is because these were not used frequently or long enough that there were enough patients being treated with these therapies such that a clinical trial evaluating them directly could be conducted. Neither calculates actual dose delivery to the tumor, although this can be done, again, therapies have not been used often enough that more advanced applications were clinically developed.

16.12.4 Non-myeloablative Trials

There are several prognostic factors which can be used to predict the responsiveness of patients to therapy, and these include non-bulky disease, no bone marrow involvement, fewer prior regimens, normal serum lactate dehydrogenase levels, higher total body radiation dose, and no prior history of transplant. Patients usually perform better with the fewer prior therapies they have had. Long-term follow-up of the patients treated in the initial phase I/II trials indicated that 24% of the responding patients had a TTP of more than 3 years and some were over 5 years out without needing further treatment [82, 109].

RIT with $[^{131}I]$I-tositumomab and $[^{90}Y]Y$-IT has also been explored beyond a single therapeutic administration. In a small patient series for relapsed follicular NHL, $[^{131}I]$I-tositumomab given to previous responders as a repeat therapy in patients at least 3 months after initial treatment, it was shown that the response after second treatment was similar to the first, with ~55% of responders having a longer duration of response than the first one and over 1.8 years in 5 of them. The rates of HAMA development were similar but with ~12% noted to have elevated thyroid-stimulating hormone (TSH) values [110]. Reviews of using repeat dosing of [^{90}Y]Y-IT also showed similar response rates and toxicity profiles for second therapies compared to the first. Furthermore, it was shown that the response rates were better with the fewer prior treatments received and were useful even in the cases of transformation. Median TTP fell from 12.6–15.4 months after initial relapse to 7.9–9.2 months after multiple prior treatments for relapse [111]. Some cases and anecdotal reports suggest that patients treated with one agent and then crossed over to the second agent for the subsequent treatment also appear to respond in the same manner as patients who have had multiple prior treatments [112].

Beyond refractory disease, RIT has also been explored in the frontline and consolidation settings. When used as a frontline agent, a single dose of [^{131}I]I-tositumomab showed >95% response rate, 75% complete response (CR), with estimated median PFS rate at 5 years of 59%, and PFS of 6.1 years. Again, the relapse rate appears to depend upon the quality of initial response and progressively decreased with time after treatment [105]. When used in a consolidative setting, the results showed tolerability, but not clear superiority, for the addition of RIT. A phase III trial using either R-CHOP regimen (rituximab, cyclophosphamide, doxorubicin, vincristine, and prednisone) versus a single dosage of RIT delivered after six cycles of CHOP (RIT-CHOP) showed no difference in either PFS or overall survival (OS) [113].

One of the earlier studies evaluated the use of [^{131}I]I-tositumomab as part of the initial chemotherapy regimen following three cycles of fludarabine in stage III and IV follicular lymphomas. The ORR was 97%, CR 76%, and median PFS was >48 months and had still not been reached >58 months of follow-up. The minimum PFS was 27 months for these patients. HAMA was noted in 6% of the patients [114]. When [^{90}Y]Y-IT was used in the consolidation setting, the PFS improved by 3 years over patients who did not receive consolidative RIT after initial chemotherapy who achieved at least a PR. The number of patients who had been initially at PR that later converted to CR improved by ~60%, and the TTNT also improved by almost 5 years between the two groups, although the response to second therapy and 8-year survival was similar in both groups; however, RIT has not been compared to the use of rituximab in these studies as with the [^{131}I]I-tositumomab study; hence, it is unclear how [^{90}Y]Y-IT would have performed in that comparison [104, 115].

Additional newer therapies are now being explored and thus moving beyond R-CHOP. Trials have studied the effect of adding [^{90}Y]Y-IT to more modern therapeutic regimens to see if that might make a difference. A phase I study with synthetic oligodeoxynucleotide, CpG, appears to show good tolerance and feasibility to the combination with [^{90}Y]Y-IT [116]. The most recent study to date evaluates [^{90}Y]Y-IT in a consolidative setting as a frontline therapy following bendamustine and rituximab, which is an established regimen superior to R-CHOP. In this phase II trial, the overall response (OR) was ~95% with CR/CR unconfirmed (CRu) ~77% in the intention-to-treat analysis. Following RIT, 81% of the patients converted from PR to CR/CRu. PFS was 71% after a median follow-up of 45 months. These results are encouraging given that 82% of the patients had an intermediate or high-risk follicular lymphoma international prognostic index (FLIPI) score, and 15% were grade IIIa. Nevertheless, the study is not a direct comparison against other frontline therapies, maintenance rituximab, or other newer strategies such as the use of newer anti-CD20 antibodies like obinutuzumab [117]. Possibilities of combining chimeric antigen receptor T (CAR-T) with programmed death ligand 1 (PD-L1) inhibitors might be another avenue for treating resistant disease in the future, and RIT will have to prove its worth against or complementary to these newer combination therapies [118].

Toxicities, specifically the hemotoxicity, in the frontline and consolidative settings are milder than when RIT had been used in the recurrent settings. The incidence of HAMA occurrence, many of whom had symptoms, was higher in these settings, and this group has been suggested to have a decreased PFS [105, 113]. In reviews of studies using RIT followed by up to seven cycles of chemotherapies and radiation therapies, toxicities subsequently appear to be similar to after RIT [119, 120]. Whether repeating therapies or following up after other prior hematotoxic therapies, one should consider time from last treatment, baseline hematologic profile, previous hematologic toxicity, and time to recovery in deciding the type and timing of the next therapy.

RIT is also being investigated as part of a combined-modality approach with conventional radiation therapy and other newer therapies. In a phase II trial [Southwest Oncology Group (SWOG) 0313] patients received consolidative [^{90}Y]Y-IT following CHOP and external beam radiation for limited stage aggressive B-cell NHL. The results in outcomes and toxicities appear to compare favorably with historical cohorts and could be used for future intensification of therapy in aggressive disease [121]. Additionally, RIT has been studied in combination with bortezomib, a biologic response modifier, in a phase I study in advanced and heavily pre-treated NHL, again with favorable and tolerable responses and toxicities, respectively [122].

16.12.5 Myeloablative Trials

Autologous and allogeneic stem cell transplants (ASCT) have also been performed, with adequate stem cell collection occurring after RIT. The concept of myeloablative therapy with stem cell transplant was tested in 1993 in a phase I dose escalation trial of anti-CD20 and anti-CD37 antibodies labeled with iodine-131 in patients with relapsed B-cell lymphoma. In these studies, high-dose RIT was followed by ASCT once bone marrow doses have decreased to less than 5 cGy to allow engraftment to take place. A total of 19 out of 43 patients underwent an escalated dose regimen with total dose ranging between 10–30 Gy. Out of a total 19 patients, 15 required stem cell transplants. There was CR in 16 patients, 2 had PR, and 1 had a minor response (40% reduction in the size of the tumor without regrowth for

18 months). The median duration of response exceeded 11 months for patients receiving ^{131}I-labeled B1 and 7 months for all patients. Myelosuppression was severe, but it was manageable with autologous marrow reinfusion, treatment with granulocyte-macrophage colony-stimulating factor, antibiotic therapy, and transfusions [50].

Further analysis of these phases I and II trials with ^{131}I-labeled anti CD20 revealed a PFS of 62% and an OS of 93% with a median follow-up of 2 years. The response rates (RR) were significantly improved, with overall response rate (ORR) reaching 86–95% and CR of 79–84%. Moreover, 39% of the patients had a recurrence-free survival for 5–10 years without any further therapy. It was concluded that ^{131}I-anti-CD20 (B1) antibody therapy produces CR of long duration in most patients with relapsed B-cell lymphomas when given at maximally tolerated doses with ASCT rescue [91]. Follow-up at 42 months showed 68% overall survival and 42% PFS. A subsequent long-term follow-up showed 48% of patients in continued remission [123]. Nevertheless, approximately 60% were noted to have thyrotoxicity as demonstrated by an elevated TSH, and two patients developed non-myelodysplastic malignancies. Other trials looking at myeloablative doses have also been shown to be feasible although not commonly used currently [124].

Likewise, a phase I/II study demonstrated that high-dose [^{90}Y]Y-IT can be safely given in combination with high-dose etoposide and cyclophosphamide in an ASCT setting for NHL without additional transplantation-related toxicity. Although the highest dosage given was 3.7 GBq with the median dosage of 2.65 GBq for [^{90}Y] Y-IT, the Kaplan-Meier estimated 2-year recurrence-free survival (RFS) and OS are 78% and 92%, respectively. This study further evaluated survival based on histopathology and concluded that if aggressive histopathologies like mantle cell lymphomas are excluded, survival is up to 100% [125]. Many clinical trials have shown excellent efficacy with low or comparable toxicity of myeloablative RIT regimens followed by ASCT as monotherapy or in combination with chemotherapy. This seems to be an innovative myeloablative regimen with unprecedented short-term and long-term toxicity profile. One study showed 90% CR and 92% ORR, with a 5-year PFS and OS of 63% and 73%, respectively [126, 127]. However, myeloablative RIT has not been incorporated in routine clinical setup, partly because of the low usage of RIT, as well as the complex logistics involved in it, limiting to performing the procedure at select institutions.

Alternate approaches and regimens have been looked at in several different studies. A multivariate cohort comparing patients receiving ASCT following either high-dose RIT versus high-dose chemotherapy with whole-body radiation therapy showed improved ORR of 67% versus 53% and PFS of 48% versus 29%, respectively. The 100-day mortality rate for high-dose RIT was 3.7% and for conventional high-dose therapy was 11%, suggesting that high-dose RIT could improve outcomes while also decreasing morbidities [128]. A subsequent trial evaluated the use of modified high-dose [^{131}I]I-tositumomab radiation absorbed dose escalation in combination with high-dose etoposide and cyclophosphamide. There was an objective improvement in ORR and PFS, but decreased symptoms otherwise related to transplant-related toxicities [129]. Patients who have failed bone marrow transplant have also had remarkable responses to RIT [89].

Older patients of more than 60 years of age are often not candidates for high-dose curative intent therapies and yet the majority of relapses fall into this category. A high-dose phase II trial in this group using [^{131}I]I-tositumomab with ASCT rescue reported encouraging OS of 59% with PFS of 51% at 3 years. It was also found that the organ dose limits were tolerated with similar toxicities to groups of less than 60 years of age, and stem cell engraftment occurred without significant complication [92]. Likewise, reduced intensity conditioning regimens have also been precisely developed to cater to elderly patients, as well as those with other comorbid conditions. Studies using [^{90}Y]Y-IT have shown that when added to non-myeloablative ASCT preceded by fludarabine and 2 Gy whole-body irradiation, there was objective OR in the majority of high-risk patients and that the regimen was also feasible with acceptable toxicities, even in the elderly and heavily pre-treated patients [130, 131].

Since the initial studies in 1993, a number of studies have attempted myeloablative RIT regimen with and without ASCT support. A subsequent phase I trial concluded that dose-escalated [^{90}Y]Y-IT may be safely combined with high-dose etoposide, arabinoside, cytarabine, and melphalan (BEAM) with autologous transplantation and has the potential to be more effective than the standard-dose RIT. However, this study recommended careful patient-specific dosimetry to avoid toxicity and under-treatment [132]. A GLEA (Groupe d'Etudes des Lymphomes de l'Adulte) trial was designed to evaluate the safety and efficacy of a conventional dose of [^{90}Y]Y-IT combined with the BEAM regimen before ASCT in chemosensitive relapsed or refractory low-grade B-cell lymphomas. In 77 prospective follicular lymphoma (FL) patients, 2-year event-free survival (EFS) and OS were 63% and 97%, respectively. This study concluded that Z-BEAM (Zevalin plus BEAM chemotherapy regimen) appeared safe and needed to be further evaluated in a randomized trial [133]. A study looking at the effect of RIT plus high-dose chemotherapy concluded that augmenting BEAM conditioning with RIT is safe and does not lead to long-term toxicity. Indeed, this favorable safety signal was used as a rationale for two ongoing trials of [^{90}Y]Y-IT based RIT plus high-dose chemotherapy in T-cell lymphoma and Hodgkin lymphoma (NCT 02342782, 01476839) [134]. Although these initial results appeared promising, a subsequent study randomizing patients to receive BEAM conditioning with either RIT or rituximab showed similar toxicities and side effects, without a difference in OS [135].

Standard and myeloablative doses have been used for conditioning with [^{131}I]I-tositumomab, and initial phase II trials also appeared to show some advantages for the use of RIT in this setting [136]. A subsequent phase III clinical trial evaluated standard-dose RIT with a chemotherapy-based transplantation regimen followed by autologous hematopoietic cell transplantation versus rituximab with the same regimen in patients with relapsed diffuse large B-cell lymphoma (DLBCL). A total of 234 patients were randomly recruited to receive R-BEAM (rituximab plus BEAM chemotherapy regimen prior to stem cell transplant) and B-Beam ([^{131}I] I-tositumomab plus BEAM prior to stem cell transplant). The OS and EFS and 2-year PFS were similar between the two arms. This study concluded that there was no added advantage of introducing [^{131}I]I-tositumomab as compared to rituximab [137]. Nevertheless, it is important to note that RIT was performed at lower than maximum dosages and could in part explain the failure of the combination of RIT with BEAM conditioning to improve overall outcomes, but further work would be needed to see if that would be advantageous without significant problems with toxicity.

16.12.6 Miscellaneous B-Cell Lymphomas

Since their initial introduction, there have been uses seen in other indications for lymphomas with CD20 surface expression. These mAbs have shown to have activity in mantle cell lymphoma (MCL) and Hodgkin's lymphoma, among other pathologies. Many of the trials looking beyond the standard single dose regimens, in fact, have looked at patients beyond low-grade follicular lymphomas. When used in the setting of transformed but indolent lymphoma in patients with an otherwise poor prognosis, RIT achieved an observed ORR of 39% and a CR of 25%, with a median duration of 36 months for CR [138].

MCL is an aggressive heterogeneous type of lymphoma characterized by the chromosomal translocation t(11; 14) (q13; q32). Owing to its aggressive nature, no single therapy has proven to be effective, and there are recurrence and relapse after conventional therapies. RIT has been used in MCL based on the rationale that MCL expresses surface CD20 and is radiosensitive and thus a good candidate for potential RIT; however, published literature has shown diverse results. RIT has been used as first-line therapy and secondary therapy in relapsed and/or refractory cases,

with or without ASCT [139]. [^{131}I]I-tositumomab has been explored in the role of sequential RIT cytoreduction followed by CHOP chemotherapy as initial therapy. The ORR to RIT was 83%, and at the completion of delivered therapy, the ORR was 86%. The median follow-up was 2.1 years. The median EFS was 1.4 years. However, the therapy was not able to effectively target minimal residual disease [140].

In a phase II study where [^{90}Y]Y-IT was used upfront as consolidation therapy after brief initial therapy with four cycles of R-CHOP in patients with MCL, the ORR was 82%, and the median time to treatment failure (TTF) was 34.2 months after a 10-year follow-up. The authors reported that the regimen was well tolerated and should be applicable to most patients with this disease [141]. These patients had a 93% OS at 18 months with 55% CR/CRu [142]. Another phase II trial used [^{90}Y]Y-IT in 34 patients with relapsed or refractory MCL. The results showed that 31% of the study population achieved CR or PR with a median EFS duration of 6 months and median OS of 7.9 years [143].

Trials have also been performed using high-dose RIT with ASCT. One such trial evaluated high-dose [131I]I-tositumomab with high-dose chemotherapy (etoposide and cyclophosphamide) followed by ASCT support, in 16 patients that had a conventionally measurable relapsed or refractory to treatment disease. The ORR was 100%, with CR of 91%, and of the total that were treated, almost 94% were alive at the time of reporting, with 75% having no progression of disease at 6–57 months from transplantation and 16–97 months from diagnosis. OS at 3 years from transplantation is estimated at 93% and PFS at 61%, which when compared to other high-risk clinical trial groups, was an improvement in treatment response over conventional therapy [144]. The major toxicities involve transient hematologic cytopenias with nadirs occurring usually from 4–6 weeks posttreatment and recovery to grade II by 8–9 weeks following therapy. Grade IV toxicities were observed in 2–17% of patients, which were mostly neutropenias. HAMA elevations occurred in about 9% of patients who had prior chemotherapy, but in 65% when it was administered as first-line therapy.

Since a few of these trials were using [^{131}I] I-tositumomab, there are no further results available since the discontinuation of the product by the manufacturer; however, [^{90}Y]Y-IT has also been used in patients with untreated MCL. A study delivering [^{90}Y]Y-IT following four cycles of rituximab with CHOP chemotherapy regimen resulted in a 75% RR, 43% CR, and 93% OS rate at 18 months [141]. The European MCL Network conducted a prospective, multicenter phase II trial evaluating a single dose of [^{90}Y]Y-IT as salvage induction or consolidation therapy in patients with relapsed/refractory MCL after ASCT or those unsuitable for high-dose therapies. The ORR was 61%, including a CR rate of 32% and a PR of 29%. The results of this trial are not yet published; however, in a communiqué, the authors concluded that [^{90}Y]Y-IT therapy has the potential for benefiting the MCL patients, particularly older age patients [145].

There have also been studies using RIT in mucosa-associated lymphoid tissue (MALT) lymphomas. The therapies for marginal zone lymphomas (MZL) are not well defined. A phase II trial has looked at using [^{90}Y]Y-IT in untreated, non-gastric, extranodal disease. The results were encouraging, showing ORR at 12 weeks post-therapy of 88%, with CR in 50%/CRu in 6% and PR in 31% of patients. The median PFS was 47.6 months with a median follow-up of 65.6 months, and median OS was not reached. The 5-year PFS was 40%, with 5-year OS at 72%, with tolerable toxicities [146]. A review of studies performed with [^{90}Y]Y-IT concluded that RIT was a safe and effective possibility, with few side effects in untreated as well as refractory/recurrent disease, and a good alternative to chemotherapy in elderly patients, especially when avoiding surgical options. It also performed well in chemorefractory and highly pre-treated individuals, as well as patients with widespread bulky disease [147].

Of great interest is the potential use of RIT in high-grade aggressive lymphomas. Again, many of the trials with RIT have included DLBCL as part of the cohort of patients, but some studies have been performed specifically looking at this

group. A multicenter phase II study evaluated 55 elderly high-risk untreated DLBCL patients who were given a short course of R-CHOP, followed by [^{90}Y]Y-IT. At a median 7 years of follow-up, the ORR was 80% with a CR of 73%. Disease-free survival was ~43%, PFS was ~36%, and the OS at almost 8 years was ~39%. Deaths were primarily due to the progression of the disease, with two patients developing secondary hematologic malignancies [148]. In another study of relapsed DLBCL following treatment with chemotherapy with or without rituximab and not eligible for ASCT, 104 patients were treated with [^{90}Y]Y-IT. The ORR was 44% with a median OS of 22 months for the group previously treated with chemotherapy alone and 4.6 months for those who had failed chemotherapy with rituximab [149]. Another phase II dose escalation trial using [^{90}Y]Y-IT with reduced intensity conditioning for allogeneic transplant was performed in a mixed set of patients with CLL, DLBCL, MCL, and FL, showing the feasibility of dose escalation and favorable results [150].

16.13 Rituximab

Rituximab is a chimeric IgG1 kappa anti-CD20 monoclonal antibody. The proposed mechanisms of cytotoxicity are complement-dependent cytotoxicity and cellular toxicity, antibody-dependent cytotoxicity, and apoptosis [151]. The target agent for rituximab is CD20, and it is most extensively used in immunotherapy alone or in conjunction with chemotherapy, radiation therapy, and RIT. It is approved as immunotherapy by the FDA for the treatment of B-cell non-Hodgkin's lymphomas, chronic lymphocytic leukemia (CLL), and rheumatoid arthritis. It has also been used in various other pathologies. Since its initial phase I/II clinical trials, it has been extensively used as monotherapy and in conjunction with other chemotherapeutic regimens. The availability of this mAb has revolutionized the management of refectory and indolent lymphomas [152]. The indications and contraindications for the administration of radiolabeled rituximab are demonstrated in Table 16.3.

Table 16.3 Indications and contraindications for radio-labeled rituximab (anti-CD20 antigen therapy) [23]

Indications (adult patients)
- Relapsed or refractory lymphomas
  - Follicular lymphomas
  - Mantle cell lymphomas (MCL)
  - Mucosa-associated lymphoid tissue (MALT) lymphomas
  - Small lymphocytic lymphomas
- Aged more than 18 years
- World Health Organization performance status of less than 3
- Life expectancy of more than 3 months
- Patients who had received previous rituximab if more than 6 months had elapsed from prior treatment

Contraindications
- Pregnancy and continuing breastfeeding
- Children and adolescents under 18 years of age
- Marked bone marrow suppression (<1.5 × 10^9/L leukocytes; <100 × 10^9/L thrombocytes)
- Significant impairment in cardiac, renal, or hepatic function

The main drawback of FDA-approved murine anti-CD20 mAb [^{90}Y]Y-IT and [^{131}I]I-tositumomab was potential HAMA. This drawback limited the role of FDA approval of the mAb in repeat dosing [110]. Freedom from HAMA is especially important if first-line RIT is planned as HAMA may limit repeat dosing. Due to barriers in the usage of [^{90}Y]Y-IT and [^{131}I]I-tositumomab as RIT agents in the relapsed and refractory treatment and as first-line therapy in indolent lymphoma, an alternate was sought in the form of rituximab labeled with iodine-131. An early experience of RIT with rituximab labeling with iodine-131 was described in 2002–2003 [153, 154]. Data from this study showed that it has significantly longer organ retention (88 h) as compared to available RIT agents. This study gave insight not only about the successful labeling of rituximab with an available radioisotope but also elaborated radioimmunoconjugate transit inside the target and nontarget organ. This study recommended the use of dosimetry for the treatment of lymphoma prior to [^{131}I]I-rituximab treatment [153].

Another pilot study was conducted where rituximab was labeled with iodine-131 using the chloramine T method with >98% labeling efficiency. The study showed that rituximab immunoconjugate has similar results compared to radiolabeled tositumomab and ibritumomab. In the total study population, ORR was 71% over a median follow-up period of 14 months (range 4–28 months). CR was achieved in 54% of patients over a median duration of 20 months [154]. The first large cohort study on [^{131}I]I-rituximab RIT was reported from Australia. This study recruited 90 patients with refractory or recurrent low-grade lymphomas. Patients received a whole-body absorbed dose of 0.75 Gy with administered activities of 1.36–5.34 GBq [^{131}I]I-rituximab (median, 2.4 GBq). The ORR was 76%, the median PFS for the entire cohort was 1.1 years, and 53% of the study population attained CR. About 14% of patients had no relapse beyond 4 years. With a 2-year median follow-up (range 4–58 months), the estimated median survival was 50 months, with a 4-year actuarial survival rate of 59% ± 10%. Higher ORR had a significant association with stage I/II disease and fewer than two prior chemotherapy regimens. While age ≤60, stage I/II disease, and low FLIPI score had an association with a significantly higher CR/CRu rate ($p \leq 0.012$), this therapeutic regimen showed similar outcomes when compared with the contemporary [^{90}Y]Y-IT and [^{131}I]I-tositumomab RIT [155]. A 10-year clinical experience of [^{131}I]I-rituximab in 142 patients of low-grade lymphomas showed 67% ORR, PFS of 18 months overall, and 32 months in CR or CRu patients, with CR in 50%, median OS of 32 months, and 8-year OS of 48%. Toxicity was mostly hematologic like neutropenia or thrombocytopenia. Comparison with contemporary RIT conjugates like [^{131}I]I-tositumomab and [^{90}Y]Y-IT showed similar efficacy, utility, safety, and outcomes [156].

[^{131}I]I-rituximab has not been used in the United States. Most of the trials and published studies are from Australia. A few sporadic studies from Korea and Europe have been published in the literature. One such study recruited 24 patients for a single treatment dose of [^{131}I]I-rituximab. The ORR was 29%. The response assessment was carried out between two groups of lymphomas, and it was seen that low-grade lymphomas have a better OS (46%) and median PFS (4.5 months) as compared with DLCBL (1.3 months, $p = 0.0007$). After a median follow-up of 55 months, the median PFS for all the patients was 2.2 months. The median OS was 11.3 months [157]. Another study in Germany investigated the safety, toxicity, and therapeutic response of non-myeloablative RIT using [^{131}I]I-rituximab in B-cell non-Hodgkin's lymphoma (B-NHL) patients. A total of 10 patients underwent [^{131}I]I-rituximab RIT. These patients were heavily treated with either multiple chemotherapeutic agents and/or rituximab. Four out of 10 patients had CR while 2 patients partially responded to the therapy. RIT was less efficient in patients with bulky disease and elevated lactate dehydrogenase (LDH). The authors concluded that [^{131}I]I-rituximab therapy is another option for heavily treated recurrent or refractory lymphoma patients [158].

A study involving 31 FL patients, who required treatment according to the Groupe d'Etude des Lymphomes Folliculaires (GELF) criteria, received [^{131}I]I-rituximab as first-line or salvage therapy. The study population was a heterogeneous group of patients having various stages of the disease. All patients were followed up for a period of 12 years by a single hematologist. RR in this study population was 97%, and 2-[^{18}F] FDG PET documented complete remission in 24 (77%) patients. This study also described three duodenal lymphoma patients who had complete remission for a period of 3–4 years [159].

The administration scheme for rituximab therapy is illustrated in Fig. 16.2.

An investigation explored the safety of [^{131}I] I-rituximab outpatient RIT in 200 consecutive patients who received therapeutic activities between 1 and 4.5 GBq (mean 2.29 GBq) and studied radiation exposure to adult caregivers. The exposures ranged from <0.01 to 3.67 mSv (mean 0.48 mSv) and from <0.01 to 1.2 mSv (mean 0.23 mSv) to other co-residing family members. The excreted urinary activity was typically <25% of the administered activity. Release

dose rates of less than 25 µSv/h at 1 m were attained within 1 week of therapy [160]. The results showed that this therapy was not a hazard to the general population, including people in the more immediate vicinity of the treated patient.

16.13.1 Rituximab Myeloablative Trials

[^{131}I]I-tositumomab and [^{90}Y]Y-IT myeloablative RIT has been extensively used in phase I/II clinical trials with and without chemotherapy and ASCT. The feasibility, efficacy, safety, risk factors, and outcome of tandem therapy approach have also been investigated in studies of [^{131}I] I-rituximab myeloablative RIT followed by high-dose chemotherapy with ASCT support in heavily pre-treated patients with relapsed or refractory B-cell NHL. This phase I/II prospective study of myeloablative RIT and high-dose BEAM conditioning regimen prior to ASCT in patients with 9.5 years of follow-up determined the PFS of 47.5 months and OS of 43% (10/23 patients). Thirty-nine percent of patients were in complete remission (CR) after a median follow-up of 9.5 years. However, this trial could not find a statistically significant difference in OS and PFS when compared RIT alone versus RIT with high-dose chemotherapy with or without a second ASCT. The tandem approach showed hematologic and non-hematologic toxicities, albeit non-hematologic toxicities were higher than compared to the RIT group alone. An additional worrisome outcome was the development of treatment-related secondary malignancies in three patients [161, 162]. Another study recruited 16 patients with relapsed, refractory, aggressive B-cell NHL. Fifteen patients out of the total population showed CR while 1 patient underwent PR. Twelve out of 16 patients remained alive and disease free at a median of 44 months (range 4–108 months) post-ASCT. This study suggested that the addition of [^{131}I]I-rituximab RIT to BEAM conditioning, before ASCT, improves survival compared with BEAM conditioning alone, without significant additional toxicity [163].

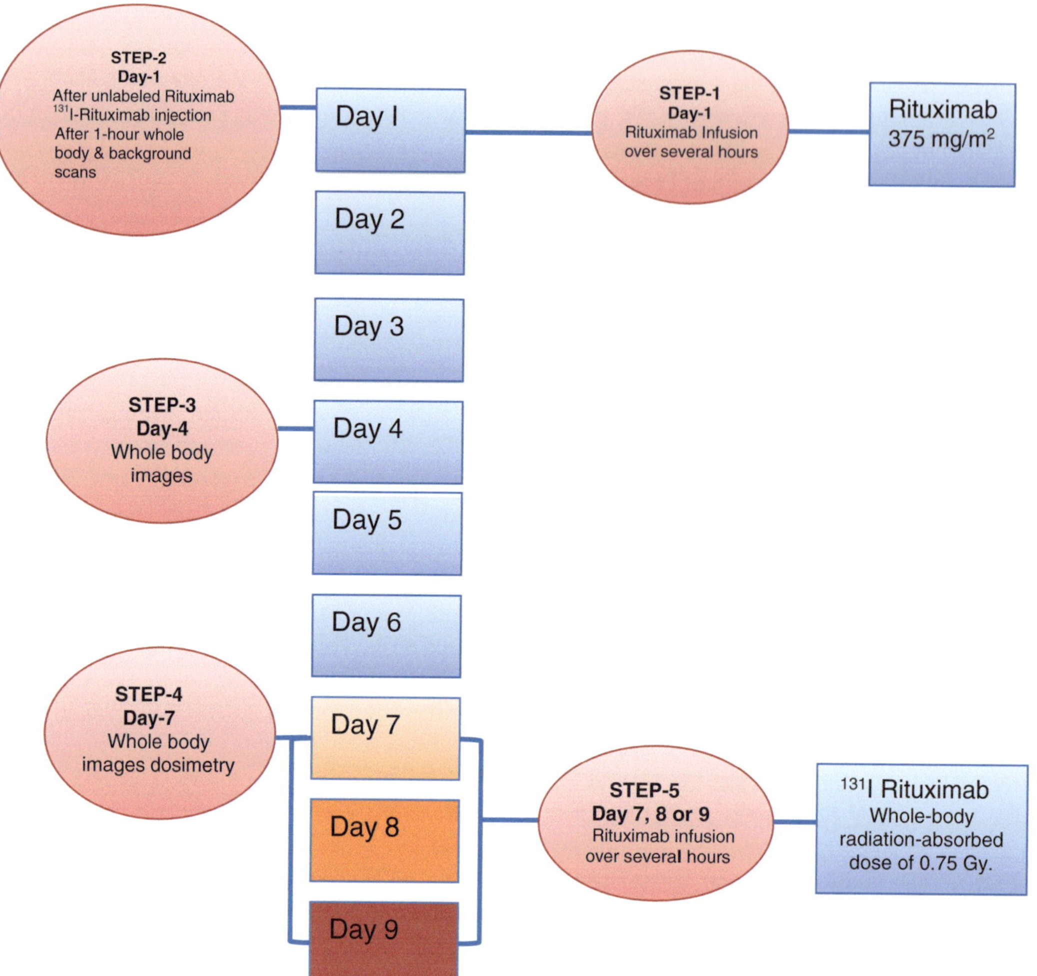

Fig. 16.2 Administration scheme for rituximab therapy

16.14 Hodgkin's Disease

Hodgkin's lymphoma (HL) is a relatively uncommon lymphoid malignancy, originating from B cells. It mostly affects the young adult population (5–6% of all childhood malignancies) and is more prevalent in males than females, with an annual incidence of 2–3 per 100,000. Multiple factors, namely, age, sex, socioeconomic status, ethnicity, and geographical locations, have an impact on its incidence [164, 165]. The clinical presentation follows a bimodal curve with the peak incidence in young adults and the elderly population [166]. Hodgkin's disease almost always presents in the form of generalized or solitary lymphadenopathy [14]. Histologically, it is characterized by the presence of an abnormal cell type called Reed-Sternberg cells (RS cells). RS cells are large malignant B cells found in tissues involved in HL. The evidence of disease is mainly found in lymph nodes or spleen. The bulk of the lymph node regions involved belong to the cervical and mediastinal areas.

Among all the hematologic malignancies, HL shows a remarkably good prognosis, and with sound and efficacious treatment methodology, the 5-year OS rate of more than 95% has been reported [167–170]. The mainstay of treatment for HL is chemoradiation therapy, although recurrent disease can be more resistant. The radiosensitivity of HL has enabled RIT to be a good treatment option. Some attempts have been made to use it in low-grade Hodgkin's disease, which similarly has indolent courses to low-grade follicular NHL and can be done instead of rituximab or chemotherapy as an alternative. A phase I/II dose escalation trial using [131I] I-tositumomab has been performed in recurrent lymphocytic-predominant Hodgkin's lymphoma, found similar toxicity profile to NHL, and overall appeared to be feasible [171].

Other radiolabeled compounds have also been developed as RIT agents. Antiferritin has been radiolabeled with both iodine-131 and yttrium-90 and has been used for the treatment of Hodgkin's lymphoma. Thymus-derived lymphocytes in the tumor microenvironment synthesize and secrete ferritin [172, 173]. The radioimmunoconjugates bind to the ferritin to exert their action. However, radiolabeled antiferritin should be used prior to chemotherapy or EBRT as these modalities decrease intratumoral ferritin concentration [174]. The largest phase II study of iodine-131 labeled antiferritin in patients with relapsed HL showed a 40% ORR among 37 patients while 1 patient achieved a CR [175]. The results with yttrium-90-labeled antiferritin in 39 patients with heavily pre-treated relapsed/refractory HL showed a 51% ORR and a median OS of 6 months [176]. Radiolabeled antiferritin only targets lesions >1 cm and those which have abundant ferritin. In cases where it is used, it should be prior to chemotherapy or external beam radiotherapy as these modalities decrease ferritin concentration in cells [174].

CHT-25 is an iodine-131 radiolabeled anti-CD25 conjugate. HL cells frequently express CD25 [177, 178]. A phase I study using this drug in 11 patients with relapsed/refractory HL resulted in an ORR of 45% [179]. Iodine-131 Ki-4 is an agent consisting of a radiolabeled murine anti-CD30 monoclonal antibody. In a study of 22 patients with relapsed/refractory CD30+ HL, treatment with iodine-131 Ki4 resulted in a 27% OS rate and 1 case of complete remission [180]; however, grade IV hematologic toxicity developed in 32% of patients, discouraging further investigation of this agent.

16.15 T-Cell Lymphoma

NHLs are subdivided on the basis of their originating cells; they can either be B-cell lymphoma or T-cell lymphoma. The commonest type is B-cell lymphoma comprising about 80–85% of NHL. The difference between these two types is due to their origins. T-cells mature in the thymus while B cells are located and mature in bone marrow. T-cells have a longer life span and secrete lymphokines while B cells secrete antibodies and have shorter life spans.

T-cell NHL represents approximately 10–15% of all lymphomas in Western countries. Patients with T-cell NHLs are often treated similarly as intermediate grade B-cell lymphomas. Survival rates are dependent on the type of pathology, and some adult T-cell lymphomas and leukemia have been associated with very poor 5-year survival rates (10–30%) [181]. Since B-cell therapies do not show good outcomes in T-cell lymphomas/leukemia, many new therapies have been tested in clinical studies. Many new agents target monoclonal antibodies or monoclonal antibodies conjugates with CD30, CD52, CD4, and chemokine receptor 4 (CCR4) (e.g., brentuximab vedotin, alemtuzumab, lenalidomide); histone deacetylase inhibitors (romidepsin, belinostat); antifolates (pralatrexate); fusion proteins (denileukin diftitox); nucleoside analogs (pentostatin, gemcitabine); and other agents (e.g., alisertib, plitidepsin, bendamustine, bortezomib) which have been used for the treatment of T-cell malignancies [182].

RIT in T-cell lymphomas has a limited role to play. Since the target constructs currently used mostly target CD20, which is expressed on B cells, their efficacy in T-cell lymphomas is questionable. Nevertheless, other targets have been developed for which some trials have been conducted with radiolabeled constructs. An experiment evaluated immunohistochemistry (IHC) expression of tenascin-C in T-cell NHL using the mAb tenatumomab. The clinical feasibility of targeting tenascin-C expressed in the microenvironment of B cells has been shown to be active in NHL and HL, but this study just confirmed the expression of tenascin-C in T-cell NHL. The expression of tenascin-C is variable in various histopathological types of T-cell lymphomas. However, this has shown the potential of tenascin-C in radiolabeled tenatumomab therapy in T-cell lymphomas [183].

The surface density of CD45 on T-NHL lines and T-NHL patient tumor samples was measured to figure out whether CD45 expression would be sufficient to serve as a target for RIT and whether subsequent animal models using T-NHL lines would be representative of clinical T-cell lymphoma [184].

A radiolabeled murine monoclonal antibody (T101) was used for imaging and therapy of six cases of cutaneous T-cell lymphoma. Imaging was performed with a 207–485 MBq [^{131}I]I-T101 preparation (9.6–10.5 mg). The treatment dose of 3.72–5.55 GBq on 9.9–16.9 mg of antibody was administered to five patients, with subsequent retreatment following plasmapheresis in three patients at the time of disease progression. All patients responded to their initial therapy, and two patients responded to retreatment. The duration of response ranged from 3 weeks to 3 months. Myelosuppression was the dose-limiting toxicity. Although it was suggested that this regimen has the potential for T-cell NHL therapy, this was not further explored [185]. Another study described five cutaneous T-cell lymphoma (CTCL) patients which were also given this radiolabeled murine monoclonal antibody. All patients developed a HAMA 2 weeks after the primary antibody infusion. HAMA responses persisted more than 22 months after [^{131}I]I-T101 treatment [186]. A subsequent report from the same group summarized the retreatment of three patients at the time of disease progression, including the utility of plasmapheresis and the effect of residual HAMA on antibody clearance rates and subsequent response to retreatment [187].

16.16 Posttransplant Lymphoproliferative Disorder

RIT has also been used in posttransplant lymphoproliferative disorder (PTLD). A small study using [^{90}Y]Y-IT in the salvage setting for CD20$^+$ PTLD patients who had failed rituximab and were ineligible for CHOP or other similar chemotherapy showed an ORR of 62.5% and CR of 50% at 37-month posttreatment, with no evidence of rejection seen, even though immunosuppression was reduced after PTLD was diagnosed [188]. Again, this showed that RIT was feasible in this patient population and could be explored in the future.

16.17 Pediatric Lymphoma

Pediatric malignancies, in particular, hematologic malignancies, in general tend to be radiosensitive. Many of these diseases are treated with high-dose immunosuppressive chemotherapy and/or radiation. While these are effective in many cases, in patients that the regimen is curative, there is a concern for the development of later complications, in particular, second malignancies, in part due to the increased tissue sensitivity to cytotoxic therapies in the pediatric population compared to adults and the longer longevity over which such complications can develop. Many of the same adult targets such as CD20–22 and HLA-DR are present in some of the pediatric lymphomas. There are many additional targets against acute leukemias but are beyond the scope of the current chapter. RIT provides a cytotoxic therapy but could theoretically reduce acute and long-term toxicities and complications by potentially reducing or eliminating the need for some of the other types of therapies. While the results of studies have shown promise, there has not been widespread development in the field of pediatrics for the use of RIT in hematologic disorders outside the acute leukemias. Nevertheless, there have been some limited trials of RIT in the pediatric population, although they have never made it to routine clinical use.

The prognosis for recurrent CD20$^+$ lymphomas is poor in this population. A phase I trial has been conducted using [^{90}Y]Y-IT in 5 children (4 DLBCL, 1 Burkitt's lymphoma) at 14.8 MBq/kg in 3 patients, and at 3.7 MBq/kg in 2 patients with poor marrow function. Toxicities included grade III–IV marrow cytopenias as well as a grade

III infection. Although neither CR nor PR was observed, a follow-up positron emission tomography (PET) scan showed evidence of disease stabilization [189]. There was a case report of a 6-year-old patient, heavily pre-treated for anaplastic large cell lymphoma, who underwent a pre-targeted antibody-guided RIT with yttrium-90-labeled anti-tenascin monoclonal antibody, which showed CR with a good quality of life 10 months after therapy [190]. Other targets in other hematologic disorders such as the various histiocytoses are theoretically possible. Preclinical studies had shown this to be promising but have not progressed to clinical trials [191, 192].

16.18 Multiple Myeloma

Multiple myeloma (MM) is a B-cell clonal disorder with a history of natural progression. The conventional treatment has a high relapse and recurrence rate. Only high-dose chemotherapy with ASCT will result in an improved PFS, remission rate, and OS. Multiple myelomas are radiosensitive, and in cases of extensive disease, total body irradiation (TBI) is used; however, this results in an enormous radiation burden without any substantial survival benefit. Hence, targeted therapy approaches have been explored in the treatment of myelomas, though the main treatment remains various forms of chemotherapy.

RIT may have a limited part in the treatment of multiple myeloma. The presence of CD20+ cells is limited, and [^{131}I]I-tositumomab use has been reported in this setting [193]. A phase II trial enrolling 16 patients who have failed at least a third-line therapy, of which only 6 were CD20+, was carried out. [^{131}I]I-tositumomab was administered as per the standard clinical procedure. The results showed the regimen was well tolerated by patients despite having prior therapies, with CR seen. ORR was 67% versus 10% ($p = 0.036$). Achievement of response was delayed compared to what is observed with standard therapy [194]. Another phase I trial with dosage escalation of [^{90}Y]Y-IT followed by ASCT has been conducted in 30 patients. Dose-limiting toxicities have been seen in 3 patients, with ORR in 22

patients, CR in a total of 7 patients, and PR in 15 patients. A median PFS of 16.5 months and OS of 63.4 months have been observed. The maximum tolerated dose was 18 Gy to the liver [195].

The chemokine receptor CXCR4 (C-X-C chemokine receptor type 4) is a transmembrane receptor, which is widely expressed in the human body throughout embryonic development. Chemokine receptor CXCR4's overexpression and activation by stromal cell-derived factor 1 binding are postulated to be triggers for tumor growth, survival, progression, invasion, and metastasis. The overall level of the expression of this chemokine receptor is predictive of metastatic potential of many tumors. The CXCR-4 has been associated with many pathological conditions. It has particularly high expression in hematologic malignancies. C-X-C motif chemokine ligand 12 (CXCL12)-CXCR4 axis has been used as a promising molecular target for future specific cancer therapies. Among them, the bicyclam AMD3100 (Plerixafor/Mozobil™) is the only compound that has been approved by the FDA (in 2008) for the mobilization of stem cells and for the treatment of hematologic malignancies and other cancers.

CXCR4-directed endoradiotherapy constitutes a highly promising targeted therapeutic concept. ^{177}Lu- and ^{90}Y-pentixather were recently developed as endoradiotherapeutic vectors. The first-in-human experience in three pre-treated patients with multiple myeloma undergoing CXCR4-directed endoradiotherapy showed promising results as a treatment option in combination with cytotoxic chemotherapy and autologous stem cell transplantation. A recently published paper showed that CXCR4-directed endoradiotherapy with pentixather showed a favorable toxicity profile. The most common toxicity was seen in the hemopoietic system in form of cytopenias. One patient showed acute kidney failure due to tumor lysis syndrome. Other higher-grade adverse events were either transient and resolved or easily manageable. This study concluded that RIT with radiolabeled pentixather appears to be well tolerated and easily applicable when preceding conventional conditioning regimens for hematopoietic stem cell transplantation [196–198].

Another approach has been to treat with bone-seeking radiopharmaceuticals to specifically target bone lesions, such as strontium-89 chloride (^{89}Sr), [^{153m}Sm]Sm-EDTMP (samarium-153-methylenediamine-tetramethylenephosphonic acid), and [^{166}Ho]Ho-DOTMP (holmium-166 1,4,7,10-tetraazcyclododecane-1,4,7,10-tetramethylenephosphonate) and [^{166}Ho]Ho-EDTMP. These are all β-emitters, with the advantage that samarium-153 and holmium-166 are also γ-emitters, which makes them excellent theranostic agents for imaging, dosimetry, and therapy. Samarium-153 has a β-decay with a high energy of 0.81 MeV and a half-life of 46.3 h. Holmium-166 also has a β-decay with a high energy of 1.85 MeV and a relatively shorter half-life of 26.8 h. These radiopharmaceuticals target active osteoblasts around the site of a metastatic focus, thus concentrating a radiation dose to the site, and have been used clinically for palliating pain from metastases. Yet, they have never been shown to have influenced clinical outcomes when used as monotherapies. Other than bone pain palliation, samarium-153 has been tried in the settings of bone involvement in myeloma initially in animal experimental models [199]. In another preclinical study, the orthotopic, syngeneic 5TGM1 myeloma model was studied and compared to the outcome of samarium-153 treatment with and without proteasome inhibitor PS-341. The results showed that proteasome inhibitor PS-341 is a good option as a radiation sensitizer in multiple myeloma treatment settings [200].

Samarium-153 was later tried in clinical settings through a phase I/II clinical trial. This trial explored the side effects and best dose of samarium-153 when given together with high-dose melphalan in treating patients with multiple myeloma undergoing stem cell transplantation. In this trial, a total of 46 patients were treated with targeted absorbed radiation dose to the red marrow of 40 Gy based on a trace-labeled infusion 1 week prior to the therapy. The [^{153}Sm]Sm-EDTMP infusion was followed by high-dose melphalan and peripheral blood stem cell transplant (PBSCT). There was no significant difference in CR rates, OS, or PFS among patients treated with or without [^{153}Sm]Sm-EDTMP. The 6-year OS rates were 54% versus 43% for the study and control groups, respectively. The authors concluded that the addition of high-dose [^{153}Sm]Sm-EDTMP to melphalan conditioning appears to be safe, well tolerated, and worthy of further study in the context of novel agents and in the phase III setting [201].

For hematologic malignancies, most of the holmium-166 utility has been in bone marrow ablation in multiple myeloma. The first preclinical study in multiple myeloma was in 1993 in dogs [202]. It concluded that a dose of 0.37 GBq/kg can be successfully given to dogs to fully ablate the bone marrow. Subsequently, dose escalation studies were done to measure the absorbed dose distribution to the bone marrow of multiple myeloma patients who received [^{166}Ho]Ho-DOTMP by gamma camera images and MIRD dosimetry method. Their estimated dose to bone marrow ranged from 15.0 to 46.3 Gy. They tried a dosage up to 2.7 GBq in their study population, which showed a decrease in myeloma proteins, bone pain palliation, and a variable disease-free survival (up to 5 years) [203, 204].

A phase I/II study was conducted on 32 patients to see pharmacokinetics, biodistribution, and dose escalation. The [^{166}Ho]Ho-DOTMP was used with melphalan and ASCT. The authors concluded that [^{166}Ho]Ho-DOTMP has a preferential uptake in bones/bone marrow, and rapid clearance through kidneys makes it a suitable agent for myeloablative therapy in multiple myeloma patients [205]. Another phase I/II trial was conducted to see the efficacy and safety of [^{166}Ho]Ho-DOTMP. There were 83 patients with varying doses of radio-conjugate in conjunction with various doses of melphalan. Out of 83 patients, 81 responded to the treatment while two patients died within initial 60 days. Patients receiving more than 30 Gy dose were more susceptible to grade III–IV hematopoietic and other toxicities, but 35% of patients had complete remission at the end of 23 months follow-up period. The authors concluded that it is a safe and effective therapy in combination with melphalan and ASCT [206]. The same group did a retrospective analysis on 104 patients with multiple myeloma to see the potential impact of this radionuclide therapy on disease outcome. A total of 41 patients had melphalan and [^{166}Ho]Ho-DOTMP while 63 patients had melphalan alone. Patients treated in the radiopharmaceutical arms were further divided into two categories: receiving <2.4 GBq versus >2.4 GBq. Univariate analysis of the patients showed that EFS, CR, and OS at 5 years were better in patients having low-dose [^{166}Ho]Ho-DOTMP along with melphalan compared to high-dose holmium-166 or melphalan-alone arms [207].

Not many phase III clinical trials were documented using [^{166}Ho]Ho-DOTMP after 2007. However, there was an animal study published in Iran about the production [^{166}Ho]Ho-DOTMP and its utility in mouse cell lines. It was concluded that [^{166}Ho]Ho-DOTMP produced had a good safety profile, biodistribution, stability, imaging characteristics, and pharmacokinetics. Authors concluded that [^{166}Ho]Ho-DOTMP has promising features suggesting good potential for efficient use of this radiopharmaceutical for bone marrow ablation in different hematologic malignancies including multiple myeloma [208].

16.19 Chronic Leukemia

Chronic leukemias, such as chronic lymphocytic leukemia (CLL), can be indolent and low grade, unless undergoing Richter syndrome, which is defined as the transformation of CLL into an aggressive lymphoma, most commonly DLBCL. Richter syndrome occurs in approximately 2–10% of CLL patients during the course of their disease, with a transformation rate of 0.5–1% per year. Other transformations into HL, multiple myeloma, promyelocytic leukemia, and even acute myelogenous leukemias (AML) have also been observed. Chronic myelogenous leukemia (CML) may undergo blast crises and progress to acute lymphoblastic leukemia (ALL). Whereas the mainstay of treatment of the transformed forms primarily depends upon chemotherapy, tyrosine kinase inhibitors, etc., the role of radionuclide-based therapies has also been explored in the past for the more indolent forms of these diseases.

Before the advent of chemotherapy, phosphorus-32 was used for chronic leukemias. It demonstrated activity in CML as initially only external beam radiation (EBRT) was available for treatment. The aim was to decrease symptoms, WBC levels, and splenic size; however, the OS seemed to be similar between the groups treated by phosphorus-32 and EBRT. With the advent of modern chemotherapy, phosphorus-32 has not been used anymore, though no specific comparison trials exist to evaluate its efficacy, which is intriguing given that phosphorus-32 is associated with virtually no side effects compared to conventional chemotherapy. Chemotherapy trials performed decades later made historic comparisons to phosphorus-32, but again given that overall medical care had significantly evolved over that time, no valid comparisons could be made [67]. Patients were initially treated to control symptoms. Early treatments had similar clinical endpoints in CLL and showed some efficacy with regards to the improvement of patient symptoms.

CLL is more radiosensitive than CML and thus amenable to better responses. Nevertheless, phosphorus-32 is not considered the standard of care, and its already rare use is almost nonexistent in this setting. Still, there have been therapy trials evaluating the use in CLL and small lymphocytic lymphoma (SLL) that express the CD20 antigen. These typically have a low density of antigen expression, but the use of RIT has been a concern since there is usually extensive marrow involvement, which usually precludes the use of RIT. There is frequently a problem of relapse and minimal residual disease for which RIT would be suitable. [^{131}I]I-tositumomab has been used in CLL and SLL for patients in CR or PR or those who had minimal residual disease after induction chemotherapy. Three months following standard protocol [^{131}I]I-tositumomab treatment, CR was achieved or sustained in 75% of patients, and minimal residual disease was eliminated in 33%. Aside from the expected hematologic toxicities, 2/16 patients developed myelodysplastic syndrome (MDS) 17–20 months after consolidation. In conclusion, [^{131}I]I-tositumomab consolidation after induction for the first remission appeared feasible, with the added benefit of potentially converting PR to CR, and eliminating minimal residual disease [209]. Conversely, a phase II study with standard protocol [^{90}Y]Y-IT showed grade III–IV hematologic toxicity in 92% of the evaluable patients, with myelosuppression lasting a median of 37 days, with 38% of the patients having persistent thrombocytopenia beyond 3 months after treatment. The group concluded that treatment with RIT led to unacceptably high myelotoxicities, even in CLL with relatively low marrow involvement [210].

16.20 PET and Theranostics in RIT

16.20.1 PET-CT Staging, Interim Evaluation, and Follow-Up

Imaging as a tool for assessing staging, prognosis, and response has been present for several decades and has been crucial in the management of patients with hematologic disorders and specifically in lymphomas. Initially, gallium-67 citrate (^{67}Ga) was investigated and used as the agent of choice to not only determine the stage of the disease but also to gather other prognostic information along with the treatment response assessment [211–217].

With the advent of 2-[^{18}F]FDG PET scanning, standalone PET was employed at the turn of this century [218]. This functional imaging was indeed of great value, but lack of ancillary anatomical information was a great limitation until the computed tomography (CT) component was finally incorporated by 2001 for use in a single study. Over the years, 2-[^{18}F]FDG PET-CT imaging has not only been employed with the imaging part of lymphomas but has had a profound role in staging and response assessment [219, 220]. The Lugano classification identifies 2-[^{18}F]FDG PET-CT (non-contrast-enhanced) as the choice of scanning for staging all 2-[^{18}F]FDG avid or non-avid lymphomas. The unique aspect of metabolic imprint attained by 2-[^{18}F]FDG PET-CT, in comparison to CT, has well established its efficacy and sensitivity in not only picking up the suspected lesions for staging purposes [221] but also monitoring its treatment management and disease recurrence [222].

The accuracy of 2-[^{18}F]FDG PET-CT to identify bone marrow involvement has alleviated the need for a marrow biopsy especially in HL as multiple investigators have shown that the results of bone marrow involvement, proven by biopsy, are, in the majority of the cases, concordant with the imaging results of PET-CT studies. Lugano classification does not recommend a marrow biopsy in HL when a PET-CT has been performed based on its high sensitivity to detect bone marrow involvement [223–228]. The introduction of 2-[^{18}F]FDG PET has an impact on initial lymphoma staging that ultimately up- or down-stages the disease, thus resulting in a treatment plan that carries more beneficial outcomes for the patient. Multiple investigators have established that in approximately 8–48% of cases, a 2-[^{18}F]FDG PET study could bring a change in staging and result in changes of management [220, 224–228].

In a post-therapy scenario, anatomical imaging is grossly limited due to the inability to detect any viable and metabolically active tumor in residual mass, but the unique feature to detect the tumor viability by 2-[^{18}F]FDG PET scan imparts valuable clinical information in terms of prognosis. However, a negative post-therapy PET scan cannot accurately negate the presence of residual micrometastases owing to the limited resolution capability of the PET scanner. This becomes more into consideration in a negative scan with or without a residual mass [229–235]. Nevertheless, it has been used in multiple studies to evaluate the effectiveness of therapies. A set of 109 newly diagnosed patients with DLBCL underwent interim PET-CT scans, which noted a remarkable difference in OS between interim PET-CT negative and positive groups, showing that despite limitations, a negative scan still afforded a good prognosis as compared to a positive study. They concluded that interim PET-CT can play a pivotal role in identifying nonresponders on the basis of the international prognostic index (IPI) score [236].

Several studies have specifically used 2-[^{18}F] FDG PET in the setting of RIT as it is useful to predict response and outcome in patients treated with RIT independent of anatomical criteria. When utilized for assessment of treatment response, 2-[¹⁸F]FDG PET findings are significantly associated with PFS and OS in subjects with NHL treated with RIT [237]. Similarly, a multicenter trial of 59 relapsed or refractory FL patients treated with [⁹⁰Y]Y-IT in four different PET centers showed that disease extension before treatment and response to RIT, as assessed by 2-[¹⁸F]FDG PET, resulted as main predictors of PFS, with the post-RIT PET result being the only independent predictive factor [238]. An interesting study showed that the ORR was equivalent in both [⁹⁰Y]Y-IT and [¹³¹I]I-tositumomab groups. As a group, transformed lymphomas tended to have a better response, and mantle cell lymphomas had the least response [239].

Another phase II study from Australia described the outcome of 68 patients with indolent NHL who underwent [¹³¹I]I-rituximab first-line therapy in conjunction with rituximab and maintenance therapy for 1 year. Patients were followed up for 7 years with a median follow-up period of 4 years. Patients' prognosis and response assessment of therapy were done with baseline and follow-up of 2-[¹⁸F]FDG PET as reported using Deauville criteria. The median time to next therapy was significantly different for patients in Deauville category 1–3 versus category 4–5. The investigators concluded that iodine-131 anti-CD20 therapy is an effective, practical, and affordable alternative in newly diagnosed, advanced stage, and symptomatic follicular NHL based on the 2-[¹⁸F]FDG PET findings [240].

The imaging window to assess treatment response needs to be optimized. Since individual patients may have a varying response to the therapy offered, an early scan may be relevant for an early responder, but may not be able to accommodate the slow responders. Multiple studies have also argued that an appropriate time for a post-RIT scan should be around 3 months [238, 240–244]. On the contrary, a few investigators performed both early and delayed interim scans 1–8 weeks post-RIT, and the findings showed that scans performed later correlated well in terms of treatment response prediction [245–248].

Imaging had a pivotal role in myeloma staging workup, follow-up, and prognostica-

tion. Conventional whole-body radiography remained the backbone of multiple myeloma imaging armamentarium for the last four decades. With the technological advances, the whole-body computed tomography has replaced conventional radiography. It has the advantage of being more sensitive, fast, and able to identify bone as well as soft tissue involvement. Whole-body magnetic resonance imaging (MRI) has been found to be more accurate in staging, follow-up, and evaluating response to treatment having higher sensitivity and lesion detection [249–252]. The International Myeloma Working Group (IMWG) has declared MRI as the imaging modality of choice based on the findings indicating that it has higher sensitivity and detects marrow infiltration much earlier than other imaging modalities [253, 254].

Initial studies on the utility of PET and PET-CT in the diagnosis and staging of myeloma showed good sensitivity (~90%) and specificity (~70–100%) [255, 256]. It was also found that PET-CT can accurately differentiate between intra- and extramedullary involvement and shows an increased number of lesions compared with conventional radiography and those out of the field of MR imaging [257]. MRI, despite having excellent sensitivity and superiority over other imaging modalities, lacks the prognostic and survival implications. 2-[¹⁸F]FDG PET-CT has emerged as a modality, which has overcome this disadvantage. Various studies like TT3, TT5, and TT6 evaluated a large cohort of myeloma patients and concluded that the presence of more than three PET focal lesions is a bad prognostic indicator and its persistence at day 7 scan is associated with inferior OS, PFS, and event-free survival. These trials also concluded that 2-[¹⁸F]FDG PET-CT can be used for therapy adaptation [258–260]. Extramedullary uptake was also associated with decreased OS and worse prognosis [261, 262]. Multiple small-scale studies proved the utility of PET as a predictor of response to therapy and PFS with greater accuracy in determining remission in comparison with MRI [263–265]. A study conducted between 2002 and 2012 in 282 multiple myeloma patients showed that that post-ASCT PET status was an independent prognostic factor of PFS. The study showed that that PET negativity has a positive impact on PFS and OS [266–268]. Few small populations showed that >3, >10, or >6 focal lesions with high standardized uptake value (SUV) and extramedullary disease were associated with longer time to progression (TTP) and independent prognostic factors for PFS and OS. Similarly, the SUV of greater than 15.9 was a prognostic indicator for decreased PFS and OS [267–269].

The major reported drawback of PET-CT imaging in multiple myeloma is that there are no standardized definitions of evaluation criteria in published clinical studies. A multicentric French IMAJEM study is underway which is evaluating the role of MRI and PET-CT in bone lesion detection, and researchers as part of this study have also evaluated the prognostic value of interim 2-[^{18}F]FDG PET analysis using decrease in maximum standardized uptake value (SUVmax) versus visual analysis in patients with multiple myeloma [270]. Two more clinical trials are underway to standardize the prognostic cutoffs, complete metabolic response (CMR), and minimal residual disease criteria. The preliminary results of these two trials in 236 patients were shared in the HE American Society of Hematology meeting in 2018 [271, 272]. Reproducible, standardized reporting criteria are also lacking in 2-[^{18}F]FDG PET-CT. For this purpose, a recent study from Italy proposed IMPeTUs criteria (Italian Myeloma Criteria for PET Use) which were demonstrated as highly reproducible [273]. Another shortcoming in 2-[^{18}F]FDG PET evaluation is that a small cohort of myeloma patients have deranged the hexokinase 2 gene, resulting in reduced 2-[^{18}F]FDG uptake and false-negative studies.

Other than multiple myeloma, the role of 2-[^{18}F]FDG PET-CT in plasma cell disorders, particularly plasmacytoma, has been explored less extensively. Few published studies have limited data on its usage. PET-CT has been used as an imaging technique in extramedullary plasmacytoma (EMP) and solitary bone plasmacytoma (SBP). Diagnosis of plasmacytoma needs a biopsy-proven bone or soft tissue lesion with evidence of clonal plasma cells, normal bone marrow with or without any evidence of clonal plasma cells, and absence of end-organ damage as seen in multiple myeloma. Imaging with skeletal survey or MRI remained an important part of diagnostic protocols. The first study reported in the literature which compared 2-[^{18}F]FDG PET-CT with MRI reported better sensitivity (98% vs. 93%), specificity (99% vs. 94%), positive predictive value (PPV) (93% vs. 84%), and negative predictive value (NPV) (99% vs. 98%) in the baseline staging of plasmacytoma, respectively. In therapy assessment, PET-CT fared better than MRI as well [274]. Subsequently, many published studies explored and shared the utility of PET-CT in the diagnostic algorithm of plasmacytoma. These studies emphasized that PET-CT usually resulted in the upstaging of disease and eventual change in management [275–278].

This utility was further reiterated by a joint statement of the International Myeloma Working Group in 2017 with emphasis on its utility in settings where MRI and whole-body PET are either unavailable or cannot be performed. Its role in distinguishing between inactive and smoldering multiple myeloma was also emphasized in this paper [279]. Since its initial evaluation, many other PET-CT indications were further explored in both subgroups of plasmacytomas, EMP, and SBP. Since 10–20% of EMP cases can transform into multiple myeloma, the early detection of single EMP lesions with PET-CT is highly recommended as in early stage, and EMP is highly amenable to local treatments such as external beam radiotherapy. A study conducted on 21 patients concluded that PET-CT scanning has value for staging and radiotherapy planning [280].

PET-CT findings were also used to predict prognosis and the transformation of plasmacytoma to multiple myeloma. A study evaluated 62 patients in 29 of whom there was transformation to myeloma. This study evaluated factors which were predictive of the transformation, and it concluded that transformation was more likely in patients having bone disease and 2-[^{18}F]FDG avid lesions. Additionally, SUV lean body mass (SUVlbm) of more than 5.2 and SUV body surface area (SUVbsa) of more than 1.7 were predictors for time to multiple myeloma (TTMM) [281]. Another study evaluating EMP refuted the impression that SUVs of 2-[^{18}F]FDG have an effect on PFS. This study concluded that lesion size of greater than 4 cm and partial response to therapy were strong prognostic predictors [278].

Similar results were shown in 21 SBP patients who underwent PET-CT immediately after radiotherapy treatment. This study showed that low SUV values have suboptimal specificity; however, high SUV values seem to have a strong predictive potential for disease progression [282]. Another study explored the utility of PET-CT in the prediction of progression to multiple myeloma in 43 patients and concluded that at least more than two 2-[^{18}F]FDG avid hypermetabolic lesions and abnormal involved serum-free light chain (sFLC) value are predictors of shortened TTMM [283].

16.20.2 PET-MRI

So far, 2-[^{18}F]FDG PET imaging has proven its utility in lymphomas providing valuable knowledge in the form of a baseline, interim to finally posttreatment scan to address disease progression or recurrence. The issue of false-positive studies owing to inflammation can still hamper the clinical utility of the results. Additionally, the interpretation of SUVmax readings can be problematic due to the aggressive or indolent nature of the tumor. To address such concerns, there is always a need to develop novel tracers and technology, such as PET-MRI studies, that can effectively address these technical issues.

PET-MRI is an innovative and relatively newer technique that appears promising to benefit both patients and treating physicians. The technical aspects related to crispier image quality secondary to enhanced MRI-based motion correction [284] and low radiation exposure are the most favorable characteristics of this technique. As a novel advanced MRI technique, diffusion-weighted imaging (DWI) that indirectly measures cell density has shown some promising results in lymphomas and may become an alternative to 2-[^{18}F]FDG PET-CT in some cases, particularly in pediatric patients, for treatment

response evaluation [285, 286]. For the latter, this is advantageous because by replacing the CT component with MRI, a lower radiation dose to the patient can be obtained. Given that image quality could also improve, lower dosages of tracer could be utilized, further reducing patient radiation exposure.

The unique principle of high tissue contrast of MR imaging allows it to be the ideal technique employed in the regional studies of the brain and spine. However, other than central nervous system (CNS) studies, there have been a couple of hindrances that may limit its use in lymphoma. Studies have suggested that the optimal performance of CT in lung scans has so far not been matched by MR [287]; likewise, lymphoma evaluation in bone marrow studies has reported high sensitivity [288]. However, relatively low sensitivity has been reported in posttreatment cohorts owing to bone marrow inflammation and regeneration [289]. To address the posttreatment drop in sensitivity, various MR sequences combinations can be used, and it was demonstrated that T1-weighted images have the highest sensitivity (92%), while the highest specificity can be seen in DWI, fat saturation, and Short-TI Inversion Recovery (STIR) combination (up to 92.5%). A combination of T1-weighted images with STIR was the best possible combination (sensitivity of 85% and specificity of 97%) [290].

The combination of both PET and MR modalities as a single unit has enabled researchers and clinicians to evaluate the glycolytic function of a tumor along with the estimation of cell density. Multiple researchers have established the fact that decreased glycolytic activity and a decrease in cell density can be well studied after a few cycles of chemotherapy [219, 291–294]. In lymphoma, the alteration in cellular glycolytic metabolism and cell density can be picked up by 2-[^{18}F]FDG PET-MR within 2–3 days of treatment [295]. The question of which modality can be employed earlier in the treatment stage to observe the glycolytic pattern and tumor cell density has gathered much interest in recent years. Some studies have reported no significant correlation between apparent diffusion coefficient (ADC) and SUVmax in a set of 27 lymphoma patients [296]. This would suggest that the two modalities do not have sufficient information to supplant one another, and there could be a role specific to each one.

In specific subsets of lymphomas, MALT for instance, the accurate estimation of disease extent can be limited with conventional CT scanning [297], and this can be coupled with the fact that MALT lymphomas may exhibit a decreased glycolytic uptake that in turn limit the effective utility of 2-[^{18}F]FDG PET imaging [291]. Although in such clinical scenarios whole-body diffusion-weighted MRI can be employed as a sound imaging tool, its incorporation in the management paradigm for diagnosis and staging needs further assessment [298, 299]. Thus, the combination of each of these modalities could improve the overall utility in these areas. An investigation into the prospective role of PET-MRI in 36 patients with MALT lymphomas concluded that it is a reasonable measure for the disease with considerably good tumor/background ratio [300].

Despite being a novel technique in oncological imaging, PET-MRI still faces a few technical hurdles in its development process. The segment-based attenuation correction method employed in MRI studies underestimated the SUV values in comparison to PET-CT, especially in areas in or adjacent to cortical bones [301]. The architectural placement of certain patient positioning devices such as headphones used for brain MRI can also be a source of under calculation of SUV values using the current segmentation based attenuation correction [302].

With the advent of PET-MR, recent studies have been using this modality to overcome PET-CT shortcomings, showing comparable sensitivity to PET-CT in multiple myeloma evaluation [303, 304]. The supremacy of PET-MRI in identifying skeletal lesions is better than PET-CT and boosts the diagnostic confidence [305]. Focal or diffuse bone marrow involvement can feasibly be studied with MRI in myeloma. Although it is a very sensitive modality for marrow changes, in scenarios of low tumor burden, the MRI findings may tend to be normal [306]. Recent results from a study presented at the society of nuclear medicine and molecular imaging

(SNMMI) conference showed that not only there is concordance between PET-CT and PET-MR results, but also PET-MR provides incremental information about the spinal involvement and the extent of disease [307]. Another study presented at the 2018 SNMMI conference showed similar results in PET-MR and PET-CT studies in osseous lesions; however, 21% of the study cohort had PET-MR abnormalities which were not 2-[^{18}F]FDG avid [308].

16.20.3 PET Imaging Beyond 2-[^{18}F]FDG

Lymphoma has been studied with alternate metabolic tracers. [^{18}F]Fluorodeoxythymidine (FLT), a synthetic amino acid, has been investigated clinically in patients with lymphoma, and the results have been promising so far. Data have suggested that it can be beneficial as a mid-treatment interim scan [309] and its sensitivity is comparable to 2-[^{18}F]FDG [310]. The uptake of FLT is directly related to the tumor proliferation rate, and thus it can assist in distinguishing between low- and high-grade tumors [310, 311]. Several studies have also highlighted the possible beneficial role that FLT can play in assessing early response to treatment in lymphoma [312–315]. Whereas a negative scan may potentially help design risk-adapted therapies in patients with aggressive lymphomas, the positive predictive value remains too low to justify changes in patient management [316]. [^{11}C]C-Methionine (MET) is another radiolabeled amino acid that has attained wide acceptability in lymphoma imaging. The basis of its uptake in tumor cells is attributed to their increased amino acid uptake and rapid rate of cell proliferation that in turn depicts relatively low uptake in non-neoplastic cellular entities. An advantage of MET over 2-[^{18}F]FDG is that the former appears to be more sensitive in the detection of a wide variety of malignancies, whereas 2-[^{18}F]FDG is better suited for detecting higher-grade malignancies [317].

The continuous advancement and the characteristic property of mAbs to target the specific surface antigens have gained the attention of nuclear medicine investigators to devise protocols that can effectively evaluate their benefits in both in vivo and in vitro models. Target expression levels are key factors for the success of any RIT, and this can be well-assessed in vivo with immuno-PET. Noninvasiveness and the ability to acquire whole-body imaging are positive points of this technique. Since the advent of the theranostic molecular imaging approach, a number of RIT techniques are showing promising results.

Although 2-[^{18}F]FDG has been a mainstay in the diagnostic algorithm of lymphomas, more differentiated lymphomas have compromised sensitivity and specificity with 2-[^{18}F]FDG PET-CT.

In recent trials, we have seen gallium-68 being used as an imaging agent in less common varieties/differentiated lymphomas. Those papers reported the use of CXCR (pentixafor) for anchoring gallium-68, showing its utility as a diagnostic agent. One of the recent reports showed its utility in marginal cell and indolent lymphomas in humans. When comparing the utility of gallium-68 pentixafor with standard 2-[^{18}F] FDG PET-CT in 21 marginal zone lymphoma patients, the former picked more lesions than the latter (95.2% vs. 42.9%) leading to the conclusion that gallium-68 pentixafor PET seemed to be a more accurate tool for staging marginal lymphoma patients [318]. In another study, the diagnostic ability of [^{68}Ga]Ga-pentixafor was studied for Waldenström macroglobulinemia/lymphoplasmacytic lymphoma, an indolent B-cell lymphoma. Comparison of imaging results in 17 patients found that [^{68}Ga]Ga-pentixafor PET identified bone marrow, lymph nodes, and other extramedullary involvement significantly better than the standard 2-[^{18}F]FDG PET [319]. Another recently published study showed the utility of [^{68}Ga]Ga-pentixafor in primary and secondary lymphomas in 11 patients compared with standard MRI imaging. The authors concluded that gallium-68-labeled pentixafor showed good uptake by the lymphoma tissue and its initial uptake was helpful in predicting the treatment response as well [320].

The limited specificity of 2-[^{18}F]FDG has led to the exploration of many other compounds to be used as PET imaging agents. Some of them have been tested as novel PET imaging probes in lymphomas. Fluorine-18-labeled fludarabine is one of these promising agents. Fludarabine is an adenine nucleoside analog which was synthesized and used in preclinical trials with success [321–325]. Its first human trial included 10 untreated patients of DLBCL and CLL, and the results were compared with 2-[^{18}F]FDG scans. This "proof of concept" study showed better performance of [^{18}F]F-fludarabine in DLBCL patients [326].

Zirconium-89 (^{89}Zr)-labeled mAb has also been a subject of interest in CD20$^+$ B-cell lymphomas. They are of great interest due to their potential use in theranostics. There have been reports of a higher positive lymph node detection rate than 2-[^{18}F]FDG [327]. The ability of this immuno-PET technique has also been found to be useful in other nonmalignant pathologies that involve B-cell-related immunological responses [328–330]. Recently, zirconium-89 was labeled to rituximab to produce an imaging probe. This compound was used in relapsed/refractory DLBCL patients. Imaging performed at 0, 3, and 6 days showed a positive correlation between tumor uptake and CD20 tumor expression, and this pilot study showed its potential to be used as an imaging biomarker [331]. Given its radiochemistry and relatively long half-life (78.4 h), the radioisotope is desirable in its ability to perform extended imaging and thereby derive pharmacokinetics and dosimetry of the ligand it is labeled to. The fact that it is a PET agent makes it more accurate to calculate such values over single photon emission computed tomography (SPECT)-CT-based parameters. Hence, the development of these types of imaging agents could provide companion products to the therapeutic versions, which is in parallel to the developments taking place in targeted radionuclide-based therapies in neuroendocrine tumors, prostate cancer, etc.

In multiple myeloma, few other tracers like MET, [^{11}C]C-choline, [^{18}F]F-choline, and [^{11}C] C-acetate have been tried beyond 2-[^{18}F]FDG in the evaluation of patients [332–334]. In an online published case report, the uptake of [^{68}Ga]Ga-PSMA was also documented in multiple plasmacytomas in bone lesions. This utility can be further explored in prospective clinical trials [335].

As in lymphoma, ^{68}Ga-labeled CXCR (pentixafor) has also been used in diagnosing multiple myeloma and to establish the utility of endoradiotherapy. The first study in the literature which tried this imaging in human compared 14 multiple myeloma patients and found that [^{68}Ga]Ga-CXCR identified 10/14 while 2-[^{18}F]FDG detected lesions in 9/14 patients. The authors concluded that this seems to be a promising agent with potential superiority over conventional PET in multiple myeloma cohort [336]. Another study of 30 patients compared [^{68}Ga]Ga-CXCR with standard 2-[^{18}F]FDG PET in newly diagnosed multiple myeloma patients [337]. The [^{68}Ga]Ga-CXCR not only had a higher positive rate (93.3% vs. 53.3%, $p = 0.0005$), but the quantitative parameters of [^{68}Ga]Ga-CXCR PET like total bone marrow uptake, SUVmax, and SUVmean correlated well with clinical, pathological, staging, and laboratory parameters of the disease, while in the case of 2-[^{18}F]FDG PET, only SUVmean positively correlated with the clinical, pathological, and laboratory findings. Then again in a study of 35 patients, the tracer was able to identify lesions in 66% of patients irrespective of myeloma type, cytogenetic, or heterogeneity. In some patients, there were 2-[^{18}F]FDG images available for comparison, and in this subset, there was significant discordance in performance for lesion detection. The authors concluded that [^{68}Ga]Ga-CXCR is a potential imaging agent with more utility as a decision-maker for subsequent [^{177}Lu]Lu-CXCR endoradiotehrapeutic regimen [338].

16.21 Pre-targeting Methodologies

Despite having an excellent outcome, RIT in lymphomas has never been disseminated to a larger extent. There are multiple reasons for the low spread of RIT. On a technological front, the most exhaustively discussed reasons are low therapeutic index, hematologic side effects related to prolonged serum half-life, and heterogeneous tumor distribution of radioimmunoconjugates. To overcome these hurdles, several strategies have been developed, like design changes in the antibody constructs, pre-targeting or pre-sensitization, fractionation, etc. Antibody engineering leads to smaller sized antibodies. There were better tumor penetration and pharmacokinetics compared to the larger sized antibodies, but tumor residence time and tumor uptake were compromised. Additionally, smaller sized molecules still could not overcome the impediments encountered before their uptake in target tumor cells. Hence, it was deducted that alteration in size is not the only solution, and other approaches would also need to be considered.

The concept of pre-targeting is binding of unlabeled tumor antibodies at avid sites, followed by a waiting period of 24–48 h. This delay allows accretion of antibody into the tumor and clearance of unattached antibodies spontaneously or aided by a clearing agent. This is followed by the injection of a small-sized radiolabeled agent, which has a high affinity for bound antibodies on target cells, thus concentrating radiation, leading to the ablation of the tumor. Due to its smaller size, the unbound fraction rapidly clears from the background, hence resulting in improved tumor to background ratios and improved dosimetry.

This concept was proposed in 1986 and described mAb hapten radiopharmaceutical delivery through chelators binding of mAb with tumor antigen and radiopharmaceuticals [339, 340]. Many pre-targeting approaches have been developed so far: streptavidin (SA)-biotin system, affinity enhancement system, hapten-based pre-targeting, bispecific mAb pre-targeting, click chemistry approach, DNA/DNA approach, etc. [341, 342]. Most of these pre-targeting approaches have been used in experimental settings in solid tumors. In hematologic malignancies, these have been mostly used in preclinical settings focusing on CD20, CD22, CD25, CD38, HLA-DR, etc. Early experimental studies on lymphoma xenografts showed that there is a significant improvement in the therapeutic index using the pre-targeting approach [343–345]. Two experimental studies compared the performance of different target constructs in xenograft lymphoma setting with a pre-targeting approach and concluded that HLA-DR and CD20 have better efficacy compared to CD22 [79, 346]. Some studies focused on efficacy and safety of the pre-targeting approach targeting CD20 in the lymphoma xenograft model [347] while a few studies explored bismuth-213 (^{213}Bi) labeling with the SA-biotin pre-targeted radioimmunotherapy (PRIT) in T-cell lymphoma mouse model [348] and SA-Biotin targeting CD20 NHL xenograft model. The latter study concluded that there was significantly increased tumor uptake with this experimental PRIT technique (16.5% ± 7.0% vs. 2.3% ± 0.9%). There was a significant disease response as well in the form of delays in tumor growth [349]. PRIT was also tried in multiple myeloma model targeting CD38, and there was 300 folds increased accumulation in the tumor as compared to the background [350].

SA-biotin pre-targeting approach was used in a phase I/II study, in 10 relapsed refractory NHL patients. Researchers used a chimeric anti-CD20 antibody-labeled C2B8/rituximab, which was further conjugated to SA and administered to patients with NHL. After a waiting period of 34 h, a biotin clearing agent was injected to clear the unbound SA-antibody complex. Subsequently, biotin-DOTA labeled with yttrium-90 and/or indium-111 was injected for binding with SA complex. The tumor to background ratio was 38:1, mean tumor dose was 7.84 ± 6.22 Gy/GBq, and the average whole-body dose was 0.21 ± 0.08 Gy/GBq. The hematologic toxicities were grade I–II. All patients showed an excellent response to the therapy. This study described higher tumor uptake with low hematologic toxicities [351].

Another phase I/II clinical trial in 15 NHL patients evaluated the efficacy, dosimetry, safety, and outcome of SA-Biotin PRIT using B9E9FP antibody developed against CD20 and subsequently labeled with yttrium-90. The tumor to background ratio achieved in this study was 49:1.

The OS in the study population was 21%, with two patients showing CR, one having PR, and two patients showing stable disease during the study period. Two doses of the conjugate were evaluated at 160 and 320 mg/m^2. Eleven out of 14 patients showed no significant hematologic toxicity while 2 patients had grade I–II toxicity, and 1 patient progressed to grade IV toxicity. HAMA response was lower as compared to the PRIT in solid tumors; however, all patients having higher dosages did show transient HAMA response [352].

16.22 Future Directions in Radioimmunotherapy in Lymphoma and Hematologic Disorders

With novel advancements in the understanding of cancer biology, researchers have devised potentially promising techniques of RIT. The methodology involves delivering radiation therapy using radionuclides directly to the tumor cell surface antigens using engineered mAbs. The strategy not only ensures that high-dose radiation is imparted to the cancer cells but also reduces exposure to the healthy tissues to a great extent. Further developments include advancements in modeling, dose measurements, and software to be able to evaluate better delivery and response. Few such clinical trials have been discussed in Table 16.4 obtained from multiple recently finalized and ongoing clinical trials.

Advances in genomics and proteomics have resulted in an enormous increase in novel target constructs, targets, and molecules for RIT. In RIT, the most challenging aspects are delivery and therapeutic efficacy of the radioimmunoconjugate, while minimizing toxicity. Various approaches have been investigated to achieve this. These advances include structural modifications (such as reducing the size of the carrier), pre-targeting, multidosing, locoregional administration, and using a cocktail of radiolabeled monoclonal antibodies for targeting multiple antigens simultaneously.

Table 16.4 Ongoing clinical trials (accessed from https://clinicaltrials.gov in 2019)

Isotope	Antibody	Target	Indication	Clinical phase	Primary objective
Yttrium-90	Anti-CD25 monoclonoal antibody Basiliximab	CD25	T-cell NHL	Phase I	To determine: 1. Safety of [^{90}Y]Y-basiliximab plus standard BEAM conditioning for autologous hematopoietic stem cell transplantation 2. MTD
Yttrium-90	Daclizumab	CD25	HL	Phase I/II	To determine: 1. MTD of [^{90}Y]Y-daclizumab + BEAM + ASCT 2. Adverse events rate 3. Dose-limiting toxicity
Yttrium-90	Epratuzumab Unlabeled veltuzumab	CD22 CD20	NHL, aggressive NHL, DLBCL	Phase I/II	Safety/dose-limiting toxicity
Yttrium-90	[^{90}Y]Y-HAT	CD25	Hodgkin's lymphoma, NHL, lymphoid leukemia	Phase I/II Completed 87 patients	1. MTD of [^{90}Y]Y-HAT 2. Clinical response measured by 2-[^{18}F]FDG PET and CT
Lutetium-177	Lilotomab	CD37	Relapsed, diffuse large B-cell lymphoma Refractory diffuse large B-cell lymphoma	Phase I/II 4 arms	To determine: 1. Phase I: MTD 2. Phase IIa: Tumor response rates 3. Phase IIb: Overall response rate
Lutetium-177	Lilotomab	CD37	Relapsed, diffuse large B-cell lymphoma Refractory diffuse large B-cell lymphoma	Phase I/II 2 arms	Dosimetry Estimation of individual tumor/organ uptake and retention of radioactivity
Lutetium-177	Lilotomab	CD37	Relapsed, diffuse large B-cell lymphoma Refractory diffuse large B-cell lymphoma	Phase I	To determine the MTD

CD cluster of differentiation, *MTD* maximum tolerated dose, *NHL* non-Hodgkin's lymphoma, *DLBCL* diffuse large B-cell lymphoma, *ASCT* autologous stem cell transplant, *PET* positron emission tomography, *CT* computed tomography, *BEAM* regimen consisting of etoposide, arabinoside, cytarabine, and melphalan, *FDG* fluorodeoxyglucose

16.22.1 Structural Advances in Target Antibody

Optimization of antibody design is being achieved through genetically engineering antibody constructs, which have improved the capability of delivering radiation to the target tumor.

Various antigen constructs have been engineered having a molecular weight ranging from small, monovalent 25 kDa to bivalent and multivalent constructs in the 80–150 kDa range. The varying size and weight of these conjugates have the potential advantage of improved clearance rates. Large-sized intact antibodies have a relatively prolonged blood clearance, which contributes to marrow dose and dose-limiting hematologic toxicity. Small monovalent constructs (25–50 kDa) clear much more rapidly from blood, but that also results in lower tumor uptake and shorter retention of uptake at the tumor site, making them unsuitable for therapy. Intermediate molecular weight in the 80–100 kDa range seems to be ideal as it would retain reasonably high tumor targeting but still have significantly increased clearance from the blood compared to an intact 150 kDa antibody.

16.22.2 Advances in Dose Delivery and Modeling

Several clinical trials have looked at fractionated approaches to dosing to try and improve response rates. A phase II trial enrolled 74 patients for fractionated treatment of [^{90}Y]Y-IT, of which 55 patients tolerated side effects enough to go on for a second dosage. After the first round, ORR was ~94%, CR was ~58%, and 9 patients improved their response after the second dose. The 3-year OS was 95%, and the median PFS was 3.4 years. Grade III–IV toxicities were slightly higher in percentage and duration after the second dosage [353]. Another phase II trial looked to determine the maximum tolerated dose (MTD) of two rapidly sequenced doses of [^{90}Y]Y-IT. Dose-limiting hematologic toxicity was seen in those receiving a second dosage at 7.4 MBq/kg [354].

Initial strategies were based on the observation of the relationship of the whole-body absorbed dose to tumor response, but the problem was that a consistent dose-response relationship was never clearly achieved. Observed doses have varied by ten-fold in tumors, and responses were variable and not necessarily linear; however, the responses appear more predictable at the extreme dose ranges [355, 356]. Newer methods have tried to model tumor response to lesional dosimetry. This is due to the development of more accurate and sophisticated techniques, models, and software that allowed such analysis. Moreover, this modeling also tries to consider combining two different RIT therapies but can also be extrapolated to combining other modalities such as EBRT. The approach attempts at limiting toxicities while utilizing the advantage of each modality, ideally synergistically [357]. Modeling has also led to theoretic considerations of instances where each type of RIT may be slightly more advantageous than the other. Monte Carlo simulations suggested that [^{131}I]I-tositumomab could be more efficacious in the treatment of lung nodules, especially those smaller than 2 cm in size as compared to [^{90}Y]Y-IT. This would be important in scenarios where the tumors were small, those adjacent to normal tissue, the involvement of bone marrow by disease, etc. [358].

The utility of three-dimensional imaging for dosimetry was emphasized in initial preclinical studies using conventional iodine-131. Early immunoimaging focused either on planar images or SPECT. Due to the low accuracy of these techniques for the determination of lesion and organ sizes, dosimetric quantitation never gained widespread use. Initial immunoimaging was also suboptimal, due to the immunoreactivity of murine antibodies and nonavailability of radioisotopes with a longer half-life and physical characters optimal for doing biodistribution studies. The subsequent introduction of fusion of stand-alone CT and SPECT images to obtain attenuation maps and CT-based volume of interest for iodine-131 lymphoma treatment dosimetry seems to substantially improve organ dosage calculation; however, quantitation with SPECT-CT is still an area undergoing development and refinement, and its accuracy is limited and not optimal especially for smaller lesions [359].

Recently, immunoimaging has had a new boost with the introduction of PET imaging utilizing new radioisotopes with an optimally longer half-lives, like zirconium-89, yttrium-86, iodine-124, copper-64, etc. PET-based radioisotopes like zirconium-89 have been extensively used in preclinical models as it improves the sensitivity of the experimental settings. Zirconium-89-labeled ibritumomab tiuxetan has been used in mouse models to see the ability of PET to evaluate the biodistribution and dosimetric calculation. The authors concluded that zirconium-89 can be successfully used as a surrogate label for quantification of [^{90}Y]Y-IT in treatment settings [360]. These initial results encouraged many researchers to modify and improve its radiochemical yield, purity, immunoreactivity, and stability. For this purpose, many molecules have been tried for radioconjugation, including desferrioxamine-p-SCN (Df-Bz-NCS)-rituximab [361] and p-isothiocyanatobenzyl-desferrioxamine (Df-Bz-NCS) [362]. Subsequently, many preclinical studies were performed to evaluate the zirconium-89 immuno-PET for dosimetry and biodistribution [363–365]. Next generation humanized anti-CD20 antibodies ofatumumab and obinutuzumab have better characteristics than currently available constructs and which have also been labeled with zirconium-89 to evaluate their biodistribution and tumor uptake as a potential theranostic agent in hematologic malignancies [366].

16.23 Radiomic Applications

Medical imaging modalities including CT, PET, or MRI are mandatory in the diagnosis, staging, treatment planning, postoperative surveillance, and response evaluation in the management of cancer. These modalities provide essential anatomical information, and in the case of PET, physiologic information can also be obtained. The interpretation of all these modalities is essentially visual; however, there are features within each image that cannot be apprehended by the naked eye. Moreover, when images are assessed in a more quantitative manner, standard region of interest analysis might provide a mean parameter value, e.g., Hounsfield unit (HU) on CT, signal intensity (SI) on MRI, or standardized uptake value (SUV) on PET, but these do not typically describe the underlying spatial distribution [367].

Tumors are heterogeneous both on genetic and histopathological levels. Despite the fact that tumors usually originate from a single cell, human cancers frequently display substantial intratumoral heterogeneity in virtually all distinguishable phenotypic features, such as cellular morphology, gene expression (including the expression of cell surface markers and growth factor and hormonal receptors), metabolism, motility, and angiogenic, proliferative, immunogenic, and metastatic potential [368–371]. This genetic heterogeneity translates into phenotypic heterogeneity evident as spatial variation within the tumor. Tumors with high intratumoral heterogeneity have been shown to have a poorer prognosis, which could be secondary to intrinsic aggressive biology or treatment resistance [372, 373]. This variability can give rise to altered tumor behavior in response to therapy and prog-

nostic criteria and forms the basis of personalized medicine. A thorough analysis of each patient's tumoral heterogeneity can help in deciding a specific therapy for that tumor.

The identification of tumor heterogeneity can be helpful in effective lesion characterization and treatment planning. It is not possible to assess intratumoral heterogeneity with biopsy as it is a probe into a very small volume of tumor, and does not give information about the full extent of phenotypic and genetic variation within the tumor [374]. Therefore, a noninvasive imaging method for assessing the tumor heterogeneity is of utmost importance as this can help in selecting patients with poor prognosis, and an attempt can be made in redesigning the treatment which is a vital part of personalized therapy. This particular approach gives rise to radiomics. The field of radiomics involves the processes where a large amount of data is extracted from clinical images applying highly advanced quantitative imaging features [375]. In recent times, the emphasis has been put on radiomics and multiple studies involving many tumors have been brought forward. Quantification of spatial variation has helped to find cell clusters involved in disease progression, differentiation and therapy resistance.

Radiomics is a complex analysis requiring dedicated software, where the input is in the form of clinical images and quantitative data is mathematically extracted at variable complexities. Different methods of information extraction involve analysis of the spatial arrangement of variable intensities at the level of voxels (as data is analyzed in the form of volumes of interest) such as voxel intensity histograms and application of transform functions. Data on various orders are obtained. First-order statistics features describe the distribution of individual voxel values independent of neighboring intensities [376]. These are histogram-based and examples of first-order features include mean, median, maximum, and minimum values of the voxel intensities on the image, as well as their skewness (asymmetry), kurtosis (flatness), uniformity, and randomness (entropy). Second-order statistics features include textural features which are obtained by calculating the statistical interrelationships between neighboring voxels [376]. They are very good depicters of intratumoral heterogeneity. They are usually obtained through analysis of the gray-level co-occurrence matrix (GLCM) or the gray-level run-length matrix (GLRLM). Examples include homogeneity, dissimilarity, and correlation. Higher-order statistics features are obtained by statistical methods after applying filters or mathematical transforms to the images, calculated using neighborhood gray-tone-difference matrices (NGTDM), which examine the spatial relationship among three or more pixels, for example, coarseness, contrast, and busyness [377, 378].

Numerous studies show the positive application of radiomics and textural analysis of clinical images for predicting the outcome of various therapies. Several published articles have investigated the beneficial information that can be extracted from the analysis of tumor heterogeneity. More than 70% of the articles involve MR and ultrasonography. Since the last decade, the interest in exploring tumor heterogeneity using PET has gained momentum and is being explored worldwide owing to the role of PET in oncology. Established work in radiomics includes enhanced improvement in therapy planning, outcome, survival, and pre-therapy response prediction in many cancers, such as esophageal, lung, brain, prostate, breast, and neuroendocrine tumors.

Radiomics is also being applied for hematologic malignancies as an attempt for risk stratification, prediction of treatment refractoriness, and personalized management. In the case of classical HL, de-intensified therapeutic regimens are in practice to minimize undesirable side effects, and most patients have a good prognosis [167]. However, a small minority of patients develop relapsed or refractory disease, which may be fatal. Primary refractory disease is associated with particularly poor outcomes [379]. For patients with refractory disease, therapy should not be minimized [380]. Therefore, risk stratification is essential for patients predicted to be treatment refractory. Most recently, measurements that reflect both the three-dimensional disease volume and metabolic activity, such as metabolic tumor volume (MTV) and total lesion glycolysis

(TLG), have been associated with patient outcomes in HL [381, 382].

The first study to demonstrate an association between advanced PET radiomic features and refractory disease status in early-stage HL patients showed that first-order radiomic features, such as MTV and TLG, are associated with disease progression. It was hypothesized that a model incorporating first- and second-order radiomic features would more accurately predict outcome than MTV or TLG alone. Radiomic features were extracted from a cohort of 251 patients, and it was concluded that the PET radiomic model may improve upfront stratification of early-stage HL patients with the mediastinal disease and thus contribute to risk-adapted, individualized management [383]. Another study analyzed the usability of interim 2-[^{18}F]FDG PET as a prognostic factor for clinical outcome in HL. This was conducted with the purpose to assess the applicability of the pre-treatment PET-based textural analysis (TA) in a cohort of early-stage HL and its correlation with early response to chemotherapy, as early response prediction could enhance the better outcome by enabling personalization of therapy. After the application of textural analysis, it was concluded that these parameters held great promise for the early prediction of tumor outcome analysis. Interestingly, the results showed that lymph nodes which appeared coarser on pre-treatment PET images had a higher probability of being positive at interim PET. Four features are able to predict interim PET response with statistical significance ($p < 0.02$) [384].

In the debate regarding the utility of PET-based radiomics analysis and their potential superiority to anatomical imaging modalities, a study was conducted to determine the diagnostic performance of three-dimensional (3D) TA of contrast-enhanced computed tomography (CE-CT) images for treatment response assessment in patients with Hodgkin's lymphoma (HL), compared with 2-[^{18}F]FDG PET-CT [385]. It was seen that the combination of TA and CT imaging achieved an accuracy of 83.3%, a sensitivity of 86.2%, and a specificity of 78.9%. 3D-TA of CE-CT images was found to be potentially useful to identify nodal residual disease in HL, with a performance comparable to that of classical CT parameters. The best results were achieved when TA and classical CT features were combined.

In a recently published, very informative, and interesting study, the analysis of CT-based textural parameters was taken a step forward. The aim of the study was to test the hypothesis that both indolent and aggressive CLL can be differentiated from DLBCL of RS by CT texture analysis (CTTA) of involved lymph nodes [386]. Multiple textural features like entropy, uniformity, mean intensity, mean average, and number nonuniformity gray-level dependence matrix (NGLDM) showed statistically significant differences. It was propounded that CTTA characteristics of ultrastructure and vascularization considerably differ in CLL compared to that in DLBCL of Richter syndrome, allowing complementary to visual characteristics for noninvasive differentiation by CE-CT.

Apart from HL, textural analysis is also being used for analyzing the behaviors of other types of lymphomas. A study [387] was conducted to investigate whether the textural features of pre-treatment 2-[^{18}F]FDG PET images can predict prognosis for nasal-type extranodal natural killer/T-cell lymphoma (ENKTL). Dissimilarity and low-intensity short-zone emphasis (LISZE) were acknowledged as independent predictors of PFS. It was suggested that dissimilarity and LISZE were the noteworthy predictors of disease progression in patients with nasal-type ENKTL and can improve their prognostic classification. Another study [388] aimed at examining the application of MRI-based textural parameters in response monitoring during chemotherapy for NHL patients. Texture characteristics of MRI data were classified successfully, and this proved texture analysis to be potentially a quantitative means of representing lymphoma tissue changes during chemotherapy response monitoring.

Analysis of PET textural features for prognostication has been performed in multiple myeloma patients as well. In a study, radiomic features such as heterogeneity, texture, and energy were analyzed as additional predictors of PFS in an investigation conducted as part of a prospective multicenter French IMAJEM trial. Energy seemed to be the only important prognostic feature for the predication of PFS. These avenues are still under further exploration and were presented in the Seventh International Workshop on PET in Lymphoma and myeloma in 2018 [389].

Radiomic analysis has been applied for the evaluation of yttrium-90 microspheres radioembolization therapy for hepatic tumors. In a study [390], an assessment was made of the textural parameters in CT images. The study suggested that hepatic texture signatures generated from tumor regions on pre-treatment triphasic CT studies were highly accurate in distinguishing subjects in terms of serologic response and survival. Similarly, a study was conducted with the aim to determine pre-therapy 2-[^{18}F]FDG PET and CT imaging parameters to facilitate the identification of patients who would benefit most from yttrium-90 microspheres radioembolization therapy [391]. The results showed that the model was able to predict a patient with liver cancer as a responder or nonresponder to radioembolization therapy with a sensitivity of 79.1% using extracted invariant imaging features from the pre-therapy 2-[^{18}F]FDG PET-CT test. The sensitivity increased to 82.1% when combining extracted invariant image features with variable features of tumor volume. Similar approaches can be applied in radioimmunotherapies specified for hematologic malignancies for better pre-therapy risk stratification, evaluation of therapy response, and outcome.

Currently, immune checkpoint blockade therapy is gaining wide momentum for various malignancies. However, it is optimal to identify patients who can have the potential benefit of immunotherapy in an effort to decrease immune-related toxicities. Programmed cell death ligand 1 (PD-L1) has been used as a biomarker to identify patients who can benefit from immunotherapy [392], but it has not proved to be very reliable mainly due to the above discussed spatial heterogeneity of tumors. A phase III trial [393] that compared immune checkpoint blockade and immunotherapy showed no difference between these treatments in the OS of patients with overexpression of PD-L1. Quantitative image analysis can give a better assessment of patient outcomes in such scenarios taking into account the inter- and intratumoral textural heterogeneities. A four feature radiomic model has been developed which was predictive of the OS of lung cancer patients having surgery for treatment [394]. Using immunohistochemistry and automated cell counting, the excised primary tumors were then quantified for percent tumor PD-L1 expression and density of tumor-infiltrating lymphocyte (via CD3 count). The radiomics analysis was significantly associated with OS. Specifically, a favorable outcome group was identified characterized by low CT intensity and high heterogeneity that exhibited low PD-L1 and high CD3 infiltration, suggestive of a favorable immune activated state. Similarly, in a recent and also interesting study [395], the aim was to develop and independently validate a radiomic-based biomarker of tumor-infiltrating CD8[+] cells in patients included in phase I trials of anti-programmed cell death protein (PD)-1 or anti-programmed cell death ligand 1 (PD-L1) monotherapy. The association between the biomarker and tumor immune phenotype and clinical outcomes of these patients were also analyzed. The radiomic signature of CD8[+] cells was validated in three independent cohorts. This imaging predictor provided a promising way to predict the immune phenotype of tumors and to infer clinical outcomes for patients with cancer who had been treated with anti-PD-1 and PD-L1. The imaging biomarker could help estimating CD8[+] cell count and predicting clinical outcomes of patients undergoing immunotherapy, when validated by further prospective randomized trials. The results can be further strengthened by the application of radiomics in multimodalities.

In a recently published abstract (European Association of Nuclear Medicine Annual Meeting, 2019), in 94 MCL patients, radiomic features predictive of bone marrow involvement were analyzed. The study described 16 co-occurrence matrix radiomic features which were inferred from pre-therapeutic 2-[^{18}F] FDG PET-CT metabolic tumor volumes. These radiomic features were then read in combination with the histopathological and laboratory parameters, and it was concluded that radiomic features

of metabolic tumor volume are predictive of bone marrow involvement in MCL patients, alone and in conjunction with the laboratory features [396]. Another abstract focused on patients undergoing checkpoint inhibitor treatment. PET-derived radiomic features in these patients affected by refractory HL were derived using LifeX, a free software. Six radiomic features were used for prediction modeling, namely, SUVmean, TLG, NGLDM_Coarseness, GLRLM_LRLGE, GLZLM_GLNU, and GLZLM_ZP. A total of 56 patients were studied in 2 cohorts (training and prediction). Radiomics successfully predicted the outcome in all 21 patients studied in the prediction cohort [397].

As very appropriately mentioned [398], this technique of "digital biopsy" as provided by radiomics may have the potential to allow for a personalized approach for cancer patients treated with immunotherapy. Further vigorous research is in order to identify the corresponding patterns between tumoral quantitative parameters and immunotherapy mediated responses. It will be highly beneficial to incorporate these studies in the evaluation of RIT as well, which is an already established, greatly specialized and highly targeted treatment option for patients with hematologic malignancies.

Likewise, metabolomics can be applied in looking at its utility in RIT in hematologic malignancies and the use of PET in personalized medicine. In a research project [399], 2-[^{18}F]FDG PET was used for predicting response to ^{90}Y-labeled mAbs for patients with NHL. Preliminary results indicated that pre-therapy 2-[^{18}F]FDG PET functional parameters such as SUVmax and TLG may help predict a more accurate response to single agent ^{90}Y-based RIT. However, radiomics analysis was not applied in this study.

Image analysis can also be further involved using techniques such as deep learning and neural networks. Heterogeneity on [^{68}Ga]Ga-CXCR scan uptake has been analyzed with deep learning methods employing automated neural networks on phantoms and then on actual [^{68}Ga]Ga-CXCR scans of myeloma patients. The authors concluded that these deep learning methods can be used for automated identification of scan findings, thus enhancing the diagnostic ability beyond the visual analysis of human readers [400].

16.24 Optical Coherence Imaging

Intraocular lymphomas can arise in various parts of the eyes with two basic types of uveal and vitreoretinal lymphomas. The mainstay of diagnosis is biopsy from the primary lesions either through vitrectomy or fine needle aspiration. Noninvasive auxiliary testing could be useful to determine the extent of disease and evaluate treatment response; however, conventional imaging modalities have a limited role due to their limited resolution in this setting where the lesions are very small. Optical ultrasound is a noninvasive imaging modality, but it has the limitation of measuring thinner lesion. Optical coherence imaging, also known as optical coherence tomography (OCT), is a newer developed imaging modality and is a valuable diagnostic tool for evaluation of tissue architecture of retina and choroid, especially in ocular oncology.

Since its introduction in 1991 by a team from the Massachusetts Institute of Technology (MIT), it has been used extensively in transparent weakly scattering media like the eye, especially the posterior compartment [401]. With the advancement in techniques, it was later used to image nontransparent tissue with improved spatial resolution up to 10 µm [402]. Intraocular or peri-vitreoretinal lymphomas (PVRL) are extranodal presentations of lymphomas, which are mostly B-cell types. Although ocular lymphomas are mostly localized, there have been reports of extraocular spread and involvement of this disease [403]. Retinal or fornical involvement in these lymphomas can be diagnosed with the help of OCT guided biopsy. Moreover, these lymphomas have been successfully imaged with the OCT technique [404]. OCT has been used in diagnosis, monitoring, and response assessment of PVRLs [405–407]. Typical findings include vertical hyper-reflective lesions, hyper-reflective foci in the subretinal space or posterior vitreous. The hyper-reflective infiltration in the inner layers of the retina, subretinal pigmented epithelial deposits, retinal pigment epithelium (RPE), undulations, and clumps of vitreous cells are noted in many patients as well [408, 409]. Of all these aforementioned findings, hyper-reflective subretinal infiltrates seem to be unique for the PVRLs [407].

16.25 Newer Radioisotopes

Iodine-131 has been extensively used for labeling immunoconjugates because of the vast experience, easy availability, clinically suitable half-life, simpler radiolabeling chemistry, and imageable gamma emissions. However, unnecessary radiation exposure, and inability to image in the case of yttrium-90, lead to the exploration of new radioisotopes with better physical and chemical properties. Furthermore, alternate types of radioisotopes with more desirable therapeutic properties could be used to try and improve overall clinical outcomes and toxicities.

16.25.1 Alpha Emitters

Among the promising strategies to treat hematologic malignancies, mAbs and radioimmunoconjugates using β-emitting radioisotopes are of particular importance, as mentioned above. Because of their long range (0.8–5 mm), β-particles usually cause a field effect which can result in the killing of normal bystander cells in addition to the targeted cells. In contrast to this, the path length of α-particles is just 50–80 µm, and their linear energy transfer (LET) (100 keV/µm) is almost 500 times that of a β-particle (0.2 keV/µm) [410]. Hence, there is a better killing of target cells with minimal damage to normal surrounding cells. The specificity and efficacy of targeted α-particle immunotherapy with bismuthh-212 and bismuth-213, astatine-211 (^{211}At), and actinium-225 (^{225}Ac) have been reported in several experimental models [411–414]. The potential of having higher LET is a tool of great cytotoxic latency. The in vitro and mice studies have shown that α-particles carry a much greater property of inducing cytotoxic lesions in a single tumor cell in comparison with β-particles [414].

Bismuth-213 has gained more popularity as a RIT agent in recent years. It has been investigated comprehensively in a number of animal studies and in vitro models. In an experimental study, the relative biological efficacy (RBE) of α-RIT was compared to external γ-irradiation. Induction of apoptosis in B-chronic lymphocytic leukemia (B-CLL) and induction of chromosomal damage in healthy donor B- and T-lymphocytes were determined. The total absorbed dose was calculated in samples by using binding assays. Apoptosis scoring was done using flow cytometric analyses of the cells stained with annexin V-FITC and 7-AAD. Apoptosis was expressed as percent excess over spontaneous apoptosis in control samples. The late toxicity was assessed by the micronucleus yield in lymphocytes of healthy volunteers. While γ-radiation induced a steady increase in micronucleus yields in B and T-cells, the damage triggered by bismuth-213 was more dramatic. Full-dose range experiments demonstrated bismuth-213 conjugated CD20 antibody to be more effective than equivalent doses of external γ-irradiation [415].

An experimental study indicated the capability of an α-emitter conjugated to a chimeric anti-CD20 monoclonal antibody to kill human B-lymphoma cells selectively in vitro. A high tumor cell to normal bone marrow cell toxicity ratio was observed (4.1 to 1.0 log cell kill). Biodistribution studies of [^{211}At]At-rituximab in Balb/c mice revealed similar stability as that of the iodinated analogue. The data indicated that testing of [^{211}At]At-rituximab in human patients is warranted [416].

Thorium-227 (^{227}Th), the precursor of radium-223 (^{223}Ra), has favorable physical and chemical properties for RIT. It has a half-life of 18.7 days and is produced from actinium-227, which in turn is generated by thermal neutron irradiation of radium-226. The longer half-life of thorium-227 is conducive for conjugation, administration, and targeting of a thorium-227-labeled radioimmunoconjugates before a significant amount of radium-223 is generated.

The longer half-life increases the residence time inside the target organ, whereas the short range of thorium-227 decreases the likelihood of bone marrow toxicity at relevant levels. In an investigation with an α-emitting radioimmunoconjugate [^{227}Th]Th-DOTA-p-benzyl-rituximab, which explored the immunoreactivity, in vivo stability and biodistribution and the impact on in vitro cell growth, the immunoreactive fraction of [^{227}Th]Th-DOTA-p-benzyl-rituximab was found to be 56–65%. During the 28 days after injection of radioimmunoconjugates only, very modest amounts of the thorium-227 had detached from DOTA-p-benzyl-rituximab, signifying relevant stability in vivo. The half-life of [^{227}Th]Th-DOTA-p-benzyl-rituximab in blood was 7.4 days. This was then tested in an animal model, where the response to the radioimmunoconjugate dosing was complete tumor regression in up to 60% of nude mice bearing B-lymphoma xenografts at Becquerel per gram (Bq/g) levels without apparent toxicity. Therapy with [^{227}Th]Th-rituximab was compared with [^{227}Th]Th-trastuzumab and the standard β-emitting radioimmunoconjugates for CD20$^+$ lymphoma [^{90}Y]Y-IT, and it was found to be significantly more effective than these control radioimmunoconjugates. Authors concluded that thorium-227-based constructs may provide a novel approach for targeted therapy against a wide variety of cancers [417].

Radium-223 has been studied in conjunction with immunotherapies. Bortezomib restores the impaired osteoblastic activity in multiple myeloma. Given that radium-223 is taken up by active osteoblastic activity, it is a desirable radiopharmaceutical to use in combination with bortezomib. A nude mouse preclinical study has demonstrated that both bortezomib and radium-223 demonstrated therapeutic activity independently but that this increased significantly when the two were used in combination [418]. This entered phase Ib/II human clinical trials, accrued seven patients, but no results have been published.

Terbium-149 (^{149}Tb) is also under investigation for its potential use as an α-immunotherapy agent. It has been used in a few preclinical studies. Coupled to rituximab, it was effective in controlling lymphoma in nude mice [419]. Owing to its longer half-life (4.12 h) and shorter range (28 μm in tissues), it can be used as an α-emitter for targeted therapy provided that easy availability is ensured. In this mouse model experimental study, rituximab was labeled with terbium-149 using CHX-A-DTPA as a chelator. After intravenous injection of 5 million Daudi cells (human Burkitt lymphoma cells) in 89% of the treated mice, the therapy resulted in tumor-free survival of more than 4 months and a significant increase in survival time as compared to the other groups. Untreated animals developed signs of Burkitt lymphoma. Animals treated with a high dose of rituximab (300 μg per mouse) resulted in increased median survival of 100 days. Preliminary dose estimation for humans revealed that a therapeutic activity of 5 GBq [^{149}Tb]Tb-rituximab would result in a bone marrow radiation dose far below the critical level [419].

Despite the beneficial study results, there a number of factors that hamper the utility of these emitters. The relatively shorter half-life of bismuth-213 (45.6 min) poses an issue with both its clinical use and conjugate preparation. The unfavorable high energy may result in undesirable effects due to irradiation of the surrounding healthy tissues which in turn warrants the development of selective and very high-affinity antibodies against the target cells. The logistical availability of astatine-211 can be problematic as it requires an accelerator for its production, and its half-life (7.2 h) provides only a limited radius over which any product can be shipped from the manufacturing facility. Likewise, terbium-149 has a relatively short half-life for the purposes of shipping over long distances, but with the increasing availability of radiopharmacies, these issues could be of less concern, provided that these products are used frequently enough. A potential problem with thorium-227 is that its breakaway product, radium-223, has a relatively long half-life (11.4 days), is taken up by the active bone, and is the reason why it is used for the treatment of bone metastases in prostate cancer; however, for other malignancies, especially where there is no evidence for bone metastases, this provides a prolonged and nonspecific radiation exposure to the bone and marrow, increasing potential toxicity. Hence, it might be better suited for situations where bone metastases are demonstrated, but this also might not be a significant problem if α-therapy proves to be clinically superior to β-emitter therapies.

The anti-CD33 monoclonal antibody (HuM195) has displayed promising results in mice models. The therapeutic potential and in vitro studies in leukemia have prompted encouraging results [420]. Actinium-225 has also been a subject of research recently. Its half-life of approximately 10 days is well suited for RIT protocols. Clinical trials using [^{225}Ac]Ac-HuM195 in advanced myeloid leukemia are underway [410].

16.25.2 Auger Electron Emitters

These radionuclides decay by either electron capture or internal conversions that result in the release of Auger electrons. These electrons have relatively low energy, thus travel distances in orders of few nanometers only. Examples of auger emitters are iodine-125 and tin-117m (^{117m}Sn). Like α-emitters, Auger emitters can theoretically spare surrounding normal tissue from irradiation. The biggest challenge with this therapy technique is mostly related to its physical parameters that include dense ionization leading to high toxicity to the target site, but owing to its short range, it has to be incorporated within the nucleus of the target cells to be effective. Hence, some advantages from radionuclide therapy, such as bystander effects, are less likely to take place. The most beneficial results could be sought in treating micrometastatic disease [421, 422].

Avoiding a bystander effect can also be an advantage. Few large-scale clinical studies have been performed with Auger emitters. A trial using iodine-125 in Graves' disease was conducted in the 1970s in 367 patients, with the hopes that post-therapy hypothyroidism could be avoided. Although initial results were promising, long-term follow-up showed no advantages compared to standard iodine-131 therapy [423]. Of note, the trial did not account for the long-term pathophysiology of the disease itself which results in hypothyroidism if left untreated, but the initial results did prove that the concept worked in the short run.

More recently, Monte Carlo simulations have been done using radioiodine isotopes, iodine-131, iodine-125, and iodine-123, for the treatment of B-cell lymphomas. These showed that the ideal isotopes would be the Auger emitters, with the highest dose resulting from iodine-125, whereas iodine-123 provided the highest dose rate. When using a more realistic model, iodine-123 provided the best overall dosimetry in both the absorbed dose and dose rates [424]. These findings thus show that very specific disease characteristics have to be present to gain full advantage of such radioisotopes, so it will need to be proven that Auger emitters will provide a clear clinical benefit over other standard isotopes, which will include the outcomes, cost, and logistics.

16.25.3 Newer Beta Emitter

Lutetium-177 has been able to secure its prime acceptability as a RIT agent due to its optimum physical properties, as comparable to iodine-131, and relatively higher specific index in comparison to ^{90}Y-labeled antibodies. The potency of lutetium-177 has been found to be slightly lower than iodine-131, but this property has not hampered its value as an agent of choice in clinical management. In vivo stability of the antibody-labeled radionuclide may be a field of research interest as it carries a notable in vivo halogenation [425, 426].

There are several theoretical advantages of lutetium-177 over traditional iodine-131 and yttrium-90 radioisotopes. Given its relatively short half-life, ^{90}Y-radiolabeled mAbs often cannot be shipped as a final product over remote distances but may have to be reconstituted at more locally, or at the hospital radiopharmacy. This not only limits the product being able to be delivered in places where such services have to be available but may also put a financial burden on the institution to perform the work and can be an additional cost to the procedure itself. In the United

States, the cost of the drug reimbursement has not necessarily included these costs in the past, so some institutions might not have been able to recoup the total costs associated with the delivery of this therapy since the drug reimbursement did not cover this additional step, and it may not have been reimbursed as a part of the procedure as well. Given the additional logistics involved, the distribution of such products could be more easily disrupted, which occasionally prevented the timely administration of the therapy. All these factors have additionally contributed to discouraging clinicians and hospitals from using such products in the past. Whereas ^{131}I-labeled mAb did not have these issues, the main problem has been the radiation safety precautions that patients, and their significant others would have to take as a result of its administration. ^{177}Lu-radiolabeled mAbs thus have the advantage of having a long enough half-life that they can be shipped as a final product to the sites of administration and probably recoup all costs associated with more simplified financials compared to yttrium-90 but also not have the radiation safety issues associated with ^{131}I-mAbs. The product could also be administered at the sites that have simpler radiopharmacy setups where complex reconstitutions would not be needed. Conversely, commercial radiopharmacies are more readily available, and the distribution of ^{90}Y-labeled products is less problematic than it has been in the past, but the logistics could still remain more challenging than lutetium-177.

16.26 Other Potential Theranostic Agents

Theranostics has been extensively used in neuroendocrine tumors and prostate cancers more recently, with remarkable results. They have utilized ^{68}Ga-labeled compounds for pre-therapy imaging with PET and lutetium-177 labeling of the same compound for therapy and post-therapy imaging with SPECT. This pair has revolutionized the theranostic concept, and a multitude of trials and studies in various malignancies have been published to date.

With the successful utility of [^{68}Ga]Ga-CXCR in various lymphomas, the compound could conceivably be labeled with lutetium-177 or yttrium-90 for therapeutic purposes in lymphomas, since it has been successfully used in multiple myeloma already [193–195]. However, these DOTA CXCR complexes need different precursors for imaging probes as opposed to the therapeutic ^{177}Lu-labeled complexes. Since CXCR scaffold has a predilection for smaller molecules, other compounds have been tried and labeled instead of DOTA with varying success and have a theoretical edge.

The recent focus on CXCR4 targeting led to many radionuclides labeling this conjugate, such as copper-64, using alternate chelators. The copper-64 pentixather NOTA compounds have already been successfully labeled and tried in multiple myeloma. Recently, synthesized conjugates of ^{64}Cu-labeled NOTA- and NODAGA- analogues of pentixather showed better in vivo and in vitro stability and biodistribution in small animal PET studies [427]. The biodistribution and tumor uptake of [^{64}Cu]Cu-NOTA-obinutuzumab-F(ab′)2 or [^{64}Cu]Cu-NOTA-IgG-F(ab′)2 in a Ramos lymphoma model concluded that these compounds have the potential to be used in humans [428]. These constructs could also be labeled with lutetium-177 or copper-67 for therapy in the future. Thus, CXCR-labeled NOTA and NOGADA compounds can revive the utility of copper-67 as a therapeutic agent in hematologic malignancies.

Whereas many of the theranostic aspects of hematologic malignancies are primarily based on targeting specific immunologic antigens, there are other approaches that are being developed that show some promise. Radioiodinated CLR1404 (Cellectar Biosciences, Inc.: Florham Park, NJ; USA) is a novel alkylphosphocholine analogue that capitalizes on the overabundance of phospholipid ethers present in most cancer cells and exploits the selective uptake and retention of phospholipid ethers by tumor cells, thus targeting specific lipid molecules in the cell membrane. It has been developed into a targeted radiotherapeutic and sees activity in a wide range of malignancies in both hematologic (multiple myeloma, NHL, etc.) and solid malignancies (melanoma, bronchogenic lung carcinoma, breast cancers, etc.) [429]. It has been imaged with iodine-124, showing good uptake in various tumors, and thus demonstrated that dosimetry could also be performed using this agent. An advantage of such agents over 2-[^{18}F]FDG is that they are more specific for tumors, less sensitive to nonspecific uptakes such as in inflammation and infections, and covers a wider variety of tumors than 2-[^{18}F]FDG. An analogue CLR131 radiolabeled with iodine-131 is undergoing phase I clinical trials in relapsed or refractory multiple myeloma, with single dosages escalating from 0.46 to 1.16 GBq/m^2, as well as in fractionated dosages from 1.16 to 1.48 GBq/m^2 [430]. The results of four patients in one of the cohorts have shown PR in 2 patients and minimal response (MR) in the other 2. Grade III–IV hematologic toxicities were noted, but they all recovered by an average of 2 weeks after their nadir, and dose escalation continues. This approach is also being tried on B-cell lymphomas in a phase II trial, and a company press release of the results of the initial 10 patients showed a 30% ORR [431]. This also brings up the possibility of using Auger emitters such as iodine-125 in this or other cancers [432].

Another class of agents is quinolone derivatives which act as fibroblast activation protein inhibitors (FAPI). Fibroblast activation protein is overexpressed by cancer-associated fibroblasts of several tumor entities and has been radiolabeled to form a tumor imaging agent. This seems to show that FAPI may have uptake in a wider range of malignancies than 2-[^{18}F]FDG, again potentially with greater specificity. Moreover, FAPI could be radiolabeled in theory, and the hope is this could be turned into a theranostic agent [433].

16.27 Newer Clinical Antibody Constructs

16.27.1 Epratuzumab

Epratuzumab is a novel humanized antihuman CD22 IgG1 antibody and is the humanized version of the mouse antibody, LL2. The first clinical study on anti-CD22 was performed three decades back with ^{131}I-labeled LL2 IgG (anti-CD22) which was used in varying doses to see distribution, pharmacokinetics, dosimetry, toxicity, tumor targeting, and efficacy. Dosimetry analysis showed that the tumor gets 3–4 times more dose than other organs. Few of the treated patients showed HAMA response, and there was a marked decrease in B-lymphocytes attributed to radiation-related effect [434]. Another phase I/II clinical trial was conducted to determine the toxicity and efficacy of the ^{131}I-labeled CD22 monoclonal antibody ([131I]I-MAb-LL2). The investigators experimented with escalating dose and concluded that there were mild non-hematologic side effects and ORR was 33% in the study cohort. These two clinical trials conducted with chimeric antibody showed HAMA response in the study population; hence, later humanized anti-CD22 LL2 was developed later on for therapeutic purposes [435]. This humanized form was studied in fractionated weekly 185 MBq/m^2 [^{90}Y]Y-epratuzumab doses in 16 patients. These fractionated doses were well tolerated by the patients with improved RR of 62% across all types of lymphoma. The authors concluded that three consecutive doses of [^{90}Y] Y-epratuzumab were well tolerated with a favorable RR and durable CR [436].

The idea of combining labeled and unlabeled target constructs for treatment of NHL was being practiced for many years on the premise of preventing uptake by normal B cells and sequestration of labeled radioimmunoconjugates in the normal B-cell sink. For this purpose, unlabeled rituximab and radiolabeled [^{90}Y]Y-IT and [^{131}I] I-tositumomab combinations have been extensively used. However, researchers used a combination of labeled and unlabeled anti-CD20 antibodies combinations only. There was a concern based on the original studies that the standard unlabeled antibodies being delivered were diminishing radiation dose delivery of the radiolabeled antibody. It was thus postulated that combining an unlabeled anti-CD20 antibody with a radiolabeled antibody to a different target, such as CD22, could increase the efficacy of RIT. The novel idea of combining different antibody domains such as anti-CD20 and anti-CD22

was tested in a preclinical trial in 2004 [437]. Further advancement in this preclinical concept came by combining the unlabeled antibody construct with radioimmunoconjugates [438]. This concept eventually translated into a phase I clinical trial, and the investigators treated 18 patients with treatment refractory lymphomas with a combination of [^{90}Y]Y-epratuzumab tetraxetan (anti-CD22) along with once-weekly 200 mg/m^2 veltuzumab for 4 weeks. The aim of this clinical trial was to determine the acceptable dosage of [^{90}Y]Y-epratuzumab tetraxetan. The dosimetry was done using [^{111}In]In-epratuzamab. The maximum tolerable activity (MTA) was 222 MBq/m^2, and OR was seen in 53% of the study population. One of the recent phase II trials used fractionated [^{90}Y]Y-epratuzumab tetraxetan as consolidation after six cycles of R-CHOP. This multicenter trial evaluated 75 patients. The estimated 2-year event-free survival was 75% (95% CI 63–84), and 79–84% of study population showed grade III–IV thrombocytopenia and neutropenia. One patient, later on, developed MDS and another had AML [439].

Finally, this antibody has been radiolabeled with α-particles to improve therapeutic response. Phase I trials have been completed with [^{227}Th] Th-epratuzumab in NHL, but no data has been published at the time of writing this chapter.

16.27.2 Daclizumab

CD25 is not expressed by most normal cells, with the exception of regulatory T cells (Tregs). A minority of RS cells may also express it, but it is mostly expressed by polyclonal T cells rosetting around RS cells. Anti-TAC was developed in 1981 and was used in pathologies where interleukin-2 receptor (IL-2R) alpha expression was demonstrated in cells like adult T-cell leukemia (ATL), cutaneous T-cell lymphoma, anaplastic large cell lymphoma, hairy cell B-cell leukemia, HL, as well as acute and chronic granulocytic leukemia cells [440]. Initially, murine anti-TAC was used in ATL patients [441, 442]. Daclizumab is a humanized form of anti-TAC which identifies the alpha subunit of the IL-2R and blocks the interaction of this cytokine with its growth factor receptor [372]. Daclizumab has been used in lymphoid malignancies expressing IL-2 receptor and is being evaluated in clinical trials of patients with CD25-expressing ATL. The efficacy of unconjugated antibody was not very encouraging; hence, it was conjugated with *Pseudomonas* exotoxin A (PE38) linked genetically to the Fv region of anti-TAC and evaluated in clinical trials in patients [443].

A study focused on 46 patients with refractory and relapsed HL which were administered up to seven infusions of the radiolabeled anti-CD25 antibody [^{90}Y]Y-daclizumab. The response and effect were assessed by measuring phosphory-lated H2AX as a bioindicator of the effects of radiation exposure. Out of 46 patients, 23 showed remission, 14 had stable disease, and only 9 had progressive disease. Six patients showed transient bone marrow suppression and myelodysplastic syndrome. It was concluded by the authors that [^{90}Y]Y-daclizumab seems to be a feasible RIT in select HL patients [444].

16.27.3 Radretumab

Antibodies are large proteins and as such tend to have slow clearances from the vasculature. This can be a disadvantage for any form of radioim-munotherapy as it increases the residence time in the blood, thereby increasing the radiation dose to the marrow and resulting in higher hemato-logic toxicities. This can be both an advantage and a problem in hematologic malignancies. Newer constructs of smaller immunoproteins not only have a high affinity for target sites but also have increased vasculature clearance and conse-quently improve radiation delivery of target regions while decreasing toxicities, including in hematologic malignancies. Radretumab ([^{131}I] I-L19SIP) is an ^{131}I-radiolabeled human recombi-nant antibody fragment consisting of the variable regions in the small immunoprotein format that binds with high affinity to the extradomain-B splice variant of fibronectin, which is expressed during angiogenesis. Hence, the molecule targets tumor neovasculature, and thus cannot only be used in hematologic malignancies, but also in solid cancers as well as other inflammatory non-malignant conditions. A trial with 18 patients with relapsed HL, DLBCL, or multiple myeloma, who were treated with radretumab, and demon-strated ORR 40%, with uncomplicated grade III–IV thrombocytopenia or leukocytopenia observed in 5 patients lasting 4–129 days [445]. There is overall good uptake in malignant lesions with a low absorbed dose to red marrow, which helps optimize therapy.

16.27.4 [^{177}Lu]Lu-Lilotomab Satetraxetan

CD37 has been generating interest as an alterna-tive to CD20. It is a glycoprotein which is a mem-ber of the Tetraspan internalizing transmembrane protein. CD37 is strongly expressed (>90%) on mature B-lymphocytes of normal as well as can-cerous cells. Due to the overexpression in B-lymphocytes, it was considered as an alternate target for RIT especially in relapsed and refrac-tory patients to rituximab therapy. Initial labeling of anti-CD37 (MB1) was done with iodine-131 and was used in some preclinical studies [50, 53, 59]. However, this initial interest in ant-CD37 never gained much popularity. There were few other studies which focused on new target con-structs like otlertuzumab (TRU-016) with and without bendamustine [446–448].

In recent times the interest in ant-CD37 was rekindled, and a murine mAb HH1 against CD37 was labeled through DOTA chelates with lutetium-177. This beta-emitting radioimmu-noconjugate is available as [^{177}Lu]Lu-lilotomab satetraxetan ([^{177}Lu]Lu-LS, Betalutin® Nordic Nanovector; Oslo, Norway). After many pre-clinical trials established strong binding of this compound to CD37, its biodistribution, and effi-cacy, [^{177}Lu]Lu-LS went into phase I/II clinical trial LYMRIT-37-01. The main aim of the trial was to determine the safety, toxicity, biodistribu-tion, pharmacokinetics, efficacy, dosing regimen, and MTD of [^{177}Lu]Lu-LS in indolent follicular lymphoma. The patients were recruited under four arms with varying doses, with and without pre-dosing of unlabeled HH1. Interim results of these trials have been presented at various international forums and in journal publications. The latest results presented at the American Society of Hematology in December 2018 reported 74 recruited patients (FL, 57; MZL, 9; MCL, 7; SLL, 1) with an OS of 61%, CR of 28%, PR of 32%, and stable disease in 19%, while 20% of patients showed progressive disease. Out of 74 patients, 46 showed >50% shrinkage in tumor volume. Only 7/74 patients showed an increase in tumor volume. The most common adverse event was grade III/IV reversible transient neutropenia and thrombocytopenia. [^{177}Lu]Lu-LS was well tolerated with only 19% of patients showing serious adverse events (SAEs). SAEs include atrial fibrillation ($N > 2$), thrombocytopenias, NHL progression, and sepsis ($N = 2$). There was no drug related death during the study period. The median duration of response was 20.5 months [449, 450].

During the initial assessment of recruited LYMRIT trial, two patients showed dose-limiting toxicities in the 15 MBq/kg group which did not receive HH1 pre-dosing. Based on these observation, phase IIb recruitment was done under the PARADIGME study. This study introduced new pre-dosing regimens with a higher quantity of HH1 or rituximab [451]. Recently published data has shown excellent outcomes in pre-dosing with rituximab in preclinical models [452, 453]. This open-label dose escalation study was run in many centers in Europe and later on was registered in the United States (NCT01796171, NCT02657447, NCT02658968) and is currently running in 23 countries. Due to its excellent results, it has received fast track agent by the US Food and Drug Administration in June 2018. Furthermore, preclinical studies have shown that [^{177}Lu]Lu-LS has the potential of reversing rituximab resistance and improving antitumor activity in mice [454].

An attractive aspect of this radiopharmaceutical is that it uses a different target than CD20. Hence, in those patients who have failed rituximab, being able to have therapeutic at an alternate target, in theory, could boost responses, and ideally, the agents could be used synergistically.

The agent has the simplicity of [^{90}Y]Y-mAbs and could be more popular than [^{131}I]I-mAbs for radiation safety issues and due to the lack of added complexity of the dosimetric analysis which routinely had to be done for [^{131}I]I-tositumomab. Despite logistical advantages in product delivery of [^{131}I]I-tositumomab, there was no clear advantage in toxicities or outcomes compared to [^{90}Y]Y-IT, which also provided a hindrance in its adaptation. Even if [^{177}Lu]Lu-LS turns out not to show any outcomes advantages like its predecessors, it still offers logistical advantages that could make it more palatable to use as discussed previously. Currently, a dosimetric approach is not being evaluated as a part of clinical development. That being said, in theory, a dosimetric approach is still possible if needed to start evaluating advanced areas such as with high-dose myeloablative therapies since lutetium-177 is a theranostic radioisotope, possessing both therapeutic and imaging capabilities.

16.28 Photo Dynamic Therapy

Photo dynamic therapy (PDT) is a treatment option using a specific wavelength of light after giving a photosensitizing agent. This agent has a matching absorbance band which facilitates the absorption of certain wavelengths of light. This light eventually causes microvascular and inflammatory changes via free radical production and leads to cell death. Since the light cannot pass through the thick layer of tissue, its main utility is in cancer that is present superficially on surfaces, such as just under the skin or cavity linings. So far it has been used in precancerous lesions; esophageal, non-small cell lung, and skin cancers; and few types of lymphomas. This treatment modality is only useful in small volume local disease, and large or metastasized tumors cannot be treated with this kind of therapy.

PDT was discovered about a decade back by an accident and eventually was used for treatment in the 1990s [455]. Interestingly, this first non-oncological application was discovered in 1907, but other radiation treatment modalities like internal and external radiotherapy outmoded it, and PDT application in oncology never gained popularity until the 1990s [456–458].

PDT has been used in primary cutaneous B- and C-cell lymphomas for many decades. The first case report which came out was in 1999 where few cases of conventional therapy resistant B- and T-cell lymphomas were successfully treated with PDT [459]. Subsequently, many case reports were published but had very few patients, and no standardized protocol and outcome were described [460–464].

For instance, one of the case report series with 12 patients described an objective response in 75% of patients after clinical and histological response assessment [465]. In another case series, 10 patients treated with PDT had 5 and 2 patients showing complete and partial remission, respectively, and 6/7 treated patients had stable remission [466]. Almost all of the reported case series used aminolevulinate-based photodynamic therapy (ALA-PDT). In a recently published preclinical study on cell line, the authors have suggested the use of methotrexate (MTX) as a sensitizer for augmentation in PDT [467].

There were two reported clinical trials on PDT in cutaneous T-cell lymphomas (CTCL). One of the trials, initiated in 2003 (NCT00030589), used photosensitizing drugs, such as methoxsalen with PDT. So far, no results of this trail have been shared [468]. However, recently very promising results were shared on another clinical trial "FLASH [Fluorescent Light Activated Synthetic Hypericin] Clinical Study: Topical SGX301 (Synthetic Hypericin) for the Treatment of Cutaneous T-Cell Lymphoma." The open-label treatment of the pivotal phase III FLASH study had two cycles. A total of 169 patients were enrolled in the study and were randomized to receive either SGX301 or placebo in cycle 1. A total of 16% of the patients who received SGX301 achieved at least a 50% reduction in their lesions according to the Composite Assessment of Index Lesion Severity (CAILS) scoring method of dermatological scoring, compared to only 4% of patients in the placebo group ($p = 0.04$) during the first treatment cycle. In the second cycle, all patients received SGX301 treatment of their index lesions. In total, 155 patients were evaluated in this cycle, and patients were either getting 12 weeks of SGX301 treatment or 6 weeks of the same treatment. The response rate was better by 40% in the 12-week group demonstrating a statistically significant improvement ($p < 0.0001$) between the two groups [469]. PDT, therefore, seems to be a promising treatment option in CTCL and the final outcome of the FLASH trial may prove it as a standard of care.

16.29 Quality of Life and Medical Economics

The use of target radionuclide therapies and specifically RIT in hematologic disorders has been demonstrated to have benefits beyond medical health, with improvements in quality of life, and is cost-effective compared to conventional therapy and/or nonuse of RIT. Given the longer durable responses, quality of life surveys have shown to be similar to that of the general population for health [470]. Additionally, RIT is considered cost-effective because despite initial costs being higher, RIT involves fewer visits compared to other therapies such as maintenance rituximab, as well as additional adverse events from the other therapies [471]. These are further compounded when accounting for all the additional expenses of dealing with side effects from chemotherapy versus RIT and accounting for additional overhead for each visit for chemotherapy for personnel, pre-treatment drugs, follow-up laboratory studies, etc. It would thus appear surprising that this therapy is not being frequently used and has in fact its use declining. This is partly evident by the discontinuation of the commercial availability of [^{131}I]I-tositumomab. There are some more recent obvious reasons for this. The paradigm for treatments of lymphomas has been changing, going from the decades-old R-CHOP approach, now instead of using newer frontline therapies, such as bendamustine and rituximab, among others. The data for RIT is compared to the standard old regimens, with little or no data with the new ones. Hence, it is unknown if the efficacy of RIT will be as good as when it was compared to R-CHOP or similar treatments in terms of response and toxicities. Worldwide, some other barriers have limited the use of RIT. For one, the financial models are different in various regions, and who should bear the cost as well as reap the benefit is an issue. In many countries, radiation regulations can be restrictive as hospitals frequently have quotas as to how much radioactive waste they can generate. This can be a burden when considering [^{131}I]NaI is already a mainstay of many thyroid therapies, and adding on newer agents can be challenging.

Although there are also other reasons that are cited—such as the overestimated risk for MDS, logistic and regulatory restrictions, the availability of multiple competing targeted agents, and cost of therapy—one of the most important factors in the United States appears to be nonmedical in nature, i.e., loss of financial incentive by referring oncologists, particularly in the private setting [472, 473]. On the nuclear medicine side, there has been a reluctance by many physicians outside academic centers to offer this therapy due to lack of confidence in their being able to handle its complexities [474]. Private oncologists were additionally unwilling to refer their patients to larger academic centers due to fear of loss of patient control and even the patients themselves to the center. It should be noted that outside the United States, there is no option for nonnuclear physicians to deliver this therapy, and these reasons are seldom reported by those referring physicians as being an obstacle for referrals, so these arguments could be somewhat overstated in the United States. More importantly, no healthcare delivery model developed between nuclear medicine and referring oncologists that allayed the fears of the latter or entering a partnership where referring physicians might have additional incentives to refer their patients. Private nuclear medicine clinics are virtually nonexistent in the United States, and those that do exist are radiology-based models and are themselves not incentivized to deliver therapies. Moreover, they are often incapable of handling the significant finances involved with performing these treatments. Of the physicians trained in the field, there are even fewer of them that specialize in the delivery of therapeutic radiopharmaceuticals.

Those that are trained are currently concentrated in academic centers but where even their roles are primarily expected to maintain diagnostic imaging work over therapeutics.

Nevertheless, the landscape has changed considerably since the initial clinical introduction of RIT in lymphomas. At the time, the only successful radionuclide-based therapies were [^{131}I] NaI for benign and malignant thyroid diseases. Phosphorus-32 for PCV/ET was being phased out in favor of hydroxyurea and newer drugs, and bone pain palliation therapies (strontium-89 chloride and [^{153m}Sm]Sm-EDTMP) had no demonstrable survival benefit beyond palliation and yet were also commonly associated with marrow toxicities. There was also no clear indication of when to use RIT at the time of release. There were additional concerns about limited availability since RIT was performed mostly in academic centers, complicating logistics of scheduling a referral and therapy. Sometimes there was uncertainty of delivery of the radiopharmaceutical if there was a disruption at any point in the supply chain. These factors appear to have contributed to RIT falling out of favor with many clinicians.

Newer agents have been successfully introduced since that era, such as [^{223}Ra]radium dichloride for prostate cancer bone metastases, and [^{177}Lu]Lu-DOTATATE and [^{131}I]mIBG for neuroendocrine tumors. These have been shown to have definite survival advantages and have a more reliable delivery system so that referring clinicians are less concerned about referring for these therapies. As a result, clinicians appear to have opened up to the idea of radiolabeled therapies. Despite the loss of [^{131}I]I-tositumomab from commercial availability and a decline in the use of [^{90}Y]Y-IT, there appears to have been renewed interest in RIT for lymphomas in places such as Canada and Japan, where the radiopharmaceuticals are finding their way back into clinical use. Commercial companies are still dedicated to the development of [^{90}Y]Y-IT and [^{177}Lu]Lu-LS, perhaps initially as lower lines of therapies, and then bring them to more frontline indications as familiarity increases.

There has also been a shift in the medical makeup in the US system in more recent years.

Most of the private oncology practices have been consolidated and affiliated with hospitals and large academic centers. As a result, nuclear medicine facilities are more accessible to clinicians, and there is less fear of loss of the patient to the large centers. This has also improved the ability to coordinate the treatment steps needed to administer RIT. Furthermore, the concept of a multidisciplinary approach to treating diseases is recognized as a better way to benefit the patient. Hence, there is an opportunity for the nuclear medicine community to initiate change now with the advent of the newer therapies that have begun to emerge clinically in other malignancies, combine it with their knowledge of RIT in hematologic disorders, and reach out to the community and academic clinicians. Some newer collaborative models between nuclear medicine and medical oncologists have started forming that appear to encourage the use of theranostics and where a renaissance of RIT also appears to be taking place.

There is also a move to try and simplify treatment regimens, again as demonstrated as the loss of the ability to do pre-therapy [^{111}In] In-ibritumomab tiuxetan imaging, and not do imaging for [^{177}Lu]Lu-LS treatments despite the ability being present, as well as expand the pool of physicians who can deliver such therapies beyond those who specialize in this field, to deal with some of the problems outlined above; however, this itself also severely limits the capabilities of the field. As pointed out earlier in this chapter, studies have not only shown that RIT has been effective in the routine clinical approaches, but it is also useful when dealing with high-dose myeloablative approaches. The latter requires the use of theranostics in the way of pre-therapy imaging, dosimetry, and more sophisticated approaches of using radiomics and metabolomics. This also requires experts in the field specifically trained to deal with complex applications, which cannot be accomplished with an expanded physician pool of authorized users. The full potential of these therapies cannot be fully realized until not only newer models of multidisciplinary approaches develop towards the common good of improving patient outcomes and by involving expertise of the various specialties involved in patient care, but also ensuring that no single group is also financially compromised by referring patients for the most appropriate therapy.

16.30 Conclusion

RIT in lymphomas is not only as effective but also better tolerated, cost-effective, and with an improvement in the quality of life as compared to traditional chemotherapy. It has great responses and toxicities as much or better than other therapies. Long-term concerns of MDS are of concern, but again have not borne out to be more problematic than traditional treatments. Moreover, they are also more convenient, since one infusion of RIT appears to perform as well as several rounds of maintenance treatments. Nevertheless, there continue to be evaluations of looking to improve its performance, whether in combination with traditional chemotherapy or newer immunotherapies or other modalities such as EBRT. RIT itself may be optimized by utilizing different mAb constructs. Potency may further be increased by using pre-targeting methods or introducing newer radioisotopes such as lutetium-177 or ideally auger or β-emitters. The therapy can also be personalized to the patient by performing patient-specific dosimetry for high-dose ablations or the arising promise of radiomics and metabolomics, which could potentially help pick patients in whom these therapies would be most beneficial. In theory, theranostic agents could be used in combination with RIT and other ligands that could target tumors in different ways, leading to more effective therapies. In all, these require a multidisciplinary approach so that the most appropriate therapy is delivered in an optimized fashion in a cost-effective way that is most beneficial to the patient in terms of both quality of life and outcomes.

Acknowledgments We would like to thank Nordic Nanovector, Servier Pharmaceuticals, Mundipharma, and Acrotech Biopharma in being willing to share their own commercial perspectives on the current status and future prospects of RIT in lymphomas. We would also like to thank Dr. Samuel Mehr, MD, of Nebraska Cancer

Specialists for being willing to discuss newer clinical models in the multidisciplinary approach to the delivery of RIT.

References

1. Ferlay J, Soerjomataram I, Ervik M, Dikshit R, Eser S, Mathers C, Rebelo M, Parkin DM, Forman D, Bray F. Globocan 2012: estimated cancer incidence, mortality and prevalence worldwide in 2012. 2012. Retrieved from http://globocan.iarc.fr/Pages/fact_sheets_cancer.aspx.

2. Bray F, Ferlay J, Soerjomataram I, Siegel RL, Torre LA, Jemal A. Global cancer statistics 2018: GLOBO-CAN estimates of incidence and mortality worldwide for 36 cancers in 185 countries. CA Cancer J Clin. 2018;68(6):394–424.

3. Non-Hodgkin's lymphoma statistics. CRUK. 2012.

4. Boffetta PI. Epidemiology of adult non-Hodgkin lymphoma. Ann Oncol. 2011;22(4):iv27–31.

5. Allemani C, Matsuda T, Di Carlo V, Harewood R, Matz M, Nikšić M, et al. Global surveillance of trends in cancer survival 2000–14 (CONCORD-3): analysis of individual records for 37 513 025 patients diagnosed with one of 18 cancers from 322 population-based registries in 71 countries. Lancet. 2018;391(10125):1023–75.

6. Morton LM, Slager SL, Cerhan JR, Wang SS, Vajdic CM, Skibola CF, et al. Etiologic heterogeneity among non-Hodgkin lymphoma subtypes: the interlymph non-Hodgkin lymphoma subtypes project. J Natl Cancer Inst Monogr. 2014;2014(48):130–44.

7. Plummer M, de Martel C, Vignat J, Ferlay J, Bray F, Franceschi S. Global burden of cancers attributable to infections in 2012: a synthetic analysis. Lancet Glob Health. 2016;4(9):e609–16.

8. Shiels MS, Engels EA. Evolving epidemiology of HIV-associated malignancies. In: Current opinion in HIV and AIDS, vol. 12. London: Lippincott Williams and Wilkins; 2017. p. 6–11.

9. Miranda-Filho A, Piñeros M, Znaor A, Marcos-Gragera R, Steliarova-Foucher E, Bray F. Global patterns and trends in the incidence of non-Hodgkin lymphoma. Cancer Causes Control. 2019;30(5): 489–99.

10. Bardia A. Johns Hopkins patients' guide to lymphoma. Sudbury, MA: Jones and Bartlett; 2010. p. 6.

11. The lymphoma guide information for patients and caregivers. White Plains, NY: Leukemia and Lymphoma Society; 2013.

12. WHO. World cancer report 2014. Geneva: WHO; 2015. p. 2015.

13. Walter JB, Talbot I. General pathology. 7th ed. Edinburgh: Churchill Livingstone; 1996. p. 535–55.

14. Brady LW. Hodgkin's disease. In: Chao CKS, Perez CA, editors. Radiation oncology management decisions. 2nd ed. Philadelphia, PA: Lippincott Williams and Wilkins; 2002. p. 575–87.

15. Jaffe ES, Harris NL, Vardiman JW, Campo E, Arber D. Hematopathology. 1st ed. Philadelphia, PA: Elsevier Saunders; 2011.

16. Campo E, Swerdlow SH, Harris NL, Pileri S, Stein H, Jaffe ES. The 2008 WHO classification of lymphoid neoplasms and beyond: evolving concepts and practical applications. Blood. 2011;117:5019–32.

17. Pouget J-P, Navarro-Teulon I, Bardiès M, Chouin N, Cartron G, Pèlegrin A, et al. Clinical radioimmunotherapy—the role of radiobiology. Nat Rev Clin Oncol. 2011;8(12):720–34.

18. Liang Y, Buckley TR, Tu L, Langdon SD, Tedder TF. Structural organization of the human MS4A gene cluster on chromosome 11q12. Immunogenetics. 2001;53(5):357–68.

19. Cragg MS, Walshe CA, Ivanov AO, Glennie MJ. The biology of CD20 and its potential as a target for mAb therapy. Curr Dir Autoimmun. 2005;8:140–74.

20. Kennedy AD, Beum PV, Solga MD, DiLillo DJ, Lindorfer MA, Hess CE, et al. Rituximab infusion promotes rapid complement depletion and acute CD20 loss in chronic lymphocytic leukemia. J Immunol. 2004;172(5):3280–8.

21. Beum PV, Kennedy AD, Williams ME, Lindorfer MA, Taylor RP. The shaving reaction: rituximab/CD20 complexes are removed from mantle cell lymphoma and chronic lymphocytic leukemia cells by THP-1 monocytes. J Immunol. 2006;176(4): 2600–9.

22. Press OW, Appelbaum F, Ledbetter JA, Martin PJ, Zarling J, Kidd P, et al. Monoclonal antibody 1F5 (anti-CD20) serotherapy of human B cell lymphomas. Blood. 1987;69(2):584–91.

23. Singh V, Gupta D, Arora R, Tripathi RP, Almasan A, Macklis RM. Surface levels of CD20 determine anti-CD20 antibodies mediated cell death in vitro. PLoS One. 2014;9(11):e111113.

24. Lim SH, Beers SA, French RR, Johnson PWM, Glennie MJ, Cragg MS. Anti-CD20 monoclonal antibodies: historical and future perspectives. Haematologica. 2010;95(1):135–43.

25. McLaughlin P, Grillo-López AJ, Link BK, Levy R, Czuczman MS, Williams ME, et al. Rituximab chimeric anti-CD20 monoclonal antibody therapy for relapsed indolent lymphoma: half of patients respond to a four-dose treatment program. J Clin Oncol. 1998;16(8):2825–33.

26. Glennie MJ, Van De Winkel JGJ. Renaissance of cancer therapeutic antibodies. Drug Discov Today. 2003;8:503–10.

27. Naeim F, Nagesh Rao P, Song SX, Grody WW. Principles of immunophenotyping. In: Atlas of hematopathology. Burlington: Elsevier; 2013. p. 25–46.

28. Sgroi D, Stamenkovic I. CD22. Encycl Immunol. 1998;479–81.

29. Xu-Monette ZY, Li L, Byrd JC, Jabbar KJ, Manyam GC, De Winde CM, et al. Assessment of CD37 B-cell antigen and cell of origin significantly improves risk prediction in diffuse large B-cell lymphoma. Blood. 2016;128(26):3083–100.

30. Pusey WA. Cases of sarcoma and of hodgkin's disease treated by exposures to X-rays—a preliminary report. J Am Med Assoc. 1902;XXXVIII(3):166–9.

31. Senn N. Therapeutical value of roentgen ray in treatment of pseudoleukemia. New York Med J. 1903;77:665–8.

32. DeVita VT, DeVita-Raeburn E, Moxley JH. Intensive combination chemotherapy and X-irradiation in Hodgkin's disease. Cancer Res. 2016;76(6): 1258–63.

33. Strebhardt K, Ullrich A. Paul Ehrlich's magic bullet concept: 100 years of progress. Nat Rev Cancer. 2008;8:473–80.

34. Reichert JM. Antibodies to watch in 2016 (Accepted manuscript). MAbs. 2016;862:197–204.

35. Ecker DM, Jones SD, Levine HL. The therapeutic monoclonal antibody market. MAbs. 2015;7:9–14.

36. Pressman D, Korngold L. The in vivo localization of anti-Wagner-osteogenic-sarcoma antibodies. Cancer. 1953;6(3):619–23.

37. Sugiura K, Stock CC. Studies in a tumor spectrum. I. Comparison of the action of methylbis (2-chloroethyl)amine and 3-bis(2-chloroethyl) aminomethyl-4-methoxymethyl-5-hydroxy-6-methylpyridine on the growth of a variety of mouse and rat tumors. Cancer. 1952;5(2):382–402.

38. Köhler G, Milstein C. Continuous cultures of fused cells secreting antibody of predefined specificity. Nature. 1975;174(5):2453–5.

39. Nadler LM, Stashenko P, Antman KH, Schlossman SF. Serotherapy of a patient with a monoclonal antibody directed against a human lymphoma-associated antigen. Cancer Res. 1980;40(9):3147–54.

40. Goldenberg DM, Deland F, Kim E, Bennett S, Primus FJ, Van Nagell JR, et al. Use of radio-labeled antibodies to carcinoembryonic antigen for the detection and localization of diverse cancers by external photoscanning. N Engl J Med. 1978;298(25):1384–6.

41. Press OW. Radioimmunotherapy for non-Hodgkin's lymphomas: a historical perspective. Semin Oncol. 2003;30:43–60.

42. Press OW, Rasey J. Principles of radioimmunotherapy for hematologists and oncologists. Semin Oncol. 2000;27:62–73.

43. Press OW, Shan D, Howell-Clark J, Eary J, Appelbaum FR, Matthews D, et al. Comparative metabolism and retention of iodine-125, yttrium-90, and indium-111 radioimmunoconjugates by cancer cells. Cancer Res. 1996;56(9):2123–9.

44. Humm JL. Problems and advances in the dosimetry of radionuclide targeted therapy. Recent Results Cancer Res. 1996;141:37–65.

45. Suzuki K, Yamashita S. Radiation-induced bystander response: mechanism and clinical implications. Adv Wound Care. 2014;3(1):16–24.

46. Knox SJ. Overview of studies on experimental radioimmunotherapy. Cancer Res. 1995;55(23 Suppl):5832s–6s.

47. Knox SJ, Goris ML, Wessels BW. Overview of animal studies comparing radioimmunotherapy with dose equivalent external beam irradiation. Radiother Oncol. 1992;23(2):111–7.

48. Travis EL, Peters LJ, McNeill J, Thames HD, Karolis C. Effect of dose-rate on total body irradiation: lethality and pathologic findings. Radiother Oncol. 1985;4:341–51.

49. Knox SJ, Goris ML, Tempero M, Weiden PL, Gentner L, Breitz H, et al. Phase II trial of yttrium-90-DOTA-biotin pretargeted by NR-LU-10 antibody/streptavidin in patients with metastatic colon cancer. Clin Cancer Res. 2000;6(2):406–14.

50. Press OW, Eary JF, Appelbaum FR, Martin PJ, Badger CC, Nelp WB, et al. Radiolabeled-antibody therapy of B-cell lymphoma with autologous bone marrow support. N Engl J Med. 1993;329(17):1219–24.

51. Spiess C, Zhai Q, Carter PJ. Alternative molecular formats and therapeutic applications for bispecific antibodies. Mol Immunol. 2015;67(2 Pt A):95–106.

52. DeNardo SJ, DeNardo GL, O'Grady LF, Macey DJ, Mills SL, Epstein AL, et al. Treatment of a patient with B cell lymphoma by I-131 LYM-1 monoclonal antibodies. Int J Biol Markers. 1987;2(1):49–53.

53. Press OW, Eary JF, Badger CC, Martin PJ, Appelbaum FR, Levy R, et al. Treatment of refractory non-Hodgkin's lymphoma with radiolabeled MB-1 (anti-CD37) antibody. J Clin Oncol. 1989;7(8):1027–38.

54. Goldenberg DM, DeLand F, Kim E, Bennett S, Primus FJ, van Nagell JR, et al. Use of radiolabeled antibodies to carcinoembryonic antigen for the detection and localization of diverse cancers by external photoscanning. N Engl J Med. 1978;298(25):1384–6.

55. Scheinberg DA, Straus DJ, Yeh SD, Divgi C, Garin-Chesa P, Graham M, et al. A phase I toxicity, pharmacology, and dosimetry trial of monoclonal antibody OKB7 in patients with non-Hodgkin's lymphoma: effects of tumor burden and antigen expression. J Clin Oncol. 1990;8(5):792–803.

56. Knox SJ, Levy R, Miller RA, Uhland W, Schiele J, Ruehl W, et al. Determinants of the antitumor effect of radiolabeled monoclonal antibodies. Cancer Res. 1990;50(16):4935–40.

57. Juweid M, Sharkey RM, Markowitz A, Behr T, Swayne LC, Dunn R, et al. Treatment of non-Hodgkin's lymphoma with radiolabeled murine, chimeric, or humanized LL2, an anti-CD22 monoclonal antibody. Cancer Res. 1995;55(23 Suppl):5899s–907s.

58. Juweid ME, Stadtmauer E, Hajjar G, Sharkey RM, Suleiman S, Luger S, et al. Pharmacokinetics, dosimetry, and initial therapeutic results with 131I- and (111)In-/90Y-labeled humanized LL2 anti-CD22 monoclonal antibody in patients with relapsed, refractory non-Hodgkin's lymphoma. Clin Cancer Res. 1999;5(10 Suppl):3292s–303s.

59. Kaminski MS, Fig LM, Zasadny KR, Koral KF, Del-Rosario RB, Francis IR, et al. Imaging, dosimetry, and radioimmunotherapy with iodine 131-labeled anti-CD37 antibody in B-cell lymphoma. J Clin Oncol. 1992;10(11):1696–711.

60. Czuczman MS, Straus DJ, Divgi CR, Graham M, Garin-Chesa P, Finn R, et al. Phase I dose-escalation

trial of iodine 131-labeled monoclonal antibody OKB7 in patients with non-Hodgkin's lymphoma. J Clin Oncol. 1993;11(10):2021–9.

61. Vose JM, Zelenetz AD, Rohatiner A, Knox S, Stagg R, Kroll S TG. Iodine I 131 tositumomab for patients with follicular non-Hodgkin's lymphoma (NHL): overall clinical trial experience by histology. [Internet]. 2000 [cited 2021 Sep 14]. Available from: https://www.cancernetwork.com/view/iodine-i-131-tositumomab-patients-follicular-nonhodgkins-lymphoma-nhl-overall-clinical-trial.

62. Knox SJ, Sutherland W, Goris ML. Determinants of low dose rate effects associated with radioimmunotherapy. Antibod Immunoconj Radiopharm. 1993;6:197–207.

63. Parker BA, Vassos AB, Halpern SE, Miller RA, Hupf H, Amox DG, et al. Radioimmunotherapy of human B-cell lymphoma with 90Y-conjugated antiidiotype monoclonal antibody. Cancer Res. 1990;50(3 Suppl):1022s–8s.

64. Fisher RI, Gaynor ER, Dahlberg S, Oken MM, Grogan TM, Mize EM, et al. Comparison of a standard regimen (CHOP) with three intensive chemotherapy regimens for advanced non-Hodgkin's lymphoma. N Engl J Med. 1993;328(14):1002–6.

65. Davis TA, Grillo-López AJ, White CA, McLaughlin P, Czuczman MS, Link BK, et al. Rituximab anti-CD20 monoclonal antibody therapy in non-Hodgkin's lymphoma: safety and efficacy of re-treatment. J Clin Oncol. 2000;18(17):3135–43.

66. Murray IPCEP. Nuclear medicine in clinical diagnosis and treatment. Edinburgh: Churchill Livingstone; 1994.

67. Rozman C, Feliu E, Giralt M, Rubio D, Cortés MT. Life expectancy of patients with chronic non-leukemic myeloproliferative disorders. Cancer. 1991;67(10):2658–63.

68. Najean Y, Rain JD. The very long-term evolution of polycythemia vera: an analysis of 318 patients initially treated by phlebotomy or 32P between 1969 and 1981. Semin Hematol. 1997;34(1):6–16.

69. Najean Y, Rain JD. Treatment of polycythemia vera: the use of hydroxyurea and pipobroman in 292 patients under the age of 65 years. Blood. 1997;90(9):3370–7.

70. Balan KK, Critchley M. Outcome of 259 patients with primary proliferative polycythaemia (PPP) and idiopathic thrombocythaemia (IT) treated in a regional nuclear medicine department with phosphorus-32—a 15 year review. Br J Radiol. 1997;70(839):1169–73.

71. Berk PD, Goldberg JD, Silverstein MN, Weinfeld A, Donovan PB, Ellis JT, et al. Increased incidence of acute leukemia in polycythemia vera associated with chlorambucil therapy. N Engl J Med. 1981;304(8):441–7.

72. Meuret G, Hoffmann G, Gmelin R. [Experiences with radioactive phosphorus therapy in cases of polycythemia vera (author's transl)]. Strahlentherapie. 1975;149(1):49–54.

73. Harbert JC. Phosphorous-32 therapy in the myeloproliferative diseases. In: Nuclear medicine therapy. New York: Thieme Medical Publishers; 1986. p. 193–205.

74. Epstein AL, Marder RJ, Winter JN, Stathopoulos E, Chen FM, Parker JW, et al. Two new monoclonal antibodies, Lym-1 and Lym-2, reactive with human B-lymphocytes and derived tumors, with immunodiagnostic and immunotherapeutic potential. Cancer Res. 1987;47(3):830–40.

75. Epstein AL, Zimmer AM, Spies SM, Mills D, Denardo G, Denardo S. Radioimmunodetection of human B-cell lymphomas with a radiolabeled tumor-specific monoclonal antibody (Lym-1). In: Malignant lymphomas and Hodgkin's disease: experimental and therapeutic advances. Boston, MA: Springer; 1985. p. 569–77.

76. O'Donnell RT, Shen S, Denardo SJ, Wun T, Kukis DL, Goldstein DS, et al. A phase I study of 90Y-2IT-BAD-Lym-1 in patients with non-Hodgkin's lymphoma. Anticancer Res. 2000;20(5 C):3647–55.

77. O'Donnell RT, DeNardo GL, Kukis DL, Lamborn KR, et al. 67Copper-2-iminothiolane-6-[p-(bromoacetamido)benzyl]-TETA-Lym-1 for radioimmunotherapy of non-Hodgkin's lymphoma. Clin Cancer Res. 1999;5(10 Suppl):3330s–6s.

78. DeNardo GL, Kukis DL, Shen S, DeNardo DA, Meares CF, DeNardo SJ. 67Cu- versus 131I-labeled Lym-1 antibody: comparative pharmacokinetics and dosimetry in patients with non-Hodgkin's lymphoma. Clin Cancer Res. 1999;5(3):533–41.

79. Pagel JM, Orgun N, Hamlin DK, Wilbur DS, Gooley TA, Gopal AK, et al. A comparative analysis of conventional and pretargeted radioimmunotherapy of B-cell lymphomas by targeting CD20, CD22, and HLA-DR singly and in combinations. Blood. 2009;113(20):4903–13.

80. Buchsbaum DJ, Kaminski MS. Improved delivery of radiolabeled anti-B1 monoclonal antibody to Raji lymphoma xenografts by predosing with unlabeled anti-B1 monoclonal antibody. Cancer Res. 1992;52:637–42.

81. Knox SJ, Goris ML, Trisler K, Negrin R, Davis T, Liles TM, et al. Yttrium-90-labeled anti-CD20 monoclonal antibody therapy of recurrent B-cell lymphoma. Clin Cancer Res. 1996;2(3):457–70.

82. Witzig TE, Gordon LI, White CA, Emmanouilides C, et al. Phase I/II trial of IDEC-Y2B8 radioimmunotherapy for treatment of relapsed or refractory CD20+ B-cell non-Hodgkin's lymphoma. J Clin Oncol. 1999;17(12):3793–803.

83. Witzig TE, Gordon LI, Cabanillas F, Czuczman MS, Emmanouilides C, Joyce R, et al. Randomized controlled trial of yttrium-90-labeled ibritumomab tiuxetan radioimmunotherapy versus rituximab immunotherapy for patients with relapsed or refractory low-grade, follicular, or transformed B-cell non-Hodgkin's lymphoma. J Clin Oncol. 2002;20(10):2453–63.

84. Horning SJ, Younes A, Jain V, Kroll S, Lucas J, Podoloff D, et al. Efficacy and safety of tositumomab and iodine-131 tositumomab (Bexxar) in B-cell lymphoma, progressive after rituximab. J Clin Oncol. 2005;23:712–9.

85. Vose JM, Wahl RL, Saleh M, Rohatiner AZ, Knox SJ, Radford JA, et al. Multicenter phase II study of iodine-131 tositumomab for chemotherapy-relapsed/refractory low-grade and transformed low-grade B-cell non-Hodgkin's lymphomas. J Clin Oncol. 2000;18(6):1316–23.

86. Horning SJ, Younes ALJ. Rituximab treatment failures: tositumomab and iodine I-131 tositumomab (Bexxar) can produce meaningful durable responses | OncoLink. Poster. 2002 [cited 2019 Sept 1]. Available from: https://www.oncolink.org/conferences/coverage/scientific-meetings/oncolink-at-ash-2002/saturday-december-7-2002/rituximab-treatment-failures-tositumomab-and-iodine-i-131-tositumomab-bexxar-can-produce-meaningful-durable-responses.

87. Witzig TE, Flinn IW, Gordon LI, Emmanouilides C, Czuczman MS, Saleh MN, et al. Treatment with ibritumomab tiuxetan radioimmunotherapy in patients with rituximab-refractory follicular non-Hodgkin's lymphoma. J Clin Oncol. 2002;20(15):3262–9.

88. Kaminski MS, Zasadny KR, Francis IR, Milik AW, Ross CW, Moon SD, et al. Radioimmunotherapy of B-cell lymphoma with [131I]anti-B1 (anti-CD20) antibody. N Engl J Med. 1993;329(7):459–65.

89. Vose JM, Bierman PJ, Loberiza FR, Bociek RG, Matso D, Armitage JO. Phase I trial of (90)Y-ibritumomab tiuxetan in patients with relapsed B-cell non-Hodgkin's lymphoma following high-dose chemotherapy and autologous stem cell transplantation. Leuk Lymphoma. 2007;48(4):683–90.

90. Conti PS, White C, Pieslor P, Molina A, Aussie J, Foster P. The role of imaging with 111In-ibritumomab tiuxetan in the ibritumomab tiuxetan (Zevalin) regimen: results from a Zevalin imaging registry. J Nucl Med. 2005;46(11):1812–8.

91. Press OW, Appelbaum F, Martin PJ, Matthews DC, Bernstein ID, Eary JF, et al. Phase II trial of 131I-B1 (anti-CD20) antibody therapy with autologous stem cell transplantation for relapsed B cell lymphomas. Lancet. 1995;346(8971):335–40.

92. Gopal AK, Rajendran JG, Gooley TA, Pagel JM, Fisher DR, Petersdorf SH, et al. High-dose [131I] tositumomab (anti-CD20) radioimmunotherapy and autologous hematopoietic stem-cell transplantation for adults > or = 60 years old with relapsed or refractory B-cell lymphoma. J Clin Oncol. 2007;25(11):1396–402.

93. Eary J. Non-Hodgkin's lymphoma high dose therapy. In: Baum RP, editor. Therapeutic nuclear medicine. Berlin: Springer-Verlag; 2014. p. 535–42.

94. Juweid ME. Radioimmunotherapy of B-cell non-Hodgkin's lymphoma: from clinical trials to clinical practice. J Nucl Med. 2002;43(11):1507–29.

95. Cremonesi M, Ferrari M, Grana CM, Vanazzi A, Stabin M, Bartolomei M, et al. High-dose radioimmunotherapy with 90Y-ibritumomab tiuxetan: comparative dosimetric study for tailored treatment. J Nucl Med. 2007;48(11):1871–9.

96. Wiseman GA, Leigh BR, Dunn WL, Stabin MG, White CA. Additional radiation absorbed dose estimates for Zevalin™ radioimmunotherapy. Cancer Biother Radiopharm. 2003;18:253–8.

97. Garsi JP, Schlumberger M, Rubino C, Ricard M, et al. Therapeutic administration of 131I for differentiated thyroid cancer: radiation dose to ovaries and outcome of pregnancies. J Nucl Med. 2008;49:845–52.

98. Garsi JP, Schlumberger M, Ricard M, Labbé M, Ceccarelli C, Schvartz C, et al. Health outcomes of children fathered by patients treated with radioiodine for thyroid cancer. Clin Endocrinol (Oxf). 2009;71:880–3.

99. Kylstra JW, Witzig TE, Huang M, Emmanouilides E, Hagenbeek A, Tidmarsh GF. Discriminatory power of the 111-indium scan (111-In) in the prediction of altered biodistribution of radio-immunoconjugate in the 90-yttrium ibritumomab tiuxetan therapeutic regimen: meta-analysis of five clinical trials and 9 years of post-approval safety data. J Clin Oncol. 2011;29(15 suppl):8048. Abstract.

100. Kaminski MS, Zelenetz AD, Press OW, Saleh M, Leonard J, Fehrenbacher L, et al. Pivotal study of iodine I 131 tositumomab for chemotherapy-refractory low-grade or transformed low-grade B-cell non-Hodgkin's lymphomas. J Clin Oncol. 2001;19(19):3918–28.

101. Davis TA, Kaminski MS, Leonard JP, Hsu FJ, Wilkinson M, Zelenetz A, et al. The radioisotope contributes significantly to the activity of radioimmunotherapy. Clin Cancer Res. 2004;10(23):7792–8.

102. Czuczman MS, Emmanouilides C, Darif M, Witzig TE, Gordon LI, Revell S, et al. Treatment-related myelodysplastic syndrome and acute myelogenous leukemia in patients treated with ibritumomab tiuxetan radioimmunotherapy. J Clin Oncol. 2007;25(27):4285–92.

103. Witzig TE, White CA, Gordon LI, Wiseman GA, Emmanouilides C, Murray JL, et al. Safety of yttrium-90 ibritumomab tiuxetan radioimmunotherapy for relapsed low-grade, follicular, or transformed non-Hodgkin's lymphoma. J Clin Oncol. 2003;21(7):1263–70.

104. Morschhauser F, Radford J, Van Hoof A, Vitolo U, Soubeyran P, Tilly H, et al. Phase III trial of consolidation therapy with yttrium-90-ibritumomab tiuxetan compared with no additional therapy after first remission in advanced follicular lymphoma. J Clin Oncol. 2008;26(32):5156–64.

105. Kaminski MS, Tuck M, Estes J, Kolstad A, Ross CW, Zasadny K, et al. 131I-tositumomab therapy as initial treatment for follicular lymphoma. N Engl J Med. 2005;352(5):441–9.

106. Bexxar Package Insert. 2012.

107. Jacene HA, Filice R, Kasecamp W, Wahl RL. Comparison of 90Y-ibritumomab tiuxetan and 131I-tositumomab in clinical practice. J Nucl Med. 2007;48(11):1767–76.

108. Tennvall J, Fischer M, Bischof Delaloye A, Bombardieri E, Bodei L, Giammarile F, et al. EANM procedure guideline for radio-immunotherapy for B-cell lymphoma with 90Y-radiolabelled ibritumomab tiuxetan (Zevalin). Eur J Nucl Med Mol Imaging. 2007;34:616–22.

109. Gordon LI, Molina A, Witzig T, Emmanouilides C, Raubtischek A, Darif M, et al. Durable responses after ibritumomab tiuxetan radioimmunotherapy for CD20+ B-cell lymphoma: long-term follow-up of a phase 1/2 study. Blood. 2004;103(12):4429–31.

110. Kaminski MS, Radford JA, Gregory SA, Leonard JP, Knox SJ, Kroll S, et al. Re-treatment with I-131 tositumomab in patients with non-Hodgkin's lymphoma who had previously responded to I-131 tositumomab. J Clin Oncol. 2005;23(31):7985–93.

111. Emmanouilides C, Witzig TE, Gordon LI, Vo K, Wiseman GA, Flinn IW, et al. Treatment with yttrium 90 ibritumomab tiuxetan at early relapse is safe and effective in patients with previously treated B-cell non-Hodgkin's lymphoma. Leuk Lymphoma. 2006;47(4):629–36.

112. Rana TM. Post Bexxar relapse in NHL responds to Zevalin and can be safely accomplished. [Abstract]. Proc Am Soc Clin Oncol. 2003;22:613.

113. Press OW, Unger JM, Rimsza LM, Friedberg JW, LeBlanc M, Czuczman MS, et al. Phase III randomized intergroup trial of CHOP plus rituximab compared with CHOP chemotherapy plus 131iodine-tositumomab for previously untreated follicular non-hodgkin lymphoma: SWOG S0016. J Clin Oncol. 2013;31(3):314–20.

114. Leonard JP, Coleman M, Kostakoglu L, Chadburn A, Cesarman E, Furman RR, et al. Abbreviated chemotherapy with fludarabine followed by tositumomab and iodine I 131 tositumomab for untreated follicular lymphoma. J Clin Oncol. 2005;23(24):5696–704.

115. Morschhauser F, Radford J, Van Hoof A, Botto B, Rohatiner AZS, Salles G, et al. 90Yttrium-ibritumomab tiuxetan consolidation of first remission in advanced-stage follicular non-hodgkin lymphoma: updated results after a median follow-up of 7.3 years from the international, randomized, phase III first-line indolent trial. J Clin Oncol. 2013;31(16):1977–83.

116. Witzig TE, Wiseman GA, Maurer MJ, Habermann TM, Micallef INM, Nowakowski GS, et al. A phase I trial of immunostimulatory CpG 7909 oligodeoxynucleotide and 90yttrium ibritumomab tiuxetan radioimmunotherapy for relapsed B-cell non-Hodgkin lymphoma. Am J Hematol. 2013;88(7):589–93.

117. Lansigan F, Costa CA, Zaki B, Yen S, Winer EP, Ryan H, et al. Multicenter, open label, phase II study of bendamustine and rituximab followed by 90-yttrium (Y) ibritumomab tiuxetan for untreated follicular lymphoma (Fol-BRITe). Clin Cancer Res. 2019;25:6073–9.

118. Jacobson CA, Locke FL, Miklos DB, Herrera AF, Westin JR, Lee J, et al. End of phase 1 results from Zuma-6: axicabtagene ciloleucel (Axi-Cel) in combination with atezolizumab for the treatment of patients with refractory diffuse large B cell lymphoma. Blood. 2018;132(Supplement 1):4192.

119. Ansell SM, Ristow KM, Habermann TM, Wiseman GA, Witzig TE. Subsequent chemotherapy regimens are well tolerated after radioimmunotherapy with Yttrium-90 ibritumomab tiuxetan for non-Hodgkin's lymphoma. J Clin Oncol. 2002;20(18):3885–90.

120. Dosik AD, Coleman M, Kostakoglu L, Furman RR, Fiore JM, Muss D, et al. Subsequent therapy can be administered after tositumomab and iodine I-131 tositumomab for non-Hodgkin lymphoma. Cancer. 2006;106(3):616–22.

121. Persky DO, Miller TP, Unger JM, Spier CM, Puvada S, Dino Stea B, et al. Ibritumomab consolidation after 3 cycles of CHOP plus radiotherapy in high-risk limited-stage aggressive B-cell lymphoma: SWOG S0313. Blood. 2015;125(2):236–41.

122. Beaven A, Shea TC, Moore DT, Feldman T, Ivanova A, Ferraro M, et al. A phase I study of bortezomib (Velcade®) plus 90yttrium labeled ibritumomab tiuxetan (Zevalin®) in patients with relapsed or refractory B-cell non-Hodgkin lymphoma (NHL). Blood. 2008;112(11):4944.

123. Liu SY, Eary JF, Petersdorf SH, Martin PJ, Maloney DG, Appelbaum FR, et al. Follow-up of relapsed B-cell lymphoma patients treated with iodine-131-labeled anti-CD20 antibody and autologous stem-cell rescue. J Clin Oncol. 1998;16(10):3270–8.

124. Rajendran JG, Gopal AK, Fisher DR, Durack LD, Gooley TA, Press OW. Myeloablative 131I-tositumomab radioimmunotherapy in treating non-Hodgkin's lymphoma: comparison of dosimetry based on whole-body retention and dose to critical organ receiving the highest dose. J Nucl Med. 2008;49(5):837–44.

125. Nademanee A, Forman S, Molina A, Fung H, Smith D, Dagis A, et al. Aphase 1/2 trial of high-dose yttrium-90-ibritumomab tiuxetan in combination with high-dose etoposide and cyclophosphamide followed by autologous stem cell transplantation in patients with poor-risk or relapsed non-Hodgkin lymphoma. Blood. 2005;106(8):2896–902.

126. Devizzi L, Guidetti A, Tarella C, Magni M, Matteucci P, Seregni E, et al. High-dose yttrium-90-ibritumomab tiuxetan with tandem stem-cell reinfusion: an outpatient preparative regimen for autologous hematopoietic cell transplantation. J Clin Oncol. 2008;26(32):5175–82.

127. Devizzi L, Guidetti A, Seregni E, Passera R, Maccauro M, Magni M, et al. Long-term results of autologous hematopoietic stem-cell transplantation after high-dose90Y-ibritumomab tiuxetan for patients with poor-risk non-Hodgkin lymphoma not eligible for high-dose BEAM. J Clin Oncol. 2013;31: 2974–6.

128. Gopal AK, Gooley TA, Maloney DG, Petersdorf SH, Eary JF, Rajendran JG, et al. High-dose radioimmunotherapy versus conventional high-dose therapy and autologous hematopoietic stem cell

transplantation for relapsed follicular non-Hodgkin lymphoma: a multivariable cohort analysis. Blood. 2003;102(7):2351–7.

129. Press OW, Eary JF, Gooley T, Gopal AK, Liu SY, Rajendran JG, et al. A phase I/II trial of iodine-131-tositumomab (anti-CD20), etoposide, cyclophosphamide, and autologous stem cell transplantation for relapsed B-cell lymphomas. Blood. 2000;96(9):2934–42.

130. Gopal AK, Guthrie KA, Rajendran J, Pagel JM, Oliveira G, Maloney DG, et al. 90Y-Ibritumomab tiuxetan, fludarabine, and TBI-based nonmyeloablative allogeneic transplantation conditioning for patients with persistent high-risk B-cell lymphoma. Blood. 2011;118(4):1132–9.

131. Bethge WA, Lange T, Meisner C, Von Harsdorf S, Bornhaeuser M, Federmann B, et al. Radioimmunotherapy with yttrium-90-ibritumomab tiuxetan as part of a reduced-intensity conditioning regimen for allogeneic hematopoietic cell transplantation in patients with advanced non-Hodgkin lymphoma: results of a phase 2 study. Blood. 2010;116(10):1795–802.

132. Winter JN, Inwards DJ, Spies S, Wiseman G, Patton D, Erwin W, et al. Yttrium-90 ibritumomab tiuxetan doses calculated to deliver up to 15 Gy to critical organs may be safely combined with high-dose BEAM and autologous transplantation in relapsed or refractory B-cell non-Hodgkin's lymphoma. J Clin Oncol. 2009;27(10):1653–9.

133. Decaudin D, Mounier N, Tilly H, Ribrag V, Ghesquières H, Bouabdallah K, et al. 90Y ibritumomab tiuxetan (Zevalin) combined with BEAM (Z-BEAM) conditioning regimen plus autologous stem cell transplantation in relapsed or refractory low-grade CD20-positive B-cell lymphoma. A GELA phase II prospective study. Clin Lymphoma Myeloma Leuk. 2011;11:212–8.

134. Krishnan AY, Palmer J, Nademanee AP, Chen R, Popplewell LL, Tsai NC, et al. Phase II study of yttrium-90 ibritumomab tiuxetan plus high-dose BCNU, etoposide, cytarabine, and melphalan for non-Hodgkin lymphoma: the role of histology. Biol Blood Marrow Transplant. 2017;23(6):922–9.

135. Berger MD, Branger G, Klaeser B, Taleghani BM, Novak U, Banz Y, et al. Zevalin and BEAM (Z-BEAM) versus rituximab and BEAM (R-BEAM) conditioning chemotherapy prior to autologous stem cell transplantation in patients with mantle cell lymphoma. Hematol Oncol. 2016;34(3):133–9.

136. Gisselbrecht C, Vose J, Nademanee A, Gianni AM, Nagler A. Radioimmunotherapy for stem cell transplantation in non-Hodgkin's lymphoma: in pursuit of a complete response. Oncologist. 2009;12(Suppl 2):41–51.

137. Vose JM, Carter S, Burns LJ, Ayala E, Press OW, Moskowitz CH, et al. Phase III randomized study of rituximab/carmustine, etopo-side, cytarabine, and melphalan (BEAM) compared with iodine-131 tositumomab/BEAM with autologous hematopoietic cell transplantation for relapsed diffuse large B-cell lymphoma: results from the BMT. J Clin Oncol. 2013;31(13):1662–8.

138. Zelenetz AD, Saleh M, Vose J, et al. Patients with transformed low grade lymphoma attain durable responses following outpatient radioimmunotherapy with tositumomab and iodine I-131 tositumomab (Bexxar). Blood. 2002;357a:100.

139. Skarbnik AP, Smith MR. Radioimmunotherapy in mantle cell lymphoma. Best Pract Res Clin Haematol. 2012;25:201–10.

140. Zelenetz AD, Noy A, Pandit-Taskar N, Scordo M, Rijo IV, Zhou Y, et al. Sequential radioimmunotherapy with tositumomab/Iodine I131 tositumomab followed by CHOP for mantle cell lymphoma demonstrates RIT can induce molecular remissions. J Clin Oncol. 2006;24(18):7560.

141. Smith MR, Li H, Gordon L, Gascoyne RD, Paietta E, Forero-Torres A, et al. Phase II study of rituximab plus cyclophosphamide, doxorubicin, vincristine, and prednisone immunochemotherapy followed by yttrium-90-ibritumomab tiuxetan in untreated mantle-cell lymphoma: Eastern Cooperative Oncology Group study E1499. J Clin Oncol. 2012;30(25):3119–26.

142. Smith MR, Hong F, Li H, Gordon LI, Gascoyne RD, Paietta EM, et al. Mantle cell lymphoma initial therapy with abbreviated R-CHOP followed by 90Y-ibritumomab tiuxetan: 10-year follow-up of the phase 2 ECOG-ACRIN study E1499. Leukemia. 2017;31(2):517–9.

143. Wang M, Oki Y, Pro B, Romaguera JE, Rodriguez MA, Samaniego F, et al. Phase II study of yttrium-90-ibritumomab tiuxetan in patients with relapsed or refractory mantle cell lymphoma. J Clin Oncol. 2009;27(31):5213–8.

144. Gopal AK, Rajendran JG, Petersdorf SH, Maloney DG, Eary JF, Wood BL, et al. High-dose chemoradioimmunotherapy with autologous stem cell support for relapsed mantle cell lymphoma. Blood. 2002;99(9):3158–62.

145. Ferrero S, Pastore A, Scholz CW, Forstpointner R, Pezzutto A, Bergmann L, et al. Radioimmunotherapy in relapsed/refractory mantle cell lymphoma patients: final results of a European MCL Network Phase II Trial. Leukemia. 2016;30(4):984–7.

146. Lossos IS, Fabregas JC, Koru-Sengul T, Miao F, Goodman D, Serafini AN, et al. Phase II study of 90Y Ibritumomab tiuxetan (Zevalin) in patients with previously untreated marginal zone lymphoma. Leuk Lymphoma. 2015;56(6):1750–5.

147. Zinzani PL, Broccoli A. Possible novel agents in marginal zone lymphoma. Best Pract Res Clin Haematol. 2017;30:149–57.

148. Stefoni V, Casadei B, Bottelli C, Gaidano G, Ciochetto C, Cabras MG, et al. Short-course R-CHOP followed by (90)Y-Ibritumomab tiuxetan in previously untreated high-risk elderly diffuse large B-cell lymphoma patients: 7-year long-term results. Blood Cancer J. 2016;6:e425.

149. Morschhauser F, Illidge T, Huglo D, Martinelli G, Paganelli G, Zinzani PL, et al. Efficacy and safety of yttrium-90 ibritumomab tiuxetan in patients with relapsed or refractory diffuse large B-cell lymphoma not appropriate for autologous stem-cell transplantation. Blood. 2007;110(1):54–8.

150. Bethge WA, Von Harsdorf S, Bornhauser M, Federmann B, Stelljes M, Trenschel R, et al. Dose-escalated radioimmunotherapy as part of reduced intensity conditioning for allogeneic transplantation in patients with advanced high-grade non-Hodgkin lymphoma. Bone Marrow Transplant. 2012;47(11):1397–402.

151. Reff ME, Carner K, Chambers KS, Chinn PC, Leonard JE, Raab R, et al. Depletion of B cells in vivo by a chimeric mouse human monoclonal antibody to CD20. Blood. 1994;15(83):435–45.

152. Maloney DG, Grillo-López AJ, Bodkin DJ, White CA, Liles TM, Royston I, et al. Idec-c2b8: results of a phase I multiple-dose trial in patients with relapsed non-Hodgkin's lymphoma. J Clin Oncol. 1997;15(10):3266–74.

153. Scheidhauer K, Wolf I, Baumgartl HJ, Von Schilling C, Schmidt B, Reidel G, et al. Biodistribution and kinetics of 131I-labelled anti-CD20 MAB IDEC-C2B8 (rituximab) in relapsed non-Hodgkin's lymphoma. Eur J Nucl Med. 2002;29(10): 1276–82.

154. Turner JH, Martindale AA, Boucek J, Claringbold PG, Leahy MF. 131I-anti CD20 radioimmunotherapy of relapsed or refractory non-Hodgkins lymphoma: a phase II clinical trial of a nonmyeloablative dose regimen of chimeric rituximab radiolabeled in a hospital. Cancer Biother Radiopharm. 2003;18(4):513–24.

155. Leahy MF, Seymour JF, Hicks RJ, Turner JH. Multicenter phase II clinical study of iodine-131-rituximab radioimmunotherapy in relapsed or refractory indolent non-Hodgkin's lymphoma. J Clin Oncol. 2006;24(27):4418–25.

156. Leahy MF, Turner JH. Radioimmunotherapy of relapsed indolent non-Hodgkin lymphoma with 131I-rituximab in routine clinical practice: 10-year single-institution experience of 142 consecutive patients. Blood. 2011;117(1):45–52.

157. Kang HJ, Park YH, Cheon GJ, Choi TH, Lee SS, Kim S, et al. Radioimmunotherapy in refractory B-cell non-Hodgkin's lymphoma with I-131-labeled chimeric anti-CD20 C2B8 (I-131 rituximab): preliminary results. J Nucl Med. 2006;47(1): 484P.

158. Bienert M, Reisinger I, Srock S, Humplik BI, Reim C, Kroessin T, et al. Radioimmunotherapy using 131I-rituximab in patients with advanced stage B-cell non-Hodgkin's lymphoma: initial experience. Eur J Nucl Med Mol Imaging. 2005;32(10): 1225–33.

159. Kruger PC, Joske DJL, Turner JH. Iodine-131 rituximab radioimmunotherapy: durable control of follicular lymphoma. J Nucl Med Radiat Ther. 2014;5:4.

160. Calais PJ, Turner JH. Outpatient 131I-rituximab radioimmunotherapy for non-Hodgkin lymphoma: a study in safety. Clin Nucl Med. 2012;37(8): 732–7.

161. Wagner JY, Schwarz K, Schreiber S, Schmidt B, Wester HJ, Schwaiger M, et al. Myeloablative anti-CD20 radioimmunotherapy +/− high-dose chemotherapy followed by autologous stem cell support for relapsed/refractory B-cell lymphoma results in excellent long-term survival. Oncotarget. 2013;4(6):889–910.

162. Deshayes E, Kraeber-Bodéré F, Vuillez J-P, Bardiès M, Teulon I, Pouget J-P. Tandem myeloablative 131I-rituximab radioimmunotherapy and high-dose chemotherapy in refractory/relapsed non-Hodgkin lymphoma patients. Immunotherapy. 2013;5(12):1283–6.

163. Kruger PC, Cooney JP, Turner JH. Iodine-131 rituximab radioimmunotherapy with BEAM conditioning and autologous stem cell transplant salvage therapy for relapsed/refractory aggressive non-Hodgkin lymphoma. Cancer Biother Radiopharm. 2012;27(9):552–60.

164. Salati M, Cesaretti M, Macchia M, El Mistiri M, Federico M. Epidemiological overview of Hodgkin lymphoma across the Mediterranean basin. Mediterr J Hematol Infect Dis. 2014;6:e2014048.

165. Thomas RK, Re D, Zander T, Wolf J, Diehl V. Epidemiology and etiology of Hodgkin's lymphoma. Ann Oncol. 2002;13(4):147–52.

166. Yahalom JSD. Hodgkin's lymphoma. In: Pazdur R, Coia LR, Hoskins WJ, et al., editors. Cancer management: a multidisciplinary approach medical, surgical and radiation oncology. 9th ed. New Delhi: Jaypee Brothers; 2005. p. 675–96.

167. Engert A, Plütschow A, Eich HT, Lohri A, Dörken B, Borchmann P, et al. Reduced treatment intensity in patients with early-stage Hodgkin's lymphoma. N Engl J Med. 2010;363(7):640–52.

168. Engert A, Haverkamp H, Kobe C, Markova J, Renner C, Ho A, et al. Reduced-intensity chemotherapy and PET-guided radiotherapy in patients with advanced stage Hodgkin's lymphoma (HD15 trial): a randomised, open-label, phase 3 non-inferiority trial. Lancet. 2012;379(9828):1791–9.

169. Böll B, Görgen H, Fuchs M, Pluetschow A, Eich HT, Bargetzi MJ, et al. ABVD in older patients with early-stage hodgkin lymphoma treated within the german hodgkin study group HD10 and HD11 trials. J Clin Oncol. 2013;31(12):1522–9.

170. Borchmann S, Von Tresckow B, Engert A. Current developments in the treatment of early-stage classical Hodgkin lymphoma. Curr Opin Oncol. 2016;28:377–83.

171. Jacene HA, Kasamon YL, Ambinder RF, Kasecamp W, Serena D, Wahl RL. Phase I/II dose-escalation study of tositumomab and iodine I 131 tositumomab for relapsed/refractory classical or lymphocyte-predominant Hodgkin's lymphoma: feasibility and initial safety. Blood. 2008;112(11):3059.

172. Sarcione EJ, Smalley JR, Lema MJ, Stutzman L. Increased ferritin synthesis and release by Hodgkin's disease peripheral blood lymphocytes. Int J Cancer. 1977;20(3):339–46.

173. Eshhar Z, Order SE, Katz DH. Ferritin, a Hodgkin's disease associated antigen. Proc Natl Acad Sci U S A. 1974;71(10):3956–60.

174. Vriesendorp HM, Quadri SM, Andersson BS, Wyllie CT, Dicke KA. Recurrence of Hodgkin's disease after indium-111 and yttrium-90 labeled antiferritin administration. Cancer. 1997;80(12):2721–7.

175. Lenhard RE, Order SE, Spunberg JJ, Asbell SO, Leibel SA. Isotopic immunoglobulin: a new systemic therapy for advanced Hodgkin's disease. J Clin Oncol. 1985;3(10):1296–300.

176. Herpst JM, Klein JL, Leichner PK, Quadri SM, Vriesendorp HM. Survival of patients with resistant Hodgkin's disease after polyclonal yttrium 90-labeled antiferritin treatment. J Clin Oncol. 1995;13(9):2394–400.

177. Sheibani K, Winberg CD, van De Velde S, Blayney DW, Rappaport H. Distribution of lymphocytes with interleukin-2 receptors (TAC antigens) in reactive lymphoproliferative processes, Hodgkin's disease, and non-Hodgkin's lymphomas: an immunohistologic study of 300 cases. Am J Pathol. 1987;127(1):27–37.

178. Agnarsson BA, Kadin ME. The immunophenotype of reed-Sternberg cells. A study of 50 cases of Hodgkin' disease using fixed frozen tissues. Cancer. 1989;1(63):2083–7.

179. Dancey G, Violet J, Malaroda A, Green AJ, Sharma SK, Francis R, et al. A phase I clinical trial of CHT-25 a 131 I-labeled chimeric anti-CD25 antibody showing efficacy in patients with refractory lymphoma. Clin Cancer Res. 2009;15(24):7701–10.

180. Schnell R, Dietlein M, Staak JO, Borchmann P, Schomaecker K, Fischer T, et al. Treatment of refractory Hodgkin's lymphoma patients with an iodine-131-labeled murine anti-CD30 monoclonal antibody. J Clin Oncol. 2005;23(21):4669–78.

181. Vose J, Armitage J, Weisenburger D, International T-Cell Lymphoma Project. International peripheral T-cell and natural killer/T-cell lymphoma study: pathology findings and clinical outcomes. J Clin Oncol. 2008;26(25):4124–30.

182. Coiffier B, Federico M, Caballero D, Dearden C, Morschhauser F, Jäger U, et al. Therapeutic options in relapsed or refractory peripheral T-cell lymphoma. Cancer Treat Rev. 2014;40:1080–8.

183. Gritti G, Gianatti A, Petronzelli F, De Santis R, Pavoni C, Rossi RL, et al. Evaluation of tenascin-C by tenatumomab in T-cell non-Hodgkin lymphomas identifies a new target for radioimmunotherapy. Oncotarget. 2018;9(11):9766–75.

184. Gopal AK, Pagel JM, Fromm JR, Wilbur S, Press OW. 131I anti-CD45 radioimmunotherapy effectively targets and treats T-cell non-Hodgkin lymphoma. Blood. 2009;113:5905–10.

185. Rosen ST, Zimmer AM, Goldman-Leikin R, Gordon LI, Kazikiewicz JM, Kaplan EH, et al. Radioimmunodetection and radioimmunotherapy of cutaneous T cell lymphomas using an 131I-labeled monoclonal antibody: an Illinois cancer council study. J Clin Oncol. 1987;5(4):562–73.

186. Goldman-Leikin RE, Kaplan EH, Zimmer AM, Kazikiewicz J, Manzel LJ, Rosen ST. Long-term persistence of human anti-murine antibody responses following radioimmunodetection and radioimmunotherapy of cutaneous T-cell lymphoma patients using 131I-T101. Exp Hematol. 1988;16(10):861–4.

187. Zimmer AM, Rosen ST, Spies SM, Goldman-Leikin R, Kazikiewicz JM, Silverstein EA, et al. Radioimmunotherapy of patients with cutaneous T-cell lymphoma using an iodine-131-labeled monoclonal antibody: analysis of retreatment following plasmapheresis. J Nucl Med. 1988;29(2):174–80.

188. Rossignol J, Terriou L, Robu D, Willekens C, Hivert B, Pascal L, et al. Radioimmunotherapy (90Y-ibritumomab tiuxetan) for posttransplant lymphoproliferative disorders after prior exposure to rituximab. Am J Transplant. 2015;15(7):1976–81.

189. Cooney-Qualter E, Krailo M, Angiolillo A, Fawwaz RA, Wiseman G, Harrison L, et al. A phase I study of 90yttrium-ibritumomab-tiuxetan in children and adolescents with relapsed/refractory CD20-positive non-Hodgkin's lymphoma: a Children's Oncology Group study. Clin Cancer Res. 2007;13(18 Pt 2):5652s–60s.

190. Palumbo G, Grana CM, Cocca F, De Santis R, Del Principe D, Baio SM, et al. Pretargeted antibody-guided radioimmunotherapy in a child affected by resistant anaplastic large cell lymphoma. Eur J Haematol. 2007;79(3):258–62.

191. Jekunen AP, Kairemo KJ, Paavonen T. Imaging of Hand-Schüller-Christian syndrome by a monoclonal antibody. Clin Nucl Med. 1997;22(11):771–4.

192. Murray S, Rowlinson-Busza G, Morris JF, Chu AC. Diagnostic and therapeutic evaluation of an anti-Langerhans cell histiocytosis monoclonal antibody (NA1/34) in a new xenograft model. J Invest Dermatol. 2000;114(1):127–34.

193. Jakubowiak AJ, Hari M, Kendall T, Khaled Y, Mineishi S, Al-Zoubi A, et al. Elimination of CD20-expressing cells in multiple myeloma by iodine I-131 tositumomab (Bexxar®) correlates with response to therapy. Blood. 2008;112(11):5176.

194. Lebovic D, Kaminski MS, Anderson TB, Detweiler-Short K, Griffith KA, Jobkar TL, et al. A phase II study of consolidation treatment with iodine-131 tositumomab (Bexxar™) in multiple myeloma (MM). Blood. 2012;120(21):1854.

195. Dispenzieri A, D'Souza A, Gertz MA, Laumann K, Wiseman G, Lacy MQ, et al. A phase 1 trial of 90Y-Zevalin radioimmunotherapy with autologous stem cell transplant for multiple myeloma. Bone Marrow Transplant. 2017;52(10):1372–7.

196. Schottelius M, Osl T, Poschenrieder A, Hoffmann F, Beykan S, Hänscheid H, et al. [177 Lu]pentixather:

comprehensive preclinical characterization of a first CXCR4-directed endoradiotherapeutic agent. Theranostics. 2017;7(9):2350–62.

197. Herrmann K, Schottelius M, Lapa C, Osl T, Poschenrieder A, Hänscheid H, et al. First-in-human experience of CXCR4-directed endoradiotherapy with 177 Lu-and 90 Y-labeled pentixather in advanced-stage multiple myeloma with extensive intra-and extramedullary disease. J Nucl Med. 2016;57(2):248–51.

198. Maurer S, Herhaus P, Lippenmeyer R, Hänscheid H, Kircher M, Schirbel A, et al. Side effects of CXC-chemokine receptor 4 directed endoradiotherapy with Pentixather prior to hematopoietic stem cell transplantation. J Nucl Med. 2019;60(10):1399–405.

199. Appelbaum R, Sandmaier B, Brown PDK, et al. Myelosuppression and mechanism of recovery following administration of samarium-EDTMP. Antibod Immunoconj Radiopharm. 1988;1:263–8.

200. Goel A, Dispenzieri A, Geyer SM, Greiner S, Peng KW, Russell SJ. Synergistic activity of the proteasome inhibitor PS-341 with non-myeloablative 153-Sm-EDTMP skeletally targeted radiotherapy in an orthotopic model of multiple myeloma. Blood. 2006;107(10):4063–70.

201. Dispenzieri A, Wiseman GA, Lacy MQ, Hayman SR, Kumar SK, Buadi F, et al. A phase II study of 153Sm-EDTMP and high-dose melphalan as a peripheral blood stem cell conditioning regimen in patients with multiple myeloma. Am J Hematol. 2010;85(6):409–13.

202. Parks NJ, Kawakami TG, Avila MJ, White R, Cain GR, Raaka SD, et al. Bone marrow transplantation in dogs after radio-ablation with a new Ho-166 amino phosphonic acid bone-seeking agent (DOTMP). Blood. 1993;82(1):318–25.

203. Bayouth JE, Macey DJ, Kasi LP, Garlich JR, McMillan K, Dimopoulos MA, et al. Pharmacokinetics, dosimetry and toxicity of holmium-166-DOTMP for bone marrow ablation in multiple myeloma. J Nucl Med. 1995;36(5):730–7.

204. Bavouth JE, Macey DJ, Boyer AL, Champlin RE. Radiation dose distribution within the bone marrow of patients receiving holmium-166-labeled-phosphonate for marrow ablation. Med Phys. 1995;22:743–53.

205. Rajendran JG, Eary JF, Bensinger W, Durack LD, Vernon C, Fritzberg A. High-dose 166Ho-DOTMP in myeloablative treatment of multiple myeloma: pharmacokinetics, biodistribution, and absorbed dose estimation. J Nucl Med. 2002;43(10):1383–90.

206. Giralt S, Bensinger W, Goodman M, Podoloff D, Eary J, Wendt R, et al. 166Ho-DOTMP plus melphalan followed by peripheral blood stem cell transplantation in patients with multiple myeloma: results of two phase 1/2 trials. Blood. 2003;102(7):2684–91.

207. Christoforidou AV, Saliba RM, Williams P, Qazilbash M, Roden L, Aleman A, et al. Results of a retrospective single institution analysis of targeted skeletal radiotherapy with 166Holmium-DOTMP as conditioning regimen for autologous stem cell transplant for patients with multiple myeloma. Impact on transplant outcomes. Biol Blood Marrow Transplant. 2007;13(5):543–9.

208. Bagheri R, Jalilian AR, Bahrami-Samani A, Mazidi M, Ghannadi-Maragheh M. Production of holmium-166 DOTMP: a promising agent for bone marrow ablation in hematologic malignancies. Iran J Nucl Med. 2011;19(1):12–20.

209. Shadman M, Gopal AK, Kammerer B, Becker PS, Maloney DG, Pender B, et al. Radioimmunotherapy consolidation using 131I-tositumomab for patients with chronic lymphocytic leukemia or small lymphocytic lymphoma in first remission. Leuk Lymphoma. 2016;57(3):572–6.

210. Jain N, Wierda W, Ferrajoli A, Wong F, Lerner S, Keating M, et al. A phase 2 study of yttrium-90 ibritumomab tiuxetan (Zevalin) in patients with chronic lymphocytic leukemia. Cancer. 2009;115(19):4533–9.

211. Adler S, Parthasarathy KL, Bakshi SP, Stutzman L. Gallium 67 citrate scanning for the localization and staging of lymphomas. J Nucl Med. 1975;16(4):255–60.

212. Even-Sapir E, Bar-Shalom R, Israel O, Frenkel A, Iosilevsky G, Haim N, et al. Single-photon emission computed tomography quantitation of gallium citrate uptake for the differentiation of lymphoma from benign hilar uptake. J Clin Oncol. 1995;13(4):942–6.

213. Front D, Bar-Shalom R, Mor M, Haim N, Epelbaum R, Frenkel A, et al. Hodgkin disease: prediction of outcome with 67Ga scintigraphy after one cycle of chemotherapy. Radiology. 1999;210(2):487–91.

214. Front D, Bar-Shalom R, Mor M, Haim N, Epelbaum R, Frenkel A, et al. Aggressive non-Hodgkin lymphoma: early prediction of outcome with 67Ga scintigraphy. Radiology. 2000;214(1):253–7.

215. Israel O, Front D, Lam M, Ben-Haim S, Kleinhaus U, Ben-Shachar M, et al. Gallium 67 imaging in monitoring lymphoma response to treatment. Cancer. 1988;61(12):2439–43.

216. Israel O, Mor M, Epelbaum R, Frenkel A, Haim N, Dann EJ, et al. Clinical pretreatment risk factors and Ga-67 scintigraphy early during treatment for prediction of outcome of patients with aggressive non-Hodgkin lymphoma. Cancer. 2002;94(4):873–8.

217. Janicek M, Kaplan W, Neuberg D, Canellos GP, Shulman LN, Shipp MA. Early restaging gallium scans predict outcome in poor-prognosis patients with aggressive non-Hodgkin's lymphoma treated with high-dose CHOP chemotherapy. J Clin Oncol. 1997;15(4):1631–7.

218. Kuwabara Y, Ichiya Y, Otsuka M, Miyake Y, Gunasekera R, Hasuo K, et al. High [18F]FDG uptake in primary cerebral lymphoma: a PET study. J Comput Assist Tomogr. 1988;12(1):47–8.

219. Barrington SF, Mikhaeel NG, Kostakoglu L, Meignan M, Hutchings M, Müeller SP, et al. Role of imaging in the staging and response assessment of lymphoma: consensus of the international con-

ference on malignant lymphomas imaging working group. J Clin Oncol. 2014;32(27):3048–58.

220. Kostakoglu L, Cheson BD. Current role of FDG PET/CT in lymphoma. Eur J Nucl Med Mol Imaging. 2014;41(5):1004–27.

221. la Fougère C, Hundt W, Bröckel N, Pfluger T, Haug A, Scher B, et al. Value of PET/CT versus PET and CT performed as separate investigations in patients with Hodgkin's disease and non-Hodgkin's lymphoma. Eur J Nucl Med Mol Imaging. 2006;33(12): 1417–25.

222. Wright CL, Maly JJ, Zhang J, Knopp MV. Advancing precision nuclear medicine and molecular imaging for lymphoma. PET Clin. 2017;12:63–82.

223. Cheson BD, Fisher RI, Barrington SF, Cavalli F, Schwartz LH, Zucca E, et al. Recommendations for initial evaluation, staging, and response assessment of Hodgkin and non-Hodgkin lymphoma: the lugano classification. J Clin Oncol. 2014;32:3059–67.

224. Carr R, Barrington SF, Madan B, O'Doherty MJ, Saunders CAB, Van Der Walt J, et al. Detection of lymphoma in bone marrow by whole-body positron emission tomography. Blood. 1998;91(9): 3340–6.

225. El-Galaly TC, d'Amore F, Mylam KJ, de Nully BP, Bøgsted M, Bukh A, et al. Routine bone marrow biopsy has little or no therapeutic consequence for positron emission tomography/computed tomography-staged treatment-naive patients with Hodgkin lymphoma. J Clin Oncol. 2012;30(36):4508–14.

226. Moulin-Romsee G, Hindié E, Cuenca X, Brice P, Decaudin D, Bénamor M, et al. 18 F-FDG PET/CT bone/bone marrow findings in Hodgkin's lymphoma may circumvent the use of bone marrow trephine biopsy at diagnosis staging. Eur J Nucl Med Mol Imaging. 2010;37(6):1095–105.

227. Moog F, Bangerter M, Kotzerke J, Guhlmann A, Frickhofen N, Reske SN. 18-F-fluorodeoxyglucose-positron emission tomography as a new approach to detect lymphomatous bone marrow. J Clin Oncol. 1998;16(2):603–9.

228. Moog F, Bangerter M, Diederichs CG, Guhlmann A, Merkle E, Frickhofen N, et al. Extranodal malignant lymphoma: detection with FDG PET versus CT. Radiology. 1998;206(2):475–81.

229. Jochelson M, Mauch P, Balikian J, Rosenthal D, Canellos G. The significance of the residual mediastinal mass in treated Hodgkin's disease. J Clin Oncol. 1985;3(5):637–40.

230. Jerusalem G, Beguin Y, Fassotte MF, Najjar F, Paulus P, Rigo P, et al. Whole-body positron emission tomography using18F-fluorodeoxyglucose for post-treatment evaluation in Hodgkin's disease and non-Hodgkin's lymphoma has higher diagnostic and prognostic value than classical computed tomography scan imaging. Blood. 1999;94(2):429–33.

231. Naumann R, Vaic A, Beuthien-Baumann B, Bredow J, Kropp J, Kittner T, et al. Prognostic value of positron emission tomography in the evaluation of post-treatment residual mass in patients with Hodgkin's disease and non-Hodgkin's lymphoma. Br J Haematol. 2001;115(4):793–800.

232. Spaepen K, Stroobants S, Dupont P, Van Steenweghen S, Thomas J, Vandenberghe P, et al. Prognostic value of positron emission tomography (PET) with fluorine-18 fluorodeoxyglucose ([18F]FDG) after first-line chemotherapy in non-Hodgkin's lymphoma: is [18F]FDG-PET a valid alternative to conventional diagnostic methods? J Clin Oncol. 2001;19(2):414–9.

233. Spaepen K, Stroobants S, Dupont P, Thomas J, Vandenberghe P, Balzarini J, et al. Can positron emission tomography with [(18)F]-fluorodeoxyglucose after first-line treatment distinguish Hodgkin's disease patients who need additional therapy from others in whom additional therapy would mean avoidable toxicity? Br J Haematol. 2001;115(2):272–8.

234. Zinzani PL, Magagnoli M, Chierichetti F, Zompatori M, Garraffa G, Bendandi M, et al. The role of positron emission tomography (PET) in the management of lymphoma patients. Ann Oncol. 1999;10(10):1181–4.

235. Weihrauch MR, Re D, Bischoff S, Dietlein M, Scheidhauer K, Krug B, et al. Whole-body positron emission tomography using 18F-fluorodeoxyglucose for initial staging of patients with Hodgkin's disease. Ann Hematol. 2002;81(1):20–5.

236. Nyilas R, Farkas B, Bicsko RR, Magyari F, Pinczes LI, Illes A, et al. Interim PET/CT in diffuse large B-cell lymphoma may facilitate identification of good-prognosis patients among IPI-stratified patients. Int J Hematol. 2019;110(3):331–9.

237. Coughlan K, Dadparvar S, Pampaloni M, Chong EYJ, et al. Correlation of clinical outcome with FDG-PET based response of non-Hodgkin's lymphoma (NHL) to radioimmunotherapy (RIT). J Nucl Med. 2008;49(1):338.

238. Lopci E, Santi I, Derenzini E, Fonti C, Savelli G, Bertagna F, et al. FDG-PET in the assessment of patients with follicular lymphoma treated by ibritumomab tiuxetan Y 90: multicentric study. Ann Oncol. 2010;21(9):1877–83.

239. Shrikanthan S, Berkowitz A, Srinivas S, Hochhold J, Zhuang H, Newberg A, et al. FDG PET in evaluation of bone marrow involvement in patients with lymphoma correlation with subtypes and bone marrow biopsy patterns. J Nucl Med. 2006;47(1):452p.

240. McQuillan AD, Macdonald WBG, Turner JH. Phase II study of first-line 131I-rituximab radioimmunotherapy in follicular non-Hodgkin lymphoma and prognostic 18F-fluorodeoxyglucose positron emission tomography. Leuk Lymphoma. 2015;56(5):1271–7.

241. Jacene HA, Filice R, Kasecamp W, Wahl RL. 18F-FDG PET/CT for monitoring the response of lymphoma to radioimmunotherapy. J Nucl Med. 2009;50(1):8–17.

242. Storto G, De Renzo A, Pellegrino T, Perna F, De Falco T, Erra P, et al. Assessment of metabolic response to radioimmunotherapy with 90Y-ibritu-

momab tiuxetan in patients with relapsed or refractory B-cell non-Hodgkin lymphoma. Radiology. 2010;254(1):245–52.

243. Grgic A, Nestle U, Scheidhauer K, Puskas C, Ballek E, Hohloch K, et al. Retrospective web-based multicenter evaluation of 18F-FDG-PET and CT derived predictive factors: Radioimmunotherapy with yttrium-90-ibritumomab tiuxetan in follicular non Hodgkin's lymphoma. Nuklearmedizin. 2011;50(1):39–47.

244. Kesavan M, Boucek J, MacDonald W, McQuillan A, Turner JH. Imaging of early response to predict prognosis in the first-line management of follicular non-Hodgkin lymphoma with iodine-131-rituximab radioimmunotherapy. Diagnostics (Basel, Switzerland). 2017;7(2):26.

245. Bodet-Milin C, Kraeber-Bodéré F, Dupas B, Morschhauser F, Gastinne T, Le Gouill S, et al. Evaluation of response to fractionated radioimmunotherapy with 90Y-epratuzumab in non-Hodgkin's lymphoma by 18F-fluorodeoxyglucose positron emission tomography. Haematologica. 2008;93:390–7.

246. Jacene H, Crandall J, Kasamon YL, Ambinder RF, Piantadosi S, Serena D, et al. Initial experience with tositumomab and I-131-labeled tositumomab for treatment of relapsed/refractory Hodgkin lymphoma. Mol Imaging Biol. 2017;19(3):429–36.

247. Lim I, Park JY, Kang HJ, Hwang JP, Lee SS, Kim KM, et al. Prognostic significance of pretreatment F-FDG PET/CT in patients with relapsed/refractory B-cell non-Hodgkin's lymphoma treated by radioimmunotherapy using 131I-rituximab. Acta Haematol. 2013;130(2):74–82.

248. Torizuka T, Zasadny KR, Kison PV, Rommelfanger SG, Kaminski MS, Wahl RL. Metabolic response of non-Hodgkin's lymphoma to131I-anti-B1 radioimmunotherapy: evaluation with FDG PET. J Nucl Med. 2000;41(6):999–1005.

249. Lecouvet FE, Vande Berg BC, Michaux L, Malghem J, Maldague BE, Jamart J, et al. Stage III multiple myeloma: clinical and prognostic value of spinal bone marrow MR imaging. Radiology. 1998;209(3):653–60.

250. Walker R, Barlogie B, Haessler J, Tricot G, Anaissie E, Shaughnessy JD, et al. Magnetic resonance imaging in multiple myeloma: diagnostic and clinical implications. J Clin Oncol. 2007;25(9):1121–8.

251. Dinter DJ, Neff WK, Klaus J, Böhm C, Hastka J, Weiss C, et al. Comparison of whole-body MR imaging and conventional X-ray examination in patients with multiple myeloma and implications for therapy. Ann Hematol. 2009;88(5):457–64.

252. Gleeson TG, Moriarty J, Shortt CP, Gleeson JP, Fitzpatrick P, Byrne B, et al. Accuracy of whole-body low-dose multidetector CT (WBLDCT) versus skeletal survey in the detection of myelomatous lesions, and correlation of disease distribution with whole-body MRI (WBMRI). Skelet Radiol. 2009;38(3):225–36.

253. Dimopoulos M, Terpos E, Comenzo RL, Tosi P, Beksac M, Sezer O, et al. International Myeloma Working Group consensus statement and guidelines regarding the current role of imaging techniques in the diagnosis and monitoring of multiple myeloma. Leukemia. 2009;23:1545–56.

254. Rajkumar SV, Dimopoulos MA, Palumbo A, Blade J, Merlini G, Mateos MV, et al. International Myeloma Working Group updated criteria for the diagnosis of multiple myeloma. Lancet Oncol. 2014;15:e538–48.

255. Schirrmeister H, Bommer M, Buck A, Müller S, Messer P, Bunjes D, et al. Initial results in the assessment of multiple myeloma using 18F-FDG PET. Eur J Nucl Med. 2002;29(3):361–6.

256. Weng WW, Dong MJ, Zhang J, Yang J, Xu Q, Zhu YJ, et al. A systematic review of MRI, scintigraphy, FDG-PET and PET/CT for diagnosis of multiple myeloma related bone disease—which is best? Asian Pac J Cancer Prev. 2014;15(22):9879–84.

257. Nanni C, Zamagni E, Farsad M, Castellucci P, Tosi P, Cangini D, et al. Role of 18F-FDG PET/CT in the assessment of bone involvement in newly diagnosed multiple myeloma: preliminary results. Eur J Nucl Med Mol Imaging. 2006;33(5):525–31.

258. Bartel TB, Haessler J, Brown TLY, Shaughnessy JD, Van Rhee F, Anaissie E, et al. F18-fluorodeoxyglucose positron emission tomography in the context of other imaging techniques and prognostic factors in multiple myeloma. Blood. 2009;114(10):2068–76.

259. Usmani SZ, Mitchell A, Waheed S, Crowley J, Hoering A, Petty N, et al. Prognostic implications of serial 18-fluoro-deoxyglucose emission tomography in multiple myeloma treated with total therapy 3. Blood. 2013;121(10):1819–23.

260. Davies FE, Rosenthal A, Rasche L, Petty NM, McDonald JE, Ntambi JA, et al. Treatment to suppression of focal lesions on positron emission tomography-computed tomography is a therapeutic goal in newly diagnosed multiple myeloma. Haematologica. 2018;103(6):1047–53.

261. Zamagni E, Patriarca F, Nanni C, Zannetti B, Englaro E, Pezzi A, et al. Prognostic relevance of 18-F FDG PET/CT in newly diagnosed multiple myeloma patients treated with up-front autologous transplantation. Blood. 2011;118(23):5989–95.

262. Haznedar R, Akı SZ, Akdemir ÖU, Özkurt ZN, Çeneli Ö, Yağcı M, et al. Value of 18 F-fluorodeoxyglucose uptake in positron emission tomography/computed tomography in predicting survival in multiple myeloma. Eur J Nucl Med Mol Imaging. 2011;38(6):1046–53.

263. Spinnato P, Bazzocchi A, Brioli A, Nanni C, Zamagni E, Albisinni U, et al. Contrast enhanced MRI and 18F-FDG PET-CT in the assessment of multiple myeloma: a comparison of results in different phases of the disease. Eur J Radiol. 2012;81(12):4013–8.

264. Nanni C, Zamagni E, Celli M, Caroli P, Ambrosini V, Tacchetti P, et al. The value of 18F-FDG PET/CT after autologous stem cell transplantation (ASCT) in patients affected by multiple myeloma

(MM): experience with 77 patients. Clin Nucl Med. 2013;38(2):e74–9.

265. Derlin T, Peldschus K, Münster S, Bannas P, Herrmann J, Stübig T, et al. Comparative diagnostic performance of 18F-FDG PET/CT versus whole-body MRI for determination of remission status in multiple myeloma after stem cell transplantation. Eur Radiol. 2013;23(2):570–8.

266. Zamagni E, Nanni C, Mancuso K, Tacchetti P, Pezzi A, Pantani L, et al. PET/CT improves the definition of complete response and allows to detect otherwise unidentifiable skeletal progression in multiple myeloma. Clin Cancer Res. 2015;21(19):4384–90.

267. Lapa C, Lückerath K, Malzahn U, Samnick S, Einsele H, Buck AK, et al. 18FDG-PET/CT for prognostic stratification of patients with multiple myeloma relapse after stem cell transplantation. Oncotarget. 2014;5(17):7381–91.

268. Jamet B, Bailly C, Carlier T, Planche L, Touzeau C, Kraeber-Bodéré F, et al. Added prognostic value of FDG-PET/CT in relapsing multiple myeloma patients. Leuk Lymphoma. 2019;60:222–5.

269. Abe Y, Narita K, Kobayashi H, Kitadate A, Takeuchi M, O'uchi T, et al. Medullary abnormalities in appendicular skeletons detected with 18F-FDG PET/CT predict an unfavorable prognosis in newly diagnosed multiple myeloma patients with high-risk factors. AJR Am J Roentgenol. 2019;213(4): 918–24.

270. Bailly C, Carlier T, Jamet B, Eugene T, Touzeau C, Attal M, et al. Interim PET analysis in first-line therapy of multiple myeloma: prognostic value of ΔSUVmax in the FDG-avid patients of the IMAJEM study. Clin Cancer Res. 2018;24(21):5219–24.

271. Jamet B, Bailly C, Carlier T, Touzeau C, Nanni C, Zamagni E, et al. Interest of pet imaging in multiple myeloma. Front Med. 2019;6:69.

272. Zamagni E, Nanni C, Dozza L, Carlier T, Tacchetti P, Versari A. Standardization of 18F-FDG PET/CT according to deauville criteria for MRD evaluation in newly diagnosed transplant eligible multiple myeloma patients: joined analysis of two prospective randomized phase III trials. In: Oral communication ASH annual meeting, San Diego, CA, 2018.

273. Nanni C, Versari A, Chauvie S, Bertone E, Bianchi A, Rensi M, et al. Interpretation criteria for FDG PET/ CT in multiple myeloma (IMPeTUs): final results. IMPeTUs (Italian myeloma criteria for PET USe). Eur J Nucl Med Mol Imaging. 2018;45(5):712–9.

274. Salaun PY, Gastinne T, Frampas E, Bodet-Milin C, Moreau P, Bodéré-Kraeber F. FDG-positron-emission tomography for staging and therapeutic assessment in patients with plasmacytoma. Haematologica. 2008;93:1269–71.

275. Grammatico S, Scalzulli E, Petrucci MT. Solitary plasmacytoma. Mediterr J Hematol Infect Dis. 2017;9(91):1–14.

276. Lu YY, Chen JH, Lin WY, Liang JA, Wang HY, Tsai SC, et al. FDG PET or PET/CT for detecting intramedullary and extramedullary lesions in multiple myeloma: a systematic review and meta-analysis. Clin Nucl Med. 2012;37:833–7.

277. Dammacco F, Rubini G, Ferrari C, Vacca A, Racanelli V. 18F-FDG PET/CT: a review of diagnostic and prognostic features in multiple myeloma and related disorders. Clin Exp Med. 2014;15(1):1–18.

278. Zhang L, Zhang X, He Q, Zhang R, Fan W. The role of initial 18F-FDG PET/CT in the management of patients with suspected extramedullary plasmocytoma. Cancer Imaging. 2018;18(1):19.

279. Cavo M, Terpos E, Nanni C, Moreau P, Lentzsch S, Zweegman S, et al. Role of 18F-FDG PET/CT in the diagnosis and management of multiple myeloma and other plasma cell disorders: a consensus statement by the International Myeloma Working Group. Lancet Oncol. 2017;18:e206–17.

280. Kim PJ, Hicks RJ, Wirth A, Ryan G, Seymour JF, Prince HM, et al. Impact of 18F-fluorodeoxyglucose positron emission tomography before and after definitive radiation therapy in patients with apparently solitary plasmacytoma. Int J Radiat Oncol Biol Phys. 2009;74(3):740–6.

281. Albano D, Bosio G, Treglia G, Giubbini R, Bertagna F. 18F–FDG PET/CT in solitary plasmacytoma: metabolic behavior and progression to multiple myeloma. Eur J Nucl Med Mol Imaging. 2018;45(1):77–84.

282. Alongi P, Zanoni L, Incerti E, Fallanca F, Mapelli P, Papathanasiou N, et al. ^{18}F-FDG PET/CT for early postradiotherapy assessment in solitary bone plasmacytomas. Clin Nucl Med. 2015;40(8):e399–404.

283. Fouquet G, Guidez S, Herbaux C, Van De Wyngaert Z, Bonnet S, Beauvais D, et al. Impact of initial FDG-PET/CT and serum-free light chain on transformation of conventionally defined solitary plasmacytoma to multiple myeloma. Clin Cancer Res. 2014;20(12):3254–60.

284. Catalano OA, Masch WR, Catana C, Mahmood U, Sahani DV, Gee MS, et al. An overview of PET/ MR, focused on clinical applications. Abdom Radiol (NY). 2017;42:631–44.

285. Lin C, Luciani A, Itti E, Haioun C, Safar V, Meignan M, et al. Whole-body diffusion magnetic resonance imaging in the assessment of lymphoma. Cancer Imaging. 2012;12:403–8.

286. Sun M, Cheng J, Zhang Y, Wang F, Meng Y, Fu X. Application value of diffusion weighted whole body imaging with background body signal suppression in monitoring the response to treatment of bone marrow involvement in lymphoma. J Magn Reson Imaging. 2016;44(6):1522–9.

287. Cieszanowski A, Lisowska A, Dabrowska M, Korczynski P, Zukowska M, Grudzinski IP, et al. MR imaging of pulmonary nodules: detection rate and accuracy of size estimation in comparison to computed tomography. PLoS One. 2016;11(6):e015627.

288. Kwee TC, Kwee RM, Verdonck LF, Bierings MB, Nievelstein RAJ. Magnetic resonance imaging for the detection of bone marrow involvement in malignant lymphoma. Br J Haematol. 2008;141(1):60–8.

289. Daldrup-Link HE, Henning T, Link TM. MR imaging of therapy-induced changes of bone marrow. Eur Radiol. 2007;17:743–61.

290. Yasumoto M, Nonomura Y, Yoshimura R, Haraguchi K, Ito S, Ohashi I, et al. MR detection of iliac bone marrow involvement by malignant lymphoma with various MR sequences including diffusion-weighted echo-planar imaging. Skelet Radiol. 2002;31(5):263–9.

291. Mayerhoefer ME, Karanikas G, Kletter K, Prosch H, Kiesewetter B, Skrabs C, et al. Evaluation of diffusion-weighted MRI for pretherapeutic assessment and staging of lymphoma: results of a prospective study in 140 patients. Clin Cancer Res. 2014;20(11):2984–93.

292. Mayerhoefer ME, Karanikas G, Kletter K, Kiesewetter B, Weber M, Rausch I, et al. Can interim 18 F-FDG PET or diffusion-weighted MRI predict end-of-treatment outcome in FDG-Avid MALT lymphoma after rituximab-based therapy? Clin Nucl Med. 2016;41(11):837–43.

293. Furth C, Steffen IG, Amthauer H, Ruf J, Misch D, Schönberger S, et al. Early and late therapy response assessment with [18F]fluorodeoxyglucose positron emission tomography in pediatric Hodgkin's lymphoma: analysis of a prospective multicenter trial. J Clin Oncol. 2009;27(26):4385–91.

294. Itti E, Meignan M, Berriolo-Riedinger A, Biggi A, Cashen AF, Véra P, et al. An international confirmatory study of the prognostic value of early PET/CT in diffuse large B-cell lymphoma: comparison between Deauville criteria and ΔSUVmax. Eur J Nucl Med Mol Imaging. 2013;40(9):1312–20.

295. Mayerhoefer ME, Raderer M, Jaeger U, Staber P, Kiesewetter B, Senn D, et al. Ultra-early response assessment in lymphoma treatment: [18F]FDG PET/MR captures changes in glucose metabolism and cell density within the first 72 hours of treatment. Eur J Nucl Med Mol Imaging. 2018;45(6):931–40.

296. Hagtvedt T, Seierstad T, Lund KV, Løndalen AM, Bogsrud TV, Smith H-J, et al. Diffusion-weighted MRI compared to FDG PET/CT for assessment of early treatment response in lymphoma. Acta Radiol. 2015;56(2):152–8.

297. Zucca E, Copie-Bergman C, Ricardi U, Thieblemont C, Raderer M, Ladetto M. Gastric marginal zone lymphoma of MALT type: ESMO clinical practice guidelines for diagnosis, treatment and follow-up. Ann Oncol. 2013;24(6):vi114–8.

298. Ruskoné-Fourmestraux A, Fischbach W, Aleman BMP, Boot H, Du MQ, Megraud F, et al. EGILS consensus report. Gastric extranodal marginal zone B-cell lymphoma of MALT. Gut. 2011;60(6):747–58.

299. Dreyling M, Thieblemont C, Gallamini A, Arcaini L, Campo E, Hermine O, et al. Esmo consensus conferences: guidelines on malignant lymphoma. Part 2: marginal zone lymphoma, mantle cell lymphoma, peripheral T-cell lymphoma. Ann Oncol. 2013;24(4):857–77.

300. Haug AR, Leisser A, Wadsak W, Mitterhauser M, Pfaff S, Kropf S, et al. Prospective non-invasive evaluation of CXCR4 expression for the diagnosis of MALT lymphoma using [68Ga]Ga-pentixafor-PET/MRI. Theranostics. 2019;9(12):3653–8.

301. Aznar MC, Sersar R, Saabye J, Ladefoged CN, Andersen FL, Rasmussen JH, et al. Whole-body PET/MRI: the effect of bone attenuation during MR-based attenuation correction in oncology imaging. Eur J Radiol. 2014;83(7):1177–83.

302. Ferguson A, McConathy J, Su Y, Hewing D, Laforest R. Attenuation effects of MR headphones during brain PET/MR studies. J Nucl Med Technol. 2014;42(2):93–100.

303. Shah SN, Oldan JD. PET/MR imaging of multiple myeloma. Magn Reson Imaging Clin N Am. 2017;25:351–65.

304. Sachpekidis C, Hillengass J, Goldschmidt H, Mosebach J, Pan L, Schlemmer H-P, et al. Comparison of (18)F-FDG PET/CT and PET/MRI in patients with multiple myeloma. Am J Nucl Med Mol Imaging. 2015;5(5):469–78.

305. Beiderwellen K, Huebner M, Heusch P, Grueneisen J, Ruhlmann V, Nensa F, et al. Whole-body [18F]FDG PET/MRI vs. PET/CT in the assessment of bone lesions in oncological patients: initial results. Eur Radiol. 2014;24(8):2023–30.

306. Dimopoulos MA, Hillengass J, Usmani S, Zamagni E, Lentzsch S, Davies FE, et al. Role of magnetic resonance imaging in the management of patients with multiple myeloma: a consensus statement. J Clin Oncol. 2015;33(6):657–64.

307. Tuli A, Ayache JB, Samir P, Thamnirat K, Chari A, Kostakoglu L, et al. Comparison of sequential PET/CT and PET/MR in previously treated multiple myeloma patients. J Nucl Med. 2017;58(1):187.

308. Zhang H, Jhanwar Y, Dutruel S, Chabbra S, Kim JA, Goldsmith S. PET MRI in patients with multiple myeloma. J Nucl Med. 2018;59(1):18.

309. Mena E, Lindenberg ML, Turkbey BI, Shih J, Logan J, Adler S, et al. A pilot study of the value of 18F-fluoro-deoxy-thymidine PET/CT in predicting viable lymphoma in residual 18F-FDG avid masses after completion of therapy. Clin Nucl Med. 2014;39(10):874–81.

310. Buck AK, Bommer M, Stilgenbauer S, Juweid M, Glatting G, Schirrmeister H, et al. Molecular imaging of proliferation in malignant lymphoma. Cancer Res. 2006;66(22):11055–61.

311. Kasper B, Egerer G, Gronkowski M, Haufe S, Lehnert T, Eisenhut M, et al. Functional diagnosis of residual lymphomas after radiochemotherapy with positron emission tomography comparing FDG- and FLT-PET. Leuk Lymphoma. 2007;48(4):746–53.

312. Buck AK, Kratochwil C, Glatting G, Juweid M, Bommer M, Tepsic D, et al. Early assessment of therapy response in malignant lymphoma with the thymidine analogue [18F]FLT. Eur J Nucl Med Mol Imaging. 2007;34(11):1775–82.

313. Herrmann K, Buck AK, Schuster T, Rudelius M, Wester H-J, Graf N, et al. A pilot study to evaluate 3′-deoxy-3′-18F-fluorothymidine pet for initial and early response imaging in mantle cell lymphoma. J Nucl Med. 2011;52(12):1898–902.

314. Herrmann K, Buck AK, Schuster T, Junger A, Wieder HA, Graf N, et al. Predictive value of initial18F-FLT uptake in patients with aggressive non-hodgkin lymphoma receiving R-CHOP treatment. J Nucl Med. 2011;52(5):690–6.

315. Graf N, Herrmann K, den Hollander J, Fend F, Schuster T, Wester HJ, et al. Imaging proliferation to monitor early response of lymphoma to cytotoxic treatment. Mol Imaging Biol. 2008;10(6):349–55.

316. Schoder H, Zelenetz AD, Hamlin P, Gavane S, Horwitz S, Matasar M, et al. Prospective study of 3′-deoxy-3′-18F-fluorothymidine PET for early interim response assessment in advanced-stage B-cell lymphoma. J Nucl Med. 2016;57(5):728–34.

317. Leskinen-Kallio S, Ruotsalainen U, Någren K, Teräs MJH. Uptake of carbon-11-methionine and fluorodeoxyglucose in non-Hodgkin's lymphoma: a PET study. J Nucl Med. 1991;6(32):1211–8.

318. Viering O, Kircher M, Lapaand C, Buck A. 68Ga-Pentixafor PET/CT is superior to [18F]FDG PET/CT in newly diagnosed marginal zone lymphoma. J Nucl Med. 2019;60(1):614.

319. Lou Y, Cao X, Pan Q, Li J, et al. 68Ga-Pentixafor PET/CT for imaging of chemokine receptor 4 expression in Waldenström macroglobulinemia/lymphoplasmacytic lymphoma: comparison to 18F-FDG PET/CT. J Nucl Med. 2019;60(12):1724–9.

320. Herhaus P, Lipkova J, Lammer F, Slotta-Huspenina J, Wiestler B, Vag T, et al. CXCR4-targeted positron emission tomography imaging of central nervous system B-cell lymphoma. Blood. 2019;134(Suppl 1):2900.

321. Guillouet S, Patin D, Tirel O, Delamare J, Gourand F, Deloye JB, et al. Fully automated radiosynthesis of 2-[18F]fludarabine for PET imaging of low-grade lymphoma. Mol Imaging Biol. 2014;16(1):28–35.

322. Dhilly M, Guillouet S, Patin D, Fillesoye F, Abbas A, Gourand F, et al. 2-[18F]fludarabine, a novel positron emission tomography (PET) tracer for imaging lymphoma: a micro-PET study in murine models. Mol Imaging Biol. 2014;16(1):118–26.

323. Hovhannisyan N, Guillouet S, Fillesoye F, Dhilly M, Patin D, Galateau F, et al. Evaluation of the specificity of [18F]fludarabine PET/CT in a xenograft model of follicular lymphoma: comparison with [18F]FDG and impact of rituximab therapy. EJNMMI Res. 2015;5(1):23.

324. Hovhannisyan N, Dhilly M, Guillouet S, Leporrier M, Barré L. Comparative analysis between [18F]Fludarabine-PET and [18F]FDG-PET in a murine model of inflammation. Mol Pharm. 2016;13:2136–9.

325. Hovhannisyan N, Dhilly M, Fidalgo M, Fillesoye F, Guillouet S, Sola B, et al. [F]Fludarabine-PET in a murine model of multiple myeloma. PLoS One. 2017;12(5):e0177125.

326. Barré L, Hovhannisyan N, Bodet-Milin C, Kraeber-Bodéré F, Damaj G. [18F]-fludarabine for hematological malignancies. Front Med. 2019;6:77.

327. Muylle K, Flamen P, Vugts DJ, Guiot T, Ghanem G, Meuleman N, et al. Tumour targeting and radiation dose of radioimmunotherapy with 90Y-rituximab in CD20+ B-cell lymphoma as predicted by 89Zr-rituximab immuno-PET: impact of preloading with unlabelled rituximab. Eur J Nucl Med Mol Imaging. 2015;42(8):1304–14.

328. Bugatti S, Vitolo B, Caporali R, Montecucco C, Manzo A. B cells in rheumatoid arthritis: from pathogenic players to disease biomarkers. Biomed Res Int. 2014;2014:678–81.

329. Möller B, Aeberli D, Eggli S, Fuhrer M, Vajtai I, Vögelin E, et al. Class-switched B cells display response to therapeutic B-cell depletion in rheumatoid arthritis. Arthritis Res Ther. 2009;11(3):R62.

330. Thurlings RM, Vos K, Wijbrandts CA, Zwinderman AH, Gerlag DM, Tak PP. Synovial tissue response to rituximab: mechanism of action and identification of biomarkers of response. Ann Rheum Dis. 2008;67(7):917–25.

331. Jauw YWS, Zijlstra JM, De Jong D, Vugts DJ, Zweegman S, Hoekstra OS, et al. Performance of 89Zr-labeled-rituximab-PET as an imaging biomarker to assess CD20 targeting: a pilot study in patients with relapsed/refractory diffuse large B cell lymphoma. PLoS One. 2017;12(1):e0169828.

332. Nanni C, Zamagni E, Cavo M, Rubello D, Tacchetti P, Pettinato C, et al. 11C-choline vs. 18F-FDG PET/CT in assessing bone involvement in patients with multiple myeloma. World J Surg Oncol. 2007;5:68.

333. Cassou-Mounat T, Balogova S, Nataf V, Calzada M, Huchet V, Kerrou K, et al. 18F-fluorocholine versus 18F-fluorodeoxyglucose for PET/CT imaging in patients with suspected relapsing or progressive multiple myeloma: a pilot study. Eur J Nucl Med Mol Imaging. 2016;43(11):1995–2004.

334. Ho CL, Chen S, Leung YL, Cheng T, Wong KN, Cheung SK, et al. 11C-Acetate PET/CT for metabolic characterization of multiple myeloma: a comparative study with 18F-FDG PET/CT. J Nucl Med. 2014;55(5):749–52.

335. Alabed YZ. Multiple solitary Plasmacytomas with multifocal bone involvement diagnosed with 68Ga–prostate-specific membrane antigen PET/CT. Clin Nucl Med. 2020;45:e51–2.

336. Philipp-Abbrederis K, Herrmann K, Knop S, Schottelius M, Eiber M, Lückerath K, et al. In vivo molecular imaging of chemokine receptor CXCR 4 expression in patients with advanced multiple myeloma. EMBO Mol Med. 2015;7(4):477–87.

337. Pan Q, Cao X, Luo Y, Li J, Feng J, Li F. Chemokine receptor-4 targeted PET/CT with 68Ga-Pentixafor in assessment of newly diagnosed multiple myeloma: comparison to 18F-FDG PET/CT. Eur J Nucl Med Mol Imaging. 2020;47(3):537–46.

338. Lapa C, Schreder M, Schirbel A, Samnick S, Kortüm KM, Herrmann K, et al. 68Ga-Pentixafor-PET/CT for imaging of chemokine receptor CXCR4 expression in multiple myeloma—comparison to [18F]FDG and laboratory values. Theranostics. 2017;7(1):205–12.

339. Goodwin DA, Meares CF, David GF, McTigue M, McCall MJ, Frincke JM, et al. Monoclonal antibodies as reversible equilibrium carriers of radiopharmaceuticals. Int J Radiat Appl Instrum. 1986;13(4):383–91.

340. Goodwin DA, Mears CF, McTigue M, David GS. Monoclonal antibody hapten radiopharmaceutical delivery. Nucl Med Commun. 1986;7(8):569–80.

341. Goldenberg DM, Sharkey RM, Paganelli G, Barbet J, Chatal JF. Antibody pretargeting advances cancer radioimmunodetection and radioimmunotherapy. J Clin Oncol. 2006;24:823–34.

342. Sharkey RM, Van Rij CM, Karacay H, Rossi EA, Frielink C, Regino C, et al. A new tri-fab bispecific antibody for pretargeting trop-2-expressing epithelial cancers. J Nucl Med. 2012;53(10):1625–32.

343. Walter RB, Press OW, Pagel JM. Pretargeted radioimmunotherapy for hematologic and other malignancies. Cancer Biother Radiopharm. 2010;25:125–42.

344. Pagel JM, Hedin N, Subbiah K, Meyer D, Mallet R, Axworthy D, et al. Comparison of anti-CD20 and anti-CD45 antibodies for conventional and pretargeted radioimmunotherapy of B-cell lymphomas. Blood. 2003;101(6):2340–8.

345. Green DJ, Pagel JM, Nemecek ER, Lin Y, Kenoyer A, Pantelias A, et al. Pretargeting CD45 enhances the selective delivery of radiation to hematolymphoid tissues in nonhuman primates. Blood. 2009;114:1226–35.

346. Pagel JM, Pantelias A, Hedin N, Wilbur S, Saganic L, Lin Y, et al. Evaluation of CD20, CD22, and HLA-DR targeting for radioimmunotherapy of B-cell lymphomas. Cancer Res. 2007;67(12):5921–8.

347. Subbiah K, Hamlin DK, Pagel JM, Wilbur DS, Meyer DL, Axworthy DB, et al. Comparison of immunoscintigraphy, efficacy, and toxicity of conventional and pretargeted radioimmunotherapy in CD20-expressing human lymphoma xenografts. J Nucl Med. 2003;44(3):437–45.

348. Zhang M, Zhang Z, Garmestani K, Schultz J, Axworthy DB, Goldman CK, et al. Pretarget radiotherapy with an anti-CD25 antibody-streptavidin fusion protein was effective in therapy of leukemia/lymphoma xenografts. Proc Natl Acad Sci U S A. 2003;100(4):1891–5.

349. Park SI, Shenoi J, Page JM, Hamlin DK, Wilbur DS, Orgun N, et al. Conventional and pretargeted radioimmunotherapy using bismuth-213 to target and treat non-Hodgkin lymphomas expressing CD20: a preclinical model toward optimal consolidation therapy to eradicate minimal residual disease. Blood. 2010;116(20):4231–9.

350. Green DJ, Orgun NN, Jones JC, Hylarides MD, Pagel JM, Hamlin DK, et al. A preclinical model of CD38-pretargeted radioimmunotherapy for plasma cell malignancies. Cancer Res. 2014;74(4):1179–89.

351. Weiden PL, Breitz HB, Press O, Appelbaum JW, Bryan JK, Gaffigan S, et al. Pretargeted radioimmunotherapy (PRIT) for treatment of non-Hodgkin's lymphoma (NHL): initial phase I/II study results. Cancer Biother Radiopharm. 2000;15(1):15–29.

352. Forero A, Weiden PL, Vose JM, Knox SJ, LoBuglio AF, Hankins J, et al. Phase 1 trial of a novel anti-CD20 fusion protein in pretargeted radioimmunotherapy for B-cell non-Hodgkin lymphoma. Blood. 2004;104(1):227–36.

353. Illidge TM, Mayes S, Pettengell R, Bates AT, Bayne M, Radford JA, et al. Fractionated 90Y-ibritumomab tiuxetan radioimmunotherapy as an initial therapy of follicular lymphoma: an international phase II study in patients requiring treatment according to GELF/BNLI criteria. J Clin Oncol. 2014;32(3):212–8.

354. Witzig TE, Wiseman WG, Geyer SM, et al. A phase I trial of two-sequential doses of ZEVALIN radioimmunotherapy for relapsed low grade B-cell non-Hodgkins lymphoma [abstract]. Blood. 2003;102(406a):1475.

355. Meredith RF, Buchsbaum DJ, Knox SJ. Radionuclide dosimetry and radioimmunotherapy of cancer. In: Abrams PG, Fritzberg AR, editors. Radioimmunotherapy of cancer. New York: Marcel Dekker; 2000.

356. Dewaraja YK, Schipper MJ, Shen J, Smith LB, Murgic J, Savas H, et al. Tumor-absorbed dose predicts progression-free survival following 131I-tositumomab radioimmunotherapy. J Nucl Med. 2014;55(7):1047–53.

357. Hobbs RF, Wahl RL, Frey EC, Kasamon Y, Song H, Huang P, et al. Radiobiologic optimization of combination radiopharmaceutical therapy applied to myeloablative treatment of non-hodgkin lymphoma. J Nucl Med. 2013;54(9):1535–42.

358. Song H, Du Y, Sgouros G, Prideaux A, Frey E, Wahl RL. Therapeutic potential of 90Y- and 131I-labeled anti-CD20 monoclonal antibody in treating non-Hodgkin's lymphoma with pulmonary involvement: a Monte Carlo-based dosimetric analysis. J Nucl Med. 2007;48(1):150–7.

359. Koral K, Zasadny KR, Kaminski MS, Wahl RL, Francis IR. CT-SPECT fusion plus conjugate views for determining dosimetry in iodine-131-monoclonal antibody therapy of lymphoma patients. J Nucl Med. 1994;35(10):1714–20.

360. Perk LR, Visser OJ, Stigter-van Walsum M, Vosjan MJWD, Visser GWM, Zijlstra JM, et al. Preparation and evaluation of (89)Zr-Zevalin for monitoring of (90)Y-Zevalin biodistribution with positron emission tomography. Eur J Nucl Med Mol Imaging. 2006;33(11):1337–45.

361. Natarajan A, Habte F, Gambhir SS. Development of a novel long-lived immunoPET tracer for monitoring lymphoma therapy in a humanized transgenic mouse model. Bioconjug Chem. 2012;23(6):1221–9.

362. Vosjan MJWD, Perk LR, Visser GWM, Budde M, Jurek P, Kiefer GE, et al. Conjugation and radiolabeling of monoclonal antibodies with zirconium-89 for PET imaging using the bifunctional chelate p-isothiocyanatobenzyl-desferrioxamine. Nat Protoc. 2010;5(4):739–43.

363. Zettlitz KA, Tavaré R, Knowles SM, Steward KK, Timmerman JM, Wu AM. ImmunoPET of malignant and normal B cells with 89Zr- and 124I-labeled obinutuzumab antibody fragments reveals differential CD20 internalization in vivo. Clin Cancer Res. 2017;23(23):7242–52.

364. Jauw YWS, Bensch F, Brouwers AH, Hoekstra OS, Zijlstra JM, Pieplenbosch S, et al. Interobserver reproducibility of tumor uptake quantification with 89Zr-immuno-PET: a multicenter analysis. Eur J Nucl Med Mol Imaging. 2019;46(9):1840–9.

365. Rizvi SNF, Visser OJ, Vosjan MJWD, van Lingen A, Hoekstra OS, Zijlstra JM, et al. Biodistribution, radiation dosimetry and scouting of 90Y-ibritumomab tiuxetan therapy in patients with relapsed B-cell non-Hodgkin's lymphoma using 89Zr-ibritumomab tiuxetan and PET. Eur J Nucl Med Mol Imaging. 2012;39(3):512–20.

366. Yoon JT, Longtine MS, Marquez-Nostra BV, Wahl RL. Evaluation of next-generation anti-CD20 antibodies labeled with 89Zr in human lymphoma xenografts. J Nucl Med. 2018;59(8):1219–24.

367. Davnall F, Yip CSP, Ljungqvist G, Selmi M, Ng F, Sanghera B, et al. Assessment of tumor heterogeneity: an emerging imaging tool for clinical practice? Insights Imaging. 2012;3:573–89.

368. Fidler IJ, Hart IR. Biological diversity in metastatic neoplasms: origins and implications. Science. 1982;217:998–1003.

369. Dick JE. Stem cell concepts renew cancer research. Blood. 2008;112:4793–807.

370. Nicolson GL. Generation of phenotypic diversity and progression in metastatic tumor cells. Cancer Metastasis Rev. 1984;3(1):25–42.

371. Heppner GH. Tumor heterogeneity. Cancer Res. 1984;44:2259–65.

372. Höckel M, Schlenger K, Aral B, Mitze M, Schäffer U, Vaupel P. Association between tumor hypoxia and malignant progression in advanced cancer of the uterine cervix. Cancer Res. 1996;56(19):4509–15.

373. Yang Z, Tang LH, Klimstra DS. Effect of tumor heterogeneity on the assessment of Ki67 labeling index in well-differentiated neuroendocrine tumors metastatic to the liver: implications for prognostic stratification. Am J Surg Pathol. 2011;35(6):853–60.

374. Gerlinger M, Rowan AJ, Horswell S, Larkin J, Endesfelder D, Gronroos E, et al. Intratumor heterogeneity and branched evolution revealed by multiregion sequencing. N Engl J Med. 2012;366(10):883–92.

375. Lee G, Lee HY, Ko ES, Jeong WK. Radiomics and imaging genomics in precision medicine. Precis Fut Med. 2017;1(1):10–31.

376. Jain A, Tuceryan M. Handbook of pattern recognition and computer vision. River Edge, NJ: World Sci Publishing Co.; 1998. p. 996.

377. Amadasun M, King R. Texural features corresponding to texural properties. IEEE Trans Syst Man Cybern. 1989;19(5):1264–74.

378. Srinivasan GN, Shobha G. Statistical texture analysis. Proc World Acad Sci Eng Technol. 2008;36:1264–9.

379. Bonfante V, Santoro A, Viviani S, Devizzi L, Balzarotti M, Soncini F, et al. Outcome of patients with Hodgkin's disease failing after primary MOPP-ABVD. J Clin Oncol. 1997;15(2):528–34.

380. Allen PB, Gordon LI. Frontline therapy for classical Hodgkin lymphoma by stage and prognostic factors. Clin Med Insights Oncol. 2017;11:1179554917731072.

381. Akhtari M, Milgrom SA, Pinnix CC, Reddy JP, Dong W, Smith GL, et al. Reclassifying patients with early-stage Hodgkin lymphoma based on functional radiographic markers at presentation. Blood. 2018;131(1):84–94.

382. Song MK, Chung JS, Lee JJ, Jeong SY, Lee SM, Hong JS, et al. Metabolic tumor volume by positron emission tomography/computed tomography as a clinical parameter to determine therapeutic modality for early stage Hodgkin's lymphoma. Cancer Sci. 2013;104(12):1656–61.

383. Milgrom SA, Elhalawani H, Lee J, Wang Q, Mohamed ASR, Dabaja BS, et al. A PET radiomics model to predict refractory mediastinal Hodgkin lymphoma. Sci Rep. 2019;9(1):1322.

384. Fama A, Ciammella P, Casali M, Barbolini E, Podgornii A, Iori M, et al. PET-based textural analysis assessment in early stage hodgkin lymphoma treated with standard combined approach. Blood. 2015;126:3949.

385. Thomas K, Karem ER, Michael W, Georgios K, Erik MM. Three-dimensional texture analysis of contrast enhanced CT images for treatment response assessment in Hodgkin lymphoma: comparison with F-18-FDG PET. Med Phys. 2014;41:121904.

386. Reinert CP, Federmann B, Hofmann J, Bösmüller H, Wirths S, Fritz J, et al. Computed tomography textural analysis for the differentiation of chronic lymphocytic leukemia and diffuse large B cell lymphoma of Richter syndrome. Eur Radiol. 2019;29:6911–21.

387. Ko KY, Liu CJ, Ko CL, Yen RF. Intratumoral heterogeneity of pretreatment 18F-FDG PET images predict disease progression in patients with nasal type extranodal natural killer/T-cell lymphoma. Clin Nucl Med. 2016;41(12):922–6.

388. Harrison LC, Luukkaala T, Pertovaara H, Saarinen TO, Heinonen TT, Järvenpää R, et al. Non-Hodgkin lymphoma response evaluation with MRI texture classification. J Exp Clin Cancer Res. 2009;28:87.

389. Carlier T, Jamet B, Bailly C, Touzeau C, Moreau P, Bodet-Milin C. Preliminary results of prognostic added value of PET textural features at diagnosis in multiple myeloma with a long-term follow-up. In:

7th international workshop on PET in lymphoma and myeloma, 2018.

390. Gensure RH, Foran DJ, Lee VM, Gendel VM, Jabbour SK, Carpizo DR, et al. Evaluation of hepatic tumor response to Yttrium-90 radioembolization therapy using texture signatures generated from contrast-enhanced CT images. Acad Radiol. 2012;19(10):1201–7.

391. Mehta R, Cai K, Kumar N, Knuttinen MG, Anderson TM, Lu H, et al. A lesion-based response prediction model using pretherapy PET/CT image features for Y90 radioembolization to hepatic malignancies. Technol Cancer Res Treat. 2017;16(5):620–9.

392. McLaughlin J, Han G, Schalper KA, Carvajal-Hausdorf D, Pelekanou V, Rehman J, et al. Quantitative assessment of the heterogeneity of PD-L1 expression in non-small-cell lung cancer. JAMA Oncol. 2016;2(1):46–54.

393. Carbone DP, Reck M, Paz-Ares L, Creelan B, Horn L, Steins M, et al. First-line nivolumab in stage IV or recurrent non-small-cell lung cancer. N Engl J Med. 2017;376:2415–26.

394. Tang C, Hobbs B, Amer A, Li X, Behrens C, Canales JR, et al. Development of an immune-pathology informed radiomics model for non-small cell lung cancer. Sci Rep. 2018;8:1922.

395. Sun R, Limkin EJ, Vakalopoulou M, Dercle L, Champiat S, Han SR, et al. A radiomics approach to assess tumour-infiltrating CD8 cells and response to anti-PD-1 or anti-PD-L1 immunotherapy: an imaging biomarker, retrospective multicohort study. Lancet Oncol. 2018;19(9):1180–91.

396. Mayerhoefer M, Riedel C, Schöder H. Radiomic features of glucose metabolism enable prediction of bone marrow involvement in mantle cell lymphoma. Eur J Nucl Med Mol Imaging. 2019;46(1):S139.

397. Sollini M, Kirienko M, Cozzi L, Torrisi C, Antunovic LE, et al. Value of FDG-PET/CT radiomic features in predicting response to anti-programmed death 1 (PD-1) antibodies treatment in refractory Hodgkin Lymphoma patients. Eur J Nucl Med Mol Imaging. 2019;46(1):S154.

398. Banna GL, Olivier T, Rundo F, Malapelle U, Fraggetta F, Libra M, et al. The promise of digital biopsy for the prediction of tumor molecular features and clinical outcomes associated with immunotherapy. Front Med. 2019;6:172.

399. Cazaentre T, Morschhauser F, Vermandel M, Betrouni N, Prangère T, Petyt G, et al. Pre-therapy 18F-FDG PET quantitative parameters help in predicting the response to radioimmunotherapy in non-Hodgkin lymphoma. Med Nucl. 2010;37(3):494–504.

400. Xu L, Tetteh G, Lipkova J, Zhao Y, Li H, Christ P, et al. Automated whole-body bone lesion detection for multiple myeloma on 68 Ga-Pentixafor PET/CT imaging using deep learning methods. Contrast Media Mol Imaging. 2018;2018:2391925.

401. Huang D, Swanson EA, Lin CP, Schuman JS, Stinson WG, Chang W, et al. Optical coherence tomography. Science. 1991;254(5035):1178–81.

402. Shields CL, Materin MA, Shields JA. Review of optical coherence tomography for intraocular tumors. Curr Opin Ophthalmol. 2005;16:141–54.

403. Gao S, Zhou Y, Jin X, Lin Z, Zhong Y, Shen X. Primary vitreoretinal natural killer/T-cell lymphoma with breast involvement: a case report and review of the literature. Surv Ophthalmol. 2019;64:225–32.

404. Say EAT, Shah SU, Ferenczy S, Shields CL. Optical coherence tomography of retinal and choroidal tumors. J Ophthalmol. 2012;2012:385058.

405. Saito T, Ohguro N, Iwahashi C, Hashida N. Optical coherence tomography manifestations of primary vitreoretinal lymphoma. Graefes Arch Clin Exp Ophthalmol. 2016;254(12):2319–26.

406. Lavine JA, Singh AD, Sharma S, Baynes K, Lowder CY, Srivastava SK. Ultra-widefield multimodal imaging of primary vitreoretinal lymphoma. Retina. 2019;39(10):1861–71.

407. Barry RJ, Tasiopoulou A, Murray PI, Patel PJ, Sagoo MS, Denniston AK, et al. Characteristic optical coherence tomography findings in patients with primary vitreoretinal lymphoma: a novel aid to early diagnosis. Br J Ophthalmol. 2018;102(10):1362–6.

408. Zhao H, Wang X, Mao Y, Peng X. Longitudinal observation of OCT imaging is a valuable tool to monitor primary vitreoretinal lymphoma treated with intravitreal injections of methotrexate. BMC Ophthalmol. 2020;20(1):10.

409. Deák GG, Goldstein DA, Zhou M, Fawzi AA, Jampol LM. Vertical hyperreflective lesions on optical coherence tomography in vitreoretinal lymphoma. JAMA Ophthalmol. 2019;137(2):194–8.

410. Miederer M, McDevitt MR, Sgouros G, Kramer K, Cheung NKV, Scheinberg DA. Pharmacokinetics, dosimetry, and toxicity of the targetable atomic generator,225Ac-HuM195, in nonhuman primates. J Nucl Med. 2004;45(1):129–37.

411. McDevitt MR, Finn RD, Ma D, Larson SM, Scheinberg DA. Preparation of α-emitting 213Bi-labeled antibody constructs for clinical use. J Nucl Med. 1999;40(10):1722–7.

412. Zalutsky MR, Schuster JM, Garg PK, Archer GE, Dewhirst MW, Bigner DD. Two approaches for enhancing radioimmunotherapy: alpha emitters and hyperthermia. Recent Results Cancer Res. 1996;141:101–22.

413. Zalutsky MR, Garg PK, Friedman HS, Bigner DD. Labeling monoclonal antibodies and F(ab')2 fragments with the α-particle-emitting nuclide astatine-211: preservation of immunoreactivity and in vivo localizing capacity. Proc Natl Acad Sci U S A. 1989;86(18):7149–53.

414. Couturier O, Supiot S, Degraef-Mougin M, Faivre-Chauvet A, Carlier T, Chatal JF, et al. Cancer radioimmunotherapy with alpha-emitting nuclides. Eur J Nucl Med Mol Imag. 2005;32:601–14.

415. Vandenbulcke K, De Vos F, Offner F, Philippé J, Apostolidis C, Molinet R, et al. In vitro evaluation of 213Bi-rituximab versus external gamma irradiation for the treatment of B-CLL patients: relative biologi-

cal efficacy with respect to apoptosis induction and chromosomal damage. Eur J Nucl Med Mol Imaging. 2003;30(10):1357–64.

416. Aurlien E, Larsen RH, Kvalheim G, Bruland S. Demonstration of highly specific toxicity of the α-emitting radioimmunoconjugate 211At-rituximab against non-Hodgkin's lymphoma cells. Br J Cancer. 2000;83(10):1375–9.

417. Dahle J, Borrebæk J, Jonasdottir TJ, Hjelmerud AK, Melhus KB, Bruland ØS, et al. Targeted cancer therapy with a novel low-dose rate α-emitting radioimmunoconjugate. Blood. 2007;110(6):2049–56.

418. Suominen MI, Rissanen JP, Luostarinen A, Fagerlund KM, Sjöholm B, Alhoniemi E, et al. Abstract 5202: Additive benefits of radium-223 dichloride and bortezomib combination in a syngeneic 5TGM1 multiple myeloma mouse model. In: American Association for Cancer Research (AACR); 2017. p. 5202.

419. Beyer GJ, Miederer M, Vranješ-Durić S, Čomor JJ, Künzi G, Hartley O, et al. Targeted alpha therapy in vivo: direct evidence for single cancer cell kill using 149Tb-rituximab. Eur J Nucl Med Mol Imaging. 2004;31(4):547–54.

420. Jurcic JG, Larson SM, Sgouros G, McDevitt MR, Finn RD, Divgi CR, et al. Targeted α particle immunotherapy for myeloid leukemia. Blood. 2002;100:1233–9.

421. Charlton DE, Booz J. A Monte Carlo treatment of the decay of 125 I. Radiat Res. 1981;87(1):10–23.

422. Behr TM, Béhé M, Löhr M, Sgouros G, Angerstein C, Wehrmann E, et al. Therapeutic advantages of auger electron-over β-emitting radiometals or radioiodine when conjugated to internalizing antibodies. Eur J Nucl Med. 2000;27(7):753–65.

423. McDougall IR, Greig WR. 125I therapy in Graves' disease. Long term results in 355 patients. Ann Intern Med. 1976;85(6):720–3.

424. Bousis C, Emfietzoglou D, Nikjoo H. Monte Carlo single-cell dosimetry of I-131, I-125 and I-123 for targeted radioimmunotherapy of B-cell lymphoma. Int J Radiat Biol. 2012;88:908–15.

425. Goldenberg DM, Sharkey RM. Advances in cancer therapy with radiolabeled monoclonal antibodies. Q J Nucl Med Mol Imaging. 2006;50(4):248–64.

426. Michel RB, Andrews PM, Rosario AV, Goldenberg DM, Mattes MJ. 177Lu-antibody conjugates for single-cell kill of B-lymphoma cells in vitro and for therapy of micrometastases in vivo. Nucl Med Biol. 2005;32(3):269–78.

427. Poschenrieder A, Schottelius M, Osl T, Schwaiger M, Wester H-J. [64Cu]NOTA-pentixather enables high resolution PET imaging of CXCR4 expression in a preclinical lymphoma model. EJNMMI Radiopharm Chem. 2017;2(1):2.

428. Kang L, Jiang D, Wei W, NI D, Ferreira C, Engle J, et al. In vivo PET imaging of CD20 using 64Cu-labeled F(ab)2 fragment of obinumumab in lymphoma models. J Nucl Med. 2018;59(1):1123.

429. Weichert JP, Clark PA, Kandela IK, Vaccaro AM, Clarke W, Longino MA, et al. Alkylphosphocholine analogs for broad-spectrum cancer imaging and therapy. Sci Transl Med. 2014;6(240):240ra75.

430. Longcor J, Ailawadhi S, Oliver K, Callander N, Stiff P. CLR 131 demonstrates high rate of activity in a phase 1, dose escalation study in patients with relapsed or refractory multiple myeloma (RRMM). In: Poster SP-305, 17th international Myeloma workshop (IMW), Boston, Massachusetts, 2019.

431. Park F. Cellectar reports positive top-line response rate of 30% from R/R multiple myeloma cohort in ongoing phase 2 study of CLR 131. Cellectar Biosciences. 2019.

432. Grudzinski J, Marsh I, Titz B, Jeffery J, Longino M, Kozak K, et al. CLR 125 Auger electrons for the targeted radiotherapy of triple-negative breast cancer. Cancer Biother Radiopharm. 2018;33(3):87–95.

433. Kratochwil C, Flechsig P, Lindner T, Abderrahim L, Altmann A, Mier W, et al. 68Ga-FAPI PET/CT: tracer uptake in 28 different kinds of cancer. J Nucl Med. 2019;60(6):801–5.

434. Goldenberg DM, Horowitz JA, Sharkey RM, Hall TC, Murthy S, Goldenberg H, et al. Targeting, dosimetry, and radioimmunotherapy of B-cell lymphomas with iodine-131-labeled LL2 monoclonal antibody. J Clin Oncol. 1991;9(4):548–64.

435. Leung SO, Goldenberg DM, Dion AS, Pellegrini MC, Shevitz J, Shih LB, et al. Construction and characterization of a humanized, internalizing, B-cell (CD22)-specific, leukemia/lymphoma antibody, LL2. Mol Immunol. 1995;32(17–18):1413–27.

436. Lindén O, Hindorf C, Cavallin-Ståhl E, Wegener WA, Goldenberg DM, Horne H, et al. Dose-fractionated radioimmunotherapy in non-Hodgkin's lymphoma using DOTA-conjugated, 90Y-radiollabeled, humanized anti-CD22 monoclonal antibody, epratuzumab. Clin Cancer Res. 2005;15(11):5215–22.

437. Stein R, Qu Z, Chen S, Rosario A, Shi V, Hayes M, et al. Characterization of a new humanized anti-CD20 monoclonal antibody, IMMU-106, and its use in combination with the humanized anti-CD22 antibody, epratuzumab, for the therapy of non-Hodgkin's lymphoma. Clin Cancer Res. 2004;10(8):2868–78.

438. Mattes MJ, Sharkey RM, Karacay H, Czuczman MS, Goldenberg DM. Therapy of advanced B-lymphoma xenografts with a combination of 90Y-anti-CD22 IgG (epratuzumab) and unlabeled anti-CD20 IgG (veltuzumab). Clin Cancer Res. 2008;14(19): 6154–60.

439. Kraeber-Bodere F, Pallardy A, Maisonneuve H, Campion L, Moreau A, Soubeyran I, et al. Consolidation anti-CD22 fractionated radioimmunotherapy with 90Y-epratuzumab tetraxetan following R-CHOP in elderly patients with diffuse large B-cell lymphoma: a prospective, single group, phase 2 trial. Lancet Haematol. 2017;4(1):e35–45.

440. Waldmann TA. The structure, function, and expression of interleukin-2 receptors on normal and malignant lymphocytes. Science. 1986;232(4751):727–32.

441. Waldmann TA, Goldman CK, Bongiovanni KF, Sharrow SO, Davey MP, Cease KB, et al. Therapy

of patients with human T-cell lymphotrophic virus I-induced adult T-cell leukemia with anti-Tac, a monoclonal antibody to the receptor for interleukin-2. Blood. 1988;72(5):1805–16.

442. Waldmann TA, White JD, Carrasquillo JA, Reynolds JC, Paik CH, Gansow OA, et al. Radioimmunotherapy of interleukin-2Rα-expressing adult T-cell leukemia with Yttrium-90-labeled anti-Tac. Blood. 1995;86(11):4063–75.

443. Kreitman RJ, Wilson WH, White JD, Stetler-Stevenson M, Jaffe ES, Giardina S, et al. Phase I trial of recombinant immunotoxin anti-Tac(Fv)-PE38 (LMB-2) in patients with hematologic malignancies. J Clin Oncol. 2000;18(8):1622–36.

444. Janik JE, Morris JC, O'Mahony D, Pittaluga S, Jaffe ES, Redon CE, et al. 90Y-daclizumab, an anti-CD25 monoclonal antibody, provided responses in 50% of patients with relapsed Hodgkin's lymphoma. Proc Natl Acad Sci U S A. 2015;112(42):13045–50.

445. Erba PA, Sollini M, Orciuolo E, Traino C, Petrini M, Paganelli G, et al. Radioimmunotherapy with radretumab in patients with relapsed hematologic malignancies. J Nucl Med. 2012;53(6):922–7.

446. Gopal AK, Tarantolo SR, Bellam N, Green DJ, Griffin M, Feldman T, et al. Phase 1b study of otlertuzumab (TRU-016), an anti-CD37 monospecific ADAPTIR™ therapeutic protein, in combination with rituximab and bendamustine in relapsed indolent lymphoma patients. Investig New Drugs. 2014;32(6):1213–25.

447. Robak T, Hellmann A, Kloczko J, Loscertales J, Lech-Maranda E, Pagel JM, et al. Randomized phase 2 study of otlertuzumab and bendamustine versus bendamustine in patients with relapsed chronic lymphocytic leukaemia. Br J Haematol. 2017;176(4):618–28.

448. Heider KH, Kiefer K, Zenz T, Volden M, Stilgenbauer S, Ostermann E, et al. A novel Fc-engineered monoclonal antibody to CD37 with enhanced ADCC and high proapoptotic activity for treatment of B-cell malignancies. Blood. 2011;118(15):4159–68.

449. Kolstad A, Madsbu U, Beasley M, Bayne M, Illidge TM, O'Rourke N, et al. 177 Lu-Lilotomab satetraxetan, a novel CD37-targeted antibody-radionuclide conjugate in relapsed non-Hodgkin's lymphoma (NHL): updated results of an ongoing phase I/II study (LYMRIT 37-01). Blood. 2017;130(Suppl 1):2769.

450. Kolstad A, Madsbu U, Beasley M, Bayne M, Illidge TM, O'Rourke N, et al. LYMRIT 37-01: a phase I/II study of 177lu-Lilotomab Satetraxetan (Betalutin®) antibody-radionuclide-conjugate (ARC) for the treatment of relapsed non-Hodgkin's lymphoma (NHL) — analysis with 6-month follow-up. Blood. 2018;132(Suppl 1):2879.

451. Stokke C, Blakkisrud J, Løndalen A, Dahle J, Martinsen ACT, Holte H, et al. Pre-dosing with lilotomab prior to therapy with 177Lu-lilotomab satetraxetan significantly increases the ratio of tumor to red marrow absorbed dose in non-Hodgkin lymphoma patients. Eur J Nucl Med Mol Imaging. 2018;45(7):1233–41.

452. Repetto-Llamazares AHV, Malenge MM, O'Shea A, Eiríksdóttir B, Stokke T, Larsen RH, et al. Combination of 177Lu-lilotomab with rituximab significantly improves the therapeutic outcome in preclinical models of non-Hodgkin's lymphoma. Eur J Haematol. 2018;101(4):522–31.

453. Hicks SW, Lai KC, Gavrilescu LC, Yi Y, Sikka S, Shah P, et al. The antitumor activity of IMGN529, a CD37-targeting antibody-drug conjugate, is potentiated by rituximab in non-Hodgkin lymphoma models. Neoplasia (United States). 2017;19(9):661–71.

454. Malenge MM, Patzke S, Ree AH, Stokke T, Ceuppens P, Middleton B, et al. 177 Lu-lilotomab satetraxetan has the potential to counteract resistance to rituximab in non-Hodgkin's lymphoma. J Nucl Med. 2020; https://doi.org/10.2967/jnumed.119.237230.

455. Kato H. History of photodynamic therapy-past, present and future. Gan To Kagaku Ryoho. 1996;23(1):8–15.

456. von Tappeiner H, Joldlbauer A. The sensitizing action of fluorescent substances. An overall account of investigations on photodynamic phenomena. Lepzig: Vogel FCW; 1907.

457. Dougherty TJ. A brief history of clinical photodynamic therapy development at Roswell Park Cancer Institute. J Clin Laser Med Surg. 1996;14(5):219–21.

458. Allison RR, Bagnato VS, Sibata CH. Future of oncologic photodynamic therapy. Future Oncol (Lond, Engl). 2010;6:929–40.

459. Eich D, Eich HT, Otte H-G, Ghilescu V, Stadler R. Photodynamische therapie kutaner T-Zell-lymphome in besonderer lokalisation. Hautarzt. 1999;50(2):109–14.

460. Orenstein A, Haik J, Tamir J, Winkler E, Trau H, Malik Z, et al. Photodynamic therapy of cutateneous lymphoma using 5-aminolevulinic acid topical application. Dermatol Surg. 2000;26(8):765–70.

461. Díez Recio E, Zambrano B, Alonso ML, De Eusebio E, Martín M, Cuevas J, et al. Topical 5-aminolevulinic acid photodynamic therapy for the treatment of unilesional mycosis fungoides: a report of two cases and review of the literature. Int J Dermatol. 2008;47(4):410–3.

462. Pileri A, Sgubbi P, Agostinelli C, Infusino SD, Vaccari S, Patrizi A. Photodynamic therapy: an option in mycosis fungoides. Photodiagn Photodyn Ther. 2017;20:107–10.

463. Mori M, Campolmi P, Mavilia L, Rossi R, Cappugi P, Pimpinelli N. Topical photodynamic therapy for primary cutaneous B-cell lymphoma: a pilot study. J Am Acad Dermatol. 2006;54(3):524–6.

464. Coors EA, Von Den Driesch P. Topical photodynamic therapy for patients with therapy-resistant lesions of cutaneous T-cell lymphoma. J Am Acad Dermatol. 2004;50(3):363–7.

465. Quéreux G, Brocard A, Saint-Jean M, Peuvrel L, Knol AC, Allix R, et al. Photodynamic therapy

with methyl-aminolevulinic acid for paucilesional mycosis fungoides: a prospective open study and review of the literature. J Am Acad Dermatol. 2013;69(6):890–7.

466. Kim ST, Kang DY, Kang JS, Baek JW, Jeon YS, Suh KS. Photodynamic therapy with methyl-aminolaevulinic acid for mycosis fungoides. Acta Derm Venereol. 2012;92(3):264–8.

467. Salva KA, Kim YH, Rahbar Z, Wood GS. Epigenetically enhanced PDT induces significantly higher levels of multiple extrinsic pathway apoptotic factors than standard PDT, resulting in greater extrinsic and overall apoptosis of cutaneous T-cell lymphoma. Photochem Photobiol. 2018;94(5):1058–65.

468. Chemotherapy and photodynamic therapy in treating patients with cutaneous T-cell lymphoma—F. 2003. ClinicalTrials.gov.

469. Soligenix I. Soligenix announces positive top-line results for its pivotal phase 3 FLASH trial evaluating SGX301 in treatment of cutaneous T-cell lymphoma [news release].

470. Andrade-Campos MM, Montes-Limón AE, Soro-Alcubierre G, Lievano P, López-Gómez L, Baringo T, et al. Patients older than 65 years with non-Hodgkin lymphoma are suitable for treatment with 90yttrium-ibritumumab tiuxetan: a single-institution experience. Clin Lymphoma Myeloma Leuk. 2015;15(8):464–71.

471. Otte A, Thompson SL. Practical and clinical benefits of radioimmunotherapy lead to advantages in cost-effectiveness in the treatment of patients with non-hodgkin's lymphoma. Nucl Med Commun. 2006;27:753–6.

472. Schaefer NG, Ma J, Huang P, Buchanan J, Wahl RL. Radioimmunotherapy in non-Hodgkin lymphoma: opinions of U.S. medical oncologists and hematologists. J Nucl Med. 2010;51(6):987–94.

473. Chen Q, Ayer T, Nastoupil LJ, Rose AC, Flowers CR. Comparing the cost-effectiveness of rituximab maintenance and radioimmunotherapy consolidation versus observation following first-line therapy in patients with follicular lymphoma. Value Health. 2015;18(2):189–97.

474. Schaefer NG, Huang P, Buchanan JW, Wahl RL. Radioimmunotherapy in non-Hodgkin lymphoma: opinions of nuclear medicine physicians and radiation oncologists. J Nucl Med. 2011;52(5):830–8.

Radioimmunotherapy of Acute Leukemia

17

Roland B. Walter and Johnnie Orozco

Contents

R. B. Walter (✉)
Clinical Research Division, Fred Hutchinson Cancer Research Center, Seattle, WA, USA

Division of Hematology, Department of Medicine, University of Washington, Seattle, WA, USA
e-mail: rwalter@fredhutch.org

J. Orozco
Clinical Research Division, Fred Hutchinson Cancer Research Center, Seattle, WA, USA

Division of Medical Oncology, Department of Medicine, University of Washington, Seattle, WA, USA
e-mail: jorozco@fredhutch.org

17.1 Introduction

Allogeneic hematopoietic cell transplantation (HCT) may provide the best curative potential for aggressive hematologic malignancies such as acute myeloid leukemias and myelodysplastic syndromes (MDS). However, HCT outcomes for patients with high-risk leukemias or MDS are not optimal and are significantly inferior to outcomes for patients with more favorable risk disease, largely because of higher rates of relapse after HCT for high-risk disease. Therefore, approaches

© Springer Nature Switzerland AG 2022
S. Harsini et al. (eds.), *Nuclear Medicine and Immunology*,
https://doi.org/10.1007/978-3-030-81261-4_17

to increase the cytotoxic effect from treatment have been investigated to decrease the rates of relapse. Because hematologic malignancies are exquisitely sensitive to radiation, increased doses of total body irradiation (TBI) in conditioning chemotherapy regimens for HCT have indeed decreased relapse rates, but this has been associated with increases in treatment-related toxicities and mortality, resulting in no net survival benefit. Targeted radiation delivery via radioimmunotherapy, or target-specific antibodies labeled with radionuclides, has been developed to deliver radiation to sites of disease while sparing normal organs to mitigate some of the toxicities from higher TBI doses on normal organs. In this chapter, we describe some of these RIT efforts to improve outcomes of HCT for high-risk leukemias and MDS, the acute myeloid leukemia (AML)-related targets that have been pursued to deliver radiation to sites of disease, as well as the relative merits and limitations of investigated radionuclides, including alpha- and beta-emitters. To close, novel preclinical studies to improve the efficacy of RIT such as pretargeted RIT approaches are reviewed.

17.2 Leukemia-Associated Target Antigens for RIT

17.2.1 Ideal Characteristics for RIT Targets

The ideal target for leukemia-directed RIT has a variety of desired characteristics. To minimize off-target toxicity, the target antigen should be expressed selectively on the cell surface of tumor cells but not on normal cells or tissues. Expression on tumor cells at high copy number should maximize the accumulation of radioimmunoconjugates at the target tissues or cells [1]. Ideally, the antigen is neither internalized (as this may reduce its cell surface density) nor shed. If the number of binding sites is relatively low (say, less than 10,000/cell), saturation may occur at lower radioimmunoconjugate doses. However, as each antibody can be labeled with a limited number of radionuclides before target binding or immunoreactivity is compromised, and many antibody mol-

ecules are in fact not conjugated with radionuclides, RIT efficacy may be reduced. Lower cell surface densities of target antigens are less problematic for alpha- than beta-emitters. This is because for lethal DNA damage to occur, fewer high-energy alpha-particles than beta-particles are required to bind to the target cell. In addition to leading to reduced binding site availability, internalization of target antigens may also impact the efficacy and/or toxicity of bound radioimmunoconjugates. For iodine-131 (^{131}I)-labeled antibodies, this is problematic because of rapid lysosomal metabolism and release of free iodine-131 and/or [^{131}I]I-tyrosine [2, 3]. This contrasts with antibodies labeled with the radiometals yttrium-90 (^{90}Y) and lutetium-177 (^{177}Lu) that retain cationic metabolites within lysosomes [4].

17.2.2 Leukemia-Associated Antigen Targets

While the ideal target may be difficult to find for RIT of acute leukemias, lineage-specific cell surface antigens have been effectively pursued for this purpose. Particularly for beta-emitter-based RIT, delivering a radiation payload to hematopoietic antigens or myeloid or lymphoid differentiation antigens may increase the likelihood of destroying neoplastic hematopoietic cells because of bystander effects, i.e., radiation from nearby antigen-positive cells that have bound radioimmunoconjugates [5]. Because of its broad expression on at least a subset of AML blasts in almost all patients, and possibly expression on underlying leukemia stem cells in some, CD33 was one of the earliest RIT targets for the treatment of acute leukemia. As a myeloid differentiation antigen, however, its expression is not AML specific. Rather, CD33 is also displayed on normal immature and mature myeloid cells. Initial RIT applications with iodine-131 were limited by the short residence time of ^{131}I-anti-CD33 radioimmunoconjugates after endocytosis and catabolism. As will be highlighted, CD33 has met more success when targeted with alpha-emitters.

As stably expressed myeloid cell surface proteins, CD66 antigens have also been explored as targets for RIT. CD66 antigens are found on members of the carcinoembryonic-antigen-related cell-adhesion molecule (CEACAM) family of proteins that play a role in cellular adhesion and signaling important for cell growth and differentiation [6]. Some of these targets, CD66a, CD66b, CD66c, and CD66d, are expressed on hematopoietic cells but are also expressed on epithelial or endothelial cells. CD66 targets are found on myeloid cells, from late myeloblast or early promyelocyte to metamyelocyte stages, but not on early myeloid precursors or hematopoietic stem cells [7, 8]. CD66 antigens are only occasionally found on AML blasts.

A broader pan-hematopoietic-specific target, CD45, is expressed on nearly all hematopoietic cells except mature erythrocytes and platelets and some of their precursors. This cell surface glycoprotein with tyrosine phosphatase activity is expressed on most hematologic malignancies, including 85–90% of acute leukemias [9–11]. CD45 is expressed at a high copy number (~200,000/cell) with limited internalization and no substantive shedding after ligand binding. Although several CD45 isoforms exist, antibodies capable of binding all isoforms have been successfully developed for RIT. Because CD45 is expressed on both benign and malignant cells, anti-CD45 antibodies labeled with an appropriate long effective path-length radionuclide will cause bystander effects and allow killing of CD45-negative neoplastic cells if surrounded by normal CD45-expressing hematopoietic cells.

17.2.3 Antibody Binding Kinetics

In addition to target expression patterns, antibody avidity and binding kinetics are other considerations for optimal target choice. The extent of immunoreactivity will impact the concentration of radiation payload and targeting of radiation; antibodies with low immunoreactivity may not focus radiation at target sites, resulting in non-specific biodistribution patterns. On the other hand, high-avidity binding could be disadvantageous if the radiation dose cannot be adequately managed. When RIT is used in conjunction with HCT, concentrating high doses of radiation to the marrow may be tolerable because of the hemato-

poietic rescue with the stem cell graft, but in non-HCT settings, ensuing myelosuppression could be dose limiting.

The strength of antibody-target interactions is captured through avidity, and initially for RIT applications, high-avidity antibodies were thought to be ideal. However, radiolabeled antibodies with high avidity were found to preferentially bind peripherally at readily accessible sites. As shown in nonhuman primate models, antibodies with lower avidity circulated slightly longer and yielded higher uptakes in less accessible sites such as lymph nodes [12].

Another strategy to increase radioimmunoconjugate uptake at less accessible sites is to use antibody fragments. Smaller antibody fragments, whether produced by enzymatic digestion into Fab or F[ab′]₂ or molecular cloning approaches, can more readily diffuse into tumor sites [13, 14]. Unfortunately, their smaller size results in faster clearance compared to regular antibodies, which may limit retention times and uptake at target sites [15–17].

A final consideration is the origin of the antibody. Many antibodies used for RIT are of murine origin and have the potential to elicit an immunological response with the production of a therapy neutralizing human anti-mouse antibody (HAMA). Although many patients with hematologic malignancies may have an altered, dysfunctional immune system, they may still be able to produce HAMA within a matter of weeks after antibody exposure, precluding the possibility of repeat RIT administration. Strategies to minimize the production of HAMAs include the use of fully human, humanized, or chimeric antibodies or antibody fragments.

17.3 Types of Radionuclides

17.3.1 Beta-Emitters

A variety of radionuclide properties such as ease of antibody conjugation chemistry, and decay characteristics like type of particle emitted and their associated effective path lengths and decay energies need consideration for RIT (Table 17.1). The majority of initial efforts with RIT to treat

Table 17.1 RIT radionuclides and their characteristics

Element	Isotope	Particle(s) emitted	Half-life ($t_{1/2}$)	Path length	Median decay energy (MeV)
Iodine-131	^{131}I	β, γ	8 days	0.8 mm	0.66 (β)
Yttrium-90	^{90}Y	β	2.7 days	2.7 mm	2.3 (β)
Lutetium-177	^{177}Lu	β, γ	6.7 days	0.9 mm	0.5 (β)
Rhenium-188	^{188}Re	β, γ	17 h	2.4 mm	2.1 (β)
Copper-67	^{67}Cu	β	2.6 days	0.4–0.8 mm	0.6 (β)
Bismuth-213	^{213}Bi	1α, 2β	46 min	84 µm	5.8 (α)
Astatine-211	^{211}At	1α	7.2 h	60 µm	5.9 (α)
Actinium-225	^{225}Ac	4α, 2β	10 days	50–80 µm	5.8–8.4 (α)

leukemias took advantage of a radionuclide previously used in medical settings, iodine-131 (^{131}I). Iodine-131 decays via beta-particles and gamma rays, with a beta-decay energy of 0.66 MeV and a half-life of 8.1 days. Compared to other radionuclides, iodine-131 is relatively abundant and inexpensive to produce, helping its popularity and detailed characterization with regard to methods to conjugate it to proteins and antibodies. The gamma component of iodine-131 enables imaging that can be used for dosimetry to tailor individualized radiation doses. Iodine-131 was extensively studied as RIT for non-Hodgkin lymphoma (NHL) and received regulatory approval in the form of tositumomab, a ^{131}I-labeled anti-CD20 antibody, for the treatment of relapsed or refractory B-cell NHL [18]. Unfortunately, tositumomab was discontinued and marketing approval withdrawn in February 2014 for a variety of reasons. Iodine-131 has important limitations, most notably the need for radiation isolation for patients treated at high therapeutic doses because of the high-energy gamma rays (364 keV) that pose a safety risk to caregivers and healthcare professionals. In addition, internalized ^{131}I-labeled antibodies can be metabolized, leading to the release of [^{131}I] I-tyrosine and/or free iodine-131 which will decrease the residence time of the radionuclide at its target site and its therapeutic efficacy [3, 19].

To address some of the shortcomings of iodine-131, yttrium-90 (^{90}Y) has been studied as alternative for RIT. The radiometal yttrium-90 decays by emitting beta-particles that have a higher decay energy (2.3 MeV) than iodine-131. Compared to iodine-131, yttrium-90 has a shorter half-life (2.7 days) and deposits energy over a longer path length. Because of these properties, yttrium-90 was incorporated into the only other FDA-approved RIT drug, [^{90}Y]ibritumomab, similarly targeting CD20. Unlike iodine-131, yttrium-90 is considered a pure beta-emitter and hence does not require radiation isolation, but lack of gamma decay also precludes imaging via gamma cameras. Instead, dosimetry studies require the use of a surrogate radionuclide, indium-111 (^{111}In), which emits gamma rays. Yttrium-90 is less abundant than iodine-131 and therefore more costly. As another disadvantage, unless stably conjugated to targeting protein, free ^{90}Y can accumulate in the liver and bone [20].

Because of the interest in imaging for dosimetry purposes and tailoring radiation doses to individual patients, the lanthanide radiometal lutetium-177 (^{177}Lu) is another radionuclide that has been explored for RIT applications as an alternative to iodine-131. These radionuclides share some similarities: the decay energy of the beta-emission of lutetium-177 (0.5 MeV) is comparable to that of iodine-131 (0.66 MeV), as are the decay half-lives (6.7 days for lutetium-177 and 8.1 days for iodine-131) and path lengths (0.9 mm for lutetium-177 and 0.8 mm for iodine-131). As a major difference, lutetium-177 does not emit high-energy gamma rays that would require radiation isolation as with high-dose iodine-131 therapies. Still, low-energy gamma emission makes lutetium-177 amenable to gamma camera imaging for dosimetry calculations. Finally, ^{177}Lu-labeled radioimmunoconjugates can be produced at high specific activity (i.e., high relative ratio of radioactivity to the amount of carrier protein), rendering lutetium-177 appealing when the delivery of high amounts of radiation is desired.

Rhenium-188 (^{188}Re) is another beta-emitting radionuclide that, like lutetium-177, has a high decay energy from beta-emissions (2.1 MeV) but lower-energy gamma rays that can be exploited for imaging. Its conjugation chemistry is well understood, and its short half-life of 17 h can support therapeutic applications. Its effective path length of 2.4 mm is comparable to the path length of yttrium-90. Despite these characteristics, its limited availability makes large-scale applications challenging. Like the radiometals yttrium-90 and lutetium-177 that are retained intracellularly after internalization, copper-67 (^{67}Cu) is a radionuclide with both therapeutic beta-emissions (0.57 MeV) and photon emissions that can be imaged via positron emission tomography (PET). The half-life of copper-67 (2.6 days) is comparable to that of yttrium-90. Since its path length is shorter (0.4–0.8 mm), the potential for off-target cell toxicities may be reduced. However, limited availability and high costs associated with copper radionuclides have impeded rapid research advances and therapeutic applications.

17.3.2 Alpha-Emitters

Unlike beta-emitters that decay via electrons and/or energy waves, alpha-emitters are radionuclides that decay via the release of a helium nucleus. The substantially higher mass of alpha-particles, about 7000 times that of beta-particles, translates into more powerful decay energies in the order of 3–13 times that of beta-emitters and higher linear energy transfer (LET), i.e., the number of ionizations per unit distance traveled by the decay particle. Deposition of higher amounts of energy over shorter path lengths (usually <0.1 mm) because of the interference from the mass of the alpha-particle translates into higher LET for alpha-emitters (~100 keV/μm) than beta-emitters (~0.2 keV/μm). Higher LETs and shorter path lengths are responsible for more effective cell kill of alpha-emitters compared to beta-emitters and better sparing of surrounding non-targeted cells

and tissues. Consequently, alpha-emitters do not produce a bystander effect. Hence, conceptually, they may be more ideal than beta-emitters for the specific eradication of individual tumor cells or small tumor cell clusters, as may be seen in individuals with leukemia and low residual disease burden. On the other hand, they may be less suited for the treatment of bulky tumors, e.g., lymphomas or solid tumors [21, 22].

A small number of alpha-emitters have been investigated for RIT, including bismuth-213 (^{213}Bi), astatine-211 (^{211}At), and actinium-225 (^{225}Ac). The higher decay energies of bismuth-213 and astatine-211 (5.84 and 5.87 MeV average, respectively) are among the highest studied for RIT and render them particularly appealing for the eradication of measurable ("minimal") residual disease (MRD). While bismuth-213 and astatine-211 have short half-lives (45.6 min and 7.2 h, respectively), actinium-225 has a longer half-life (10 days) and decays via the production of four daughter alpha-particles. This can be problematic when considering patient applications. Beyond use as antileukemic therapeutics, these higher-energy alpha-emitters have been studied as replacement for total body irradiation (TBI) for conditioning before allogeneic hematopoietic cell transplantation in canine and murine models [23, 24]. In the latter, bismuth-213 and astatine-211 were compared to each other for their ability to deliver radiation to hematopoietic tissues via CD45, and astatine-211 was found more myelosuppressive and less toxic [25]. While bismuth-213 can be produced by bombarding radium with a linear particle accelerator, efficient production of astatine-211 currently requires a cyclotron, which limits its availability.

17.4 AML-Directed RIT

Early RIT as primary treatment for AML included efforts at Memorial Sloan Kettering Cancer Center (MSKCC) in which CD33 was targeted with a murine antibody (M195) radiolabeled with iodine-131. The initial phase I trial with [^{131}I] I-M195 enrolled 24 patients with AML, MDS, or chronic myeloid leukemia (CML) in blast crisis who were treated with divided doses of the radio-immunoconjugate to maximize antibody delivery to this internalizing antigen [26]. Nearly all patients (90%) had a decrease in peripheral and marrow leukemic blasts. With higher iodine-131 doses, significant cytopenias developed, and 8 patients were thus subjected to autologous or allogeneic HCT.

MSKCC investigators subsequently developed a humanized M195 (HuM195; also known as SGN-CD33 or lintuzumab) antibody to overcome some of the limitations of the parent murine antibody. HuM195 was then conjugated to bismuth-213, and this radioimmunoconjugate was tested in an early study of 18 patients with relapsed or refractory AML or CML [27]. All patients experienced profound myelosuppression and absorbed dose ratios at sites of disease (spleen, bone marrow, and liver) and whole body were 1000-fold higher than what could have been achieved with beta-emitters. Again, most patients experienced a decrease of blasts in the blood (93%) or marrow (78%), but no complete remissions (CRs) were achieved. A maximum tolerated dose was not reached because doses beyond 37 MBq/kg could not be delivered because of limited production capacity and costs.

In another dose-escalation study conducted at MSKCC, 31 patients with untreated or relapsed AML were given [^{213}Bi]-HuM195 following cytarabine [28]. Among the 25 patients treated at or above the MTD, 2 patients achieved a CR, 2 patients achieved a CR with incomplete hematologic recovery (CRi), and 2 patients obtained a partial response for an overall response rate of 24%.

More recently, HuM195 has been conjugated to actinium-225 (^{225}Ac-lintuzumab). In a phase I trial, monotherapy with ^{225}Ac-lintuzumab led to elimination of peripheral blood blasts in 10/16 adults with relapsed/refractory AML, and 3 patients treated with doses ≥0.037 MBq/kg achieved marrow blasts of ≤5% [29, 30]. A subsequent phase I/II study used ^{225}Ac-lintuzumab with low-dose cytarabine (LDAC) in older adults with previously untreated AML. In this trial, a response rate of 69% was observed among 13

patients treated with a dose of 0.074 MBq/kg, providing strong evidence for substantial antileukemic efficacy of alpha-emitter-based RIT. However, consistent with on-target, off-leukemia cell toxicity, many patients suffered from prolonged, severe thrombocytopenia and neutropenia, leading to deaths from infections in some and necessitating reduction to 0.0555 MBq/kg/dose for further evaluation [31]. At 0.0555 MBq/kg/dose, objective responses were much lower (4/18 treated patients) when the study was closed [32]. This observation highlights the importance of on-target, off-leukemia cell toxicities as key clinical limitation of such therapeutics, at least potentially if used without hematopoietic stem cell rescue.

17.5 Incorporating RIT into Transplant Conditioning Regimens for High-Risk Leukemias and MDS

17.5.1 Initial Efforts with Iodine-131

To augment transplant conditioning regimens for patients with high-risk myeloid neoplasms via integration of radioimmunoconjugates, initial studies at the Fred Hutchinson Cancer Research Center (Fred Hutch) used a murine anti-CD33 antibody (P67) conjugated to iodine-131. Only four of the nine patients enrolled in the first trial were found to have a favorable biodistribution of the radiolabeled antibody after dosimetry infusion, with preferential delivery of radiation to the bone marrow and spleen compared to other organs [33]. These patients received a therapeutic dose of ^{131}I-P67 in combination with high-dose cyclophosphamide and myeloablative doses of TBI. While the treatment was well tolerated, three of these four patients subsequently relapsed. Suboptimal residence time of the ^{131}I-anti-CD33 antibody in the marrow due to internalization and metabolism of antibody-receptor complexes with production of free iodine-131 and [^{131}I]I-tyrosine may have contributed to these poor outcomes. While this study was ultimately halted, it proved feasibility and tolerability of RIT in the context of a conditioning regimen before HCT.

Investigators at MSKCC also incorporated anti-CD33 RIT into a conditioning regimen, initially using the 131I-labeled M195 antibody together with myeloablative doses of busulfan and cyclophosphamide. Among 19 patients with relapsed or refractory AML treated with this regimen, engraftment was uniform, and 18 of the 19 patients achieved a decrease in marrow blasts [34]. HAMA responses were noted in 37% of patients. Subsequent studies used ^{131}I-labeled HuM195 instead. Three phase I studies using ^{131}I-HuM195 with busulfan and cyclophosphamide for patients with relapsed/refractory AML ($n = 16$), accelerated or blast phase CML ($n = 14$), or high-risk MDS ($n = 1$) reported a combined median overall survival (OS) of 4.9 months after HCT across all patients [35]. Although myeloablative conditioning with RIT was well tolerated and the RIT component appeared to add little toxicity beyond what could be attributed to the preparative chemotherapy backbone, higher amounts of iodine-131 at higher specific activity negatively impacted binding affinity of the antibody, requiring multiple antibody infusions to achieve delivery of myeloablative doses of radiation to the marrow.

As an alternative to CD33, RIT investigators at Fred Hutch have focused on targeting CD45. In initial studies, a murine anti-CD45 antibody (BC8) was conjugated to iodine-131 and combined with high-dose cyclophosphamide and high-dose TBI before HCT for patients with AML, acute lymphoblastic leukemia (ALL), or MDS [36]. Compared to the prior experience with ^{131}I-labeled anti-CD33 antibodies, ^{131}I-BC8 showed favorable biodistributions in 37 of 41 patients (90%), 34 of whom were able to receive therapeutic doses of the radioimmunoconjugate. Among 25 patients with AML or MDS, 7 were disease-free at 15–89 months (median 65 months) after HCT. Even though patients had received myeloablative doses of TBI together with cyclophosphamide, substantial doses of additional radiation could be delivered to the bone marrow (total estimated average of 24 Gy) and spleen

(total estimated average of 50 Gy) via the radioimmunoconjugate.

Having shown the feasibility and safety of additional targeted radiation delivery via anti-CD45 RIT, ^{131}I-BC8 was then combined with myeloablative doses of busulfan and cyclophosphamide before allogeneic HCT for patients with AML in first CR [37]. As before, the majority of 59 enrollees (88%) showed a favorable biodistribution after dosimetry infusions, and 46 of these then receive a therapeutic dose of the radioimmunoconjugate. Among these 46 patients, the estimated 3-year OS and DFS were 63% and 61%, respectively. ^{131}I-BC8 delivered an average of 11 Gy to the bone marrow and nearly 30 Gy to the spleen. The estimated relapse probability was remarkably low (19% at 3 years) and compared favorably to a control group of 509 patients with AML in first CR from CIBMTR who were conditioned with busulfan and cyclophosphamide. Despite the younger median age of the control patients (28 vs. 39 years), survival was better for patients treated with RIT (hazard ratio = 0.65 [95% confidence interval: 0.39–1.08]; $p = 0.09$).

The intensity of myeloablative conditioning regimens limits their use to younger adults without substantial comorbidities, even without addition of radioimmunoconjugates. Consequently, reduced- or minimal-intensity conditioning regimens have been developed using lower doses of chemotherapy and/or TBI for individuals who are older and/or are medically less fit [38–40]. Such conditioning platforms are amenable to augmentation via RIT. This was demonstrated in a study conducted at Fred Hutch in which adults ≥50 years with AML beyond first remission or MDS with ≥5% marrow blasts were treated with increasing doses of ^{131}I-BC8 in conjunction with minimal-intensity conditioning with fludarabine and 2 Gy TBI [41]. It is worth noting that 86% of the 58 enrolled patients had refractory disease or significant disease burden (>5% blasts in the bone marrow) at the time of transplant and were considered not eligible for standard transplant protocols. All patients achieved a complete response (<5% blasts in the bone marrow) at 1 month after HCT, and all patients showed evidence of engraftment. Despite the older patient age (median 63 years), the day 100 non-relapse mortality rate was relatively low (12% at day 100 and 22% at 1 year). Many of the adverse events observed were attributable to known toxicities of minimal-intensity conditioning. Infusion reactions were the most common side effect of ^{131}I-BC8. In this trial, the maximum tolerated dose of radiation delivered via RIT was estimated to be 24 Gy to the liver as dose-limiting organ, yielding 36 and 102 Gy estimated absorbed radiation dose to the marrow and spleen, respectively. Analyzing outcomes for patients treated at the MTD, the median OS and DFS were estimated to be 206 and 189 days, respectively, with a probability of 1-year survival of 48%.

Based on these encouraging results with ^{131}I-anti-CD45 RIT in older adults with high-risk myeloid neoplasms, a randomized, multicenter phase III trial (SIERRA) was launched to compare Iomab-B (^{131}I-BC8) before HCT in adults ≥55 years of age with relapsed or refractory AML against standard of care (SOC) chemotherapy with the option of crossing over for SOC patients who do not achieve CR with chemotherapy alone (**NCT02665065**). This trial is currently ongoing with no outcomes data reported to date. However, preliminary safety data have been reported, indicating feasibility of this approach [42]. Of the initial 38 patients, 19 were randomized to each arm. As with prior RIT trials, patients had significant disease burden, with a median percentage of bone marrow blasts of 30% and 47% in the Iomab-B and SOC arm, respectively. In the RIT arm, engraftment after HCT with matched related donors did not appear impaired or delayed, with a median time to engraftment of 13 (range: 9–22) days for neutrophils and 17 (range: 13–26) days for platelets. Donor chimerism of ≥95% within 100 days after HCT was achieved in 9 of 10 evaluable patients in the Iomab-B arm and in 8 of 9 evaluable patients who crossed over to RIT after being assigned to the SOC arm. There were no grade ≥3 infusion-related reactions, and the most common non-hematologic grade ≥3 adverse events noted in >10% of patients were neutropenic fever (34.2%), stomatitis (15.8%), and malnutrition (13.2%), all adverse events well described with standard HCT

conditioning therapy. Rapid reductions of peripheral blasts were noted among these initial trial patients. Specifically, among 16 patients with data available (7 from the Iomab-B arm, 9 from crossover to Iomab-B from the SOC arm), peripheral blasts were reduced by 98% on day 3, with 100% reduction on day 8 after Iomab-B infusion [43]. A total of 150 patients are targeted for accrual on this trial to evaluate the primary endpoint of durable complete response rate at 6 months.

While reduced- and minimal-intensity conditioning approaches have traditionally been used primarily for older and less-fit patients, another study assessed the impact of ^{131}I-anti-CD45 RIT before minimal-intensity conditioning with fludarabine and 2 Gy TBI in patients younger than 50 years of age [44]. On this trial, 15 patients with advanced AML or high-risk MDS received escalating doses of ^{131}I-BC8 up to a maximum of 28 Gy delivered to the liver without reaching dose-limiting toxicities. To avoid stromal damage, radiation to the bone marrow was capped at 43 Gy, even though no graft failure as potential evidence of stromal damage was noted. In this younger patient population, the estimated 1-year survival was 73%, with no nonrelapse mortality observed. As in other studies, relapse was the primary cause of treatment failure and was experienced by 8 of the 15 patients, with a median time to relapse of only 54 (range: 26–1364) days, highlighting the need for further improvements of the antileukemic efficacy of this transplantation platform.

Another setting where reduced-intensity conditioning approaches could be successfully combined with RIT is with the posttransplant cyclophosphamide platform for HCT with human leukocyte antigen (HLA)-haploidentical donors. Many of the earlier RIT-based conditioning regimens were used for allogeneic HCT with HLA-matched related or unrelated donors. This is an important limitation because many potentially curable patients do not have a suitable HLA-matched donor available. This is an especially challenging hurdle for patients from ethnic minority backgrounds, with data from the National Marrow Donor Program and cord blood unit registry indicating that Blacks of South or Central American ancestry have a 16% chance of finding an optimal donor as compared to 75% for white patients of European heritage [45]. Because most patients should have at least one related donor with one identical HLA haplotype (parent, sibling, or child), HCT approaches using haploidentical donors have been used to extend this potentially lifesaving treatment strategy to patients with leukemias and MDS. One such study enrolled 25 patients with high-risk AML (21 patients), ALL (3 patients), or high-risk MDS (1 patient) who then received ^{131}I-BC8 in escalating doses before fludarabine and 2 Gy TBI. Following infusion of stem cells from a haploidentical donor, graft-versus-host disease prophylaxis was given with posttransplant cyclophosphamide, tacrolimus, and mycophenolate mofetil. No MTD was reached, and no unexpected adverse events were observed. Among 21 AML patients, 10 had active disease (6–20% blasts in the bone marrow) and 9 were in remission but had MRD detectable (0.03–5.4% abnormal blasts by flow cytometry) [46]. The estimated overall survival and progression-free survival at 1 year were 42% and 40%, respectively, with relapse accounting for the majority of deaths, where twelve patients relapsed on this trial.

17.5.2 RIT Prior to HCT Utilizing Higher-Energy Emitters

A commonality of most of the trials discussed so far is that administration of the radiolabeled antibody was generally well tolerated but relapses were common. In an attempt to improve the antitumor efficacy of RIT-based treatments, investigators have pursued other radionuclides capable of delivering higher radiation payloads. In a phase I/II dose-escalation study, 15 adults with high-risk acute leukemias or MDS received ^{90}Y-anti-CD45 RIT in escalating doses before proceeding to minimal-intensity conditioning with fludarabine and 2 Gy TBI. Peripheral blood HCT from matched related or unrelated donors was performed about 12 days after RIT infusion

[47]. Patients on this study were mostly older (median age 62 [range: 37–76] years), with 9 of them having refractory disease and 6 having MRD-positive remissions at the time of HCT. The maximum dose of 28 Gy to the liver was achieved without dose-limiting toxicity. Only 2 patients had persistent disease 28 days after HCT, with the remaining 13 achieving a CR. All patients engrafted, but 6 patients experienced relapse after a median of 59 (range: 6–351) days, yielding a 1-year estimate of relapse of 41%. The overall survival and progression-free survival at 1 year were estimated at 66% and 46%, respectively. To treat patients with high-risk neoplasms and those with higher-level disease burdens, investigators have now turned to delivering higher radiation payloads with astatine-211, with two early phase clinical trials ongoing at our institution investigating ^{211}At-BC8 when integrated in a minimal-intensity conditioning HCT platform for patients with high-risk leukemias and MDS undergoing HCT with HLA-matched or haploidentical donors.

Another alternative to iodine-131 that has been explored in targeted radiation delivery prior to HCT is rhenium-188, as it has a higher beta-decay energy of 2.1 MeV. One of the earliest trials studied 12 patients with advanced leukemias, treated with ^{188}Re-anti-CD66, followed by standard conditioning chemotherapy and T-cell-depleted allogeneic graft [48]. Having demonstrated favorable biodistributions [49], with a median of 14 Gy delivered to the bone marrow, a subsequent study enrolled 36 patients with high-risk AML or MDS [50]. The majority (31 patients) received an allogeneic graft, 1 a syngeneic graft, and 4 autologous grafts. In these studies, the normal organ receiving the highest dose was the kidney, unlike other $[^{131}$I] I-anti-CD45 RIT trials where the liver was the dose-limiting organ. Nonetheless, with the kidneys as dose-limiting organ, there were no surprising additional adverse effects aside from the expected toxicities associated with conditioning regimens, but six patients did experience some nephrotoxicity possibly associated with radiation between 6 and 12 months after HCT. The DFS was estimated at 45% at a median follow-up of

18 months and, not unexpectedly, was better for patients undergoing HCT in remission (67%) than those not in remission at the time of HCT (31%). Congruently, relapse rates were lower for patients transplanted in remission (20%) than those transplanted while not in remission (30%).

Another trial enrolled 21 patients with high-risk AML or MDS, treated with [188]Re-anti-CD66 RIT followed by myeloablative conditioning with busulfan and cyclophosphamide in 11 patients, and reduced-intensity conditioning in the remaining 10 patients [51]. The DFS for all patients was estimated at 43% with a median follow-up of 42 months. Treatment-related mortality was estimated at 28.6% with 6 patients dying from veno-occlusive disease, acute graft-versus-host disease (GVHD), and infections between day +30 and day +213. Another 6 patients experienced relapse between day +41 and day +367 from transplant, specifically 3 of the 13 patients undergoing HCT in CR, and 3 of the 8 patients with relapsed/refractory disease who received minimal-intensity conditioning.

[188]Re-anti-CD66 RIT was also investigated in elderly patients with high-risk AML or MDS [52]. A total of 58 patients received [188]Re-anti-CD66 RIT before fludarabine and busulfan combined with alemtuzumab at one of two doses to probe the question of whether in vivo T-cell depletion could improve leukemia-free survival and relapse rates. Relapse rates were similar between the two alemtuzumab doses (38% vs. 35%, $p = 0.81$) as was nonrelapse mortality (46% vs. 27%, $p = 0.31$). The DFS at 2 years was not statistically different between the two alemtuzumab doses (16% lower and 38% higher doses, $p = 0.38$), and the median overall survival was 13 months in the higher alemtuzumab dose group compared to 12 months ($p = 0.38$). The nonrelapse mortality rate at 2 years was 46% in the lower dose group compared to 27% in the higher alemtuzumab dose group at 2 years, with the majority of deaths due to relapse and infectious complications.

Although not designed to compare the different radionuclides, a different study enrolled 20 elderly patients with advanced acute leukemias or MDS, and were treated with anti-CD66 anti-body radiolabeled with either rhenium-188 or yttrium-90. Patients then received reduced-intensity conditioning with fludarabine and anti-thymocyte globulin (ATG) in transplants using matched related donors, or with additional melphalan in transplants using matched unrelated donors [53]. A comparison of the two radionuclides showed a higher bone marrow dose and lower kidney dose favoring yttrium-90 possibly because of the higher in vivo stability of ^{90}Y-labeled radioimmunoconjugate utilizing a chelator, whereas rhenium-188 is directly attached to the antibody. Toxicities were low with only two patients experiencing grade 3 organ toxicities, and one of those attributed to cyclosporine use. The nonrelapse mortality was estimated at 25% at 2 years, and relapse incidence at 55% at 30 months after HCT. In this older patient cohort, RIT infusions were well tolerated, but relapse was still an issue, as 60% of patients not in remission at the time of HCT relapsed, compared to 42% of patients in first or second remission, with an overall relapse rate of 55% at 30 months. Relapse occurred in 6 of the 8 patients treated with the [188]Re-labeled anti-CD66 antibody and in 3 of the 12 patients treated with ^{90}Y-labeled anti-CD66 antibody. The probability of survival was estimated at 70% at 1 year and 52% at 2 years. This early study showed the feasibility of increasing radiation delivery to site of disease using [188]Re- or ^{90}Y-labeled anti-CD66 antibody in the elderly patient population without significant increasing toxicity. This report also suggests that increasing the radiation payload may improve outcomes by decreasing relapse rates.

17.6 Future Directions

17.6.1 Pretargeted RIT (PRIT) to Further Reduce Off-Target Toxicities

Despite the additional cytoreductive radiation payloads that are delivered to sites of leukemia involvement, relapse remains the main limitation of current RIT approaches (Fig. 17.1a). Motivated by the belief that increasing the radiation payload

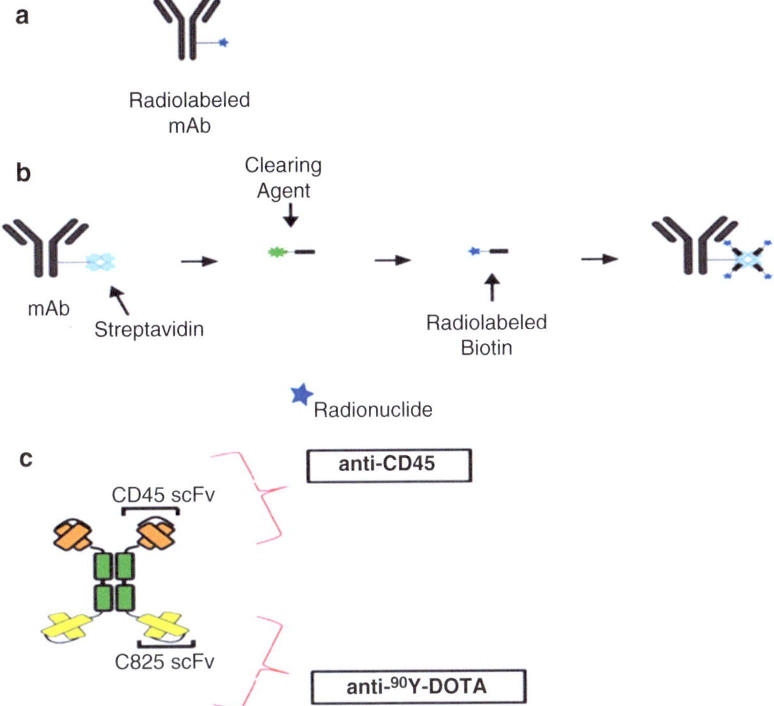

Fig. 17.1 Directly labeled antibody RIT compared to streptavidin-biotin and bispecific antibody PRIT approaches. (**a**) Initial constructs utilized direct radiolabeling of antibody with radionuclide, sometimes directly as with ^{131}I, and others via a chelator like DOTA. (**b**) Streptavidin-biotin PRIT relies on first step infusion of antibody-streptavidin conjugate, followed by clearing agent to clear unbound, freely circulating first step, then infusion of therapeutic radiolabeled biotin. (**c**) Model of bispecific antibody targeting antihuman CD45 and radiometal ligand ^{90}Y-DOTA. The bispecific antibody (anti-hCD45 x anti-Y-DOTA) was engineered by incorporating the region coding for the single-chain variable fragment (scFv) of the BC8 Ab specific for hCD45 and the scFv of the DOTAY-specific C825 Ab onto a hIgG1 Fc hinge (green)

would improve outcomes by providing more effective antileukemic therapy, additional toxicity-reducing strategies have been developed in which radiation delivery is separated from the targeting step via pretargeted RIT (PRIT). One PRIT strategy is employing the streptavidin-biotin (SA-biotin) system (Fig. 17.1b), in which the targeting antibody is conjugated to SA and delivered as a nonradioactive first step [54]. Any unbound conjugated antibody is then cleared from circulation via a clearing agent, followed by administration of the therapeutic radiolabeled ligand such as biotin conjugated to DOTA-chelate for capture of the radiometal [55, 56]. Radiobiotin can then bind to the pretargeted antibody-SA conjugate that is already bound to the target antigen. Any unbound radiobiotin is quickly excreted

via the kidneys, reducing any non-target radiation exposure that would otherwise occur with directly labeled antibody. This approach has been explored in numerous preclinical leukemia models and found to lead to substantially improved tumor-to-normal organ ratios compared to conventional RIT. For example, in a murine leukemia model [57], athymic mice harboring HEL human leukemia xenografts were treated with either conventional RIT (anti-CD45 DOTA-antibody labeled with fluorophore) or PRIT (anti-CD45 antibody-SA followed by biotinylated fluorophore). There was higher fluorescence in the blood pool in RIT-treated mice compared to PRIT-treated mice, which had the majority of fluorescent activity localized at the tumor 12 h after injection. In disseminated murine leukemia models, over three times more radiation could be delivered to hematologic tissues via CD45-targeting PRIT compared to CD45-targeting RIT [58]. Tumor-to-normal organ ratios provide an indication of the targeting of radiation to target organs. In syngeneic murine leukemia models, significantly prolonged survival was observed after anti-CD45 PRIT compared to directly labeled anti-CD45 RIT.

To further increase radiation payloads, PRIT has been pursued using alpha-emitters in murine leukemia models [59]. BALB/c mice bearing human leukemia xenografts were given anti-CD45 antibody-SA first step, followed by a clearing agent and administration of ^{213}Bi-DOTA-biotin. Biodistribution studies confirmed favorable localization of ^{213}Bi-DOTA-biotin to tumors with minimal localization to normal organs. In therapeutic applications, 29.6 MBq of ^{213}Bi-DOTA-biotin given 24 h after first step anti-CD45 antibody-SA resulted in median leukemia-free survival for >100 days with minimal toxicities, whereas untreated mice succumbed to leukemia within 20–40 days.

Despite the promise of SA-biotin PRIT approaches, alternatives to the SA-biotin approach have been explored because of the concern of immunogenicity with SA and the potential interference from endogenous biotin from a normal diet. One such alternative is the use of bispecific antibody fragments (Fig. 17.1c), where one arm of the single chain is structured to detect a tumor antigen (e.g., CD45), whereas the other arm captures the radiolabeled ligand (e.g., DOTA-biotin) [60, 61]. Successful preclinical development of bispecific antibody-based PRIT approaches has been reported for several hematologic malignancies, including non-Hodgkin lymphoma [62], multiple myeloma [63], and AML [64]. To treat the latter, an anti-CD45 scFv fusion protein was engineered onto a high-affinity anti-Y-DOTA scFv fusion protein to bind both CD45$^+$ target cells and ^{90}Y-DOTA-biotin. When HEL-bearing mice were sequentially injected with this PRIT reagent, a clearing agent, and the radiolabeled ^{90}Y-DOTA-biotin ligand, uptake at target tumors was demonstrated as early as 4 h after injection, with peak uptake at 24 h and minimal uptake in non-target organs like the kidneys. In therapeutic studies, similarly treated athymic mice bearing subcutaneous HEL xenografts received 29.6–55.5 MBq of ^{90}Y-DOTA-biotin. The group of mice treated with 51.8 MBq of [^{90}Y]Y-DOTA-biotin had 6 of 10 mice survive past 170 days post radioligand injection. In contrast, untreated mice and mice treated with non-targeting negative control bispecific antibody required euthanasia by days 26 and 32, respectively, because of excessive tumor size.

Approaches to treat leukemia in disseminated models, more closely resembling the clinical setting of patients with AML, are currently being pursued. In addition to innovative approaches just described, other innovations include developing pretargeted approaches with the alpha-emitter astatine-211. The overall goal continues to be to develop well tolerated therapies with minimal off-target toxicities that will reduce relapse rates to improve outcomes for patients with acute leukemias.

References

1. Shockley TR, Lin K, Sung C, Nagy JA, Tompkins RG, Dedrick RL, et al. A quantitative analysis of tumor specific monoclonal antibody uptake by human melanoma xenografts: effects of antibody immunological properties and tumor antigen expression levels. Cancer Res. 1992;52(2):357–66.
2. Press OW, Hansen JA, Farr A, Martin PJ. Endocytosis and degradation of murine anti-human CD3 monoclonal antibodies by normal and malignant T-lymphocytes. Cancer Res. 1988;48(8):2249–57.
3. Geissler F, Anderson SK, Venkatesan P, Press O. Intracellular catabolism of radiolabeled anti-μ antibodies by malignant B-cells. Cancer Res. 1992;52(10):2907–15.
4. van der Jagt RHC, Badger CC, Appelbaum FR, Press OW, Matthews DC, Eary JF, et al. Localization of radiolabeled antimyeloid antibodies in a human acute leukemia xenograft tumor model. Cancer Res. 1992;52(1):89–94.
5. Nourigat C, Badger CC, Bernstein ID. Treatment of lymphoma with radiolabeled antibody: elimination of tumor cells lacking target antigen. J Natl Cancer Inst. 1990;82(1):47–50. https://doi.org/10.1093/jnci/82.1.47.
6. Gray-Owen SD, Blumberg RS. CEACAM1: contact-dependent control of immunity. Nat Rev Immunol. 2006;6(6):433–46. https://doi.org/10.1038/nri1864.

7. Wahren B, Gahrton G, Hammarström S. Nonspecific cross-reacting antigen in normal and leukemic myeloid cells and serum of leukemic patients. Cancer Res. 1980;40(6):2039–44.

8. Watt S, Sala-Newby G, Hoang T, Gilmore D, Grunert F, Nagel G, et al. CD66 identifies a neutrophil-specific epitope within the hematopoietic system that is expressed by members of the carcinoembryonic antigen family of adhesion molecules. Blood. 1991;78(1):63–74.

9. Andres TL, Kadin ME. Immunological markers in the differential-diagnosis of small round cell tumors from lymphocytic lymphoma and leukemia. Am J Clin Pathol. 1983;79(5):546–52.

10. Nakano A, Harada T, Morikawa S, Kato Y. Expression of leukocyte common antigen (CD45) on various human leukemia lymphoma cell-lines. Acta Pathol Jpn. 1990;40(2):107–15.

11. Taetle R, Ostergaard H, Smedsrud M, Trowbridge I. Regulation of CD45 expression in human leukemia-cells. Leukemia. 1991;5(4):309–14.

12. Matthews DC, Appelbaum FR, Eary JF, Hui TE, Fisher DR, Martin PJ, et al. Radiolabeled anti-CD45 monoclonal antibodies target lymphohematopoietic tissue in the macaque. Blood. 1991;78(7):1864–74.

13. Colcher D, Bird R, Roselli M, Hardman KD, Johnson S, Pope S, et al. In vivo tumor targeting of a recombinant single-chain antigen-binding protein. J Natl Cancer Inst. 1990;82(14):1191–7. https://doi.org/10.1093/jnci/82.14.1191.

14. Larson SM. Improved tumor targeting with radiolabeled, recombinant, single-chain, antigen-binding protein. J Natl Cancer Inst. 1990;82(14):1173–4. https://doi.org/10.1093/jnci/82.14.1173.

15. Matthews DC, Badger CC, Fisher DR, Hui TE, Nourigat C, Appelbaum FR, et al. Selective radiation of hematolymphoid tissue delivered by anti-CD45 antibody. Cancer Res. 1992;52(5):1228–34.

16. King DJ, Turner A, Farnsworth APH, Adair JR, Owens RJ, Pedley RB, et al. Improved tumor targeting with chemically cross-linked recombinant antibody fragments. Cancer Res. 1994;54(23):6176–85.

17. Nieroda CA, Milenic DE, Carrasquillo JA, Schlom J, Greiner JW. Improved tumor radioimmunodetection using a single-chain Fv and γ-interferon: potential clinical applications for radioimmunoguided surgery and γ scanning. Cancer Res. 1995;55(13):2858–65.

18. Horning SJ, Younes A, Jain V, Kroll S, Lucas J, Podoloff D, et al. Efficacy and safety of tositumomab and iodine-131 tositumomab (Bexxar) in B-cell lymphoma, progressive after rituximab. J Clin Oncol. 2005;23(4):712–9. https://doi.org/10.1200/jco.2005.07.040.

19. Press OW, Shan D, Howell-Clark J, Eary J, Appelbaum FR, Matthews D, et al. Comparative metabolism and retention of iodine-125, yttrium-90, and indium-111 radioimmunoconjugates by cancer cells. Cancer Res. 1996;56(9):2123–9.

20. Wilder RB, DeNardo GL, DeNardo SJ. Radioimmunotherapy: recent results and future directions. J Clin Oncol. 1996;14(4):1383–400. https://doi.org/10.1200/jco.1996.14.4.1383.

21. Zhang M, Yao Z, Garmestani K, Axworthy DB, Zhang Z, Mallett RW, et al. Pretargeting radioimmunotherapy of a murine model of adult T-cell leukemia with the α-emitting radionuclide, bismuth 213. Blood. 2002;100(1):208–16. https://doi.org/10.1182/blood-2002-01-0107.

22. McDevitt MR, Ma D, Lai LT, Simon J, Borchardt P, Frank RK, et al. Tumor therapy with targeted atomic nanogenerators. Science. 2001;294(5546):1537–40. https://doi.org/10.1126/science.1064126.

23. Bethge WA, Wilbur DS, Storb R, Hamlin DK, Santos EB, Brechbiel MW, et al. Radioimmunotherapy with bismuth-213 as conditioning for nonmyeloablative allogeneic hematopoietic cell transplantation in dogs: a dose deescalation study. Transplantation. 2004;78(3):352–9.

24. Sandmaier BM, Bethge WA, Wilbur DS, Hamlin DK, Santos EB, Brechbiel MW, et al. Bismuth 213–labeled anti-CD45 radioimmunoconjugate to condition dogs for nonmyeloablative allogeneic marrow grafts. Blood. 2002;100:318–26.

25. Nakamae H, Wilbur DS, Hamlin DK, Thakar MS, Santos EB, Fisher DR, et al. Biodistributions, myelosuppression, and toxicities in mice treated with an anti-CD45 antibody labeled with the alpha-emitting radionuclides bismuth-213 or astatine-211. Cancer Res. 2009;69(6):2408–15. https://doi.org/10.1158/0008-5472.can-08-4363.

26. Caron PC, Jurcic JG, Scott AM, Finn RD, Divgi CR, Graham MC, et al. A phase-1b trial of humanized monoclonal-antibody M195 (anti-CD33) in myeloid leukemia—specific targeting without immunogenicity. Blood. 1994;83(7):1760–8.

27. Sgouros G, Ballangrud ÅM, Jurcic JG, McDevitt MR, Humm JL, Erdi YE, et al. Pharmacokinetics and dosimetry of an α-particle emitter labeled antibody: 213Bi-HuM195 (anti-CD33) in patients with leukemia. J Nucl Med. 1999;40(11):1935–46.

28. Rosenblat TL, McDevitt MR, Mulford DA, Pandit-Taskar N, Divgi CR, Panageas KS, et al. Sequential cytarabine and alpha-particle immunotherapy with bismuth-213-lintuzumab (HuM195) for acute myeloid leukemia. Clin Cancer Res. 2010;16(21):5303–11. https://doi.org/10.1158/1078-0432.ccr-10-0382.

29. Jurcic JG. Targeted alpha-particle immunotherapy for acute myeloid leukemia. Am Soc Clin Oncol Educ Book. 2014;34:e126–31. https://doi.org/10.14694/EdBook_AM.2014.34.e126.

30. Jurcic JG, Rosenblat TL, McDevitt MR, Pandit-Taskar N, Carrasquillo JA, Chanel SM, et al. Phase I trial of the targeted alpha-particle nano-generator actinium-225 (Ac-225)-lintuzumab (anti-CD33; HuM195) in acute myeloid leukemia (AML). Blood. 2011;118(21):348–9.

31. Finn LE, Levy M, Orozco JJ, Park JH, Atallah E, Craig M, et al. A phase 2 study of actinium-225 (^{225}Ac)-lintuzumab in older patients with previously untreated acute myeloid leukemia (AML) unfit for

intensive chemotherapy. Blood. 2017;130(Suppl 1):2638.

32. Atallah EL, Orozco JJ, Craig M, Levy MY, Finn LE, Khan SS, et al. A phase 2 study of actinium-225 (Ac-225)-lintuzumab in older patients with untreated acute myeloid leukemia (AML)—interim analysis of 1.5 mu ci/kg/dose. Blood. 2018;132:4. https://doi.org/10.1182/blood-2018-99-111951.

33. Appelbaum FR. The use of radiolabeled anti-CD33 antibody to augment marrow irradiation prior to marrow transplantation for acute myelogenous leukemia. Transplantation. 1992;54(5):829–33. https://doi.org/10.1097/00007890-199211000-00012.

34. Schwartz MA, Lovett DR, Redner A, Finn RD, Graham MC, Divgi CR, et al. Dose-escalation trial of M195 labeled with iodine 131 for cytoreduction and marrow ablation in relapsed or refractory myeloid leukemias. J Clin Oncol. 1993;11(2):294–303. https://doi.org/10.1200/jco.1993.11.2.294.

35. Burke JM, Caron PC, Papadopoulos EB, Divgi CR, Sgouros G, Panageas KS, et al. Cytoreduction with iodine-131-anti-CD33 antibodies before bone marrow transplantation for advanced myeloid leukemias. Bone Marrow Transplant. 2003;32(6):549–56. https://doi.org/10.1038/sj.bmt.1704201.

36. Matthews DC, Appelbaum FR, Eary JF, Fisher DR, Durack LD, Hui TE, et al. Phase I study of I-131-anti-CD45 antibody plus cyclophosphamide and total body irradiation for advanced acute leukemia and myelodysplastic syndrome. Blood. 1999;94(4):1237–47.

37. Pagel JM, Appelbaum FR, Eary JF, Rajendran J, Fisher DR, Gooley T, et al. I-131-anti-CD45 antibody plus busulfan and cyclophosphamide before allogeneic hematopoietic cell transplantation for treatment of acute myeloid leukemia in first remission. Blood. 2006;107(5):2184–91. https://doi.org/10.1182/blood-2005-06-2317.

38. Giralt S, Estey E, Albitar M, van Besien K, Rondón G, Anderlini P, et al. Engraftment of allogeneic hematopoietic progenitor cells with purine analog-containing chemotherapy: harnessing graft-versus-leukemia without myeloablative therapy. Blood. 1997;89(12):4531–6.

39. Slavin S, Nagler A, Naparstek E, Kapelushnik Y, Aker M, Cividalli G, et al. Nonmyeloablative stem cell transplantation and cell therapy as an alternative to conventional bone marrow transplantation with lethal cytoreduction for the treatment of malignant and nonmalignant hematologic diseases. Blood. 1998;91(3):756–63.

40. Gyurkocza B, Storb R, Storer BE, Chauncey TR, Lange T, Shizuru JA, et al. Nonmyeloablative allogeneic hematopoietic cell transplantation in patients with acute myeloid leukemia. J Clin Oncol. 2010;28(17):2859–67. https://doi.org/10.1200/jco.2009.27.1460.

41. Pagel JM, Gooley TA, Rajendran J, Fisher DR, Wilson WA, Sandmaier BM, et al. Allogeneic hematopoietic cell transplantation after conditioning with I-131-anti-CD45 antibody plus fludarabine and low-dose total body irradiation for elderly patients with advanced acute myeloid leukemia or high-risk myelodysplastic syndrome. Blood. 2009;114(27):5444–53. https://doi.org/10.1182/blood-2009-03-213298.

42. Agura E, Gyurkocza B, Nath R, Litzow MR, Tomlinson BK, Abhyankar S, et al. Targeted conditioning of Iomab-B (^{131}I-anti-CD45) prior to allogeneic hematopoietic cell transplantation versus conventional care in relapsed or refractory acute myeloid leukemia (AML): preliminary feasibility and safety results from the prospective, randomized phase 3 Sierra trial. Blood. 2018;132(Suppl 1):1017. https://doi.org/10.1182/blood-2018-99-111914.

43. Bea T. Rapid reduction of peripheral blasts in older patients with refractory acute myeloid leukemia (AML) using reinduction with single agent anti-CD45 targeted iodine (131I) apamistamab [Iomab-B] radioimmunotherapy in the phase III SIERRA trial. J Clin Oncol. 2019;37:abstract 7048.

44. Mawad R, Gooley TA, Rajendran JG, Fisher DR, Gopal AK, Shields AT, et al. Radiolabeled anti-CD45 antibody with reduced-intensity conditioning and allogeneic transplantation for younger patients with advanced acute myeloid leukemia or myelodysplastic syndrome. Biol Blood Marrow Transplant. 2014;20(9):1363–8. https://doi.org/10.1016/j.bbmt.2014.05.014.

45. Gragert L, Eapen M, Williams E, Freeman J, Spellman S, Baitty R, et al. HLA match likelihoods for hematopoietic stem-cell grafts in the U.S. Registry. N Engl J Med. 2014;371(4):339–48. https://doi.org/10.1056/NEJMsa1311707.

46. Orozco JJ, Gooley T, Rajendran JG, Fisher DR, Deeg HJ, Storb RF, et al. Anti-CD45 radioimmunotherapy followed by haploidentical allogeneic hematopoietic cell transplantation for advanced acute leukemia or high-risk MDS. Blood. 2017;130(Suppl 1):2048.

47. Vo PT, Gooley T, Rajendran JG, Fisher DR, Orozco JJ, Green DJ, et al. Safety and efficacy of yttrium-90-labeled anti-CD45 antibody (Y-90-DOTA-BC8) followed by a standard reduced-intensity hematopoietic stem cell transplant (HCT) regimen for patients with refractory/relapsed leukemia or high-risk myelodysplastic syndrome (MDS). Blood. 2018;132:3. https://doi.org/10.1182/blood-2018-99-111915.

48. Seitz U. Preparation and evaluation of the rhenium-188-labelled anti-NCA antigen monoclonal antibody BW 250/183 for radioimmunotherapy of leukaemia. Eur J Nucl Med. 1999;26(10):1265–73. https://doi.org/10.1007/s002590050582.

49. Kotzerke J, Glatting G, Seitz U, Rentschler M, Neumaier B, Bunjes D, et al. Radioimmunotherapy for the intensification of conditioning before stem cell transplantation: differences in dosimetry and biokinetics of 188Re- and 99mTc-labeled anti-NCA-95 MAbs. J Nucl Med. 2000;41(3):531–7.

50. Bunjes D, Buchmann I, Duncker C, Seitz U, Kotzerke J, Wiesneth M, et al. Rhenium 188-labeled anti-CD66 (a, b, c, e) monoclonal antibody to intensify the con-

ditioning regimen prior to stem cell transplantation for patients with high-risk acute myeloid leukemia or myelodysplastic syndrome: results of a phase I-II study. Blood. 2001;98(3):565–72. https://doi.org/10.1182/blood.V98.3.565.

51. Koenecke C, Hofmann M, Bolte O, Gielow P, Dammann E, Stadler M, et al. Radioimmunotherapy with [188Re]-labelled anti-CD66 antibody in the conditioning for allogeneic stem cell transplantation for high-risk acute myeloid leukemia. Int J Hematol. 2008;87(4):414–21. https://doi.org/10.1007/s12185-008-0043-1.

52. Schneider S, Strumpf A, Schetelig J, Wunderlich G, Ehninger G, Kotzerke J, et al. Reduced-intensity conditioning combined with 188Rhenium radioimmunotherapy before allogeneic hematopoietic stem cell transplantation in elderly patients with acute myeloid leukemia: the role of in vivo T cell depletion. Biol Blood Marrow Transplant. 2015;21(10):1754–60. https://doi.org/10.1016/j.bbmt.2015.05.012.

53. Ringhoffer M, Blumstein N, Neumaier B, Glatting G, von Harsdorf S, Buchmann I, et al. 188Re or 90Y-labelled anti-CD66 antibody as part of a dose-reduced conditioning regimen for patients with acute leukaemia or myelodysplastic syndrome over the age of 55: results of a phase I–II study. Br J Haematol. 2005;130(4):604–13. https://doi.org/10.1111/j.1365-2141.2005.05663.x.

54. Paganelli G, Grana C, Chinol M, Cremonesi M, De Cicco C, De Braud F, et al. Antibody-guided three-step therapy for high grade glioma with yttrium-90 biotin. Eur J Nucl Med. 1999;26(4):348–57. https://doi.org/10.1007/s002590050397.

55. Pagel JM, Orgun N, Hamlin DK, Wilbur DS, Gooley TA, Gopal AK, et al. A comparative analysis of conventional and pretargeted radioimmunotherapy of B-cell lymphomas by targeting CD20, CD22, and HLA-DR singly and in combinations. Blood. 2009;113(20):4903–13. https://doi.org/10.1182/blood-2008-11-187401.

56. Weiden PL. Pretargeted radioimmunotherapy (PRIT) for treatment of non-Hodgkin's lymphoma (NHL): initial phase I/II study results. Cancer Biother Radiopharm. 2000;15(1):15–29. https://doi.org/10.1089/cbr.2000.15.15.

57. Pagel JM, Matthews DC, Kenoyer A, Hamlin DK, Wilbur DS, Fisher DR, et al. Pretargeted radioimmunotherapy using anti-CD45 monoclonal antibodies to deliver radiation to murine hematolymphoid tissues and human myeloid leukemia. Cancer Res. 2009;69(1):185–92. https://doi.org/10.1158/0008-5472.can-08-2513.

58. Pagel JM, Hedin N, Drouet L, Wood BL, Pantelias A, Lin YK, et al. Eradication of disseminated leukemia in a syngeneic murine leukemia model using pretargeted anti-CD45 radioimmunotherapy. Blood. 2008;111(4):2261–8. https://doi.org/10.1182/blood-2007-06-097451.

59. Pagel JM, Kenoyer AL, Back T, Hamlin DK, Wilbur DS, Fisher DR, et al. Anti-CD45 pretargeted radioimmunotherapy using bismuth-213: high rates of complete remission and long-term survival in a mouse myeloid leukemia xenograft model. Blood. 2011;118(3):703–11. https://doi.org/10.1182/blood-2011-04-347039.

60. Green DJ, Press OW. Whither Radioimmunotherpay: To Be or Not to Be? Cancer Res. 2017;77(9): 2191–6. https://doi.org/10.1158/0008-5472.CAN-16-2523.

61. Sharkey RM, Rossi EA, McBride WJ, Chang C-H, Goldenberg DM. Recombinant bispecific monoclonal antibodies prepared by the dock-and-lock strategy for pretargeted radioimmunotherapy. Semin Nucl Med. 2010;40(3):190–203. https://doi.org/10.1053/j.semnuclmed.2009.12.002.

62. Green DJ, Frayo SL, Lin Y, Hamlin DK, Fisher DR, Frost SHL, et al. Comparative analysis of bispecific antibody and streptavidin-targeted radioimmunotherapy for B-cell cancers. Cancer Res. 2016;76(22):6669–79. https://doi.org/10.1158/0008-5472.can-16-0571.

63. Green DJ, O'Steen S, Lin Y, Comstock ML, Kenoyer AL, Hamlin DK, et al. CD38-bispecific antibody pretargeted radioimmunotherapy for multiple myeloma and other B-cell malignancies. Blood. 2018;131(6):611–20. https://doi.org/10.1182/blood-2017-09-807610.

64. Orozco JJ, Kenoyer AL, Lin Y, O'Steen S, Guel R, Nartea ME, et al. Therapy of Myeloid Leukemia using Novel Bispecific Fusion Proteins Targeting CD45 and 90Y-DOTA. Mol Cancer Ther. 2020; 19(12);2575–84. https://doi.org/10.1158/1535-7163.MCT-20-0306.

Targeted Radionuclide Therapy and Immunotherapy of Metastatic Prostate Cancer

Hossein Jadvar

Contents

18.1   Introduction

Prostate cancer is the most common non-cutaneous cancer and the second most common cause of cancer death after lung cancer in men in the United States. The 2019 estimated new cases and estimated deaths were 174,650 men (9.9% of all new cancer cases) and 31,620 men (5.2% of all cancer deaths), respectively. In 2016, there were an estimated 3,110,403 men living with prostate cancer in the United States. The lifetime risk of developing prostate cancer is one in seven men (approximately 12%) at a median age of 66 years. The percentages of cases by stage at diagnosis are 77% for localized, 13% for regional (spread to regional lymph nodes), 6% distant disease sites, and 4% unknown [1].

The National Comprehensive Cancer Network (NCCN) clinical practice guideline provides information on risk-adapted treatment options in patients with prostate cancer in primary, locally recurrent, and metastatic settings [2]. Regardless of the clinical setting, the treatment options continue to evolve as new data becomes available with the ultimate goal to improve patient outcome and reduce toxicity in a cost-effective manner. The clinical space for therapy regimens in patients with metastatic disease has particularly been recently active with many novel agents with different modes of action that include androgen axis inhibitors, targeted radionuclide therapy, chemotherapy, and immunotherapy. In this chapter, we focus on targeted radionuclide therapy

H. Jadvar (✉)
Division of Nuclear Medicine, Department of Radiology, Keck School of Medicine, University of Southern California, Los Angeles, CA, USA
e-mail: jadvar@med.usc.edu

© Springer Nature Switzerland AG 2022
S. Harsini et al. (eds.), *Nuclear Medicine and Immunology*,
https://doi.org/10.1007/978-3-030-81261-4_18

and radioactive or nonradioactive immunotherapy of patients with advanced prostate cancer.

18.2 Targeted Radionuclide Therapy

Delivering local therapy with radioactive particles (alpha, beta, auger) is efficacious and generally associated with low incidence and severity of treatment-induced adverse events. Earlier, such treatments targeted the metastatic bone lesions primarily for bone pain palliation. These agents included beta-emitting radiopharmaceuticals $[^{89}Sr]SrCl_2$ and $[^{153}Sm]Sm$-EDTMP that were approved by the US Food and Drug Administration (FDA) in 1993 and 1997, respectively [3].

18.2.1 $[^{223}Ra]RaCl_2$

It was not until the approval of the first-in-class alpha-emitter $[^{223}Ra]RaCl_2$ (Xofigo™, previously Alpharadin, Bayer Healthcare) on May 15, 2013, when a targeted radiopharmaceutical became available for the treatment of osseous metastases in metastatic castration-resistant prostate cancer (mCRPC) with demonstration of overall survival benefit, decrease in skeletal events, and low toxicity. The final approval of $[^{223}Ra]RaCl_2$ was based on the results of the randomized, double-blind, placebo-controlled phase 3 ALSYMPCA (Alpharadin in Symptomatic PC) trial [4]. In this investigation, 921 patients who had received, were ineligible to receive, or declined docetaxel chemotherapy were randomized in a 2:1 ratio to receive 6 injections (50 kBq/kg) of $[^{223}Ra]RaCl_2$ at intervals of 4 weeks plus best standard of care versus placebo (saline) plus best standard of care with the primary outcome of overall survival (OS). There were a number of secondary outcome endpoints including time to the first symptomatic skeletal event. The prescribed interim analysis showed the outcome superiority of $[^{223}Ra]RaCl_2$ over that with a placebo. The final analysis of 921 patients confirmed the $[^{223}Ra]RaCl_2$ OS benefit over placebo (median 14.9 months vs. 11.3 months; hazard ratio (HR),

0.70; 95% confidence interval (CI), 0.58–0.83; $p < 0.001$). The OS benefit was demonstrated regardless of prior docetaxel use. The median OS benefit was 4.6 months in patients without prior docetaxel therapy, while the median OS benefit was 3.1 months in patients who received docetaxel. Similarly, there was a 5.8-month benefit (delay) in time to first skeletal-related events with $[^{223}Ra]RaCl_2$ compared to that with placebo (15.6 months vs. 9.8 months; HR, 0.66; 95% CI, 0.52–0.83; $p < 0.001$). The adverse events with $[^{223}Ra]RaCl_2$ were generally mild and manageable. The most common symptomatic adverse events were nausea, diarrhea, vomiting, and peripheral edema. The most common hematologic abnormalities were anemia, leukopenia, neutropenia, and thrombocytopenia. A recent interim analysis of a global, prospective, non-interventional study to assess the long-term safety of $[^{223}Ra]RaCl_2$ in 564 patients with mCRPC and a median follow-up of 7 months, entitled REASSURE (Radium-223 alpha Emitter Agent in non-intervention Safety Study in mCRPC popUlation for long-teRm Evaluation), further demonstrated the safety of the treatment. It was also observed that no prior chemotherapy was associated with lower burden of disease and improved tolerability for $[^{223}Ra]RaCl_2$ continuation to completion [5, 6].

A decline in serum alkaline phosphatase level is more common than a decline in serum PSA level [7]. Advancing soft tissue disease, which is unaffected by $[^{223}Ra]RaCl_2$ therapy, is the primary reason for cessation of therapy [8]. A recent investigation reported that PSA flare may occur during the first 2 months of $[^{223}Ra]RaCl_2$ therapy and that this event is associated with favorable outcome in comparison with patients who do not show PSA flare (OS 23.9 months vs. 11.5 months, respectively) [9]. Re-treatment with $[^{223}Ra]RaCl_2$ has also been investigated. The first experience from an international open-label, phase 1/2 study showed that re-treatment with the second course of six $[^{223}Ra]RaCl_2$ reinjections after disease progression is well tolerated, with minimal hematologic toxicity and low radiographic bone progression rates [10]. Moreover, a phase 1 dose escalation/randomized phase 2a trial has shown that combination of [²²³Ra]RaCl₂ (55 kBq/kg every 6 weeks for 5 doses) and docetaxel (60 mg/m² every 3 weeks for 10 doses) therapy is associated with longer PSA and alkaline phosphatase suppression [11]. The NCCN guideline (version 3.2013) incorporates [²²³Ra]RaCl₂ in the treatment strategy of patients with mCRPC.

18.3 Radioligand Therapy

A great sense of excitement has been generated over the past several years upon the development and initial encouraging clinical results with radioligands targeting specific biomarkers for imaging and treatment (theranostics) of prostate cancer [12, 13]. These include, but are not limited to, targets such as the gastrin-releasing peptide receptor (GRPR) and the external moiety of the prostate-specific membrane antigen (PSMA). Most investigations have focused on PSMA which is overexpressed in metastatic and androgen-independent prostate cancer. Also known as folate hydrolase I or glutamate carboxypeptidase II, PSMA is a type II transmembrane protein (100–120 kDa) anchored in the prostate epithelial cells. PSMA is neither specific for prostate tissue nor for cancer. However, despite the overall nonspecificity, accumulated experience suggests that PSMA-based radioligands will likely play a major role in prostate cancer theranostics [14, 15].

Ahmadzadehfar and colleagues from Germany reported two-center data on the safety and efficacy of [¹⁷⁷Lu]Lu-PSMA-617 RLT (mean administered activity 5.6 GBq, range 4.1–61 GBq) in 10 patients with hormone- and/or chemo-refractory patients with metastatic prostate cancer [16]. A PSA decline of more than 50% was noted in half of the patients, 8 weeks after RLT. Three patients showed PSA increase. Grade III or IV hematotoxicity occurred in only one patient, and there was no grade III or IV nephrotoxicity. The authors concluded that [¹⁷⁷Lu]Lu-PSMA-617 RLT has a low early side-effect profile with overall good efficacy. In another retrospective investigation, the same group of investigators reported a low toxicity profile with [¹⁷⁷Lu]Lu-PSMA-617 RLT in 24 patients with mCRPC [17]. These authors also assessed the outcome of and response pattern to multiple cycles [¹⁷⁷Lu]Lu-PSMA-617 RLT in 52 patients with mCRPC [18]. PSA decline was seen in 80.8% of patients after only one cycle of therapy with 44.2% showing a PSA decline of equal to or more than 50%. Half of the patients who did not have a PSA response after the first cycle of therapy demonstrated response after second and third therapy cycles. The median overall survival was longer in patients who responded after the first cycle compared to patients without a decrease in PSA level (68 weeks vs. 33 weeks). The potential for delayed response has also been noted by other investigators; in one retrospective study, about one-third of nonresponders to the first therapy cycle responded to additional therapy cycles [19].

The efficacy of [¹⁷⁷Lu]Lu-PSMA-617 RLT has been documented in challenging clinical settings of multiple prior non-efficacious therapies including androgen deprivation therapy, chemotherapy, and [²²³Ra]RaCl₂ therapy [20]. Rahbar et al. reported on the efficacy of 50 [¹⁷⁷Lu]Lu-PSMA therapies in 28 patients with mCRPC who had exhausted all conventional therapies [21]. A PSA decline of 50% or more was noted in 32% of patients after one cycle and 50% of patients after two cycles of therapy. The estimated overall survival benefit over historical data for the best supportive care was 9.7 weeks. All side effects were mild and manageable. In a multicenter retrospective analysis, the response and tolerability of a single dose of [¹⁷⁷Lu]Lu-PSMA-617 were evaluated in 74 mCRPC patients with a complete dataset [22]. In this clinical setting, a PSA decline of 50% or greater was seen in about one-third of the patients. Progressive disease (defined as PSA level rise by more than 25%) despite receiving a single dose of radioligand therapy was noted in about one-quarter of the patients. There were no significant changes in hemoglobin, white blood cell count, creatinine, or renal tubular extraction, and only a mild decline in platelet count was noted.

Rahbar and colleagues reported on a German multicenter study of 145 patients with mCRPC who underwent [¹⁷⁷Lu]Lu-PSMA-617 radioligand therapy at 12 centers across Germany [23]. These patients underwent a total of 248 therapy cycles ranging from 1 to 4 cycles per patient with an activity range of 2–8 GBq per cycle. The overall biochemical response rate was 45% after all cycles. Grade III–IV anemia, leukopenia, and thrombocytopenia occurred in 10%, 3%, and 4% of the patients, respectively. Xerostomia occurred in 8% of the patients. Negative predictive factors for PSA decline were elevated alkaline phosphatase (proxy for total osseous metastatic load) and the presence of visceral metastasis. The favorable predictive parameter was the total number of therapy cycles received. The German investigators also performed a retrospective study of 104 heavily pretreated patients who received [177Lu]Lu-PSMA-617 radioligand therapy [24]. The median OS was 56 weeks. Any initial PSA decline, initial alkaline phosphate <220 U/L, and cumulative injected activity $\geq$18.8 GBq were associated with longer survival. The multivariate analysis showed that PSA decline $\geq$20.87% was an independent prognosticator of improved OS.

Radiation dosimetry has been studied in 30 patients with mCRPC undergoing 1–3 cycles of [177Lu]Lu-PSMA-617 radioligand therapy [25]. Dosimetry showed doses of 0.75, 0.03, and 1.4 Gy/GBq to the kidney, red marrow, and salivary gland, respectively. The mean tumor-absorbed dose was between 6 and 22 Gy/GBq during the first cycle of therapy. Baum et al. from Bad Berka, Germany, reported similar values with median absorbed of 3.3 Gy/GBq to tumor doses of 3.3, 0.8 Gy/GBq to kidneys and 1.3 Gy/GBq to parotid glands [26]. These authors also reported both biochemical and radiological responses in some patients, a significant decline in pain severity in about one-third of patients, and no long-term untoward side effects [27].

A systematic review and meta-analysis of 17 studies and 744 patients supported the notion that [177Lu]Lu-PSMA radioligand therapy is effective (pooled proportion of 46% (95% CI, 40–53%), PSA decline of 50% or greater) in mCRPC that is refractory to standard treatment regimens (docetaxel, cabazitaxel chemotherapy, and first- and second-generation androgen deprivation therapies) and has a low and manageable toxicity profile (median 23% hematotoxicity, 14.2% leukopenia, 15% thrombocytopenia, 9.5% nephrotoxicity, and 14.5% xerostomia) [28]. A procedure guideline has recently been published with the following statement that "the guideline is to assist nuclear medicine specialists to deliver PSMA radioligand therapy as an *unproven intervention in clinical practice*, in accordance with the best currently available knowledge" [29].

Given the aforementioned exciting results and evidence for the safety and efficacy of [177Lu]Lu-PSMA-617 radioligand therapy, efforts have been initiated and/or are underway to perform controlled randomized investigations (e.g., the VISION trial) to further assess the comparative utility of this targeted radionuclide therapy in the clinical setting of mCRPC [30]. A recent single-center, single-arm, phase 2 trial from Australia was an important step toward justifying additional clinical trials [31]. In this investigation, 30 patients who had previously been treated with at least one line of chemotherapy, second-line androgen deprivation therapy, or both underwent [177Lu]Lu-PSMA-617 radioligand therapy with a mean administered radioactivity of 7.5 GBq per cycle. A PSA decline of 50% or greater occurred in 57% of patients. Objective response in the nodal or visceral disease was observed in 82% of patients with measurable disease. The most common side effect was grade I xerostomia in 87% of patients. Grade III or IV thrombocytopenia was seen in 13% of patients. An important feature of Hofman et al.'s phase 2 study and other similar reports is that patients with discordant 2-deoxy-2-[18F]fluoro-D-glucose (2-[18F]FDG)-positive lesions were excluded in order to optimize therapy efficacy in patients who only harbor suffiecintly PSMA positive tumors [32]. Other encouraging results have been reported that re-treatment with [177Lu]Lu-PSMA-617 radioligand therapy upon progression may be feasible and associated with higher response rates than other systemic therapies [33].

The potential efficacy of alpha-particle actinium-225 (^{225}Ac)-labeled or bismuth-213 (^{213}Bi)-labeled PSMA-targeted treatment of patients with mCRPC has been exhibited in a small number of cases, typically in patients who have been heavily pretreated and have failed those therapies. These reports have been encouraging with few exceptionally favorable responses in individual patients with xerostomia as the major limiting adverse event [34, 35]. Kratochwil and colleagues from Germany reported on dosimetry estimates and empiric dose finding for targeted therapy of mCRPC with [^{225}Ac]Ac-PSMA-617 reporting that a treatment activity of 100 kBq/kg of [^{225}Ac]Ac-PSMA-617 per cycle every 8 weeks was an optimal trade-off between xerostomia and biochemical efficacy in terms of PSA decline [36]. Recently, the South African investigators reported on the efficacy and outcome in 73 men with mCRPC who were treated with 210 cycles of [^{225}Ac]Ac-PSMA-617 [37]. A PSA decline of greater than or equal to 50% from pre-therapy baseline level was noted in 70% of patients. In 29% of patients, all lesions were resolved as evidenced on [^{68}Ga]Ga-PSMA-11 positron emission tomography (PET). A PSA decline of greater than or equal to 50% after treatment with [^{225}Ac]Ac-PSMA-617 was significantly associated with OS and progression-free survival (PFS) in a multivariate analysis. With regard to adverse events, xerostomia was seen in 85% of patients but was not severe enough to discontinue treatment. Renal failure (grade III/IV) was only seen in a few patients with baseline renal impairment. The same group of researchers performed a pilot clinical trial of [^{225}Ac]Ac-PSMA-617 radioligand therapy in 17 chemotherapy naïve patients with advanced prostate cancer [38]. More than 90% decline in serum PSA level was noted in 82% of these patients, and in 41% of patients, PSA became undetectable for 1 year. This interesting investigation suggested that [^{225}Ac]Ac-PSMA-617 RLT can be quite efficacious earlier in the spectrum of metastatic prostate cancer and in fact may be a contender to conventional chemotherapy.

18.4 Immunotherapy

One of the hallmarks of cancer is the evasion of the immune system. Recent key discoveries in understanding the interactions between cancer and immune cells have provided unprecedented opportunities for drug development unleashing the intrinsic power of the immune system to fight against cancer [39]. An initial drug relevant to prostate cancer in this space was sipuleucel-T approved by the US FDA in 2010 [40–42]. Sipuleucel-T is an activated cellular immunotherapy that targets prostatic acid phosphatase. The approval was based on the results of the IMPACT clinical trial that randomized 512 mCRPC patients 2:1 to receive either sipuleucel-T or placebo with OS as the primary outcome [43]. The median OS was 25.8 months in the drug arm versus 21.7 months in the placebo arm (HR, 0.77; $p = 0.02$) without a statistically significant difference in time to progression. This personalized treatment regimen involves leukapheresis to harvest autologous peripheral blood mononuclear cells which are then activated with recombinant protein consisting of prostatic acid phosphatase and GM-CSF followed by reinfusion to the patient after 3 days, with this procedure repeated every 2 weeks for a total of 3 cycles [44].

More recently, there have been a number of clinical studies of checkpoint inhibitors in prostate cancer. These studies have been relatively less efficacious than those with other cancers such as melanoma and lung cancer, probably because the generally slow-growing prostate cancer is less infiltrated with T cells (relatively "cold" tumor microenvironment), expresses fewer checkpoint molecules, and produces lower antigen load [45]. The degree of infiltration of inflammatory T cells within the tumor is positively prognostic with less T-cell infiltration in high-grade prostate cancer associated with less favorable prognosis [46]. For example, in a few phase 1/2 studies, ipilimumab (the first approved fully human immunoglobulin (Ig) G1 monoclonal antibody directed against the checkpoint molecule, cytotoxic T-lymphocyte-associated protein 4 (CTLA-4)) studies did not result in meeting the primary endpoint of prolonging OS despite observations of declines in serum PSA levels in a minority of patients [47, 48]. A phase 3 randomized clinical trial of a single dose of bone-directed radiation followed by either placebo or ipilimumab (10 mg/kg every 3 weeks for up to 4 cycles) in mCRPC patients with at least one bone metastasis who had failed docetaxel chemotherapy demonstrated a 0.9-month PFS benefit and a PSA response benefit of 7.9% in the ipilimumab arm but without OS benefit [49].

The programmed death-1 (PD-1)/programmed death ligand-1 (PD-L1) axis is also a relevant biological pathway in the regulation of T-cell activity against tumor cells. PD-1 is a transmembrane glycoprotein T-cell co-inhibitory receptor expressed on activated CD4$^+$ and CD8$^+$ T cells among other inflammatory cells. PD-L1 is overexpressed in tumor microenvironment cells (tumor, stroma, lymphocytes). The ultimate effect of PD-1/PD-L1 overexpression and biological activity is to dampen the immune system against the tumor and support tumor growth. Phase 1 investigations with anti-PD-1 antibodies, nivolumab and pembrolizumab, in patients with mCRPC have not revealed robust objective responses, although a few patients demonstrated partial responses or their disease remained stable [50, 51]. Preliminary results of a phase 2 study of durvalumab (an anti-PD-L1 antibody) plus olaparib (inhibiting poly adenosine diphosphate ribose polymerase, or PARP), an enzyme involved in DNA repair showed favorable PSA responses and were well tolerated in all mCRPC patients regardless of prior therapies [52, 53]. Interestingly, preclinical data also suggest that targeted radionuclide therapy with [^{223}Ra]RaCl$_2$ may also have immunotherapy (abscopal) effects [54].

In summary, after approval of sipuleucel-T and other immune system-directed drug regimens, the interest in the use of immunotherapy (or radioimmunotherapy) either as a single agent or as multiple immunotherapies and in combination with other traditional treatments (e.g., hormonal therapy, chemotherapy, radiotherapy) has increased in the clinical space of metastatic prostate cancer. The interested reader is referred to excellent reviews on this rapidly evolving topic including antigen-specific vaccines, immune checkpoint inhibition, and combination therapy approaches [55–58]. Important unmet clinical needs in this arena are the development of robust methods (imaging and non-imaging biomarkers)

to predict and evaluate the response and adverse events with immunotherapy, the timing of immunotherapy along the natural history of the disease, optimal sequencing and combination of various therapies with immunotherapy to achieve therapeutic synergism, and strategies to enhance the immunogenicity of prostate cancer [59].

18.5 Conclusion

In this chapter, we discussed the current utility, limitations, and outlook for targeted radionuclide therapy and immunotherapy in men with metastatic prostate cancer. The approval of the first alpha-particle therapy with the calcium mimetic [^{223}Ra]RaCl$_2$ and the anticipated approval for PSMA-targeted radioligand therapy in the foreseeable future paves the way for employing this new class of effective and safe therapeutics in the clinical space of metastatic prostate cancer. The approval of sipuleucel-T was also the first step in personalized immunotherapy in these patients. While the initial investigations with the CTLA-4 and the PD-1/PD-L1 axis have been less enthusiastic, further research is warranted to harness the innate power of the human immune system to combat metastatic prostate cancer.

References

1. National Cancer Institute Surveillance, Epidemiology, and End Results Program. https://seer.cancer.gov/statfacts/html/prost.html. Accessed 31 Dec 2019.
2. Mohler JL, Antonarakis ES, Armstrong AJ, et al. NCCN clinical practice guidelines in oncology: prostate cancer, version 2.2019. J Natl Compr Cancer Netw. 2019;17:479–505.
3. Iagaru AH, Mittra E, Colletti PM, Jadvar H. Bone-targeted imaging and radionuclide therapy in prostate cancer. J Nucl Med. 2016;57:19S–24S.
4. Parker C, Nilsson S, Heinrich D, et al. Alpha emitter radium-223 and survival in metastatic prostate cancer. N Engl J Med. 2013;369:213–23.
5. Dizdarevic S, Petersen PM, Essler M, et al. Interim analysis of the REASSURE (Radium-223 alpha emitter agent in non-intervention safety study in mCRPC popUlation for long-teRm Evaluation) study: patient characteristics and safety according to prior use of chemotherapy in routine clinical practice. Eur J Nucl Med Mol Imaging. 2019;46:1102–10.

6. Dizdarevic S, McCready R, Vinjamuri S. Radium-223 dichloride in prostate cancer: proof of principle for the use of targeted alpha treatment in clinical practice. Eur J Nucl Med Mol Imaging. 2020;47:192–217.

7. Etchebehere EC, Milton DR, Araujo JC, et al. Factors affecting [223]Ra therapy: clinical experience after 532 cycles from a single institution. Eur J Nucl Med Mol Imaging. 2016;43:8–20.

8. Jadvar H, Quinn DI, Conti PS. One-year postapproval clinical experience with radium-223 dichloride in patients with metastatic castrate-resistant prostate cancer. Cancer Biother Radiopharm. 2015;30:195–9.

9. Castello A, Macapinlac H, Lopci E, Santos EB. Prostate-specific antigen flare induced by [223]RaCl$_2$ in patients with metastatic castration-resistant prostate cancer. Eur J Nucl Med Mol Imaging. 2018;45:2256–63.

10. Sartor O, Heinrich D, Mariados N, et al. Re-treatment with radium-223: first experience from an international, open-label, phase I/11 study in patients with castration-resistant prostate cancer and bone metastases. Ann Oncol. 2017;28:2464–71.

11. Morris MJ, Loriot Y, Sweeney CJ, et al. Radium-223 in combination with docetaxel in patients with castration-resistant prostate cancer and bone metastases: a phase 1 escalation/randomized phase 2a trial. Eur J Cancer. 2019;114:107–16. [Epub ahead of print].

12. Jadvar H, Chen X, Cai W, Mahmood U. Radiotheranostics in cancer diagnosis and management. Radiology. 2018;286:388–400.

13. Bouchelouche K, Tagawa ST, Goldsmithe SJ, et al. PET/CT imaging and radioimmunotherapy of prostate cancer. Semin Nucl Med. 2011;41:29–44.

14. Osmany S, Zaheer S, Bartel T, et al. Gallium-68-labeled prostate-specific membrane antigen-11 PET/CT of prostate and nonprostate cancers. AJR Am J Roentgenol. 2019;213:286–99.

15. Rahbar K, Afshar-Oromieh A, Jadvar H, Ahmadzadefar H. PSMA theranostics: current status and future directions. Mol Imaging. 2018;17 https://doi.org/10.1177/1536012118776068.

16. Ahmadzadehfar H, Rahbar K, Kurpig S, et al. Early side effects and first results of radioligand therapy with (177)Lu-DKFZ-617 PSMA of castrate-resistant metastatic prostate cancer: a two center study. EJNMMI Res. 2015;5(1):114.

17. Ahmadzadehfar H, Eppard E, Kurpig S, et al. Therapeutic response and side effects of repeated radioligand therapy with ^{177}Lu-PSMA-DKFZ-617 of castrate-resistant metastatic prostate cancer. Oncotarget. 2016;7(11):12477–88.

18. Ahmadzadehfar H, Wegen S, Yordanova A, et al. Overall survival and response pattern of castration-resistant metastatic prostate cancer to multiple cycles of radioligand therapy using [177Lu] Lu-PSMA-617. Eur J Nucl Med Mol Imaging. 2017;44(9):1448–54.

19. Rahbar K, Bogeman M, Yordanova A, et al. Delayed response after repeated (177)Lu-PSMA-617 radioligand therapy in patients with metastatic castra-tion resistant prostate cancer. Eur J Nucl Med Mol Imaging. 2018;45(2):243–6.

20. Ahmadzadehfar H, Zimbelmann S, Yordanova A, et al. Radioligand therapy of metastatic prostate cancer using ^{177}Lu-PSMA-617 after radiation exposure to 223Ra-dichloride. Oncotarget. 2017;8(33):55567–74.

21. Rahbar K, Bode A, Weckesser M, et al. Radioligand therapy with ^{177}Lu-PSMA-617 as a novel therapeutic option in patients with metastatic castration resistant prostate cancer. Clin Nucl Med. 2016;41(7):522–8.

22. Rahbar K, Schmidt M, Heinzel A, et al. Response and tolerability of a single dose of 177Lu-PSMA-617 in patients with metastatic castration-resistant prostate cancer: a multicenter retrospective analysis. J Nucl Med. 2016;57(9):1334–8.

23. Rahbar K, Ahmadzadehfar H, Kratochwil C, et al. German multicenter study investigating ^{177}Lu-PSMA-617 radioligand therapy in advanced prostate cancer patients. J Nucl Med. 2017;58(1):85–90.

24. Rahbar K, Boegemann M, Yordanova A, et al. PSMA targeted radioligand therapy in metastatic castration resistant prostate cancer after chemotherapy, abiraterone and/or enzalutamide. A retrospective analysis of overall survival. Eur J Nucl Med Mol Imaging. 2018;45(1):12–9.

25. Kratochwil C, Giesel FL, Stefanova M, et al. PSMA-targeted radionuclide therapy of metastatic castration-resistant prostate cancer with ^{177}Lu-labeled PSMA-617. J Nucl Med. 2016;57:1170–6.

26. Baum RP, Kulkarni HR, Schuchardt C, et al. ^{177}Lu-labeled prostate-specific membrane antigen radioligand therapy of metastatic castration-resistant prostate cancer: safety and efficacy. J Nucl Med. 2015;7:1006–13.

27. Kulkarni HR, Singh A, Schuchardt C, et al. PSMA-based radioligand therapy for metastatic castration-resistant prostate cancer: the Bad Berka experience since 2013. J Nucl Med. 2016;57:97S–104S.

28. Yadav MP, Ballal S, Sahoo RK, et al. Radioligand therapy with ^{177}Lu-PSMA for metastatic castration-resistant prostate cancer: a systematic review and meta-analysis. AJR Am J Roentgenol. 2019;213:275–85.

29. Kratochwil C, Fendler WP, Eiber M, et al. EANM procedure guidelines for radionuclide therapy with ^{177}Lu-labelled PSMA-ligands (^{177}Lu-PSMA-RLT). Eur J Nucl Med Mol Imaging. 2019;46:2536–44.

30. Rahbar K, Bodei L, Morris MJ. Is the vision of radioligand therapy for prostate cancer becoming a reality? An overview of the phase III VISION trial and its importance for the future of theranostics. J Nucl Med. 2019;60:1504–6.

31. Hofman MS, Violet J, Hicks RJ, et al. [177Lu]-PSMA-617 radioligand therapy in patients with metastatic castration-resistant prostate cancer (LuPSMA trial): a single-center, single-arm, phase 2 study. Lancet Oncol. 2018;19:825–33.

32. Emmett L, Crumbaker M, Ho B, et al. Results of a prospective phase 2 pilot trial of ^{177}Lu-PSMA-617 therapy for metastatic castration-resistant prostate

Cancer including imaging predictors of treatment response and patterns of progression. Clin Genitourin Cancer. 2019;17(1):15–22.

33. Violet J, Sandhu S, Iravani A, et al. Long-term follow-up and outcomes of re-treatment in an expanded 50 patient single-center phase II prospective trial of Lutetium-177 (^{177}Lu) PSMA-617 theranostics in metastatic castrate-resistant prostate cancer. J Nucl Med. 2020;61:857–65. [Epub ahead of print].

34. Kratochwil C, Bruchertseifer F, Giesel FL, et al. ^{225}Ac-PSMA-617 for PSMA-targeted α-radiation therapy of metastatic castration resistant prostate cancer. J Nucl Med. 2016;57:1941–4.

35. Sathekge M, Knoesen O, Meckel M, et al. ^{213}Bi-PSMA-617 targeted alpha-radionuclide therapy in metastatic castration-resistant prostate cancer. Eur J Nucl Med Mol Imaging. 2017;44:1099–100.

36. Kratochwil C, Bruchertseifer F, Rathke H, et al. Targeted a-therapy of metastatic castration-resistant prostate cancer with ^{225}Ac-PSMA-617: dosimetry estimates and empiric dose finding. J Nucl Med. 2017;58:1624–31.

37. Sathekge M, Bruchertseifer F, Voster M, et al. Predictive of overall survival and disease-free survival in metastatic castration-resistant prostate cancer patients receiving ^{225}Ac-PSMA-617 radioligand therapy. J Nucl Med. 2020;61:62–9.

38. Sathekge M, Brucherseifer F, Knoesen O, et al. ^{225}Ac-PSMA-617 in chemotherapy-naïve patients with advanced prostate cancer: a pilot study. Eur J Nucl Med Mol Imaging. 2019;46:129–38.

39. Ye Z, Qian Q, Jin H, Qian Q. Cancer vaccine: learning from immune checkpoint inhibitors. J Cancer. 2018;9:263–8.

40. Thara E, Dorff TB, Averia-Suboc M, et al. Immune response to sipuleucel-T in prostate cancer. Cancers. 2012;4:420–41.

41. Singh H, Gulley JL. Immunotherapy and therapeutic vaccines in prostate cancer: an update on current strategies and clinical implications. Asian J Androl. 2014;16:364–71.

42. Tse BW-C, Jovanovic L, Nelson CC, et al. From bench to bedside: immunotherapy for prostate cancer. Biomed Res Int. 2014;2014:981434.

43. Kantoff PW, Higano CS, Shore ND, et al. Sipuleucel-T immunotherapy for castration-resistant prostate cancer. N Engl J Med. 2010;363:411–22.

44. Bilusic M, Madan RA, Gulley JL. Immunotherapy of prostate cancer: facts and hopes. Clin Cancer Res. 2017;23:6764–70.

45. Vitkin N, Nersessian S, Siemens DR, Koti M. The tumor immune contexture of prostate cancer. Front Immunol. 2019;10:603.

46. Modena A, Ciccarese C, Iacovelli R, et al. Immune checkpoint inhibitors and prostate cancer: a new frontier? Oncol Rev. 2016;10:2931.

47. Kittai A, Meshikhes M, Aragon-Ching JB. Ipilimumab: a potential immunologic agent in the treatment of metastatic castration-resistant prostate cancer. Cancer Biol Ther. 2014;15:1299–300.

48. Beer TM, Kwon ED, Drake CC, et al. Randomized double-blind phase III trial of ipilimumab versus placebo in asymptomatic or minimally symptomatic patients with metastatic chemotherapy-naïve castration-resistant prostate cancer. J Clin Oncol. 2017;35:40–7.

49. Kwon ED, Drake CG, Scher HI, et al. Ipilimumab versus placebo after radiotherapy in patients with metastatic castration-resistant prostate cancer that had progressed after docetaxel chemotherapy (CA184-043): a multicenter, randomized, double-blind, phase 3 trial. Lancet Oncol. 2014;15:700–12.

50. Hansen A, Massard C, Ott P. Pembrolizumab for patients with advanced prostate adenocarcinoma: preliminary results from KEYNOTE-028 study. Ann Oncol. 2016;27:725PD.

51. Topalian SL, Hodi FS, Brahmer JR, et al. Safety, activity, and immune correlates of anti-PD-1 antibody in cancer. N Engl J Med. 2012;366:2443–54.

52. Karazi F, Madan RA, Owens H, et al. A phase II study of the anti-programmed death ligand-1 antibody durvalumab in combination with PARP inhibitor, olaparib, in metastatic castration-resistant prostate cancer (mCRPC). J Clin Oncol. 2017;35:abstr 162.

53. Karzai F, VanderWeele D, Madan RA, et al. Activity of durvalumab plus olaparib in metastatic castration-resistant prostate cancer in men with and without DNA damage mutations. J Immunother Cancer. 2018;6:141.

54. Malmas AS, Gameiro SR, Knudson KM, et al. Sublethal exposure to alpha radiation (223Ra dichloride) enhances various carcinoma's sensitivity to lysis by antigen-specific cytotoxic T-lymphocytes through calreticulin-mediated immunogenic modulation. Oncotarget. 2016;7:86937–47.

55. Schweizer MT, Drake CG. Immunotherapy for prostate cancer—recent developments and future challenges. Cancer Metastasis Rev. 2014;33:641–55.

56. Surdacki G, Szudy-Szczyrek A, Goracy A, et al. The role of immune checkpoint inhibitors in prostate cancer. Ann Agric Environ Med. 2019;26:120–4.

57. Madan RA, Gulley JL, Kantoff PW. Demystifying immunotherapy in prostate cancer: understanding current and future treatment strategies. Cancer J. 2013;19:50–8.

58. Schepisi G, Farolfi A, Conteduca V, et al. Immunotherapy for prostate cancer: where we are headed. Int J Mol Sci. 2017;18:2627.

59. Slovin SF. Emerging treatments in management of prostate cancer: biomarker validation and endpoints for immunotherapy clinical trial design. Immunotargets Ther. 2014;3:1–8.

Radioimmunotherapy and Targeted Radiotherapy of Squamous Cell Carcinoma of the Head and Neck

19

Siroos Mirzaei and Heying Duan

Contents

19.1 Introduction

Head and neck squamous cell carcinoma (HNSCC) is the seventh most common cancer worldwide with an annual incidence rate of more than 600,000 [1] and the ninth most fatal cancer [2]. It originates from multiple anatomical subsites in the head and neck region including the oropharynx, hypopharynx, larynx, and oral cavity. Besides the well-known risk factors such as tobacco smoking and alcohol consumption, the incidence of human papillomavirus (HPV)-related HNSCC has risen, especially in the oropharynx, known as oropharyngeal squamous cell carcinoma (OPSCC) [3, 4].

HPV are DNA viruses infecting the epithelium of the deep tonsillar crypts. These crypts are immune-privileged sites able to tolerate new antigens without launching an immune response. The consequence is an inhibition of the effector function of HPV-specific T cells and thus facilitates immune evasion at the time of initial HPV infection [5]. A multicenter study consisting of 25,500 patients demonstrated that tobacco is a major risk

S. Mirzaei (✉)
Institute of Nuclear Medicine with PET-Center, Wilhelminen Hospital, Vienna, Austria
e-mail: siroos.mirzaei@gesundheitsverbund.at

H. Duan
Department of Radiology, Stanford University, Stanford, CA, USA
e-mail: heying@stanford.edu

© Springer Nature Switzerland AG 2022
S. Harsini et al. (eds.), *Nuclear Medicine and Immunology*,
https://doi.org/10.1007/978-3-030-81261-4_19

factor for head and neck and oropharynx carcinoma [6]. On the other hand, patients with HPV-positive tumors are generally nonsmokers [7]. It seems that there has been an epidemiologic shift towards OPSCC with the decline of cigarette smoking. Nonetheless, smoking is still a major risk factor but has less impact on HPV-related cancers. Thirty percent of OPSCC patients are nonsmokers as opposed to 5% of HNSCC patients [8].

The treatment option for early-stage disease is either surgery or radiotherapy with a reported 5-year survival rate ranging from 40% to 50% in the past three decades [9–11]. The cure rates are above 90% and 70% for stages I and II, respectively [10, 12]. For patients with advanced, metastatic, or relapsed HNSCC in stage III or IV, the treatment landscape is complex and requires a multimodality approach comprising of surgery, radiation therapy, and chemotherapy in various combinations depending on the extent of the disease [13, 14]. Overall, the prognosis is poor with a median survival of less than a year and marginally longer for patients with OPSCC [15, 16]. However, all these standard therapy regimens bear significant side effects involving vital functions such as breathing, swallowing, and talking, thus narrowing the patient's quality of life (QoL).

A targeted treatment approach and personalized precision medicine should be the goal of treating cancer. It is important to identify a target structure that is expressed in abundance on the tumor cell but is rare on the healthy cell. In HNSCC, targeting immunological structures of the tumor cell has been shown to be efficacious. In order to assess whether a patient would benefit from the so-called immunotherapy (IT), accurate diagnostic imaging should be performed. Immuno-imaging using single photon emission computed tomography (SPECT) or positron emission tomography (PET), best when combined with computed tomography (CT), are the methods of choice. A diagnostic radionuclide is bound to the drug, such as monoclonal antibodies (mAbs), and injected intravenously. This allows for imaging and stratification for radioimmunotherapy (RIT). For RIT, a therapeutic radionuclide is chelated to the same agent and binds specifically to the immune target of the tumor. That way, the radiation dose to the tumor can be maximized while sparing healthy, normal tissue [17, 18]. However, the challenges are to identify suitable targets and to develop a tracer which is specific and radiochemically stable. Immunotherapy targets the same immunological structure on the tumor cell but is not bound to radiation. The most common agent are mAbs. For better outcome results, it is often given in combination with radiotherapy [14, 19]. However, the treatment response is not as satisfactory, compared to the disease in the early stages [20].

RIT and IT are not referred to as standard treatments in the therapy landscape of HNSCC. They interact with different immune reactions and are well tolerated. Combined with standard therapy, the outcome is promising.

19.2 Current Development in Treatment Options

For many years, standard therapy consisted of surgery, radiation therapy, and chemotherapy. They bear a significant amount of side effects impacting the patient's QoL. Particularly, concurrent radiochemotherapy may cause mucositis, dermatitis, and dysphagia and is frequently accompanied by leukopenia and thrombocytopenia, which increases the risk of infection or bleeding [12]. Late complications include sensorineural hearing loss, polyneuropathy caused by chemotherapy, permanent xerostomia, and impaired swallowing [12]. Unsatisfactory outcomes of the standard HNSCC treatment regimen with a high toxicity profile raised a demand for novel therapeutic options. Targeted drugs consist of inactivating specific target molecules required for oncogenesis and tumor growth [21].

Novel treatment methods are on the rise. Advances in radiotherapy techniques like the implementation of intensity-modulated radiotherapy (IMRT) allow a more accurate dose delivery to the tumor while sparing surrounding healthy structures to minimize side effects. Surgical techniques have expanded to new technologies, such as robot-assisted surgeries and laser surgery. They show promising results, are well tolerated with minimal side effects. Over the next years, there will be a shift from standard therapies towards a personalized therapeutic approach like IT and RIT to optimize oncological outcome while keeping toxicity low and maintaining QoL in patients with HNSCC/OPSCC.

Despite the major differences in the pathogenesis of HNSCC and OPSCC [22, 23], the recommended treatment options are the same. Therapies are dependent on the tumor stage, potential metastases and the patient's comorbidities and preferences. Early-stage disease is usually treated with a single modality such as surgery or radiotherapy alone. For locoregionally advanced oropharyngeal cancer, a dual-modality approach with either trans-oral robotic surgery (TORS) and postoperative radiotherapy or chemotherapy or combined radiochemotherapy is applied. In cancers of the tonsil and tongue base, radiochemotherapy is more frequently used [24, 25].

The long-term toxicity following radiochemotherapy has elucidated TORS as a primary treatment option. Comparable oncological outcomes with TORS and IMRT have been reported, but functional outcomes *may* be better with TORS. However, it should be noted that the follow-up times have been relatively short and that the TORS studies included more early-stage OPSCC patients than the IMRT studies [26].

19.3 Immunotherapy (IT)

In HNSCC patients with unresectable, advanced disease, a combination therapy modalities only achieved suboptimal disease control with a 5-year survival rate of less than 10% [27]. Therefore, there has been a demand for novel treatment options to improve clinical outcome and with a better toxicity profile. IT may be the answer. There are several indications that the pathogenesis of HNSCC is based on an immunosuppressive process. Jie et al. reported that HNSCC patients have overall lower white blood cell counts which consist more of suppressive regulatory T cells (Tregs) upregulating immunosuppressive molecules [28]. Tregs control autoreactive lympho-

cytes, but also downregulate the immune response to tumor-associated antigens. Furthermore, tumor-infiltrating lymphocytes (TILs) comprise of a larger population of Tregs as compared to the periphery. Immunosuppressive tumor cells, therefore, evade the detection by the immune system and consecutively cannot be destroyed [29, 30]. These findings strongly suggest that there is an interaction between tumor development and the immune system, bearing potential therapeutic targets [31]. Tregs have been regularly described among TILs and in the peripheral circulation in various solid tumors [32–35].

There are several target points for IT. For one, immune checkpoint inhibitors which inhibit proteins made to keep T cells from attacking cancer cells. The most investigated and promising immune checkpoint inhibitors are nivolumab, pembrolizumab, durvalumab, atezolizumab, and avelumab. Pembrolizumab and nivolumab received US Food and Drug Administration (FDA) approval in the recurrent and metastatic setting of HNSCC. The majority of current studies is assessing the efficacy of immune checkpoint inhibitors or their combination with other treatments in the advanced disease stage [36]. Fewer trials explore the use of IT in the primary setting with curative intent. Monoclonal antibodies are immunoglobulins produced by hybrid cell lines (hybridomas) derived from the fusion of B lymphocytes from previously immunized animals with myeloma cells adapted for growing in culture [12]. At first, all mAbs were obtained from murine hybridomas. This posed certain obstacles to their use in humans—first and foremost, these mAbs induced a human-antibody reaction to the alien protein, a phenomenon known as the human anti-mouse antibody (HAMA) response. This was one of the driving forces behind the development of second-generation mAbs, especially for therapeutic use [12].

Second-generation mAbs, or recombinant antibodies, are molecules produced with molecular biology techniques and recombinant DNA—that is, the mAbs are generated by immortalizing the genes that code for immunoglobulin molecule rather than the cell that produces the antibody, as in the case of the first-generation mAbs. In recombinant antibodies, the variable region of murine immunoglobulin can be retained, while the constant region (Fc) is human (chimeric antibodies). Alternatively, just the hypervariable murine region can be retained, keeping the remainder human (humanized antibodies). This has resulted in better patient response to treatment with mAbs and a marked reduction in adverse reactions [13].

Monoclonal antibodies have extremely high specificity, and this stands as a very useful property, as monoclonal and recombinant antibodies can be produced binding specifically to an antigen molecule. Two other characteristics contribute to their success. First, they can be prepared in pure form in large quantities under tightly controlled conditions. Second, they are chemically well-defined substances with well-known nature and structure, making it possible to formulate stable preparations, thereby facilitating their conjugation to tracers such as fluorescent substances, enzymes, and radioisotopes [12, 13].

A majority of immune checkpoint inhibitors act on the programmed cell death 1 (PD-1) and its ligand, programmed cell death ligand 1, (PD-L1) axis [32]. This pathway is applicable for HNSCC and OPSCC since the oropharynx is known to be an immune-privileged site and it has been demonstrated that the reticulated epithelium of the deep tonsillar crypts expresses PD-L1 [37, 38]. When PD-1 binds to PD-L1, the cytotoxic T cell response is suppressed, which plays a role against excessive inflammation but, in the case of HNSCC, leads to evasion of the immune response and/or persistent HPV infection [39]. Pembrolizumab is an anti-PD-1 mAb that has been approved by the FDA for the treatment of chemotherapy refractory, recurrent, and metastatic HNSCC. In the study leading to the FDA approval of pembrolizumab, it was well tolerated and showed a better outcome in OPSCC than HNSCC with a progression-free survival (PFS) of 17.2 weeks versus 8.1 weeks in HNSCC as well as overall survival (OS) not reached versus 9.5 months for HNSCC [40]. Currently, the efficacy of pembrolizumab is being evaluated in multiple studies as first-line therapy in recurrent and metastatic disease or in comparison with the standard of care regimen.

Epidermal growth factor receptor (EGFR) is another immune target which is addressed by EGFR mAb (cetuximab, panitumumab, zalutumumab, and nimotuzumab), EGFR tyrosine kinase inhibitors (TKI) (gefitinib, erlotinib, lapatinib, afatinib, and dacomitinib), vascular endothelial growth factor (VEGF) inhibitor (bevacizumab) or vascular endothelial growth factor receptor (VEGFR) inhibitors (sorafenib, sunitinib, and vandetanib), and inhibitors of phosphatidylinositol 3-kinase/serine/threonine-specific protein kinase/mammalian target of rapamycin. There are also various inhibitors of other pathways and targets requiring more investigation in further studies. EGFR is the best-studied target for HNSCC and is overexpressed in more than 90% of HNSCC [41–43]. Overexpression of EGFR is associated with poor prognosis, increased tumor growth, metastases, and resistance to chemotherapy and radiation therapy [44]. Despite the high hopes for agents addressing EGFR, the results are controversial [45–48]. However, as monotherapy, TKI and mAb against EGFR showed only limited efficacy in HNSCC [49–51].

A key role player of the immune system in control of tumor growth and progression has been elucidated [52, 53]. The lymphocytic infiltrate of tumors is known to be associated with the prognosis of malignant tumors [54–56]. In HNSCC, a high density of TILs is associated with improved outcome [57, 58]. A correlation with outcome has mainly been demonstrated for CD8+ lymphocytes [59]. The rate of CD8+ infiltrating effector lymphocytes is higher in OPSCC, which might be an explanation for the improved clinical outcome observed [59, 60].

19.4 Immuno-Imaging

Most tumor cells sequester or overexpress specific antigens that differentiate them from adjacent healthy tissue. These antigens can be found in blood or on the tumor cell surface and constitute tumor markers. Immuno-imaging with scintigraphy and PET underlies this principle. The corresponding mAb to the tumor antigen is bound to a radioisotope (known as the radiolabeling process). The radioisotope used for scintigraphy is most commonly a gamma emitter with a short half-life such as technetium-99m

(^{99m}Tc) and for PET a positron emitter such as copper-64 (^{64}Cu). The patient receives the radiolabeled antibody, also called tracer, intravenously. In the body, the tracer finds its way to its specific antigen on the tumor surface and binds to it. The labeled radionuclide will emit radioactivity which is captured by a gamma camera or PET scanner revealing the tumor location and extent. This method is very specific since the antibody binds only to its corresponding antigen on the tumor cell surface [14].

Scintigraphy can produce both planar and tomographic images (SPECT). SPECT, especially combined with CT (SPECT/CT), provides a better contrast since superimposed layers are separated and allow for anatomical correlation to be more precise in locating the lesion and have a better estimate of size. PET, especially combined with CT (PET/CT), has significant advantages over scintigraphy as it has a higher spatial resolution and sensitivity. Song et al. prepared an anti-EGFR antibody radiolabeled with copper-64 for imaging or lutetium-177 (^{177}Lu) for RIT. In an esophageal squamous cell carcinoma (ESCC) model, they showed EGFR expression in the tumor on [^{64}Cu]Cu-cetuximab immuno-PET and [^{177}Lu]Lu-cetuximab RIT effectively inhibited tumor growth [61]. These findings are sustained in further studies evaluating [^{64}Cu]Cu-labeled cetuximab as an immuno-PET imaging agent in tumor-bearing mouse models [62, 63].

Copper-64 is a well-suited radionuclide for imaging as it provides high resolution with a short half-life of 12.7 h. Lutetium-177 has low-energy beta-emission with only minimal tissue penetration, making it an appropriate radioisotope for therapy, especially of small and metastatic tumors [64]. Studies with other positron-emitting radionuclides (gallium-68, fluoride-18, yttrium-86, zirconium-89, iodine-124) have been conducted [65–67]. It appears that the only radioisotope suitable would be zirconium-89 (^{89}Zr). However, ^{89}Zr-labeled antibodies showed an eight-times higher whole-body dose (40 mSv/74 MBq in zirconium-89 vs. 5 mSv/130 MBq in copper-64) compared to ^{64}Cu-labeled antibodies [68], making it less desirable.

Immuno-imaging is an effective and specific diagnostic imaging tool that helps in the delin-eation of primary and recurrent disease extent, especially in cases with clinical suspicion and/or elevated tumor markers and when other imaging techniques fail [13, 14]. Moreover, it allows for stratification for RIT.

19.5 Radioimmunotherapy

The first IT approved by the FDA was rituximab (MabThera, Rituxan) in 1997. It is a chimeric antibody that targets CD20 antigen in B cells and was initially used for the treatment of refractory or recurrent low-grade follicular non-Hodgkin lymphoma [15]. Nowadays, it is routinely given as first-line monotherapy or added to a chemotherapy regimen consisting of various drugs as it improves OS by 15% [56]. Given these results, rituximab was radiolabeled to yttrium-90 (^{90}Y), a beta radiation emitter, to enhance its therapeutic effect by aiming high doses of radiation directly at the CD20 antigen on tumor cell surfaces [20]. RIT is a targeted therapy which not only delivers a high radiation dose to the tumor cells but also has the "crossfire effect," a phenomenon of radiation-induced cell death of adjacent tumor cells which do not have a specific bond to the mAb. As opposed to conventional radiation therapy, the radiation applied is continuous and decreases over time, and the treatment duration is shorter. Compared to standard antitumoral therapy, the toxicity profile is low [69]. Currently, yttrium-90 and lutetium-177 have been the most frequently used radionuclides. Especially, lutetium-177 is suitable for RIT due to its low tissue penetration range (~2 mm) and the additional emission of gamma radiation allowing for post-therapeutic imaging with scintigraphy enhanced by CT. The dose-limiting factor is myelotoxicity. A study in nude mice bearing human ovarian cancer receiving [^{177}Lu]Lu-CC49 RIT showed that four out of nine mice survived after receiving 13.5 MBq, whereas all mice tolerated 12.95 MBq [70]. However, it has also been demonstrated that the bone marrow dose is acceptable and does not limit further administration of currently used doses of chemotherapy. Supportive therapy with bone marrow blood cell precursors harvested prior to RIT and reimplanted after 12–18 days can minimize myelotoxicity. Its efficacy for HNSCC has been demonstrated through multiple clinical trials [67, 69–72].

Cetuximab is a chimeric anti-EGFR mAb and has been approved by the FDA for HNSCC, initially in combination with radiation therapy [73–75], but further studies have shown promising results in combination with chemotherapy, leading to its approval for initial therapy [76, 77]. It is important to couple cetuximab with other treatment modalities since it has been shown that there is a drug resistance leaving many HNSCC unresponsive to EGFR-targeted therapy [78]. RIT using radiolabeled anti-EGFR antibodies has shown promising results compared to IT alone in preclinical HNSCC xenograft models [79, 80].

Song et al. investigated the efficacy of [^{177}Lu] Lu-PCTA-cetuximab RIT in an HNSCC tumor model [81]. In the group treated with saline, time-dependent tumor growth was observed. After a single dose of cetuximab, tumor development was slightly delayed or inhibited, but regrowth was noted with an increased average tumor volume up until day 30. A single dose of [^{177}Lu]Lu-PCTA-cetuximab showed a significant decrease in tumor volume by 55% on day 30. No observable toxicity could be detected in this mouse model [81]. This group also focused on dosimetry which is important to spare vital organs like the bone marrow, kidneys, or liver. Regarding these organs, they found low radiation doses, whereas the tumor-absorbed radiation dose was high (bone marrow 8.2 E^{-04} mGy/MBq vs. HNSCC tumor 67.2 ± 14.6 Gy/12.95 MBq) [79].

19.6 Targeted Radiotherapy of Squamous Cell Carcinoma of the Head and Neck

Radiotherapy is one of the keystones in the treatment of HNSCC. For early-stage disease, surgery and radiotherapy are the first-line therapies with a curative approach, and in advanced stages, radiotherapy is combined with other treatment modalities. Initially, two-dimensional radiotherapy (2DRT) was performed. With this technique, a large amount of healthy tissue were irradiated, which leads to severe side effects, oftentimes involving vital functions manifesting with dysphagia, xerostomia, skin fibrosis, and speech difficulties. Advances in radiotherapeutic methods improved the toxicity profile by zooming the radiation beam closer around the tumor [82]. Three-dimensional conformal radiotherapy (3DCRT) was implemented in the 1980s taking advantage of anatomical information provided by CT. Despite these advances, the head and neck region with its small anatomical structures still remains a challenge.

Over the years, with technical improvements of appliances and combining radiotherapy with chemotherapy, an improved outcome has been observed by a number of studies [83]. Chemotherapy protocols were either platinum-based or combined with other agents. Several large phase III trials showed a significantly better outcome of locoregional tumor control and overall survival (OS) for patients receiving combination therapies [84–86]. However, a combination with chemotherapy led to a higher rate of acute side effects, especially mucosal-related. Late toxicity was comparable [87]. A large meta-analysis with more than 17,000 patients in 25 trials confirmed the results and showed a consistent survival benefit of 6.5% for concurrent chemoradiation [88].

Currently, functional imaging is embedded in treatment planning to pursue a personalized treatment approach with an individual dose. Intensification of therapy therefore seems to lead to an improved outcome in patients with advanced HNSCC. Fractionation of radiotherapy is an effective method of escalating treatment dose while protecting surrounding normal tissue. Conventional fractionation protocols for HNSCC are defined by smaller "treatment fractions" given once a day up to an individualized total dose [87]. With a better radiobiological understanding and the development of various treatment techniques like computerized three-dimensional (3D) treatment planning and IMRT, both the fraction dose and the daily radiation frequency can be modified. This underlies the radiobiological principle that normal tissue cells will recover fully from radiation-induced DNA damage within 6 h. Hyper-fractionation is defined by splitting the total dose into small fraction sizes (1.2 Gy) as opposed to acceleration where bigger daily doses (2.5 Gy) are given. Pure acceleration means that higher single doses (1.8–2 Gy) are applied twice a day or more than five times per week. A combination of these protocols is known as hybrid acceleration. They have all been proven effective in randomized clinical trials in locoregional tumor control and survival [89]. A meta-analysis consisting of 6,515 patients revealed a survival benefit of 3.4% for hyperfractionated and accelerated protocols versus an 8% benefit for pure hyperfractionation. The benefit in controlling the primary tumor was 6.4% for the hyperfractionated and accelerated protocol and was more pronounced in younger patients (<50 years). Although acute treatment-related toxicity of accelerated protocols was significantly elevated in most studies, chronic toxicity was not significantly affected [90].

Tumor hypoxia substantially reduces radio-sensitivity, and necrotic and hypoxic lymph node metastases in HNSCC are common. Overcoming tumor hypoxia may hence improve radiotherapeutic response. A phase II trial investigated the hypoxic modifier nimorazole with radiotherapy and cisplatin in 227 patients with stage III and IV HNSCC and revealed good tolerability and promising tumor control and survival rates [91].

A phase II trial comparing radiotherapy alone and in combination with the EGFR antagonist cetuximab revealed a clear advantage for combination treatment with a 9% survival difference after 5 years [92, 93].

The incidence of OPSCC has risen since 1988 [94], stratifying OPSCC as a distinct tumor entity [95]. Although it shows more aggressive tumor biology, especially in advanced lymph node spread, local tumor control, PFS, and OS are clearly better than in HNSCC [85]. This seems to be independent of the treatment modalities such as the addition of IT to radiotherapy, intensified protocols in radiochemotherapy, intensified chemotherapy followed by concurrent radiochemotherapy, or surgery [96–98].

IMRT has become the standard radiotherapy protocol in HNSCC. This technique provides an accurate dose application to the tumor. The dose intensity can also be altered. This method results in inhomogeneous radiation delivery to the tumor allowing the possibility of a simultaneous boost and dose escalation in preferred areas of the tumor [87]. Areas of hypoxia would, for instance, benefit from escalated radiation doses as tumor hypoxia is a major cause of radioresistance. PET/CT with the hypoxiaavid tracer [^{18}F] fluoromisonidazole (FMISO) aids delineating hypoxic tumor areas for radiation planning [99].

Volumetric modulated arc therapy (VMAT) is a novel radiation technique which includes advanced treatment planning algorithms and computerized treatment application to further improve accuracy of radiation therapy, resulting in an improved sparing of adjacent healthy tissue and fewer side effects [100]. Especially, radiation of HNSCC can cause damage to the parotid and submandibular glands, resulting in xerostomia. Pow et al. [101] compared 2DRT to IMRT in patients with nasopharyngeal cancers. At 1-year follow-up, 24 patients treated with IMRT showed significantly better stimulated whole salivary as well as stimulated parotid salivary flow rates than the 21 patients treated with 2DRT. The salivary flow decreased in both groups after treatment, but after IMRT, salivary function improved, whereas limited improvement was noted after 2DRT. A study consisting of 91 HNSCC patients undergoing VMAT sparing the parotid gland showed significantly less grade II xerostomia compared to conventional 3D-planned treatment [102].

Irradiation of the oral cavity can cause mucositis which can be worsened in combination with chemotherapy. Mucositis leads to decreased oral intake and hence weight loss and impact on QoL. Gupta et al. [103] found no significant difference in acute mucositis between 3DCRT and IMRT treatments in a randomized controlled trial comprising of 60 patients with HNSCC. The conclusion drawn from this and comparable studies shows that the occurrence of mucositis is determined by the area of irradiation and not the technique used [82]. Ghosh-Laskar et al. [104] investigated weight loss which often occurs as a result of radiation-induced side effects such as mucositis and dysphagia. A significant substantial weight loss was observed in patients receiving 3DCRT as opposed to treatment with IMRT (50% vs. 21%, $p = 0.038$). This difference was not significant in the acute setting, although there was a similar trend. Hypothyroidism is another postradiation side effect. Murthy et al. reported an incidence of hypothyroidism after radiochemotherapy for HNSCC in 122 patients. Patients who received IMRT showed significantly more subclinical hypothyroidism than 3DCRT (51.1% vs. 27.3%, $p = 0.021$). However, the incidence is high following radiation therapy, and the dose to the thyroid gland should be kept to a minimum [105]. Concerning the effect of conventional radiation therapy and IMRT on voice and speech, no data from randomized controlled trials are available. However, some authors found that there was a significantly better outcome in speech and voice in favor of IMRT [82]. All these side effects affect the patient's QoL. Pow et al. [101] were the first to conduct a randomized controlled trial to compare QoL in patients treated with 2DRT or IMRT for nasopharyngeal cancer. IMRT showed overall better QoL than conventional radiotherapy.

Modern linear accelerators allow for image-guided radiotherapy as the CT images acquired during radiotherapy allows to adjust to anatomical changes such as tumor shrinkage or due to acute weight loss. That way, the treatment dose and beam delivery can be modified and adapted to the patient's needs. This is also known as adaptive radiotherapy (ART). However, ART is time-consuming and costly and does not apply to all patients and should only be performed in patients who will have a clinical benefit [82, 87].

19.7 Adjuvant Radiotherapy

Adjuvant radiotherapy is given to patients having unfavorable prognostic factors like extracapsular lymph node extension or close or positive margins of the primary tumor or perineural invasion, resulting in a high risk of relapse after surgery [106, 107]. This underlies the principle that postoperative radiotherapy destroys microscopic tumor cells in the tumor bed as well as the lymphoid tissue which could cause recurrent disease [85]. There

are multiple prospective studies demonstrating the efficacy of adjuvant radiotherapy not only for local tumor control but also for OS [85].

19.8 Conclusion

For patients with advanced, metastatic or relapsed HNSCC in stage III or IV, the treatment landscape is complex with poor prognosis, and requires a multimodality approach comprising of surgery, radiation therapy, and chemotherapy in various combinations depending on the extent of disease. A targeted treatment approach and personalized precision medicine should be the goal of treating these patients to improve their outcome. RIT using radiolabeled anti-EGFR antibodies has shown promising results compared to IT alone in preclinical HNSCC xenograft models. Hereby, the therapeutic radionuclide is chelated to the agent and binds specifically to the immune target of the tumor. That way, the radiation dose to the tumor can be maximized while sparing healthy, normal tissue.

References

1. Jemal A, Bray F, Center MM, Ferlay J, Ward E, Forman D. Global cancer statistics. CA Cancer J Clin. 2011;61:69–90.
2. Kozakiewicz P, Grzybowska-Szatkowska L. Application of molecular targeted therapies in the treatment of head and neck squamous cell carcinoma. Oncol Lett. 2018;15:7497–505.
3. Gillison ML, Chaturvedi AK, Anderson WF, Fakhry C. Epidemiology of human papillomavirus-positive head and neck squamous cell carcinoma. J Clin Oncol. 2015;33(29):3235–42.
4. Ang KK, Harris J, Wheeler R, Weber R, Rosenthal DI, Nguyen-Tân PF, et al. Human papillomavirus and survival of patients with oropharyngeal cancer. N Engl J Med. 2010;363(1):24–35.
5. Best SR, Niparko KJ, Pai SI. Biology of human papillomavirus infection and immune therapy for HPV-related head and neck cancers. Otolaryngol Clin N Am. 2012;45(4):807–22.
6. Winn DM, Lee YC, Hashibe M, et al. The INHANCE consortium: toward a better understanding of the causes and mechanisms of head and neck cancer. Oral Dis. 2015;21(6):685–93.
7. Lindel K, Beer KT, Laissue J, et al. Human papillomavirus positive squamous cell carcinoma of the

oropharynx: a radiosensitive subgroup of head and neck carcinoma. Cancer. 2001;92(4):805–13.

8. Hong AM, Martin A, Chatfield M, et al. Human papillomavirus, smoking status and outcomes in tonsillar squamous cell carcinoma. Int J Cancer. 2013;132(12):2748–54.

9. Shanti RM, O'Malley BW Jr. Surgical management of oral cancer. Dent Clin N Am. 2018;62(1):77–86.

10. Hashibe M, Brennan P, Chuang SC, Boccia S, Castellsague X, Chen C, Curado MP, Dal Maso L, Daudt AW, Fabianova E, et al. Interaction between tobacco and alcohol use and the risk of head and neck cancer: pooled analysis in the international head and neck cancer epidemiology consortium. Cancer Epidemiol Biomark Prev. 2009;18:541–50.

11. Pignon JP, Bourhis J, Domenge C, Designé L. Chemotherapy added to locoregional treatment for head and neck squamous-cell carcinoma: three meta-analyses of updated individual data. MACH-NC Collaborative Group. Meta-analysis of chemotherapy on head and neck cancer. Lancet. 2000;355(9208):949–55.

12. Fung C, Grandis JR. Emerging drugs to treat squamous cell carcinomas of the head and neck. Expert Opin Emerg Drugs. 2010;15:355–73.

13. Adelstein D, Gillison ML, Pfister DG, Spencer S, Adkins D, Brizel DM, Burtness B, Busse PM, Caudell JJ, Cmelak AJ, et al. NCCN guidelines insights: head and neck cancers, version 2.2017. J Natl Compr Cancer Netw. 2017;15:761–70. https://doi.org/10.6004/jnccn.2017.0101.

14. Brierley JD, Gospodarowicz MK, Wittekind CH. TNM classification of malignant tumours. 8th ed. Chichester: John Wiley & Sons, Inc.; 2017.

15. Argiris A, Li S, Ghebremichael M, Egloff AM, Wang L, Forastiere AA, et al. Prognostic significance of human papillomavirus in recurrent or metastatic head and neck cancer: an analysis of Eastern Cooperative Oncology Group trials. Ann Oncol. 2014;25(7):1410–6.

16. Fakhry C, Zhang Q, Nguyen-Tan PF, Rosenthal D, El-Naggar A, Garden AS, et al. Human papillomavirus and overall survival after progression of oropharyngeal squamous cell carcinoma. J Clin Oncol. 2014;32(30):3365–73. https://doi.org/10.1200/JCO.2014.55.1937.

17. Zukotynski K, Jadvar H, Capala J, Fahey F. Targeted radionuclide therapy: Practical applications and future prospects. Biomark Cancer. 2016;8(Suppl 2):35–8.

18. Dash A, Knapp FF, Pillai MR. Targeted radionuclide therapy—an overview. Curr Radiopharm. 2013;6:152–80.

19. Pignon JP, le Maitre A, Maillard E, Bourhis J, MACH-NC Collaborative Group. Meta-analysis of chemotherapy in head and neck cancer (MACH-NC): an update on 93 randomised trials and 17,346 patients. Radiother Oncol. 2009;92:4–14.

20. Argiris A, Karamouzis MV, Raben D, Ferris RL. Head and neck cancer. Lancet. 2008;371:1695–709.

21. NCI dictionary of cancer terms: definition of targeted therapy. National Cancer Institute, 2016. https://www.cancer.gov/publications/dictionaries/cancer-terms?cdrid=270742.

22. Ang KK, Harris J, Wheeler R, et al. Human papillomavirus and survival of patients with oropharyngeal cancer. N Engl J Med. 2010;363(1):24–35.

23. Iyer NG, Dogan S, Palmer F, et al. Detailed analysis of clinicopathologic factors demonstrate distinct difference in outcome and prognostic factors between surgically treated HPV-positive and negative oropharyngeal cancer. Ann Surg Oncol. 2015;22:4411–21.

24. Calais G, Alfonsi M, Bardet E, et al. [Stage III and IV cancers of the oropharynx: results of a randomized study of Gortec comparing radiotherapy alone with concomitant chemotherapy]. Bull Cancer. 2000;87:48–53.

25. Marur S, D'Souza G, Westra WH, et al. HPV-associated head and neck cancer: a virus-related cancer epidemic. Lancet Oncol. 2010;11(8):781–9.

26. Hay A. Recent advances in the understanding and management of oropharyngeal cancer. Version 1. F1000Res. 2018;7:F1000 Faculty Rev-1362.

27. Argiris A, Stenson KM, Brockstein BE, Mittal BB, Pelzer H, Kies MS, Jayaram P, Portugal L, Wenig BL, Rosen FR, Haraf DJ, Vokes EE. Neck dissection in the combined-modality therapy of patients with locoregionally advanced head and neck cancer. Head Neck. 2004;26:447–55.

28. Jie HB, Gildener-Leapman N, Li J, et al. Intratumoral regulatory T cells upregulate immunosuppressive molecules in head and neck cancer patients. Br J Cancer. 2013;109:2629–35.

29. Allen CT, Judd NP, Bui JD, et al. The clinical implications of antitumor immunity in head and neck cancer. Laryngoscope. 2012;122:144–57.

30. Whiteside TL. Immunobiology of head and neck cancer. Cancer Metastasis Rev. 2005;24:95–105.

31. Ferris RL. Immunology and immunotherapy of head and neck cancer. J Clin Oncol. 2015;33:3293–304.

32. Woo EY, Yeh H, Chu CS, Schlienger K, Carroll RG, Riley JL, et al. Cutting edge: regulatory T cells from lung cancer patients directly inhibit autologous T cell proliferation. J Immunol. 2002;168(9):4272–6.

33. Woo EY, Chu CS, Goletz TJ, Schlienger K, Yeh H, Coukos G, et al. Regulatory CD4(+)CD25(+) T cells in tumors from patients with early-stage non-small cell lung cancer and late-stage ovarian cancer. Cancer Res. 2001;61(12):4766–72.

34. Liyanage UK, Moore TT, Joo H-G, Tanaka Y, Herrmann V, Doherty G, et al. Prevalence of regulatory T cells is increased in peripheral blood and tumor microenvironment of patients with pancreas or breast adenocarcinoma. J Immunol. 2002;169(5):2756–61.

35. Wolf AM, Wolf D, Steurer M, Gastl G, Gunsilius E, Grubeck-Loebenstein B. Increase of regulatory T cells in the peripheral blood of cancer patients. Clin Cancer Res. 2003;9(2):606–12.

36. Dogan V, Rieckmann T, Münscher A, et al. Current studies of immunotherapy in head and neck cancer. Clin Otolaryngol. 2018;43(1):13–21.

37. Strome SE, Dong H, Tamura H, et al. B7-H1 blockade augments adoptive T-cell immunotherapy for squamous cell carcinoma. Cancer Res. 2003;63:6501–5.

38. Tsushima F, Tanaka K, Ostuki N, et al. Predominant expression of B7-H1 and its immunoregulatory roles in oral squamous cell carcinoma. Oral Oncol. 2006;42:268–74.

39. Lyford-Pike S, Peng S, Young GD, et al. Evidence for a role of the PD-1:PD-L1 pathway in immune resistance of HPV-associated head and neck squamous cell carcinoma. Cancer Res. 2013;73(6):1733–41.

40. Chow LQ, Burtness B, Weiss J, et al. A phase Ib study of pembrolizumab (Pembro; MK-3475) in patients (Pts) with human papilloma virus (HPV)-positive and negative head and neck cancer (HNC). Ann Oncol. 2014;25:1–41.

41. Dassonville O, Formento JL, Francoual M, Ramaioli A, Santini J, Schneider M, Demard F, Milano G. Expression of epidermal growth factor receptor and survival in upper aerodigestive tract cancer. J Clin Oncol. 1993;11:1873–8.

42. Rubin Grandis J, Melhem MF, Barnes EL, Tweardy DJ. Quantitative immunohistochemical analysis of transforming growth factor-alpha and epidermal growth factor receptor in patients with squamous cell carcinoma of the head and neck. Cancer. 1996;78:1284–92.

43. Rubin Grandis J, Melhem MF, Gooding WE, Day R, Holst VA, Wagener MM, Drenning SD, Tweardy DJ. Levels of TGF-alpha and EGFR protein in head and neck squamous cell carcinoma and patient survival. J Natl Cancer Inst. 1998;90:824–32.

44. Cohen EE, Kane MA, List MA, Brockstein BE, Mehrotra B, Huo D, Mauer AM, Pierce C, Dekker A, Vokes EE. Phase II trial of gefitinib 250 mg daily in patients with recurrent and/or metastatic squamous cell carcinoma of the head and neck. Clin Cancer Res. 2005;11:8418–24.

45. Giralt J, Trigo J, Nuyts S, et al. Panitumumab plus radiotherapy versus chemoradiotherapy in patients with unresected, locally advanced squamous-cell carcinoma of the head and neck (CONCERT-2): A randomised, controlled, open-label phase 2 trial. Lancet Oncol. 2015;16:221–32.

46. Mesía R, Henke M, Fortin A, et al. Chemoradiotherapy with or without panitumumab in patients with unresected, locally advanced squamous-cell carcinoma of the head and neck (CONCERT-1): a randomised, controlled, open-label phase 2 trial. Lancet Oncol. 2015;16:208–20.

47. Argiris A, Ghebremichael M, Gilbert J, et al. Phase III randomized, placebo-controlled trial of docetaxel with or without gefitinib in recurrent or metastatic head and neck cancer: an eastern cooperative oncology group trial. J Clin Oncol. 2013;31:1405–14.

48. Bonner JA, Harari PM, Giralt J, et al. Radiotherapy plus cetuximab for locoregionally advanced head and neck cancer: 5-year survival data from a phase 3 randomised trial, and relation between cetuximab-induced rash and survival. Lancet Oncol. 2010;11:21–8.

49. Vermorken JB, Trigo J, Hitt R, Koralewski P, Diaz-Rubio E, Rolland F, Knecht R, Amellal N, Schueler A, Baselga J. Open-label, uncontrolled, multicenter phase II study to evaluate the efficacy and toxicity of cetuximab as a single agent in patients with recurrent and/or metastatic squamous cell carcinoma of the head and neck who failed to respond to platinum-based therapy. J Clin Oncol. 2007;25:2171–7.

50. Bernier J, Bentzen SM, Vermorken JB. Molecular therapy in head and neck oncology. Nat Rev Clin Oncol. 2009;6:266–77.

51. Boeckx C, Baay M, Wouters A, Specenier P, Vermorken JB, Peeters M, Lardon F. Anti-epidermal growth factor receptor therapy in head and neck squamous cell carcinoma: focus on potential molecular mechanisms of drug resistance. Oncologist. 2013;18:850–64.

52. Hanahan D, Weinberg RA. Hallmarks of cancer: the next generation. Cell. 2011;144(5):646–74.

53. Vesely MD, Kershaw MH, Schreiber RD, Smyth MJ. Natural innate and adaptive immunity to cancer. Annu Rev Immunol. 2011;29(1):235–71.

54. Gooden MJM, de Bock GH, Leffers N, Daemen T, Nijman HW. The prognostic influence of tumour-infiltrating lymphocytes in cancer: a systematic review with meta-analysis. Br J Cancer. 2011;105(1):93–103.

55. Ogino S, Nosho K, Irahara N, Meyerhardt JA, Baba Y, Shima K, et al. Lymphocytic reaction to colorectal cancer is associated with longer survival, independent of lymph node count, microsatellite instability, and CpG island methylator phenotype. Clin Cancer Res. 2009;15(20):6412–20.

56. de Miranda NFCC, Goudkade D, Jordanova ES, Tops CMJ, Hes FJ, Vasen HFA, et al. Infiltration of Lynch colorectal cancers by activated immune cells associates with early staging of the primary tumor and absence of lymph node metastases. Clin Cancer Res. 2012;18(5):1237–45.

57. Balermpas P, Michel Y, Wagenblast J, Seitz O, Weiss C, Rödel F, et al. Tumour-infiltrating lymphocytes predict response to definitive chemoradiotherapy in head and neck cancer. Br J Cancer. 2014;110(2):501–9.

58. Ward MJ, Thirdborough SM, Mellows T, Riley C, Harris S, Suchak K, et al. Tumour-infiltrating lymphocytes predict for outcome in HPV-positive oropharyngeal cancer. Br J Cancer. 2014;110(2):489–500.

59. Näsman A, Romanitan M, Nordfors C, Grün N, Johansson H, Hammarstedt L, et al. Tumor infiltrat-

ing CD8+ and Foxp3+ lymphocytes correlate to clinical outcome and human papillomavirus (HPV) status in tonsillar cancer. PLoS One. 2012;7(6):e38711.

60. Partlová S, Bouček J, Kloudová K, Lukešová E, Zábrodský M, Grega M, et al. Distinct patterns of intratumoral immune cell infiltrates in patients with HPV-associated compared to non-virally induced head and neck squamous cell carcinoma. OncoImmunology. 2015;4(1):e965570.

61. Song IH, Lee TS, Park YS, et al. Immuno-PET imaging and radioimmunotherapy of 64Cu-/177Lu-labeled anti-EGFR antibody in esophageal squamous cell carcinoma model. J Nucl Med. 2016;57:1105–11.

62. Cai W, Chen K, He L, Cao Q, et al. Quantitative PET of EGFR expression in xenograft-bearing mice using 64Cu-labeled cetuximab, a chimeric anti-EGFR monoclonal antibody. Eur J Nucl Med Mol Imaging. 2007;34:850–8.

63. Niu G, Sun X, Cao Q, et al. Cetuximab-based immunotherapy and radioimmunotherapy of head and neck squamous cell carcinoma. Clin Cancer Res. 2010;16:2095–105.

64. Dash A, Pillai MR, Knapp FF Jr. Production of 177Lu for targeted radionuclide therapy: available options. Nucl Med Mol Imaging. 2015;49:85–107.

65. Fischer E, Grünberg J, Cohrs S, et al. L1-CAM-targeted antibody therapy and 177Lu-radioimmunotherapy of disseminated ovarian cancer. Int J Cancer. 2012;130:2715–21.

66. Knowles SM, Wu AM. Advances in immuno-positron emission tomography: antibodies for molecular imaging in oncology. J Clin Oncol. 2012;30:3884–92.

67. Trousil S, Hoppmann S, Nguyen QD, Kaliszczak M, Tomasi G, Iveson P, Hiscock D, Aboagye EO. Positron emission tomography imaging with 18F-labeled ZHER2: 2891 affibody for detection of HER2 expression and pharmacodynamic response to HER2-modulating therapies. Clin Cancer Res. 2014;20:1632–43.

68. Lamberts LE, Williams SP, Terwisscha van Scheltinga AG, Lub-de Hooge MN, Schroder CP, Gietema JA, Brouwers AH, de Vries EG. Antibody positron emission tomography imaging in anticancer drug development. J Clin Oncol. 2015;33:1491–504.

69. Suh Y, Amelio I, Urbano Guerrero T, Tavassoli M. Clinical update on cancer: molecular oncology of head and neck cancer. Cell Death Dis. 2014;5:e1018.

70. Scholm J, Siler K, Milenic DE, et al. Monoclonal antibody-based therapy of a human tumor xenograft with a 177lutetium-labeled immunoconjugate. Cancer Res. 1991;51:2889–96.

71. Goerner M, Seiwert TY, Sudhoff H. Molecular targeted therapies in head and neck cancer—an update of recent developments. Head Neck Oncol. 2010;2:8.

72. Song J, Chen C, Raben D. Emerging role of EGFR-targeted therapies and radiation in head and neck cancer. Oncology (Williston Park). 2004;18(14):1757–67, 1771–2, 1777.

73. Robert F, Ezekiel MP, Spencer SA, Meredith RF, Bonner JA, Khazaeli MB, Saleh MN, Carey D, LoBuglio AF, Wheeler RH, Cooper MR, Waksal HW. Phase I study of anti-epidermal growth factor receptor antibody cetuximab in combination with radiation therapy in patients with advanced head and neck cancer. J Clin Oncol. 2001;19:3234–43.

74. Dattatreya S, Goswami C. Cetuximab plus radiotherapy in patients with unresectable locally advanced squamous cell carcinoma of head and neck region—a open labelled single arm phase II study. Indian J Cancer. 2011;48:154–7.

75. Bonner JA, et al. Radiotherapy plus cetuximab for squamous-cell carcinoma of the head and neck. N Engl J Med. 2006;354(6):567–78.

76. Burtness B, et al. Phase III randomized trial of cisplatin plus placebo compared with cisplatin plus cetuximab in metastatic/recurrent head and neck cancer: an Eastern Cooperative Oncology Group Study. J Clin Oncol. 2005;23(34):8646–54.

77. Vermorken JB, et al. Platinum-based chemotherapy plus cetuximab in head and neck cancer. N Engl J Med. 2008;359(11):1116–27.

78. Vermorken JB, Herbst RS, Leon X, Amellal N, Baselga J. Overview of the efficacy of cetuximab in recurrent and/or metastatic squamous cell carcinoma of the head and neck in patients who previously failed platinum-based therapies. Cancer. 2008;112:2710–9.

79. Niu G, Sun X, Cao Q, Courter D, Koong A, Le QT, Gambhir SS, Chen X. Cetuximab-based immunotherapy and radioimmunotherapy of head and neck squamous cell carcinoma. Clin Cancer Res. 2010;16:2095–105.

80. Liu Z, Ma T, Liu H, Jin Z, Sun X, Zhao H, Shi J, Jia B, Li F, Wang F. 177Lu-labeled antibodies for EGFR-targeted SPECT/CT imaging and radioimmunotherapy in a preclinical head and neck carcinoma model. Mol Pharm. 2014;11:800–7.

81. Song IH, Noh Y, Kwon J, Jung JH, Lee BC, Kim KI, Lee YJ, Kang JH, Rhee CS, Lee CH, Lee TS, Choi IJ. Immuno-PET imaging based radioimmunotherapy in head and neck squamous cell carcinoma model. Oncotarget. 2017;8(54):92090–105.

82. van der Veen J, Nuyts S. Can intensity-modulated-radiotherapy reduce toxicity in head and neck squamous cell carcinoma? Cancers (Basel). 2017;9(10):135.

83. Adelstein DJ, Lavertu P, Saxton JP, Secic M, Wood BG, Wanamaker JR, Eliachar I, Strome M, Larto MA. Mature results of a phase III randomized trial comparing concurrent chemoradiotherapy with radiation therapy alone in patients with stage III and IV squamous cell carcinoma of the head and neck. Cancer. 2000;88:876–83.

84. Budach V, Stuschke M, Budach W, Baumann M, Geismar D, Grabenbauer G, Lammert I, Jahnke K, Stueben G, Herrmann T, Bamberg M, Wust P, Hinkelbein W, Wernecke KD. Hyperfractionated accelerated chemoradiation with concurrent

fluorouracil-mitomycin is more effective than dose-escalated hyperfractionated accelerated radiation therapy alone in locally advanced head and neck cancer: final results of the radiotherapy cooperative clinical trials group of the German Cancer Society 95-06 prospective randomized trial. J Clin Oncol. 2005;23:1125–35.

85. Denis F, Garaud P, Bardet E, Alfonsi M, Sire C, Germain T, Bergerot P, Rhein B, Tortochaux J, Calais G. Final results of the 94-01 French Head and Neck Oncology and Radiotherapy Group randomized trial comparing radiotherapy alone with concomitant radiochemotherapy in advanced-stage oropharynx carcinoma. J Clin Oncol. 2004;22:69–76.

86. Semrau R, Mueller RP, Stuetzer H, Staar S, Schroeder U, Guntinas-Lichius O, Kocher M, Eich HT, Dietz A, Flentje M, Rudat V, Volling P, Schroeder M, Eckel HE. Efficacy of intensified hyperfractionated and accelerated radiotherapy and concurrent chemotherapy with carboplatin and 5-fluorouracil: updated results of a randomized multicentric trial in advanced head-and-neck cancer. Int J Radiat Oncol Biol Phys. 2006;64:1308–16.

87. Semrau R. The role of radiotherapy in the definitive and postoperative treatment of advanced head and neck cancer. Oncol Res Treat. 2017;40:347–52.

88. Pignon JP, le Maitre A, Maillard E, Bourhis J. Meta-analysis of chemotherapy in head and neck cancer (MACH-NC): an update on 93 randomised trials and 17,346 patients. Radiother Oncol. 2009;92:4–14.

89. Deloch L, Derer A, Hartmann J, Frey B, Fietkau R, Gaipl US. Modern radiotherapy concepts and the impact of radiation on immune activation. Front Oncol. 2016;6:141.

90. Bourhis J, Overgaard J, Audry H, Ang KK, Saunders M, Bernier J, Horiot JC, Le Maitre A, Pajak TF, Poulsen MG, O'Sullivan B, Dobrowsky W, Hliniak A, Skladowski K, Hay JH, Pinto LH, Fallai C, Fu KK, Sylvester R, Pignon JP. Hyperfractionated or accelerated radiotherapy in head and neck cancer: a meta-analysis. Lancet. 2006;368:843–54.

91. Bentzen J, Toustrup K, Eriksen JG, Primdahl H, Andersen LJ, Overgaard J. Locally advanced head and neck cancer treated with accelerated radiotherapy, the hypoxic modifier nimorazole and weekly cisplatin. Results from the DAHANCA 18 phase II study. Acta Oncol. 2015;54:1001–7.

92. Bonner JA, Harari PM, Giralt J, Cohen RB, Jones CU, Sur RK, Raben D, Baselga J, Spencer SA, Zhu J, Youssoufian H, Rowinsky EK, Ang KK. Radiotherapy plus cetuximab for locoregionally advanced head and neck cancer: 5-year survival data from a phase 3 randomised trial, and relation between cetuximab-induced rash and survival. Lancet Oncol. 2010;11:21–8.

93. Bonner JA, Harari PM, Giralt J, Azarnia N, Shin DM, Cohen RB, Jones CU, Sur R, Raben D, Jassem J, Ove R, Kies MS, Baselga J, Youssoufian H, Amellal N, Rowinsky EK, Ang KK. Radiotherapy plus cetuximab for squamous-cell carcinoma of the head and neck. N Engl J Med. 2006;354:567–78.

94. Chaturvedi AK, Engels EA, Pfeiffer RM, et al. Human papillomavirus and rising oropharyngeal cancer incidence in the United States. J Clin Oncol. 2011;29(32):4294–301.

95. Klussmann JP, Weissenborn SJ, Wieland U, Dries V, Kolligs J, Jungehuelsing M, Eckel HE, Dienes HP, Pfister HJ, Fuchs PG. Prevalence, distribution, and viral load of human papillomavirus 16 DNA in tonsillar carcinomas. Cancer. 2001;92:2875–84.

96. Rosenthal DI, Harari PM, Giralt J, Bell D, Raben D, Liu J, Schulten J, Ang KK, Bonner JA. Association of human papillomavirus and p16 status with outcomes in the IMCL-9815 phase III registration trial for patients with locoregionally advanced oropharyngeal squamous cell carcinoma of the head and neck treated with radiotherapy with or without cetuximab. J Clin Oncol. 2016;34:1300–8.

97. Fakhry C, Westra WH, Li S, Cmelak A, Ridge JA, Pinto H, Forastiere A, Gillison ML. Improved survival of patients with human papillomavirus-positive head and neck squamous cell carcinoma in a prospective clinical trial. J Natl Cancer Inst. 2008;100:261–9.

98. Klussmann JP, Gultekin E, Weissenborn SJ, Wieland U, Dries V, Dienes HP, Eckel HE, Pfister HJ, Fuchs PG. Expression of p16 protein identifies a distinct entity of tonsillar carcinomas associated with human papillomavirus. Am J Pathol. 2003;162:747–53.

99. Tamaki N, Hirata K. Tumor hypoxia: a new PET imaging biomarker in clinical oncology. Int J Clin Oncol. 2016;21(4):619–25. Review.

100. Wu Q, Mohan R, Morris M, Lauve A, Schmidt-Ullrich R. Simultaneous integrated boost intensity-modulated radiotherapy for locally advanced head-and-neck squamous cell carcinomas. I: dosimetric results. Int J Radiat Oncol Biol Phys. 2003;56:573–85.

101. Pow EH, Kwong DL, McMillan AS, Wong MC, Sham JS, Leung LH, Leung WK. Xerostomia and quality of life after intensity-modulated radiotherapy vs. conventional radiotherapy for early-stage nasopharyngeal carcinoma: initial report on a randomized controlled clinical trial. Int J Radiat Oncol Biol Phys. 2006;66:981–91.

102. Nutting CM, Morden JP, Harrington KJ, Urbano TG, Bhide SA, Clark C, Miles EA, Miah AB, Newbold K, Tanay M, Adab F, Jefferies SJ, Scrase C, Yap BK, A'Hern RP, Sydenham MA, Emson M, Hall E. Parotid-sparing intensity modulated versus conventional radiotherapy in head and neck cancer (PARSPORT): a phase 3 multicentre randomised controlled trial. Lancet Oncol. 2011;12:127–36.

103. Gupta T, Agarwal J, Jain S, Phurailatpam R, Kannan S, Ghosh-Laskar S, Murthy V, Budrukkar A, Dinshaw K, Prabhash K, et al. Three-dimensional conformal radiotherapy (3D-CRT) versus intensity modulated radiation therapy (IMRT) in squamous

cell carcinoma of the head and neck: a randomized controlled trial. Radiother Oncol. 2012;104:343–8.

104. Ghosh-Laskar S, Yathiraj PH, Dutta D, Rangarajan V, Purandare N, Gupta T, Budrukkar A, Murthy V, Kannan S, Agarwal JP. Prospective randomized controlled trial to compare 3-dimensional conformal radiotherapy to intensity-modulated radiotherapy in head and neck squamous cell carcinoma: long-term results. Head Neck. 2016;38:1481–7.

105. Murthy V, Narang K, Laskar SG, Gupta T, Budrukkar A. Hypothyroidism after 3-dimensional conformal radiotherapy and intensity-modulated radiotherapy for head and neck cancers: Prospective data from 2 randomized controlled trials. Head Neck. 2014;36:1573–80.

106. Huang DT, Johnson CR, Schmidt-Ullrich R, Grimes M. Postoperative radiotherapy in head and neck carcinoma with extracapsular lymph node extension and/or positive resection margins: a comparative study. Int J Radiat Oncol Biol Phys. 1992;23:737–42.

107. Langendijk JA, Ferlito A, Takes RP, Rodrigo JP, Suárez C, Strojan P, Haigentz M Jr, Rinaldo A. Postoperative strategies after primary surgery for squamous cell carcinoma of the head and neck. Oral Oncol. 2010;46:577–85.

Judy Nguyen, Carina Mari Aparici,
Sundeep Nayak, and Benjamin L. Franc

Contents

20.1 Introduction

Immunotherapy has revolutionized the way cancer is treated and has rapidly taken a prominent position with other key anticancer strategies including surgery, radiation, chemotherapy, and molecular targeted therapies. Immune-based therapies radically differ from these other treatment modalities, relying entirely upon a patient's own immune system to recognize and kill cancer cells.

Given this novel pathway to achieve the ultimate effect on the cancer cell, new methods of

J. Nguyen · C. M. Aparici · B. L. Franc (✉)
Department of Radiology, Division of Nuclear Medicine and Molecular Imaging, Stanford University School of Medicine, Stanford, CA, USA
e-mail: Dr.JudyNguyen@stanford.edu; drmari@stanford.edu; benster@stanford.edu

S. Nayak
Kaiser Permanente Santa Rosa Medical Center, Santa Rosa, CA, USA
e-mail: sundeep.m.nayak@kp.org

© Springer Nature Switzerland AG 2022
S. Harsini et al. (eds.), *Nuclear Medicine and Immunology*,
https://doi.org/10.1007/978-3-030-81261-4_20

interrogating the intended effect of immunotherapy in vivo are required. Traditional imaging methods are incapable of determining whether the therapy triggered the intended molecular pathway, nor can they provide insight into the level of immune response in the region of the tumor or systemically. Likewise, traditional methods of measuring the cancer's response to therapy based on changes in size and volume on imaging are known to not necessarily correlate with patient outcomes and may, in some cases, provide misleading information.

This chapter focuses on the use of positron emission tomography (PET) to predict the effectiveness of immunotherapies and to evaluate the response of cancers to immunotherapy. In the first section, we will review the utilization of PET in immune checkpoint inhibitor strategies. This section will start with a focus on the use of the PET radiopharmaceutical 2-[^{18}F]fluoro-2-deoxy-D-glucose (2-[^{18}F]FDG), followed by the use of other PET radiopharmaceuticals. Then, we will address the current use of PET in evaluating the response and monitoring of other immune-based strategies. And finally, we will explore some promising advances in PET tracer development and image analysis, potentially improving our ability to evaluate the mechanism and efficacy of various immune-based therapies in the not too distant future.

20.2 Anti-PD-L1/Anti-CTLA-4-Based Therapies

Immunomodulatory monoclonal antibodies directly enhance the antitumor immune response or block immunological checkpoints that would otherwise restrain effective anticancer immunity. The ever-increasing use of the immunomodulatory strategy of immune checkpoint inhibitors (ICIs), including those targeting the programmed death-ligand 1 (PD-L1) or cytotoxic T-lymphocyte-associated protein 4 (CTLA-4) receptors on T cells, is predicated on results in managing select cases of melanoma and non-small cell lung cancer. The use of immunomodulatory therapies has made rapid

strides, resulting in numerous validated indications for their application alone or in combination with other conventional chemotherapies. In select histologies and tissue types, this has translated into durable response and survival benefit.

20.2.1 2-[^{18}F]FDG PET-Based Strategies to Evaluate the Efficacy of ICI Therapy

20.2.1.1 Predicting Who Will Respond

Many questions still exist around how best to optimize ICI utilization, particularly in light of their high cost and potential side effects. Depending on the type of cancer being treated, ICIs can cost hundreds of thousands of dollars per quality-adjusted life-year (QALY) [1]. The toxicities of ICIs mainly are a manifestation of their ability to activate the entire immune system, causing unintended consequences for normal tissues. Ranging from less serious to highly serious immune-related adverse events (IRAEs), side effects include colitis, skin rash, pruritus, hepatitis, hypophysitis, thyroiditis, and more rarely episcleritis, uveitis, pancreatitis, nephritis, myasthenia gravis, autoimmune autonomic ganglionopathy, Guillain-Barré syndrome (GBS), other neuropathies, sarcoidosis-like reactions, autoimmune thrombocytopenia, toxic epidermal necrolysis, and Stevens-Johnson-like syndromes [2]. When compared to traditional chemotherapy, fatal adverse events are relatively rare during treatment with ICIs and are estimated to range from 0.3% to 1.3% [3].

No specific criteria have been established as an accurate predictive indicator for the efficacy of ICIs. 2-[^{18}F]FDG imaging with positron emission tomography itself may, in some settings, be capable of differentiating those patients who will respond to regimens limited to ICIs from those who may not, solely based on the whole-body metabolic tumor volume (wMTV) [4].

Evaluation of the gut biome on initial 2-[^{18}F]FDG PET imaging has also been explored as a means of predicting immunotherapy response. Animal models have suggested an association between the presence of specific gut microbiota and level of response to immunomodulating regimens. Higher physiologic colonic 2-[^{18}F] FDG uptake has been associated with lower total colonic bacterial load, and, in fact, a low total physiologic colonic maximum standardized uptake value (SUVmax) has been found to be associated with a poor immunotherapeutic clinical outcome. The basis of this association has been hypothesized to be due to a shift from short-chain fatty acid metabolism by colonic bacteria to glycolysis, further suggesting that a minimum bacterial load and diversity of gut microbiota is required to promote an immune response [5].

20.2.1.2 Defining the Level of Response and Predicting Treatment Outcomes

Once an ICI treatment strategy has been chosen, a means of evaluating the efficacy of therapy must be available. As experience with ICIs has grown, so has the realization of the limitations of anatomic-based imaging modalities in assessing for and predicting therapeutic response of the targeted tumors [6]. Due to its ability to reveal underlying functional and biochemical signals that could potentially be associated with mechanisms or manifestations of therapeutic response, the potential role for 2-[^{18}F]FDG PET in the assessment of therapeutic response has been explored extensively in the setting of immunotherapy [7].

Several response criteria have been developed and used to assess the response of solid tumors to immunotherapies based on checkpoint inhibition. Given the initial indications for the use of these therapies, the bulk of experience in the use of 2-[^{18}F]FDG PET for response assessment is in the setting of melanoma or non-small cell lung cancer (NSCLC) [8]. Response criteria have focused on describing a combination of changes in size and/or functional metrics of one or more malignant index lesions on 2-[^{18}F]FDG PET, though developing approaches have also used measures of total metabolically active tumor volume rather than focus on a select set of index lesions to evaluate response or predict patient outcome [9, 10]. There is also recognition that changes in functional indices of benign lymphoid tissues may provide a complementary window into the effectiveness of immunotherapy in harnessing a response [11–13]. As discussed above, 2-[^{18}F]FDG uptake related to the gut biome has been explored as a means to predict response to immunotherapy [5].

20.2.1.3 Response Evaluation Criteria in Solid Tumors (RECIST)

Assessing the change in tumor burden is a meaningful endpoint in clinical trials as well as for the real-world assessment of tumor shrinkage (or absence of shrinkage) and disease progression. To achieve those ends, the Response Evaluation Criteria in Solid Tumors (RECIST) workgroup developed and published objective criteria in 2000 as applicable to anatomic changes in tumor burden. This was followed by RECIST 1.1 in 2009, a revision of the original RECIST criteria resulting in the reduction in the number of lesions assessed, guidelines to classify lymph nodes as pathologic or normal based on measurement, and additional methodologies to improve measurement of disease progression (Table 20.1) [14].

20.2.1.4 European Organization for Research and Treatment of Cancer (EORTC)

With the evolution of functional oncological imaging, it was time to migrate to modifying the original criteria to accommodate 2-[^{18}F]FDG imaging with positron emission tomography as complementary to determining the trajectory of response assessment for solid tumors in the oncological canon. In 1999, the "EORTC PET" criteria standardized response assessment using 2-[^{18}F]FDG PET imaging [15]. In fact, complete metabolic response on 2-[^{18}F]FDG PET, as defined by the EORTC criteria, has been shown to predict ongoing tumor response and long-term benefit of immunotherapy in patients with metastatic melanoma (Fig. 20.1) [16].

The "EORTC PET" criteria have been further refined by PET Response Criteria in Solid Tumors (PERCIST), each resulting in very similar classi-

Table 20.1 Comparison of RECIST 1.0 to RECIST 1.1—major changes

	RECIST 1.0	RECIST 1.1

Minimum measurable lesion size	10 mm CT
	LN: Not included
		10 mm CT
		LN:
		  ≥15 mm short axis (target)
		  10–15 mm (nontarget)
		  <10 mm is non-pathological

Overall tumor burden	10 lesions (max 5/organ)	5 lesions (max 2/organ)
Response criteria for target disease	CR node not mentioned PD is 20% increase over least sum on study **OR** new lesion(s)	CR node must be <10 mm SA PD is 20% increase over least sum on study (including baseline if least sum) **AND** at least 5 mm increase **OR** new lesion(s)
Response criteria for non-target disease	Unequivocal progression considered PD	Unequivocal progression should not usually trump target disease status but should be representative of overall disease status change, not increase in a singular lesion
New lesion	–	New section on this item
Overall response assessment	Integration of target and nontarget lesions in a single table	Separate tables integrating (1) target and nontarget and (2) nontarget only

CT computed tomography, *max* maximum, *CR* complete response, *SA* short axis, *PD* progressive disease, *LN* lymph node

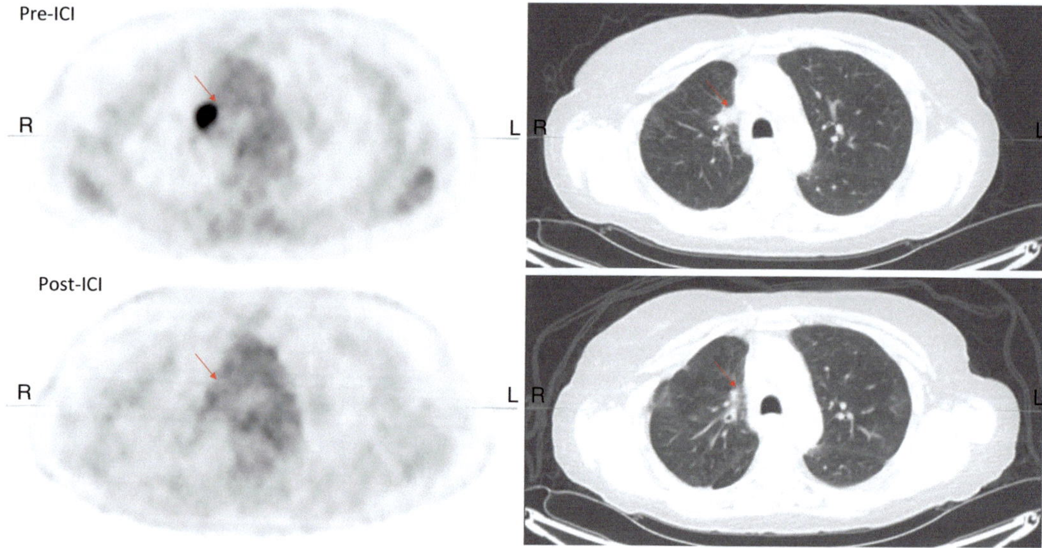

Fig. 20.1 Partial response of non-small cell lung carcinoma to immune checkpoint inhibitor (ICI) therapy in an 88-year-old woman who was classified as a poor surgical candidate due to concomitant medical conditions. 2-[^{18}F]FDG PET/CT prior to immunotherapy demonstrates a large hypermetabolic primary lung cancer (top row, arrow). Six months later, following completion of ICI therapy, 2-[^{18}F]FDG PET/CT demonstrates complete resolution of 2-[^{18}F]FDG uptake within a target lesion that has demonstrated a decrease in metabolic volume >30%, reduction of SULpeak >30% and an absolute drop of 0.8 SULpeak units, and greater than 25% reduction in the sum of SUVmax (bottom row, arrow)

fications of response assessment with preliminary data suggesting that PERCIST use is better correlated with outcomes and thus could prove a superior predictor for the efficacy of novel oncological therapies. For example, in a small pilot study of ten patients, PERCIST criteria have been used to successfully predict complete response using 2-[^{18}F]FDG PET 2 weeks after initiation of the programmed cell death protein 1 (PD-1) therapy in patients with stage IV melanoma (Table 20.2) [17].

Table 20.2 Comparison of EORTC and PERCIST criteria

	EORTC	PERCIST
CMR	Complete resolution of 2-[^{18}F]FDG uptake in all lesions	
PMR	Greater than 25% reduction in the sum of SUVmax of 2-[^{18}F]FDG uptake after more than 1 cycle of therapy	Minimum of 30% reduction of SULpeak of 2-[^{18}F]FDG uptake **AND** an absolute drop of 0.8 SULpeak units
PMD	More than 25% increase in the sum of SUVmax of 2-[^{18}F]FDG uptake **OR** appearance of new 2-[^{18}F]FDG-avid lesion(s)	More than 30% increase in SULpeak of 2-[^{18}F]FDG uptake **AND** absolute increase of 0.8 SULpeak **OR** appearance of new 2-[^{18}F]FDG-avid lesion(s)
SD	Does not qualify for any of CMR, PMR, or PMD	

EORTC European Organization for Research and Treatment of Cancer, *PERCIST* PET Response Criteria in Solid Tumors, *CMR* complete metabolic response, *PMR* partial metabolic response, *PMD* progressive metabolic disease, *SD* stable disease, *SUVmax* maximum standardized uptake value, *SULpeak* peak lean body mass SUV

20.2.1.5   Immune PET Response Criteria in Solid Tumors (iPERCIST)

Owing to the systemic paradigm of cancer and the complexities inherent to evaluating response over prolonged courses of immunotherapy, response assessment in solid tumors became challenging using conventional criteria. In addition, complexities to measuring response based on metabolism are inherent in the mechanisms of immunomodulating therapies; for example, pseudoprogression occurs when previously undetected disease is discovered on PET, not because it is truly new, but because metabolic activity related to immune reactions around the site of malignancy makes it detectable (Fig. 20.2) [18]. This can occur in soft tissue or bone [19]. Even more confounding, it can be difficult to differentiate between pseudo-progression and true progression that somehow later responds to immune system manifestations of the immunotherapy [20]. To address these challenges to traditional criteria, immune PET Response Criteria in Solid Tumors (iPERCIST)

was conceived as a hybrid of both PERCIST and immune Response Evaluation Criteria in Solid Tumors (iRECIST). iPERCIST employs a second interim time point in the case of apparent progressive disease on the first 2-[^{18}F]FDG PET performed to assess response. Thus, "unconfirmed progressive metabolic disease" (UPMD) is thus re-evaluated 4 weeks later to confirm or reject true progression status (Table 20.3) [21].

20.2.1.6   2-[^{18}F]FDG PET/CT Criteria for Early Prediction of Response to Immune Checkpoint Inhibitor Therapy (PECRIT)

Further refinement of 2-[^{18}F]FDG PET-based response criteria yielded the predictive criteria for response assessment to immune checkpoint inhibitor (ICI) therapy (PECRIT). PECRIT proposed 2-[^{18}F]FDG PET responses for classification as clinical or no clinical benefit. CT-based antitumor responses between baseline and response assessment 2-[^{18}F]FDG PET studies were classified as complete response (CR), partial response (PR), stable disease (SD), or progressive disease (PD) according to RECIST 1.1 and immune complete response (iCR), immune partial response (iPR), immune stable disease (iSD), immune progressive disease (iPD), and immune unconfirmed progressive disease (iUPD) according to iRECIST. 2-[^{18}F]FDG PET-based response assessment was classified as complete metabolic response (CMR), partial metabolic response (PMR), stable metabolic disease (SMD), or progressive metabolic disease (PMD) according to PERCIST 1.0 (Table 20.4).

Based upon 2-[^{18}F]FDG PET results, three classes of treatment response are defined according to each criteria:

1. Responder (R) which includes CR/PR/SD, iCR/iPR/iSD, and CMR/PMR/SMD/non-PMD for RECIST 1.1, iRECIST, and PERCIST 1.0 criteria, respectively.
2. Nonresponder (NR) which includes PD, iPD, and PMD for these three criteria.
3. Indeterminate: immune unconfirmed progressive disease (iUPD).

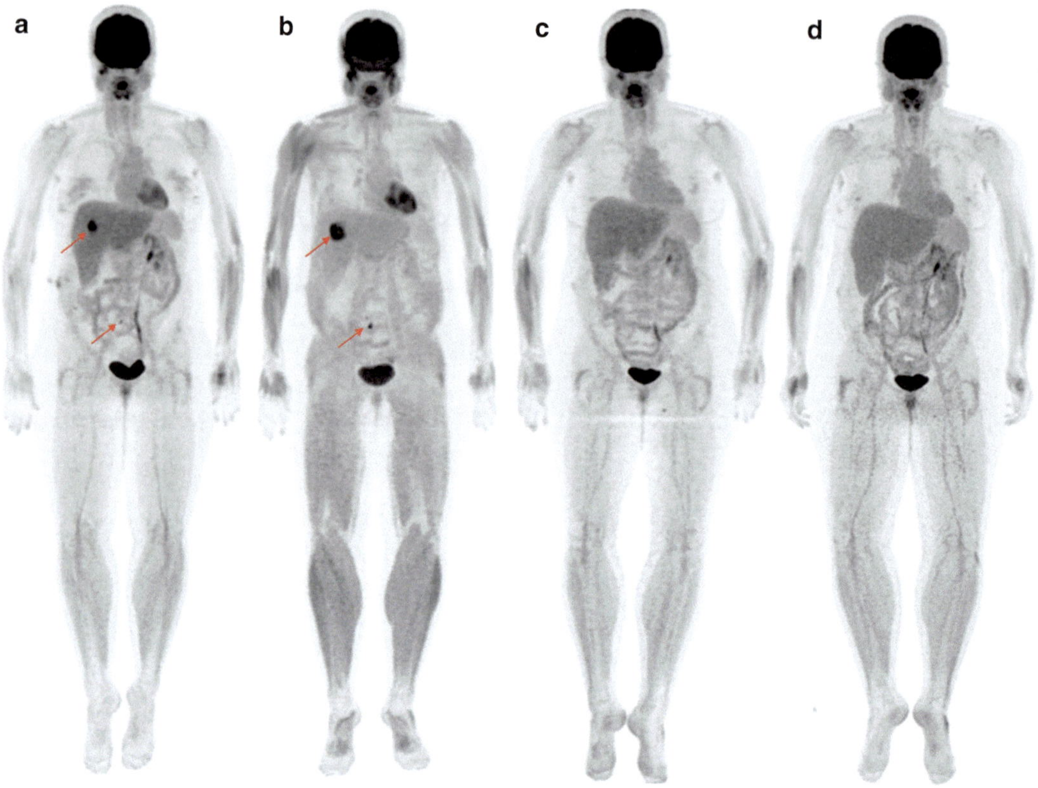

Fig. 20.2 Pseudoprogression of metastatic melanoma on PET in a 48-year-old patient treated with pembrolizumab. Pre-ICI treatment PET demonstrates hypermetabolic metastases in the liver and in an aortocaval lymph node (**a**, arrows). Following 3 months of ICI therapy, PET demonstrates an increase in the metabolically active tumor volume at both metastatic locations (**b**, arrows). However, PET acquired 3 months later (after a total of 6 months of ICI therapy) demonstrates complete metabolic response of the metastatic sites (**c**) that persisted 3 months later (after a total of 9 months of ICI therapy) (**d**)

These three classes are also applied for progression-free survival (PFS) and overall survival (OS) categories. In addition, pseudoprogression is defined as a decrease or stabilization of tumoral activity (or tumor growth) of an initially evaluated disease progression.

Limited data is available comparing the utility of PECRIT versus other response assessments, though at least one small retrospective study has suggested that PERSIST criteria remain more valuable in predicting the outcome of patients with advanced melanoma to ICIs [22].

20.2.1.7 PET Response Evaluation Criteria for Immunotherapy (PERCIMT)

Finally, the more recently proposed PERCIMT criteria [23] incorporate both the functional size and number of new lesions on PET. Its proponents suggest that it can be a more sensitive method of predicting clinical response [24, 25]. The addition of quantitative and semiquantitative methods of evaluating response on PET showed no additional value to the use of PERCIMT alone in a small cohort of patients undergoing immuno-

Table 20.3 Comparison of RECIST 1.1, iRECIST, PERCIST, and iPERCIST criteria for immunotherapy response evaluation

	RECIST 1.1	iRECIST	PERCIST	iPERCIST
CR	Disappearance of all target and nontarget lesions LN must regress to <10 mm in SA		Complete resolution of 2-[^{18}F]FDG uptake within target lesion	
PR	≥30% decrease in tumor burden compared to baseline (largest diameter in axial plane)		≥30% decrease in target tumor 2-[^{18}F]FDG SULpeak	
DP	≥20% + 5 mm absolute increase in tumor burden compared with nadir Appearance of new lesion(s) or progression of nontarget lesions	≥20% + 5 mm absolute increase in tumor burden compared with nadir Appearance of new lesion(s) or progression of nontarget lesions (iUPD) Need to be confirmed 4–8 weeks later (iCPD) If progression is followed by tumor shrinkage, the bar is reset Clinical stability is considered when deciding whether treatment is continued after iUPD	≥30% increase in SULpeak **OR** appearance of new 2-[^{18}F]FDG-avid lesion(s)	≥30% increase in SULpeak **OR** appearance of new 2-[^{18}F]FDG-avid lesions (UPMD) Need to be confirmed 4–8 weeks later (CPMD); if progression slowed by PMR or SMD, the bar is reset Clinical stability is considered when deciding whether treatment is continued after UPMD
SD	None of CR, PR, or DP			

CR complete response, *PR* partial response, *SD* stable disease, *DP* disease progression, *SA* short axis, *SULpeak* peak lean body mass SUV with 2-[^{18}F]FDG PET, *iUPD* immune unconfirmed progressive disease, *iCPD* immune confirmed progressive disease, *UPMD* unconfirmed progressive metabolic disease, *CPMD* confirmed progressive metabolic disease, *LN* lymph node

Table 20.4 Comparison of PET-based criteria for treatment response

	PERCIST 1.0	PECRIT
CR	Complete resolution of 2-[^{18}F]FDG uptake within measurable TL AND disappearance of all other lesions to BBP levels	Resolution of all TLs and NLs All LNs <10 mm SA » Clinical benefit (CR at 4 months)
PR	>30% RD **AND** >0.8 AD in SULpeak of HL	≥30% decrease in SoD of TL NL may persist but not unequivocally progress » Clinical benefit (CT at 4 months)
DP	>305 RI **AND** >0.8 AI in SULpeak of HL **OR** unequivocal progression of 2-[^{18}F]FDG-avid NL **OR** appearance of new 2-[^{18}F]FDG-avid lesion(s)	≥20% increase in SoD of TL **OR** unequivocal progression of NL OR appearance of new lesion(s) » **NO** clinical benefit
SD	Not meeting criteria for CR, PR, or DP	Neither sufficient TR nor TG to qualify for PR or PD Percent change in SULpeak per PERCIST criteria at 3–4 weeks If SULpeak ≤15.5% » **NO** clinical benefit If SULpeak >15.5% » Clinical benefit

CR complete response, *PR* partial response, *SD* stable disease, *DP* disease progression, *SA* short axis, *SULpeak* average SUV corrected by lean body mass within a 1 cm^3 spherical volume of interest, *iUPD* immune unconfirmed progressive disease, *iCPD* immune confirmed progressive disease, *UPMD* unconfirmed progressive metabolic disease, *CPMD* confirmed progressive metabolic disease, *TL* target lesion, *BBP* background blood pool, *NL* nontarget lesion, *LN* lymph node, *RD* relative decrease, *RI* relative increase, *AD* absolute decrease, *AI* absolute increase, *HL* hottest lesion, *SoD* sum of diameters, *TR* tumor regression, *TG* tumor growth

Table 20.5 Proposed criteria for assessing tumor response to immunotherapy

	PECRIT		PERCIMT	
CR	Disappearance of all TLs LN: Reduction in SA to <1 cm No new lesion	Clinical benefit	Complete resolution of all pre-existing 2-[^{18}F]FDG-avid lesions No new 2-[^{18}F]FDG-avid lesion(s)	Clinical benefit
PR	Decrease in target lesion SoD >30%	Clinical benefit	Complete resolution of some pre-existing 2-[^{18}F]FDG-avid lesions No new 2-[^{18}F]FDG-avid lesion(s)	Clinical benefit
DP	Increase in TL SoD >20% **AND** at least 5 mm **OR** new lesion(s)	**NO** clinical benefit	Four or more new 2-[^{18}F]FDG-avid lesions of <1 cm in functional diameter **OR** 3 or more new 2-[^{18}F]FDG-avid lesions of >1 cm in functional diameter **OR** 2 or more 2-[^{18}F]FDG-avid lesions of >1.5 cm in functional diameter	**NO** clinical benefit
SD	Not meeting criteria for CR, PR, or DP	Change in SULpeak of HL >15%: Clinical benefit Change in SULpeak of HL ≤15%: **NO** clinical benefit	Not meeting criteria for CR, PR, or DP	Clinical benefit

CR complete response, *PR* partial response, *SD* stable disease, *DP* disease progression, *TL* target lesion, *LN* lymph node, *SA* short axis, *SoD* sum of diameters, *SULpeak* average SUV corrected by lean body mass within a 1 cm^3 spherical volume of interest, *HL* hottest lesion

therapy for metastatic melanoma [26]. However, the most versatile and accurate means of assessing response of these agents using PET remains of considerable debate (Table 20.5) [27, 28].

20.2.1.8 "Location-Specific" and "Histology-Specific" Response Criteria

There is some evidence of the use of 2-[^{18}F]FDG PET in several different cancer types [29–31], and, as clinical trials expand into these new applications, specific response criteria continue to be adapted [32]. Given that the implementation of ICIs in the management of cancer patients other than those with melanoma or lung cancer is relatively nascent, the relationship between 2-[^{18}F]FDG PET response criteria and outcomes is not well understood.

Lymphomas are a class of malignancies in which "histology-specific" response assessment criteria have been employed in the setting of immunotherapy. Such response criteria include, but are not limited to, the Lugano 2014 criteria for assessing 2-[^{18}F]FDG PET in lymphoma [33]. In 1999, the National Cancer Institute (NCI) Lymphoma International Working Group (IWG) first published imaging and clinical response guidelines for non-Hodgkin lymphoma (NHL), commonly invoked as the Cheson 1999 criteria [34], which were updated in 2007 when the IWG published revised response criteria for malignant lymphoma (Cheson 2007 criteria). These last criteria incorporate bone marrow immunohistochemistry, flow cytometry, and the 2-[^{18}F]FDG PET for visualizing the presence and distribution of lymphoma burden [35]. Despite some challenges from the potential for ambiguity in the interpretation of lesion positivity owing to a binary response system, these criteria remained the standard for evaluating lymphoma (both Hodgkin and NHL) until 2014 when the most recent revised criteria integrated Deauville criteria with input from the follow-up IWG workshop conferences of 2011 and 2013 (Table 20.6) [33, 36].

Adaptation of these existing lymphoma-specific response criteria to the setting of immunotherapy has been successfully demonstrated in Hodgkin lymphoma [37]. Due to the potential for phenomenon such as "flare response" whereby increases in metabolism and/or lymph node size secondary to immune activation can be mistaken for disease nonresponse or progression, it is difficult to fit any early response criteria to the immunotherapy or any prolonged therapy where response may follow long periods of treatment administration [36]. With advances in genome sequencing studies and identification of tumor histology-agnostic driver genetic mutations, it is increasingly critical to align lymphoma response criteria with the response evaluation criteria used in solid tumors, such as RECIST. The new response evaluation criteria in lymphoma (RECIL) were introduced and approved at the International Workshop on Non-Hodgkin Lymphoma (iwNHL) in September 2016 [38]. In many cases of chronic medication administration (such as with immunotherapy), the best durable response may only be achieved after prolonged administration, and hence an initial designation

of SD should not be a basis for premature termination especially if well tolerated; also, they may derive benefit from a given therapy even if an imaging response is not achieved. Appearance of a new 2-[^{18}F]FDG-avid focus that is smaller than RECIL thresholds should be closely monitored, and, whenever feasible, tissue sampling may be considered if clinically indicated (Tables 20.7 and 20.8).

20.2.1.9 Limitations of Response Criteria

There are a number of limitations in using a relatively traditional model of response criteria adapted to the case of functional imaging with 2-[^{18}F]FDG PET, as well as to the novel and relatively indirect cancer-killing approach represented by immunomodulating agents.

For example, existing response criteria also do not explicitly take into consideration the possibility of hyperprogression, a rapid increase in tumor growth after initiation of immunotherapy. Hyperprogression confers extremely poor prognosis and is one of the most concerning adverse effects associated with, and distinctive to, immunotherapy [39]. Hyperprogression occurs in a subset of cancer patients when ICI administration appears to result in acceleration of the malignancy [40–42], usually defined as a RECIST 1.1 progression at the first evaluation and as a ≥2-fold increase of the tumor growth kinetic rate (TGKR) compared with pre-immunotherapy. There is no

Table 20.6 Determination of Lugano response assessment criteria in lymphoma

Lesion 5PS	Change from baseline study	New lesion(s)	Lugano response
1, 2, or 3	Decrease	No	CMR
4 or 5	Decrease	No	PMR
	No change	No	NMR
	Increase	Yes/no	PMD
Any	Any	Yes	PMD

5PS 5-point scale "Deauville score", *CMR* complete metabolic response, *PMR* partial metabolic response, *NMR* no metabolic response, *PMD* progressive metabolic disease

Table 20.7 RECIL 2017 response categories based on assessment of target lesions

	% Change SoD from baseline	2-[^{18}F]FDG PET	Bone marrow involvement	New lesion(s)
CR	Disappearance of all TLs All LNs with LA <10 mm ≥30% decrease in SoD of TL with normalization of 2-[^{18}F] FDG PET	Deauville 1–3	Uninvolved	No
PR	≥30% decrease in SoD of TL but not CR	Deauville 4–5	Any	No
MR	10–30% decrease in SoD of TL but not PR	Any	Any	No
PD	>20% increase in SoD of TL For LN <15 mm post-therapy, minimum AI of 5 mm **AND** LA 15 mm **OR** appearance of new lesion(s)	Any	Any	Yes **OR** no
SD	<10% decrease or ≤20% increase in SoD of TL	Any	Any	No

CR complete response, *PR* partial response, *MR* minor response, a provisional category, *PD* progressive disease, *SD* stable disease, *DP* disease progression, *TL* target lesion, *LN* lymph node, *LA* long axis, *SoD* sum of diameters, *AI* absolute increase

Table 20.8 Comparison between RECIST 1.1, Lugano, and RECIL 2017

	RECIST 1.1	Lugano	RECIL 2017
Number of TLs	Up to 5	Up to 6	Up to 3
Measurement method	Unidimensional: LA of non-LN lesions; SA of LN	Bidimensional: Perpendicular diameters	Unidimensional: LA of any TL
Incorporates 2-[^{18}F] FDG PET findings to describe CR	May be considered to confirm CR and/or to declare PD based on detecting new lesion(s)	Yes	Yes
Minor response	N/A	N/A	Yes Reduction in SoD between 10% and 30%
Stable disease	−29% to +20%	−50% to +50%	Decrease <10% to increase ≥20%
PD	Increase in SoD by 20%	Increase in the sum of products of perpendicular diameters by >50% **OR** any single lesion by >50%	Increase in SoD by 20% For relapse from CR, at least one lesion should measure 2 cm in LA without/with 2-[^{18}F]FDG-avidity

CR complete response, *PR* partial response, *MR* minor response, a provisional category, *PD* progressive disease, *SD* stable disease, *DP* disease progression, *TL* target lesion, *LN* lymph node, *LA* long axis, *SA* short axis, *SoD* sum of diameters, *AI* absolute increase

consensus regarding the definition or mechanism of hyperprogression (Fig. 20.3) [41, 43, 44].

20.2.1.10 Evolving Methodologies of ICI Response Assessment and Prediction Using 2-[^{18}F] FDG PET

Measures of the Total Metabolically Active Volume of Tumor

Measuring total lesion glycolysis (TLG) rather than a single SUV value or measuring metabolic tumor volume (MTV) rather than evaluation of a limited subset of index lesions may offer additional ability to evaluate response or predict patient outcome, independent of established response criteria [9, 10]. In non-small cell lung cancer, in particular, TLG can provide independent predictive value of patient outcome [45].

Changes in Metabolism of Benign Lymphoid Tissue as a Harbinger of Systemic Immune-Mediated Response

There has been a recognition that changes in functional indices of benign lymphoid tissues may provide a complementary window into the effectiveness of the immunotherapy in harnessing a response [11–13]. Increases in activity within benign lymphoid tissues may reflect the flared immune activity that is needed to promulgate an antitumor effect. One of the most common patterns on 2-[^{18}F]FDG PET indicating an "immune flare" response is symmetric hilar and mediastinal lymphadenopathy similar to what is seen in sarcoidosis. The other common pattern is diffuse splenic uptake. Such responses can be misinterpreted on 2-[^{18}F]FDG PET as disease progression if not carefully correlated with the clinical setting [12].

Detection of Immune-Related Adverse Events (IRAEs)

Development of other concurrent immune-mediated processes triggered by immunotherapy itself [46, 47] or an unrelated development or recurrence of an immune-mediated disease should be recognized on 2-[^{18}F]FDG PET [48]. The side effects associated with upregulating the immune system by ICIs often resemble autoimmune diseases and are known collectively as IRAEs. Management is challenging and unique from that of conventional chemotherapy given the wide variety of organ systems that can be involved including the gastrointestinal tract, lungs, liver, skin, nervous system, and musculoskeletal system. Thus, early recognition, even in the subclini-

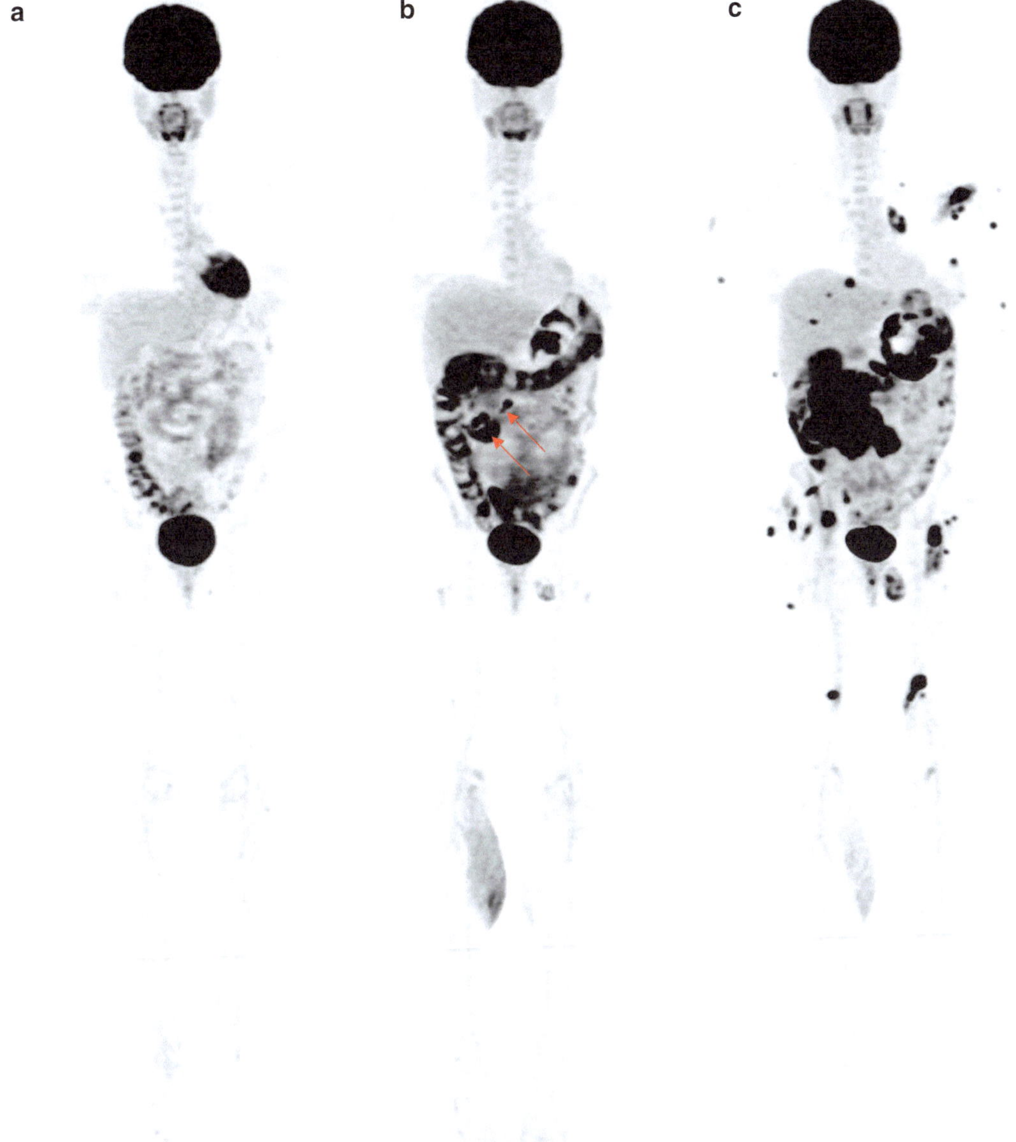

Fig. 20.3 Hyperprogression in a 38-year-old woman with metastatic melanoma. Following initial treatment, the patient was under surveillance by 2-[^{18}F]FDG PET every 3–4 months without clinical evidence of disease (**a**) until, 8 months later, adrenal and intra-abdominal metastases were identified on PET (**b**, arrows). She began ICI therapy (ipilimumab) and underwent a PET 3 months later (**c**) that demonstrated progression to new sites and a >2-fold increase in the tumor growth kinetic rate compared with the pre-immunotherapy period (the period of time between **a** and **b**)

cal stage, is crucial both for proper treatment and management of IRAEs [49].

An association between IRAEs and improved clinical response to immunotherapy has also been described. IRAEs may reflect an extreme manifestation of the flared immune activity that is needed to promulgate an anti-tumor effect. The utility of IRAEs to predict favorable response to immunotherapy has been explored with differing results among investigators [50]. In a study by Sachpekidis and colleagues, increased 2-[^{18}F]FDG uptake in organs classically affected by IRAEs correlated with improved response to treatment and long-term outcome. In particular, in that specific study, colitis and arthritis were the most frequent IRAEs associated with significantly longer progression-free survival than those without IRAEs ($p = 0.036$) [51].

20.2.2 PET-Based Strategies Using Radiopharmaceuticals with Targets Other Than Glucose Metabolism to Evaluate the Efficacy of ICI Therapy

20.2.2.1 Predicting Who Will Respond

Expression of the targets PD-L1 or CTLA-4, quantity of tumor-infiltrating lymphocytes (TILs), detection of interferon-gamma (IFN-γ), detection of mismatch repair deficiencies, and multiplex detection methods combining driver mutations and markers of the immune environment have all been explored as means of identifying patients whose cancer will respond to ICIs [52]. Some of these same biologic processes, as well as others, have been explored as potential targets for imaging-based response prediction using PET (Fig. 20.4).

Expression of PD-L1 in pretreatment melanoma biopsy samples correlates with level of response rate, progression-free survival, and overall survival [53]. The ability of noninvasive imaging to better characterize the entirety of a tumor volume's PD-L1 status more accurately than a single tumor sample remains to be tested. However, the outcome of immune checkpoint inhibitor therapy appears to be, in some cases, unrelated to the level of PD-L1 or CTLA-4 expression [54]. In fact, patients with PD-L1-negative tumors can still respond to anti-PD-L1 therapy [53].

Thus far, several PET agents have been developed to identify and quantify PD-L1 expression in vivo. Truillet and colleagues have developed a novel ^{89}Zr-labeled PET imaging agent based on a recombinant human immunoglobulin (Ig) G1 that binds to an extracellular epitope on human and mouse PD-L1. This agent has shown a high sensitivity to identify PD-L1 in vivo and can detect acute changes in its expression during chemotherapy in small animal cancer models [55]. Similarly, [^{64}Cu]Cu-NOTA-ipilimumab and [^{64}Cu]Cu-NOTA-ipilimumab-F(ab')2 have been developed and tested in animal models with the goal of monitoring the CTLA-4$^+$ target and

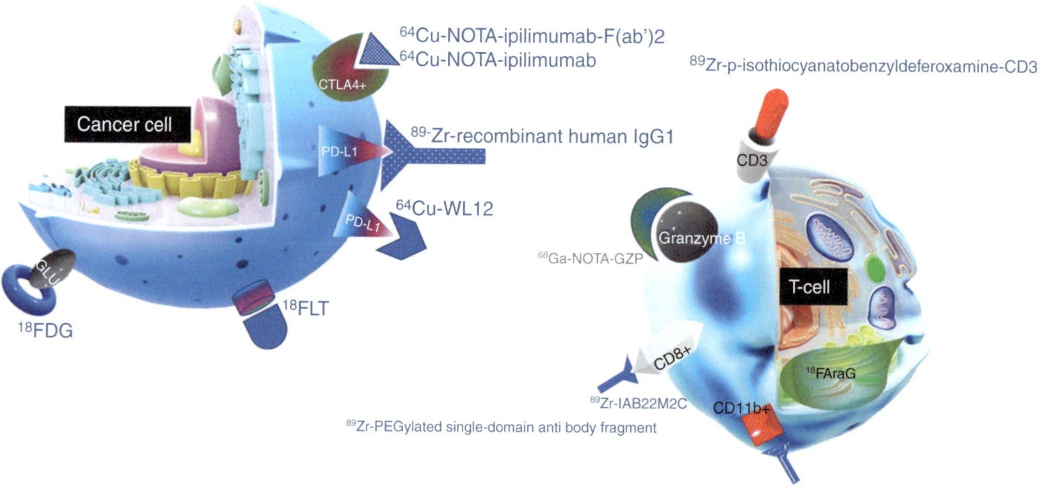

Fig. 20.4 Several targets of PET-based strategies present on cancer cells and T cells to predict responders and assess response to ICI therapies

thereby eventually potentially stratifying patients for CTLA-4+-mediated ICI therapy [56]. With a focus on eventual clinical translation, Chatterjee and colleagues have developed a ^{64}Cu-labeled imaging probe using a highly specific PD-L1-binding peptide, WL12, which is able to provide rapid binding to PD-L1 sites and rapid washout from background soft tissues [57].

20.2.2.2 Defining the Level of Response and Predicting Treatment Outcomes

Due to the mechanism of 2-[^{18}F]FDG uptake, its use to evaluate response to immunotherapy may not be pertinent to certain clinical settings where the immune response may be altered, such as postoperative or instances where the patient may be on corticosteroids or other inflammation-altering medications [32]. In addition, the complex interactions between tumor cells and numerous different immune cell types complicate the interpretation of the signal from 2-[^{18}F]FDG PET as uptake of 2-[^{18}F]FDG may be associated with increases in metabolism in any of the cell types [58].

3′-Deoxy-3′-[^{18}F]-fluorothymidine (FLT), a ^{18}F-labeled version of the DNA nucleoside thymidine, is preferentially concentrated in proliferating cells. Small studies exploring the use of FLT in cancer patients have demonstrated heterogeneous results, with no change in tumoral uptake of FLT during anti-CTLA therapy in melanoma patients but changes in FLT uptake in some intracranial melanoma lesions treated with other immunotherapeutics [59, 60]. Changes in FLT uptake were also observed within the tumor during combined anti-PD-L1/vaccine therapy in prostate cancer patients where greater increase in tumor SUVmean during therapy was predictive of shorter progression-free survival [61].

A different approach to defining the level of response and predicting outcome has focused on assessing the ability of the patient's immune system to recruit tumor-infiltrating lymphocytes in response to administration of the ICI. The level of cluster of differentiation (CD)3, a marker of T lymphocytes, around a murine xenograft tumor model was shown to separate CTLA-4 therapy

responders from nonresponders in vivo using a CD3 PET probe ([^{89}Zr]Zr-p-isothiocyanatobenzyldeferoxamine-CD3) administered and imaged after the third therapeutic administration of CTLA-4 [62].

In order to achieve rapid clearance of a PET imaging probe targeting T lymphocytes and thereby optimize its use for imaging, Tavare and colleagues engineered a ^{89}Zr-labeled minibody against CD8+ T cells ([^{89}Zr]Zr-IAB22M2C) [63, 64]. This minibody-based tracer has demonstrated promise clinically, having shown uptake in CD8+-rich tissues and some tumor sites in a first-in-human trial [65]. Longitudinal assessment of the pattern of T-cell infiltration in tumors by imaging a CD8-specific ^{89}Zr-labeled PEGylated single-domain antibody fragment in animals with PET has also demonstrated the ability to separate those who will respond to CTLA-4 therapy from those who will not [66].

A somewhat different approach focuses on identifying activated T cells (rather than all T cells) using the ^{18}F-labeled analogue of arabino-furanosylguanine (AraG), an agent that is phosphorylated by cytoplasmic deoxycytidine kinase (dCK) and deoxyguanosine kinase (dGK), both enzymes with activity upregulated in activated T cells. Following phosphorylation, [^{18}F]F-AraG is trapped intracellularly, thereby concentrating in activated T cells [67]. In murine models, [^{18}F]F-AraG PET has demonstrated its ability to report changes in the levels of T-cell activation around tumors during ICI treatment as well as diagnose acute graft-versus-host disease following allogeneic hematopoietic cell transplantation [68]. As of the writing of this chapter, [^{18}F]F-AraG is undergoing initial study of predicting response in human cancer patients undergoing ICI therapy (Fig. 20.5).

As important as it is for ICI therapy to result in the recruitment of a sufficient level of T lymphocytes from the periphery, the ability for those T cells to infiltrate the tumor itself is also critical in determining the ultimate level of therapeutic response. Localization within the tumor can be blocked by CD11b+ myeloid-derived suppressor cells, the presence of which is associated with tumor growth, differentiation, and metasta-

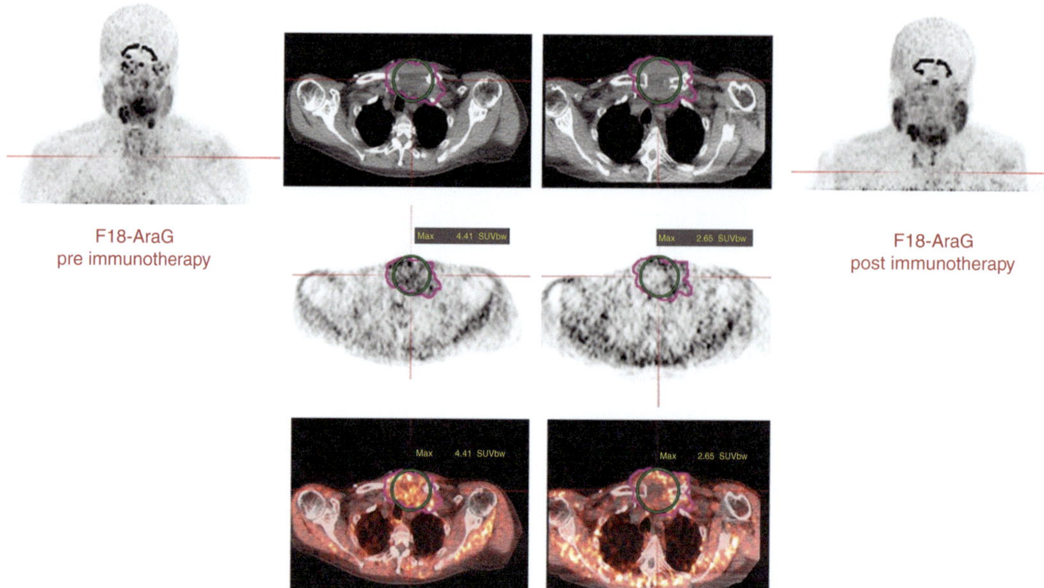

Fig. 20.5 A 65-year-old male with a history of T4N3M1 squamous cell carcinoma of the tongue, p16 positive, with metastatic anterior mediastinal and cervical LN. The patient was considered a candidate to receive immunotherapy. [^{18}F]F-AraG PET/CT imaging of the head and neck was obtained at baseline before the start of immunotherapy ([^{18}F]F-AraG pre-immunotherapy) and after 2 cycles ([^{18}F]F-AraG post-immunotherapy). The images demonstrate MIP (maximum intensity projection) images of the head and neck and cross-sectional images at the level of the anterior mediastinum. Volumes of interest (VOI) were placed around the patient's known metastatic mediastinal lesion, and SUVmax values were obtained before and after 2 cycles of immunotherapy. The quantification study demonstrates a decrease in SUVmax values in the mediastinal lesion with a ~50% reduction in SUVmax activity of AraG. Findings were consistent with a decrease in activated T cells at the metastatic site. The patient did not respond to immunotherapy and passed away a few months later

sis. Using ^{89}Zr-labeled PEGylated anti-CD8 and anti-CD11b single-domain antibody fragments to monitor the dynamics of cytotoxic T cells and CD11b^{+} cells during treatment with anti-PD-1 therapy, Rashidian and colleagues showed that anti-PD-1 administration resulted in recruitment of T cells from the tumor periphery to a more central location and complete resolution of the tumor occurred only when the tumor was completely infiltrated by CD8^{+} T cells. Interestingly, CD11b^{+} cells were present in all tumors but tended to congregate in the center of those tumors that showed response to ICI therapy [69]. These results point to the importance of the spatial location of the immune mediator's signal on PET (intratumoral versus around the tumor periphery) rather than measurement of the amplitude of the signal alone.

Granzyme B (GZP), a serine protease released by active cytotoxic T cells, is involved in tumor apoptosis. Because ICI treatment induces increased expression of granzyme B, PET strategies to detect levels of granzyme B have been studied as potential means to detect response early in the course of ICI therapy [70]. [^{68}Ga] Ga-NOTA-GZP, a GZP-targeting peptide labeled with the positron emitter gallium-68, can be used with PET to detect granzyme B and may offer early insight into tumor response to immune checkpoint inhibition [71]. Using small animal tumor models, Larimer and colleagues have demonstrated GZP PET's high accuracy (93% sensitivity, 94% negative predictive value) for predicting response to ICIs. In these same studies, GZP signal was also able to provide insight into the efficacy of specific changes in ICI sequencing, suggesting GZP PET could prove to be a critical biomarker for ICI management and determining dosing regimens; however, as of now, this approach has yet to enter human clinical trials [72].

20.3 Predicting/Evaluating the Efficacy of Other Immune-Based Therapies

PET has shown promise in evaluating the effectiveness of other immune-based therapies. Metabolic response of tumor tissue to immune-based therapies using 2-[^{18}F]FDG PET has been associated with improvement in other malignant marker levels and favorable prognosis in select malignancies [73]. However, the ability of activated T cells, the common effector mechanism of many immunomodulating therapeutic approaches, to increase glucose consumption and thereby be capable of detection using 2-[^{18}F]FDG PET has also been recognized and used to evaluate the efficacy of various approaches early in the therapeutic timeline [74].

20.3.1 Vaccines

A number of promising vaccine therapies have been developed, including those based on oncolytic virus activity, vaccines based on dendritic cells, and vaccines against cancer RNA. Tools such as 2-[^{18}F]FDG PET have been explored as means to monitor cutaneous or subcutaneous melanoma lesions or lymph node metastases treated using intralesionally administered talimogene laherparepvec (TVEC), a herpes simplex virus (I) modified by the deletion of neurovirulence gene (ICP34.5), deletion of the immunogenicity gene (ICP47), and addition of the gene-encoding human granulocyte-macrophage colony-stimulating factor (GM-CSF) [75, 76].

20.3.2 Stem Cell Transplant and T-Cell Infusions

Autologous and allogeneic stem cell transplants (SCTs) are well-established tools in the treatment of hematologic malignancies. As such, 2-[^{18}F]FDG PET has been utilized to monitor the response of myelomatous lesions to such transplants [77].

Antineoplastic strategies based on the infusion of engineered immune cells are relatively new, but have rapidly gained momentum in their use, creating an urgent need for noninvasive methods to evaluate their efficacy. Chimeric antigen receptors (CARs) are non-native receptors that link an antigen-binding domain to cell signaling domain(s). When T cells are engineered to express CARs (CAR T cells), they are capable of major histocompatibility complex (MHC)-unrestricted antigen specificity. CD19 is a transmembrane protein expressed by B cells from the time of immunoglobulin rearrangement through B-cell development and maturation until it is lost with terminal plasma cell differentiation [78]. Over the past decade, numerous trials using CAR T cells targeting CD19 have demonstrated high response rates in patients with B-cell malignancies [79–82]. Responses following CD19-CAR therapy for B-cell acute lymphoblastic leukemia (ALL) occur rapidly, with maximal response observed within 28 days following infusion. The magnitude and duration of the therapeutic effect achieved by the expansion of the CD19-CAR T cells in vivo are affected by distinct costimulatory domains [80, 81, 83].

Although experience in utilizing 2-[^{18}F]FDG PET to evaluate response to CD19-CAR treatment is quite limited, Shah et al. reported an association between total metabolic tumor volume on 2-[^{18}F]FDG PET 1 month following CD19-CAR T infusion and prognosis, in a population of patients with diffuse large B-cell lymphoma and follicular lymphoma. Notably, interpretation of the 2-[^{18}F]FDG PET images was not confounded by pseudoprogression or cytokine release syndrome (CRS) [84]. Very early work in treating malignancies with NKG2D natural killer cells engineered to express CARs has been promising, demonstrating complete metabolic response of malignant lesions on 2-[^{18}F]FDG PET in human subjects [85].

Direct monitoring of genetically altered T cells has been recognized as a potentially important component of adoptive T-cell therapy in patients. The ability to visualize their trafficking and targeting, as well as their proliferation and retention in vivo in a way that does not itself create immunogenicity, will be critical in assessing and improving the efficacy of these immunotherapy strategies. Monitoring of specific populations of transferred cells in vivo using ex vivo by means of radiolabeling has been described [86]. Several highly sensitive PET reporter systems that may be incorporated into DNA of human T cells via transduction with retroviral vectors have been developed and characterized. These PET reporter systems include the reporter/imaging agent combinations of human norepinephrine transporter (hNET)/meta-[^{18}F]fluorobenzylguanidine ([^{18}F]MFBG), human sodium iodide symporter (hNIS)/[^{124}I]iodide, human deoxycytidine kinase double mutant (hdCKDM)/[^{18}F]fluoro-5-ethyl-1-β-D-arabinofuranosyluracil ([^{18}F]FEAU), and herpes simplex virus type 1 thymidine kinase (hsvTK)/[^{18}F]FEAU, of which hNET/[^{18}F]MFBG appears most sensitive according to one recently published study [87].

20.3.3 Antibody-Based Therapies and Radioimmunotherapy

Active exploration of PET's potential roles in the selection of patients for radioimmunotherapy (RIT), performing pre- and post-therapy dosimetry, and evaluating response to RIT continue. In a recent Japanese study of patients with non-Hodgkin lymphoma treated with [^{90}Y]Y-ibritumomab, 2-[^{18}F]FDG PET findings 6 weeks after radioimmunotherapy administration provided accurate determination of response to therapy and prediction of prognosis [88].

There is also a resurgent interest in the development of new antibody-based radiolabeled therapeutic and theranostic agents and strategies [89], many of which are based on antibody-based drugs using monoclonal antibodies (mAbs), angiogenic inhibitors, immune checkpoint inhibitors, bispecific T-cell engagers, antibody-drug conjugates, and engineered antibody structures (such as minibodies, diabodies, and nanobodies) previously approved by the FDA or the European Medicines Agency (EMA) [90].

20.4 Future Advances

20.4.1 New Tracer Development

At the end of the day, activation of the T cell is the critical result of many immunomodulating strategies. As such, [^{64}Cu]Cu-DOTA-AbOX40 is a new PET tracer focused on reliable detection and tracking of T-cell activation in vivo. Alam et al. demonstrated longitudinal PET imaging of OX40, a cell-surface marker of T-cell activation, following in situ vaccination tumor treatment strategy in mice [91]. Also, a ^{18}F-fluorinated version of interleukin-2 (IL-2) may potentially be useful for PET imaging of the upregulation of IL-2 receptors that occurs on T lymphocytes upon activation [92].

Another factor in immunomodulation occurs within the microenvironment surrounding cancer cells and involves the activation of the indoleamine 2,3-dioxygenase (IDO)-mediated kynurenine pathway which breaks down tryptophan, an essential amino acid that supports T-cell activation and proliferation [93, 94]. The resulting decrease in tryptophan and increase in kynurenine suppress effector T and natural killer cell functions by activating T regulatory cells and myeloid-derived suppressor cells, and cancer therapeutics targeting this pathway have been developed, some of which are in clinical trials [95]. PET imaging of IDO pathway activity has been accomplished using various radiolabeled forms of tryptophan, including [^{18}F]F-tryptophan whose radiochemistry has evolved significantly over the past decade [96, 97].

Tumor-associated macrophages (TAMs) have also been implicated in modulation of responses to immunotherapies targeting cancer as well as in tumor progression itself. Generally, TAMs suppress function in the tumor microenvironment and TAM-depleting therapies combined with more conventional antineoplastic therapies have shown promise [98]. Given the affinity of high-density lipoprotein (HDL) particles and polyglucose nanoparticles for macrophages, PET using zirconium-89 (^{89}Zr)-labeled HDL nanoparticles or copper-64 (^{64}Cu)-labeled dextran nanoparticles has been explored as a method of monitoring treatments focused on TAMs [99, 100].

Chemokines and cytokines offer additional targets for PET imaging probes as these small molecules are intimately involved in migration and homing patterns of a variety of immune effectors [7]. Monitoring of multiple response indicators may be achieved using multimodal imaging such as PET/magnetic resonance imaging (MRI) or combined nuclear/optical imaging approaches [70]. A key part of the future development of any molecular imaging probe will be ensuring that the imaging probe itself does not inadvertently interfere with normal immune cell functionality [101].

In immune-based strategies other than those involving T cells or immunomodulation, selection of appropriate immunotherapies to treat malignancies remains an area where continued innovation in PET radiotracers is needed. For example, new tracers targeting the cell membrane glycolipid GD2, expressed by some osteosarcomas and most neuroblastomas, have been developed to enable targeting of anti-GD2 immunotherapy to only those tumors that highly express the glycolipid [102].

20.4.2 Advances in Quantitative Imaging and Radiomics

The semiquantitative measure of standardized uptake value (SUV) has been central to clinical PET reporting and studies of associations between semiquantitative measurement of metabolism and patient response to therapy and/or prognosis. Because glucose uptake is associated with inflammation and infection as well as malignancy, measurement of the sheer magnitude of 2-[^{18}F]FDG uptake in the setting of immune-mediated treatment for malignancy may provide an overall picture of several underlying molecular processes.

Radiomics, a rapidly developing field in quantitative imaging, entails the process of uncovering signals and patterns within imaging data that provide new information related to structure, underlying functional and molecular processes, and therapeutic response over what might be possible using traditional approaches to radio-

logic interpretation and quantitation [103, 104]. By using data from baseline CT and genomics data from tumor biopsy, Sun and colleagues developed a radiomics signature for CD8 cell infiltration that, when validated in patients with solid cancers treated with anti-PD-1 or anti-PD-L1 immunotherapy, demonstrated the ability to identify immune-desert versus inflamed tumors and to thereby infer clinical outcomes and predict prognosis [105]. Development of such approaches using molecular imaging techniques faces significant hurdles, such as differences in image acquisition timing and techniques, among others [7]. However, initial results evaluating the ability of tumor heterogeneity index from 2-[^{18}F] FDG PET imaging to predict overall survival in a small cohort of patients with metastatic melanoma treated with immunotherapy are encouraging [106]. More recently, Mu and colleagues were able to successfully train a multiparametric radiomics signature (mpRS) model on 2-[^{18}F] FDG PET/CT imaging data to identify patients who would receive durable clinical benefit from checkpoint blockade immunotherapy for non-small cell lung cancer as well as to estimate progression-free and overall survival [107]. As expression of PD-L1 varies markedly within individual tumors, future radiomics investigations using PET tracers with greater immune specificity than 2-[^{18}F]FDG could potentially yield even greater ability to predict outcomes [108].

20.5 Conclusion

While much of the current literature on the use of PET to manage immunomodulatory therapies in cancer patients focuses on 2-[^{18}F]FDG PET using a variety of response criteria, the development of more quantitative methodologies, including radiomics approaches, holds promise to uncover additional signals to more accurately predict tumor response. In addition, there are numerous additional molecular targets that may be used to elucidate various key steps in eliciting an immune response, and their use as targets for molecular imaging with PET may enable increased precision in characterization of the body's response to immunomodulating drugs. PET will undoubtedly remain a key modality to interrogate the complex network of signals that underlie the immune response, and with greater knowledge of the meaning of these signals, PET will hopefully enable personalized approaches to cancer therapies using immune-based approaches in the future.

References

1. Verma V, Sprave T, Haque W, Simone CB 2nd, Chang JY, Welsh JW, et al. A systematic review of the cost and cost-effectiveness studies of immune checkpoint inhibitors. J Immunother Cancer. 2018;6(1):128. https://doi.org/10.1186/s40425-018-0442-7.
2. Martins F, Sofiya L, Sykiotis GP, Lamine F, Maillard M, Fraga M, et al. Adverse effects of immune-checkpoint inhibitors: epidemiology, management and surveillance. Nat Rev Clin Oncol. 2019;16(9):563–80. https://doi.org/10.1038/s41571-019-0218-0.
3. Wang DY, Salem JE, Cohen JV, Chandra S, Menzer C, Ye F, et al. Fatal toxic effects associated with immune checkpoint inhibitors: a systematic review and meta-analysis. JAMA Oncol. 2018;4(12):1721–8. https://doi.org/10.1001/jamaoncol.2018.3923.
4. Ito K, Schoder H, Teng R, Humm JL, Ni A, Wolchok JD, et al. Prognostic value of baseline metabolic tumor volume measured on (18)F-fluorodeoxyglucose positron emission tomography/computed tomography in melanoma patients treated with ipilimumab therapy. Eur J Nucl Med Mol Imaging. 2019;46(4):930–9. https://doi.org/10.1007/s00259-018-4211-0.
5. Boursi B, Werner TJ, Gholami S, Margalit O, Baruch E, Markel G, et al. Physiologic colonic fluorine-18-fluorodeoxyglucose uptake may predict response to immunotherapy in patients with metastatic melanoma. Melanoma Res. 2019;29(3):318–21. https://doi.org/10.1097/CMR.0000000000000566.
6. Rossi S, Toschi L, Castello A, Grizzi F, Mansi L, Lopci E. Clinical characteristics of patient selection and imaging predictors of outcome in solid tumors treated with checkpoint-inhibitors. Eur J Nucl Med Mol Imaging. 2017;44(13):2310–25. https://doi.org/10.1007/s00259-017-3802-5.
7. Shields AF, Jacobs PM, Sznol M, Graham MM, Germain RN, Lum LG, et al. Immune modulation therapy and imaging: workshop report. J Nucl Med. 2018;59(3):410–7. https://doi.org/10.2967/jnumed.117.195610.
8. Aide N, Hicks RJ, Le Tourneau C, Lheureux S, Fanti S, Lopci E. FDG PET/CT for assessing tumour response to immunotherapy: report on the EANM symposium on immune modulation and recent review of the literature. Eur J Nucl Med Mol Imaging. 2019;46(1):238–50. https://doi.org/10.1007/s00259-018-4171-4.
9. Evangelista L, Cuppari L, Menis J, Bonanno L, Reccia P, Frega S, et al. 18F-FDG PET/CT in non-small-cell lung cancer patients: a potential predictive biomarker of response to immunotherapy. Nucl Med Commun. 2019;40(8):802–7. https://doi.org/10.1097/MNM.0000000000001025.
10. Nakamoto R, Zaba LC, Rosenberg J, Reddy SA, Nobashi TW, Davidzon G, et al. Prognostic value of volumetric PET parameters at early response evaluation in melanoma patients treated with immunotherapy. Eur J Nucl Med Mol Imaging. 2020; https://doi.org/10.1007/s00259-020-04792-0.
11. Tsai KK, Pampaloni MH, Hope C, Algazi AP, Ljung BM, Pincus L, et al. Increased FDG avidity in lymphoid tissue associated with response to combined immune checkpoint blockade. J Immunother Cancer. 2016;4:58. https://doi.org/10.1186/s40425-016-0162-9.
12. Sachpekidis C, Larribere L, Kopp-Schneider A, Hassel JC, Dimitrakopoulou-Strauss A. Can benign lymphoid tissue changes in (18)F-FDG PET/CT predict response to immunotherapy in metastatic melanoma? Cancer Immunol Immunother. 2019;68(2):297–303. https://doi.org/10.1007/s00262-018-2279-9.
13. Seban RD, Nemer JS, Marabelle A, Yeh R, Deutsch E, Ammari S, et al. Prognostic and theranostic 18F-FDG PET biomarkers for anti-PD1 immunotherapy in metastatic melanoma: association with outcome and transcriptomics. Eur J Nucl Med Mol Imaging. 2019;46(11):2298–310. https://doi.org/10.1007/s00259-019-04411-7.
14. Eisenhauer EA, Therasse P, Bogaerts J, Schwartz LH, Sargent D, Ford R, et al. New response evaluation criteria in solid tumours: revised RECIST guideline (version 1.1). Eur J Cancer. 2009;45(2):228–47. https://doi.org/10.1016/j.ejca.2008.10.026.
15. Young H, Baum R, Cremerius U, Herholz K, Hoekstra O, Lammertsma AA, et al. Measurement of clinical and subclinical tumour response using [18F]-fluorodeoxyglucose and positron emission tomography: review and 1999 EORTC recommendations. European Organization for Research and Treatment of Cancer (EORTC) PET Study Group. Eur J Cancer. 1999;35(13):1773–82. https://doi.org/10.1016/s0959-8049(99)00229-4.
16. Tan AC, Emmett L, Lo S, Liu V, Kapoor R, Carlino MS, et al. FDG-PET response and outcome from anti-PD-1 therapy in metastatic melanoma. Ann Oncol. 2018;29(10):2115–20. https://doi.org/10.1093/annonc/mdy330.
17. Seith F, Forschner A, Schmidt H, Pfannenberg C, Guckel B, Nikolaou K, et al. 18F-FDG-PET detects complete response to PD1-therapy in melanoma patients two weeks after therapy start. Eur J Nucl Med Mol Imaging. 2018;45(1):95–101. https://doi.org/10.1007/s00259-017-3813-2.
18. Chiou VL, Burotto M. Pseudoprogression and immune-related response in solid tumors. J Clin Oncol. 2015;33(31):3541–3. https://doi.org/10.1200/JCO.2015.61.6870.

19. Comito F, Ambrosini V, Sperandi F, Melotti B, Ardizzoni A. Osteoblastic bone response mimicking bone progression during treatment with pembrolizumab in advanced cutaneous melanoma. Anti-Cancer Drugs. 2018;29(10):1026–9. https://doi.org/10.1097/CAD.0000000000000689.

20. Eshghi N, Lundeen TF, Kuo PH. Dynamic adaptation of tumor immune response with nivolumab demonstrated by 18F-FDG PET/CT. Clin Nucl Med. 2018;43(2):114–6. https://doi.org/10.1097/RLU.0000000000001934.

21. Goldfarb L, Duchemann B, Chouahnia K, Zelek L, Soussan M. Monitoring anti-PD-1-based immunotherapy in non-small cell lung cancer with FDG PET: introduction of iPERCIST. EJNMMI Res. 2019;9(1): 8. https://doi.org/10.1186/s13550-019-0473-1.

22. Amrane K, Le Goupil D, Quere G, Delcroix O, Gouva S, Schick U, et al. Prediction of response to immune checkpoint inhibitor therapy using 18F-FDG PET/CT in patients with melanoma. Medicine (Baltimore). 2019;98(29):e16417. https://doi.org/10.1097/MD.0000000000016417.

23. Dimitrakopoulou-Strauss A. Monitoring of patients with metastatic melanoma treated with immune checkpoint inhibitors using PET-CT. Cancer Immunol Immunother. 2019;68(5):813–22. https://doi.org/10.1007/s00262-018-2229-6.

24. Anwar H, Sachpekidis C, Winkler J, Kopp-Schneider A, Haberkorn U, Hassel JC, et al. Absolute number of new lesions on (18)F-FDG PET/CT is more predictive of clinical response than SUV changes in metastatic melanoma patients receiving ipilimumab. Eur J Nucl Med Mol Imaging. 2018;45(3):376–83. https://doi.org/10.1007/s00259-017-3870-6.

25. Sachpekidis C, Anwar H, Winkler J, Kopp-Schneider A, Larribere L, Haberkorn U, et al. The role of interim (18)F-FDG PET/CT in prediction of response to ipilimumab treatment in metastatic melanoma. Eur J Nucl Med Mol Imaging. 2018;45(8):1289–96. https://doi.org/10.1007/s00259-018-3972-9.

26. Sachpekidis C, Anwar H, Winkler JK, Kopp-Schneider A, Larribere L, Haberkorn U, et al. Longitudinal studies of the (18)F-FDG kinetics after ipilimumab treatment in metastatic melanoma patients based on dynamic FDG PET/CT. Cancer Immunol Immunother. 2018;67(8):1261–70. https://doi.org/10.1007/s00262-018-2183-3.

27. Ito K, Teng R, Schoder H, Humm JL, Ni A, Michaud L, et al. (18)F-FDG PET/CT for monitoring of ipilimumab therapy in patients with metastatic melanoma. J Nucl Med. 2019;60(3):335–41. https://doi.org/10.2967/jnumed.118.213652.

28. Wong ANM, McArthur GA, Hofman MS, Hicks RJ. The advantages and challenges of using FDG PET/CT for response assessment in melanoma in the era of targeted agents and immunotherapy. Eur J Nucl Med Mol Imaging. 2017;44(Suppl 1):67–77. https://doi.org/10.1007/s00259-017-3691-7.

29. Keating M, Giscombe L, Tannous T, Hartshorn K. Prolonged treatment response to pembrolizumab in a patient with pretreated metastatic colon cancer and lynch syndrome. Case Rep Oncol Med. 2019;2019:3847672. https://doi.org/10.1155/2019/3847672.

30. Paoluzzi L, Cacavio A, Ghesani M, Karambelkar A, Rapkiewicz A, Weber J, et al. Response to anti-PD1 therapy with nivolumab in metastatic sarcomas. Clin Sarcoma Res. 2016;6:24. https://doi.org/10.1186/s13569-016-0064-0.

31. Eshghi N, Lundeen TF, MacKinnon L, Avery R, Kuo PH. 18F-FDG PET/CT for monitoring response of Merkel cell carcinoma to the novel programmed cell death ligand 1 inhibitor avelumab. Clin Nucl Med. 2018;43(5):e142–e4. https://doi.org/10.1097/RLU.0000000000002051.

32. Johnson DR, Guerin JB, Ruff MW, Fang S, Hunt CH, Morris JM, et al. Glioma response assessment: classic pitfalls, novel confounders, and emerging imaging tools. Br J Radiol. 2019;92(1094):20180730. https://doi.org/10.1259/bjr.20180730.

33. Cheson BD, Fisher RI, Barrington SF, Cavalli F, Schwartz LH, Zucca E, et al. Recommendations for initial evaluation, staging, and response assessment of Hodgkin and non-Hodgkin lymphoma: the Lugano classification. J Clin Oncol. 2014;32(27):3059–68. https://doi.org/10.1200/JCO.2013.54.8800.

34. Cheson BD, Horning SJ, Coiffier B, Shipp MA, Fisher RI, Connors JM, et al. Report of an international workshop to standardize response criteria for non-Hodgkin's lymphomas. NCI Sponsored International Working Group. J Clin Oncol. 1999;17(4):1244. https://doi.org/10.1200/JCO.1999.17.4.1244.

35. Cheson BD, Pfistner B, Juweid ME, Gascoyne RD, Specht L, Horning SJ, et al. Revised response criteria for malignant lymphoma. J Clin Oncol. 2007;25(5):579–86. https://doi.org/10.1200/JCO.2006.09.2403.

36. Cheson BD, Ansell S, Schwartz L, Gordon LI, Advani R, Jacene HA, et al. Refinement of the Lugano classification lymphoma response criteria in the era of immunomodulatory therapy. Blood. 2016;128(21):2489–96. https://doi.org/10.1182/blood-2016-05-718528.

37. Chen A, Mokrane FZ, Schwartz L, Morschhauser F, Stamatoullas A, Schiano de Colella JM, et al. Early (18)F-FDG PET/CT response predicts survival in Relapsed/Refractory Hodgkin Lymphoma treated with Nivolumab. J Nucl Med. 2019; https://doi.org/10.2967/jnumed.119.232827.

38. Younes A, Hilden P, Coiffier B, Hagenbeek A, Salles G, Wilson W, et al. International Working Group consensus response evaluation criteria in lymphoma (RECIL 2017). Ann Oncol. 2017;28(7):1436–47. https://doi.org/10.1093/annonc/mdx097.

39. Fuentes-Antras J, Provencio M, Diaz-Rubio E. Hyperprogression as a distinct outcome after immunotherapy. Cancer Treat Rev. 2018;70:16–21. https://doi.org/10.1016/j.ctrv.2018.07.006.

40. Champiat S, Dercle L, Ammari S, Massard C, Hollebecque A, Postel-Vinay S, et al. Hyperprogressive dis-

ease is a new pattern of progression in cancer patients treated by anti-PD-1/PD-L1. Clin Cancer Res. 2017;23(8):1920–8. https://doi.org/10.1158/1078-0432.CCR-16-1741.

41. Kato S, Goodman A, Walavalkar V, Barkauskas DA, Sharabi A, Kurzrock R. Hyperprogressors after immunotherapy: analysis of genomic alterations associated with accelerated growth rate. Clin Cancer Res. 2017;23(15):4242–50. https://doi.org/10.1158/1078-0432.CCR-16-3133.

42. Saada-Bouzid E, Defaucheux C, Karabajakian A, Coloma VP, Servois V, Paoletti X, et al. Hyperprogression during anti-PD-1/PD-L1 therapy in patients with recurrent and/or metastatic head and neck squamous cell carcinoma. Ann Oncol. 2017;28(7):1605–11. https://doi.org/10.1093/annonc/mdx178.

43. Kato S, Kurzrock R. Genomics of immunotherapy-associated hyperprogressors-response. Clin Cancer Res. 2017;23(20):6376. https://doi.org/10.1158/1078-0432.CCR-17-1990.

44. Tachihara M, Nishimura Y. Who will suffer from hyperprogressive disease in patients with advanced non-small cell lung cancer treated with PD-1/PD-L1 inhibitors. J Thorac Dis. 2019;11(Suppl 9):S1289–91. https://doi.org/10.21037/jtd.2019.04.76.

45. Kaira K, Higuchi T, Naruse I, Arisaka Y, Tokue A, Altan B, et al. Metabolic activity by (18)F-FDG-PET/CT is predictive of early response after nivolumab in previously treated NSCLC. Eur J Nucl Med Mol Imaging. 2018;45(1):56–66. https://doi.org/10.1007/s00259-017-3806-1.

46. Lang N, Dick J, Slynko A, Schulz C, Dimitrako-poulou-Strauss A, Sachpekidis C, et al. Clinical significance of signs of autoimmune colitis in (18) F-fluorodeoxyglucose positron emission tomography-computed tomography of 100 stage-IV melanoma patients. Immunotherapy. 2019;11(8):667–76. https://doi.org/10.2217/imt-2018-0146.

47. Ganatra S, Neilan TG. Immune checkpoint inhibitor-associated myocarditis. Oncologist. 2018;23(8):879–86. https://doi.org/10.1634/theoncologist.2018-0130.

48. Fakhri G, Akel R, Salem Z, Tawil A, Tfayli A. Pulmonary sarcoidosis activation following neoadjuvant Pembrolizumab plus chemotherapy combination therapy in a patient with non-small cell lung Cancer: a case report. Case Rep Oncol. 2017;10(3):1070–5. https://doi.org/10.1159/000484596.

49. Bajwa R, Cheema A, Khan T, Amirpour A, Paul A, Chaughtai S, et al. Adverse effects of immune checkpoint inhibitors (programmed death-1 inhibitors and cytotoxic T-lymphocyte-associated protein-4 inhibitors): results of a retrospective study. J Clin Med Res. 2019;11(4):225–36. https://doi.org/10.14740/jocmr3750.

50. Nobashi T, Baratto L, Reddy SA, Srinivas S, Torii-hara A, Hatami N, et al. Predicting response to immunotherapy by evaluating tumors, lymphoid cell-rich organs, and immune-related adverse events using FDG-PET/CT. Clin Nucl Med. 2019;44(4):e272–e9. https://doi.org/10.1097/RLU.0000000000002453.

51. Sachpekidis C, Kopp-Schneider A, Hakim-Meibodi L, Dimitrakopoulou-Strauss A, Hassel JC. 18F-FDG PET/CT longitudinal studies in patients with advanced metastatic melanoma for response evaluation of combination treatment with vemurafenib and ipilimumab. Melanoma Res. 2019;29(2):178–86. https://doi.org/10.1097/CMR.0000000000000541.

52. Teng F, Meng X, Kong L, Yu J. Progress and challenges of predictive biomarkers of anti PD-1/PD-L1 immunotherapy: a systematic review. Cancer Lett. 2018;414:166–73. https://doi.org/10.1016/j.canlet.2017.11.014.

53. Daud AI, Wolchok JD, Robert C, Hwu WJ, Weber JS, Ribas A, et al. Programmed death-ligand 1 expression and response to the anti-programmed death 1 antibody pembrolizumab in melanoma. J Clin Oncol. 2016;34(34):4102–9. https://doi.org/10.1200/JCO.2016.67.2477.

54. Liu X, Yao J, Song L, Zhang S, Huang T, Li Y. Local and abscopal responses in advanced intrahepatic cholangiocarcinoma with low TMB, MSS, pMMR and negative PD-L1 expression following combined therapy of SBRT with PD-1 blockade. J Immunother Cancer. 2019;7(1):204. https://doi.org/10.1186/s40425-019-0692-z.

55. Truillet C, Oh HLJ, Yeo SP, Lee CY, Huynh LT, Wei J, et al. Imaging PD-L1 expression with ImmunoPET. Bioconjug Chem. 2018;29(1):96–103. https://doi.org/10.1021/acs.bioconjchem.7b00631.

56. Ehlerding EB, Lee HJ, Jiang D, Ferreira CA, Zahm CD, Huang P, et al. Antibody and fragment-based PET imaging of CTLA-4+ T-cells in humanized mouse models. Am J Cancer Res. 2019;9(1):53–63.

57. Chatterjee S, Lesniak WG, Miller MS, Lisok A, Sikorska E, Wharram B, et al. Rapid PD-L1 detection in tumors with PET using a highly specific peptide. Biochem Biophys Res Commun. 2017;483(1):258–63. https://doi.org/10.1016/j.bbrc.2016.12.156.

58. Jeong H, Kim S, Hong BJ, Lee CJ, Kim YE, Bok S, et al. Tumor-associated macrophages enhance tumor hypoxia and aerobic glycolysis. Cancer Res. 2019;79(4):795–806. https://doi.org/10.1158/0008-5472.CAN-18-2545.

59. Nguyen NC, Yee MK, Tuchayi AM, Kirkwood JM, Tawbi H, Mountz JM. Targeted therapy and immunotherapy response assessment with F-18 fluoro-thymidine positron-emission tomography/magnetic resonance imaging in melanoma brain metastasis: a pilot study. Front Oncol. 2018;8:18. https://doi.org/10.3389/fonc.2018.00018.

60. Ribas A, Benz MR, Allen-Auerbach MS, Radu C, Chmielowski B, Seja E, et al. Imaging of CTLA4 blockade-induced cell replication with (18)F-FLT PET in patients with advanced melanoma treated with tremelimumab. J Nucl Med. 2010;51(3):340–6. https://doi.org/10.2967/jnumed.109.070946.

61. Scarpelli M, Zahm C, Perlman S, McNeel DG, Jeraj R, Liu G. FLT PET/CT imaging of metastatic prostate cancer patients treated with pTVG-HP DNA vaccine and pembrolizumab. J Immunother Cancer.

2019;7(1):23. https://doi.org/10.1186/s40425-019-0516-1.

62. Larimer BM, Wehrenberg-Klee E, Caraballo A, Mahmood U. Quantitative CD3 PET imaging predicts tumor growth response to anti-CTLA-4 therapy. J Nucl Med. 2016;57(10):1607–11. https://doi.org/10.2967/jnumed.116.173930.

63. Tavare R, Escuin-Ordinas H, Mok S, McCracken MN, Zettlitz KA, Salazar FB, et al. An effective immuno-PET imaging method to monitor CD8-dependent responses to immunotherapy. Cancer Res. 2016;76(1):73–82. https://doi.org/10.1158/0008-5472.CAN-15-1707.

64. Tavare R, McCracken MN, Zettlitz KA, Knowles SM, Salazar FB, Olafsen T, et al. Engineered antibody fragments for immuno-PET imaging of endogenous CD8+ T cells in vivo. Proc Natl Acad Sci U S A. 2014;111(3):1108–13. https://doi.org/10.1073/pnas.1316922111.

65. Pandit-Taskar N, Postow M, Hellmann M, Harding J, Barker C, O'Donoghue J, et al. First-in-human imaging with (89)Zr-Df-IAB22M2C anti-CD8 minibody in patients with solid malignancies: preliminary pharmacokinetics, biodistribution, and lesion targeting. J Nucl Med. 2019; https://doi.org/10.2967/jnumed.119.229781.

66. Rashidian M, Ingram JR, Dougan M, Dongre A, Whang KA, LeGall C, et al. Predicting the response to CTLA-4 blockade by longitudinal noninvasive monitoring of CD8 T cells. J Exp Med. 2017;214(8):2243–55. https://doi.org/10.1084/jem.20161950.

67. Levi J, Lam T, Goth SR, Yaghoubi S, Bates J, Ren G, et al. Imaging of activated T cells as an early predictor of immune response to anti-PD-1 therapy. Cancer Res. 2019;79(13):3455–65. https://doi.org/10.1158/0008-5472.CAN-19-0267.

68. Ronald JA, Kim BS, Gowrishankar G, Namavari M, Alam IS, D'Souza A, et al. A PET imaging strategy to visualize activated T cells in acute graft-versus-host disease elicited by allogenic hematopoietic cell transplant. Cancer Res. 2017;77(11):2893–902. https://doi.org/10.1158/0008-5472.CAN-16-2953.

69. Rashidian M, LaFleur MW, Verschoor VL, Dongre A, Zhang Y, Nguyen TH, et al. Immuno-PET identifies the myeloid compartment as a key contributor to the outcome of the antitumor response under PD-1 blockade. Proc Natl Acad Sci U S A. 2019;116(34):16971–80. https://doi.org/10.1073/pnas.1905005116.

70. Du Y, Jin Y, Sun W, Fang J, Zheng J, Tian J. Advances in molecular imaging of immune checkpoint targets in malignancies: current and future prospect. Eur Radiol. 2019;29(8):4294–302. https://doi.org/10.1007/s00330-018-5814-3.

71. Larimer BM, Wehrenberg-Klee E, Dubois F, Mehta A, Kalomeris T, Flaherty K, et al. Granzyme B PET imaging as a predictive biomarker of immunotherapy response. Cancer Res. 2017;77(9):2318–27. https://doi.org/10.1158/0008-5472.CAN-16-3346.

72. Larimer BM, Bloch E, Nesti S, Austin EE, Wehrenberg-Klee E, Boland G, et al. The effectiveness of checkpoint inhibitor combinations and administration timing can be measured by granzyme B PET imaging. Clin Cancer Res. 2019;25(4):1196–205. https://doi.org/10.1158/1078-0432.CCR-18-2407.

73. Ranki T, Pesonen S, Hemminki A, Partanen K, Kairemo K, Alanko T, et al. Phase I study with ONCOS-102 for the treatment of solid tumors—an evaluation of clinical response and exploratory analyses of immune markers. J Immunother Cancer. 2016;4:17. https://doi.org/10.1186/s40425-016-0121-5.

74. Pektor S, Hilscher L, Walzer KC, Miederer I, Bausbacher N, Loquai C, et al. In vivo imaging of the immune response upon systemic RNA cancer vaccination by FDG-PET. EJNMMI Res. 2018;8(1):80. https://doi.org/10.1186/s13550-018-0435-z.

75. Covington MF, Curiel CN, Lattimore L, Avery RJ, Kuo PH. FDG-PET/CT for monitoring response of melanoma to the novel oncolytic viral therapy talimogene laherparepvec. Clin Nucl Med. 2017;42(2):114–5. https://doi.org/10.1097/RLU.0000000000001456.

76. Franke V, van der Hiel B, van de Wiel BA, Klop WMC, Ter Meulen S, van Akkooi ACJ. Positron emission tomography/computed tomography evaluation of oncolytic virus therapy efficacy in melanoma. Eur J Cancer. 2018;90:149–52. https://doi.org/10.1016/j.ejca.2017.11.007.

77. Patriarca F, Carobolante F, Zamagni E, Montefusco V, Bruno B, Englaro E, et al. The role of positron emission tomography with 18F-fluorodeoxyglucose integrated with computed tomography in the evaluation of patients with multiple myeloma undergoing allogeneic stem cell transplantation. Biol Blood Marrow Transplant. 2015;21(6):1068–73. https://doi.org/10.1016/j.bbmt.2015.03.001.

78. Wang K, Wei G, Liu D. CD19: a biomarker for B cell development, lymphoma diagnosis and therapy. Exp Hematol Oncol. 2012;1(1):36. https://doi.org/10.1186/2162-3619-1-36.

79. Davila ML, Riviere I, Wang X, Bartido S, Park J, Curran K, et al. Efficacy and toxicity management of 19-28z CAR T cell therapy in B cell acute lymphoblastic leukemia. Sci Transl Med. 2014;6(224):224ra25. https://doi.org/10.1126/scitranslmed.3008226.

80. Maude SL, Frey N, Shaw PA, Aplenc R, Barrett DM, Bunin NJ, et al. Chimeric antigen receptor T cells for sustained remissions in leukemia. N Engl J Med. 2014;371(16):1507–17. https://doi.org/10.1056/NEJMoa1407222.

81. Lee DW, Kochenderfer JN, Stetler-Stevenson M, Cui YK, Delbrook C, Feldman SA, et al. T cells expressing CD19 chimeric antigen receptors for acute lymphoblastic leukaemia in children and young adults: a phase 1 dose-escalation trial. Lancet. 2015;385(9967):517–28. https://doi.org/10.1016/S0140-6736(14)61403-3.

82. Kochenderfer JN, Dudley ME, Kassim SH, Somerville RP, Carpenter RO, Stetler-Stevenson M, et al. Chemotherapy-refractory diffuse large B-cell lymphoma and indolent B-cell malignancies can be effectively treated with autologous T cells expressing an anti-CD19 chimeric antigen receptor. J Clin Oncol. 2015;33(6):540–9. https://doi.org/10.1200/JCO.2014.56.2025.

83. Long AH, Haso WM, Shern JF, Wanhainen KM, Murgai M, Ingaramo M, et al. 4-1BB costimulation ameliorates T cell exhaustion induced by tonic signaling of chimeric antigen receptors. Nat Med. 2015;21(6):581–90. https://doi.org/10.1038/nm.3838.

84. Shah NN, Nagle SJ, Torigian DA, Farwell MD, Hwang WT, Frey N, et al. Early positron emission tomography/computed tomography as a predictor of response after CTL019 chimeric antigen receptor -T-cell therapy in B-cell non-Hodgkin lymphomas. Cytotherapy. 2018;20(12):1415–8. https://doi.org/10.1016/j.jcyt.2018.10.003.

85. Xiao L, Cen D, Gan H, Sun Y, Huang N, Xiong H, et al. Adoptive transfer of NKG2D CAR mRNA-engineered natural killer cells in colorectal cancer patients. Mol Ther. 2019;27(6):1114–25. https://doi.org/10.1016/j.ymthe.2019.03.011.

86. Moroz MA, Zanzonico P, Lee JT, Ponomarev V. Ex vivo radiolabeling and in vivo PET imaging of T cells expressing nuclear reporter genes. Methods Mol Biol. 1790;2018:153–63. https://doi.org/10.1007/978-1-4939-7860-1_12.

87. Moroz MA, Zhang H, Lee J, Moroz E, Zurita J, Shenker L, et al. Comparative analysis of T cell imaging with human nuclear reporter genes. J Nucl Med. 2015;56(7):1055–60. https://doi.org/10.2967/jnumed.115.159855.

88. Kitajima K, Okada M, Kashiwagi T, Yoshihara K, Tokugawa T, Sawada A, et al. Early evaluation of tumor response to (90)Y-ibritumomab radioimmunotherapy in relapsed/refractory B cell non-Hodgkin lymphoma: what is the optimal timing for FDG-PET/CT? Eur Radiol. 2019;29(7):3935–44. https://doi.org/10.1007/s00330-019-06134-7.

89. Houghton JL, Membreno R, Abdel-Atti D, Cunanan KM, Carlin S, Scholz WW, et al. Establishment of the in vivo efficacy of pretargeted radioimmunotherapy utilizing inverse electron demand Diels-Alder click chemistry. Mol Cancer Ther. 2017;16(1):124–33. https://doi.org/10.1158/1535-7163.MCT-16-0503.

90. Moek KL, Giesen D, Kok IC, de Groot DJA, Jalving M, Fehrmann RSN, et al. Theranostics using antibodies and antibody-related therapeutics. J Nucl Med. 2017;58(Suppl 2):83S–90S. https://doi.org/10.2967/jnumed.116.186940.

91. Alam IS, Mayer AT, Sagiv-Barfi I, Wang K, Vermesh O, Czerwinski DK, et al. Imaging activated T cells predicts response to cancer vaccines. J Clin Invest. 2018;128(6):2569–80. https://doi.org/10.1172/JCI98509.

92. Di Gialleonardo V, Signore A, Glaudemans AW, Dierckx RA, De Vries EF. N-(4-18F-fluorobenzoyl) interleukin-2 for PET of human-activated T lymphocytes. J Nucl Med. 2012;53(5):679–86. https://doi.org/10.2967/jnumed.111.091306.

93. Eleftheriadis T, Pissas G, Antoniadi G, Liakopoulos V, Stefanidis I. Indoleamine 2,3-dioxygenase depletes tryptophan, activates general control nonderepressible 2 kinase and down-regulates key enzymes involved in fatty acid synthesis in primary human CD4+ T cells. Immunology. 2015;146(2):292–300. https://doi.org/10.1111/imm.12502.

94. Lee GK, Park HJ, Macleod M, Chandler P, Munn DH, Mellor AL. Tryptophan deprivation sensitizes activated T cells to apoptosis prior to cell division. Immunology. 2002;107(4):452–60. https://doi.org/10.1046/j.1365-2567.2002.01526.x.

95. Liu M, Wang X, Wang L, Ma X, Gong Z, Zhang S, et al. Targeting the IDO1 pathway in cancer: from bench to bedside. J Hematol Oncol. 2018;11(1):100. https://doi.org/10.1186/s13045-018-0644-y.

96. Xin Y, Cai H. Improved radiosynthesis and biological evaluations of L- and D-1-[(18)F]Fluoroethyl-tryptophan for PET imaging of IDO-mediated kynurenine pathway of tryptophan metabolism. Mol Imaging Biol. 2017;19(4):589–98. https://doi.org/10.1007/s11307-016-1024-z.

97. Giglio BC, Fei H, Wang M, Wang H, He L, Feng H, et al. Synthesis of 5-[(18)F]Fluoro-alpha-methyl tryptophan: new Trp based PET agents. Theranostics. 2017;7(6):1524–30. https://doi.org/10.7150/thno.19371.

98. Brown JM, Recht L, Strober S. The promise of targeting macrophages in cancer therapy. Clin Cancer Res. 2017;23(13):3241–50. https://doi.org/10.1158/1078-0432.CCR-16-3122.

99. Mason C, Kossatz S, Carter L, Pirovano G, Brand C, Guru N, et al. A (89)Zr-HDL PET tracer monitors response to a CSF1R inhibitor. J Nucl Med. 2019; https://doi.org/10.2967/jnumed.119.230466.

100. Kim HY, Li R, Ng TSC, Courties G, Rodell CB, Prytyskach M, et al. Quantitative imaging of tumor-associated macrophages and their response to therapy using (64)cu-labeled macrin. ACS Nano. 2018;12(12):12015–29. https://doi.org/10.1021/acsnano.8b04338.

101. Mayer KE, Mall S, Yusufi N, Gosmann D, Steiger K, Russelli L, et al. T-cell functionality testing is highly relevant to developing novel immuno-tracers monitoring T cells in the context of immunotherapies and revealed CD7 as an attractive target. Theranostics. 2018;8(21):6070–87. https://doi.org/10.7150/thno.27275.

102. Butch ER, Mead PE, Amador Diaz V, Tillman H, Stewart E, Mishra JK, et al. Positron emission tomography detects in vivo expression of disialoganglioside GD2 in mouse models of primary and metastatic osteosarcoma. Cancer Res. 2019;79(12):3112–24. https://doi.org/10.1158/0008-5472.CAN-18-3340.

103. Shaikh F, Franc B, Allen E, Sala E, Awan O, Hendrata K, et al. Translational radiomics: defining the

strategy pipeline and considerations for application-part 1: from methodology to clinical implementation. J Am Coll Radiol. 2018;15(3 Pt B):538–42. https://doi.org/10.1016/j.jacr.2017.12.008.

104. Liu G, Huang SY, Franc B, Seo Y, Mitra D. Unsupervised learning in PET Radiomics. IEEE Nucl Sci Symp Conf Rec (1997). 2017;2017 https://doi.org/10.1109/NSSMIC.2017.8532959.

105. Sun R, Limkin EJ, Vakalopoulou M, Dercle L, Champiat S, Han SR, et al. A radiomics approach to assess tumour-infiltrating CD8 cells and response to anti-PD-1 or anti-PD-L1 immunotherapy: an imaging biomarker, retrospective multicohort study. Lancet Oncol. 2018;19(9):1180–91. https://doi.org/10.1016/S1470-2045(18)30413-3.

106. Sanli Y, Leake J, Odu A, Xi Y, Subramaniam RM. Tumor heterogeneity on FDG PET/CT and immunotherapy: an imaging biomarker for predicting treatment response in patients with metastatic melanoma. AJR Am J Roentgenol. 2019:1–9. https://doi.org/10.2214/AJR.18.19796.

107. Mu W, Tunali I, Gray JE, Qi J, Schabath MB, Gillies RJ. Radiomics of (18)F-FDG PET/CT images predicts clinical benefit of advanced NSCLC patients to checkpoint blockade immunotherapy. Eur J Nucl Med Mol Imaging. 2019; https://doi.org/10.1007/s00259-019-04625-9.

108. Rasmussen JH, Lelkaitis G, Hakansson K, Vogelius IR, Johannesen HH, Fischer BM, et al. Intratumor heterogeneity of PD-L1 expression in head and neck squamous cell carcinoma. Br J Cancer. 2019;120(10):1003–6. https://doi.org/10.1038/s41416-019-0449-y.

Moving Forward: Expected Opportunities for the Development of New Therapeutic Agents

21

Philip F. Cohen, Tassia R. M. de Godoy, and Kalevi Kairemo

Contents

P. F. Cohen (✉) · T. R. M. de Godoy
Department of Radiology, University of British
Columbia, Vancouver, BC, Canada
e-mail: Philip.Cohen@vch.ca

K. Kairemo
Department of Nuclear Medicine, University of Texas
MD Anderson Cancer Center, Houston, TX, USA

© Springer Nature Switzerland AG 2022
S. Harsini et al. (eds.), *Nuclear Medicine and Immunology*,
https://doi.org/10.1007/978-3-030-81261-4_21

21.1 Introduction

Radionuclide therapy was impossible before 1896 until the discovery of radioactivity by Henri Becquerel. The first attempts at radiotherapy were limited to the few radioactive elements available, namely, radium used first in 1913 to treat various diseases, and George de Hevesy using radioactive isotopes of bismuth-214 (^{214}Bi) and lead-210 (^{210}Pb) for the first tracer studies. The invention of the cyclotron by Ernest Lawrence in the 1930s ushered in a new era of abundance of novel radionuclides. In 1936, John H. Lawrence, the brother of Ernest, became the first person to use artificial radioactivity when he used phosphorus-32 (^{32}P) to treat a patient with leukemia. This was followed by Joseph Gilbert Hamilton and Robert Spencer Stone administering sodium-24 (^{24}Na) to a leukemia patient [1].

In 1941, the therapeutic isotope iodine-130 (^{130}I) was administered to a patient by Saul Hertz. This was shortly followed in 1946 with pioneers at the Massachusetts General Hospital treating a patient with thyroid cancer with iodine-131 (^{131}I), an "atomic cocktail." Iodine-131 and phosphorus-32 were used in therapeutic nuclear medicine for the next 74 years [2], but very few therapeutic radionuclides followed. Radiosotopes, which had shown such initial promise for treatment, became increasingly more interesting as new "diagnostic radiotracers", as new diagnostic scanners, gamma cameras, and then positron emission tomography (PET) scanners allowed the visualization of hitherto invisible physiologic processes in the intact human body. Nuclear medicine, which had started as a therapeutic discipline, quickly morphed into a primarily diagnostic modality and then as a branch of diagnostic imaging/radiology. Nuclear medicine, which by the 1970s had witnessed tremendous growth due to the arrival of myriad new radionuclides and had become a recognized separate medical specialty, suddenly became challenged by new diagnostic modalities of real-time ultrasound, computed tomography

(CT), magnetic resonance imaging (MRI), and interventional radiology. This lessened the appeal of radioisotopes, and interest of new medical school graduates in nuclear medicine declined. By 2015, a proposal to disband the American Board of Nuclear Medicine and merge it into the American Board of Radiology was proposed, although not approved [3].

In recent years, however, a renaissance in nuclear medicine therapies has been underway. Theranostics, the combination of "therapies and diagnostics," has entered the nuclear medicine vocabulary. The first theranostic had been iodine-131 in the 1940s for the diagnosis and treatment of thyroid cancer and hyperthyroidism. This was based on the unique properties of the thyroid gland, including differentiated thyroid cancers of the thyroid gland, to trap and organify iodine. No real competitor to radioiodine was developed for decades, although different iodine radionuclides were introduced, such as iodine-123 for imaging, iodine-124 for PET imaging, and iodine-125 for imaging and therapy in preclinical applications, and iodine-131 first for imaging and then for radiotherapies [4].

The understanding and discovery of novel molecular targets, beginning in the 1960s and 1970s, led to the use of somatostatin receptors (SSTR), prostate-specific membrane antigen (PSMA), or cell integrins. These new molecular targets could be pinpointed by ligands carrying novel therapeutic radionuclides such as lutetium-177 (^{177}Lu) and actinium-225 (^{225}Ac). The concept of theranostic pairs using the same targeting agent, such as gallium-68 (^{68}Ga) PSMA or fluorine-18-DCFPyL (2-(3-{1-carboxy-5-[(6-^{18}F-fluoro-pyridine-3-carbonyl)-amino]-pentyl}-ureido)-pentanedioic acid), to image the target, then followed by [^{177}Lu]Lu-PSMA or [^{225}Ac]Ac-PSMA meant that on the molecular level, physicians could both "see what they treat and treat what they see" at the microscopic level. The introduction of 2-[^{18}F]fluoro-2-deoxy-D-glucose (2-[^{18}F]FDG) as a diagnostic PET agent, first in neurology and then in oncology and cardiology, began the era of molecular imaging. Unfortunately, 2-[^{18}F]FDG could not be used

as a theranostic agent, since it targeted normal brain and heart, despite high level of uptake in tumors and infection, and the glucose molecule could not be labeled readily with any therapeutic radionuclide, although several attempts to do so were made.

The use of selective theranostic molecular pairs began earnestly in the 1970s with the realization that pheochromocytomas and neuroendocrine tumors could be targeted with meta-iodo-benzylguanidine (MIBG) using iodine-123 for imaging and iodine-131 for radiotherapy. Later, it was observed that many of these tumors also contained somatostatin receptors, which could be imaged first using [^{111}In]In-octreotide and then treated using much larger doses of [^{111}In]In-octreotide. [^{111}In]In-octreotide had limited success as a therapeutic, but was followed by the more powerful beta emitter yttrium-90 octreotide. Significant renal toxicity limited the use of [^{90}Y]Y-octreotide, which was supplanted with a newer agent [^{177}Lu]Lu-DOTATATE and [^{177}Lu]Lu-DOTATOC. The NETTER-1 trial (2017) showed improved survival compared to chemotherapy. Prostate cancer had been targeted beginning with [^{111}In]In-PSMA (ProstaScint) with little commercial success, but followed in this decade by [^{68}Ga]Ga-PSMA and novel [^{18}F]F-PSMA ligands, and most recently by PSMA therapeutics such as [^{177}Lu]Lu-PSMA, [^{213}Bi]Bi-PSMA, and [^{225}Ac]Ac-PSMA [5].

A plethora of novel molecular targets are now in preclinical and clinical development (Table 21.1). Once the molecular target is identified, a ligand can be developed to bind to the target. The ligand can be an antibody, a peptide, a nanoparticle, an aptamer or a pretargeting compound, a simple protein, or other constructs. The targeting ligand can then deliver a radiotherapeutic—which can be an alpha particle, beta particle, conversion, or Auger electron. The delivery can also be passive, by using a particle, colloid, or radiotherapy coating.

Whatever the tissue, specific molecular therapies are now emerging which will change the traditional diagnostic strategy. Rather than comparing nuclear medicine diagnostic studies

Table 21.1 Summary of new radiotheranostics in clinical trials or recently approved (adapted in 2019)

Radiopharmaceutical	Radioisotope	Major emission	E_{max} (keV)	E_{avg} (keV)	$E_{main}\ \gamma$ component (keV)	Half-life	Production	Compound ± chelator	Type of compound	Cancer biomarker/ target	Therapy form	Clinical development phase	Indications
[225]Ac (Actimab-A CD33)	Actinium-225	α	–	5830	99.8	10.0 d	Nuclear reactor/ cyclotron	HuM195	Monoclonal antibody	CD33	Targeted alpha therapy	Phase 2	Newly diagnosed patients with acute myelogenous leukemia over the age of 60
[225]Ac (Actimab-A-CD33 and venetoclax)	Actinium-225	α	–	5830	99.8	10.0 d	Nuclear reactor/ cyclotron		Monoclonal antibody	CD33	Targeted alpha therapy	Phase 1	Relapsed/refractory acute myelogenous leukemia
[225]Ac (Actimab-M-CD33)	Actinium-225	α	–	5830	99.8	10.0 d	Nuclear reactor/ cyclotron		Monoclonal antibody	CD33	Targeted alpha therapy	Phase 1	Multiple myeloma (penta-refractory) patients aged 18 and above
[225]Ac (Actimab-MDS-CD33)	Actinium-225	α	–	5830	99.8	10.0 d	Nuclear reactor/ cyclotron		Monoclonal antibody	CD33	Targeted alpha therapy	Phase 2	Myelodysplastic syndrome (MDS); myeloablation prior to bone marrow transplantation for high-risk MDS patients
[225]Ac-FPI-1434	Actinium-225	α	–	5830	99.8	10.0 d	Nuclear reactor/ cyclotron	FPI-1434	Monoclonal antibody	Insulin-like growth factor-1 receptor (IGF-1R)	Targeted alpha therapy	Phase 1	Multiple tumor types that express IGF-1R
[225]Ac (Iomab-ACT)	Actinium-225	α	–	5830	99.8	10.0 d	Nuclear reactor/ cyclotron	Apamis-tamab-I-131	Monoclonal antibody	CD45	Targeted alpha therapy	Phase 1	Produce myeloablation to facilitate a bone marrow transplantation
[225]Ac (Iomab-B-CD45)	Actinium-225	α	–	5830	99.8	10.0 d	Nuclear reactor/ cyclotron	^{131}I-BC8	Monoclonal antibody	CD45	Targeted alpha therapy	Phase 3 (SIERRA)	Myeloablation prior to bone marrow transplantation for patients over the age of 55 with relapsed or refractory acute myelogenous leukemia

[225]Ac-DOTATOC	Actinium-225	α	–	5830	99.8	10.0 d	Nuclear reactor/ cyclotron	DOTATOC	Peptide	Somatostatin receptor subtype-2 (SSTR2)	Peptide target alpha therapy	First-in-human experience	Progressive/ metastatic neuroendocrine neoplasms
[225]Ac-DOTAGA-SP	Actinium-225	α	–	5830	99.8	10.0 d	Nuclear reactor/ cyclotron	DOTAGA-SP	Peptide	Neurokinin-1 receptor	Peptide target alpha therapy	Clinical studies	Locoregional treatment of grade 2–4 gliomas
[213]Bi-DOTA-SP	Bismuth-213	α	1390	425	441	45.6 min	Nuclear reactor	DOTA-SP	Peptide	Neurokinin-1 receptor	Peptide target alpha therapy	Clinical studies	Locoregional treatment of grade 2–4 gliomas
[213]Bi-DOTATOC	Bismuth-213	α	1390	425	441	45.6 min	Nuclear reactor	DOTATOC	Peptide	SSTR2	Peptide target alpha therapy	First-in-human experience	Metastatic neuroendocrine neoplasms
[213]Bi-DTPA-PAN-622	Bismuth-213	α	1390	425	441	45.6 min	Nuclear reactor	DTPA-PAN-622	Monoclonal antibody	Human aspartyl (asparaginyl) β-hydroxylase (HAAH)	Radioim-muno-therapy	Pilot study	Metastatic breast cancer
[213]Bi-HuM195	Bismuth-213	α	1390	425	441	45.6 min	Nuclear reactor	HuM195	Monoclonal antibody	CD33	Targeted alpha therapy	Phase 1	Myeloid leukemia
[64]CuCl$_2$	Copper-64	β+, β−	580	560	–	12.7 h	Cyclotron	N/A	Small molecule	Human copper transporter 1 (hCTR1)	Molecular therapy	Clinical study for imaging	Potentially for prostate cancer
[64]CuCl$_2$	Copper-64	β+, β−	580	560	–	12.7 h	Cyclotron	N/A	Small molecule	hCTR1	Molecular therapy	Preclinical	Potentially for tumors that express high levels of hCtr1, like melanomas and hepatocellular carcinomas
[64]Cu-CB-TE2A-AS1411	Copper-64	β+, β−	580	560	–	12.7 h	Cyclotron	CB-TE2A-AS1411	Aptamer	Large nucleolin complex		Preclinical	Potentially for lung cancer
[64]Cu-BAT-2IT-1A3	Copper-64	β+, β−	580	560	–	12.7 h	Cyclotron	BAT-2IT-1A3	Monoclonal antibody	Ephrin type B receptor 4 (EphB4)	Radioim-muno-therapy	Phase 1/2 clinical study for diagnosis	Potentially for colorectal cancers

(continued)

Table 21.1 (continued)

Radiopharmaceutical	Radioisotope	Major emission	E_{max} (keV)	E_{avg} (keV)	$E_{main}\,\gamma$ component (keV)	Half-life	Production	Compound ± chelator	Type of compound	Cancer biomarker/ target	Therapy form	Clinical development phase	Indications
[64]Cu-DOTA-trastuzumab	Copper-64	β+, β−	580	560	–	12.7 h	Cyclotron	DOTA-trastuzumab	Monoclonal antibody	HER2+ and HER2−	Radioimmuno-therapy	Clinical studies	Breast cancer (HER2+ and HER2−)
[67]Cu (SARTATE™ kids)	Copper-67	β−, γ	600	141	186	2.58 d	Nuclear reactor/ cyclotron	DOTATATE	Peptide	SSTR2	Peptide receptor radionuclide therapy	Phase 2a (meningioma); phase 1-2a (neuroblastoma)	Neuroendocrine tumors, meningioma, neuroblastoma, and other children's cancers that express SSTR2
[67]Cu (SAR-BBN)	Copper-67	β−, γ	600	141	186	2.58 d	Nuclear reactor/ cyclotron	BBN (bombesin)	Peptidomimetic	Gastrin-releasing peptide receptor (GRPR)	Peptide receptor radionuclide therapy	–	Prostate, breast, ovarian, small-cell lung cancers, glioblastoma, gastrointestinal stromal tumors, and tumoral vessels of urinary cancers
[67]Cu (SAR-PSMA)	Copper-67	β−, γ	600	141	186	2.58 d	Nuclear reactor/ cyclotron	PSMA	Peptidomimetic	Prostate-specific membrane antigen (PSMA)	Peptide receptor radionuclide therapy	–	Metastatic prostate cancer
^{68}Ga-GRPR antagonists RM2 and NeoBOMB1	Gallium-68	β+, β−	1900	890	–	68 min	Generator	GRPR/RM2 and NeoBOMB1	Peptide	GRPR	Peptide receptor radionuclide therapy	Clinical studies	Currently under clinical evaluation in prostate cancer and gastrointestinal stromal tumor; potentially in estrogen receptor-positive breast tumors
^{68}Ga-GRPR antagonists × ^{68}Ga-PSMA analogs	Gallium-68	β+, β−	1900	890	–	68 min	Generator	GRPR/PSMA	Peptide × peptidomimetic	GRPR/PSMA	Peptide receptor radionuclide therapy	Clinical studies	Understand the role of each radiotracer in the management of prostate cancer patients

^{68}Ga-pentixafor/^{177}Lu/^{90}Y-pentixather	Gallium-68	β+, β−	1900	890	–	68 min	Generator	Pentixafor/pentixather	Peptide	CXCR4	Peptide receptor radionuclide therapy	Clinical studies	Hematologic malignancies, such as multiple myeloma, leukemia, and non-Hodgkin's lymphoma, and in some solid cancers (e.g., lung cancer, adrenocortical cancer, and high-grade neuroendocrine neoplasms)
^{68}Ga-NODAGA-THERANOST™	Gallium-68	β+, β−	1900	890	–	68 min	Generator	NODAGA	Peptidomimetic	$\alpha_v\beta_3$ integrin receptor	Peptide receptor radionuclide therapy	Current clinical trials only for imaging/diagnosisa	Potentially for glioblastomas, melanomas, myelomas, ovarian, breast, and prostate cancers
^{68}Ga-satoreotide trizoxetan (^{68}Ga-OPS202 or ^{68}Ga NODAGA-JR11)	Gallium-68	β+, β−	1900	890	–	68 min	Generator	OPS202/NODAGA-JR11	Peptide	SSTR	Peptide receptor radionuclide therapy	Phase 1/2	Gastroenteropancreatic neuroendocrine tumor
^{68}Ga-OPS202 + Lutetium-177-OPS201	Gallium-68	β+, β−	1900	890	–	68 min	Generator	OPS202/OPS201	Peptide	SSTR	Peptide receptor radionuclide therapy	Phase 1/2	Metastatic breast and small-cell lung cancers
												–	Cholangiocarcinoma and hepatic tumors
^{131}I-di-DTPA-indium hapten and hMN-14 × m734	Iodine-131	β−, γ	606	181	364	8.04 d	Nuclear reactors	DTPA-indium/hMN-14 × m734	Monoclonal antibody	CEA	Radioimmunotherapy	Phase 1	Potentially for progressive medullary thyroid cancer, CEA-expressing tumors
^{131}I-TX101	Iodine-131	β−, γ	606	181	364	8.04 d	Nuclear reactors	TX101	Small molecule	L-type amino acid transporter (LAT-1)	Molecular therapy	Phase 1	Glioblastoma multiforme

(continued)

Table 21.1 (continued)

Radiopharmaceutical	Radioisotope	Major emission	E_{max} (keV)	E_{avg} (keV)	$E_{main\ \gamma}$ component (keV)	Half-life	Production	Compound ± chelator	Type of compound	Cancer biomarker/target	Therapy form	Clinical development phase	Indications
^{177}Lu-PP-F11N/^{111}In-CP04/^{177}Lu-CP04/^{90}Y-CP04	Multiple	–	–	–	–	–	–	PP-F11N/CP04	Peptide	Cholecystokinin 2 receptor	Peptide receptor radionuclide therapy	Clinical studies	Recurrent or metastatic medullary thyroid cancer
^{177}Lu-DOTA-F(ab')2-trastuzumab	Lutetium-177	β–	497	140	208	6.65 d	Nuclear reactors	DOTA-F(ab')2-trastuzumab	Monoclonal antibody	HER2+	Radioimmunotherapy	–	HER2-positive breast cancer
^{177}Lu-DOTA-PEG7-Tz	Lutetium-177	β–	497	140	208	6.65 d	Nuclear reactors	DOTA-PEG7-Tz	Monoclonal antibody	SSTR	Radioimmunotherapy	Preclinical	Pancreatic cancer
^{177}Lu-DOTA0-Tyr3-octreotate (^{177}Lu-oxodotreotide)[b]	Lutetium-177	β–	497	140	208	6.65 d	Nuclear reactors	DOTATATE	Peptide	SSTR	Peptide receptor radionuclide therapy	Phase 3 (NETTER-1)	Advanced, progressive, somatostatin receptor-positive midgut neuroendocrine tumors
^{177}Lu-DOTATOC (^{177}Lu-edotreotide)	Lutetium-177	β–	497	140	208	6.65 d	Nuclear reactors	DOTATOC	Peptide	SSTR	Peptide receptor radionuclide therapy	Phase 3 (COMPETE)	Inoperable, progressive gastroenteropancreatic neuroendocrine neoplasms
^{177}Lu-OPS201	Lutetium-177	β–	497	140	208	6.65 d	Nuclear reactors	OPS201	Peptide	SSTR	Peptide receptor radionuclide therapy	Phase 1/2	Inoperable or metastatic neuroendocrine neoplasms that overexpress somatostatin receptors
^{177}Lu-PSMA-617	Lutetium-177	β–	497	140	208	6.65 d	Nuclear reactors	PSMA-617	Peptidomimetic	PSMA	Peptide receptor radionuclide therapy	Phase 2	Advanced prostate cancer and positive uptake on PSMA imaging
^{177}Lu-TX250	Lutetium-177	β–	497	140	208	6.65 d	Nuclear reactors	TX250	Monoclonal antibody	Carbonic anhydrase IX(CA-IX)	Radioimmunotherapy	Phase 2a	Clear cell renal carcinomas

^{177}Lu-TX591	Lutetium-177	β−	497	140	208	6.65 d	Nuclear reactors	TX591 (derived from the huJ591 humanized mAb)	Monoclonal antibody	PSMA	Radioimmuno-therapy	Phase 2a	Metastatic prostate cancers
[212]Pb-DOTAMTATE	Lead-212	α	570	100	238	10.64 h	Nuclear reactors	DOTAM-TATE	Peptide	SSTR	Peptide target alpha therapy	Phase 1	Metastatic neuroen-docrine neoplasm
[224]Ra (alpha DaRT®)	Radium-224	α	5690	–	241	3.66 d	Generator	N/A	Particle (seeds)		Diffusing α-emitters radiation therapy	Clinical studies	Squamous cell carcinoma of the head and neck, cutaneous and mucosal malignant neoplasia
[188]Re-SCT® (ONCOBETA®)	Rhenium-188	β−, γ	2120	795	155	17.0 h	Nuclear reactor/generator	Sterile precipitate of carrier	Nanocol-loid		Epidermal radioiso-tope therapy	–	Basal and squamous cell carcinomas of the skin, and keloid
[117m]Sn-DOTA-aminobenzyl	Tin-117m	ce	–	127–152	159	14.0 d	Nuclear reactors	Aminobenzyl-DOTA	Colloid	CD206 receptor	Radiosyn-oviorthesis	Phase 1/2	Canine and equine osteoarthritis, human rheumatoid arthritis, and other inflammatory conditions (such as atherosclerosis)
[117m]Sn-DOTA-annexin	Tin-117m	ce	–	127–152	159	14.0 d	Nuclear reactors	Annexin V-DOTA	molecule	Phosphatidyl-serine (PS)	Endarter-ectomy	Phase 2	Treating vulnerable plaques
^{90}Y-DOTA-biotin	Yttrium-90	β−	2280	934	–	2.67 d	Nuclear reactors	DOTA-biotin	Monoclonal antibody	CEA, tenascin, and ep-CAM	Radioimmuno-therapy	Clinical studies	Glioblastomas, anaplastic gliomas, and lymphoma
												Phase 3	Relapsed/refractory follicular non-Hodgkin's lymphoma

ce conversion electrons, *d* days, *min* minutes, *h* hours, *CEA* carcinoembryonic antigen, *CD* cluster of differentiation, *HER2* human epidermal growth factor receptor 2, *mAb* monoclonal antibody, *CXCR4* C-X-C chemokine receptor type 4

[a]Copper-64 and gallium-68 are radioisotopes used only for imaging

[b]Marketing authorization throughout the European Union

against traditional imaging modalities in terms of specificity or sensitivity, the standard by which most imaging modalities are judged, with a theranostic, it will simply be necessary and sufficient to know whether a molecular target is present or not, using a radiodiagnostic tracer. If the target is present, then the only determination is whether the proposed radiotherapy will be effective or not against this target.

This chapter will review the emerging new radiotherapies now in clinical trials or just emerging as novel radiotherapies.

21.2 Target Delivery for Imaging and Therapy

The evolving strategy in radiotherapy has been to couple a molecular ligand, which can be thought of as a missile, to a molecular target on the surface of a cell of interest (cancer cell, neuro-receptor, inflammatory cell) coupled to a "warhead"—either a diagnostic radionuclide for single photon emission computed tomography (SPECT) or PET imaging, or a therapeutic radionuclide (alpha, beta, or Auger emitter) for cell death (Fig. 21.1).

The strategy can be enhanced by pretargeting or choosing a target on the cell surface, where the ligand and radionuclide are internalized inside the cell. Increasingly, the term "theranostics" has evolved into the concept of a "theranostic pair"—one radionuclide for diagnosis and a similar radionuclide for therapy, ideally using the same ligand or "missile." The reference theranostic remains iodine-123 or iodine-124 for imaging thyroid cancer and iodine-131 for therapy. However, as mentioned, recent successes have centered around somatostatin ligands as the target, with [^{111}In]In-octreotide, then [^{68}Ga]Ga-octreotide, and [^{18}F]F-octreotide agents for imaging neuroendocrine tumors, and analogs of [^{177}Lu]Lu-DOTATATE or [^{225}Ac]Ac-DOTATATE for therapy. Similarly, recent success has been achieved with [^{68}Ga]Ga-PSMA or [^{18}F]F-PSMA for imaging prostate cancer and [^{177}Lu]Lu-PSMA or [^{225}Ac]Ac-PSMA or [^{213}Bi]Bi-PSMA for therapy of prostate cancer [6].

Ideally, as with thyroid cancer, the theranostic would be the same element and would differ only in whether it was used for diagnosis or therapy. Several "theranostic pairs" have been proposed, in addition to iodine.

21.3 True Theranostic Pairs

Table 21.2 represents some examples of theranostic pairs of metallic radionuclides.

The term theranostic is defined to "combine diagnostic and therapeutic capabilities into a *single* agent" where the entire molecular targeting

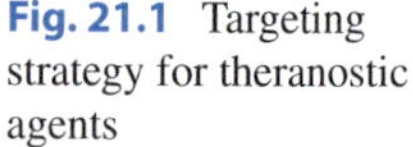

Fig. 21.1 Targeting strategy for theranostic agents

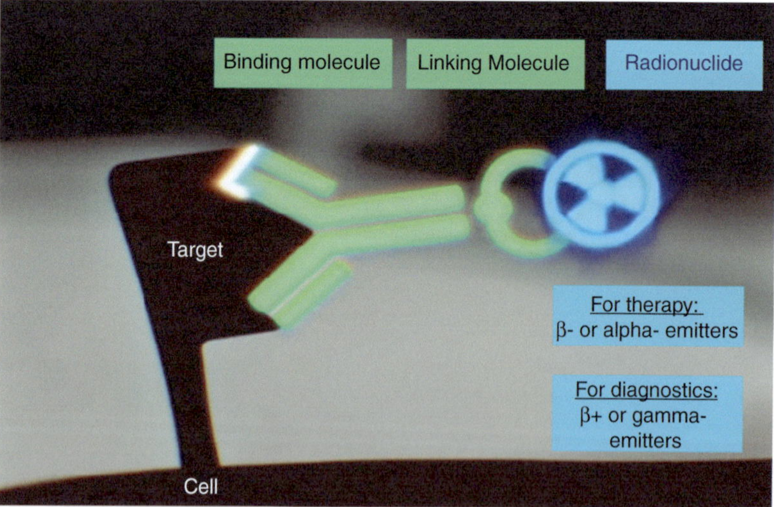

Table 21.2 Examples of theranostic pairs of metallic radionuclides

Radionuclide pair (imaging/ therapeutic)	Half-life	Therapeutic particle	E_{avg} (keV)
Copper-64/copper-67	12.7 h/2.58 days	β^-	141
Iodine-124/iodine-131	4.2 days/8.04 days	β^-	181
Gallium-68/gallium-67	68 min/3.26 days	Auger/conversion electron	82–291
Scandium-44/scandium-47	3.97 h/3.35 days	β^-	162
Strontium-83/strontium-89	32.4 h/50.5 days	β^-	1460
Terbium-152/terbium-161	17.5 h/6.89 days	β^-	154
Yttrium-86/yttrium-90	14.7 h/2.67 days	β^-	934

compound, including the radioisotope, must be *chemically identical*. Apart from a few select isotope pairs noted above that interchangeably permit PET or SPECT and therapeutic applications (e.g., [86]Y/^{90}Y), the use of a single element for diagnosis and targeted therapy has been impractical. Due to this difficulty, a pair of radiometals is often used. For example, DOTATATE, which is labeled with gallium-68 for diagnosis and lutetium-177 for therapy, is commonly considered to be a theranostic. Yet whereas the peptide-chelator is identical, the two isotopes differ in their chemistry. The affinity of [^{68}Ga]Ga-DOTATATE has been reported to be up to 20-fold higher than that of [^{177}Lu]Lu-DOTATATE. In human studies, these differences may account for noted discordance in lesion detection whereby lesions are revealed by one tracer but not the other, and vice versa [5, 7].

Similar discrepancies are observed with PSMA-617: in vitro, the affinity of the ^{68}Ga-chelate is twice that of the ^{177}Lu-chelate; in mice, tumor uptake values and tumor-to-non-tumor ratios differ substantially between the two chelates. Finally, for DOTA-PEG4-LLP2A, the Ki value of the ^{68}Ga-chelate is half that of the ^{177}Lu-chelate. To meet the challenge of designing a true theranostic agent, an attractive solution has been the production of "hot-cold/cold-hot" paired isotopologs (e.g., fluorine-18/natural lutetium and natural fluorine/lutetium-177) that are absolutely identical in *chemical* composition. In this scheme, a peptide designed for diagnosis is bound via chelation to a nonradioactive metal cation, also labeled with fluorine-18, whereas when designed for radiotherapy, the peptide is bound via chelation to unlabeled trifluorate and a radioactive metal cation. This concept expands the choices of radioactive therapeutic metals for treatment while simultaneously (1) allowing fluorine-18 to remain the isotope of choice for diagnostic PET, helping to alleviate the supply problems associated with gallium-68, and (2) preventing the dissimilarity in chelation chemistries arising from the use of two different radiometals for PET and therapy [7].

Going through various theranostic pairs, two elements that are of particular interest are scandium and terbium. Scandium has three radioisotopes for theranostic application. Scandium-43 ([43]Sc) ($T1/2 = 3.9$ h) and scandium-44 ($T1/2 = 4.0$ h) are positron emitters and can be used diagnostically in PET imaging, while scandium-47 ($T1/2 = 3.35$ days) is a beta emitter, suitable for radiotherapy, but also has a 159 keV gamma emission suitable for SPECT imaging. Currently, scandium-44 is most advanced in terms of production, and with preclinical investigations, and has been employed in proof-of-concept investigations in patients. In PC-3 PIP/flu tumor-bearing mice, [[44]Sc]Sc-PSMA-617 demonstrated high tumor uptake and fast renal excretion, similar to that of [^{177}Lu]Lu-PSMA-617. [[44]Sc]Sc-PSMA-617 enabled distinct visualization of PC-3 PIP tumor xenografts shortly after injection. Due to the almost fourfold longer half-life of scandium-44, as compared to gallium-68, centralized production of [[44]Sc]Sc-PSMA-617 would enable distribution to satellite PET imaging centers. Production of scandium-44 can be from titanium-44 ([44]Ti) with its long half-life of almost 60 years, which provides a cyclotron-independent source of scandium-44 for several decades. Initial human studies with [[44]Sc]Sc-DOTATOC PET-CT imaging of somatostatin receptor-positive liver metastases in a patient at 40 min postinjection demonstrated comparable findings to [^{68}Ga]Ga-DOTATATE at 90 min postinjection in the same patient [8].

The production of scandium-43 as a therapeutic part of the theranostic pair may be more challenging, but it would be advantageous due to the absence of high-energy γ-ray emission. The development of scandium-47 is still in its infancy. However, its therapeutic potential has been demonstrated preclinically [9].

Another potentially useful new radiotherapy involves the element terbium. There are four medically useful radioisotopes, terbium-155 (^{155}Tb) ($T1/2 = 5.32$ days), that can be used for SPECT, while terbium-152 (^{152}Tb) ($T1/2 = 17.5$ h) is a potential PET radionuclide. Both have undergone preclinical studies, but terbium-152 has been used (as [^{152}Tb]Tb-DOTATOC) in a patient with a neuroendocrine tumor. Both isotopes could potentially be used to determine dosimetry prior to radio-lanthanide therapy. The decay properties of terbium-161 (^{161}Tb) ($T1/2 = 6.89$ days) are similar to lutetium-177, but the co-emission of Auger electrons makes it attractive for a combined β⁻/Auger electron therapy, which was depicted to be effective in preclinical experiments. Terbium-149 ($T1/2 = 4.1$ h) is an alpha emitter which can be used for α therapy but has decays with a positron, adding the possibility of PET imaging. In terms of production, terbium-161 and terbium-155 are most promising to be made available at the large quantities suitable for future clinical translation [10].

Therapies using yttrium-90 (^{90}Y) can utilize the sister isotope yttrium-86 (^{86}Y) as an intriguing alternative to indium-111 (^{111}In) for pre-treatment imaging and dosimetry. In preclinical studies, the superiority of yttrium-86 over indium-111 has been demonstrated. However, yttrium-86 itself has some limitations such as the high-energy gamma emission and a lack of adequate commercial availability (as compared to indium-111). More than 65% of yttrium-86 decays are accompanied by additional gamma rays with energies from 200 to 3000 keV that are mostly emitted simultaneously with positron emissions and the subsequent annihilation photons resulting in increased scatter and random events, degrading image resolution [11].

21.3.1 Copper-64/Copper-67 Theranostic Agents

The copper-64 (^{64}Cu) and PET imaging can be used to verify where the target vector goes into the body and confirm targeting. For therapies, copper-67 can be used taking advantage of the 2.58-day half-life and the 184 keV gamma ray and the 150 keV average energy of the beta particles and conversion electors. This has led to the commercial development of several targeted agents, most notably ^{64}Cu/^{67}Cu chelate (SARTATE) with PSMA for prostate cancer, somatostatin receptor for neuroendocrine tumors, and gastrin-releasing peptide (GRP) bombesin analogs for prostate cancer [12, 13].

Radiolabeled octreotate using alpha or beta emitters is now recognized as an effective treatment for somatostatin receptor 2 (SSTR2)-expressing neuroendocrine malignancies. The diagnostic and therapeutic characteristics of the copper isotopes, copper-64 and copper-67, respectively, deliver the potential for using a single SSTR2-targeted peptide conjugate as a theranostic agent. Copper-Sartate, consisting of a bifunctional chelator, MeCOSar, conjugated to (Tyr)-octreotate, was successfully trialed as an imaging agent and a potential prospective dosimetry tool in ten patients with NETs [13].

A number of copper agents are currently being assessed in clinical trials such as "imaging CXCR4 expression in subjects with cancer using [^{64}Cu]Cu-plerixafor," "evaluation of a new radiotracer ([^{64}Cu]Cu-DOTA-AE105) for diagnosing aggressive cancer with positron emission tomography," "[^{64}Cu]Cu-DOTA-trastuzumab PET-CT in studying patients with gastric cancer," "[^{64}Cu]Cu-DOTA-trastuzumab positron emission tomography in women with advanced HER2-positive breast cancer," "[^{64}Cu]Cu-DOTA-trastuzumab PET in predicting response to treatment with ado-trastuzumab emtansine," "use of [^{64}Cu]Cu-Anti-CEA mAbs M5A PET in diagnosing patients with CEA-positive cancer," and "image-derived prediction of response to chemo-radiation in glioblastoma ([^{64}Cu]Cu-ATSM)" [14, 15].

21.4 Targeting Vectors

21.4.1 Simple Physical Carriers: Microspheres

Microsphere classification depends on particle size. Particles in the submicrometer size range (10–1000 nm) are called nanoparticles, whereas larger particles are called microparticles or microspheres. The term "colloid particle" is, in nuclear medicine, often used for both nanoparticles and small microparticles (less than a few micrometers). By definition, colloid particles in suspension are small enough not to form sediment but large enough to scatter the incoming light [16].

After intravenous or intra-arterial injection or injection into a joint cavity, particles in the size range of about 5 nm to 2 μm will be rapidly cleared from the bloodstream by macrophages of the reticuloendothelial system (RES). Particles larger than 7 μm will be mechanically entrapped in the lung capillaries.

The simplest approach has been to attach a radionuclide- to attach a radionuclide—either for therapy or diagnosis to a simple inert molecule, such as glass or resin microspheres, or a colloid, and let the physical property of the molecule take the agent to the organ of interest. Delivery can be by blood flow (albumin, glass or plastic spheres), where the targeting moiety wimply occludes the first capillary it encounters, or in the case of colloids, where the agent is simply phagocytosed by reticuloendothelial cells. Many different kinds of microparticles are used for both diagnostic and therapeutic medical applications. Microparticles or microspheres are defined as small spheres made of any material ranging in size from about 10 nm to about 2000 μm. In contrast to microparticles, the term nanospheres is applied to smaller spheres (sized 10–500 nm) to distinguish them from larger microspheres. Ideally, microspheres are completely spherical [16, 17].

Due to delayed detection of hepatic tumors and poor underlying liver function, only 10% of patients with liver metastases currently qualify for curative therapies such as ablation, segmental resection, and transplantation [18].

Agents which are already approved for the treatment of hepatic metastases, Therasphere® (BTG Interventional Medicine; London, UK), made of glass, and SIR-Spheres® (Sirtex Medical Limited; New South Wales, Australia), are made of resin. These agents are injected under angiographic fluoroscopy into the hepatic artery and preferentially occlude the capillary beds or arterioles of hepatic tumors or hepatic metastases, as these are highly vascular. QuiremSpheres® using holmium-166-embedded microspheres were developed as a competitive alternative to yttrium-90 microspheres for treating unresectable liver tumors, a procedure known as "selective internal radiation therapy" (SIRT). Holmium-166 microspheres can be imaged with SPECT and MR, with high sensitivity and resolution, respectively. Labeling of Lipiodol or microspheres with rhenium-188 (^{188}Re) offers an alternative treatment option for patients with colorectal liver metastases or hepatocellular carcinomas. As a generator product, rhenium-188 has excellent availability, which permits on-site labeling. The long shelf life of 3–5 months results in low costs, especially if it is used for other therapeutic modalities, such as bone pain palliation, intravascular radionuclide therapy, or labeling of antibodies.

Rhenium-188 microspheres are proposed to have several advantages over current yttrium-90 agents. Current microspheres labeled with yttrium-90 cannot be labeled instead with a diagnostic radioisotope, such as technetium-99m (^{99m}Tc). Instead, to rule out the deposition of microspheres in undesired organs, patients first undergo a hepatic perfusion study, where macroaggregated albumin (MAA) is labeled with technetium-99m. [^{99m}Tc]Tc-MAA and yttrium-90 microspheres ([^{90}Y]Y-MS) do not have the same size and distribution, and [^{99m}Tc]Tc-MAA is prone to disaggregation, potentially leading to misdiagnosis.

One of the major advantages of [^{90}Y]Y-MS is size and uniformity. Compared to prior

[90]Y-agents, which may bypass the liver and deposit in the lungs due to arterial/portal shunting of tumor blood flow, [90Y]Y-MS are retained in the patient's capillary bed indefinitely as they are made of nonbiodegradable materials, preventing reopening of the embolized capillaries after treatment [17].

Imaging of yttrium-90 β^- particles is not straightforward, as only bremsstrahlung photons can be used to create images using single photon emission computed tomography (SPECT). But such bremsstrahlung images are very poor for diagnostic imaging and are not useful for quantitation. It is possible, however, to use the limited positron decay in yttrium-90 for PET imaging, by exploiting its low-yield internal pair production. This allows quantitative images that could subsequently be used for dosimetry calculations. PET systems, however, are relatively unavailable. Rhenium-188, in comparison, decays with a half-life of 17.0 h to stable osmium-188 (^{188}Os) by the emission of β^- particles with maximum and mean energies of 2.12 and 0.76 MeV, respectively. These β^- particles with a maximum and a mean penetration distance in the tissue of 11.0 and 3.8 mm, respectively, are very similar to yttrium-90. Rhenium-188 also emits 155 keV γ photons with an abundance of 15.6%, so patients treated with rhenium-188 can be imaged simultaneously by SPECT, allowing for simultaneously specific dosimetry calculations and biodistribution studies [19].

21.4.1.1 Rhenium-188 Lipiodol Therapy of Hepatocellular Carcinoma

[^{188}Re]Re-Lipiodol has been studied in several early phase clinical trials in patients with hepatocellular carcinoma (HCC), advanced cirrhosis, or those with extensive portal vein thrombosis in second-line therapy as a way of managing recurrences or to stabilize patients waiting for liver transplants.

To assess the maximum tolerated dose (MTD), several dose-escalation studies have been carried out. The main at-risk organs are the lungs and healthy liver. The International Atomic Energy Agency (IAEA) phase 1 and 2 clinical trials were coordinated in several countries. The overall results demonstrated favorable responses and potential usefulness of [^{188}Re]Re-Lipiodol for the therapy of HCC, which is now almost routinely used in several centers in India. One limitation of these studies is that, except for the IAEA-sponsored trials, all other trials included a very small number of patients, making it difficult to be conclusive. Another limitation was the low labeling yields and high urinary excretion (more than 40% at 72 h). The next generation compounds, such as [^{188}Re]ReN-DEDC and [^{188}Re]Re-SSS, demonstrated higher yields and higher in vivo stabilities [20].

21.4.2 Simple Physical Carriers: Colloids

Colloids have been used since the earliest days of nuclear medicine, first to target the reticuloendothelial cells in the liver/spleen/bone marrow and then to target lymph nodes during lymphoscintigraphy—in both cases mainly for diagnosis.

Historically, radiolabeled colloids are also used for therapy, e.g., [90Y]Y-citrate and [90Y]Y-silicate colloids have been used in the treatment of pleural and peritoneal carcinosis, while intra-articular treatment has been used for the treatment of rheumatoid arthritis of the knees, and colloidal gold-198 (^{198}Au) has been used in the past for intrathecal treatment of leukemia. Radiocolloids which have been used in the therapy of rheumatoid arthritis, were originally with ^{198}Au-colloids, and then with colloids of yttrium-90, rhenium-186, and erbium-187 (^{187}Er), using the term "radiosynoviorthesis." The rationale of using therapuetic radionuclides with colloids for treating arthritis is that bound to colloids, they will be phagocytosed in the inflamed synovial membrane in the affected joint, and by destroying the inflamed synovial cells, reduce the inflammation and halt the destruction of the joint cartilage. Synovial inflammation is implicated in many signs and symptoms of osteoarthritis (OA), including joint swelling and effusion [21].

Radiation synovectomy was first used by Fellinger and Schmid in 1952 as a therapeutic method to cure chronic synovitis in hemophilia, orthopedic troubles, or rheumatoid arthritis. Kamaleshwaran and co-workers described the first case report of the use of [^{90}Y]Y-albumin particulates in a 33-year-old male who presented with diffuse pigmented villonodular synovitis (PVNS) of the knee joint as a primary modality of treatment. PVNS is a joint disease characterized by both inflammation and thickening of the joint lining. Treatment of PVNS demonstrated that [^{90}Y]Y-albumin could potentially become an ideal agent for radiosynovectomy of the joints. Davarpanah et al. were the first to optimize the routine use of ^{90}Y-human albumin (HA) for radiosynovectomy. The first human study in the treatment of painful synovitis and recurrent effusion of knee joints in rheumatoid arthritis using ^{177}Lu-labeled HA was reported by Shinto and co-workers. The preparation and preliminary biological assessment of ^{177}Lu-labeled HA as a promising agent for radiation synovectomy of small joints were formerly portrayed by Chakraborty et al. The use of [^{153}Sm]Sm-HA for knee synovectomy in hemophilia was reported by Calegaro et al. Effectiveness of radiation synovectomy with yttrium-90 and samarium-153 (^{153}Sm) particulate hydroxyapatite in rheumatoid arthritis patients with knee synovitis was reported by dos Santos and co-workers [22].

A novel agent for radiosynoviorthesis is tin-117m (^{117m}Sn). Tin-117m (T1/2 = 14 days) is an interesting radionuclide for the development of theranostic radiopharmaceuticals. Tin-117m decays via isomeric transition, with the emission of three major monoenergetic conversion electrons, unlike most radiotherapeutic beta emitters. These have energies of 127, 129, and 152 keV, with an abundance of 65%, 12%, and 26%, respectively. The conversion electrons have a very high linear energy transfer (LET), and short discrete penetrations, ranging between 0.22 mm (127 keV) and 0.29 mm (152 keV) in water [23].

In osteoarthritis, the synovium exhibits both inflammation and destruction in response to macrophages. The effects are cytokine driven, through the action of interleukin (IL)-1 and tumor necrosis factor (TNF)α. The production of these cytokines induces synovial cells and chon-drocyte production of IL-6, IL-8, and leukocyte inhibitory factor, as well as stimulating protease (matrix metalloproteinases (MMPs) and aggre-canases) and prostaglandin production. Therapy with tin-117m suggests that radio-destruction of macrophage function in OA decreases both inflammatory synovitis and the production of degradative enzymes of importance for the progression of the disease [24].

A veterinary product using tin-117m is currently being commercialized to treat canine osteoarthritis. Human clinical trials are expected to start, treating human osteoarthritis and rheumatoid arthritis, and are expected to have several advantages over the traditional beta emitters [25, 26].

The ^{117m}Sn-colloid gamma ray (159 keV), similar to Tc-99m (140 keV), allows confirmation of the presence of the radiocolloid in the joint space. The tin-117m colloid is large enough to stay in the joint, but small enough for macrophage engulfment and not leak out of the joint (Fig. 21.2). The colloid is retained in the patient's joint with no need for splinting.

In addition to serving as a potential therapy for osteoarthritis and rheumatoid arthritis, tin-117m is being investigated as a possible therapeutic in other diseases. It also shows promise for the noninvasive molecular imaging and treatment of active atheromatous disease, especially vulnerable plaque (VP). Thin-cap fibroatheroma in the coronary arteries and other areas of vasculature has been treated in animals through the use of coronary stents electroplated with tin-117m and in human trials using specific ^{117m}Sn-labeled molecules systemically targeted to vulnerable plaque components. Additionally, human phase 1 and 2 trials have been completed using [^{117m}Sn]Sn-diethylenetriaminepentaacetic acid (DTPA) for the treatment of metastatic bone pain, which appears likely to be involved in additional new clinical trials [27, 28].

21.4.3 Simple Physical Carriers: Calcium Analogs

The principle of alpha radiotherapy is to induce double-stranded breaks in DNA. Radium-223

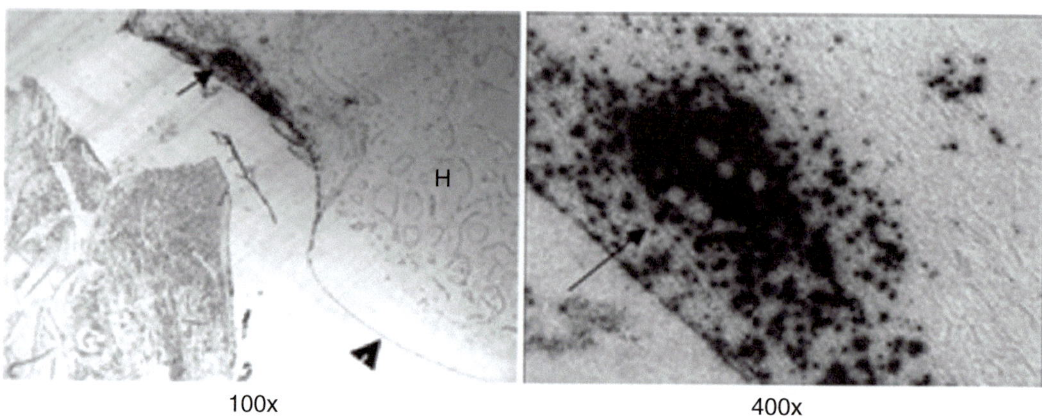

Fig. 21.2 Targeting of tin-117m colloids in the synovium. Radioactive colloidal particles are collected on the synovial lining and then transported deeper into the synovial tissue. The arrow indicates an area of inflammation in the autoradiographs

(^{223}Ra) is a bone-seeking alpha emitter which has been studied extensively in preclinical models. Its half-life is 11.4 days. Studies of radium-223 biodistribution confirmed that in mice, the uptake was preferentially retained in the bone matrix. Radium-223 is well tolerated, with doses of 50–250 kBq/kg, and therapies are now available in symptomatic patients with castration-resistant prostate cancer with two or more bone metastases. In light of the marked retention of radium-223 in the bone matrix, a phase 1 trial was set up for osteosarcoma to determine the maximum tolerated dose. In a dose-escalation study of monthly intravenous [^{223}Ra]Ra-dichloride, 18 patients (age >15 years) with osteosarcoma were treated. The phase 1 starting intravenous dose was 50 kBq/kg [^{223}Ra]Ra-dichloride, injected over several minutes on day 1 during a 4-week cycle. Patients received between 1 and 6 cycles of [^{223}Ra]Ra-Cl$_2$. Using this protocol, subjects' cumulative doses were 6.84–57.81 MBq. Fluorine-18 sodium fluoride ([^{18}F]NaF) PET revealed more sites of metastases than did 2-[^{18}F]FDG PET. One patient showed a metabolic response on 2-[^{18}F] FDG PET and [^{18}F]NaF PET. Four patients had mixed responses, and one patient had a response in brain metastasis. The median survival was 25 weeks. Evaluation of the safety and efficacy of alpha particles in patients with osteosarcoma led to a recommended phase 2 dose for [^{223}Ra] RaCl$_2$ of 100 kBq/kg monthly in patients with

osteosarcoma (twice the dose approved for prostate cancer) with minimal hematologic toxicity, setting the stage for combination therapies [29].

21.4.3.1 Rhenium-188 Colloid

The rhenium-188 (^{188}Re) isotope is a beta-gamma emitter with a half-life of 16.98 h; the β particles have a maximal energy of 2.12 MeV and a mean energy of 764 keV. Rhenium-188 is a certified isotope easily obtained from the tungsten-188/rhenium-188 (^{188}W/^{188}Re) generator, making it very convenient for clinical use. The development of an in-house ^{188}W/^{188}Re generator has greatly increased the use of rhenium-188 for treating various diseases, such as non-Hodgkin's lymphoma (NHL), rheumatoid arthritis, peritoneal effusion, hepatocellular carcinoma, and other solid tumors, and for palliation of metastatic bone pain. Rhenium-188 is of widespread interest due to its attractive physical and chemical properties, making it suitable for labeling peptides, antibodies, and colloids to form radiopharmaceuticals. The main gamma-ray component energy of 155 keV accounts for 15% of the radiation intensity and is detectable by gamma cameras, for imaging, biodistribution, or absorbed radiation studies, also allowing excellent control of possible contamination. Moreover, the high-energy β particles of rhenium-188 are therapeutically effective only at short ranges and penetrate human tissue up to 1 cm. However, 92% of the doses are deposited in the first 2–3 mm, therefore sparing healthy tissue, unlike external electron beam devices which have a large footprint and deposit a significant dose beyond the dermis due to secondary radiation. The fact that rhenium-188 is available from a generator at a reasonable cost could lead not only to greater use in research but also great use in clinical treatments with [188]Re-labeled radiopharmaceuticals [20].

In this chapter, a nuclear medicine therapeutic option for the treatment of basal cell carcinoma (BCC), squamous cell carcinoma (SCC), and keloid is described. Non-melanoma skin cancer is the most common human malignancy, while keloids are benign dermal fibroproliferative scars developed during the process of healing at the site of surgery or trauma. Several treatment options are currently available. Surgical resection is curative and the gold standard for treating BCC and SCC. However, satisfactory surgical treatment can be very challenging for patients with large or multiple lesions. In those cases, the results may be suboptimal in terms of aesthetics and/ or function. Moreover, the conventional surgical approach can simply not be desired, such as in elderly patients with comorbidities, which makes surgery an inconvenient option. Conversely, relapse is often common in patients with keloids as the skin has the tendency to develop keloid at surgery or trauma site.

An alternative dermatological high-dose-rate beta brachytherapy using non-sealed rhenium-188 was developed for these conditions (Fig. 21.3). The treatment basically consists of superficial high-dose radiotherapy to the epidermis without damaging the underlying layers characterized by the use of radioactive beta-emitting isotopes, incorporated in a specially formulated acrylic matrix. The application product, based on this synthetic inert resin matrix containing the radioactive beta-emitting isotope, is applied on the surface of keloids, BCC, and SCC, independently from its shape, extension, and lesion site. The available matrix containing a beta emitter brachytherapy irradiation is able to adapt to every skin surface without contamination, imparting an accurate distribution of dose strictly limited to the area and depth affected by the lesion, and sparing the healthy tissue [30].

The skin to be treated is delineated with a dermatological pen including a safety margin of 3–5 mm. The lesion is protected with a thin, flex-

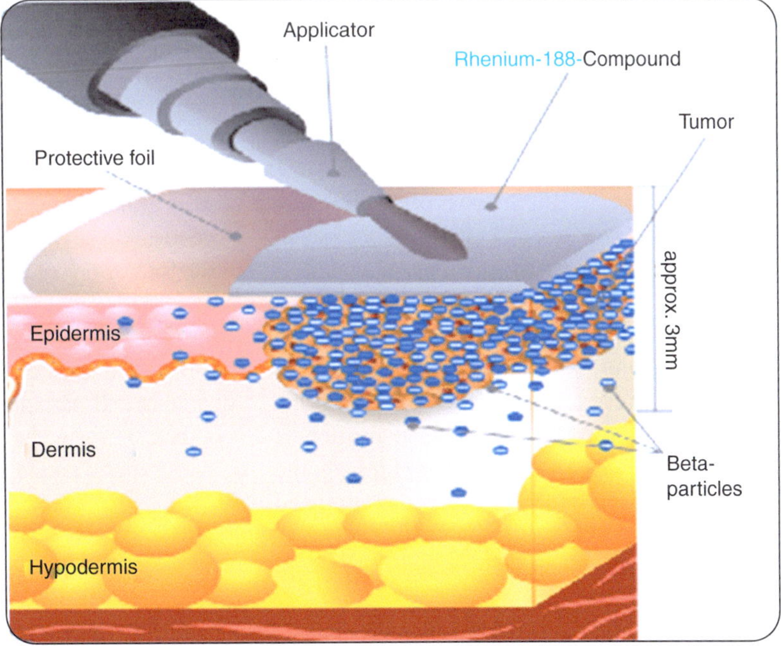

Fig. 21.3 Rhenium-188 therapy

ible, plastic foil in order to prevent direct contact of the radioactive matrix with the epidermis and minimize the risk of its incorporation through the skin or wounds. Thick tumors may need to be cleaned before the treatment by eliminating all the granulation tissue, keratinic crusts, and scabs to improve the efficacy of the treatment as the penetration path of the beta particles is short. Similarly, if surgically feasible, keloids should be reduced before the procedure to decrease both size and depth of the lesion.

The radioactive source is then applied in close proximity to the lesions above the protection layers. After some minutes, the matrix solidifies, and the radioactive mold is kept on the lesion for the time required to impart the measured dose distribution.

The thickness of matrix and protective layers is accurately measured in order to account for the beta radiation absorption effects. The total exposure (dose) to the lesion is calculated on the basis of the activity and area of the mold. For each geometry, the dose distribution depends on the initial radioactivity, isotope emission energy, the surface of the lesion, and contact time. At the end of the irradiation, the radioactive mold is easily removed, by using a specially designed dedicated remote tongs device, and is discarded.

Immediately after the treatment, faint redness is visible on the treated area and can persist for a few days. In some patients, variable erythema is present, sometimes with the emission of serum, and a crust or scab is formed. An apparent worsening of the aspect of the lesion is often observed, with the appearance of a light burn, but the bleeding, if present before the therapy, stops. It is usual to see the erythema fade after 40–120 days, although occasionally a second scab occurs, an itch may be present, but the clinical healing is much more apparent. After 60–180 days, in the majority of cases, apparent clinical healing is present, rarely with the persistence of a scab; the lesion area can become paler than the untreated skin but subsides with time.

The main advantage of the described technique lies in the usefulness in all types of BCC and SCC, without the restriction of site, dimension, clinical or histological type, and patient

clinical situation. As in most of the keloid lesions, more than one treatment on the same lesions is usually needed for complete healing. The superiority of the proposed treatment with respect to the surgery is evident for all the tumors located in high-risk areas, or difficult sites on which surgery would be difficult (nose, ears, eyelids), in patients with a high number of lesions or with relapses, in patients in whom surgery would produce functional mutilations (penis, vulva, eyelids lesions), and, generally, in older, infirm, or otherwise inoperable patients. Avoidance of scarring and of suboptimal cosmetic outcome should also be considered by patients as an important decision factor in the choice of this therapeutic path. The proposed technique is a rapid, safe treatment, mostly performed in a single therapeutic session without discomfort for the patient, and offers a complete aesthetical result [31].

21.5 Alpha Emitter Brachytherapy

Diffusing Alpha-emitters Radiation Therapy ("Alpha DaRT") is a new cancer treatment modality, which enables the treatment of solid tumors by alpha particles. The treatment inserts into the tumor an array of implantable seeds, whose surface is embedded with a low activity of radium-224. Each radium seed bombards a tumor a chain of short-lived alpha-emitting daughter atoms which can diffuse into the tumor over several millimeters, creating a continuous "kill region" of high alpha particle dose. Recently, Alpha DaRT has entered clinical trials, in the framework of a new company, Alpha TAU Medical Ltd. The first clinical trial of Alpha DaRT took place at Rabin Medical Center in Israel, in the treatment of recurrent skin and oral cavity squamous cell carcinomas, with tumor sizes of less than 5 cm in the longest diameter. Fifteen of the enrolled patients have completed followup. Tumor locations included the ear, chin, lip, tongue, forehead, nose, scalp, and parotid skin areas. Treatment based on CT-simulation pretherapy placed DaRT seeds into squamous tumors under local anesthesia, using a special applicator. Each seed was 1 cm long and 0.7 mm in diameter, carrying 2 µCi radium-224, and was placed 5–6 mm from each other. The treatment protocol was based on a prior DaRT-specific dosimetry model. Radium-224 activity administered was approximately 5 µCi/g of tumor. After 2–4 weeks, the seeds were removed. After 6 weeks, a CT scan was performed to assess tumor response. A blood test and urinalysis were also performed. A range of 7–169 seeds were inserted, and the treatment duration lasted 14–26 days. Evaluation of treatment response for a single treatment was encouraging; of 15 patients who reached the study endpoint, 73% (11/15) had a complete response to treatment, and 27% (4/15) had a partial response measured by reduction in tumor volume. The treatment was shown to be safe for both the patient and the medical staff. There were minimal side effects from the treatment, mostly erythema, swelling, and mild to moderate pain at the insertion site, which usually resolved by the time the seeds were removed. Measurements of lead-212 (^{212}Pb) in the blood, a decay product of radium-224, agreed with pre-therapy biokinetic models, which predicted negligible dose levels to distant organs. There were no clinically significant abnormalities in blood or urine laboratory tests, and no changes were observed to vital signs. Based on the successful outcomes of the first clinical trial, clinical protocols are in preparation for various indications with leading research centers worldwide, including cutaneous and mucosal neoplasia, neoadjuvant and recurrent rectal cancer, recurrent prostate cancer, inoperable breast cancer, recurrent gynecological cancer, sarcoma, and pancreatic cancer [32].

21.6 Peptide Carriers

Peptide receptor radionuclide therapy (PRRT) makes use of radiolabeled peptides to deliver destructive radiation to cancer cells. The radiolabeled peptides are able to bind specifically to peptide receptors expressed in higher density on the tumor cell membrane than in non-tumor tissues. Although antibody conjugates target the cell surface and tend to have restricted access to solid tumors, radiolabeled peptides are more

desirable due to straightforward chemical synthesis, easier radiolabeling, versatility, having more rapid clearance from the circulation, more uniform distribution, deeper penetration of tumors, and less likelihood to incite an immune response.

One challenge to the use of linear peptides is degradation by peptidases. Unfortunately, peptidase degradation decreases stability and can shorten the plasma half-life to only several minutes. Stability may be increased by shortening the peptide after identification of the essential binding sequence using an alanine scan, exchange of single amino acids, the introduction of D-amino acids, peptide cyclization, and coupling to chelators such as DOTA. Although this approach may lead to increased metabolic stability, these changes frequently cause a decrease in affinity [33].

21.7 PSMA in Prostate Cancer

Prostate cancer radioligand therapy (PRLT) with ^{177}Lu-PSMA derivatives is still considered as an investigational treatment in clinics. Prostate cancer (PCa) patients usually die not from the initial local cancer, but from advanced disease, after the cancer spreads through lymphatics or blood, or locoregional spread [34]. Targeted radionuclide therapy has become an attractive and quickly developing therapy, also in prostate cancer patients [35]. Lutetium-177 has a half-life of 6.7 days and lower beta particle emission energy than iodine-131, indicating a higher probability of fewer side effects [36].

Rahbar et al. in a multicenter study of 145 patients showed that spread to visceral organs or elevated alkaline phosphatase (ALP >22 U/L) predicted negative response to therapy [34] and reported the overall survival benefit of [^{177}Lu] Lu-PSMA-RLT in comparison to a historical cohort. The estimated median survival was found to be 29.4 weeks, which was significantly longer than the 19.7 weeks of the historical controls (hazard ratio (HR), 0.44; $p = 0.031$) [37].

The 55 patients who received at least 3 cycles of radioligand therapy (RLT) with [^{177}Lu] Lu-PSMA-617 did not show any grade 3 or 4 nephrotoxicity [38]. A significant negative effect on renal function was found for age (>65 years) ($p = 0.049$), hypertension ($p = 0.001$), and pre-existing kidney disease ($p = 0.001$). Another dosimetry study with [^{177}Lu]Lu-PSMA-617 reported a mean absorbed dose/per cycle to the bone marrow, kidneys, liver, spleen, and salivary glands of 0.012, 0.6, 0.1, 0.1, and 1.4 Gy/GBq, respectively [39].

During the last decade, six new drugs have been found to increase overall survival for patients with metastatic castration-resistant prostate cancer (mCRPC); the most important of these are abiraterone (median duration of 10.0 months), docetaxel (6.5 months), enzalutamide (6.5 months), and cabazitaxel (6.0 months), respectively [40–43]. Of PCa, poorly differentiated, metastatic, and hormone-refractory adenocarcinomas express prostate-specific membrane antigen (PSMA) [42], and [^{68}Ga]Ga-PSMA HBED-CC PET-CT detects sites of cancer lesions for most patients with mCRPC [44, 45]. Patients with a positive [^{68}Ga]Ga-PSMA HBED-CC PET-CT might be treated with [^{177}Lu]Lu-PSMA radioligand therapy [46, 47]. [^{177}Lu]Lu-PSMA RLT is mainly used as compassionate treatment of patients with end-stage mCRPC [40, 47]. Over 12 studies with a total of 669 patients have reported results with [^{177}Lu]Lu-PSMA RLT. In 44% of patients treated with [^{177}Lu]Lu-PSMA, there was a decline in blood prostate-specific antigen (PSA) levels of greater than 50%, with only transient adverse effects. Sixteen studies which enrolled 1338 patients looked at prostate cancer response to third-line treatments. Following third-line treatment with enzalutamide and cabazitaxel, the symptoms caused by adverse effects with these drugs led to discontinuation of the treatment using them in 10–23% of patients. Conversely, [^{177}Lu]Lu-PSMA RLT gave a serum PSA decline of more than 50% more frequently than drug third-line treatment (mean 44% with [^{177}Lu]Lu-PSMA versus 22% with drug third-line therapy). ^{177}Lu-PSMA RLT gave greater objective remission compared to third-line treatment (overall 31 of 109 patients versus 43 of 275 patients, $p = 0.004$) [42]. Differences in median survival proved to be longer after [^{177}Lu]Lu-PSMA RLT

than after drug third-line therapy, but the difference proved not to be statistically significant (mean 14 months for [^{177}Lu]Lu-PSMA versus chemotherapy). Adverse effects resulted in cessation of treatment more often for third-line treatment compared to ^{177}Lu-PSMA RLT (22 of 66 patients versus 0 of 469 patients, $p < 0.001$) [41].

According to the results of different published data, no severe adverse events immediately after injection have been reported to date. The most common side effect in the first 48 h after injection is mild nausea and vomiting (in up to 20% of patients), which can be easily treated with antiemetics. Fatigue is the most common complaint in patients after therapy, especially in the first 4 weeks (in up to 25% of patients) [3, 37, 41]. One of the most common reported adverse side effects from [^{177}Lu]Lu-PSMA is dry mouth, reported in up to 20% of cases, but this was transient in most patients.

[^{177}Lu]Lu-PSMA dosimetry studies revealed that the kidneys are the critical organs, receiving a radiation dose of 0.88 Gy/GBq from [^{177}Lu]Lu-PSMA-617 and 0.93 Gy/GBq from [^{177}Lu]Lu-PSMA-I&T. No studies reported any high-grade nephrotoxicity (common toxicity criteria (CTC) grade 3, 4, or 5). Regarding tumor doses, all lesions received a mean dose per cycle of 23 ± 20 Gy (3.3 Gy/GBq). Calculations of mean absorbed dose to bone, lymph node, liver, and lung metastases were 26 ± 20 Gy (3.4 Gy/GBq), 24 ± 16 Gy (3.2 Gy/GBq), 8.5 ± 4.7 Gy (1.28 Gy/GBq), and 13 ± 7.4 Gy (1.7 Gy/GBq), respectively [48, 49].

There is a clear trend toward a lower absorbed dose with an increasing number of cycles [46, 47]. A similar trend can be seen for the subgroup of bone metastases.

Severe (grade 3 and 4) bone marrow toxicity is observed in less than 10% of patients in various publications. The European meta-analysis [37] and studies in Australia demonstrated that more than two-thirds of the patients benefit from [^{177}Lu]Lu-PSMA therapies, when PCa is already in castration-resistant phase [34].

The newest forms of PRLT introduce prostate-specific membrane antigen targeting alpha therapy, such as [Ac]Ac-PSMA-617. The patient number in clinical studies is still small, but it seems to improve the excellent results of PRLT as compared to [^{177}Lu]Lu-PSMA-617. In the largest published study, 5 out of 40 patients discontinued treatment because of nonresponsiveness, and 4 because of xerostomia. In 38 patients treated with [^{225}Ac]Ac-PSMA-617, in patients who survived at least 8 weeks, 24 (63%) had a PSA decline of more than 50%, and 33 (87%) had at least a modest serum PSA decline. The median duration of tumor control under [^{225}Ac]Ac-PSMA-617 last-line therapy was 9.0 months. Five patients were reported to have an enduring response of more than 2 years. The response and promising duration of tumor control, especially considering the unfavorable prognostic profile of the selected advanced-stage patients, is very good but very similar to the results of [^{177}Lu]Lu-PSMA-617. On the contrary, [^{225}Ac]Ac-PSMA-617 seems to have a permanent side effect, xerostomia (and maybe xerophthalmia). The dry mouth is caused not only by inflammation but also by the direct effect of radiation. Xerostomia could be persistent on the basis of preliminary results in 11 patients and cannot be protected even with sialadenoscopic support [50–52]. Nevertheless, the PSMA agents are very selective in targeting—anecdotally, even eye metastases can be treated (Fig. 21.4).

21.8 PRRT

The history of targeting neuroendocrine neoplasms with radiolabeled peptides began in the late 1980s and treatments began in the late 1990s, first in the Netherlands. Extensive studies included ^{111}In- and ^{90}Y-labeled octreotide analogs. The current approved practice of neuroendocrine neoplasms (NENs) consists of lutetium-177-octreotate, also known as *[^{177}Lu]Lu-DOTA0-Tyr3-octreotate (DOTATATE)* or similar compounds, *and this peptide receptor radionuclide therapy (PRRT) is already a part of international recommendations (European Neuroendocrine Tumor Society (ENETS)/National Comprehensive Cancer Network (NCCN) guidelines).* Lutetium-177-octreotate treatment is based on *somatostatin receptors, which are present in almost all neuro-*

endocrine tumors including pheochromocytoma and paraganglioma. The carrier molecule octreotate has high affinity especially to somatostatin receptor (SSTR) 2 and (SSTR) 5. For patient selection, somatostatin receptor imaging is essential, e.g., by using gallium-68-octreotate PET imaging (or [^{111}In]In-octreotide gamma imaging) in order to confirm disease that has higher SSTR expression than the liver. Nordic guidelines recommend four treatments with 7.4 GBq (200 mCi) activity typically with 8-week intervals. In real practice, the amount of treatment cycles is dependent on response and on critical organ absorbed radiation dose, i.e., kidney and bone marrow dose. Gamma imaging allows to estimate quantitatively [^{177}Lu]Lu-octreotate uptake in metastatic sites. Figure 21.5 represents a patient who has received 5 cycles of PRRT and treatment response has been followed up with [^{68}Ga]Ga-octreotate PET. [^{177}Lu]Lu-octreotate got marketing authorization in 2017 after a randomized and controlled prospective trial (NETTER-1) and has significantly improved overall survival as compared to earlier clinical practice (long-acting somatostatin analog). The treatment itself may cause fatigue and nausea due to prophylactic hyperhydration in order to decrease kidney dose. The pain in the metastatic sites is typically related to tumor-lysis. Bone marrow depression is seldom detected. Hormonal effects are also seen, because approximately half of these tumors are functional. Therefore, blood chemistry should be followed up regularly. This treatment suits NENs with World Health Organization (WHO) class of 1–2 and proliferation index Ki-67 of less than 20%. This treatment improves the quality of life and relieves symptoms significantly.

For the theranostics concept, there are currently multiple compounds under development, both for imaging in patient selection/follow-up and therapeutic compound (Table 21.1).

For SSTR imaging, some new ^{68}Ga-PET compounds are under development, such as [^{68}Ga]Ga-satoreotide trizoxetan (^{68}Ga-OPS202). The original therapeutic compound was [^{177}Lu]Lu-DOTATOC, also called [^{177}Lu]Lu-edotreotide, and this is still widely in clinical use in multiple institutions that are allowed

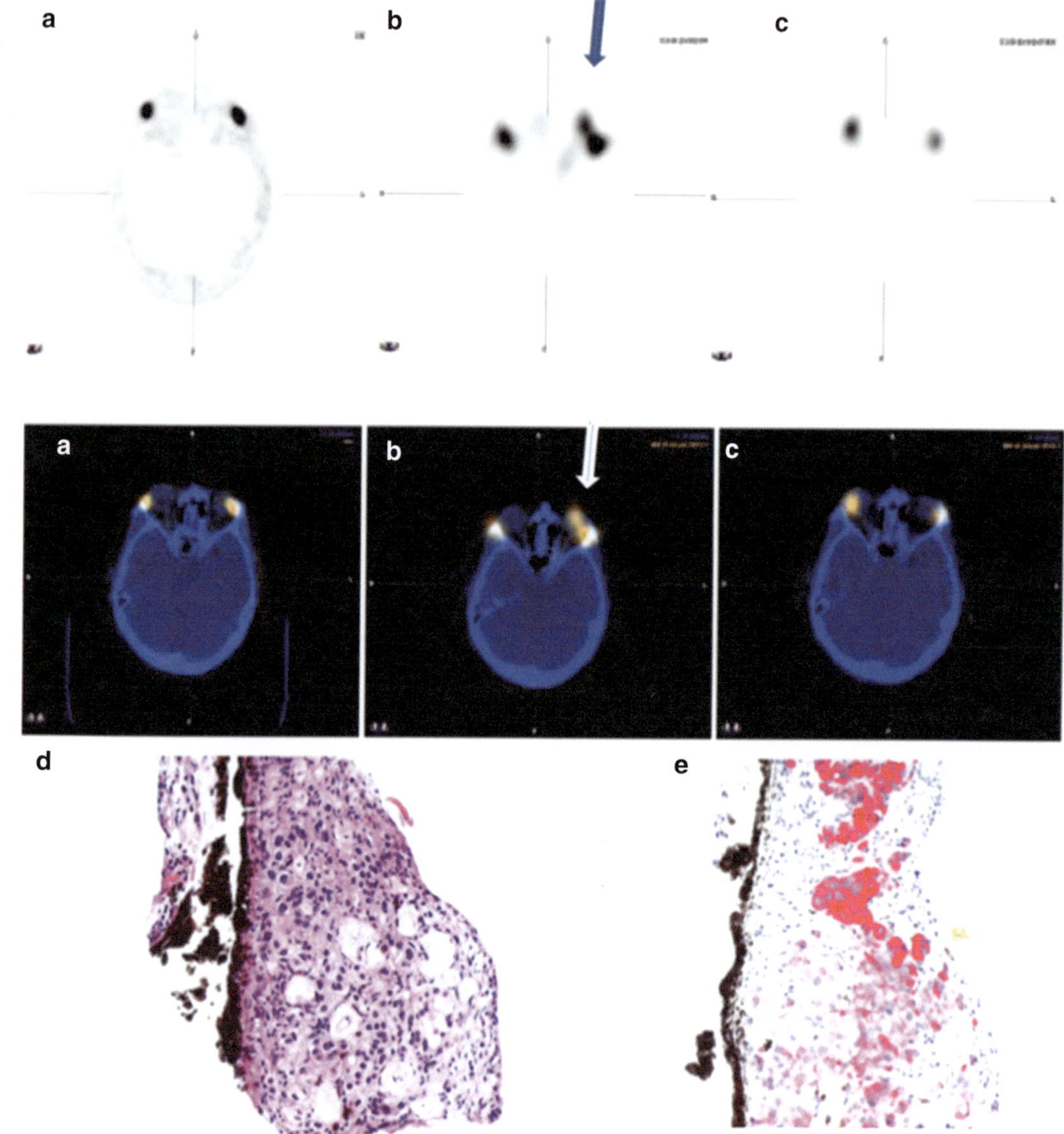

Fig. 21.4 A 60-year-old male demonstrated large PSMA-positive skeletal metastases located predominantly in the lumbosacral spine and pelvis. Metastases were seen in lung hila, mediastinal lymph nodes, and liver in the left lobe. He was decided to be treated with PRLT. In images (**A** and **a**), a cross section at eyeball level of fluorine-18-PSMA-1007-PET-CT study (PET study (**A**); PET-CT fusion image (**a**)) performed at 1 h is shown. In images (**B** and **b**), lutetium-177-PSMA-617 SPECT/CT (SPECT study (**B**); SPECT/CT fusion image (**b**)) performed 24 h after the first therapy cycle is shown; this study was performed 2 weeks later than that of (**A**). In images (**C** and **c**), the similar lutetium-177-PSMA-617 SPECT/CT study is shown after the second therapy cycle; this study was performed 4 weeks later than that of (**B**) (SPECT study (**C**); SPECT/CT fusion image (**c**)). The patient had an eye metastasis of prostate cancer, as shown in image (**D**) with hematoxylin and eosin (HE) staining and in image (**E**) with PSA immunohistochemistry, confirmed, because the eye was biopsied after the first therapy cycle due to pain. The pain disappeared as a result of treatment, and it was not anymore visible after the second cycle in image (**C**), i.e., complete response by imaging

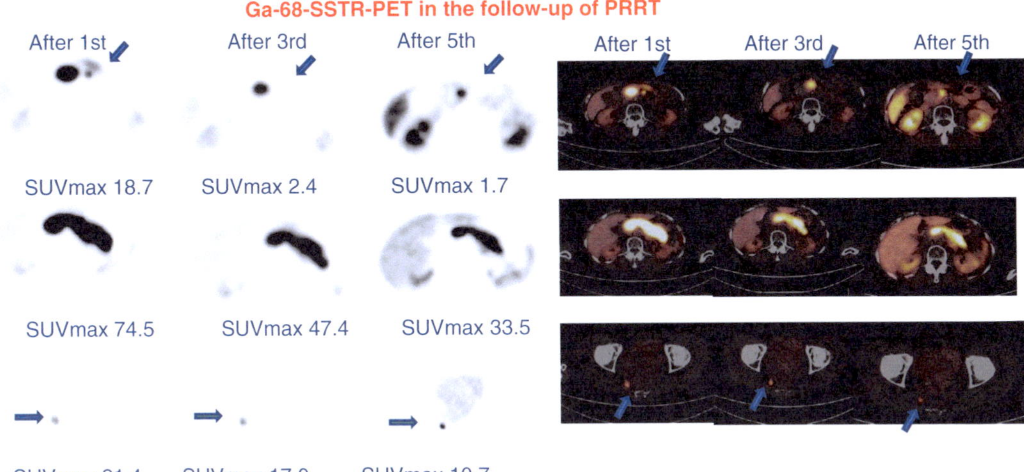

Fig. 21.5 A 70-year-old female with neuroendocrine cancer in the tail of the pancreas (Grade 2). The invasive tumor invaded the spleen, ventricle, and left adrenal gland. Lymph node metastases were seen in the upper abdomen and pelvis. She was treated with long-acting octreotide and interferon. She received five lutetium-177-peptide receptor treatments, so that the originally inoperable tumor could be removed. The images demonstrate remarkable tumor shrinkage and decrease in standardized uptake values (SUVs) by using gallium-68-octreotate PET. Chromogranin A (CgA) normalized during imaging. The cumulative absorbed radiation dose in the pancreatic tumor was 853 Gy

to use their own products. The commercial compound [^{177}Lu]Lu-DOTA0-Tyr3-octreotate (DOTATATE) is globally most widely used, but other ^{177}Lu derivatives are under development, such as [^{177}Lu]Lu-OPS201. These do not essentially differ from existing compounds, except for the fact that different chelators instead of DOTA, such as NODAGA, are used. Additionally, new indications are searched, because neuroendocrine differentiation is seen in many metastatic breast, prostate, and small-cell lung cancers besides conventional neuroendocrine tumors. New attempts include the introduction of new radionuclides, copper-67 and bismuth-213.

21.9 Gastrin in Medullary Thyroid Cancer

Different peptide receptors like somatostatin, bombesin/gastrin-releasing peptide (GRP), or vasoactive intestinal peptide (VIP) are overexpressed on cancer cells and are therefore ideal targets for the diagnosis and therapy with radiolabeled peptides in nuclear medicine. Virtually all medullary thyroid cancers (MTCs) express the cholecystokinin 2 receptor, for which the endogenous ligand is gastrin. By taking advantage of this, using peptide receptor radionuclide therapy (PRRT) with radiolabeled gastrin analogs becomes an attractive treatment paradigm for patients with recurrent or metastatic medullary thyroid cancer. Autoradiographic investigations revealed cholecystokinin (CCK)-B/gastrin receptors in over 90% of MTCs, in a high percentage of small-cell lung cancers, stromal ovarian tumors, and potentially a variety of other tumors, including gastrointestinal adenocarcinomas, neuroendocrine tumors, and malignant glioma [53]. Currently, the analogs [^{177}Lu]Lu-PP-F11N and [^{111}In]In-CP04, as a surrogate for ^{177}Lu- or ^{90}Y-labeled CP04, are in early prospective trials for medullary thyroid cancer (LUMED/NCT02088645 and GRAN-T-MTC/NCT03246659, respectively) performed for safety and to define MTD, biodistribution, and dosimetry. It was found that the stomach was the dose-limiting organ, not the kidneys, where the absorbed dose was low. Many patients given even small amounts of ^{177}Lu-radiolabeled gastrin suffered marked nausea. It is hypothesized that the use of adjuvant protease inhibitors would prevent degradation of the radiolabeled gastrin and help to improve tumor uptake of enzymatically vulnerable radiolabeled gastrin analogs [33].

In an earlier dose-escalation study, eight patients with advanced metastatic medullary thyroid cancer were injected with potentially therapeutic activities of a ^{90}Y-labeled mini-gastrin derivative at 4–6-weekly intervals (1110–1850 MBq/m^2 (30–50 mCi/m^2) per injection for a maximum of four injections). Hematologic and renal toxicities were acknowledged as the dose-limiting toxicities at the 1480 and 1850 MBq/m^2 (40 and 50 mCi/m^2) levels. Following treatment, two of the eight patients experienced partial remissions of their medullary thyroid cancer, while four had stabilization of their disease. It is hoped that CCK-B receptor ligands may become a new and useful weapon using receptor-binding proteins in patients with tumors that overexpress CCK-B receptors [53, 54].

21.10 Fibroblast Activation Protein Inhibitors

Targeting efforts against fibroblast activation protein (FAP) are becoming a promising strategy for targeting tumors. In more than 90% of epithelial cancers, fibroblasts are found to constitute a large subpopulation of tumor stroma. Because serine protease fibroblast activation protein is overexpressed in most cancers, a strategy of using inhibitors of fibroblasts labeled with radionuclides (FAPIs) was devised. FAP will be expressed in the stromal cells of most solid tumors. Overexpression is usually associated with a poor prognosis. Using radiolabeled FAP inhibitors (FAPIs), FAPI-02 and FAPI-04, the Haberkorn group at the University of Heidelberg showed that ^{68}Ga-labeled FAPI targeted various cancers on PET-CT with significantly lower background uptake in the liver and brain compared to 2-[^{18}F]FDG. To further prove this concept, a patient with metastatic breast cancer was treated with 2.9 GBq of [^{90}Y]Y-FAPI-04 and was shown to need significantly less pain medication

post-treatment. It appears that higher doses of radioactivity can be delivered while minimizing damage to healthy tissue, which may improve therapeutic outcome. FAP is a molecular target that holds great potential for tumor imaging and therapy [55, 56].

21.11 Pretargeted ^{177}Lu-Peptide in CEA-Positive Cancers

A strategy that may increase the target to background ratio is pretargeting with the first injection of an unlabeled bispecific monoclonal antibody (bsMAB), followed by a second injection of a radiolabeled bivalent hapten-peptide. The concept is that the bsMAB will attach first to the cancer cell target on the cell surface and that the radiolabeled hapten-peptide will be bound to any pretargeted bsMAB, but any radiolabeled hapten-peptide which does not find the pretargeted bsMAB will clear rapidly through the circulation. Medullary thyroid cancer cells express high amounts of CEA, and encouraging therapeutic results have been obtained using anti-CEA pretargeted [^{131}I]I-di-DTPA peptide in 2 phase 1/2 and 1 phase 2 clinical trials.

A multicenter phase 2 study of 45 medullary thyroid cancer patients assessed the chimeric hMN-14x734 bsMAB targeted to MTC cells, followed by 1.8 GBq/m^2 of [^{131}I]I-di-DTPA 4–6 days after the pretargeting. A 76.2% response rate (durable stabilization plus objective response) was noted according to the response evaluation criteria in solid tumors (RECIST) on CT. One durable complete response of at least 40 months (2.4%) and 31 durable stable diseases ≥6 months (73.8%) were observed in these patients with disease progression before radioimmunotherapy (RIT) [57].

These results have encouraged the development of newer bsMABs and bivalent peptides, based on humanized, recombinant, and even trivalent bsMABs, as well as utilizing newer hapten-peptides using histamine-succinyl-glutamine (HSG) haptens and bivalent HSG hapten-peptides. A series of bivalent HSG haptens have been synthesized, offering the possibility of labeling with different radionuclides such as lutetium-177 and yttrium-90 for therapy purposes. The first clinical results of an optimization study assessing the anti-CEA × anti-HSG bsMAB TF2 and the radiolabeled hapten-peptide, [^{177}Lu]Lu-IMP288, in patients with metastatic colorectal cancer have been reported recently. Using this pretargeting scheme, there was rapid tumor uptake within 1 h after the peptide was injected, and high tumor-to-tissue ratios were observed by 24 h. The most successful tumor targeting occurred following a 1-day pretargeting interval and 24 µg of the peptide. High activities of [^{177}Lu]Lu-IMP288 (2.5–7.4 GBq) could be injected, with some modest reactions during the injection, and only transient grade 3–4 thrombocytopenia seen in 10% of the patients. Dosimetry studies showed relatively low radiation to renal and red bone marrow following [^{177}Lu]Lu-IMP288 peptide [58].

Another target is CEA (carcinoembryonic antigen) which is expressed in 50% of lung tumors and would be susceptible to anti-CEA radioimmunotherapy. It has been shown that pretargeting with a bsMAB delivers higher radiation than simply using a labeled antibody alone. This has led to a clinical trial using pretargeted radioimmunotherapy involving a recombinant anti-CEA bsMAB and ^{177}Lu-labeled peptide to treat small-cell lung cancers (SCLC) or CEA-expressing non-small-cell lung cancer (NSCLC). In France, two multicentric prospective phase 1 clinical studies are ongoing, assessing pretargeted [^{177}Lu]Lu-IMP288 (one injection) in patients with metastatic CEA-positive lung carcinoma and fractionated injection of [^{90}Y]Y-IMP288 in metastatic colorectal patients. Other authors have suggested that the therapeutic efficacy of pretargeted radioimmunotherapy (PRIT) might be improved using α-emitting radionuclides such as bismuth-213 [59, 60].

21.12 Bombesin in Prostate and Breast Cancers

A novel target is the gastrin-releasing peptide receptor (GRPR), a glycosylated, seven-transmembrane G-protein-coupled receptor. This receptor then activates the phospholipase C signaling pathway. Gastrin-releasing peptide (GRP) itself regulates a number of physiologic processes, from the release of gastrointestinal hormones, smooth muscle contraction, and epithelial cell proliferation. This latter property likely acts as a mitogen in neoplastic tissues. The receptor is aberrantly expressed in numerous cancers such as those of the colon, prostate, lung, and breast [61].

The ^{68}Ga-labeled GRPR antagonists RM2 and NeoBOMB1 are currently under clinical evaluation in prostate cancer and gastrointestinal stromal tumor. Treatment in humans has not been reported thus far but has been examined in animal models. Interestingly, various ongoing studies compare [^{68}Ga]Ga-GRPR antagonists with [^{68}Ga]Ga-PSMA analogs (NCT03604757, NCT03606837, NCT03698370), which is essential to understand the role of each radiotracer in the management of prostate cancer patients. It appears that GRPR and PSMA are expressed in different stages of prostate cancer, and the two radiotracers show fundamentally different biodistribution. This may lead to two complementary rather than competitive theranostic approaches.

Radiolabeled GRPR antagonists may also have potential in estrogen receptor-positive breast tumors, which represent most breast cancer patients [33].

21.13 Substance P in Glioblastoma

One of the most common brain tumors is glioblastoma multiforme (GBM). GBM has been demonstrated to overexpress the neurokinin-1 (NK-1) receptor, and as a result, substance P (SP) can be used as a ligand for targeted therapy using beta or alpha emitters. ^{213}Bi-PRRT of gliomas has been investigated with the substance P analog DOTA-/DOTAGA-SP, targeting the neurokinin-1 receptor that is overexpressed in grade 2–4 gliomas. As a way of circumventing the blood-brain barrier, the ^{213}Bi-PRRT can be injected via a catheter implanted and connected to a subcutaneous access port.

Initially, the glioblastoma was targeted with yttrium-90 and lutetium-177, with some positive clinical results. Recent studies, however, focused on the alpha emitters bismuth-213 (^{213}Bi) and actinium-225 (^{225}Ac), allowing more selective tumor cell irradiation and limiting toxicity to adjacent healthy brain tissue. [^{213}Bi]Bi-DOTA-SP has been evaluated in 61 patients with grade 2–4 gliomas (up to a cumulative activity of 14.1 GBq). A subgroup analysis in seven patients with secondary glioblastoma showed a median overall survival of 18.6 months after conversion to grade 4 [33].

Fifty glioma patients of different subtypes were treated with targeted alpha therapy at the Medical University of Warsaw. Nine patients with secondary GBM were treated. Recurrent GBMs were treated by surgery, chemotherapy, and radiotherapy, and following this, by direct intra-cavitary injection of 1–6 doses of 0.9–2.3 GBq [^{213}Bi]Bi-DOTA-[Thi^8,Met(O$_2$)^{11}]-substance P ([^{213}Bi]Bi-DOTA-SP) to the GBM site at 2-month intervals. [^{68}Ga]Ga-DOTA-[Thi^8,Met(O$_2$)^{11}]-substance P ([^{68}Ga]Ga-DOTA-SP) was also injected along with the therapeutic radio-bismuth to image the biodistribution of the bismuth-213 with PET-CT. The therapeutic response was examined with MRI. Treatment with [^{213}Bi]Bi-DOTA-SP was well tolerated with only mild transient adverse reactions, mainly headaches due to transient edema reaction. Response to the alpha therapy with [^{213}Bi]Bi-DOTA-SP showed a median progression-free survival of 5.8 months and an overall survival time of 16.4 months. Two out of nine patients are still alive at 39 and 51 months, respectively, after the initiation of the therapy [62].

In another subgroup of 20 patients with recurrent glioblastoma, a median overall survival of 23.6 months was observed, compared with 14.6 months after standard therapy alone. Treatment with the longer-lived actinium-225 has been initiated and 20 glioma patients have been enrolled in a dose-escalation study (from 10 to 42 MBq) investigating the intra-tumoral or intercavitary injection of [^{225}Ac] Ac-DOTAGA-SP. The analysis of therapeutic efficacy and patient recruitment is ongoing [33].

21.14 IL-13RA2 Targeted Alpha Particle Therapy Against Glioblastomas

Chemotherapy and radiotherapy have not been completely effective as standard treatment options for patients with glioblastoma due to recurrent disease. One molecular strategy therefore has been to develop specifically targeted interleukin-13 receptor alpha 2 (IL-13RA2), a glioblastoma receptor expressed abundantly on over 75% of GBM patients.

Using Pep-1L, a peptide that binds to IL-13RA2 with high specificity, radioconjugates have been developed. Using a phage display library and bio-planning schemes in glioma cells that overexpressed or did not express IL-13RA2, three peptide ligands were identified. One of them, Pep-1L, showed the highest binding affinity to IL-13RA2. ^{64}Cu-radiolabeled Pep-1L selectively bound to IL-13RA2-expressing cells in vitro. Pep-1L was found to target GBM both in vitro and in an orthotopic model of GBM and could be monitored via PET. This study also examined conjugation of Pep-1L with an alpha particle emitter, actinium-225. Using convection-enhanced delivery, [^{225}Ac]Ac-Pep-1L improved the survival of mice compared to saline control [63, 64].

21.15 [^{131}I]Iodophenylalanine for Glioblastoma

Carrier-added 4-L-[^{131}I]iodophenylalanine ([^{131}I] IPA) is a small molecule therapeutic product that specifically targets L-type amino acid transport 1 (LAT-1), which is highly expressed in many aggressive cancers including glioblastoma and multiple myeloma.

A multicenter phase 1/2 study is underway to study its use to treat recurrent glioblastoma. The study is an international multicenter, open-label phase 1/2 dose-ranging investigation to evaluate the safety, tolerability, dosing schedule, and preliminary efficacy of carrier-added 4-L-[^{131}I] iodophenylalanine ([^{131}I]IPA), applied as single or repeated injections in patients with recurrent glioblastoma multiforme in conjunction with external radiotherapy [65].

21.16 CXCR4 in Cancer

C-X-C chemokine receptor type 4 (CXCR4) is an attractive target for theranostic interventions since it is overexpressed in hematologic malignancies, such as multiple myeloma, leukemia, and non-Hodgkin's lymphoma, and in some solid cancers (e.g., lung cancer, adrenocortical cancer, and high-grade neuroendocrine tumors). Many high-affinity ligands targeting CXCR4 have been developed, among which the theranostic pair [^{68}Ga]Ga-pentixafor/[^{177}Lu]Lu/[^{90}Y] Y-pentixather is the most advanced one.

The imaging agent, [^{68}Ga]Ga-pentixafor, was based on a cyclic pentapeptide, with a high affinity for CXCR4 and excellent stability for in vivo applications. Several radionuclides have been used in this system, attached with the metal chelator DOTA, including gallium-68, lutetium-177, and yttrium-90. Besides [^{68}Ga]Ga-pentixafor, the investigators developed [^{177}Lu]Lu- and [^{90}Y] Y-pentixather as therapeutic agents for a pilot study with three patients with multiple myeloma. All patients had been heavily treated with other standard therapies and then underwent CXCR4-targeted radionuclide therapy. Before such treatment, baseline [^{68}Ga]Ga-pentixafor PET scans were obtained to confirm the high expression of the target in these patients; 2-[^{18}F]FDG PET scans were also obtained. Excellent therapeutic efficacy was observed in two patients, evidenced with 2-[^{18}F]FDG PET, which showed much lower metabolic activity in the lesions when compared with pre-treatment scan.

It is thought that radiotherapy with alpha emitters, such as [^{213}Bi]Bi-/[^{225}Ac]Ac-pentixather, might be more successful than using beta emitters such as [^{177}Lu]Lu-pentixather, since most hematologic cancers are widely disseminated, and targeted alpha therapy (TAT) is under serious consideration [33, 66, 67].

21.17 [^{177}Lu]Lu-3BP-227 in Metastatic Pancreatic Adenocarcinoma

Ductal adenocarcinoma remains one of the deadliest cancers, with poor prognosis. It is known that neurotensin receptor 1 (NTR1) is overexpressed in ductal pancreatic cancers, and clinical trials have been conducted using this receptor. In a phase 1 trial in Germany, eligible patients were given NTR1 antagonist [^{177}Lu]Lu-3BP-227. The phase 1 study by Baum et al. offered the first clinical evidence of the feasibility of treating ductal pancreatic adenocarcinoma with a DOTA-conjugated NTR1 antagonist, 3BP-227, labeled with the radioisotope lutetium-177. Six patients with ductal pancreatic adenocarcinoma who had failed all other treatment options received [^{177}Lu] Lu-3BP-227 for assessment of NTR1 expression in vivo. Three patients received treatment activities of 5.1–7.5 GBq. [^{177}Lu]Lu-3BP-227 was well tolerated by all patients. The largest radiation dose was identified as being to the kidneys, with the most severe adverse reaction found to be a reversible grade 2 anemia. The most successful patient survived 13 months from diagnosis and 11 months after starting [^{177}Lu]Lu-3BP-227 therapy and experienced marked improvement in symptoms. The 5-year survival rate for patients with this type of cancer is less than 5% [68].

21.18 LAT1 Synthetic Iodine-131 Amino Acid Therapy in Glioblastoma

A synthetic amino acid has been developed targeting the L-type amino acid transporter 1 (LAT1), which is strongly overexpressed in many aggressive malignancies, including glioblastoma, melanoma, multiple myeloma, primary hepatocellular carcinoma (HCC), and gastric, prostate, and breast cancers. This synthetic amino acid (LAT1) has been labeled with PET agents for diagnosis and therapeutic radionuclides for therapy. It demonstrates favorable therapeutic biodistribution and kinetics and is actively transported across the intact blood-brain barrier into tumor cells. This radiolabeled synthetic amino acid potentially offers therapeutic benefit as a mono-therapy, and in conjunction with other therapeutic agents, including radiotherapies (external beam therapy, microspheres, brachytherapy, etc.), due to its radiosensitization effect [69].

2-[^{18}F]FDG is one of the most commonly used probes for the diagnosis of cancer with PET. Although 2-[^{18}F]FDG has been of assistance in the clinical diagnosis of many cancers, it sometimes showed false-positive results, especially in the brain, because even normal brain cells take up a relatively large amount of glucose. The amino acids have attracted attention as alternative probes to glucose in order to overcome this problem. If the compounds are delivered into cells specifically through LAT1, those cells are likely to be cancerous [70].

21.19 A High-Affinity Peptidomimetic for A$_V$B$_3$ Integrin Receptor Targeting in Breast Cancer

The cell adhesion motif $\alpha_v\beta_3$ arginine-glycine-aspartate (RGD) integrin receptor was discovered in fibronectin by Pytela, Pierschbacher, and Ruoslahti more than 20 years ago. The $\alpha_v\beta_3$ integrin receptor is overexpressed on endothelial cells and some tumor cells. The $\alpha_v\beta_3$ integrin is significantly overexpressed in certain types of tumor cells and almost all tumor vasculature. Integrins are intriguing targets as $\alpha_v\beta_3$ is known to be involved in neo-angiogenesis in solid tumors and is overexpressed in many different types of cancers (glioblastomas, melanomas, myelomas, ovarian tumors, breast and prostate cancers) [71].

It was hypothesized that any tumor overexpressing $\alpha_v\beta_3$ as part of angiogenesis would be able to be targeted for both imaging and therapy by a peptidomimetic. This is a small protein-like chain with properties similar to a normal peptide. Peptidomimetics cna either originate from modification of an existing peptide, or ariese from designing similar systems mimicking peptides. B-peptide natural amino acids in peptides

can be substituted by non-proteinogenic counter-parts (*proteinogenic* means "protein-building"). Such proteinogenic amino acids are able to be condensed into a polypeptide through a process known as translation. Proteinogenic amino acids are amino acids that are known to be precursors to proteins and are co-translationally (during translation to obtain drug-like targeting molecules) incorporated into proteins. The $\alpha_v\beta_3$ integrin antagonist (IAC) peptidomimetic 4-[2-(3,4,5,6-tetrahydropyrimidine-2-ylamino) ethyloxy]benzoyl-2-[*N*-(3-amino-neopenta-1-carbamyl)]-aminoethylsulfonyl-amino-β-alanine, THERANOST™, was developed to provide an alternate vector selectively targeting integrin $\alpha_v\beta_3$ receptor and clears rapidly from the whole body [71, 72].

Using this synthetic peptidomimetic for $\alpha_v\beta_3$ integrin labeled with [^{68}Ga]Ga-NODAGA, Baum et al. were able to demonstrate the superior uptake in two patients with disseminated breast cancer compared to 2-[^{18}F]FDG. A therapeutic entity using lutetium-177 in place of gallium-68 is currently in phase 1 clinical trials [72].

21.20 Antibodies

From the first report in 1975 by César Milstein and Georges J. F. Köhler describing immortal-izing hybrid B cells and mouse myeloma tumor cells, it has been possible to generate large amounts of monoclonal antibodies (mAbs) of predefined specificity. Monoclonal antibodies have revolutionized biomedical research and diagnostics and led to the generation of an arsenal of therapies for many diseases. Nuclear medicine was no exception. In fact, the emergence of monoclonal antibodies for decades generated interest initially in radiolabeling whole antibodies, then Fab fragments, single-chain antibodies, mini-bodies, and finally with humanized antibodies—the latter with only the variable portion of the antibody containing mouse proteins. Several therapeutic radiolabeled monoclonal antibodies have been developed, targeted particularly at lymphoma. Two monoclonal antibody products targeting the cluster of differentiation (CD)20 antigen have been approved, the intact murine immunoglobulins [131I]I-tositumomab (Bexxar®; GlaxoSmithKline, Mississauga, ON, USA) and [90Y]Y-ibritumomab tiuxetan (Zevalin®; Spectrum Pharmaceuticals, Henderson, NV, USA). Sales of [131I]I-tositumomab are now discontinued. [90Y] Y-ibritumomab can be incorporated in clinical practice using non-ablative activities for the treatment of patients with relapsed/refractory follicular lymphoma or has been administered following induction chemotherapy in front-line treatment in lymphoma patients [73].

It is important to know whether a monoclonal antibody or other antibodies become internalized in a cancer cell after injection, as this can lead to important dose considerations after radiolabeling. For instance, when radiometal-labeled drugs are metabolized, the metal-based radionuclide is trapped intracellularly in lysosomes through residualization. This process culminates in higher absolute uptake of the tracer and leads eventually to higher tumor-to-blood ratios [74].

21.21 [177Lu]Lu-J591 Anti-PSMA in Metastatic Prostate Cancer

Prostate-specific membrane antigen (PSMA) has emerged as the most favorable target in prostate cancer, although several targets had been previously identified, such as mucin, ganglioside, and adenocarcinoma-associated antigens. Prostate cancer is known to be radiosensitive, and most sites of prostate cancer spread such as bone marrow and lymph nodes are amenable to exposure to circulating monoclonal antibodies [75].

De-immunized J591 mAb, which targets the external domain of PSMA, seems to be the best clinical candidate for imaging and therapy of prostate cancer. In one study, 49 men were treated with fractionated doses of [177Lu]Lu-J591 ranging from 740 to 1665 MBq/m^2 (20–45 mCi/m^2) in two cycles weeks apart. The dose-limiting toxicity in the phase 1 trial was neutropenia. The recommended phase 2 doses (RP2Ds) were 1480 MBq/ m^2 (40 mCi/m^2) and 1665 MBq/m^2 (45 mCi/ m^2) × 2. At the highest RP2D of 1665 MBq/m^2

(45 mCi/m^2), 35.3% of patients were discovered to have a reversible grade 4 neutropenia and 58.8% of patients had thrombocytopenia. In addition, patients treated at this dose showed a greater drop in prostate-specific antigen (PSA)—85.5% showed some PSA decrease, 58.8% showed a greater than 30% decrease in PSA, and 29.4% showed a larger than 50% decrease. In terms of survival, the median survival was 42.3 months. Those patients who were positive with PSMA PET imaging had better responses than those patients who showed less intense upake. Those with less intense PSMA uptake tended to have poorer responses. It appears that treatment with radiolabeled and de-immunized J591 is well tolerated. There was less salivary gland toxicity with the [177Lu]Lu-J591 antibody than similar therapies with [177Lu]Lu-PSMA peptide therapies [76].

21.22 Hematologic Malignancies

An antigen known to be overexpressed on hematopoietic cancers is CD33. It is commonly associated with myeloid malignancies including acute myelogenous leukemia (AML), but recent research has shown that CD33 can also be found on malignant cells of approximately 25–35% of all multiple myeloma patients. [225Ac] Ac-lintuzumab (Actimab-A) is a radioimmunoconjugate composed of actinium-225 linked to a humanized anti-CD33 monoclonal antibody. The CD33 receptor is overexpressed in AML cells. Actinium-225 emits four α particles and has a 10-day half-life. A 53-patient multicenter phase 2 trial for patients newly diagnosed with AML aged 60 and above was conducted with [225Ac] Ac-lintuzumab developed as first-line monotherapy. The [225Ac]Ac-lintuzumab was given as two 15-min injects 7 days apart. Adverse effects included myelosuppression seen in all evaluable patients, including grade 4 thrombocytopenia with marrow aplasia for more than 6 weeks following therapy in three patients. The only reported in more than one patient, were penumonia and cellulitis were pneumonia and cellulitis. A 56% response rate was seen in older patients unfit for intensive chemotherapy. As the myelosuppression was considered to be longer than acceptable in this population, a smaller fractionation dose was felt advisable [77].

[^{225}Ac]Ac-lintuzumab is also being studied in a phase 1 clinical trial in patients who have progressing multiple myeloma disease after three prior multiple myeloma treatment regimens and are refractory to QUAD (carfilzomib, lenalidomide, pomalidomide, dexamethasone). This trial will estimate the maximum tolerated dose (MTD), assess adverse events, and measure response rates [78].

21.22.1 [^{131}I]I-Apamistamab CD45 Receptor Expressed in Leukemia and Lymphoma

Radioimmunotherapy has been used for many years in refractory/relapsed non-Hodgkin's lymphoma and shown to be effective in numerous clinical trials. The first agents were Bexxar®, a ^{131}I-radiolabeled murine monoclonal ([^{131}I]I-tositumomab) antibody, and Zevalin®, a ^{90}Y-radiolabeled murine antibody ([^{90}Y]Y-ibritumomab), both targeting CD20 receptors on the surface of lymphocytes [79].

The sale of Bexxar was terminated in February 2014 as there was a large decline in usage (fewer than 75 patients in 2012), despite the drug showing a 70% response rate; the lack of demand was because oncologists could not sell it directly to patients but had to refer patients to third parties, and because of the emergence of nonradioactive drugs that were as good, and which could be administered directly by medical oncologists.

Interest, however, has resurfaced in using anti-CD45-targeted conditioning with iodine-131 apamistamab [Iomab-B] plus allogeneic hematopoietic cell transplantation (HCT) as a safe alternative to conventional care for older patients with active relapsed/refractory AML. The treatment was shown to provide effective and tolerable therapy for ablating the patients' cancer and marrow cells. The pivotal phase trial in relapsed or refractory AML in 150 patients has been carried out as a randomized controlled clinical trial involving patients who have relapsed or refractory AML, aged 55 years and above. A durable

complete remission (dCR) was chosen as the primary endpoint in this trial, and primary endpoint in this trial, .and the secondary endpoint chosen was overall survival at 1 year. [^{131}I]I-apamistamab [Iomab-B] is intended to prepare and condition patients for a hematopoietic stem cell transplant (HSCT) as a safer and more efficacious alternative to intensive chemotherapy [80].

Another murine monoclonal antibody, lilotomab (formerly tetulomab), was developed targeting CD37, a surface glycoprotein expressed on mature human B cells. It was linked to lutetium-177 using satetraxetan, a derivative of DOTA for beta radiotherapies. The compound was developed under the trade name Betalutin ([^{177}Lu]Lu-HH1 or [^{177}Lu]Lu-lilotomab satetraxetan). The compound is being utilized in relapsed/refractory follicular lymphoma patients who have received at least two previous systemic therapies. In the LYMRIT 37-01 phase 1/2 clinical study of Betalutin® ([^{177}Lu]Lu-satetraxetan-lilotomab) in 74 evaluable patients with relapsed/refractory indolent non-Hodgkin's lymphoma (iNHL), patients with iNHL received Betalutin® in a single administration with 6 months or more of follow-up. There was an overall response rate (ORR) of 61%, with 28% of the 74 patients having a complete response (CR). Durable responses, especially for patients with a CR (20.7 months) and promising response rates (ORR and CR) for dosing regimens, have been assessed in pivotal phase 2b PARADIGME study. The compound was well tolerated with a predictable and manageable safety profile [81].

21.23 Anti-HER2 in Breast Cancer

The human epidermal growth factor 2 (HER2) has been extensively evaluated since its discovery in 1987 by Dr. Slamon and colleagues, mainly as its overexpression in tumors has been associated with more aggressive tumor types. The first humanized monoclonal antibody developed targeting HER2 in HER2-positive breast cancer patients approved by the US Food and Drug Administration (FDA) was trastuzumab (Herceptin; Genentech,

South San Francisco, CA). Pertuzumab, trastuzumab emtansine (T-DM1), and lapatinib are approved for inhibiting HER2 activity in the treatment of HER2-positive metastatic breast cancers. Pertuzumab (Perjeta; Genentech, South San Francisco, CA) is a humanized mAb version developed to bind extracellularly to domain II of the HER2 epitope. This humanized mAb works by inhibiting HER2 dimerization with other growth factor receptors, such as HER2-HER3 dimerization. Preclinical experiments showed that the combination of trastuzumab and pertuzumab enhanced the antitumor effect compared to trastuzumab or pertuzumab alone due to complementary mechanisms of action that promote tumor regression more effectively [82].

Once developed, antibodies designed for radiotherapy can be labeled with a host of tumoricidal radiotherapeutics, such as alpha, beta, and Auger electron-emitting radionuclides. Trastuzumab similarly has been labeled with a series of HER2-targeted radionuclides. This antibody has been labeled with lutetium-177 (^{177}Lu), copper-64 (^{64}Cu), indium-111 (^{111}In), thorium-227 (^{227}Th), rhenium-188 (^{188}Re), yttrium-90 (^{90}Y), and iodine-131 (^{131}I) [82, 83].

Abbas et al. performed a preliminary clinical study with [^{177}Lu]Lu-trastuzumab involving 10 patients in order to assess the localization of the [^{177}Lu]Lu-trastuzumab in primary and/or metastatic lesions and in the nontarget organs. [^{177}Lu]Lu-trastuzumab accumulated in the HER2-positive lesions, but no uptake was noted in the HER2-negative sites (as delineated by IHC). Biodistribution studies showed normal uptake in the heart, liver, spleen, and nasopharynx, but did not evaluate dose or toxicity to erythrocytes or leukocytes.

Pertuzumab has also been labeled with lutetium-177 using the chelate isothiocyanate-benzyl-CHX-A″-DTPA. One preclinical study by Persson et al. used SKOV-3 OVCa xenografted Balb/c (nu/nu) mice, showed that [^{177}Lu]Lu-DTPA-pertuzumab delivered a high tumor dose of 50.86 ± 5.57 Gy with an injected activity of 7.3 MBq. The study group treated with [^{177}Lu]Lu-pertuzumab showed a clear delay in tumor growth [83].

21.24 Targeting Hypoxic Tumor Cells with Carbonic Anhydrase IX-Specific Antibody B Radioconjugates

Because many solid tumors become hypoxic, and many cancer cells can survive under conditions of hypoxia, carbonic anhydrase IX (CA-IX) has been considered an attractive target for diagnosis and therapy of solid tumors. Under low oxygen tension, CA-IX confers cancer cell survival and is accompanied by an elevated propensity for metastasis. CA-IX is a transmembrane zinc metalloenzyme which is involved in the hydration of carbon dioxide to bicarbonate ions and hydrogen. There is an increased expression of CA-IX in many malignancies, as the tumors attempt to maintain an optimal cellular pH. For this reason, CA-IX is an ideal protein for targeting hypoxic cells, and radiolabeled antibody-targeting CA-IX has been evaluated in clinical trials [84].

A number of different targeting vectors to CA-IX have been developed, including monoclonal antibodies, peptides, small molecule inhibitors, and antibody mimetics. All have been radiolabeled for either imaging or therapeutic application, including one of the more promising, cG250, a chimeric monoclonal antibody. In early clinical trials, the effect of the mouse anti-CA-IX antibody G250 labeled with the β-emitting radionuclide iodine-131 was examined in patients with metastatic clear cell renal cell carcinoma (ccRCC). Seventeen out of 33 patients responded to this treatment resulting in stable disease, but unfortunately, patients developed human anti-mouse antibodies (HAMA), which limited further treatment. In order to prevent the HAMA response, a chimeric version of G250 (cG250 girentuximab) was developed. The chimeric antibody was labeled with iodine-131 and then administered to 12 patients with metastatic ccRCC in a low dose to document tumor uptake. Uptake in metastases was observed in nine of the patients, of whom eight received a second dose of [^{131}I]I-cG250 at 1665, 2220, or 2775 MBq/m², leading to a partial response occurring in one patient, with stable disease lasting for 3–6 months in a second patient. Fractionated dosing of [^{131}I]

I-cG250 given at a whole-body absorbed dose of 0.5, 0.75, or 1 Gy (3–7 fractions/patient) did not enhance clinical response, with 7 of the 14 patients who completed treatment showing stable disease, while the remaining 7 patients showed disease progression. In addition, administration of [^{131}I]I-cG250 given at 2220 MBq/m^2 followed 3 months later at 1110 or 1665 MBq/m^2, in 3 and 16 patients, respectively, did not improve the clinical response, with 5 patients having a stable disease and the remaining patients having progressive disease [85].

Treatment of ccRCC patients with a residualizing radionuclide (lutetium-177)-labeled cG250, compared to non-residualizing iodine-131, led to better responses in patients who underwent up to 3 cycles of treatment, with 1 partial responder and 17 out of 24 patients having stable disease 3 months after the first cycle of treatment. In a second, nonrandomized single-arm trial, 14 ccRCC patients received 2405 MBq/m^2 [^{177}Lu]Lu-cG250, culminating in 1 patient having a partial regression and 8 patients having stable disease. Of these responding patients, six patients received a second cycle of treatment, resulting in durable responses in five patients but with prolonged thrombocytopenia restricting further cycles of treatment [86].

21.25 Tumor Necrosis Therapy for Lung and Pancreatic Cancers

[^{131}I]I-ch tumor necrosis therapy (TNT) has received approval from the Chinese State Food and Drug Administration for the treatment of advanced lung cancer patients who had previous treatment failure with radiotherapy or chemotherapy. TNT utilizes the presence of degenerating and necrotic cells within tumors by exploiting mAbs directed against universal, intracellular nucleosomal determinants comprising histone H1 and DNA. The monoclonal antibody `, which increase the pharmacokinetic performance of the monoclonal antibody. The ^{131}I-TNT construct delivers iodine-131 to tumor cells and leads to the targeted imaging and/or destruction of cells

with exposed necrotic antigens. In clinical trials, patients were treated with two doses of ^{131}I-TNT and showed a favorable response rate of 34.6%. These results confirmed that the combination of tumor necrosis factor-related apoptosis-inducing ligand (TRAIL) and iodine-131 triggered apoptosis of NSCLC through caspase-9 activation [87].

Preclinically, TNT has also been studied as an antibody for targeted alpha therapy (TAT) and has been labeled with bismuth-213 for the treatment of a pancreatic cancer xenograft in this study. Antibody radioconjugate therapy was demonstrated to be more effective at controlling tumor growth with fewer side effects in comparison with gemcitabine or cisplatin. The bismuth-213 decay chain results in the emission of both α and β particles before the long-lived bismuth-209 is reached. The resulting delivery of both α and β doses would be ideal when targeting necrotic tumors for two main reasons. First, the high-energy α particles emanating from the necrotic tumor core would irradiate hypoxic cells within 2–3 cell diameters from the source located in the necrotic region, while in addition, the longer penetration of β particles can be advantageous in delivering a higher dose to well-oxygenated cancer cells, distant from the necrotic cells, and would not require as high a β dose due to the higher oxygenation [87].

21.26 Actinium-225 Insulin Growth Factor for Multiple Solid Tumors

There has been an interest in targeting type I insulin-like growth factor receptor (IGF-1R) labeled with actinium-225 to solid tumors, non-small cell lung cancers, prostate cancers, sarcomas, and breast cancers, where this growth factor is overexpressed. [^{225}Ac]Ac-FPI-1434 is a radioimmunoconjugate comprising a humanized mAb (AVE1642) that binds to the external domain of IGF-1R, a proprietary bifunctional chelate, and the alpha-emitting radionuclide actinium-225. Once internalized, the monoclonal antibody radiolabeled with actinium-225 can cause tumor cell death via double-stranded DNA breaks. An indium-111 analog [^{111}In]In-FPI-1547 has identical antibody and bifunctional chelate activity and is used for patient selection. Patients over-expressing the insulin-like growth factor can be selected based on imaging and quantitating the bound ^{111}In-antibody [88].

A phase 1 study is currently being conducted in several centers to evaluate the safety and tolerability of [^{111}In]In-FPI-1547 injection and [^{225}Ac]Ac-FPI-1434 injection in patients with advanced refractory solid tumors. It is also hoped to determine the maximum tolerated dose of a single [^{225}Ac]Ac-FPI-1434 injection. Preliminary data on tumor uptake of the [^{111}In] In-FPI-1547 compound in cancer patients is also being assessed [89].

21.27 Camelid Single Domain Antibodies (SDAB)

These single monomeric variable domain antibodies, or nanobodies, with a molecular weight of 12–15 kDa, are smaller than common antibodies by a factor of approximately 10. A group referred to as third-generation antibodies comprise two heavy chains attached to the variable domain and have been derived from dromedaries including camels, llama, alpaca, and shark. Key characteristics of the variable heavy homodimers (VHH) include high chemical and thermal stability, good solubility, a high penetration rate into tissues, low immunogenicity, and the ability to target antigenic epitopes via the long CDR3 loop on the nanobody difficult to access with conventional monoclonal antibodies. Desirable characteristics for tumor imaging include the high binding affinity for tumor antigens, rapid blood clearance of unbound nanobodies, renal elimination, high tumor-to-non-tumor ratio achieved shortly after tracer injection, and a lack of observed toxicity [90].

Radiolabeling of nanobodies with the gamma-emitting radionuclide technetium-99m via the hexahistidine tag has been performed without causing a chemical modification of the protein, and this has enabled the use of SPECT to image molecular targets such as HER2, which is a transmembrane glycoprotein overexpressed by certain tumor cells including breast cancer [91].

Xavier et al. [92] have depicted high specific contrast imaging of HER2-positive tumors in xenografts with PET-CT using gallium-68 to label the 2Rs15d nanobody utilizing the bifunctional chelating agent NOTA. Keyaerts et al. [93] reported a high accumulation in metastases of HER2-overexpressing tumor by the [^{68}Ga] Ga-anti-HER2 VHH nanobody in a phase 1 trial in patients with breast cancer. This radiolabeled nanobody has a favorable biodistribution and safety profile with no observable adverse effects at a radiation dose similar to other PET tracers with acceptable dosimetry. A phase 2 trial is currently underway using this radiotracer to characterize HER2 presence in brain metastases of breast cancer patients.

Nanobodies labeled with radionuclides other than gallium-68 have been studied. D'Huyvetter et al. [94] have shown that ^{177}Lu-labeled anti-HER2 inhibits the growth of HER2-expressing tumors in xenografted mice and suggested further investigation of [^{131}I]I-SGMIB-2Rs15d to perform dosimetry calculations prior to therapy in HER2-positive breast cancer patients [95].

Extensive research into radiolabeled nanobodies is an ongoing process with many preclinical trials investigating molecular targets such as epidermal growth factor receptor (EGFR) for skin cancer, HER3 for non-small-cell lung cancer and head and neck cancers, and CEA for colon cancer. There is preclinical evidence that anti-macrophage mannose receptor (MMR) nanobodies selectively targeting tumor-associated macrophages in vivo, anti-CD20 in CD20-positive NHL, and anti-idiotypic molecular target in multiple myeloma show promising results for future theranostic opportunities [96, 97].

The use of radiolabeled nanobodies to image atherosclerotic disease has also been investigated in preclinical trials [98] by targeting vascular cell adhesion molecule 1 (VCAM-1) and MMR to assess plaque burden in the aorta using PET-MRI to detect vessel wall inflammation, micro-calcification, and inflammatory activity [99]. The extensive preclinical work coupled with recent phase 1 and 2 trials demonstrates that an exciting future for the use of nanobodies as theranostic agents is within our grasp.

21.28 Intraperitoneal Radioimmunotherapy of Ovarian Cancer

The antibody MX35 displays uniform reactivity with 90% of human ovarian epithelial cancers, but only a limited number of normal tissues. It has been tested in a clinical phase 1 trial. The antibody MX35 is a F(ab')$_2$ which recognizes the membrane sodium transporter (NaPi2b). It was labeled with the α emitter astatine-211 ($T1/2 = 7.21$ h) and then infused via peritoneal catheters in nine women (median age of 52 years) as part of a phase 1 study. The concept was to attempt to treat micrometastases in the peritoneum. The women subjects were initially successfully treated for ovarian carcinoma but later relapsed and were treated long term with salvage chemotherapy, including Paraplatin and paclitaxel, resulting in clinically and biochemically complete remission. [^{211}At]At-MX35 F(ab')$_2$ (22.4–101 MBq/L) was infused via the peritoneal catheter over 30 min, together with 0.2 MBq of [^{125}I]I-human serum albumin (HSA), a reference for in vivo stability. The patients were given a thyroid blocking agent, which appears to have blocked any significant stomach accumulation of astatine-211. The results of the phase 1 study showed low toxicity and low dose to critical organs. There were no signs of diminished tolerability to future therapy and no signs of thyroid dysfunction. The aim of the study was not to evaluate the clinical outcome, but to evaluate the distribution and potential side effects [100].

21.29 Targeted Radiolabeled Nanoparticles

Nanoparticles (NPs) can be used for drug or radionuclide delivery either as passive or active targeting nanocarriers. Agents have been developed to improve the biodistribution, pharmacological, therapeutic, and toxicity properties in cancer diagnostics and therapeutics.

A major advantage of nanosized radioactive particles is their potential to contain numerous radioactive atoms within a single nanoparticle. Each radioactive nanoparticle can contain hundreds of radionuclides, and, consequently, by delivering one radiolabeled nanoparticle to a tumor site, hundreds of radionuclides can be transported. Conventional radiolabels using chelates allow only one tumor-avid biomolecule to carry one radioactive atom. The nanoparticles that are surface conjugated to tumor-avid biomolecules will initiate a higher ratio of radioactive particles to tumor-avid properties and daughter retention [101].

Radionuclides with therapeutic potential alpha or beta emissions have been incorporated within nano-materials for specific radiotherapies. Alternatively, gamma or PET emitters have been paired with nanoscale materials for diagnostic imaging. Particularly, 8 MeV particles (such as those produced in the decay chain of actinium-225) deliver their absorbed dose within a distance of $\sim$100 μm or approximately 10 cell diameters, thus limiting damage to nontarget cells. Recent clinical trials of bismuth-213 have used this radionuclide coupled to anti-CD33 mAb for the treatment of AML. Actinium-225 has also recently been proposed as an alternative to bismuth-213 treatment since this radionuclide has a much longer half-life ($T1/2 = 10$ days). A single atom can produce four alpha particle emissions with a total energy release of more than 27 MeV per decay, making it a potent radioisotope if all the energy is deposited at the tumor site. In comparison with single α-emitting therapies, the use of in vivo α generators within gold-contained nanoparticles holds the potential to convey a much larger biologically effective dose to target tissues. All the daughter radionuclides are released after the occurrence of initial R-decay following the attachment of actinium-225 to antibodies with conventional molecular chelators such as DOTA. When actinium-225 is encapsulated in fullerenes, the daughter radioisotopes can also be released, probably as a result of breaking the fullerene cage from the energy of nuclear decay recoil. Nevertheless, by employing $LaPO_4$ NPs to contain the radioisotopes rather than chelators, it has been shown that nearly all of the actinium-225 and almost 50% of the francium-221 and bismuth-213 daughters are retained within the NPs in vitro, indicating a dramatic improvement over conventional approaches [102].

While several radiolabeled nanoparticles have been used in preclinical work, few have currently been used thus far in human clinical trials.

21.30 Radiolabeled Aptamers

Aptamers, also known as "chemical antibodies," are short (20–100 bases) single-stranded RNA or DNA oligonucleotides, binding to targets with high selectivity and with high affinity. Aptamers are capable of folding into three-dimensional structures and bind to their target in a similar manner to their antibody protein counterpart through shape recognition. Aptamers are produced by "systematic evolution of ligands by exponential enrichment" (SELEX). This process involves iterative rounds of incubation, isolation, elution, and amplification of a randomized oligonucleotide library to a target to produce aptamers with high selectivity and specificity to the target [103, 104].

Aptamers generated by SELEX depict high affinity and specificity to a target, as the nucleic acids undergo iterative rounds of incubation, washing, isolation, and amplification. The process consists of using an initial library containing random RNA and DNA molecules, which are incubated with the target of interest, that might be biomarkers, proteins, or even entire cells. After incubation, the unbound RNA or DNA sequences are washed away, leaving only the bound sequences. To further enrich these bound sequences, they are then eluted from the sample, and using polymerase chain reaction (PCR) or reverse transcription PCR for RNA aptamers, the bound sequences are amplified. Then, this enriched pool of sequences undergoes iterative rounds of selection-amplification cycles, to

increase the affinity of the aptamers, as each consecutive round will diminish the heterogeneity of the pool. Following analysis of binding affinities, the pool with the best affinity and specificity is then cloned and sequenced [103].

Practical applications of aptamers in vivo demonstrated some challenges including susceptibility degradation by nucleases present in human serum and the fast excretion by renal filtration ribose. Fortunately, the short half-life of aptamers in human serum can be extended by modifying their exo- and endonuclease resistance. This modification can occur either pre- or post-selection via SELEX. Aptamers hold many advantages over antibodies such as the fact that they are more stable and resistant to changes in pH and temperature, also enabling them to be easily chemically modified, unlike antibodies, which cannot regain function after being denatured. While antibodies can vary significantly between production batches, aptamers are synthesized chemically and thus are more uniform. As aptamers are raised from nucleic acids rather than antibody proteins, they are generally not capable of generating immunological or toxic reactions. They are also considerably smaller than antibodies (5–15 kDa) in comparison with large monoclonal antibodies (15 kDa). As aptamers are much smaller than antibodies, they show superior tissue penetration (greater capabilities to be internalized by tumors). In addition, the smaller size gives aptamers the ability to bind to hidden epitopes which are not accessible to larger antibodies. These numerous advantages of aptamers have spurred their development as potentially more promising than antibodies [103].

Limited work has been completed in this area, but all molecular targets which have been selected for radionuclide therapy by antibodies or peptides can theoretically be considered as potential targets by radiolabeled aptamers and will provide new opportunities to treat cancer at a cellular level or at a metastatic stage, as well as providing opportunities for early diagnosis. Aptamers are emerging frontiers in medical molecular technology for cancer diagnostic and therapeutic applications [105].

21.31 Conclusion

The perspective of delivering treatments that have a more pronounced activity with specific molecular features will lead to improved benefits to patients, in ideal cases leading to palliation, control, or potentially even cure. A plethora of new cellular, intracellular, and membrane targets are adding new sensitivity to the diagnosis of diseases, particularly cancer, but also infectious diseases, atherosclerosis, and dementia. Once the diagnostic target is identified and successfully imaged, then a therapeutic radionuclide can selectively treat the diseased cells. The "molecular" ideal is to use true theranostic compounds, such as iodine-124 or iodine-123 for imaging and iodine-131 for therapy, but advances in chelation and nanoparticle therapy now make it possible to add any metal to a binding chelate for delivery to the target, and nanoparticles can potentially bind multiple diagnostic or therapeutic radionuclides. Preliminary treatments are now feasible using this approach for a large number of cancers, with extraordinary results achieved already in neuroendocrine tumors and prostate cancers, and almost certain to be followed in most other tumors. This chapter has focused on compounds already recently approved or in human clinical trials, but a plethora of other compounds are currently in preclinical animal studies and will shortly be entering human trials. For every agent in human clinical trials or awaiting approval, many more are undergoing evaluation in pre-clinical animal studies.

Targeted radionuclide therapy is not alone. In addition to the age-old therapies of surgery, external radiation, and chemotherapy, immunotherapies, microwaves, and thermal therapies are adding to the diagnostic and therapeutic toolbox becoming increasingly available to clinicians. This is the golden age of theranostic research with other cutting-edge treatments giving new hope to patients and also a new perspective to nuclear medicine physicians.

One of the main challenges facing radionuclide therapy, however, is the current shortage of trained nuclear medicine radionuclide therapists. In the past 35 years, nuclear medicine has evolved from a joint specialty of endocrinology, internal medicine, pathology, and radiology to a branch of radiology—or, in some countries, cardiology—but increasingly an "imaging" specialty. The problem is that most radiologists are not trained to do radionuclide therapy. Most of the oncology therapies, for example, are currently in the hands of radiation oncology and medical oncology. Radionuclide therapy is likely to change the specialty of nuclear imaging back to the specialty of nuclear medicine, as originally envisioned by Saul Hertz with the first radioiodine therapy.

References

1. Lawrence B. Radioactivity before the curies. Am J Phys. 1965;33:128.
2. Siegel E. The beginnings of radioiodine therapy of metastatic thyroid carcinoma: a memoir of Samuel M. Seidlin, M. D. (1895-1955) and his celebrated patient. Cancer Biother Radiopharm. 1999;14(2):71–9.
3. Arevalo-Perez J, et al. A perspective of the future of nuclear medicine training and certification. Semin Nucl Med. 2016;46(1):88–96.
4. McCready VR. Radioiodine—the success story of nuclear medicine: 75th anniversary of the first use of Iodine-131 in humans. Eur J Nucl Med Mol Imaging. 2017;44(2):179–82.
5. Turner JH. An introduction to the clinical practice of theranostics in oncology. Br J Radiol. 2018;91(1091):20180440.
6. Yordanova A, Eppard E, Kürpig S, Bundschuh RA, Schönberger S, Gonzalez-Carmona M, Feldmann G, Ahmadzadehfar H, Essler M. Theranostics in nuclear medicine practice. Onco Targets Ther. 2017;10:4821–8.
7. Roxin A, Zhang C, Hugh S, Lepage M, Zhang Z, Lin K, Bénard F, Perrin M. A metal-free DOTA-conjugated 18F-labeled radiotracer: [18F]DOTA-AMBF3-LLP2A for imaging VLA-4 over-expression in murine melanoma with improved tumor uptake and greatly enhanced renal clearance. Bioconjugate Chem. 2019:1–36. https://doi.org/10.1021/acs.bioconjchem.9b00146.
8. Muller C, et al. Therapeutic radiometals beyond (177) Lu and (90)Y: production and application of promising alpha-particle, beta(−)-particle, and Auger electron emitters. J Nucl Med. 2017;58(Suppl 2):91S–6S.
9. Huclier-Markai S, Alliot C, Kerdjoudj R, Mougin-Degraef M, Chouin N, Haddad F. Promising scandium radionuclides for nuclear medicine: a review on the production and chemistry up to in vivo proofs of concept. Cancer Biother Radiopharm. 2018;33(8):316–29.

10. Muller C, Domnanich KA, Umbricht CA, van der Meulen N. Scandium and terbium radionuclides for radiotheranostics: current state of development towards clinical application. Br J Radiol. 2018;91(1091):20180074.

11. Champion C, et al. Comparison between three promising ss-emitting radionuclides, (67)Cu, (47)Sc and (161)Tb, with emphasis on doses delivered to minimal residual disease. Theranostics. 2016;6(10): 1611–8.

12. Follacchio GA, De Feo MS, De Vincentis G, Monteleone F, Liberatore M. Radiopharmaceuticals labelled with copper radionuclides: clinical results in human beings. Curr Radiopharm. 2018;11(1):22–33.

13. Hicks RJ, Jackson P, Kong G, Ware RE, Hofman MS, Pattison DA, Akhurst TA, Drummond E, Roselt P, Callahan J, Price R, Jeffery CM, Hong E, Noonan W, Herschtal A, Hicks LJ, Hedt A, Harris M, Paterson BM, Donnelly PS. 64Cu-SARTATE PET imaging of patients with neuroendocrine tumors demonstrates high tumor uptake and retention, potentially allowing prospective dosimetry for peptide receptor radionuclide therapy. J Nucl Med. 2019;60(6):777–85.

14. Gourni E, et al. Copper-64 labeled macrobicyclic sarcophagine coupled to a GRP receptor antagonist shows great promise for PET imaging of prostate cancer. Mol Pharm. 2015;12(8):2781–90.

15. Boschi A, et al. The emerging role of copper-64 radiopharmaceuticals as cancer theranostics. Drug Discov Today. 2018;23(8):1489–501.

16. Kreuter J. Nanoparticles—a historical perspective. Int J Pharm. 2007;331(1):1–10.

17. De La Vega JC, Esquinas PL, Rodríguez-Rodríguez C, Bokharaei M, Moskalev I, Liu D, Saatchi K, Häfeli UO. Radioembolization of hepatocellular carcinoma with built-in dosimetry: first in vivo results with uniformly-sized, biodegradable microspheres labeled with 188Re. Theranostics. 2019;9(3):868–83.

18. Boas FE, Bodei L, Sofocleous CT. Radioembolization of colorectal liver metastases: indications, technique, and outcomes. J Nucl Med. 2017;58(Suppl 2):104S–11S.

19. De La Vega JC, et al. Radioembolization of hepatocellular carcinoma with built-in dosimetry: first in vivo results with uniformly-sized, biodegradable microspheres labeled with (188)Re. Theranostics. 2019;9(3):868–83.

20. Lepareur N, et al. Rhenium-188 labeled radiopharmaceuticals: current clinical applications in oncology and promising perspectives. Front Med (Lausanne). 2019;6:132.

21. Bergqvist L, Strand SE, Persson BR. Particle sizing and biokinetics of interstitial lymphoscintigraphic agents. Semin Nucl Med. 1983;13(1):9–19.

22. Schneider P, Farahati J, Reinders C. Radiosynovectomy in rheumatology, orthopedics, and hemophilia. J Nucl Med. 2005;46(Suppl 1):48S–54S.

23. Srivastava SC, Mausner LF. Therapeutic radionuclides: production, physical characteristics, and applications. In: Baum RP, editor. Therapeutic nuclear medicine. Berlin: Springer; 2014. p. 12–46.

24. Donecker JM, Stevenson NR. Radiosynoviorthesis: a new therapeutic and diagnostic tool for canine joint inflammation. In: Fox SM, editor. Multimodal management of canine osteoarthritis. 2nd ed. Boca Raton, FL: CRC Press; 2017. p. 75–80.

25. Gratz S, Gobel D, Behr TM. Radiosynoviorthesis. An efficient form of local treatment for inflammatory joint diseases. Dtsch Med Wochenschr. 2002;127(33):1704–7.

26. Lattimer JC, et al. Intraarticular injection of a Tin-117m radiosynoviorthesis agent in normal canine elbows causes no adverse effects. Vet Radiol Ultrasound. 2019;60:567–74.

27. Krishnamurthy GT, et al. Tin-117m(4+)DTPA: pharmacokinetics and imaging characteristics in patients with metastatic bone pain. J Nucl Med. 1997;38(2):230–7.

28. de Jong R, et al. The advantageous role of annexin A1 in cardiovascular disease. Cell Adhes Migr. 2017;11(3):261–74.

29. Subbiah V, Anderson P, Rohren E. Alpha emitter radium 223 in high-risk osteosarcoma: first clinical evidence of response and blood-brain barrier penetration. JAMA Oncol. 2015;1(2):253–5.

30. Sedda AF, et al. Dermatological high-dose-rate brachytherapy for the treatment of basal and squamous cell carcinoma. Clin Exp Dermatol. 2008;33(6): 745–9.

31. Carrozzo AM, et al. Dermo beta brachytherapy with 188Re in extramammary Paget's disease. G Ital Dermatol Venereol. 2014;149(1):115–21.

32. Reitkopf-Brodutch S, et al. Ablation of experimental colon cancer by intratumoral 224Radium-loaded wires is mediated by alpha particles released from atoms which spread in the tumor and can be augmented by chemotherapy. Int J Radiat Biol. 2015;91(2):179–86.

33. Nicolas GP, et al. New developments in peptide receptor radionuclide therapy. J Nucl Med. 2018; https://doi.org/10.2967/jnumed.118.213496.

34. Patrikidou A, Loriot Y, Eymard JC, Albiges L, Massard C, Ileana E, et al. Who dies from prostate cancer? Prostate Cancer Prostatic Dis. 2014;17:348–52.

35. Zechmann CM, Afshar-Oromieh A, Armor T, Stubbs JB, Mier W, Hadaschik B, Joyal J, Kopka K, Debus J, Babich JW, Haberkorn U. Radiation dosimetry and first therapy results with a (^{124})I/(^{131})I-labeled small molecule (MIP-1095) targeting PSMA for prostate cancer therapy. Eur J Nucl Med Mol Imaging. 2014;41(7):1280–92.

36. Kam BL, Teunissen JJ, Krenning EP, de Herder WW, Khan S, van Vliet EI, Kwekkeboom DJ. Lutetium-labelled peptides for therapy of neuroendocrine tumours. Eur J Nucl Med Mol Imaging. 2012;39(Suppl 1):S103–12.

37. Rahbar K, Ahmadzadehfar H, Kratochwil C, Haberkorn U, Schäfers M, Essler M, et al. German multicenter study investigating ^{177}Lu-PSMA-617

radioligand therapy in advanced prostate cancer patients. J Nucl Med. 2017;58(1):85–90.

38. Bräuer A, Grubert LS, Roll W, Schrader AJ, Schäfers M, Bögemann M, Rahbar K. ^{177}Lu-PSMA-617 radioligand therapy and outcome in patients with metastasized castration-resistant prostate cancer. Eur J Nucl Med Mol Imaging. 2017;44(10):1663–70.

39. Delker A, Fendler WP, Kratochwil C, Brunegraf A, Gosewisch A, Gildehaus FJ, et al. Dosimetry for ([177])Lu-DKFZ-PSMA-617: a new radiopharmaceutical for the treatment of metastatic prostate cancer. Eur J Nucl Med Mol Imaging. 2016;43(1):42.

40. Cornford P, Bellmunt J, Bolla M, Briers E, De Santis M, Gross T, et al. EAU-ESTRO-SIOG guidelines on prostate cancer. Part II: treatment of relapsing, metastatic, and castration-resistant prostate cancer. Eur Urol. 2017;71:630–4213.

41. von Eyben FE, Roviello G, Kiljunen T, Uprimny C, Virgolini I, Kairemo K, Joensuu T. Third-line treatment and ^{177}Lu-PSMA radioligand therapy of metastatic castration-resistant prostate cancer: a systematic review. Eur J Nucl Med Mol Imaging. 2018;45:496–508.

42. Kratochwil C, Bruchertseifer F, Rathke H, Hohenfellner M, Giesel FL, Haberkorn U, Morgenstern A. Targeted α-therapy of metastatic castration-resistant prostate cancer with [225]Ac-PSMA-617: swimmer-plot analysis suggests efficacy regarding duration of tumor control. J Nucl Med. 2018;59(5):795–802. https://doi.org/10.2967/jnumed.117.203539. Epub 2018 Jan 11.

43. Kopka K, Benesova M, Barinka C, Haberkorn U, Babich J. Glu-Ureido-based inhibitors of prostate-specific membrane antigen: lessons learned during the development of a novel class of low molecular-weight theranostic radiotracers. J Nucl Med. 2017;58:17S–26S.

44. Perera M, Papa N, Christidis D, Wetherell D, Hofman MS, Murphy DG, et al. Sensitivity, specificity, and predictors of positive ^{68}Ga-prostate-specific membrane antigen positron emission tomography in advanced prostate cancer: a systematic review and meta-analysis. Eur Urol. 2016;70:926–37.

45. Budäus L, Leyh-Bannurah SR, Salomon G, Michl U, Heinzer H, Huland H, et al. Initial experience of (68)Ga-PSMA PET/CT imaging in high-risk prostate cancer patients prior to radical prostatectomy. Eur Urol. 2016;69(3):393–6.

46. von Eyben FE, Kiljunen T, Joensuu T, Kairemo K, Uprimny C, Virgolini I. ^{177}Lu-PSMA-617 radioligand therapy for a patient with lymph node metastatic prostate cancer. Oncotarget. 2017;8:66112–6.

47. Ahmadzadehfar H, Wegen S, Yordanova A, Fimmers R, Kürpig S, Eppard E, et al. Overall survival and response pattern of castration-resistant metastatic prostate cancer to multiple cycles of radioligand therapy using [177Lu]Lu-PSMA-617. Eur J Nucl Med Mol Imaging. 2017;44(9):1448–54.

48. Baum RP, Kulkarni HR, Schuchardt C, Singh A, Wirtz M, Wiessalla S, et al. ^{177}Lu-labeled prostate-specific membrane antigen radioligand therapy of metastatic castration-resistant prostate cancer: safety and efficacy. J Nucl Med. 2016;57:1–8. https://doi.org/10.2967/jnumed.115.168443.

49. Okamoto S, Thieme A, Allmann J, D'Alessandria C, Maurer T, Retz M, et al. Radiation dosimetry for ^{177}Lu-PSMA I&T in metastatic castration-resistant prostate cancer: absorbed dose in normal organs and tumor lesions. J Nucl Med. 2017;58(3):445–50.

50. Calopedos RJS, Chalasani V, Asher R, Emmett L, Woo HH. Lutetium-177-labelled anti-prostate-specific membrane antigen antibody and ligands for the treatment of metastatic castrate-resistant prostate cancer: a systematic review and meta-analysis. Prostate Cancer Prostatic Dis. 2017;20:352–60.

51. Yordanova A, Becker A, Eppard E, Kürpig S, Fisang C, Feldmann G, et al. The impact of repeated cycles of radioligand therapy using [177Lu]Lu-PSMA-617 on renal function in patients with hormone refractory metastatic prostate cancer. Eur J Nucl Med Mol Imaging. 2017;44(9):1473–9.

52. Rathke H, Kratochwil C, Hohenberger R, Giesel FL, Bruchertseifer F, Flechsig P, et al. Initial clinical experience performing sialendoscopy for salivary gland protection in patients undergoing [225]Ac-PSMA-617 RLT. Eur J Nucl Med Mol Imaging. 2019;46(1):139–47. https://doi.org/10.1007/s00259-018-4135-8. Epub 2018 Aug 27.

53. Behe M, Behr TM. Cholecystokinin-B (CCK-B)/gastrin receptor targeting peptides for staging and therapy of medullary thyroid cancer and other CCK-B receptor expressing malignancies. Biopolymers. 2002;66(6):399–418.

54. Behr TM, Béhé M. Cholecystokinin-B/gastrin receptor-targeting peptides for staging and therapy of medullary thyroid cancer and other cholecystokinin-B receptor-expressing malignancies. Semin Nucl Med. 2002;32(2):97–109. https://doi.org/10.1053/snuc.2002.31028.

55. Malcolm J, et al. Targeted radionuclide therapy: new advances for improvement of patient management and response. Cancers (Basel). 2019;11(2):268.

56. Loktev A, et al. Development of novel FAP-targeted radiotracers with improved tumor retention. J Nucl Med. 2019;60:1421–9.

57. Bodet-Milin C, et al. Clinical results in medullary thyroid carcinoma suggest high potential of pretargeted immuno-PET for tumor imaging and theranostic approaches. Front Med (Lausanne). 2019;6:124.

58. Runcie K, Budman DR, John V, Seetharamu N. Bispecific and tri-specific antibodies—the next big thing in solid tumor therapeutics. Mol Med. 2018;24:50.

59. Frampas E, et al. Improvement of radioimmunotherapy using pretargeting. Front Oncol. 2013;3:159.

60. Heskamp S, et al. Alpha- versus beta-emitting radionuclides for pretargeted radioimmunotherapy of carcinoembryonic antigen-expressing human colon cancer xenografts. J Nucl Med. 2017;58(6):926–33.

61. Okarvi SM, Maecke HR. Radiolabelled peptides in medical imaging. In: Peptide applications in biomed-

icine, biotechnology and bioengineering. Duxford: Woodhead Publishing; 2018. p. 431–83.

62. Krolicki L, et al. Prolonged survival in secondary glioblastoma following local injection of targeted alpha therapy with (213)bi-substance P analogue. Eur J Nucl Med Mol Imaging. 2018;45(9):1636–44.

63. Sattiraju A, et al. IL13RA2 targeted alpha particle therapy against glioblastomas. Oncotarget. 2017;8(26):42997–3007.

64. Sharma P, Debinski W. Receptor-targeted glial brain tumor therapies. Int J Mol Sci. 2018;19(11):3326.

65. Israel I, et al. Validation of an amino-acid-based radionuclide therapy plus external beam radiotherapy in heterotopic glioblastoma models. Nucl Med Biol. 2011;38(4):451–60.

66. Jadvar H, et al. Radiotheranostics in cancer diagnosis and management. Radiology. 2018;286(2):388–400.

67. Lapa C, et al. CXCR4-directed endoradiotherapy induces high response rates in extramedullary relapsed multiple myeloma. Theranostics. 2017;7(6):1589–97.

68. Baum RP, et al. (177)Lu-3BP-227 for neurotensin receptor 1-targeted therapy of metastatic pancreatic adenocarcinoma: first clinical results. J Nucl Med. 2018;59(5):809–14.

69. McConathy J, et al. Radiohalogenated nonnatural amino acids as PET and SPECT tumor imaging agents. Med Res Rev. 2012;32(4):868–905.

70. Hayashi K, Anzai N. Novel therapeutic approaches targeting L-type amino acid transporters for cancer treatment. World J Gastrointest Oncol. 2017;9(1): 21–9.

71. Liu Z, Wang F, Chen X. Integrin targeted delivery of radiotherapeutics. Theranostics. 2011;1:201–10.

72. Baum RP, et al. First-in-human study demonstrating tumor-angiogenesis by PET/CT imaging with (68) Ga-NODAGA-THERANOST, a high-affinity peptidomimetic for alphavbeta3 integrin receptor targeting. Cancer Biother Radiopharm. 2015;30(4):152–9.

73. Jacene HA, Filice R, Kasecamp W, Wahl RL. Comparison of 90Y-ibritumomab tiuxetan and 131I-tositumomab in clinical practice. J Nucl Med. 2007;48:1767–76.

74. Liu G, Dou S, Yin D, Squires S, Liu X, Wang Y, Rusckowski M, Hnatowich DJ. A novel pretargeting method for measuring antibody internalization in tumor cells. Cancer Biother Radiopharm. 2007;22(1):33–9.

75. Kratochwil C, Giesel FL, Stefanova M, Benesov M, Bronzel M, Afshar-Oromieh A, Mier W, Eder M, Kopka K, Haberkorn U. PSMA-targeted radionuclide therapy of metastatic castration-resistant prostate cancer with 177Lu-labeled PSMA-617. J Nucl Med. 2016;57:1170–6.

76. Tagawa ST, et al. Phase 1/2 study of fractionated dose lutetium-177-labeled anti-prostate-specific membrane antigen monoclonal antibody J591 ((177) Lu-J591) for metastatic castration-resistant prostate cancer. Cancer. 2019;125(15):2561–9.

77. Finn LE, Levy M, Orozco JJ, Park JH, Atallah E, Craig M, Perl AE, Scheinberg DA, Cicic D, Bergonio GR, Berger MS, Jurcic JGA. Phase 2 study of actinium-225 (^{225}Ac)-lintuzumab in older patients with previously untreated acute myeloid leukemia (AML) unfit for intensive chemotherapy. Blood. 2017;130(Supplement 1):2638.

78. Jurcic JG. Clinical studies with bismuth-213 and actinium-225 for hematologic malignancies. Curr Radiopharm. 2018;11(3):192–9.

79. Iagaru A, et al. 131I-Tositumomab (Bexxar) vs. 90Y-Ibritumomab (Zevalin) therapy of low-grade refractory/relapsed non-Hodgkin lymphoma. Mol Imaging Biol. 2010;12(2):198–203.

80. Orozco JJ, et al. Anti-CD45 radioimmunotherapy without TBI before transplantation facilitates persistent haploidentical donor engraftment. Blood. 2016;127(3):352–9.

81. Blakkisrud J, et al. Biodistribution and dosimetry results from a phase 1 trial of therapy with the antibody-radionuclide conjugate (177)Lu-lilotomab satetraxetan. J Nucl Med. 2018;59(4):704–10.

82. Wang J, Xu B. Targeted therapeutic options and future perspectives for HER2-positive breast cancer. Signal Transduct Target Ther. 2019;4:34.

83. Massicano AVF, Marquez-Nostra BV, Lapi SE. Targeting HER2 in nuclear medicine for imaging and therapy. Mol Imaging. 2018;17:1536012117745386.

84. Wang J, Fang R, Wang L, Chen G, Wang H, Wang Z, Zhao D, Pavlov VN, Kabirov I, Wang Z, Guo P, Peng L, Xu W. Identification of carbonic anhydrase IX as a novel target for endoscopic molecular imaging of human bladder cancer. Cell Physiol Biochem. 2018;47(4):1565–77.

85. Stillebroer AB, Mulders PFA, Boerman OC, Oyen WJG, Oosterwijk E. Carbonic anhydrase IX in renal cell carcinoma: implications for prognosis, diagnosis, and therapy. Kidney Cancer. 2010;58(1):75–83.

86. Lau J, Lin KS, Benard F. Past, present, and future: development of theranostic agents targeting carbonic anhydrase IX. Theranostics. 2017;7(17):4322–39.

87. Yang N, Yao S, Liu D. Tumor necrosis factor-related apoptosis-inducing ligand additive with Iodine-131 of inhibits non-small cell lung cancer cells through promoting apoptosis. Oncol Lett. 2018;16(1):276–84.

88. Grinshtein N, Simms R, Hu M, Storozhuk Y, Moran M, Burak E, Forbes J, Valliant J. IGF-1R targeted alpha therapeutic FPI-1434 causes DNA double-stranded breaks and induces regression in preclinical models of human cancer proceedings from the TAT11. J Med Imaging Radiat Sci. 2019;50:S1–S42.

89. Macaulay VM, et al. Phase I study of humanized monoclonal antibody AVE1642 directed against the type 1 insulin-like growth factor receptor (IGF-1R), administered in combination with anticancer therapies to patients with advanced solid tumors. Ann Oncol. 2013;24(3):784–91.

90. Harmsen MM, De Haard HJ. Properties, production, and applications of camelid single-domain antibody fragments. Appl Microbiol Biotechnol. 2007;77: 13–22.

91. Cortez-Retamozo V, Lahoutte T, Cavaliers V, Olive L. 99mTc-labeled nanobodies: a new type of targeted

probes for imaging antigen expression. Curr Radiopharm. 2008;1(1):37–41.

92. Xavier C, et al. Synthesis, preclinical validation, dosimetry, and toxicity of 68Ga-NOTA-anti-HER2 Nanobodies for iPET imaging of HER2 receptor expression in cancer. J Nucl Med. 2013;54(5):776–84.

93. Keyaerts M, et al. Phase I study of 68Ga-HER2-nanobody for PET/CT assessment of HER2 expression in breast carcinoma. J Nucl Med. 2016;57(1):27–33.

94. D'Huyvetter M, et al. Targeted radionuclide therapy with a 177Lu-labeled anti-HER2 nanobody. Theranostics. 2014;4(7):708–20.

95. D'Huyvetter M, et al. (131)I-labeled anti-HER2 camelid sdAb as a theranostic tool in cancer treatment. Clin Cancer Res. 2017;23(21):6616–28.

96. Krasniqi A, et al. Theranostic radiolabeled anti-CD20 sdAb for targeted radionuclide therapy of non-Hodgkin lymphoma. Mol Cancer Ther. 2017;16(12):2828–39.

97. Lemaire M, et al. Imaging and radioimmunotherapy of multiple myeloma with anti-idiotypic nanobodies. Leukemia. 2014;28(2):444–7.

98. Broisat A, et al. Nanobodies targeting mouse/human VCAM1 for the nuclear imaging of atherosclerotic lesions. Circ Res. 2012;110(7):927–37.

99. Senders ML, et al. Nanobody-facilitated multiparametric PET/MRI phenotyping of atherosclerosis. JACC Cardiovasc Imaging. 2018; https://doi.org/10.1016/j.jcmg.2018.07.027.

100. Andersson H, et al. Intraperitoneal alpha-particle radioimmunotherapy of ovarian cancer patients: pharmaco kinetics and dosimetry of (211) At-MX35 F(ab')2—a phase I study. J Nucl Med. 2009;50(7):1153–60.

101. McLaughlin MF, et al. Gold coated lanthanide phosphate nanoparticles for targeted alpha generator radiotherapy. PLoS One. 2013;8(1):e54531.

102. Woodward J, et al. LaPO4 nanoparticles doped with actinium-225 that partially sequester daughter radionuclides. Bioconjug Chem. 2011;22(4):766–76.

103. Khalid U, et al. Radiolabelled aptamers for theranostic treatment of cancer. Pharmaceuticals (Basel). 2018;12(1):2.

104. Darmostuk M, Rimpelova S, Gbelcova H, Ruml T. Current approaches in SELEX: An update to aptamer selection technology. Biotechnol Adv. 2015;33(6 Pt 2):1141–61.

105. Perkins AC, Missailidis S. Radiolabelled aptamers for tumour imaging and therapy. Q J Nucl Med Mol Imaging. 2007;51(4):292–6.